Principles and Practice of
PEDIATRIC SLEEP MEDICINE

Principles and Practice of
PEDIATRIC SLEEP MEDICINE

Third Edition

Stephen H. Sheldon, DO, FAAP
Professor Emeritus
Departments of Pediatrics and Neurology
Northwestern University
Feinberg School of Medicine
Emeritus, Sleep Medicine Center
Ann and Robert H. Lurie Children's Hospital of Chicago
Chicago, Illinois

Meir Kryger, MD, FRCPC
Professor Emeritus
Department of Pulmonary Critical Care and Sleep Medicine
Yale University
New Haven, Connecticut

David Gozal, MD, MBA, PhD (Hon.)
Dean
Joan C. Edwards School of Medicine
Vice President for Health Affairs
Marshall University
Huntington, West Virginia

Craig Canapari, MD
Associate Professor
Yale University School of Medicine;
Director, Pediatric Sleep Center
Yale New-Haven Hospital
Division of Pediatric Respiratory Medicine
Yale University
New Haven, Connecticut

Temitayo O. Oyegbile-Chidi, MD, PhD
Associate Professor
Department of Neurology
University of California Davis
Davis, California;
UC Davis Health Children's Hospital
Sacramento, California

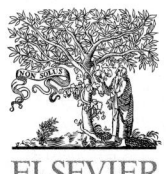

ELSEVIER

Elsevier
1600 John F. Kennedy Blvd.
Ste 1800
Philadelphia, PA 19103-2899

PRINCIPLES AND PRACTICE OF PEDIATRIC SLEEP MEDICINE, THIRD EDITION   ISBN: 978-0-323-75566-5

Previous editions copyrighted 2014 and 2005.

Content Strategist: Mary Hegeler
Senior Content Development Specialists: Priyadarshini Pandey, Sneha Kashyap
Content Development Manager: Somodatta Roy Choudhury
Publishing Services Manager: Shereen Jameel
Project Manager: Haritha Dharmarajan
Design Direction: Renee Duenow

Printed in India

Last digit is the print number: 9 8 7 6 5 4 3 2 1

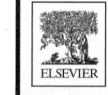
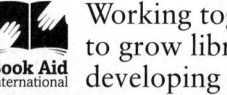

List of Contributors

Candice A. Alfano, PhD
Professor
Department of Psychology
University of Houston
Houston, Texas

W. Jerome Alonso, MD
Medical Director
Department of Sleep Medicine
Canadian Sleep Consultants
Clinical Assistant Professor
Faculty of Medicine
University of Calgary
Alberta, Canada

Raouf Samy Amin, MD
Professor of Pediatrics
Department of Pediatrics
Cincinnati Children's Hospital Medical Center
Cincinnati, Ohio

Fuad M. Baroody, MD, FACS
Professor
Department of Surgery, Section of Otolaryngology-Head
    and Neck Surgery
The University of Chicago Medicine
Department of Pediatrics
Director of Pediatric Otolaryngology
The University of Chicago Medicine and The Comer
    Children's Hospital
Chicago, Illinois

Elizabeth Berry-Kravis, MD, PhD
Professor
Departments of Pediatrics, Neurological Sciences,
    Anatomy and Cell Biology
Rush University Medical Center
Chicago, Illinois

Claire Bogan, DO
Resident Physician
Departments of Psychiatry and Human Behavior
Thomas Jefferson University Hospital
Philadelphia, Pennsylvania

Kevin Lynn Boyd, MSc, DDS
Visiting Scholar
Department of Anthropology
University of Pennsylvania
Philadelphia, Pennsylvania;
Dental Consultant
Department of Sleep Medicine
Ann & Robert H. Lurie Children's Hospital
Chicago, Illinois

Deborah Michelle Brooks, MD
Assistant Professor
Department of Psychiatry
University of Maryland School of Medicine
Baltimore, Maryland

Lee J. Brooks, MD
Clinical Professor of Pediatrics
Department of Pediatrics
Rowan University SOM
Stratford, New Jersey

Susan Calhoun, PhD
Licensed Psychologist/Associate Professor
Psychiatry
Penn State College of Medicine
Hershey, Pennsylvania

Craig Canapari, MD
Associate Professor
Yale University School of Medicine;
Director, Pediatric Sleep Center
Yale New-Haven Hospital
Division of Pediatric Respiratory Medicine
Yale University
New Haven Connecticut

John L. Carroll, MD
Professor
Department of Pediatrics
University of Arkansas for Medical Sciences
Little Rock, Arkansas

Michael S. Carroll, PhD
Director, Computational Informatics and Visualization
    Laboratory
Department of Data Analytics and Reporting
Ann & Robert H. Lurie Children's Hospital of Chicago
Assistant Professor of Pediatrics
Northwestern University Feinberg School of Medicine
Chicago, Illinois

Mary A. Carskadon, PhD
Professor
Department of Psychiatry and Human Behavior
Alpert Medical School of Brown University
Providence, Rhode Island;
Director
Chronobiology and Sleep Research Laboratory
EP Bradley Hospital
East Providence, Rhode Island

Ronald D. Chervin, MD, MS
Professor of Neurology and Director, Sleep Disorders
    Centers
Department of Neurology
University of Michigan
Ann Arbor, Michigan

Joong Ki Cho, MD
University of Illinois at Chicago College of Medicine
Chicago, Illinois

Allison Hayes Clarke, PhD
Pediatric Psychologist
Department of Psychiatry and Sleep Medicine
Ann & Robert H. Lurie Children's Hospital of Chicago
Chicago, Illinois

Anat Cohen Engler, MD
Pediatrician
Department of Pediatrics
Meir Hospital
Kfar Saba, Israel

Valerie McLaughlin Crabtree, PhD, DBSM
Chief of Psychosocial Services
Department of Psychology
St. Jude Children's Research Hospital
Memphis, Tennessee

Stephanie J. Crowley, PhD
Associate Professor
Biological Rhythms Research Laboratory
Department of Psychiatry & Behavioral Sciences
Rush University Medical Center
Chicago, Illinois

Thuan Dang, MD, MPH
Attending Physician
Department of Sleep Medicine
Ann & Robert H. Lurie Children's Hospital of Chicago
Chicago, Illinois

Sally Davidson Ward, MD
Professor of Clinical Pediatrics
Department of Pediatrics
Children's Hospital Los Angeles
Keck School of Medicine
University of Southern California
Los Angeles, California

Innessa Donskoy, MD, FAAP
Pediatric Sleep Medicine Attending
Department of Sleep Medicine
Advocate Children's Hospital
Park Ridge, Illinois;
Clinical Assistant Professor
Department of Pulmonary, Critical Care, Sleep, and
    Allergy
University of Illinois at Chicago College of Medicine
Chicago, Illinois

Jeffrey S. Durmer, MD, PhD
Sleep & Circadian Neurologist
Private Practice
Denver, Colorado

Vijayabharathi Ekambaram, MD, MPH
Child & Adolescent Psychiatry, Sleep Medicine, Integrative
    Psychiatry;
Department Chair and Psychiatry Program Director
UCF/HCA Florida Healthcare Program
Pensacola, Florida

Tamar Etzioni, MD
Deputy Director
Department of Pediatrics
Technion Faculty of Medicine
Sleep Laboratory, Carmel Medical Center
Haifa, Israel

Anna Fishbein, MD
Adjunct Associate Professor
Department of Pediatrics
Division of Allergy & Immunology
Northwestern University Feinberg School of Medicine
Ann & Robert H. Lurie Children's Hospital of Chicago
Chicago, Illinois

Aviv Goldbart, MD
Department of Pediatrics
Soroka University Medical Center
Ben Gurion University of the Negev
Beer-Sheva, Israel

David Gozal, MD, MBA, PhD (Hon.)
Dean
Joan C. Edwards School of Medicine
Vice President for Health Affairs
Marshall University
Huntington, West Virginia

Madeleine Marie Grigg-Damberger, MD
Professor of Neurology
Department of Neurology
University of New Mexico School of Medicine
Medical Director, Pediatric Sleep Medicine Services
University of New Mexico Sleep Center
University of New Mexico;
Associate Medical Director
Clinical Neurodiagnostic Laboratory
University of New Mexico Medical Center
Albuquerque, New Mexico

Paul Gringras, MRCPCH, MBChB
Professor of Paediatric Sleep Medicine
Kings Health Partners Sleep Group
Guy's and St Thomas' Hospital
London, United Kingdom

Susan M. Harding, MD
Professor of Medicine
Division of Pulmonary, Allergy & Critical Care Medicine
University of Alabama at Birmingham
Birmingham, Alabama

Rosemary S.C. Horne, BSc, MSc, PhD, BLitt, DSc
Professor
Department of Paediatrics
Monash University
Melbourne, Victoria, Australia

Anna Ivanenko, MD, PhD
Professor of Clinical Psychiatry and Behavioral Sciences
Division of Child and Adolescent Psychiatry
Ann & Robert H. Lurie Children's Hospital of Chicago
Northwestern University Feinberg School of Medicine
Chicago, Illinois;
Pediatric Sleep Medicine Director
Ascension Illinois
Elk Grove Village, Illinois

Eliot S. Katz, MD
Assistant Professor of Pediatrics
Division of Respiratory Diseases
Boston Children's Hospital; Harvard Medical School
Boston, Massachusetts

Ilya Khaytin, MD, PhD
Assistant Professor
Department of Pediatrics
Northwestern University Feinberg School of Medicine
Ann & Robert H. Lurie Children's Hospital of Chicago
Stanley Manne Children's Research Institute
Chicago, Illinois

Leila Kheirandish-Gozal, MD, MSc
Professor
Departments of Neurology and Pediatrics
University of Missouri
Columbia, Missouri

Suresh Kotagal, MD
Professor Emeritus
Department of Neurology
Mayo Clinic
Consultant in Neurology, Pediatrics, and Sleep Medicine
Mayo Clinic
Rochester, Minnesota

Jyoti Krishna, MBBS, MD, FAAP, FAASM
Director, Sleep Medicine & Associate Professor of
    Pediatrics, NEOMED
Department of Pediatrics
Akron Children's Hospital
Akron, Ohio

Meir Kryger, MD, FRCPC
Professor Emeritus
Department of Pulmonary Critical Care and Sleep
    Medicine
Yale University
New Haven, Connecticut

Theresa Annette Laguna, MD, MSCS
Professor
Department of Pediatrics
Division of Pulmonary and Sleep Medicine
University of Washington School of Medicine
Seattle, Washington

Kayla N. LaRosa, PhD, EdS, MS
Pediatric Psychology Fellow
Department of Psychology
St. Jude Children's Research Hospital
Memphis, Tennessee

Kristina Puzino Lenker, PhD
Assistant Professor
Department of Psychiatry and Behavioral Health
Penn State Hershey Medical Center
Hershey, Pennsylvania

James Luebbert, MD
Clinical Associate Professor
Department of Psychiatry and Human Behavior
Sidney Kimmel Medical College of Thomas Jefferson
    University
Philadelphia, Pennsylvania

Sonal Malhotra, MD, MPH
Assistant Professor
Department of Pulmonary and Sleep Medicine
Baylor College of Medicine
Houston, Texas

Susanna A. McColley, MD
Professor
Department of Pediatrics, Pulmonary, and Sleep Medicine
Northwestern University Feinberg School of Medicine;
Stanley Manne Children's Research Institute;
Associate Director for Child Health
Northwestern University Clinical and Translational
    Sciences Institute
Division of Pulmonary and Sleep Medicine
Ann & Robert H. Lurie Children's Hospital of Chicago
Chicago, Illinois

Jodi A. Mindell, PhD
Professor
Department of Psychology
Saint Joseph's University;
Associate Director
Sleep Center
Children's Hospital of Philadelphia
Philadelphia, Pennsylvania

Melisa Moore, PhD, DBSM
Assistant Professor
Department of Clinical Child and Adolescent Psychiatry
    and Behavioral Sciences
Children's Hospital of Philadelphia
Philadelphia, Pennsylvania

Brittany Nance, MMS, PA-C
Physician Assistant
Department of Pulmonary & Sleep Medicine
Ann & Robert H. Lurie Children's Hospital of Chicago
Chicago, Illinois

Louise M. O'Brien, PhD, MS
Professor
Division of Sleep Medicine;
Professor
Obstetrics and Gynecology;
Research Scientist
Oral & Maxillofacial Surgery
University of Michigan
Ann Arbor, Michigan

Judith A. Owens, MD, MPH
Sleep Center Senior Faculty
Department of Neurology
Boston Children's Hospital;
Professor
Department of Neurology
Harvard Medical School
Boston, Massachusetts

Temitayo O. Oyegbile-Chidi, MD, PHD
Associate Professor
Department of Neurology
University of California Davis
Davis, California;
UC Davis Health Children's Hospital
Sacramento, California

Rafael Pelayo, MD
Clinical Professor
Sleep Medicine Division
Stanford University School of Medicine
Stanford, California

Iris A. Perez, MD
Associate Professor of Clinical Pediatrics
Department of Pediatrics
Keck School of Medicine of USC
San Marino, California

Laura Petrauskas, MA, MD
Resident
Section of Otolaryngology Head & Neck Surgery
University of Chicago
Chicago, Illinois

Giora Pillar, MD, PhD
Professor of Pediatrics; Department Head
Department of Pediatrics and Sleep Clinic
Carmel Hospital
Haifa, Israel

Christian F. Poets, MD
Professor
Department of Neonatology
Tuebingen University Hospital
Tuebingen, Germany

Casey M. Rand, BS
Project Manager
Autonomic Medicine in Pediatrics
Ann & Robert H. Lurie Children's Hospital
Chicago, Illinois

Gerald M. Rosen, MD
Staff Physician
Department of Sleep Medicine
Children's Hospital of Minnesota
St Paul, Minnesota

Maria Eugenia Russi, MD
Pediatric Neurologist
Department of Neurology
Sant Joan de Deu
Barcelona, Spain

Oscar Sans Capdevila, MD
Clinical Neurophysiologist
Head of Sleep Disorders Unit
Sant Joan de Deu
Barcelona, Spain

Avani Shah, MD
Clinical Assistant Professor
Department of Pediatrics
Ann & Robert H. Lurie Children's Hospital of Chicago
Chicago, Illinois

Stephen H. Sheldon, DO, FAAP
Professor Emeritus
Department of Pediatrics & Neurology
Northwestern University
Feinberg School of Medicine;
Emeritus
Sleep Medicine Center
Ann & Robert H. Lurie Children's Hospital of Chicago
Chicago, Illinois

Susan M. Slattery, MD, MS
Physician Division of Autonomic Medicine
Department of Pediatrics
Ann & Robert H. Lurie Children's Hospital of Chicago
Physician Division of Neonatology
Department of Pediatrics
Ann & Robert H. Lurie Children's Hospital of Chicago;
Assistant Professor
Northwestern University Feinberg School of Medicine
Chicago, Illinois

Christine J. So, MA
Advanced Fellow
Department of Mental Illness Research and Treatment
Corporal Michael J. Crescenz VAMC
Philadelphia, Pennsylvania

Tracey M. Stewart, RRT
Registered Respiratory Therapist
Department of Autonomic Medicine
Ann & Robert H. Lurie Children's Hospital
Chicago, Illinois

Mary Anne Tablizo, MD
Clinical Associate Professor
Department of Pediatrics, Division of Pulmonology and
    Sleep Medicine
Stanford University
Palo Alto, California;
Pediatric Pulmonologist
Division of Pulmonary and Sleep Medicine
Valley Children's Hospital
Madera, California

Asher Tal, MD
Professor
Department of Pediatrics
Soroka Medical Center, Faculty of Health Sciences,
    Ben-Gurion University of the Negev;
Professor Emeritus
Department of Pediatrics
Faculty of Health Sciences
Ben-Gurion University of the Negev
Beer Sheva, Israel

Irina Trosman, MD
Sleep Medicine Attending
Department of Pulmonary
Ann & Robert H. Lurie Children's Hospital
Chicago, Illinois

Robert Troxler, MD
Associate Professor
Department of Pediatrics
University of Alabama
Director
Sleep Disorders Center
Children's of Alabama
Birmingham, Alabama

Kyla L. Wahlstrom, PhD
Senior Research Fellow
Department of Organizational Leadership, Policy, and
    Development
College of Education and Human Development
Senior Research Fellow
Institute for Translational Research
University of Minnesota
Minneapolis, Minnesota

Grace Wang, MD, FAAP
Director of Pediatric Sleep Medicine, Assistant Professor of
    Pediatrics
Department of Pediatrics
Penn State Health
Hershey, Pennsylvania

Debra E. Weese-Mayer, MD
Chief
Division of Pediatric Autonomic Medicine
Ann & Robert H. Lurie Children's Hospital of Chicago;
Professor
Department of Pediatrics
Northwestern University Feinberg School of Medicine
Chicago, Illinois

Merrill S. Wise, MD
Sleep Medicine Specialist
Sleep Division
Mid-South Pulmonary and Sleep Specialists, PC
Memphis, Tennessee

Manisha Witmans, MD, FRCPC, FAAP, FAASM
Associate Clinical Professor
Department of Pediatrics
University of Alberta, Edmonton
Alberta, Canada

Lisa F. Wolfe, MD
Associate Professor of Medicine
Division of Pulmonary, Critical Care, and Sleep Medicine
Northwestern University Feinberg School of Medicine
Chicago, Illinois

Amy Ruth Wolfson, PhD
Professor of Psychology
Department of Psychology
Loyola University Maryland
Baltimore, Maryland

Kai Lee Yap, PhD, FACMG
Assistant Professor of Pathology (Pediatric Pathology)
Director, Lurie Children's Molecular Diagnostic
    Laboratory
Ann & Robert H. Lurie Children's Hospital of Chicago
Chicago, Illinois

Rochelle Young, BScN, MN
Pediatric Nurse Practitioner
Department of Respiratory Medicine
University of Alberta
Edmonton, Canada

Preface

Sleep medicine is a medical specialty unique in that it concentrates on events occurring during the hours of sleep to explain various aspects of a patient's health and disease. Pediatric sleep medicine is a field holding special significance because of its concern with a state that occupies over half of a child's life during the important early years of development.

The normal maturation of sleep systems is clearly among the most important neurodevelopmental milestones. The neurologic structures responsible for sleep develop rapidly during the early months and years of life and generate sleep patterns of increasing complexity and predictability. Early disruption of these vital processes can impose major cognitive and emotional consequences. Studies have confirmed the importance of sleep for the acquisition and processing of new knowledge and for maintenance of information previously gained. Recognition of both primary and secondary sleep-related disorders has also been shown as essential to the understanding and proper treatment of many other childhood disorders.

Principles and Practice of Sleep Medicine in the Child was published as a volume separate from *Principles and Practice of Sleep Medicine* for the first time in 1995. The existence of this and other texts in pediatric sleep medicine has helped move the practice of pediatric sleep medicine away from the sphere of adult medicine practitioners to one that is overseen by professionals who have dedicated their careers to the health and well-being of the pediatric patient. The preface to that 1995 volume states, in a sentence still true today, that "a robust scientifically based body of knowledge has emerged, and the tools to diagnose and effectively treat children with sleep disorders are now available." The subsequent editions, published in 2005 and 2014 as *Principles and Practice of Pediatric Sleep Medicine*, along with this current edition hopefully represent additional meaningful steps in the development of pediatric sleep medicine as a distinct discipline.

Both the American Academy of Pediatrics and the American Board of Pediatrics have formally recognized and supported growth of this important discipline. In 2007, the American Board of Pediatrics joined several other member boards of the American Board of Medical Specialties in providing subspeciality certification in the field of sleep medicine. By so doing, these boards acknowledged that sleep-related disorders not only are distinctive but are also important in the evaluation and management of many disorders affecting children.

In diagnosing and managing sleep disorders in children, the practitioner should be aware of various possible relationships between the disorders themselves and the effects on the child and family. Three of these very important relationships are as follows:

1. A primary sleep-related pathology may directly cause important daytime symptoms and adverse health sequelae in the child, and only through treatment of the sleep disorder is resolution of these problems possible.
2. A sleep-related pathology may be a comorbid condition contributing to the daytime symptoms seen in the child. In such instances, through treatment of the sleep-related pathology, the patient becomes more responsive to treatment of the coexisting disorders.
3. A child's sleep difficulties may have greater direct impact on other family members than it does on the affected child. Thus a caretaker, for example, may be the one to become most sleep deprived and have the most medical and emotional compromise, but this compromise may include the inability to properly care for the child.

Treating the child's sleep problems can improve the lives of child and family members alike. As we continue to gain further knowledge, obtain additional evidence, and develop a better understanding of the effects of sleep and its disorders on children, major advances will be made, including insights into the often-unclear area of cause and effect. Sleep disorders in infants and children reflect an interplay among many factors, including the development and maintenance of the central nervous system, the impact of environmental influences, the effects of altered patterns of parent–child interaction, and the presence of social stress and other medical conditions.

Child-care professionals must possess a comprehensive knowledge of these interactions to deliver optimal care. This book hopefully provides both the sleep medicine specialist and the primary care practitioner with resources to enable them to provide the best possible care to their pediatric patients throughout the 24-hour day and night.

Stephen H. Sheldon, Chicago, IL
Meir Kryger, New Haven, CT
Craig Canapari, New Haven, CT
David Gozal, Huntington, WV
Temitayo O. Oyegbile-Chidi, Davis, CA

Acknowledgment

We would like to thank Sarah Barth, Mary Hegeler, Priyadarshini Pandey, and Haritha Dharmarajan for their hard work and dedication to this project.

Special thanks to Dr. Richard Ferber, whose prior contribution to this text and to pediatric sleep medicine were visionary.

—*The Editors*
Stephen H. Sheldon, DO, FAAP
Meir Kryger, MD, FRCPC
David Gozal, MD, MBA, PhD (Hon.)
Craig Canapari, MD
Temitayo O. Oyegbile-Chidi, MD, PhD

Contents

PART I

Principles

1

History of Pediatric Sleep Medicine

Stephen H. Sheldon

CHAPTER HIGHLIGHTS

- Pediatric sleep medicine has mirrored development of pediatrics as a recognized and unique medical discipline.
- Although scientific investigation of sleep and its disorders began in the early 20th century, with significant discoveries made in the 1930s and 1950s, pediatric sleep medicine has lagged behind the development of sleep medicine with a focus on adult disorders and management.
- Clinical sleep medicine emerged from research laboratories and initially focused on insomnia, but later expanded to include the evaluation and management of sleep-related breathing disorders.
- Development of standardized terminology and scoring systems for sleep stages and disorders has been crucial in advancing the field of sleep medicine. Although children are clearly different than adults, standardization of terminology and scoring systems has been required to utilize adult focused approaches to diagnosis and management that may be inadequate for assessment and treatment of the pediatric patient.
- The incorporation of pediatric criteria and the establishment of pediatric sleep medicine training programs have contributed to the recognition of pediatric sleep disorders and the importance of adequate sleep in child development, pediatric sleep health, and well-being.

Overview

Over the past quarter century, pediatric and adolescent sleep medicine (PASM) has followed remarkable parallels with the evolution of health care for infants, children, and young adults in the United States. Chronicled establishment of children's health care, as well as establishment of sleep medicine as an imperative and major medical discipline for adults, provides insight into the current position of PASM and future directions for clinical practice and research. An understanding of the evolution of sleep medicine into a research and clinical field of study and branch of knowledge will create an important perspective. Juxtaposition of disciplines will sensitize the reader to the need for state-of-the-art evaluation of sleep and its pathologies seen in infants, children, and adolescents.

Introduction

Over the past 25 years, the development of PASM as an imperative child health care discipline remarkably parallels evolution of pediatric health care in the United States. Recorded advancement of health care for children as well as establishment of sleep medicine as a recognized, necessary, and vital medical discipline for adults provides lucid insight into the current position within the child health care community of PASM and future directions for research and clinical practice.

Development of Pediatrics as a Unique Discipline

Prior to the beginning of the 20th century, health care for children and adolescents was virtually non-existent. Health care for children was principally provided by family members. Mortality rates for infants were high. More than one-third of infants died before their fifth birthday.[1] Despite this significant incidence of infant mortality, little was done to improve health care for children, and few took particular notice of the lack of professional services. Health care for children by the medical profession was provided using adult criteria, adult standards of care, adult definitions of diseases/disorders, and utilization of therapeutic techniques developed for adult patients.[2]

Medical practitioners who limited their practice to children were few and considered "baby feeders" as little was known of the cause of illness in children. Infectious diseases prevailed and diarrheal diseases resulting in dehydration affected many. It has been estimated that at the turn of the century there were fewer than 50 medical practitioners in the United States who were particularly interested in the health care of children, and less than a dozen limited their practice exclusively to children.[3] Health care facilities for clinical evaluation and management of childhood disease, specifically designed for children's needs, were non-existent.[2] Being considered the property of their parents, neither earning a living, paying taxes, nor voting, children by themselves then and now possess neither an economic nor political influence.

Childhood diseases were widespread. Prevention was the only underlying principle. Approaches to treatment of illness during childhood included tea, barley water, and protein milk. Floating hospitals and country sanatoria were occasionally utilized for the management of childhood illness because sun, fresh air, and isolation were treatments of choice and the standard of care. Nonetheless, because of the lack of children's clinics for diagnosis and management of pediatric diseases/disorders, care of children remained in the home.[4] Because of the lack of diagnostic methods, evaluation of childhood illness was based primarily on anecdotes, and clinical signs and symptoms. Even congenital malformations were thought by many child health care practitioners to be due to maternal influences.[5] Treatment was principally based on either adult medical interventions or was purely empiric. Climate therapy was common. Exposure to sunlight was prescribed for various illnesses including but not limited to tuberculosis, cutaneous abnormalities, anemia, and rickets. Some treatments were effective, but most were relatively ineffective. For example, treatment of pneumonia often included administration of digitalis, camphor, strychnia, and alcohol.

With the discovery and development of pasteurization of milk and immunizations for a variety of diseases, child health care practitioners were thrust into the forefront of preventive medicine. Use of antibiotics to treat infections and the development of corticosteroids were instrumental in decreasing high childhood mortality rates existing during the first half of the 20th century.

During the second half of the 20th century, rapid progress in pediatric medicine and surgery occurred. Practice of pediatric medicine has turned from principally treatment of infectious diseases to comprehensive preventive programs, school health, community pediatrics, developmental pediatrics, and comprehensive adolescent medicine. Extensive morbidities have been identified resulting in extensive efforts in behavioral disorders, family violence, child maltreatment, drug misuse, learning problems, school health, and developmental disabilities. Priorities have shifted and identification of many pediatric disorders requires a multidisciplinary and interdisciplinary approach to diagnosis and management.

Development of Sleep Medicine as a Unique Discipline

Although there has been a fascination with sleep since antiquity, the scientific investigation of sleep and its disorders can be traced back to 1930 when Berger first described spontaneous electroencephalogram (EEG) activity in the brains of sleeping subjects[6] and differentiation of sleep into specific and distinct states by Harvey, Loomis, and Hobart in 1937.[7] Eye movements in sleep were previously described in sleeping infants,[8] and the first description of rapid eye movement (REM) sleep was made by Aserinsky and Kleitman at the University of Chicago in 1953.[9] Five years later, Dement and Kleitman reported the cycling of REM sleep and non–rapid eye movement (NREM) sleep throughout the sleep period, proposed a classification system of NREM sleep into four distinct stages, and associated the eye movements in REM sleep with dream mentation.[10,11]

It had become clear that these discoveries ushered in the realization that it was not enough to evaluate health and disease during only waking hours, but throughout the 24-hour continuum. A new era of medical and scientific research emerged focusing on physiology, pharmacology, and pathophysiology during sleep, which differed from that during the waking state.[12] Sleep research provided the groundwork and basis for the realization that clinical evaluation and management of patients might change during sleep when compared with the awake state, resulting in the emergence of clinical sleep medicine.[13]

At first, study of sleep and its disorders began in the research laboratories. Clinical sleep medicine evolved from patient self-referrals. Initially, most sleep complaints were related to problems related to insomnia. It soon became clear that the majority of etiologies of insomnia were not purely psychiatric in origin. Obstructive sleep apnea had been identified in Europe, but there had been little notice in the United States. In 1970, Lugaresi and colleagues published the remarkable success of tracheostomy in the treatment of obstructive sleep apnea.[14] Nonetheless, similar evaluation and management of obstructive sleep apnea was not yet accepted. In 1972, remarkable results were demonstrated in managing upper airway obstruction and hypertension in a 10½-year-old boy with tracheostomy.[15] It is striking that demonstration of the first successful treatment of sequelae of obstructive sleep apnea in the United States was in a pediatric patient.

Physiologic evaluation of sleep had also progressed with the adaptation of polygraphy used in monitoring the EEG to evaluate other physiologic variables during sleep. Termed *polysomnography*, Holland and coworkers[16] changed the face of clinical assessment of sleep for adult patients. Now there were methods for both basic evaluation by history and physical examination as well as objective physiologic assessment of sleep-related complaints in a clinical laboratory setting.

By the end of the 1970s, clinical sleep disorders medicine became an accepted area of medical inquiry, although practice of sleep disorders medicine was still couched in other disciplines of pulmonology, psychiatry, neurology, and internal medicine. In 1968, *A Manual of Standardized Terminology, Techniques, and Scoring System for Sleep Stages of Human Subjects* was published.[17] This was a significant step forward in standardizing sleep stage scoring in adults and to eliminate unreliability and inconsistencies in laboratory evaluation of sleep both between laboratories and within laboratories. It was clear at that time this standardization was not appropriate for identification of sleep stages and evaluation of sleep for newborns, infants, and children. Anatomical and physiologic variables differed markedly from the adult. Similar standardization of sleep stage identification was a daunting task due to the rapid and constantly changing biology of the maturing and developing child. Therefore, the newborn infant became a starting point for a similar process that was started by Drs. Rechtschaffen and Kales in 1968.[17] Drs. Anders, Emde, and Parmelee co-chaired an ad hoc committee to provide similar standards, and the result was the publication in 1971 of *A Manual of Standardized Terminology, Techniques and Criteria for Scoring of States of Sleep and Wakefulness in Newborn Infants*.[18] Strikingly, between the publication of this manual and today (50 years later), there has been no similar unique effort for infants and children older than 2 months of age and the beginning of puberty. Many problems precluded this task. Standardization in the pediatric age group is a formidable endeavor. First, there are rapid and dynamic changes that occur during the first two decades of life. The nervous system is constantly changing structurally and functionally during this period of life. Attempting to define cross-sectional criteria for evaluation of children both within same-age subjects and between subjects is extraordinarily difficult because of normal internal and external variability. Normal ranges can be extensive. Limitations include number of evaluations required for appropriate power. External reliability and validity can also be quite difficult to establish. Several longitudinal points are often required for appropriate comparison of polysomnographic variables. This has been suggested to be termed *developmental polysomnography*.[19] This would then take into account normal progression of maturation, rather than evaluating a single polygraphic study at a single point in time. Because of these immense difficulties, little evidence-based standardized information has been available to provide accurate and reproducible normative data, despite evidence that sleep, and its normal structure and maturation, has far-reaching implications on growth, development, and learning.[20,21]

With the expansion of evaluation of the pediatric patients in adult sleep laboratories and centers, a significant need was identified for inclusion of pediatric criteria in newer editions of manuals guiding scoring and assessment of polysomnograms of children. Pediatric criteria were developed, not as a unique publication focused only on criteria for assessment of sleep of infants and children, but as variations from adult criteria juxtaposed within the context of adult-oriented sleep medicine, first in 2007[22] and regularly updated with Version 2.6 in 2020.[23] Additionally, the *International Classification of Sleep Disorders, Third Edition* (ICSD-3), has added several sections on sleep disorders unique to childhood, and comments of pediatric differences within the context of adult-oriented sleep-related diagnoses.[24] Yet there has not been a singular formal reference solely focused on unique and separate physiology of sleep and/or its disorders of infants, children, and adolescents.

Identification of effective noninvasive treatments for many sleep-related disorders developed (for example, treatment of obstructive sleep apnea in adults with nasal continuous positive airway pressure [CPAP]) and resulted in rapid development of therapeutic protocols and widespread use. A combination of a high prevalence of obstructive sleep apnea in the adult population, management of the obstructive sleep-disordered breathing with a noninvasive procedure, and effective management of sequelae led to the rapid expansion of sleep medicine into a unique medical discipline. Sleep disorders medicine has become an accepted and distinct specialty within the medical community.

Beginning in 1978, the American Board of Sleep Medicine (ABSM) provided an examination in clinical polysomnography to ensure the quality and competency of practitioners practicing sleep disorders medicine and interpreting polysomnograms. The first examination certified 21 candidates. During the next 28 years, the ABSM certified more than 3,400 individuals.[25] This examination was not specialty specific and was taken by internists, psychiatrists, psychologists, neurologists, family practitioners, and pediatricians. Successful applicants became diplomates of the ABSM. Indeed, sleep disorders medicine as a new and unique discipline became the focus of more clinical practitioners.

PASM has become an outgrowth of sleep disorders medicine practice. More pediatricians became involved in research and clinical practice, but few limited their clinical activities to the full-time practice of pediatric sleep medicine. Inspiration has come from several directions: scientific and clinical interest in sudden infant death syndrome (SIDS); identification of obstructive sleep apnea and other sleep-related breathing disorders occurring with significant prevalence in the pediatric population; identification of the importance of sleep in the origin of daytime behavioral difficulties; and the influence of sleep disorders on children's daytime performance and learning.

In the early 1980s the practice of pediatrics was a highly respected medical discipline. One of the principal textbooks utilized by most students and practitioners of health care for children was titled *Nelson's Textbook of Pediatrics*.[26] Nevertheless, the 14th edition of this text, published in 1992, had a total of *only eleven paragraphs uniquely devoted to sleep disorders in children*.

In 1985, two seminal works were published: one for parents and the other for sleep scientists. The first was the publication of Dr. Richard Ferber's book for parents titled *Solve Your Child's Sleep Problems*.[27] Based on Dr. Ferber's work at Boston Children's Hospital, this book reviewed all aspects of sleep during childhood and provided practical information in the management of many sleep-related difficulties that occur during infancy and childhood. The second publication was titled *Sleep and Its Disorders in Children* edited by Dr. Christian Guilleminault.[28] This book was a compilation of groundbreaking scientific papers on normative data providing a basis for future direction in the scientific study of sleep and sleep–wake cycles during infancy, childhood, and adolescence.

It is clear that more changes occur in anatomy, physiology, and sleep–wake patterns during the first 15 years of life than over the next four decades. Nonetheless, comparatively little evidence-based information regarding this transformation has been published. Prevalence and impact of dysfunctional sleep on the developing child requires large population-based studies. Because sleep is a neurodevelopmental process almost identical to the neuro-development of the ability to walk and the neural change required for the evolution of language, it is imperative to determine how sleep and its organization mature in infancy and early childhood. Disruption of the normal progression of neural network development during *these vastly important stages in human maturation are posited to have lifelong consequences.*

As previously suggested, clinical pediatric sleep medicine has had to rely on nosology developed for adults.[29] Adaptations have been attempted,[30] but it is clearly apparent that adapting adult criteria to infants and children can lead to many false starts and wrong turns. Most sleep-related problems in children might carry similar nomenclature, but children are different, and it is meaningfully inappropriate to apply adult sleep medicine anatomical, physiological, and pathological criteria.

Nevertheless, the general pediatric community has been very slow to grasp the significance of the entirety of pediatric sleep disorders. Child health care practitioners have been resistant to absorb the importance of sleep physiology and sleep structure to human development and behavior. However, over the past 5–10 years, pediatric pulmonologists, otolaryngologists, and neurologists have increasingly recognized the importance of sleep and its disorders and have incorporated this large portion of the child's life into clinical and academic endeavors, with particular focus on sleep-related breathing abnormalities. With the "epidemic" of obstructive sleep apnea in the adult population, this again seems to be an outgrowth of adult sleep medicine.

In 2002, the American Academy of Sleep Medicine (AASM) applied to the Accreditation Council on Graduate Medical Education (ACGME) for establishment of sleep medicine training programs under the auspices of the ACGME as part of a comprehensive plan along with the American Board of Medical Specialists (ABMS) to accept sleep medicine as an independent medical specialty. In 2003, this was approved, and a consensus plan was developed for establishment of a new multidisciplinary specialty examination in sleep medicine to be jointly offered by the American Board of Internal Medicine (ABIM), American Board of Psychiatry and Neurology (ABPN), American Board of Pediatrics (ABP), American Board of Family Medicine (ABFM), and American Board of Otolaryngology Head and Neck Surgery (ABO-HNS)[25] The first examination was administered in 2007. Considerations and disorders unique to childhood comprised only 2% of the first examination. Although pediatrics is a required portion of a sleep medicine fellowship curriculum, it is unclear how much pediatric medicine and sleep disorders in children are afforded to internists, otolaryngologists, psychiatrists, and neurologists studying general sleep medicine in these programs. It is also unclear whether training in developmental medicine and children's health care can be translated into the practice of sleep medicine without a comprehensive underpinning of pediatric medicine.

The success of incorporating a pediatric sleep medicine objective into undergraduate, graduate, and post-graduate training curricula will depend upon outcome and cost-effectiveness. First, can the provision of comprehensive sleep medicine services to children by pediatricians specializing, and devoting full time to the practice of pediatric sleep medicine, have a significant impact on comorbid medical illnesses such as sickle cell anemia, cystic fibrosis, neuromuscular disorders, craniofacial malformations, mucopolysaccharidoses, morbid obesity, or congenital/acquired cardiovascular disease? Second, what effect does early disruption of sleep and/or sleep–wake cycling have on learning, memory, and cognitive development? Is this transient and reversible or may it be permanent morbidity if not diagnosed and treated very early in life? Finally, can understanding sleep and its disorders in childhood contribute to a better understanding of behavioral disorders, problems of attention, and learning disabilities? The mystery of establishing and integrating neural networks required for early brain development and later executive functioning may be locked within the sleeping brain.

As was true of the development of pediatrics as a unique medical discipline, further appreciation of the development of sleep and its structure, as well as the effects of disruption and when in the development of the infants and small child this disruption of normal maturation occurs, might lead to improved diagnosis, treatment, and prevention of a wide variety of disorders unique to both children and adults. It is evident that the present is only the beginning of the understanding of pediatric sleep and pediatric sleep medicine.

CLINICAL PEARLS

- Clinical sleep medicine is a relatively new discipline that has rapidly evolved over the past 60 years.
- Clinical sleep medicine has evolved from the scientific study of sleep in the laboratory to a unique discipline.
- Development of pediatric sleep medicine parallels the development of pediatrics as a singular profession focused on the health and well-being of infants, children, and adolescents.

Summary

PASM has followed a similar path in its maturation to the development of pediatrics as a recognized and unique medical discipline. There has been very significant increase in evidence-based knowledge regarding sleep and its disorders in infants, children, and adolescents over the past decade. Nonetheless, what is known now about the importance of sleep in normal human development and sleep in health and disease is likely only the "tip of the iceberg." The future of PASM is truly before us, but many questions remain:

1. How important is the basic rest–activity cycle during gestation in growth and maturation of the central nervous system, neuronal migration, and neural network development?
2. What impact does disruption of normal sleep and/or its continuity during the first few years of life have on future human development and performance?
3. What effect does sleep deprivation during adolescence have on health and well-being as adults? How might this contribute to chronic illness affecting these individuals as adults?

References

1. Holt LE. Infant mortality ancient and modern, an historical sketch. *Arch Pediatr.* 1913;30:885–915.
2. Cone TE. *History of American Pediatrics.* Little Brown; 1979.
3. Smith RM. Medicine as a science: Pediatrics. *NEJM.* 1951;244(5):176–181.
4. Powers GF. Developments in pediatrics in the past quarter century. *Yale J Biol Med.* 1939;12(1):1–22.
5. Freeman RG. Fresh air in pediatric practice. *Am J Dis Child.* 1916;XII(6):590–596.
6. Berger H. Uber das Elekoenkeephalogramm des Menchen. *J Psychol Neurol.* 1930;40:160–179.
7. Harvey EN, Loomis AL, Hobart GA. Cerebral states during sleep as studied by human brain potentials. *Science.* 1937;85:443–444.
8. de Toni G. I movimenti pendolari de bulbi oculari dei bambini durante il sonno fisiologico, ed in alcuni stati morbosi. *Pediatria (Santiago).* 1933;41:489–498.
9. Aserinsky E, Kleitman N. Regularly recurring periods of eye motility, and concomitant phenomena, during sleep. *Science.* 1953;118:273–274.
10. Dement WC, Kleitman N. The relation of eye movements during sleep to dream activity: An objective method for the study of dreaming. *J Exp Psychol.* 1957;53:339–346.
11. Dement WC, Kleitman N. Cyclic variations in EEG during sleep and their relation to eye movements, body motility, and dreaming. *Electroencephalogr Clin Neurophysiol.* 1957;9:673–690.
12. Orem J, Barnes CD. *Physiology in Sleep.* Academic Press; 1980.
13. Carskadon MA, Roth T. Normal sleep and its variations. In: Kryger M, Roth T, Dement WC, eds. *Principles and Practice of Sleep Medicine.* WB Saunders; 1989:3–15.
14. Lugaresi E, Coccagna G, Mantovani M. Effects de la tracheotomie dans les hypersomnies avec respiration periodique. *Rev Neurol.* 1970;123:267–268.
15. Dement WC. In: Kryger M, Roth T, Dement WC, eds. *History of Sleep Physiology and Medicine.* 2nd ed. WB Saunders; 1994.
16. Holland V, Dement W, Raynal D. Polysomnography: Responding to a need for improved communication. In: *Presentation to the Annual Meeting of the Sleep Research Society;* 1974.
17. Rechtschaffen A, Kales A. *A Manual of Standardized Terminology, Techniques, and Scoring System for Sleep Stages of Human Subjects.* BIS/BRI. 1968.
18. Anders T, Emde R, Parmelee AH. *A Manual of Standardized Terminology, Techniques and Criteria for Scoring of States of Sleep and Wakefulness in Newborn Infants.* UCLA Brain Information Service, NINDS Neurological Information Network; 1971.
19. Sheldon SH. *Evaluating Sleep in Infants and Children.* Lippincott-Raven; 1996.
20. Karni A, Tanne D, Rubenstein BS. Dependence on REM sleep of overnight improvement of a perceptual skill. *Science.* 1994;265:679–682.
21. Wilson MA, McNaughton BL. Reactivation of hippocampal ensemble memories during sleep. *Science.* 1994;265(5172):676–679.
22. Iber C, Ancoli-Israel S, Chesson A, Quan SF, Iber C, Ancoli-Israel S, Chesson AL, Quan SF. For the American Academy of Sleep Medicine. *The AASM Manual for the Scoring of Sleep and Associated Events: Rules, Terminology and Technical Specifications.* 1st ed. American Academy of Sleep Medicine; 2007.
23. Berry R., Quan S.F., Abreu A. *The AASM Manual for the Scoring of Sleep and Associated Events: Rules, Terminology and Technical Specifications.* Version 2.6. American Academy of Sleep Medicine; 2020.
24. American Academy of Sleep Medicine. *International Classification of Sleep Disorders.* 3–TR. ed. American Academy of Sleep Medicine; 2023.
25. Quan SF, Berry RB, Buyssee D. Development and results of the first ABMS subspecialty certification examination in sleep medicine. *J Clin Sleep Med.* 2008;4(5):505–508.
26. Behrman RE, ed. *Nelson's Textbook of Pediatrics.* 14th ed. WB Saunders; 1992.
27. Ferber R. *Solve Your Child's Sleep Problems.* Simon & Schuster; 1985.
28. Guilleminault C. *Sleep and Its Disorders in Children.* Raven Press; 1987.
29. American Sleep Disorders Association Diagnostic Classification Steering Committee. *International Classification of Sleep Disorders: Diagnostic and Coding Manual.* American Sleep Disorders Association; 1990.
30. Sheldon SH, Spire JP, Levy HB. *Pediatric Sleep Medicine.* WB Saunders; 1992:185–240.

2

Development of Sleep in Infants and Children

Stephen H. Sheldon

CHAPTER HIGHLIGHTS

- Sleep is essential for growth, development, and well-being in infants and children.
- Sleep onset and structure is characterized by behavioral and physiological changes.
- Sleep microstructure and macrostructure undergoes rapid maturation during infancy, childhood, and adolescence.
- Inadequate sleep is common during adolescence and can lead to daytime sleepiness and impaired functioning.

Introduction

Sleep is an essential vital function. Its importance is critical in growth and development, as well as functional well-being. Sleep is not a passive, unitary process. Its importance is likely epitomized by the more significant amounts of sleep seen in each 24-hour cycle during the most rapid and crucial developmental periods. There are implications that a significant amount of "learning" (including but not limited to neuronal migration, dendritic branching, and synapse/neural network creation) occurs in the first months of life because so much time is spent in the sleeping state and there is limited contact with the environment.[1] Profound developmental changes occur from late in gestation throughout the life cycle; the most dramatic ontological alterations seem to occur during the first decade of life and then remain rather stable with few alterations throughout the normal life cycle. Changes in sleep of infants and children have been recorded for many decades. Nevertheless, only since the mid-1980s have physiologic variations been more completely studied and consequences of abnormal sleep (whether cause or effect) during early infancy and childhood characterized.

Sleep Onset

Sleep onset is not an isolated event. Identification of an exact moment of transition from wakefulness to sleep is somewhat difficult from both a behavioral and physiologic perspective. For practical purposes, sleep onset can be correlated with certain behavioral and physiologic changes occurring over a period of time. This time is, nonetheless, somewhat short. Behaviors typically associated with sleep include but are not limited to closed eyes, postural change, and behavioral quiescence. Additionally, there is modulation of responsiveness to auditory and visual stimuli, decrease in the ability of performance of simple tasks, and alterations in memory of events occurring several moments before sleep onset. Electroencephalogram (EEG) activity changes commonly associated with transitional sleep (N1) are not always perceived by the individual. Conversely, individuals may believe they have slept without obvious documentable changes in the EEG from the normal waking state.

Dominant posterior rhythm (DPR) varies depending upon the child's age and level of development. According to the American Academy of Sleep Medicine *Manual of Scoring Sleep Stages and Other Physiological Variables of Sleep*, DPR shows only continuous slow irregular potential changes in infants less than 3 months of age. Activity attenuates with eye opening.[2,3]

Wake

During wakefulness, DPR frequency in children less than 3 months of age ranges from 3.5 to 4.5 Hz. Frequency increases as the infant matures, reaching 5–6 Hz by 5–6 months of age, and 7–9 Hz by 3 years of age.

By 3–4 months post-gestation, about 75% of infants will have irregular 50–100 microvolt, 3–4 Hz activity over the occipital region that attenuates with eye opening. Between 5 and 6 months of age, many infants will demonstrate 50–110 microvolt activity over the occipital region at a frequency of about 5–6 Hz. This is apparent in about 70% of infants by 1 year post-gestation. This pattern of continued and consistent increase in DPR frequency and amplitude continues so that by 3 years of age, more than 80% of children have a mean occipital frequency of more than 7.5–9.5 Hz, 65% of 9-year-old children have an average frequency of 9 Hz, and by age 15 years this increases to about 10 Hz.

EEG amplitude is generally consistently greater than 50–110 microvolts. Average amplitude of the DPR during wakefulness is 50–56 microvolts in infants and children. About 10% of children have more than 100-microvolt activity between 6 and 9 years of age. Young children rarely exhibit EEG activity in the alpha range with voltage less than 30 microvolts.

Eye blinking might be seen with conjugate vertical eye movements that occur at a frequency of about 0.5–2 Hz. Chin muscle tone is high. Sucking movements may be noted and are characterized by extended rhythmic periods of increased chin muscle tone that appears to have a waxing and waning character. There may be conjugate, irregular, sharply peaked eye movements with an initial deflection lasting less than 500 milliseconds.

Transitional Sleep

T in infants 0–2 months and N1 when NREM states can be clearly differentiated. Transitional sleep in infants 0–2 months of age appears to be necessary because it is quite commonly seen, can account for 10–40% of sleep, and may be a significant marker of development and maturation.[4]

From 2 months to about 8 months of age, transitional sleep (N1) is characterized by a gradual appearance of diffuse 75- to 200-microvolt activity at a frequency of about 3–5 Hz. This amplitude is generally greater than that seen during wakefulness and is usually 1–2 Hz slower than the waking background rhythm.

By 8 months to 3 years of age, generalized runs or bursts of semirhythmic bisynchronous 75- to 200-microvolt activity in the range of 3–4 Hz characterize N1. This is maximal over the occipital region. There may also be higher amplitude 4–6 Hz activity noted maximally over the frontocentral or central regions.

After 3 years of age, N1 is characterized by slowing of the DPR by about 1–2 Hz. The DPR can also be gradually replaced by relatively lower voltage mixed frequency activity. Beginning at about 5 years of age and progressing into adolescence, rhythmic anterior theta activity (RAT) can be seen. RAT is characterized by runs of 5–7 Hz moderate voltage activity seen best over the frontal regions.

Monophasic negative broad sharp waves seen maximally over the central regions become evident during N1 (and N2) sleep at about 6 months of age. By about 16 months of age, these vertex sharp waves of about 200 milliseconds in length can occur in bursts or runs and are most often seen during transitional sleep.

A distinctive paroxysmal EEG pattern of diffuse bisynchronous 75–350 microvolt, 3–4.5 Hz activity that occurs in bursts or runs maximal over the central, frontal, or frontocentral regions during drowsiness and during N1 sleep. This activity is termed *hypnogogic hypersynchrony* (HH). This pattern occurs early during sleep and disappears during N3 sleep. It is present in about 30% of 3-month-old infants and almost all children by 6–8 months of age. HH decreases in prevalence as development progresses and is identified in only about 10% of normal healthy children over 10 years of age. It is rare after 12 years of age.

At sleep onset, the electromyogram may reveal a gradual fall in muscle tone; however, this is not always present and a discrete fall in tone below that of wake may not be appreciated. Sucking movements can be seen during wakefulness and can be sustained throughout transitional sleep. Spontaneous eye closure typically signals drowsiness and wake-to-sleep transition. Slow conjugate sinusoidal eye movements replace rapid conjugate movements. Blinking disappears, and sustained eye closure is noted.

Stage N2 Sleep

Sleep spindles typically appear between 4 and 6 weeks of age. These rudimentary spindles are noted to be maximal over the central (vertex) regions and are typically of relatively lower amplitude and slightly lower frequency, but tend to remain about 12–14 Hz. Spindles in young infants can last longer than those typically seen in adults. More than three-quarters of children less than 13 years of age show two independent locations with different frequency ranges for sleep spindles. Spindles located over the frontal regions tend to range from 10 to 12.5 Hz and those over the central or centroparietal region range from 12.5 to 14.5 Hz. Frontal sleep spindles are more prominent than centroparietal spindles in young children but abruptly decrease in EEG power and presence beginning at about age 13 years. Centroparietal spindles persist unchanged in presence or location as development continues.

K-complexes are well-defined waves characteristic of N2 sleep. These transient events consist of an initial negative sharp wave that is immediately followed by a positive wave lasting greater than or equal to 0.5 seconds. These events begin to appear as unique identifiable waveforms at about 5–6 months post-term and are maximally located over the prefrontal and frontal regions.

Electrooculogram usually shows no eye movement activity. However, there may be frontal EEG artifact noted and slow sinusoidal eye movements may continue in some children. Chin muscle electromyography (EMG) is of variable amplitude, is typically lower than during wakefulness, and on occasion may be as low as during rapid eye movement (REM) sleep.

Stage N3 Sleep

Slow-wave EEG activity during N3 sleep in the pediatric patient is typically very high voltage and can range from 100 to 400 microvolts. Activity frequency ranges from 0.5 to 2.0 Hz and is maximal over the frontal region. This slow-wave activity appears as early as 2 months of age but most often between 3 and 4.5 months of age post-term. Sleep spindles may continue during N3 sleep.

Eye movements are typically absent, and there is often slow-wave EEG activity artifact noted in the electrooculogram. Chin muscle EMG is of variable amplitude and is often lower than in N2 sleep. Sometimes it can be as low as during REM sleep. In infants and younger children, sucking artifact may also be noted. N3 sleep is noted when 20% or more of a given 30-second epoch consists of slow-wave activity (in otherwise normal children), regardless of age.

Stage REM Sleep

EEG during REM sleep in infants and children resembles that of adults. Nonetheless, the dominant frequency are slower and of higher voltage the younger the infant/child. Dominant R frequency tends to increase with age, with 3 Hz activity at 7–8 weeks post-term, 4–5 Hz activity with bursts of sawtooth waves at about 5 months of age, 4–6 Hz at 9 months of age, and prolonged runs or bursts of notched 5–7 Hz activity at 1–5 years of age. After 5 years of age, the low-voltage mixed frequency pattern of R sleep is quite similar to that of adults, although the amplitude may be somewhat higher.

Baseline chin muscle EMG is low and no higher than other stages of sleep. It is typically the nadir of activity noted throughout the recording. Irregular brief bursts of phasic muscle activity with duration less than 0.25 seconds can be superimposed on this low chin EMG tone. This phasic activity can occur in bursts and can be concomitant with similar bursts of rapid eye movements and anterior tibialis EMG twitches. Electrooculogram reveals irregular conjugate eye movements with a rapid initial deflection of signal lasting less than 500 milliseconds.

In small infants and young children, REM sleep is sometimes difficult to differentiate from wake or other sleep states. In these cases, use of other recorded variables to assist in state assignation is done. Respiration during non–rapid eye movement (NREM) sleep is classically regular and monotonous with little variation. During REM sleep, considerable respiratory instability is noted. This is characterized by variation in rate, depth, minute ventilation, brief respiratory pauses, and brief episodes of increased respiratory rate.

Normal Course of Evolution of Sleep Across The Night

Healthy Children, Adolescents, and Young Adults

Normal, healthy preschool-age children, school-age children, adolescents, and young adults transition into sleep through NREM sleep. This is in clear contrast to infants who normally transition to sleep through REM sleep. During transition, the posterior dominant EEG converts to an N1 pattern, theta activity appears, and eye movements become slow, rolling, and/or pendulous. EMG muscle tone changes little from waking levels. Arousal thresholds are low, but vary when meaning is assigned to a stimulus (e.g., a subject may respond to their name, but not to another name or a pure tone stimulus, often regardless of the amplitude, which has been shown to be age dependent). N1 sleep typically lasts briefly and is followed by transition to N2 sleep. Arousal thresholds are higher in N2 than in N1, and the same stimulus that may cause arousal or waking from N1 may cause a K-complex

to appear in N2. After approximately 5–25 minutes of N2 sleep, there is a gradual increase in the appearance of high voltage waves with a frequency ranging from 0.5 to 2 Hz. This is characteristic of N3 sleep when constituting greater than 20–50% of the recording epoch. Arousal thresholds are considerably higher in N3 sleep when compared with other sleep stages. During the first cycle of the sleep period, N3 will last about 20–40 minutes and ends with a series of body movements and ascent to a lighter/higher NREM stage.

The first REM sleep period of the night occurs about 70–110 minutes after sleep onset. The initial REM sleep period is often brief, lasting usually less than 10 minutes and is often missed during a single night of recording in the laboratory. Arousal threshold is variable during REM sleep and is generally considered to be similar to N2.

Subsequently, NREM and REM sleep cycle throughout the remainder of the sleep period at intervals of approximately 60–120 minutes. N3 sleep is most prominent during the early sleep period (first third to first half of the sleep period time), and propensity for N3 sleep decreases as the sleep period progresses. REM episodes, on the other hand, become longer and more intense throughout the sleep period, with the longest and most intense REM episode occurring in the early morning hours.

Though internal and external variability exists, volumes of sleep stages across sleep periods are relatively constant. N1 constitutes 2–5%; N2, 45–55%; N3, 13–23%; and REM, approximately 20–25%. After 5 years of age, proportions of sleep states remain remarkably constant throughout the remainder of the life cycle. Wake after sleep onset accounts for less than 5%. There are normally 4–6 cycles through various stages of sleep per night.

Newborns, Infants, and Young Children

Observation of newborns, infants, and children reveals that sleep occupies a major portion of their lives. A newborn infant spends more than 70% of every 24 hours sleeping. In contrast, adults spend 25–30% of their lives sleeping. Major "work" of the waking child has been said to be play. Because sleep occupies such a large portion of a child's life, the major work of infancy and very early childhood is more likely sleep.

Behavioral and physiologic characteristics of sleep in normal infants vary significantly from sleep in adults. Premature infants exhibit a lack of concordance between electrophysiologic parameters and behavioral observations. This may also be true in some term infants.[5] In newborn infants, electrophysiologic characteristics of sleep and waking states in infants are often difficult because traditional characteristics cannot be fulfilled. Solutions to these problems have been suggested by a number of investigators. Prechtl and Beintema[6] suggested state definition based on observable behaviors; Anders, Emde, and Parmelee[7] suggested use of behavioral and polygraphic features; and Hoppenbrouwers[8] suggested state definition based on polygraphic features, with observational criteria used only as supplemental information. Despite differences regarding state definition, it is clear that sleep in infants and children is significantly different than older children, adolescents, and adults. Sleep, therefore, most likely performs a different function in the developing human.

Observations in the Fetus and Premature Infants

Rhythmic cycling of periods of activity and quiescence can be identified in the human fetus between 28 and 32 weeks' gestation.[9] Neither quiet (NREM) nor active (REM) sleep can be identified in premature babies between 24 and 26 weeks' gestation.[5] By 28–30 weeks, active sleep can be recognized by presence of eye movements, body movements, and irregular respiratory activity. Chin muscle hypotonia is difficult to evaluate in the fetus and premature infant because there are few periods of tonic activity before 36 weeks' gestation.[9] Quiet sleep, on the other hand, cannot be clearly identified at this time and active sleep constitutes most of the sleep period. Quiet sleep does not appear to emerge significantly until approximately 36 weeks' gestation.[9] Once identifiable, this state continues to increase in proportion regularly until it becomes the dominant state at approximately 3 months of post natal life.

Spontaneous fetal movements can be identified between 10 and 12 weeks' gestation. Rhythmic cycling of quiescence and activity can be recorded in utero by 20 weeks.[10] At 28–30 weeks, brief quiet periods appear, though their period is quite unstable.[11] By 32 weeks' gestational age, body movements are absent in 53% of 20-second epochs during 2- to 3-hour sleep recordings.[9] "No movement epochs" increases to 60% at term.

Patterns of physiologic EEG activity become recognizable as early as 24 weeks' gestation. Conflicting evidence exists concerning the independence of the maturation of sleep and the EEG with respect to intrauterine stage. Very young premature infants and full-term neonates have similar EEG patterns when compared at the same conceptional age. On the other hand, it has been shown that when a premature infant reaches 40 weeks' conceptional age, they still have not attained a degree of EEG and central nervous system (CNS) organization of a comparable full-term newborn.[5] Premature infants show spindle development that is approximately 4 weeks in advance of that seen in full-term infants, and a statistical difference between the length of quiet sleep in the term and premature infant exists when measured at the same conceptional age.[12] Some conflicting reports, however, may be secondary to definition and calculation of gestational age and conceptional age, or may be actual differences precipitated by development in an extrauterine environment significantly different from the normal intrauterine milieu. Extrauterine development of the premature infant occurs either in a 24-hour "light" environment or a cycled light environment, rather than in the 24-hour "dark" conditions of the uterus. In addition, other significant medical and developmental problems often exist in the significantly preterm newborn and continuous medical interventions are often required, disrupting the natural progression of sleep-wake cycle development. The effect of constant light and medical treatment regimens on the development of the nervous system and sleep cycling has not yet been elucidated.

Term Infants: Birth to Twelve Months

By gestational term, two distinct sleep states can be identified in the term newborn: active sleep (REM) and quiet sleep (NREM). Indeterminate sleep had been a state classification defined when criteria for neither REM nor NREM can be identified.[7] However, this state has recently been reclassified as *transitional sleep* in the new visual classification criteria.[2] Sucking movements are common during active sleep. During this state fine twitches are almost continuous, and grimaces, smiles, vocalizations, and tremors also occur. Intermittent large athetoid limb movements, stretching, can be seen. Bursts of muscle movements and irregular respiration occur concomitantly with phasic eye movements. Conversely, quiet sleep is characterized by minimal movement.[7] Chin muscle tone is increased above the level seen in active sleep. Respiration is regular and monotonous. Little, if any, phasic activity is noted. Total 24-hour sleep time tends to range from 14 to 17 hours between 0 and 3 months of age.[13] REM/active sleep occupies the majority of the total sleep time before conceptional term. This rapidly declines and REM sleep occupies about 50% of the total sleep time in the term infant.

During the first 3 months of life, striking changes occur in many physiologic functions. Ten- to 12 weeks of age appears to be a critical period of CNS reorganization, when infantile sleep behavior and physiology shifts to a more mature form. Significant changes in sleep-wake patterns occur. At birth, total sleep time in each 24-hour cycle is about 14–17 hours.[9,13] Slow decrease in total sleep time occurs, generally ranging from 12 to 16 hours between 4 and 12 months of age.

Appearance of attentive behaviors occurs concomitantly with the development of quiet sleep and sustained sleep patterns. This evolution suggests continued development of inhibitory and controlling feedback mechanisms secondary to the increasing complexity of neural networks and neurochemical maturation.[9] By 3 months, maturation of these systems produces a relatively stable 24-hour distribution of sleep and wake. There is also a remarkably regular alternation of NREM and REM sleep.[8] Before 3 months of age, concordance between physiologic variables is remarkably high.[14] One explanation may be a lack of maturation of essential feedback control, and a lack of variability is occasionally seen in cardiac function when the conductive tissue of the heart fails to respond to regulatory input, resulting in a fixed rate, with almost equal beat-to-beat intervals. Periodic respiration, common in NREM sleep until 3 weeks of age, becomes rare after 7 weeks.[15]

During the first 6 months of life, consolidation and entrainment of sleep at night develops. Major changes seen are in the duration of single sleep periods and their placement in the 24-hour day. Coons has impressively described this progression.[16] Her study revealed that at 3 weeks of age, the mean length of the longest sleep period was 211.7 minutes, or 23.2% of the total sleep time during the 24-hour period. By 6 months of age, the longest sleep period was 358.0 minutes, or 48% of the total sleep time. Between 3 and 6 weeks sleep periods lengthen considerably, and by 6 weeks of age, the longest sleep period was no longer randomly distributed throughout the day. At 3 months, the pattern had become more consistent. Although sleep had begun to consolidate and establish its relation to the light/dark cycle by 6 weeks of age, the longest wake period was still randomly distributed at 3 months, becoming acceptably non-random at 4.5 months of age. Long 5- to 6-hour sleep periods at 6 weeks of age gradually lengthen to 8–9 hours and shift to nighttime, so that a diurnal pattern is relatively well established by 12–16 weeks of age.[9] At 6 months of age, the long sleep period immediately follows the longest wake period.[16] After 12 weeks of age, there is continuing development of the diurnal cycle and consolidation of daytime sleep into well-defined daytime naps.[17] Waking patterns change only slightly in comparison to sleep patterns. In the neonatal period, infants awaken about every 4 hours and stay awake for 1–2 hours. The longest period of sustained wake period increases slowly to 3–4 hours by 16 weeks of age.

Brief awakenings from sleep are more frequent during the first 2 months of life than at older ages.[8] In addition, infants 1–2 months of age are more likely to awaken from active sleep than from quiet sleep. Bowe and Anders reported that this variable helped discriminate between infant sleep at 2 and 9 months of age.[18] Good sleepers rarely woke from quiet sleep, whereas poor sleepers typically did. Sleep onset latencies in infants at 2 months were approximately 30 minutes. This was almost halved by 9 months of age. Anders and Keener have shown that 44% of 2-month-old infants and 78% of 9-month-old infants slept through the night.[19]

Striking changes occur in the EEG in the immediate newborn period. The tracé alternant EEG pattern of quiet sleep can be first identified at 32–34 weeks' gestation.[20] This pattern is fully developed at 37–38 weeks, and mature neonates show this characteristic EEG pattern. The tracé alternant pattern gradually disappears over the first month of life. Sleep spindles appear almost simultaneously with the disappearance of tracé alternant at 4–6 weeks of age. Spindles are initially rudimentary showing two spectral bands at 12–14 cycles per second (cps) and 18 cps.[15] It takes approximately 7 days for the 18 cps spindles to disappear, but the 12–14 cps spindles remain. The shape of these spindles changes impressively early in development. At 2 months of age, spindles contrast so slightly with background EEG activity that no reliable measurements are possible.[21] Long spindles are seen in the 3- to 4-month-old infant (lasting 1.8–3.4 seconds). This duration decreases continuously to an average of 0.5–0.7 seconds at the end of the second year. Spindle intervals become greater with increasing age, with a mean of 9–11 seconds at 6 months and 19–28 seconds at 24 months. After this time, the spindle interval decreases with increasing age.

True continuous delta frequency activity appears at approximately 8–12 weeks of age,[16] and quiet sleep becomes differentiated into three distinct stages characteristic of the more mature electrophysiologic pattern. At 3 months, quiet sleep is twice that of active sleep.[12] By 8 months of age, active sleep occupies approximately 30% of the total sleep time and there is a continuous but significantly slower decline until the adult proportion is reached (between 3 and 5 years of age).[8]

Sleep onset is characteristically through REM sleep in the newborn infant (i.e., the first REM period occurs within the first 15 minutes after sleep onset). During the first 12 weeks of life, this gradually changes to sleep onset through NREM. At 3 weeks of age, an infant is likely to have 64% of sleep periods beginning with REM sleep.[16] Younger infants, less than 3 months of age, manifest REM latencies that are predominantly less than 8 minutes in length.[22] Older infants produce a mixed distribution of short and long REM latencies. By 6 months, the proportion of sleep entered through REM sleep is approximately 18%.[19] The longest sleep period is equally as likely to have sleep onset through REM at 3 weeks of age. Between 4 and 13 months, the total distribution of REM latencies appears to be bimodal with latencies either shorter than 8 minutes or longer than 16 minutes.[22] In the group of older infants, the temporal distribution of latencies constitutes a diurnal rhythm, with the longest latencies appearing between noon and 4 p.m., and a tendency of short latencies to occur between 4 a.m. and 8 a.m. In the older infants, REM latency also depends upon the length of prior wakefulness. Long REM latencies are significantly more often preceded by long episodes of wakefulness than are short REM latencies. By 6 months of age, the longest sleep period is only 20% more likely to be through REM.[16] The ratio of active sleep to quiet sleep is sometimes considered an indicator of maturation.[8] Active sleep time exceeds quiet sleep time during the first months of life. A reversal of this relation is noted in 60% of infants at 3 months and 90% of infants at 6 months of age.

A specific change in REM proportion occurs during this period of development. During the first 6 months of life there is a marked reduction in the total REM sleep volume. This represents a redistribution of sleep stages, because only a relative mild decrease in the total sleep time occurs during the first year. This change is considered to be an important indicator of CNS maturation.[12] It is interesting to note that the reduction in the proportion of time spent in REM sleep is balanced by an increased proportion of the 24-hour day spent in wakefulness.

Two Years to Five Years

In contrast to the dramatic changes that take place during the first year of life, transformations during this period are ongoing but gradual. Growth and all aspects of development continue in a steady manner. Sleep becomes consolidated into a long nocturnal period of approximately 10 hours.[23–25] Children 3–5 years of age should sleep approximately

10–13 hours (including daytime naps) for optimal sleep health.[26] During the first 2–3 years, daytime sleep continues in distinct daytime naps. The first nap is ordinarily midmorning, and the second occurring in the early afternoon. Morning naps are slowly given up. This occurs in an irregular pattern similar to all other developmental processes. Often, this can be frustrating to parents due to the irregularity of nap elimination. Nonetheless, by 3–5 years of age, sleep is typically consolidated into a single long nocturnal period.

During the latter half of the first year of life, REM sleep averages about 30% of the total sleep time. Small and large body movements associated with REM sleep during infancy become less frequent. REM periods are of approximately uniform length, despite daytime naps, and are evenly distributed throughout the nocturnal sleep period. As the child develops, an ongoing change is seen in the uniformity and duration of these REM periods. The first REM period shortens, whereas succeeding periods tend to become progressively longer and more intense as the sleep period advances. There is also a slight lengthening of the overall NREM-REM cycle length.[27] Two- to 3-year-old children still show a cycle length of about 60 minutes, with the first REM period occurring approximately 1 hour after sleep onset. By 4–5 years of age, cycle length increased to about 60–90 minutes.

Between 2 and 5 years of age, REM percentage gradually decreases from 30% of the total sleep time to near the adult level of 20–25%, although the total time of each sleep state is greater than in the adult because of the longer sleep time. There appears to be a close relationship between these changes and the augmented periods of wakefulness during the daytime. Diminution of REM volume progresses until about 3–4.5 years, when daytime napping has ended. By this age, distinct differences between early and late portions of the sleep period have emerged.[27]

Typically, children in this age range have approximately seven cycles during each nocturnal sleep period.[28] Sleep onset latency averages about 15 minutes in the younger children, but lengthens to between 15 and 30 minutes in the older children in this developmental grouping. Slow-wave sleep predominantly occurs during the first third of the night,[25] and as much as 2 hours may be spent in N3. EEG voltage is also very high during this period. N2 first appears from 3 to 4 minutes after the child falls asleep, and N3 appears about 10–15 minutes after sleep onset.[29]

Distinctive characteristics of sleep occur between 2 and 5 years that may suggest stabilization and balancing of state. A relatively small number of sleep stage changes is a noticeable feature.[23] Approximately 3.5 stage shifts per hour occur, which is significantly different than that of the young adult, EEG voltage is consistently higher, and N3 is consistently longer. Another exceptional difference is the smooth progression of stages, whether moving deeper (toward N3) or lighter (toward wake). Transition is consistent and steady in contrast to the adult pattern, where there are often abrupt movements across several stages at a time when the EEG progresses toward lighter or deeper sleep.[23,25]

Five to Ten Years

Growth and development again is steady, persistent, and gradual during middle childhood. This period of development, however, is not latent. This phase is characterized by slow methodical change, searching, exploration, and increasingly sophisticated decision making. It is a time of preparation and rehearsal, trial and error.[28]

Sleep continues to coalesce into a more mature pattern. Sleep during middle childhood resembles that of older individuals. Considerable between subject variability exists. Nonetheless, an orderly sequence of sleep stages is preserved, spontaneously shifting from one stage to another. There is a certain within subject stability of pattern, a fairly consistent amount of time spent in each sleep stage, and stable number of sleep stages within nocturnal sleep periods.[29] When compared with adult sleep patterns, total sleep time in middle childhood is approximately 2.5 hours longer with equal distribution of the added time to each of the sleep stages. Stages in children of this age group tend to be longer in duration than in adults, but the sleep architecture seems to be similar. Total 24-hour sleep time ranges from 9 to 12 hours for optimal health,[26] and daytime naps are typically eliminated.

Although quite consistent, middle childhood remains a time of regular transition. After an initially long NREM period, some children will exhibit regularly spaced REM periods of equal duration (similar to the pattern seen during infancy), whereas others reveal a more mature pattern of progressively longer REM periods as sleep progresses.[16] A proportion of REM sleep approximates the adult level. But because of the decrease in total sleep time and maturation of state, there seems to be a decrease in the total number of minutes spent in REM sleep when compared with infants and younger children.

Though body movements during sleep decrease in frequency, they are generally more often seen in this age group than in adolescents and young adults. N3 sleep proportion decreases in the preschool child in the latter portion of middle childhood.[27] There does appear, however, to be a sex-related difference in the percentage of N3 sleep. Males tend to exhibit a significantly greater proportion of N3 than females of comparable age.[24,30,31]

Although naps during this period may continue, they tend to be quite irregular and sparse. Tendency to sleep during the day seems to be lowest in this age group. Consistent habitual daytime napping during middle childhood often represents an abnormal process and may be associated with unintentional daytime sleep episodes. Prepubertal children are most often significantly alert throughout the entire day. Carskadon and coworkers have shown mean daytime sleep onset latencies during the Multiple Sleep Latency Test (MSLT) of preadolescent (Tanner stage 1) children to be greater than 15 minutes,[31,32] suggesting an extremely level of alertness and low homeostatic sleep pressure.

Adolescence

Persistent maturation during middle childhood gives way to a second period of rapid change during adolescence. Not since infancy are there such quantum leaps and striking changes in physical growth, hormonal alterations, and psychologic, social, and cognitive development. Luxury of stability yields to the upheaval of navigating this transitional phase. These dramatic changes are important in assessing sleep and sleep disorders during this period of life.

By early adolescence, electrophysiologic variables of sleep have approximated normal young adult values. For some adolescents, certain elements of less mature patterns may occasionally be observed.[27] For example, body movements during sleep are usually similar to that seen in adults, but at times may be as high as in younger children. Total REM volume is at adult levels and REM periods clearly lengthen as the sleep period progresses. Total N3 sleep time approaches adult levels of approximately 45–60 minutes. Total sleep requirement decreases from 9 to 10 hours during middle childhood to approximately 8.5 hours by 16 years of age.[33,34]

Sleep habits and patterns of adolescents have been extensively studied.[32,35,36] Observations have revealed interesting tendencies in the sleep of teenagers. Considerable variation can be seen in patterns between school nights and non-school nights. Whereas total sleep time for children 10 years of age tends to be the same on school nights and non-school nights, young adolescents sleep less on school nights than non-school nights. Bedtimes and wake-times are more controlled by outside influences on school nights. Parents attempt to set bedtime limits, but homework, starting time of classes in the morning, and alarm clocks also truncate the sleep period. These influences seem to infer that sleep on non-school nights is closer to normal physiologic than sleep on school nights. Increased sleep time on non-school nights may reflect recovery from partial (although cumulative) sleep restriction during the week.

Total 24-hour sleep time ranges from 8 to 10 hours.[26] Observations by Williams and colleagues[29] have revealed a continuous decrease in total sleep time through middle and late adolescence of approximately 2 hours. If this sleep restriction is cumulative, subjective and objective evidence of increased daytime sleepiness should appear. In fact, older adolescents report greater difficulty with daytime sleepiness and nocturnal sleep than younger adolescents.[35] Various methods have been used to assess sleepiness and alertness, including pupillometry,[37] the Stanford Sleepiness Scale (a validated 7-point Likert scale measuring subjective sleepiness),[38,39] the Epworth Sleepiness Scale,[40] brainstem evoked potentials,[41] and the MSLT.[42] The MSLT, developed in the mid-1970s at the Stanford University Sleep Research Center, is the most widely used procedure for objective measurement of daytime sleep tendency. This test consists of a series of opportunities to sleep, administered at 2-hour intervals across a day using a standard procedure.[42] Sleepiness is measured as the speed of falling asleep (average sleep onset latency) across these nap opportunities. The presence of REM sleep during these naps is also noted. MSLT scores are related to a number of variables that range from the amount of sleep on one or several nights preceding the study[43,44] to pathologic states such as narcolepsy.[45] An average sleep onset latency of less than 5 minutes is a range found to be associated with performance decrements and unintentional episodes of sleep.[43]

In a series of exquisite seminal experiments by Carskadon and coworkers, manifest sleepiness during adolescence was dramatically demonstrated.[31,32,35,36,44,46] Twelve girls and 15 boys were observed longitudinally over the course of 7 years to determine sleep tendency changes that may occur during puberty. When subjects were given the opportunity to sleep for 10 hours, total sleep time did not vary significantly with adolescent maturational state, and all groups slept for a little more than 9 hours per night. One conclusion drawn from these data was that *there is not a reduced need for sleep as the adolescent matures.* Time spent in REM sleep also remained constant between each developmental stage in these subjects. N3 sleep, on the other hand, decreased dramatically (by approximately 35%) between Tanner stages 1 and 5. There was a concomitant fall in the mean sleep onset latency in mid-adolescence; indicating reduced daytime alertness, despite a constant total sleep time. This finding also suggested that *sleep requirements do not decrease as the adolescent ages and may, in fact, increase.*

Time in bed and total sleep time decreases as the adolescent ages, resulting in a cumulative sleep debt. This sleep debt becomes significant during late adolescence and is accompanied by a continued fall in daytime alertness (as measured by the MSLT) to levels that are close to being pathologic.[46] It has become clear that impact on daytime functioning may be significant. A number of normal adolescents will, therefore, have significant disturbances in daytime alertness because of normal pubertal increase in daytime sleepiness and cumulative/additive restriction of nocturnal sleep to meet expectations and obligations. Though there is considerable variability between individuals, many adolescents (particularly in the older age groups) have some degree of impairment.

Inadequate sleep is common during adolescence. Shorter than optimal total sleep time is a result of biologic, developmental, and sociologic factors.[47] These include but are not limited to normal circadian drift, blunted homeostatic sleep drive, social networking, screen time, sports and other extracurricular activities, and school start time. It has been clearly demonstrated that later school start times for high school students has a positive impact on academics, socialization, and behavior. Additionally, it has been shown that delayed school start time for adolescents increases the likelihood of motor vehicle accidents,[48,49] putatively due to a combination of inexperience driving an automobile and daytime sleepiness.

CLINICAL PEARLS

- Development of sleep in the pediatric and adolescent population rapidly changes and mirrors development of the biologic organism.
- The structure of sleep also rapidly changes with longitudinal and cross-sectional components that are independent.
- Considerable differences occur within and between individual children. Understanding these differences requires specific expertise in evaluation, diagnosis, and management of sleep-related disorders in children.
- Evaluation of management of pediatric sleep-related disorders can be best accomplished using a multidisciplinary or interdisciplinary approach.

Summary

Development of sleep in humans is not a unitary phenomenon. Sleep is a neurodevelopmental process, just as all other neurodevelopmental processes. Characteristics rapidly change as the central nervous system and all other organ systems undergo periods of exceptionally rapid development, then slow constant maturation to a relatively constant state to a point that remains generally for the rest of the life cycle. This chapter focuses on the rapid and progressive maturation of the sleep-wake continuum. The focus is on both physiologic and behavioral development of sleep across the pediatric and adolescent age spectrum.

References

1. Grigg-Damberger M. The visual scoring of sleep in infants 0 to 2 months of age. *J Clin Sleep Med.* 2016;12:429–445.
2. Berry R, Brooks R, Gamaldo C, et al. *The AASM Manual for the Scoring of Sleep and Associated Events: Rules, Terminology and Technical Specifications. Version 2.6.* 2.4 ed. American Academy of Sleep Medicine; 2020.
3. Sullivan S, Carskadon MA, Dement WC, Jackson C. Normal sleep. In: Kryger MH, Roth T, Dement WC, Goldstein C, eds. *Principles and Practice of Sleep Medicine.* 7th ed. Elsevier; 2022.
4. de Weerd A, van den Bossche R. The development of sleep during the first months of life. *Sleep Med Re.* 2003;7:179–191.
5. Dreyfus-Brisac C. Ontogenesis of sleep in human prematures after 32 weeks of conceptional age. *Dev Psychobiol.* 1970;3(2):91–121.
6. Prechtl H, Beintema D. *The neurological examination of the full term newborn infant. Clinics in Developmental Medicine.* Spastics Society and Heinemann; 1964.
7. Anders TF, Emde R, Parmelee AH. *A Manual of Standardized Terminology, Techniques and Criteria for Scoring of States of Sleep and Wakefulness in Newborn Infants.* UCLA Brain Information Service, NINDS Neurological Information Network; 1971.
8. Hoppenbrouwers T. Sleep in infants. In: Guilleminault C, ed. *Sleep and Its Disorders in Children.* Raven Press; 1987.
9. Parmelee AH, Stern E. Development of states in infants. In: Clemente CD, Purpura DP, Mayer FE, eds. *Sleep and the Maturing Nervous System.* Academic Press; 1972.xviii.
10. Sterman MB. The basic rest-activity cycle and sleep: Developmental considerations in man and cats. In: Clemente CD, Purpura DP, Mayer FE, eds. *Sleep and the Maturing Nervous System.* Academic Press; 1972.xviii.
11. Dreyfus-Brisac C. Ontogenese du sommeil chez le premature humain: Etude polygraphique. In: Minkowski A, ed. *Regional Development of the Brain in Early Life.* Blackwell; 1967:539. xii.
12. Stern E, Parmelee AH, Akiyama Y, Schultz MA, Wenner WH. Sleep cycle characteristics in infants. *Pediatrics.* 1969;43(1):65–70.
13. Hirschkowitz M, Whiton K, Albert S, et al. National Sleep Foundation's updated sleep duration recommendations: final report. *Sleep Health.* 2015;1:233–243.
14. Harper RM, Leake B, Miyahara L, Hoppenbrouwers T, Sterman MB, Hodgman J. Development of ultradian periodicity and coalescence at 1 cycle per hour in electroencephalographic activity. *Exp Neurol.* 1981;73(1):127–143.
15. Metcalf D. The ontogenesis of sleep-awake states from birth to 3 months. *Electroencephalogr Clin Neurophysiol.* 1970;28(4):421.
16. Coons S. Development of sleep and wakefulness during the first 6 months of life. In: Guilleminault C, ed. *Sleep and Its Disorders in Children.* Raven Press; 1987.
17. Parmelee AH, Jr., Wenner WH, Schulz HR. Infant sleep patterns: from birth to 16 weeks of age. *J Pediatr.* 1964;65:576–582.
18. Bowe TR, Anders TF. The use of the semi-Markov model in the study of the development of sleep-wake states in infants. *Psychophysiology.* 1979;16(1):41–48.
19. Anders TF, Keener M. Developmental course of nighttime sleep-wake patterns in full-term and premature infants during the first year of life. I. *Sleep.* 1985;8(3):173–192.
20. Nolte R, Schulte FJ, Weisse U, Gruson R. The "trace alternant" of the sleeping EEG in full-term, premature and hypotrophic neonates. *Electroencephalogr Clin Neurophysiol.* 1969;27(6):625.
21. Lenard HG. The development of sleep spindles during the first 2 years of life. *Electroencephalogr Clin Neurophysiol.* 1970;29(2):217.
22. Schulz H, Salzarulo P, Fagioli I, Massetani R. REM latency: development in the first year of life. *Electroencephalogr Clin Neurophysiol.* 1983;56(4):316–322.
23. Kohler WC, Coddington RD, Agnew Jr. HW. Sleep patterns in 2-year-old children. *J Pediatr.* Feb 1968;72(2):228–233.
24. Mattison RE, Handford HA, Vela-Bueno A. Sleep disorders in children. *Psychiatr Med.* 1986;4(2):149–164.
25. Ross JJ, Agnew HW, Jr., Williams RL, Webb WB. Sleep patterns in pre-adolescent children: an EEG-EOG study. *Pediatrics.* 1968;42(2):324–335.
26. Paruthi S, Brooks LJ, D'Ambrosio C, et al. Recommended amount of sleep for pediatric populations: a consensus statement of the American Academy of Sleep Medicine. *J Clin Sleep Med.* 2016;12(6):785–786.
27. Roffwarg H, Dement WC, Fisher C. Preliminary observations of the sleep-dream pattern in neonates, infants, children, and adults. In: Harms E, ed. *Problems of Sleep and Dreams in Children.* Macmillan; 1964.
28. Levine MD. Middle childhood. In: Levine MD, Carey WB, Crocker AC, eds. *Developmental-Behavioral Pediatrics.* 3rd ed. Saunders; 1999.xvi.
29. Williams RL, Karacan I, Hursch CJ. *Electroencephalography (EEG) of Human Sleep: Clinical Applications.* Wiley; 1974.xiv.
30. Coble PA, Kupfer DJ, Taska LS, Kane J. EEG sleep of normal healthy children. Part I: Findings using standard measurement methods. *Sleep.* 1984;7(4):289–303.

31. Carskadon MA, Keenan S, Dement W. Nighttime sleep and daytime sleep tendency in preadolescents. In: Guilleminault C, ed. *Sleep and Its Disorders in Children*. Raven Press; 1987.

32. Carskadon MA, Harvey K, Duke P, Anders TF, Litt IF, Dement WC. Pubertal changes in daytime sleepiness. *Sleep*. 1980;2(4):453–460.

33. Ames L. Sleep and dreams in childhood. In: Harms E, ed. *Problems of Sleep and Dreams in Children*. Macmillan; 1964.

34. Carskadon MA. The second decade. In: Guilleminault C, ed. *Sleep and Its Disorders in Children*. Raven Press; 1987.

35. Carskadon MA, Dement W. Sleepiness in the normal adolescent. In: Guilleminault C, ed. *Sleep and Its Disorders in Children*. Raven Press; 1987.

36. Carskadon MA, Orav EJ. Evolution of sleep and daytime sleepiness in adolescents. In: Guilleminault C, Lugaresi E, eds. *Sleep/wake Disorders: Natural History, Epidemiology, and Long-Term Evolution*. Raven Press; 1983:xvi.

37. Lowenstein O, Loewenfeld IE. Electronic pupillography; a new instrument and some clinical applications. *AMA Arch Ophthalmol*. 1958;59(3):352–363.

38. Herscovitch J, Broughton R. Sensitivity of the Stanford Sleepiness Scale to the effects of cumulative partial sleep deprivation and recovery oversleeping. *Sleep*. 1981;4(1):83–91.

39. Hoddes E, Zarcone V, Smythe H, Phillips R, Dement WC. Quantification of sleepiness: a new approach. *Psychophysiology*. 1973;10(4):431–436.

40. Johns MW. A new method for measuring daytime sleepiness: the Epworth Sleepiness Scale. *Sleep*. 1991;14(6):540–545.

41. Broughton R. Performance and evoked potential measures of various states of daytime sleepiness. *Sleep*. 1982;5(suppl 2):S135–46.

42. Carskadon MA, Dement WC, Mitler MM, Roth T, Westbrook PR, Keenan S. Guidelines for the Multiple Sleep Latency Test (MSLT): a standard measure of sleepiness. *Sleep*. 1986;9(4):519–524.

43. Carskadon MA, Dement WC. Effects of total sleep loss on sleep tendency. *Percept Mot Skills*. 1979;48(2):495–506.

44. Carskadon MA, Harvey K, Dement WC. Sleep loss in young adolescents. *Sleep*. 1981;4(3):299–312.

45. Dye TJ, Simakajornboon N. Narcolepsy in Children: Sleep disorders in children, A rapidly evolving field seeking consensus. *Pediatr Pulmonol*. 2022;57(8):1952–1962.

46. Carskadon MA, Dement WC. Cumulative effects of sleep restriction on daytime sleepiness. *Psychophysiology*. 1981;18(2):107–113.

47. Adolescent Sleep Working Group CoA, and Council on School Health. Policy statement: school start times for adolescents. *Pediatrics*. 2014;134:642–649.

48. Danner F, Phillips B. Adolescent sleep, school start times, and teen motor vehicle crashes. *J Clin Sleep Med*. 2008;4:533–535.

49. Foss R, Smith R, O'Brien N. School start times and teenage driver motor vehicle crashes. *Accid Anal Prev*. 2019;126:54–63.

3

Chronobiology and Circadian Rhythm Disorders in Children and Adolescents

Allison Hayes Clarke, Innessa Donskoy, and Stephen H. Sheldon

CHAPTER HIGHLIGHTS

- Several genes have been identified that contribute to the development of and maintenance of a continuous circadian rhythm in humans and other organisms.
- When endogenous circadian rhythms do not align with a child or adolescent's school, family, or work activities, circadian rhythm sleep-wake disorders may develop.
- In particular, DSWPD is prevalent among adolescents when the endogenous sleep-wake cycle is both delayed and lengthened, causing misalignment with school schedules.
- Consistency in daily sleep-wake schedules, timed light exposure, and timed melatonin administration can help children to better align their sleep-waking timing with daily demands.

Introduction

The development of homeostatic and circadian rhythmicity has been described in the scientific literature since the early 1950s. Theodore Hellbruegge[1] described the difficulty in studying the evolution of circadian rhythmicity in 1960. He identified three basic difficulties: (1) the human infant is not fully mature at birth compared with the anthropoid ape; (2) a precondition to the development of circadian rhythmicity is a mature neurohormonal system and the functional efficiency of the organs upon which rhythms may be measured; and (3) each day and night rhythm is bound to the function of an organ of perception, through which various synchronizing effects of zeitgebers are mediated. Since this time, there have been significant breakthroughs in the research and understanding of the underpinnings of the circadian rhythm, which were highlighted in 2017 when the Nobel Prize in physiology or medicine was awarded to Jeffrey C. Hall, Michael Rosbash, and Michael W. Young for the identification of specific genes *(PER, TIM, DBT)* that interact to maintain a continuous circadian rhythm in all living organisms. There are a number of other key genes *(CLOCK, CRY, CYCLE)* that play major roles in the functioning of an organism's circadian rhythm, and their interplay involves complex modeling with numerous paths of feedback to be self-sustaining.[2,3]

Little is known about ontogeny of circadian rhythmicity and its physiologic function before birth. Investigations have been done following delivery in premature and term newborns regarding cortisol rhythms, heart rate variability, sleep–wake/rest–activity cycling, and the effect of cycling light in the nursery. The majority of physiologic functions develop and maintain their own inherent biologic rhythmicity. Synchronization into a circadian pattern requires development and maturation of the central nervous system (CNS), receptor organ systems, establishment of zeitgebers, and time. Development of adult patterns requires integration of systems maturing at different rates, and structural pattern development. Maturation of this complex system may be likened to the development of other CNS-linked processes like sitting, walking, talking, and language development. None of these clearly observable developmental landmarks occur instantly.

Animal studies have shown that the circadian pacemaker is the suprachiasmatic nucleus (SCN) of the hypothalamus.[4] Pacemaker oscillations do not perfectly coincide with the 24-hour clock requiring resetting the clock every 24-hour period with consistently timed light exposure upon waking.[5] Without resetting, the pacemaker will drift out of phase with day and night resulting in a "free-running" state.[6] An intact pathway from the retina to the hypothalamus (the retinohypothalamic tract) is required for entrainment of the pacemaker by light/dark cycling.[6] Afferent signals from the retina via intrinsically photosensitive ganglia cells are independent of retinal visual receptors.[7]

Development and maturation of circadian rhythmicity occur in a similar manner. In this section, the classical sleep log maintained by observations of Dr. Nathaniel Kleitman will be used to exemplify, the development of this rhythmicity.[8]

During the first weeks of life in a term newborn, rhythm is typically not identifiable. Sleep–wake cycles are primarily determined by the feeding cycle. It is fairly regular throughout the 20-hour day and the cycle length lasts about 2–4 hours. Most of the 24-hour day is spent sleeping. In the term infant, about 50% of the total sleep time is equivalent to non–rapid eye movement (NREM) sleep and 50% equivalent to REM sleep. This has changed from the pattern that begins at about 28- to 30-weeks' gestation during which about 90% of the total quiet time is REM sleep and 10% of the total time quiet is NREM sleep.

Soon after delivery, the dominant influence on the sleeping habits of infants is feeding. Early in infancy there is a relatively equal distribution of feeding times throughout the 24-hour day. Between 4 and 18 weeks of life, diurnal and nocturnal rhythm becomes more pronounced. Daytime hours are used for waking and nighttime hours for sleeping. This diurnal/nocturnal periodicity develops independently from nursing functions.

Between 2 and 6–8 weeks, the pattern begins to change with the longest sleep period occurring during nocturnal hours and the longest wake periods occurring during daylight hours. The functional term is "longest," and many new parents become quite frustrated during this time because the infant is still not sleeping through the parental night. It is important to understand that "longest" does not equal "long."

Between 8 and 12 weeks of age, daytime sleep becomes shorter and is clearly consolidated into naps, usually three per daylight hours. Total 24-hour sleep time is about 16–18 hours, with the majority of sleep occurring during the dark hours.

From 12–24 weeks, another change occurs; daytime sleep becomes shorter and often one of the daytime naps is given up, and sleep during dark hours becomes longer. Parents are typically pleased during this time period because the nighttime sleep of their child will begin approximating their own sleep–wake cycle, and the baby "is finally sleeping through the night." However, an interesting development appears to occur at this time of maturation. Although there is some identifiable synchrony, it does not follow a typical entrained pattern. There appears to be a continuous sleep phase delay simulating a non–24-hour sleep–wake cycle, which is seen when there are no time cues available and is not uncommon in humans without vision or light perception.

Between 5 and 8 months of age circadian rhythm appears to be well developed, with waking occurring during about 90% of daytime hours and a considerably lower amount of waking appearing during nighttime hours.

Around 9 months of age, there is further consolidation and entrainment of a variety of other endocrine and endogenous physiologic rhythms. At this time, if there has been appropriate light cycling, the non–24-hour pattern changes and there is a progressive sleep phase advance. This advance continues between 6 and 9 months of age and seems to pass the desired time of habitual morning sleep offset. Now, habitual morning sleep offset may occur during dark hours in the morning. The infant will begin waking earlier in the morning, and daytime naps follow this pattern advancing earlier in the daylight hours. Unfortunately, parents will then tend to report their infant has begun to wake "during the night again." This, however, is not a return of nocturnal awakenings, it is shift of the time of morning sleep offset. The morning nap has also shifted. When this pattern emerges, parents will often complain in the following manner:

She was sleeping through the night until a few weeks ago and then began waking in the middle of the night again. We have tried everything, but nothing seems to work. She will wake at about 4:30 a.m. She seems to be happy and wants to eat. We change her diaper, feed her, and she stays awake and seems happy and active until about 6:00 a.m. She will then fall back to sleep and sleep until about 8:00 a.m. when she will wake, have her diaper changed, have a bottle, and remain awake and happy until her first nap at about 10:00 a.m.

What has happened is normal maturation of the development of appropriate circadian cycling. She is not "waking in the middle of the night again." The 4:00 a.m. waking is her *normal time of morning sleep offset* (she has awakened to start her day). Sleep that occurs from 6:00 a.m. is her *first morning nap*, which she is trying to give up. By consolidating that nap into the dark hours of the 24-hour cycle will support development of her circadian rhythmicity and result in her "sleeping through the night again."

Shifting to the right can be observed in sleep–wake distribution and can be seen in the development of the diurnal rhythm of the heart rate and the core body temperature. These findings support the progressive phase delay after about 18 weeks of age followed by advance of the sleep phase after about 6–8 months of age.

The data are mixed regarding the timing of circadian rhythm development outside of the womb dependent on the measure used and confounded by individual differences including varied feeding needs, how quickly infants build up sleep pressure, changing or irregular darkness/light patterns, and sound and activity patterns in the home. Higher body temperatures during daytime hours only begin to be demonstrated between 4 and 9 weeks of age, suggesting no clear rhythmicity prior to this time.[9] The temperature differential between day and night is even better demonstrated between 10 and 16 weeks of age. Changes in heart rate follow a similar pattern. Asymmetry of sleep and wakefulness appears to be already present from the third to the sixth week of life. However, actigraphy data monitoring activity and rest periods suggest that infants who were exposed to cycled lighting found evidence of circadian rhythms as early as 34 weeks postmenstrual age.[10]

The already observable increasing incidence of sleep during nighttime hours becomes more evident up to the 18th week of life. Maximum incidence of sleep between 11 p.m. and 5 a.m. appears to stabilize at about 18 weeks of age; peak values of wakefulness during the daytime increases up to the 26th week postdelivery.

Development of adult-like circadian rhythmicity is genetically and environmentally determined. This process takes time and development of the retina and development of the SNC. Throughout childhood, there is continued development of day and night patterns of sleep with a gradual decrease in the total sleep time between 1 and 5 years, along with the elimination of discrete daytime napping. In most industrialized societies, daytime napping is eliminated by the age of 6 years. Nevertheless, many cultures play close attention to the circadian influence of a midafternoon slight fall in body temperature and take advantage of an afternoon nap (siestas).

Significant changes to the circadian rhythm occur around the time of puberty. The onset of melatonin secretion becomes later with increasing age, associated with pubertal status.[11] Research has shown that the point at which humans have the largest phase delays usually occurs either during or after the final stages of gonadal development.[12] Puberty has been associated with both a delay and lengthening of the circadian rhythm.[13,14] Mechanisms for these changes include a reduced sensitivity to the phase-advancing effects of light in the morning and increased sensitivity to the phase-delaying effects of evening light exposure.[12] Moreover, research suggests that adolescents build up their sleep drive more slowly, allowing them to have more extended periods of wakefulness.[5]

The Two-Process Model

There are two main processes that are thought to underlie our sleep–wake system. The circadian system, the focus of this chapter, is also referred to as "Process C." It is our internal clock, the SNC in the hypothalamus, which dictates when in the 24-hour day an individual feels most sleepy and most alert.[15] However, its partner in sleep and wake control is the homeostatic sleep drive, or "Process S," driven by how long an individual has been awake or how much "sleep debt" they have accumulated since their last sleep period.[15] The interaction between both processes helps to determine when an individual will actually fall asleep. Recent research suggests that the interactions between these two processes are complex and continuous, supported by electrophysiologic recordings in the SCN.[15] The complex interplay of these processes can alter the timing of sleep to be significantly later than desired or expected in a way that interferes with our daily routines and can promote or perpetuate circadian rhythm disorders.

Circadian Rhythm Sleep–Wake Disorders: Diagnosis and Treatment

Introduction

Normal sleep quantity and quality at undesirable hours are the hallmarks of circadian rhythm sleep–wake disorders (CRSWDs); these are disorders associated with the timing of sleep. Work, school, or family requirements often dictate when we need to fall sleep and wake up each day. Typically, CRSWDs arise from a recurrent or chronic misalignment between the endogenous circadian clock and external schedules (e.g., school or work schedules).[16]

Unlike insomnia or obstructive sleep apnea, in CRSWDs, sleep architecture, the distribution of sleep stages, and 24-hour sleep duration are normal. Sleep is also typically refreshing. However, the timing of sleep is abnormal. Although circadian rhythms develop in infancy,[17] abnormal sleep–wake schedules may not be problematic in young children if the child does not have to engage in daily activities at set times (e.g., daycare). Often, with the introduction of school, conflicts between a child's sleep–wake schedule and school hours lead to impairments in functioning. Sleep–wake schedule preferences shift from preference to a disorder when the individual cannot sleep or wake at desired hours and suffers consequential academic or daily functioning difficulties.

The emergence of a CRSWD is thought to be the consequence of one of two underlying mechanisms. Children and adolescents may have endogenous disruption in the circadian clock system. This may be due to a genetic polymorphism, as studies have shown correlations between pediatric CRSWDs and family history of similar symptoms or chronotype.[2] Alternately, CRSWDs may emerge when external factors, such as family social schedules, school schedules, or other environmental variables, do not align with the endogenous circadian rhythm. CRSWDs resulting from this misalignment are often inadvertently maintained when children or adolescents "catch up" on sleep on weekends or by taking naps after school. For example, parents may perceive that their child is sleep deprived on school days if they struggle to fall asleep quickly at bedtime. As a result, they allow the child to sleep as late as they wish on weekends and school breaks. This leads to the child experiencing what is referred to as "social jet lag." They often struggle to initiate sleep on Sunday night or awaken Monday for school, thus leading to sleep deprivation during the school week and reinforcing this abnormal sleep–wake pattern week after week. In some children, CRSWDs emerge with the start of a school year after the child has slept abnormal hours throughout the summer or after a long school break. During the recent SARS-CoV-2 pandemic, global school closures afforded children the ability to sleep on their natural schedules throughout the week and wake naturally on "Monday morning." There were a number of children, possibly due to the true incidence of circadian rhythm sleep disorders, who reported improved sleep quality with this change.[18,19]

Biologic Clocks and Circadian Rhythms

All humans possess endogenous circadian rhythms that run slightly longer than 24 hours[16,20] (Fig. 3.1). Chronotype is defined as an individual's preference to engage in various daily activities at an early or late hour, defining when in the light–dark cycle sleep is most likely to occur. Several measures, such as the Horne-Östberg Morningness-Eveningness Questionnaire (MEQ)[3] were developed to assess chronotype. These measures help to determine an individual's chronotype, often described as morning "lark" versus night "owl." School-aged children are mostly morning chronotypes. During adolescence, many shift to evening chronotypes.[21,22] Endogenous circadian rhythms are entrained by the 24-hour cycle by numerous environmental time cues, known as zeitgebers, including light and darkness, physical activity, school, work, and social behaviors, such as,

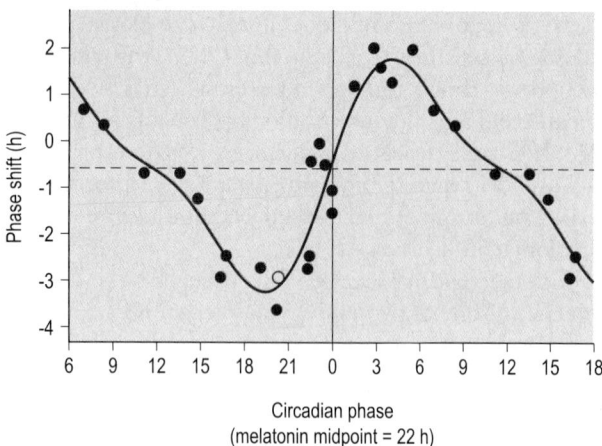

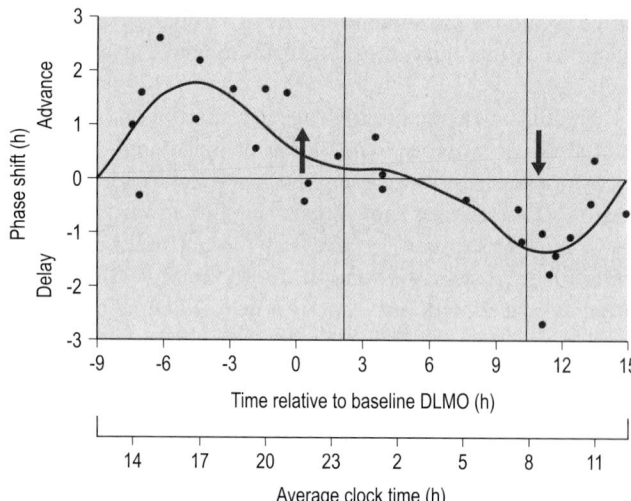

• **Fig. 3.1** The phase response curve (PRC) to the bright light stimulus using melatonin midpoints as the circadian phase marker. Phase advances (positive values) and delays (negative values) are plotted against the timing of the center of the light exposure relative to the melatonin midpoint on the prestimulus circadian rhythm (CR; defined to be 22 hours), with the core body temperature minimum assumed to occur 2 hours later at 0 hours. Data points from circadian phases 6–18 are double plotted. The filled circles represent data from plasma melatonin, and the open circle represents data from salivary melatonin in subject 18K8 from whom blood samples were not acquired. The *solid curve* is a dual harmonic function fitted through all of the data points. The *horizontal dashed line* represents the anticipated 0.54-hours average delay drift of the pacemaker between the pre- and poststimulus phase assessments. (The figure legend is from the original text.) Sat Bir S Khalsa SB, Jewett ME, Cajochen C, Czeisler C. A phase response curve to single bright light pulses in human subjects. *J Physiol.* 2003;549(3):945–952.

• **Fig. 3.2** The three pulse phase response curve (PRC) to 3 mg of exogenous melatonin generated from subjects free-running during an ultradian light–dark (LD) cycle. Phase shifts of the dim light melatonin onset (DLMO) are plotted against the time of administration of the melatonin pill relative to the baseline DLMO (*top x-axis*). The average baseline DLMO is represented by the *upward arrow*, the average baseline DLMOff by the *downward arrow*, and the average assigned baseline sleep times from before the laboratory sessions are enclosed by the *vertical lines.* Each *dot* represents the phase shift of an individual subject, calculated by subtracting the phase shift during the placebo session (free-run) from the phase shift during the melatonin session. The *curved line* illustrates the dual harmonic curve fit. The average clock time axis (*bottom x -axis*) corresponds to the average baseline sleep times. This PRC can be applied to people with different sleep schedules by moving the average clock time axis until the vertical lines align with the individual's sleep schedule. (The figure legend is from the original text.) Image and text from Burgess, HJ, Revel, VL, and Eastman, CI, A three pulse phase response curve to three milligrams of melatonin in humans, January 15, 2008 *The Journal of Physiology,* 586, 639–647[28].

mealtimes.[16,23] The strongest of these cues in mammals is light exposure. When there are challenges in synchronizing to this 24-hour clock, it can impact the relationships between the endogenous clock and lightness/darkness cycles and may result in CRSWDs. A study of preadolescent children found that those with an evening preference (chronotype) have more sleep–wake disorders, daytime sleepiness, and emotional difficulties than do those without morning or evening preference or those with a morning chronotype.[22] Moreover, later chronotype has been shown to predict future depressive episodes among adolescents.[24]

Prevalence

The prevalence of CRSWDs has been difficult to estimate due to studies using different criteria and measurements and challenges in assessing the boundaries between a chronotype and disorder. Delayed sleep–wake phase disorder (DSWPD) is by far the most common sleep–wake disorder and is estimated to effect anywhere from 3% to 16% of adolescents and young adults.[16,25,26] Advanced sleep–wake phase disorder (ASWPD) occurs much less frequently in youth, but may emerge as a concern at the age of starting school. Before school age, waking at an early hour may be alright if schedules allow them to nap during the day. Irregular sleep–wake disorder is extremely rare in children, but typically

emerges in adolescence. Non–24-hour circadian rhythm is also relatively rare and appears most often in blind individuals, including children.

Melatonin and Circadian Rhythms

The pineal gland secretes endogenous melatonin during the dark period of our 24-hour day and daylight suppresses melatonin production. The time at which melatonin concentrations rise to a certain threshold (i.e., 4 pg/mL in saliva and 10 pg/mL in blood), is called dim light melatonin onset (DLMO).[5,27] DLMO is the marker of the beginning of biological night and dim light melatonin offset is the end of biologic night. The clock hour of DLMO determines whether an individual's circadian rhythm is normal, phase advanced, or phase delayed. The phase response curve to exogenous melatonin shows its phase advance or phase delay properties (Fig. 3.2).[28]

In attempting to correct an individual's phase advance or phase delay, the biomarker employed is the shift in DLMO to an earlier or later hour, as measured by saliva or blood melatonin concentration. Advancing DLMO not only advances the time of sleep onset, but also the time of the body's core temperature minimum and the time of dim light melatonin offset, allowing the individual to awaken at an earlier hour. DLMO accurately predicts wake-up time.[13,29] The phase response curve to melatonin is the opposite of the phase response curve to light. The phase response curve shows a maximal phase advance to melatonin when it is administered 6 hours before DLMO, or 8 hours before sleep onset. Importantly, melatonin secretion is suppressed with exposure to ambient light intensities that are commonly used indoors (3,000–100,000 lux) and even lower intensities have been shown to suppress melatonin (ranging from 100–300 lux).[27,30]

Differential Diagnosis of Circadian Rhythm Sleep–Wake Disorders

Given that the most common presenting concerns among youth with CRSWD include difficulty initiating sleep and excessive sleepiness, a careful history is essential to distinguish CRSWDs from other sleep disorders. One distinguishing feature of CRSWDs is that when the child is allowed to sleep at their preferred times, sleep is normal and daytime sleepiness rapidly subsides. Children with DSWPD typically have no daytime sleepiness when allowed to sleep late on weekends. Objective measures, such as actigraphy, help to assess sleep–wake patterns over time to tease apart these factors. When not available, a detailed sleep log or diary can help to identify patterns in sleep–wake schedules. These should ideally be gathered over at least 2 weeks to capture sleep and wake data on both school and non-school days.[25] Finally, when available, physiologic circadian rhythm markers, such as salivary or plasma DLMO and urinary 6-sulfatoxymelatonin can provide additional diagnostic information.[16,25]

Youth with sleep-onset insomnia differ from children with DSWPD as they are unable to sleep in late on weekends, may struggle to fall asleep regardless of timing, and sleep is chronically nonrestorative. However, often as a result of repeatedly trying to fall asleep at a socially acceptable bedtime that does not align with their internal clock, insomnia disorders can also develop among youth with DSWPD. Children with early morning awakening insomnia differ from children with ASWPD as they are unable to initiate sleep at an early hour and as a result are chronically fatigued. Sleep disturbances are common among mental health disorders, including mood disorders, anxiety disorders, and attention-deficit/hyperactivity disorder (ADHD). It may be helpful to assess whether sleep disturbances align with changes in mood and anxiety symptoms or if the delayed sleep onset and wake time are persistently present, as is typically seen in DSWPD. Evaluating and ruling out the impact of restless legs syndrome/periodic limb movements and obstructive sleep apnea syndrome are also important as they may lead to and/or exacerbate delayed sleep onset or disrupted sleep. School avoidance may also be confused with DSWPD, and it is helpful to assess any secondary gain arising from the delayed sleep patterns. A pattern we see in practice is that children or adolescents may be allowed to miss school after a night of poor or adequate sleep. Over time, youth with a history of school anxiety, stress from the workload or social pressure, or bullying may more consistently sleep on this delayed schedule as missing school temporarily relieves these pressures. It is important to identify factors contributing to and maintaining the irregular sleep pattern, as shifting circadian rhythms often take a high level of motivation and will likely be met with resistance if these underlying challenges are not addressed.

Consequences of Circadian Rhythm Sleep–Wake Disorders

Reported consequences of CRSWD frequently include daytime sleepiness, inattention, irritability, and hyperactivity; notably, many of these symptoms mirror symptoms of ADHD. In children and adolescents with DSWPD, academic functioning, including school performance and attendance, are often primary reasons children come for treatment. Adolescents and their parents report that they are frequently late for school or do not attend at all, dropping out of school, have excessive sleepiness during the school day, and have a poor academic performance.

Evidence is strong for delaying middle school and high school start times to better align with the circadian rhythm delays that occur in adolescence. In schools who have implemented changes, there have been improvements in total sleep time, academic functioning, attendance, mental health, and a reduction in motor vehicle accidents.[31–35] However, due to political resistance, this has only been implemented in select regions and school districts to date.

Delayed Sleep–Wake Phase Disorder

In DSWPD, the sleep–wake period is delayed by one or more hours of the desired bedtime, resulting in significant academic, work, or family issues. In general, children appear to be less tolerant of sleep deprivation than adults and an hour delay in sleep onset may result in pathologic symptoms. DSWPD typically emerges in adolescence with changes to the sleep–wake schedule that are associated with puberty. DSWPD is likely much more frequent than ASWPD because the cycle length of the biologic clock exceeds 24 hours in the overwhelming majority of individuals, thus making it harder to fall asleep earlier than expected (see Fig. 3.2).

Presenting Complaints

- Bedtime struggles or difficulty falling asleep at time expected within constraints of social and environment expectations.
- Difficulty awakening at the desired time and/or excessive sleepiness in the morning.

- Falling asleep at school or being too sleepy in the morning to participate in normal activities; frequently late to or absent from school.
- Symptoms may resemble those of mental health conditions, including ADHD (e.g., difficulty sustaining attention) and depression (e.g., low energy, irritability).
- The child prefers not to eat breakfast and is hungry at or close to bedtime and/or says that they function best in the evening.

Diagnostic Criteria[25]

Diagnosis requires the following:
- A significant delay in the phase of the major sleep episode in relation to the desired or required sleep time and wake-up time, as evidenced by a chronic or recurrent complaint by the patient or a caregiver of inability to fall asleep and difficulty awakening at a desired or required clock time.
- Symptoms are present for at least 3 months.
- When patients are allowed to choose their ad libitum schedule, they will exhibit improved sleep quality and duration for age and maintain a delayed phase of the 24-hour sleep–wake pattern.
- Sleep log and, whenever possible, actigraphy monitoring for at least 7 days (preferably 14) demonstrate a delay in the timing of the habitual sleep period. Both work/school days and free days must be included within this monitoring.
- The sleep disturbance is not better explained by another current sleep disorder, medical or neurologic disorder, mental disorder, medication use, or substance use disorder.

Coexistence with Psychiatric/Behavioral Symptoms

ADHD, oppositional symptoms, conduct disorder, aggressive symptoms, and symptoms of depression all correlate with DSWPD, although we still have an incomplete understanding of causal mechanisms and associations are thought to be bidirectional. For instance, compared with 10–18% prevalence rates in youth, DSWPD is estimated to occur at rates of 62% among youth with bipolar disorder and 30% among youth with unipolar depressive disorders.[36] Among youth and adults with ADHD, delayed sleep onset and difficulty falling asleep are common with estimates between 73% and 78%.[23,37,38] Moreover, research suggests that endogenous melatonin secretion may be delayed in youth and adults with ADHD, demonstrating a possible link between ADHD and DSWPD.[39,40] In some instances, DSWPD leads to chronic sleep deprivation, which may aggravate underlying mental health predispositions.[36] Conversely, adolescents struggling with inattention are more likely to delay completing daily activities and homework and to overuse technology in the evening, both of which are thought to delay sleep onset.[40]

When psychiatric symptoms and DSWPD are present concurrently, it is important to establish whether the psychiatric symptoms are present independent of the DSWPD or only occur in conjunction with the sleep disturbance. For example, on weekends or holidays, when the child sleeps until spontaneous awakening, do psychiatric symptoms improve? If the psychiatric symptoms are isolated to periods of insufficient or irregular sleep and there are no imminent mental health concerns, sleep providers may treat the DSWPD prior to determining whether a referral for mental health treatment is warranted. If the psychiatric symptoms were present even during prior periods with sleep of adequate quality and quantity, it is best to treat both the psychiatric symptoms and the DSWPD concurrently. Some studies have demonstrated improvements in mental health symptoms with treatment for DSWPD and additional research is warranted in youth samples. For example, when adults with ADHD and DWSPD were treated with blue light therapy, they both experienced phase advances and improvements in ADHD symptoms.[23,41] Moreover, several studies have shown correlations between lower rates of ADHD and geographical places with higher sunlight intensity,[23,42,43] demonstrating the important role that sunlight may play in synchronizing the circadian rhythm.

Evaluation

Considerations among Children Presenting with Symptoms of DSWPD
- Usually have one parent with DSWPD symptoms or "night owl" preference;
- Typically feel their best and best accomplish tasks such as homework at a later hour;
- Encounter academic, emotional, and behavioral problems during morning hours;
- May require a urinary toxicology screen in cases when concerns about substance use arise;
- Should be evaluated for conditions that frequently co-occur with and/or may exacerbate DSWPD, including depression, ADHD, school refusal, conduct disorder, oppositional defiant disorder, and anxiety disorders and the impact of these conditions on sleep concerns;
- Should review sleep log including bedtime, time of sleep onset, and wake-up time for a minimum of 1 week but preferably at least 2 weeks to establish a pattern;
- Children and adolescents may present a significantly different description of their sleep habits as compared with their parents or caregivers;
- Should assess light exposure during the day and at night; and
- Should assess screen usage, especially in the few hours prior to bedtime.

The Significance of Sunday Night

Asking about challenges in falling asleep on Sunday evenings can often help to distinguish children and adolescents who may revert to a delayed sleep–wake schedule on weekends. Many children with DSWPD awaken and fall asleep at a considerably later hour on weekends, effectively "moving" to a more westward time zone. Parents expect their children or adolescents to return to a weekday schedule on Sunday night (or move east) and the child finds it nearly impossible to fall asleep. This is also called social jet lag, which commonly emerges in adolescence due to the conflict between biologically driven later chronotype and forced early awakenings on weekdays due to school start times.[23]

Impact of Electronic Device Usage on Delayed Sleep–Wake Phase Disorder

Increasing access to portable electronic devices has been postulated to be exacerbating the already delayed sleep–wake schedule associated with adolescence. Numerous studies around the world have recently been published, examining the impacts of electronic usage on sleep timing and quality (e.g.,[44–47]). Electronic devices and media use in the evening have been associated with delayed sleep onset and decreased total sleep time.[14] In addition to use of the devices replacing sleep time and increasing arousal, using devices in the hour before bed also has been shown to delay the circadian rhythm via increased light exposure.[48,49]

Treatment of Delayed Sleep–Wake Phase Disorder

Behavioral Interventions to Help Shift Sleep–Wake Schedule

A recent update by the American Academy of Sleep Medicine Task Force[50] highlighted the limited evidence we have currently available to guide evidence-based interventions for CRSWD. Overall, strategically timed melatonin administration and use of post awakening light therapy were assessed to have weak evidence in favor of their use for the treatment of DSWPD. Nonetheless, in clinical practice many treatment guidelines have been developed based on our scientific knowledge of the etiology of DSWPD and these strategies described next provide a foundation for clinical interventions at present.

Sleep Hygiene

To successfully treat DSWPD, it is important to establish a sleep environment that is quiet and relaxing and sleep habits that are conducive to easing the transition to sleep. Several behavioral changes are recommended to increase the likelihood of successful interventions including the following:

- Expose the child to dim light, or light dim enough to make reading somewhat difficult, for 2 hours preceding bedtime. Dim light permits the expression of melatonin. Normal room illumination, televisions, and computer screens suppress melatonin secretion, interfering with any attempt to help the child initiate sleep earlier. If light is needed for reading or other tasks, it is ideal to have a lamp with dim light behind the child, rather than having the light shine into their eyes.
- Along the same lines, avoid screens (i.e., phones, computers, tablets, television) in the child's bedroom. If the child uses a device as an alarm and it needs to be in the room, set a rule that the device charges overnight in a space that cannot be reached from the bed.
- Increase natural sunlight exposure in the morning by eating breakfast outside or near the windows, and walking or riding a bike to school, when possible.
- Use of a calm, consistent bedtime routine can help children and adolescents to wind down and prepare for sleep. Steps in the routine may include changing into pajamas, brushing teeth, reading books, singing bedtime songs, prayers, or telling stories.
- In children who have outgrown naps, minimize daytime sleep to optimize an earlier bedtime. Naps reduce homeostatic sleep pressure, which is problematic if the child has sleep-onset difficulties. If a child with DSWPD requires a nap, allow as little sleep as possible.
- Parents should establish a set bedtime that is consistent across weekdays, weekends, and vacations. For children with DSWPD, a consistent wake time should also be maintained 7 days a week. Other children might be able to sleep in late on weekends and still fall asleep earlier on Sunday night, but a hallmark of children with DSWPD is that they cannot do this. Children with the same wake-up time every morning do better in school[23] and have fewer behavioral and emotional problems.
- Avoid foods or beverages with caffeine, especially after the morning hours (e.g., coffee, tea, soda, chocolate).
- Make sure your child's bedroom is quiet, dark, and comfortable.

Phase Advancement

The goal of treatment for DSWPD involves first shifting the sleep–wake schedule gradually earlier and then maintaining this new schedule. This process is aided by use of the previously mentioned sleep hygiene practices, timed light exposure, strategically timed melatonin administration, and timed awakenings that are gradually earlier over time. Phase advancement is typically used when the difference between the current fall asleep time and goal fall asleep time are less than 3 hours apart. Initially, the goal may be to get the youth to maintain a consistent sleep–wake pattern. Once this is in place, they can shift the wake time by 30–60 minutes each day, utilizing the following strategies to help the circadian rhythm better align with earlier sleep and rise times. Bedtimes are often shifted more slowly (e.g., 15–30 minutes) to ensure sufficient sleep pressure has built up through the course of the day. Timing of changes to the schedule may depend on how quickly the child needs to shift their schedule and what they feel capable of sticking to for treatment to be successful.

Treatment of Delayed Sleep–Wake Phase Disorder with Optimally Timed Light Exposure

Exposure to light advances or delays affects circadian rhythms in humans more than any other zeitgeber. There is a phase response curve to bright light (see Fig. 3.1) describing the amplitude or phase advance or delay when an individual is exposed to bright light at various times throughout the day.

Light exposure at dawn signals the brain that awakening has occurred too late. It resets the SCNs to advance gene expression to occur earlier. Consequently, light exposure at the time of awakening is a powerful tool in shifting the circadian rhythm to an earlier hour, resulting in an individual becoming sleepy earlier. This is a phase advance.

Light exposure close to bedtime shifts the circadian rhythm later, causing the individual to initiate sleep later and wake up later. This is a phase delay. Both are discussed next as treatments for DSWPD and ASWPD.

Impact of Timing of Light Exposure

The timing of exposure to light determines how it impacts our circadian rhythms. Specifically, light exposure during the first half of an individual's normal sleeping hours has a phase-delaying effect.[16] Light exposure during the individual's last two or three normal sleeping hours has a phase-advancing effect. The nadir of core body temperature, or the minimum temperature in the circadian cycle, typically occurs about two-thirds of the way through the sleep cycle. A child who begins sleep at 9:00 p.m. and spontaneously awakens at 7:00 a.m. on weekends typically has a temperature minimum around approximately 3–4:00 a.m.

To illustrate this further, a child with DSWPD who begins sleep at 3:00 a.m. on weekends and awakens at 1:00 p.m. will have a temperature minimum at approximately 9–10:00 a.m. Light administered *before* the minimum causes a *phase delay*, or results in sleep occurring later, and light administered *after* the minimum causes a *phase advance*, or results in sleep occurring earlier (Fig. 3.3).

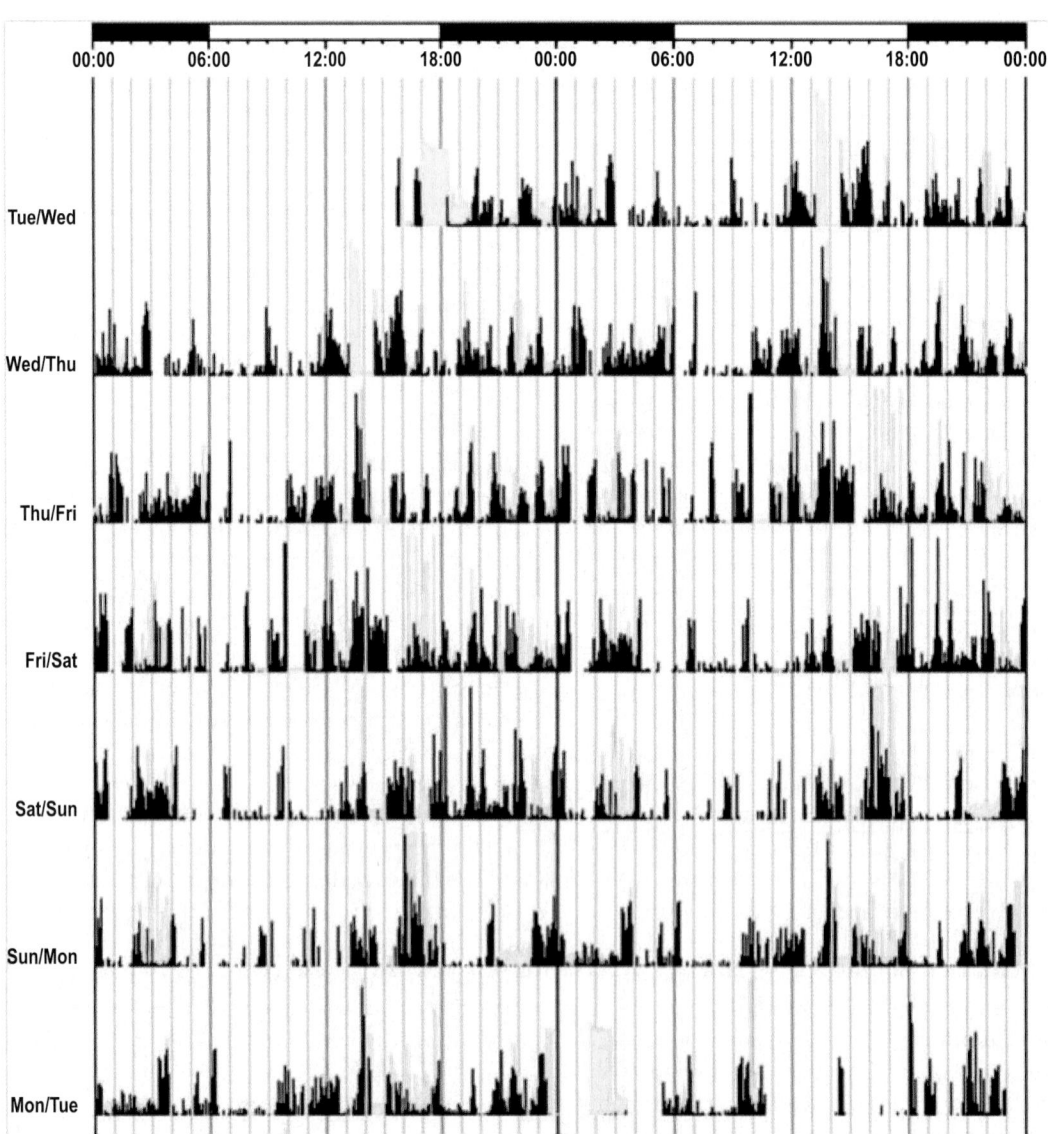

• **Fig. 3.3** Actogram obtained by actigraphy over a 7-day period from an older adult patient who has irregular sleep–wake rhythm disorder (ISWRD). The *yellow bars* indicate timing and level of ambient light exposure, and the *black bars* indicate activity levels recorded at the nondominant wrist. Note the lack of a discernible circadian sleep–wake rhythm. Sleep is characterized by nocturnal fragmentation and multiple short periods of sleeping and waking across the entire 24-hour day. *(Legend from original text.)*[51]

The timing of the temperature nadir is established by a careful history of when the child or adolescent begins sleep and awakens each day. As described previously, this information is best gathered by use of a detailed sleep diary or actigraphy for at least 1 week. In children or adolescents with phase delay, it is best to expose them to sunlight, bright light, or blue light at about the time they normally awaken and to prevent them from being exposed to morning light before their estimated temperature minimum.[50] For example, a child who awakens at noon on weekends should wear sunglasses after sunrise until the estimated time of their temperature minimum on school days.

Between the vernal and autumnal equinoxes, when day is longer than night, morning sunlight alone is extremely helpful in advancing phase. As soon as a child awakens, have them play in sunlight, preferably outdoors, but possibly indoors, in an area illuminated by sunlight. It also has a mood-elevating and antidepressant effect, as morning exposure to bright light boxes is a recognized treatment for both seasonal affective disorder (SAD) and other mild depressive disorders.[52]

Blue Light Therapy

Rods and cones were the only known photoreceptors that transduce light into a neural signal until the discovery of a third retinal photoreceptor called melanopsin.[53] Neural signals from melanopsin-containing cells are transmitted from the retina to the SCN. These cells are most sensitive to light of a blue wavelength.[54]

Bright light boxes have been replaced to a great extent by iPad-sized, blue, light-emitting diode (LED) boxes. These are lightweight, run on rechargeable batteries, and are sufficiently portable to fit in a purse, backpack, or briefcase. They have demonstrated efficacy in a number of studies.[55] It is recommended that children or adolescents with DSWPD use blue light or daylight exposure for 20 minutes to an hour soon after wake-up and avoid bright light in the hours prior to bed, as much as possible.[56] The light of dawn is extremely important in entraining circadian rhythms,[57,58] in children as well as adults. Notably, phase shifting with blue or white light has been shown to be more effective when it is associated with active play or exercise (e.g., a running wheel in rats[59]).

Treatment of Delayed Sleep–Wake Phase Disorder with Optimally Timed Melatonin Administration

Melatonin is often a misunderstood compound as it has been used both as a sedative hypnotic and as a chronobiotic (able to change the timing of sleep). The timing of administration appears to be critical to help in advancing sleep–wake schedules.[28] The pineal gland secretes approximately 300 pg (0.3 mg) of melatonin each night.[60] Over-the-counter melatonin typically is sold in quantities far exceeding this amount. Melatonin has powerful phase-shifting properties when administered in low doses. Doses exceeding

1 mg remain in the bloodstream long enough to cancel their desired effect or even delay the circadian rhythm, as they are present in blood during both the phase advance and phase delay portion of the circadian rhythm.[23]

Melatonin has the ability to shift circadian rhythms if the timing of administration accounts for the time when the pineal gland normally secretes it, approximately 2 hours before normal sleep onset. It has its most powerful effect in advancing circadian rhythms when exogenous melatonin is administered approximately 4–6 hours before its normal secretion. For an individual with DSWPD, who normally initiates sleep at 2:00 a.m., DLMO would occur at approximately midnight. To phase advance such an individual, melatonin would be administered between 6 and 8:00 p.m.

The Phase Response Curve for Melatonin and Light

The phase response curve describes when either light or melatonin has various degrees of phase-advancing or phase-delaying effects or has no effect at all. Light's maximum phase-advancing effect occurs around the time of normal awakening and its maximal delaying effect occurs around normal bedtime, or later (see Fig. 3.1). Melatonin's maximal phase-advancing effect occurs approximately 4–6 hours before normal DLMO and its maximal delaying effect occurs about the time of normal awakening (see Fig. 3.2).

Identifying Child and Family Factors That May Impact Treatment Outcomes

Making changes to the sleep–wake schedule can be challenging and requires significant motivation as waking up earlier than desired may cause frustration and daytime sleepiness in the short run. It is important to assess adolescent motivation and, in cases where intrinsic motivation is low, privileges that parents can utilize to motivate these changes. In adolescents, failure to cooperate with a plan to shift their sleep–wake schedule may be a sign of clinical depression, anxiety or school avoidance, and/or oppositional defiant symptoms. It is important to evaluate barriers to change and to help families get support in addressing underlying factors that may impact treatment readiness.

Behavioral issues frequently overlay CRSWDs. Treatment is most effective if parents and their children understand the basic principles underlying their child's inability to initiate sleep and awaken. Effective treatment of DSWPD by a sleep specialist requires that time is devoted to providing education to the child/adolescent and their family members about the nature of the disorder and the rationale for each proposed intervention. Expectations and possible resistance to treatment are best brought into the open and discussed together.

If the child is sufficiently mature, they should be encouraged to gradually take on more responsibility in working toward better aligning their sleep–wake schedule with external requirements. Given how challenging it is to maintain a wake time on weekends, sleep providers should help the family to identify and schedule fun activities for the child and a parent or peers to look forward to in the morning, such as playing outdoors, going to a neighborhood park, or going out for breakfast. Adolescents may be encouraged to set their own alarms and wake up on their own as they might soon leave their parent's household, such as when they leave for college. Although taking the initiative to do this may be challenging, adolescents may be more likely to engage in these behaviors if parents notice and praise the independent behaviors and/or allow these adolescents privileges to engage in desired activities as a reward.

Chronotherapy

Chronotherapy is a behavioral technique in which bedtime is systematically delayed, which follows the natural tendency of human biology to operate on longer than a 24-hour clock.[61] Bedtime is delayed by 3-hour increments each day, establishing a 27-hour day. The procedure is maintained until the desired bedtime is reached (say, 10 p.m.), when the normal 24-hour day is then established. This approach is favored by adolescents who are extreme night owls. It is difficult to administer, as a parent typically must be present to oversee unusual sleep and wake-up times, such as sleeping from noon to 8:00 p.m. and staying awake through the duration of the normal nighttime hours.

Successful Phase Advance Therapy

The first sign that the light and/or melatonin are having their desired effect is an earlier hour of sleep onset and fewer struggles with morning awakening. This is followed by the parents reporting the child's morning appetite to be increased.

Maintenance Phase

A strategy must be determined in advance for counteracting the natural tendency of an adolescent to slip back into a later bedtime and awakening hour on weekends. The adolescent should agree that they may remain awake late on occasion, but must still arise and be in sunlight early. The easiest way to maintain the circadian rhythm is to stick as closely as possible to a consistent wake time, even during weekends, school breaks, or summer vacations.

Advanced Sleep–Wake Phase Disorder

Presenting Complaints

ASWPD is diagnosed when an individual's major sleep episode is advanced in relation to the desired clock time. It results in compelling early sleepiness, an early sleep onset, and an awakening that is earlier than desired.

Diagnostic Criteria[25]

- Inability to stay awake until the desired bedtime or inability to remain asleep until the desired time of awakening. Children or adolescents with ASWPD fall asleep doing homework, at social events, immediately after dinner, or before dinner if it is at a late hour.

- Inability to sleep later until (desired) delayed morning hours.
- Symptoms are present for at least 3 months.
- When allowed to sleep on their own schedule (seen on weekends, vacations, prolonged breaks from school), children will do the following:
  - Fall asleep at an early hour.
  - Awaken spontaneously at an early hour.
  - Have a habitual sleep period that is of normal quality and duration.
  - Maintain stable entrainment to a 24-hour sleep–wake pattern over at least 2 weeks. Have an early DLMO.

Sleep-onset times may be as early as 5–6 p.m. and wake times 3–5 a.m. These sleep-onset and wake times occur despite the family's best efforts to delay sleep to later hours. These challenges become apparent in children and adolescents when social and academic activities stretch into evening hours. Attempts to delay sleep onset to a time later than usual may result in embarrassment due to falling asleep during social gatherings. If chronically forced to stay up later for social or vocational reasons, the physiologic early awakening could lead to chronic sleep deprivation and daytime sleepiness or napping. It is important to consider ASWPD in the workup for possible central hypersomnias.

Thorough family history is important when considering ASWPD. Several autosomal dominantly clock gene mutations have been identified as associated with familial ASWPD (*PER2, CRY2, PER3,* and *TIMELESS*).[62–65] Several of these mutations are also associated with familial migraines, depressive affect, bipolar disorder, behavioral activation, and sugar metabolism.[65]

Consequences of Advanced Sleep–Wake Phase Disorder

Data have demonstrated that morning chronotypes, "morning larks" or those who favor early sleep onset and offset like the individuals with ASWPD, fare better than evening types physically and psychologically.[66] These morning types are noted to exhibit more "constraint."[67] This results in being considered more responsible and seen in a positive light by parents and teachers, which can inform a confident sense of self. They are "early to rise" and considered diligent, hard-working, and perform better in school,[68] qualities viewed positively by society at large.

A child with ASWPD may view their symptoms as a positive character attribute. These children are frequently in a good mood following early morning awakening. With maturity and parental guidance, a child can occupy oneself and allow caretakers to sleep to a later hour. However, in early childhood when supervision is needed, the early rise can truncate parental sleep.

The late day and evening are most problematic for children with ASWPD, as they may be too sleepy to engage with homework, extracurricular activities, or family outings. This presentation overlaps with that of a hypersomnia like narcolepsy, and careful history taking regarding wake time and total sleep time is paramount.

Coexistence with Psychiatric/Behavioral Symptoms

Unlike DSWPD, which coexists with a host of psychiatric and behavioral disorders, ASWPD has not been associated with a psychiatric or behavioral disorder. Advancing the phase of an individual's circadian rhythm has been seen to improve symptoms of stress and depression[68] as well as specifically seasonal depression.[69] It is possible that the advanced sleep–wake phase may be protective against psychiatric disorders such as depression.

Age of Onset

Symptoms of ASWPD may appear as early as 12 weeks of age, when the circadian rhythm has been seen to potentially first entrain.[70]

Epidemiology

ASWPD is rare in the overall population (1%), although this may be an underestimation given the lower likelihood of individuals finding this schedule problematic.[65] This is even lower in the pediatric population. Given the autosomal dominant inheritance, it is more commonly seen in in children who have one parent with ASWPD tendencies. There is some literature to suggest that prenatal factors may also predispose children to more advanced chronotypes.[71]

Evaluation

ASWPD needs to be differentiated from other disorders producing daytime sleepiness, such as obstructive sleep apnea, disrupted nocturnal sleep, chronic sleep deprivation, or narcolepsy. Like DSWPD patients, ASWPD patients have no intrinsic sleep abnormalities; they report that sleep itself is restful and restorative when allowed to sleep on their natural schedule.

Treatment

ASWPD is treated with evening light to suppress endogenous melatonin onset and allow for later DLMO and sleep onset based on the child's phase response curve.[72,73] This can be accomplished with outdoor light exposure or use of a light box with high intensity (2,000–8,000 lux).[74]

There are no data to support melatonin use nor avoidance of light in the daytime in individuals with ASWPD.[50]

Irregular Sleep–Wake Rhythm Disorder

Irregular sleep–wake rhythm disorder (ISWRD) differs from other CRSWDs in that it appears to be the result of an impaired circadian pacemaker, as opposed to a normal pacemaker out of phase or not entrained.

Presenting Complaints

Contrary to normal circadian rhythms in which individuals have one main sleeping period and one main period of wakefulness during a typical 24-hour stretch, individuals with irregular sleep–wake rhythms have several blocks of sleep somewhat randomly during the 24-hour period, and none might be long enough to be considered the major sleep period (see Fig. 3.3).

This sleeping pattern is normal in newborn infants who accumulate and pay off sleep pressure throughout the night and day. However, this pattern is uncommon by 6 months of age by which time most infants have a major sleep period at night (of variable length), with consolidated naps during the day.[75]

Diagnostic Criteria

ISWRD can present with a complaint of insomnia, excessive daytime sleepiness, or both. Sleep logs and/or actigraphy will demonstrate at least three sleep episodes in most 24-hour periods. Nevertheless, total sleep time per 24 hours is within normal limits[25] (see Fig. 3.3).

Family Dynamics

The burden on a family with a young child with IRSWD can be high. A caretaker needs to be present continually. Planning and engaging in activities such as school, extracurricular activities, or outings can be unpredictable.

Coexistence with Psychiatric/Behavioral Symptoms

This disorder appears mostly in adults with dementia and neurodegenerative disease but may be seen in a child with developmental delay.[25]

Age of Onset

ISWRD can be seen to increase in frequency with age, given the association with progressive neuropsychiatric disorders.[51]

Evaluation

Thorough history taking and sleep monitoring over time will reveal an irregular sleep–wake pattern. While a parent may report their child having difficulty initiating sleep, carefully questioning about the daytime will reveal (importantly multiple) nap opportunities, which deplete sleep pressure, making sleep onset at a socially appropriate time at night impossible.

Treatment

ISWRD is treated with bright light daylight hours.[50] Dim light conditions at bedtime is recommended. Consistency in the timing of this light/dark cycling is important 7 days a week. Melatonin can be considered for select children with IRSWD prior to the major nocturnal sleep period to mimic endogenous melatonin onset at a consistent time, unlike their elderly or medically fragile counterparts who are at risk for falls with this therapy.[50]

Non–24-Hour Sleep–Wake Phase Disorder

Presenting Complaints

Non–24-hour sleep–wake phase disorder (N24SWPD) goes by many names. It is often called free-running or nonentrained CRSWD. It occurs when the intrinsic period of the

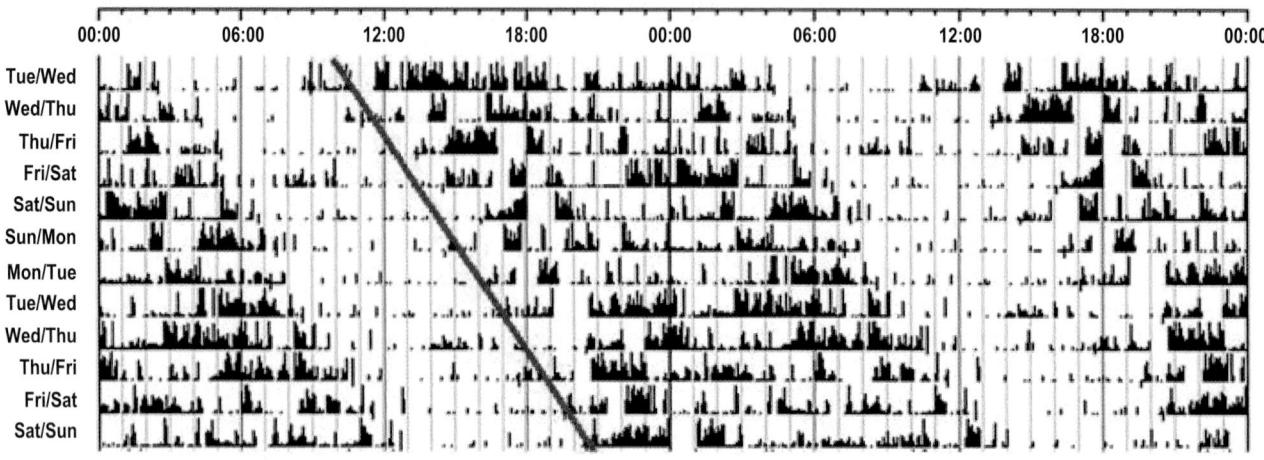

• **Fig. 3.4** Illustration of 12 days of actigraphy from a patient with non–24-hour circadian rhythm sleep–wake disorder showing a cumulative delay of 10 hours for a 24.83-hour free-running sleep–wake cycle. Data are double plotted. The patient begins monitoring beginning sleep at about 10 a.m. and ends beginning sleep at 8 p.m. From Barion A, Zee PC, A clinical approach to circadian rhythm sleep disorders. *Sleep Med.* 2007;8(6):566–577.

circadian pacemaker "free-runs" with respect to the 24-hour day. Typically, the patient has sleep onset 30 minutes to 1 hour later each day. Affected children are not able to maintain a stable sleep–wake phase. Parents initially report that their child's sleep pattern is completely random and has no pattern. They may also have fluctuating sleep complaints including insomnia and hypersomnia, dependent on which phase a child is in while presenting to care. A careful history and sleep logs and/or actigraphy for 2 weeks or more will reveal and gradually shift sleep-onset and -offset times described as a "drift" (Fig. 3.4).

When the child's endogenous rhythms are out of phase with the family and school, both insomnia and excessive daytime sleepiness are reported. Conversely, when the child's endogenous rhythm is in phase with home and school, symptoms appear to temporarily remit. The intervals between symptomatic periods may last several days to weeks. As the human pacemaker runs on a slightly longer than 24-hour period, light is needed daily to re-entrain sleep–wake rhythms.[25] Individuals with blindness to light perception are at an increased risk for N24SWPD, and 50–80% report sleep disturbance.[76,77] Some of these sleep disturbances manifest as free-running rhythms, although most demonstrate with a phase delay pattern.[25] N24SWPD has been reported in the sighted population as well, although it is challenging to discern the intrinsic and extrinsic factors of this sleep disorder in that population.[78-80] Cases of sighted children with Rett Syndrome, autism spectrum disorder, Angelman syndrome, and nonspecific neurodevelopmental disorders have also been described in the literature.[25]

Diagnostic Criteria

The International Classification of Sleep Disorders (ICSD)-3 requires a chronic complaint of insomnia, excessive sleepiness, or both, based upon a lack of synchronization between the 24-hour clock and the patient's non–24-hour sleep–wake cycle. Diagnosis is established by maintaining a sleep log and/or actigraphy for at least 14 days showing a greater than 24-hour period length for the sleep–wake schedule.

Family Dynamics

This disorder can cause a great deal of stress, confusion, and frustration to the patient's family, as the child is unable to attend school or work at designated hours but with fluctuating symptoms.

Interpersonal Dynamics

Individuals with this disorder may lack normal social relationships and do not attend school or work a normal job.[79]

Coexistence with Psychiatric/Behavioral Symptoms

The presence of N24SWPD has been shown to be associated with depression,[79,80] markedly in sighted patients. Directionality is challenging to discern, with one case report demonstrating the sleep rhythm asynchrony improving with mood control with the start of an antidepressant.[81]

Age of Onset

Onset can occur at any age, including in infancy in blind individuals.[25]

Evaluation

Diagnosis is established by a 2-week or longer diary completed daily and by concurrent actigraphy with a clear demonstrated drift of sleep–wake times. There have been reports of circadian instability in individuals with DSWPD, manifesting as shifting sleep-onset times.[82] Given reports of shared pupillary response to light between N24SWD and DSWPD, there is likely more overlap between these two disorders than is currently understood.[83]

Treatment

Timed melatonin administration has been reported to improve sleep timing in non–24-hour sleep–wake disorder, notably in blind individuals.[50] Melatonin receptor agonists have also shown to be effective in management of N24SWD in blind individuals.[84] Scheduled light exposure is not indicated for blind nor sighted individuals.[50]

Conclusion

CRSWDs can be common in children and frequently masquerade as other sleep disorders, most notably insomnia and daytime sleepiness. Many children are evaluated extensively from a medical perspective before they are referred to a sleep specialist. For the most part, history taking with a with sleep–timing-driven focus is sufficient to suggest a CRSWD diagnosis. In many cases, sleep logs are critical in confirming a suspected diagnosis, especially when a sleep-deprived caretaker perceives the child's sleep as "chaotic" and not following any pattern. Subjective or objective sleep pattern recording will often reveal the diagnosis.

Frequently, a second disorder coexists along with the CRSWD, such as depression, an anxiety disorder, or a sleep disorder such as obstructive sleep apnea or restless legs syndrome (RLS)/periodic limb movement disorder (PLMD). In these latter cases, polysomnography is required to establish the severity of a coexisting sleep disorder and treatment should be prioritized to support the behavioral interventions that will need to be in place to address the CRSWD.

If a psychiatric disorder coexists with a CRSWD, treating the CRSWD first may in fact help to lessen depressive or anxious symptoms by minimizing sleep deprivation and disruption. Bright light therapy, which is utilized in several CSWRDs, can also have an antidepressant effect on its own. Improving sleep onset and wake will also build confidence in children over their own abilities to have mastery over their schedules and alleviate anxiety and negative perceptions they may have about their sleep.

Finally, social jet lag is a term that has come to refer to a mismatch with one's internal circadian rhythm and that of the surrounding environment, without travel. This can be seen in any of the previously discussed CRSWDs. This mismatch is not only inconvenient and socially disruptive, anxiety-provoking, and confidence crushing, but there is evidence that it can be associated with cardiometabolic risk factors.[85]

Discussions with children and their families around CRSWDs can be profound. When long-standing complaints transform into clear clues to a diagnosis and logs reveal the logic behind a child's sleep–wake timing, a family becomes empowered to make impactful changes. At times, therapy as simple as timed sunshine can result in a tremendous improvement in a child's quality of life and overall physical and psychologic well-being.

CLINICAL PEARLS

- CRSWDs are a cohort of disorders with sleep and wake time that is problematic for the child and/or family. DSWPD is especially prevalent in adolescents.
- Late-night light, including room light, screens, and cell phones, worsens DSWPD.
- Light exposure promotes wake by a melatonin offset mechanism.
- Timed melatonin can mimic endogenous DLMO and promote sleep onset based on an individual's phase response curve.

References

1. Hellbruegge T. The development of circadian rhythms in infants. *Cold Spring Harb Symp Quant Biol.* 1960;25:311–323.
2. Barclay NL, Eley TC, Mill J, et al. Sleep quality and diurnal preference in a sample of young adults: Associations with 5HTTLPR, PER3, and CLOCK3111. *Am J Med Genet B Neuropsychiatr Genet.* Sep 2011;156B(6):681–690.
3. Andreani TS, Itoh TQ, Yildirim E, Hwangbo DS, Allada R. Genetics of circadian rhythms. *Sleep Med Clin.* Dec 2015;10(4):413–421.
4. Weaver DR. The suprachiasmatic nucleus: A 25-year retrospective. *J Biol Rhythms.* Apr 1998;13(2):100–112.
5. Crowley SJ, Acebo C, Carskadon MA. Sleep, circadian rhythms, and delayed phase in adolescence. *Sleep Med.* 2007;8(6):602–612.
6. Morin LP, Allen CN. The circadian visual system, 2005. *Brain Res Rev.* Jun 2006;51(1):1–60.
7. Brooks E, Canal MM. Development of circadian rhythms: Role of postnatal light environment. *Neurosci Biobehav Rev.* May 2013;37(4):551–560.
8. Kleitman N, Engelmann TG. Sleep characteristics of infants. *J Appl Physiol.* Nov 1953;6(5):269–282.
9. Glotzbach SF, Edgar DM, Boeddiker M, Ariagno RL. Biological rhythmicity in normal infants during the first 3 months of life. *Pediatrics.* Oct 1994;94(4 Pt 1):482–488.
10. Rivkees SA. Developing circadian rhythmicity in infants. *Pediatrics.* 2003;112(2):373–381.
11. Carskadon MA, Acebo C, Richardson GS, Tate BA, Seifer R. An approach to studying circadian rhythms of adolescent humans. *Journal Biol. Rhythms.* 1997;12(3):278–289.
12. Hagenauer MH, Perryman JI, Lee TM, Carskadon MA. Adolescent changes in the homeostatic and circadian regulation of sleep. *Dev Neurosci.* 2009;31(4):276–284.
13. Crowley SJ, Suh C, Molina TA, Fogg LF, Sharkey KM, Carskadon MA. Estimating the dim light melatonin onset of adolescents within a 6-h sampling window: The impact of sampling rate and threshold method. *Sleep Med.* 2016;20:59–66.
14. Tarokh L, Short M, Crowley SJ, Fontanellaz-Castiglione CE, Carskadon MA. Sleep and circadian rhythms in adolescence. *Curr Sleep Med Rep.* 2019;5(4):181–192.
15. Borbély AA, Daan S, Wirz-Justice A, Deboer T. The two-process model of sleep regulation: A reappraisal. *J Sleep Res.* 2016;25(2):131–143.
16. Zhu L, Zee PC. Circadian rhythm sleep disorders. *Neurol Clin.* Nov 2012;30(4):1167–1191.

17. Mirmiran M, Maas YG, Ariagno RL. Development of fetal and neonatal sleep and circadian rhythms. *Sleep Med Rev.* Aug 2003;7(4):321–334.

18. Staller N, Randler C. Changes in sleep schedule and chronotype due to COVID-19 restrictions and home office. *Somnologie (Berl).* 2021;25(2):131–137.

19. MacKenzie NE, Keys E, Hall WA, et al. Children's sleep during COVID-19: How sleep influences surviving and thriving in families. *J Pediatr Psychol.* Sep 27 2021;46(9):1051–1062.

20. Czeisler CA, Duffy JF, Shanahan TL, et al. Stability, precision, and near-24-hour period of the human circadian pacemaker. *Science.* Jun 25 1999;284(5423):2177–2181.

21. Randler C, Faßl C, Kalb N. From lark to owl: Developmental changes in morningness-eveningness from new-borns to early adulthood. *Sci Rep.* Apr 5 2017;7:45874.

22. Eid B, Bou Saleh M, Melki I, et al. Evaluation of chronotype among children and associations with BMI, sleep, anxiety, and depression. *Front Neurol.* 2020;11:416.

23. Arns M, Kooij JJS, Coogan AN. Review: Identification and management of circadian rhythm sleep disorders as a transdiagnostic feature in child and adolescent psychiatry. *J Am Acad Child Adolesc Psychiatry.* 2021;60(9):1085–1095.

24. Haraden DA, Mullin BC, Hankin BL. Internalizing symptoms and chronotype in youth: A longitudinal assessment of anxiety, depression and tripartite model. *Psychiatry Res.* 2019;272: 797–805.

25. American Academy of Sleep Medicine. *International Classification of Sleep Disorders: Diagnostic and Coding Manual.* 3rd ed. American Academy of Sleep Medicine; 2014.

26. Sivertsen B, Pallesen S, Stormark KM, Bøe T, Lundervold AJ, Hysing M. Delayed sleep phase syndrome in adolescents: Prevalence and correlates in a large population based study. *BMC Pub Health.* 2013;13(1).1163.

27. Pandi-Perumal SR, Smits M, Spence W, et al. Dim light melatonin onset (DLMO): A tool for the analysis of circadian phase in human sleep and chronobiological disorders. *Prog Neuropsychopharmacol Biol Psychiatry.* Jan 30 2007;31(1):1–11.

28. Burgess HJ, Revell VL, Molina TA, Eastman CI. Human phase response curves to three days of daily melatonin: 0.5 mg versus 3.0 mg. *J Clin Endocrinol Metabol.* 2010;95(7):3325–3331.

29. Crowley SJ, Acebo C, Fallone G, Carskadon MA. Estimating dim light melatonin onset (DLMO) phase in adolescents using summer or school-year sleep/wake schedules. *Sleep.* Dec 2006;29(12):1632–1641.

30. Duffy JF, Wright Jr KP. Entrainment of the human circadian system by light. *J Biol Rhythms.* Aug 2005;20(4):326–338.

31. Meltzer LJ, Plog AE, Swenka D, Reeves D, Wahlstrom KL. Drowsy driving and teen motor vehicle crashes: Impact of changing school start times. *J Adolesc.* 2022;94(5):800–805.

32. Meltzer LJ, Wahlstrom KL, Plog AE, Strand MJ. Changing school start times: Impact on sleep in primary and secondary school students. *Sleep.* Jul 9 2021;44(7):zsab048.

33. Wahlstrom KL, Berger AT, Widome R. Relationships between school start time, sleep duration, and adolescent behaviors. *Sleep Health.* Jun 2017;3(3):216–221.

34. Danner F, Phillips B. Adolescent sleep, school start times, and teen motor vehicle crashes. *J Clin Sleep Med.* Dec 15 2008;4(6):533–535.

35. Bin-Hasan S, Kapur K, Rakesh K, Owens J. School start time change and motor vehicle crashes in adolescent drivers. *J Clin Sleep Med.* 2020;16(3):371–376.

36. Robillard R, Naismith SL, Rogers NL, et al. Delayed sleep phase in young people with unipolar or bipolar affective disorders. *J Affect Disord.* 2013;145(2):260–263.

37. Van der Heijden KB, Smits MG, Gunning WB. Sleep hygiene and actigraphically evaluated sleep characteristics in children with ADHD and chronic sleep onset insomnia. *J Sleep Res.* 2006;15(1):55–62.

38. Van Veen MM, Kooij JS, Boonstra AM, Gordijn MC, Van Someren EJ. Delayed circadian rhythm in adults with attention-deficit/hyperactivity disorder and chronic sleep-onset insomnia. *Biol Psychiatry.* 2010;67(11):1091–1096.

39. Coogan AN, McGowan NM. A systematic review of circadian function, chronotype and chronotherapy in attention deficit hyperactivity disorder. *Atten Defic Hyperact Disord.* 2017;9(3):129–147.

40. Lunsford-Avery JR, Krystal AD, Kollins SH. Sleep disturbances in adolescents with ADHD: A systematic review and framework for future research. *Clin Psychol Rev.* Dec 2016;50:159–174.

41. Fargason RE, Fobian AD, Hablitz LM, et al. Correcting delayed circadian phase with bright light therapy predicts improvement in ADHD symptoms: A pilot study. *J Psychiatr Res.* 2017;91:105–110.

42. Arns M, van der Heijden KB, Arnold LE, Kenemans JL. Geographic variation in the prevalence of attention-deficit/hyperactivity disorder: The sunny perspective. *Biol Psychiatry.* 2013;74(8):585–590.

43. Arns M, van der Heijden KB, Arnold LE, Swanson JM, Kenemans JL. Reply to: Attention-deficit/hyperactivity disorder and solar irradiance: A cloudy perspective. *Biol Psychiatry.* 2014;76(8):e21–e23.

44. Olorunmoteni OE, Fatusi AO, Komolafe MA, Omisore A. Sleep pattern, socioenvironmental factors, and use of electronic devices among Nigerian school-attending adolescents. *Sleep Health.* Dec 2018;4(6):551–557.

45. Mortazavi AR, Mortazavi SMJ, Paknahad M. Late use of electronic media and its association with sleep, depression, and suicidality among Korean adolescents. *Sleep Med.* 2017;32:275–276.

46. Reynolds AC, Meltzer LJ, Dorrian J, Centofanti SA, Biggs SN. Impact of high-frequency email and instant messaging (E/IM) interactions during the hour before bed on self-reported sleep duration and sufficiency in female Australian children and adolescents. *Sleep Health.* Feb 2019;5(1):64–67.

47. Carter B, Rees P, Hale L, Bhattacharjee D, Paradkar MS. Association Between portable screen-based media device access or use and sleep outcomes: A systematic review and meta-analysis. *JAMA Pediatr.* Dec 1 2016;170(12):1202–1208.

48. Cain N, Gradisar M. Electronic media use and sleep in school-aged children and adolescents: A review. *Sleep Med.* Sep 2010;11(8):735–742.

49. Touitou Y, Touitou D, Reinberg A. Disruption of adolescents' circadian clock: The vicious circle of media use, exposure to light at night, sleep loss and risk behaviors. *J Physiol Paris.* Nov 2016;110(4 Pt B):467–479.

50. Auger RR, Burgess HJ, Emens JS, Deriy LV, Thomas SM, Sharkey KM. Clinical Practice Guideline for the Treatment of Intrinsic Circadian Rhythm Sleep-Wake Disorders: Advanced Sleep-Wake Phase Disorder (ASWPD), Delayed Sleep-Wake Phase Disorder (DSWPD), Non-24-Hour Sleep-Wake Rhythm Disorder (N24SWD), and Irregular Sleep-Wake Rhythm Disorder (ISWRD). An Update for 2015: An American Academy

of Sleep Medicine Clinical Practice Guideline. *J Clin Sleep Med.* Oct 15 2015;11(10):1199–1236.

51. Zee PC, Vitiello MV. Circadian rhythm sleep disorder: Irregular sleep wake rhythm type. *Sleep Med Clin.* Jun 1 2009;4(2):213–218.

52. Niederhofer H, von Klitzing K. Bright light treatment as monotherapy of non-seasonal depression for 28 adolescents. *Int J Psychiatry Clin Pract.* Sep 2012;16(3):233–237.

53. Provencio I, Jiang G, De Grip WJ, Hayes WP, Rollag MD. Melanopsin: An opsin in melanophores, brain, and eye. *Proc Natl Acad Sci U S A.* Jan 6 1998;95(1):340–345.

54. Enezi J, Revell V, Brown T, Wynne J, Schlangen L, Lucas RA. "melanopic" spectral efficiency function predicts the sensitivity of melanopsin photoreceptors to polychromatic lights. *J Biol Rhythms.* Aug 2011;26(4):314–323.

55. Revell VL, Molina TA, Eastman CI. Human phase response curve to intermittent blue light using a commercially available device. *J Physiol.* Oct 1 2012;590(19):4859–4868.

56. Lafrance C, Dumont M, Lesperance P, Lambert C. Daytime vigilance after morning bright light exposure in volunteers subjected to sleep restriction. *Physiol Behav.* Mar 1998;63(5):803–810.

57. Danilenko KV, Wirz-Justice A, Krauchi K, Weber JM, Terman M. The human circadian pacemaker can see by the dawn's early light. *J Biol Rhythms.* Oct 2000;15(5):437–446.

58. Clodore M, Foret J, Benoit O, et al. Psychophysiological effects of early morning bright light exposure in young adults. *Psychoneuroendocrinology.* 1990;15(3):193–205.

59. Baehr EK, Fogg LF, Eastman CI. Intermittent bright light and exercise to entrain human circadian rhythms to night work. *Am J Physiol.* Dec 1999;277(6):R1598–1604.

60. Fourtillan JB, Brisson AM, Fourtillan M, Ingrand I, Decourt JP, Girault J. Melatonin secretion occurs at a constant rate in both young and older men and women. *Am J Physiol Endocrinol Metab.* Jan 2001;280(1):E11–E22.

61. Czeisler CA, Richardson GS, Coleman RM, et al. Chronotherapy: Resetting the circadian clocks of patients with delayed sleep phase insomnia. *Sleep.* 1981;4(1):1–21.

62. Hirano A, Shi G, Jones CR, et al. A Cryptochrome 2 mutation yields advanced sleep phase in humans. *Elife.* Aug 16 2016;5:e16695.

63. Xu Y, Padiath QS, Shapiro RE, et al. Functional consequences of a CKIdelta mutation causing familial advanced sleep phase syndrome. *Nature.* Mar 31 2005;434(7033):640–644.

64. Kurien P, Hsu PK, Leon J, et al. TIMELESS mutation alters phase responsiveness and causes advanced sleep phase. *Proc Natl Acad Sci U S A.* Jun 11 2019;116(24):12045–12053.

65. Curtis BJ, Ashbrook LH, Young T, et al. Extreme morning chronotypes are often familial and not exceedingly rare: The estimated prevalence of advanced sleep phase, familial advanced sleep phase, and advanced sleep-wake phase disorder in a sleep clinic population. *Sleep.* Oct 9 2019;42(10):zsz148.

66. Knutson KL, von Schantz M. Associations between chronotype, morbidity and mortality in the UK Biobank cohort. *Chronobiol Int.* Aug 2018;35(8):1045–1053.

67. Bullock B, Murray G, Anderson JL, et al. Constraint is associated with earlier circadian phase and morningness: Confirmation of relationships between personality and circadian phase using a constant routine protocol. *Pers Individ Dif.* Jan 2017;104:69–74.

68. Facer-Childs ER, Middleton B, Skene DJ, Bagshaw AP. Resetting the late timing of "night owls" has a positive impact on mental health and performance. *Sleep Med.* Aug 2019;60:236–247.

69. Lewy AJ, Rough JN, Songer JB, Mishra N, Yuhas K, Emens JS. The phase shift hypothesis for the circadian component of winter depression. *Dialogues Clin Neurosci.* 2007;9(3):291–300.

70. Thomas KA, Burr RL, Spieker S. Light and maternal influence in the entrainment of activity circadian rhythm in infants 4–12 weeks of age. *Sleep Biol Rhythms.* Jul 2016;14(3):249–255.

71. Kennaway DJ. Programming of the fetal suprachiasmatic nucleus and subsequent adult rhythmicity. *Trends Endocrinol Metab.* Nov 2002;13(9):398–402.

72. Tahkamo L, Partonen T, Pesonen AK. Systematic review of light exposure impact on human circadian rhythm. *Chronobiol Int.* Feb 2019;36(2):151–170.

73. Shanahan TL, Kronauer RE, Duffy JF, Williams GH, Czeisler CA. Melatonin rhythm observed throughout a three-cycle bright-light stimulus designed to reset the human circadian pacemaker. *J Biol Rhythms.* Jun 1999;14(3):237–253.

74. Lam C, Chung MH. Dose-response effects of light therapy on sleepiness and circadian phase shift in shift workers: A meta-analysis and moderator analysis. *Sci Rep.* Jun 7 2021;11(1):11976.

75. Pennestri MH, Burdayron R, Kenny S, Beliveau MJ, Dubois-Comtois K. Sleeping through the night or through the nights? *Sleep Med.* Dec 2020;76:98–103.

76. Emens J, Lewy AJ, Laurie AL, Songer JB. Rest-activity cycle and melatonin rhythm in blind free-runners have similar periods. *J Biol Rhythms.* Oct 2010;25(5):381–384.

77. Sack RL, Brandes RW, Kendall AR, Lewy AJ. Entrainment of free-running circadian rhythms by melatonin in blind people. *N Engl J Med.* Oct 12 2000;343(15):1070–1077.

78. Malkani RG, Abbott SM, Reid KJ, Zee PC. Diagnostic and treatment challenges of sighted non-24-hour sleep-wake disorder. *J Clin Sleep Med.* Apr 15 2018;14(4):603–613.

79. Hayakawa T, Uchiyama M, Kamei Y, et al. Clinical analyses of sighted patients with non-24-hour sleep-wake syndrome: A study of 57 consecutively diagnosed cases. *Sleep.* Aug 1 2005;28(8):945–952.

80. Emens JS, St Hilaire MA, Klerman EB, et al. Behaviorally and environmentally induced non-24-hour sleep-wake rhythm disorder in sighted patients. *J Clin Sleep Med.* Feb 1 2022;18(2):453–459.

81. Matsui K, Takaesu Y, Inoue T, Inada K, Nishimura K. Effect of aripiprazole on non-24-hour sleep-wake rhythm disorder comorbid with major depressive disorder: A case report. *Neuropsychiatr Dis Treat.* 2017;13:1367–1371.

82. Watson LA, McGlashan EM, Hosken IT, Anderson C, Phillips AJK, Cain SW. Sleep and circadian instability in delayed sleep-wake phase disorder. *J Clin Sleep Med.* Sep 15 2020;16(9):1431–1436.

83. Abbott SM, Choi J, Wilson J, Zee PC. Melanopsin-dependent phototransduction is impaired in delayed sleep-wake phase disorder and sighted non-24-hour sleep-wake rhythm disorder. *Sleep.* Feb 12 2021;44(2).

84. Nishimon S, Nishimon M, Nishino S. Tasimelteon for treating non-24-h sleep-wake rhythm disorder. *Expert Opin Pharmacother.* Jun 2019;20(9):1065–1073.

85. Cespedes Feliciano EM, Rifas-Shiman SL, Quante M, Redline S, Oken E, Taveras EM. Chronotype, social jet lag, and cardiometabolic risk factors in early adolescence. *JAMA Pediatr.* Nov 1 2019;173(11):1049–1057.

4

Sleep During Adolescence

Stephanie J. Crowley and Mary A. Carskadon

CHAPTER HIGHLIGHTS

- A clear disparity exists between estimated sleep "need" and reported sleep duration on school nights in adolescents, especially as they get older. This reduction in sleep duration is driven by a delay in sleep onset juxtaposed with forced early school-day wake times. Later and longer sleep on non-school/weekend nights compared with school nights suggests adolescents attempt to compensate for school-week sleep restriction.
- Temporal alignment between sleep-wake homeostasis (Process S) and the circadian timing system (Process C) predicts maintenance of wakefulness and alertness during the waking day and maintenance of sleep at night. Puberty-related changes to these regulatory processes favor delayed alertness and sleep timing.
- Behavioral demands and choices alter the ideal balance between Process S and Process C. A greater biologic propensity for evening alertness paired with a reduction in parent-set bedtimes is permissive of engaging in other activities besides sleep, some of which may exacerbate evening alertness and late sleep onset. Late sleep onset is in direct conflict with school start times that begin early in many communities.

Introduction

Adolescence is often accompanied by ill-timed, insufficient, and irregular sleep patterns as sleep regulatory processes develop and the adolescent psychosocial milieu evolves. This chapter provides a broad understanding of normal adolescent sleep behavior and begins with a description of these sleep-wake pattern changes across the second decade of life. The intrinsic regulatory mechanisms of sleep and wake—the homeostatic sleep system and the circadian timing system—and our current understanding of how they change across adolescent development are also reviewed. The chapter then identifies some of the salient psychosocial factors that likely contribute to adolescent sleep-wake behavior and how they interact with maturational changes to sleep regulatory processes to modify sleep patterns.

Sleep-wake behavior changes across adolescence are the product of changing intrinsic regulatory sleep mechanisms and an evolving psychosocial milieu.[1,2] Oftentimes, these changing biologic processes regulating sleep are in direct conflict with social demands, creating a state of chronically restricted and ill-timed sleep. A description of these sleep-wake patterns begins the chapter. To understand how these patterns emerge, the intrinsic regulatory mechanisms of sleep and wake—the homeostatic sleep system and the circadian timing system—and our current understanding of how they change across adolescent development are reviewed. The chapter then identifies some of the salient psychosocial factors that likely contribute to adolescent sleep-wake behavior and how they interact with maturational changes to sleep regulatory processes to modify sleep patterns.

For the purpose of this chapter, adolescence is defined as the second decade of human life. Puberty, the process of sexual maturation and reproductive competence, usually occurs during adolescence, but is not assumed to be synonymous with adolescence. When possible, the distinction is made between these development terms.

Sleep-Wake Patterns

A hallmark behavioral change of adolescence is the tendency for sleep timing to become later. This delay of sleep patterns has been reported across the globe in preindustrial and industrial countries.[3] To start, many adolescents report going to bed later as they get older, especially on weekend and vacation nights. Self-reported school-night bedtimes in the United States range from about 9:30 p.m. to 11:30 p.m.,[4] and reported bedtimes are as late as midnight or 1 a.m. in European and Asian samples.[5] Older adolescents (ages 14–19 years) typically report later bedtimes than their younger peers (ages 11–13 years).[4,5] Wake-up times on school days remain relatively stable or get earlier across these age groups because they are dictated by school start times. The majority of U.S. schools begin before 8:15 a.m., and many start before 7:30 a.m.[6,7] School-day wake times range from about 6 a.m. to 7 a.m.,[4,5] with some reports noting a tendency for older adolescent girls to wake earlier than boys.[8]

Late bedtimes and early wake times on school nights reduce sleep opportunity time for the average teen. The range of self-reported time in bed is about 6.5 to 8.5 or 9 hours, with older adolescents usually reporting less time in bed than younger adolescents.[5,9] The majority of high school-aged adolescents (~14–18 years) report 8 hours of sleep or less, and Korean adolescents average closer to 5.5–6.5 hours of time in bed on school nights.[10,11] A meta-analysis of studies that measured sleep behavior with actigraphy in children ages 3–18 years showed a decrease of total sleep duration with age.[12] The pooled mean estimate of sleep duration on school nights for those aged 12–18 years was about 7 hours. Using actigraphy and self-reported pubertal status in a longitudinal design, Sadeh and colleagues[13] reported that delayed sleep onset and a shortening in sleep duration occurs before the manifestation of secondary sexual characteristics associated with puberty. Later sleep onset and shorter total sleep time also predicted a faster progression of self-rated puberty status. Thus the onset of puberty in this study was linked to the behavioral sleep changes observed during adolescence.

Despite this decreased time devoted to sleep on school nights, laboratory studies indicate that more mature adolescents may "need" at least the same amount of sleep compared with their younger and less mature peers. Carskadon and colleagues[14] studied youngsters aged 10–12 years old at the start longitudinally across three consecutive summers. Participants were given 10-hour nocturnal sleep opportunities (10 p.m.–8 a.m.) for 1 week before and then while in the laboratory for three consecutive nights. Polysomnography (PSG) recordings revealed that the amount of time spent asleep during these 10 hours remained constant across puberty stages (Tanner stages[a] 1–5) and averaged about 9 hours. Furthermore, the mature adolescents were often still asleep at the end of the 10-hour sleep opportunity, suggesting that these teenagers may have slept longer if permitted. Newer work using a sophisticated laboratory and analytic approach concluded that 15- to 17-year-old youth require 9.25 hours' sleep duration for optimal sustained attention when awake.[15] The disparity between this estimate of sleep "need" and reported school-night sleep duration suggests that most adolescents, especially older and more mature adolescents, are sleep restricted and likely carrying residual sleep pressure during the school week.

It remains unclear whether the sleep loss accumulated over the school week can be "recovered" on weekends. Reports indicate that many teenagers, however, exhibit behavior similar to a "behavioral sleep rebound" on weekend nights, which may indicate that adolescents try to compensate for insufficient school-week sleep by sleeping more and later on non-school nights. Weekend time in bed averages about 1–1.5 hours more on weekend nights compared with school nights, and this disparity in sleep duration increases with age.[5,16] Indeed, preteens and younger adolescents may show no weekend rebound or delays in sleep. Furthermore, a majority of mid to older adolescents typically go to sleep about 1–2 hours later on weekends compared with school nights and extend their sleep by waking 1 to as many as 4 hours later on weekend mornings.[4] Self-reported average bedtime typically ranges from about 10 p.m. to as late as 2 a.m. on weekend nights, and weekend wake times typically range between 8 a.m. and 10 a.m.[5] Standard deviations of an hour or more in some studies suggest that many teens sleep later than this average on weekend mornings. Again, older adolescents report later weekend bedtimes and wake times than their younger adolescent peers, on average.[4,5] Changes to sleep-wake timing on weekends compared with school nights result in sleep irregularity for many adolescents. A longitudinal study that followed a younger cohort (aged 9–10 years at the start) and an older cohort (aged 15–16 years at the start) across about 2.5 years showed that this weekend-weekday wake-up time difference begins to accelerate at age 11 years. Interestingly, this weekend-weekday difference in wake-up time becomes negligible after youth leave high school at about age 17 years, suggesting that the societal pressure impinging on wake-up times associated with school start time is relieved for many.[17]

COVID-19 Pandemic

The COVID-19 pandemic, which began in early 2020 and continued into 2023 in successive waves, had a dramatic effect on the sleep of children and adolescents. Remote learning, lockdowns, and stress all impacted sleep. Compared with prepandemic measures in elementary school children, screen time increased, during the pandemic physical activity decreased, sedentary behavior increased, and sleep timing shifted to about 2 hours later.[18] Adolescents exhibited more insomnia symptoms during the initial stay-at-home orders in 2020 than before the pandemic (September 2019–February 2020). Improvements in sleep during the initial lockdown, however, were also described. Bedtimes and waketimes shifted later, likely because of more flexible schedules of remote learning. Daytime sleepiness decreased and school-night sleep duration lengthened during the initial lockdown compared with prepandemic sleep behavior.[19]

As different instructional approaches were implemented at the beginning of the 2020–2021 school year in the United States, sleep behavior varied depending on the type of learning that was adopted. The Nationwide Education and Sleep in TEens During COVID (NESTED) study asked a large (n = 5,245) representative group of U.S. adolescents (13–18 years) in middle school and high school when they went to bed and woke up during the previous week, from which was derived daily sleep opportunity.[20] Adolescents also reported the type of learning they experienced each day, which included in-person, online/synchronous (online class or scheduled interaction with a teacher),

---

[a]Tanner stage, an index of pubertal development, is based on secondary sexual characteristics, including pubic hair growth and distribution, stage of genital development for boys, and stage of breast development for girls.[122]

or online/asynchronous (online, but without a live class or scheduled interaction with a teacher) instruction. They found that sleep timing was earliest on in-person learning days, and about 30 minutes later on days in which learning occurred online with a teacher (synchronous). On days with asynchronous online learning, adolescent-reported bedtimes and wake-up times were the latest. Average sleep opportunity was greatest with both types of online learning (synchronous, 8.4 hours [middle school] and 8.1 hours [high school]; asynchronous, 9.3 hours [middle school] and 9.2 hours [high school]) compared with in-person learning days (7.8 hours [middle school] and 7.4 hours [high school]). A larger percentage of students were able to obtain sufficient sleep on days when instruction was online and asynchronous; 62% of middle school students obtained at least 9 hours sleep opportunity and 81% of high school students obtained at least 8 hours sleep opportunity. Across a week, some students reported a hybrid instructional approach in which they attended school in-person on at least 1 day and the remaining days were online. These adolescents showed greater wake-time and sleep opportunity night-to-night variability across the week compared with students who were online learning.

These studies and others that examine adolescent sleep behavior during the COVID-19 pandemic further corroborate that in the absence of a socially prescribed early school start time, adolescent sleep patterns are late, but a majority of adolescents can obtain sufficient sleep on school nights. The natural experiment of learning approaches that unfolded during the pandemic and their associated impact on sleep of adolescents provides critical insights into healthy school start times.

Sleep-Wake Regulation

Borbély[21] was the first to describe a model clearly identifying the interaction between sleep-wake homeostasis and the circadian timing system. In his "Two Process Model of Sleep Regulation," he designated the homeostatic sleep-wake component as Process S and the circadian component as Process C. Since its original description, this model has been refined and variations have been developed,[22-27] and these models guide our understanding of developmental changes to sleep timing and duration across adolescence.

Homeostatic Sleep-Wake System

A simple way to characterize the homeostatic sleep-wake process is that the "pressure" to sleep increases the longer an individual is awake and dissipates as the individual sleeps. Physiologic correlates of this process have been quantified using the sleep electroencephalogram (EEG). For example, EEG slow-wave activity (SWA; power in the 0.75–4.5 Hz range) is a useful marker of "sleep pressure." SWA predominates at the beginning of the nocturnal sleep episode when sleep pressure is greatest and shows a decline across the night as sleep pressure dissipates.[21,25,28,29] The SWA decline over the course of the night can be fit with an exponential decaying function, from which the time constant of the decline gives a metric of the rate of dissipation of sleep pressure. If the system is challenged by extending wakefulness, SWA increases during subsequent sleep episodes, and this increase is proportional to the time spent awake.[28] The buildup of SWA is modeled using an exponential increasing function. The specific neuroanatomical and neurochemical factors involved in sleep-wake homeostasis are not fully understood.

Circadian Timing System

In contrast to the homeostatic sleep-wake system, the circadian system does not depend on prior sleep and wake duration, but rather is a self-sustaining system that intrinsically regulates a multitude of 24-hour rhythms, including sleep propensity. The "master clock" that organizes the timing of these rhythms in mammals has been localized to the suprachiasmatic nuclei (SCN) of the hypothalamus.[30]

Physiologic or behavioral outputs of systems regulated by the SCN can be measured over extended periods of time (hours to days), and events associated with these approximate 24-hour rhythms (e.g., when a hormone "turns on" or "turns off") are used to infer circadian time or phase. For example, melatonin, a hormone secreted by the human pineal gland, is regulated by the SCN and therefore oscillates with a circadian rhythm. Levels of the hormone are nearly absent during the day, rise in the evening, stay relatively constant during the night, and decline close to habitual wake-up time. The onset of melatonin secretion, also called the dim-light[b] melatonin onset (DLMO),[31] is the most common and reliable marker of the human circadian timing system.[32-34] The decline of melatonin, also called the dim-light melatonin offset (DLMOff) phase, is another phase marker of the circadian timing system derived from the melatonin rhythm.

Circadian rhythms oscillate with an intrinsic period slightly different from 24 hours. In adults, this period ranges from 23.5 to 24.9 hours,[35,36] and one analysis of over 150 adults reported an average period of 24.15 ± 0.2 hours.[35] The majority of people have an endogenous period longer than 24 hours; only an estimated 21% have an intrinsic period of less than 24 hours.[37] Sex[37] and race[36,38] differences in endogenous period have also been reported. The circadian timing system is capable of entrainment, the process by which the endogenous period is synchronized to the environmental 24-hour day using external time-givers, or zeitgebers. The primary entraining stimulus to the system is light and dark,[39,40] and the system shows some sensitivity to short-wavelength (~460 nm) light.[41,42] A small subset of intrinsically photosensitive retinal ganglion cells (ipRGCs) containing melanopsin and projecting to the SCN have been described in rodents.[43-45] The small percentage of ipRGCs that contain melanopsin are photosensitive,[46] are modulated by synaptic input from rods and cones,[47] and are necessary

---

[b] Melatonin synthesis is blocked by light; hence measures are taken in the presence of a dimly lit environment.

for circadian entrainment by light.[48] Light–dark cues come from the daily cycles of daylight and darkness and can also be artificially imposed in modern environments by switching an electric light on and off or by drawing a window shade.

One proposed entrainment mechanism ("discrete entrainment"[49]) describes the process as a daily phase shift in response to photic cues that corrects the difference between the endogenous period and the external solar day length. This entrainment mechanism is predicted by a phase response curve (PRC) to light. Light PRCs are experimentally derived and describe how light shifts circadian rhythms to an earlier or later time when light is presented at various times across the circadian cycle. In general, the human system responds in a systematic and predictable manner: light just before habitual bedtime or in the first half of habitual sleep shifts circadian rhythms later (phase delay), whereas light during the second half of habitual sleep or just after waking shifts circadian rhythms earlier (phase advance).[50-55] According to these general properties of the adult light PRC, morning light exposure facilitates entrainment in those with an intrinsic period greater than 24 hours, whereas evening light exposure entrains individuals with a period shorter than 24 hours. In adults, endogenous circadian period also predicts differences in how the system aligns to sleep,[56] and those with a long period have a later entrained phase (clock time) than those with a short period.[57]

Two-Process Model of Sleep Regulation

Fig. 4.1 is a schematic representation of how Process S and Process C may interact as opponent processes and is based on the models proposed by others.[26,27,58] The broad concept of "sleep pressure" is on the y-axis as a function of time on the x-axis. Sleep pressure varies across the 24-hour day (Process C, *red line*), and also depends on the amount of time awake and asleep (Process S, *blue line*). In this schematic example, sleep occurs from 10 p.m. to 7 a.m. The onset of melatonin production (DLMO phase) usually occurs before habitual bedtime and is illustrated by the *upward-facing arrow* at 9 p.m. Process S is anchored to the onset of sleep and the onset of wake. The homeostatically driven pressure to sleep decreases as sleep progresses across a night of sleep and increases with hours of wakefulness across the day. Sleep pressure dictated by the circadian timing system is greatest about 7 hours after DLMO phase, near the end of habitual sleep, and is lowest just before DLMO phase, near to habitual bedtime. According to this two-process model, the alerting signal of the circadian process opposes a wake-dependent sleep-promoting process to maintain wakefulness across the day.[26] Similarly, homeostatic sleep pressure dissipating across a night of sleep is countered by the circadian timing system as it reaches its maximal levels of sleep propensity during the second half of the habitual sleep period, thus maintaining or "protecting" the second half of nocturnal sleep.[27] Theoretically, the alignment of these two processes predicts maintenance of wakefulness and alertness

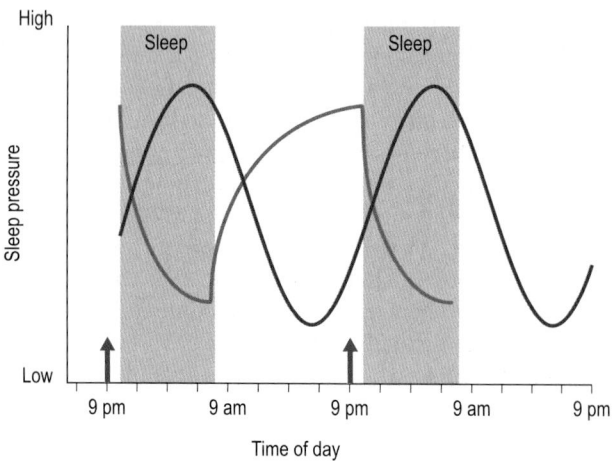

• **Fig. 4.1** A schematic representation of the Two-Process Model of Sleep Regulation. The broad concept of "sleep pressure" is illustrated on the y-axis as a function of time spanning over 2 days. An ideal sleep duration of 9 hours per night from 10 p.m. to 7 a.m. is illustrated by *shaded gray rectangles*. The *upward-facing arrow* at 9 p.m. illustrates the time of melatonin onset (DLMO phase), which usually occurs 1 to 2 hours before bedtime. Process C *(red curve)* shows sleep pressure changing with a cycle length of 24 hours. The pressure to sleep is highest approximately 7 hours after DLMO phase, and sleep pressure is lowest just before DLMO phase, and thus just before bedtime. Process S is illustrated by the *blue curve* and is dependent on the timing and duration of sleep and wake. At sleep onset, sleep pressure is highest and dissipates over the course of sleep, whereas sleep pressure is lowest at the beginning of the waking day and accumulates over the course of wakefulness. Ideally, these two processes interact with one another to maintain sleep at night and maintain alertness during the day (see text). From Crowley SJ, Kyriakos CN, and Wolfson AR. Sleep patterns and challenges. In: Brown BB, Prinstein M, eds. *Encyclopedia of Adolescence*. Elsevier; 2011.

during the daytime and maintenance of sleep at night. This ideal balance between the systems is challenged during adolescence as both processes show developmental changes and as behavioral demands and choices alter the balance.

Changes to Sleep-Wake Regulation Across Adolescence

Puberty, or the process of sexual maturation and reproductive competence, usually occurs during adolescence and is initiated with a reactivation of the hypothalamic-pituitary-gonadal axis after a dormant period during childhood. The brain also undergoes major structural reorganization during this time. One of the most prominent structural changes during development is a sharp decline of cortical synapses ("pruning") in the second decade of life. This change is further illustrated by cortical gray matter volume declining throughout the teen years. These changes to brain structure influence sleep physiology.

One of the most readily observed and striking changes to the sleep EEG is a progressive developmental decline in the amplitude of the signal across adolescence. This decline typically begins around age 9 or 10 and continues until the early 20s, though the precise timing of the beginning and termination of this decline varies across individuals and is debated.[59,60] This decline likely reflects the pruning of synapses that occurs in the healthy adolescent cortex[61,62] and is not state specific. As a result, EEG power is diminished during waking[63-65] and sleep.[66-71]

One sleep-specific change to the EEG is a redistribution of sleep-stage variables. Minutes of slow-wave sleep (SWS; sleep characterized by high-amplitude, low-frequency waves) declines by approximately 40%.[68,69,72-75] At the same time, an approximate 20% increase in stage 2 sleep is observed in both longitudinal[68] and cross-sectional[69] samples. Whether these changes are also a reflection of adolescent cortical restructuring or are of functional significance to sleep-dependent processes remains unknown. Finally, young adolescents tend to "skip" their first rapid eye movement (REM) episode.[68,74] The skipped REM episodes are characterized by the emergence from "deep" sleep stages 3 and 4 (SWS) into "lighter" stages such as stages 1 and 2 for a duration of at least 12 minutes.[69] In adults, skipped REM episodes often accompany sleep deprivation protocols, therefore some have speculated that the skipped REM episodes in young individuals may reflect increased sleep drive observed in younger individuals.[76]

The dynamics of the homeostatic system are also altered during puberty, though not involving the dissipation of Process S with sleep. One cross-sectional and two longitudinal studies have modeled the dissipation of sleep pressure across nights of sleep. All studies have found that the time constant of the decay does not change across adolescent development.[77-79] This finding lends further support to the notion that the recovery process occurring during sleep, from which some infer sleep "need," does not change across adolescent development. One cross-sectional study modeled the buildup of SWA using sleep before and after 36 hours of sleep deprivation and found an increase in the time constant of the buildup in post-pubertal versus prepubertal teens.[78] In other words, mature adolescents accumulated sleep pressure at a slower rate across a waking period compared with their younger prepubertal peers. Longer sleep onset latency near bedtime in Tanner 5 adolescents compared with Tanner 1 adolescents provides further support for this developmental difference in sleep pressure at the end of the waking day.[80] Fig. 4.2 illustrates this relative change across adolescence. Process S of the mature adolescent *(blue dashed line)* increases across the waking day at a slower rate than the immature, young adolescent *(blue solid line)*, and thus at a 10 p.m. bedtime has not reached the same level of sleep pressure as the immature adolescent. This slower accumulation of sleep pressure is thought to explain in part why mature adolescents are able to stay awake longer into the evening or night, whereas younger, prepubertal adolescents are able to, and often do, fall asleep more rapidly and earlier in the evening.

The circadian timing system is also altered during adolescence. Changes to chronotype—whether an individual is a morning/early type or an evening/late type—provided the first indication of this circadian change. Chronotype can be

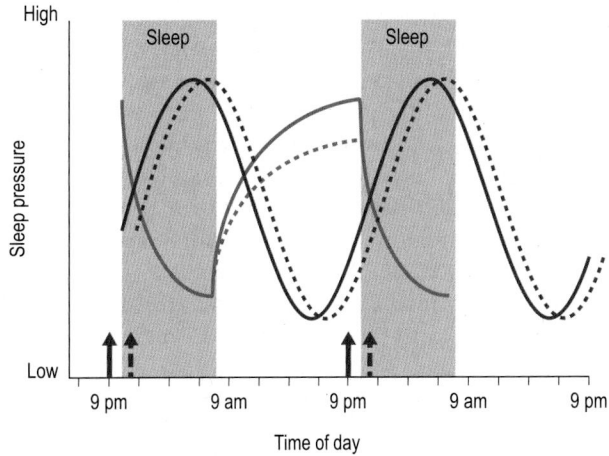

• **Fig. 4.2** A schematic representation illustrating the relative change to Process C and Process S with maturation. Illustration symbols are the same as in Fig. 4.1. Young, immature adolescents are shown in *solid lines* and mature, older adolescents are shown in *dashed lines*. The dissipation of Process S is shown as a *solid blue line* for both immature and mature adolescents because this recovery process shows little change across adolescence. A delayed Process C and a slower accumulation of Process S are permissive of later sleep times with maturation (see text).

measured via questionnaires[81-83] that ask what time of day one would choose to engage in different activities, such as when they prefer to wake up, go to bed, take a test, exercise, and so forth. The midpoint of sleep on weekend or vacation days ("free days") has also been used to assess whether an individual is a late or early chronotype.[84] Carskadon and colleagues[83] noted an association between "eveningness" and a more mature self-assessed puberty rating. This study was particularly informative because these data were sampled from a group with similar psychosocial contexts (sixth-grade students), thus reducing the potential impact of social factors driving this association between puberty and time-of-day preference. In a longitudinal study of 14-year-old Brazilian adolescents, Andrade and colleagues[85] reported sleep midpoint on weekend nights delayed in adolescents who matured from one Tanner stage to another, whereas weekend midsleep time did not change in those who remained at the same Tanner stage during the study. Others have since confirmed this change across puberty[86] and with age.[87-90] This "evening" tendency, which appears to be most pronounced during late adolescence (~20 years),[89,91] suggests that underlying properties of the adolescent circadian timing system are altered compared with children and adults. Indeed, laboratory studies show that a more mature puberty stage is associated with later onset and offset of melatonin secretion even when sleep (dark) is held fixed in young humans.[92,93] A circadian phase delay shift from prepubertal to post-pubertal development is similarly reported in other mammalian species, and several other nonhuman mammalian species are also phase delayed compared with later during adulthood.[94,95]

Similar to Process S, Process C also undergoes developmental changes that allow mature adolescents to stay awake later into the evening or night compared with younger adolescents. Fig. 4.2 shows this relative delay of the circadian system. The *dashed red curve* and *dashed red arrow* representing DLMO phase of the older adolescent is shifted later compared with the young adolescent *(red solid curve and red solid arrow)*. Thus the time of greatest pressure for sleep dictated by the circadian system in older adolescents is now closer to wake-up time, and the time when the circadian process promotes alertness (low sleep pressure) at the end of the day becomes later in the evening.

Specific factors that contribute to the developmental circadian delay during adolescence are an active area of investigation. One hypothesized mechanism includes a lengthening of the endogenous circadian period during adolescence because a longer intrinsic period length is associated with a later entrained phase in adults.[57] In a preliminary study,[96] average period in 27 adolescents aged 9–15 years was 24.27 hours. In this cross-sectional study, the sample size was too small to observe a difference among pubertal groups classified by Tanner stage; however, period measured in this group of adolescents was significantly longer than in a group of adults measured by others.[97,98] By contrast, a direct comparison of intrinsic period of older adolescents (14–17 years; Tanner 4 and 5) and adults (30–45 years) derived from the same laboratory protocol did not find a difference between the age groups.[99] More recent work with a cross-sectional and longitudinal sample provides preliminary evidence that longer circadian period may manifest in prepuberty and early puberty (Carskadon & Barker, unpublished). These analyses, however, must account for sex and ancestry as they appear to be predictors of intrinsic period.[99] Pubertal changes to intrinsic period are also observed in laboratory animals; however, the change appears to be sex dependent and does not necessarily predict the concomitant change in phase.[100]

Another hypothesized mechanism that has been proposed to explain the adolescent delay in circadian timing is a developmental difference in the circadian clock's response to light. Because most humans have an intrinsic circadian period longer than 24 hours, most entrainment occurs with discrete phase advances in response to light occurring shortly after habitual wake-up time. One suggestion is that older adolescents have an attenuated response to this phase advancing morning light. Alternatively, adolescents may develop a heightened sensitivity to delaying light in the evening. Either or both of these hypothesized differences in light sensitivity would favor a delayed circadian phase. Two studies report older adolescents showing minimal phase advances in response to 2[101] or 6[102] days of short-wavelength light exposure after waking. Preliminary animal data[103] also support the hypothesized exaggerated response to delaying light in juvenile female mice compared with adults. One report[104] directly tested the light sensitivity hypothesis by measuring melatonin suppression in response to 15, 150, and 500 lux of light compared with a dim light control (0.1 lux) condition administered on consecutive evenings (11 p.m.–midnight) or mornings (3 a.m.–4 a.m.) in prepubertal to post-pubertal adolescents. Contrary to the light-sensitivity hypothesis, prepubertal to mid-pubertal adolescents (Tanner 1, 2, and 3) showed *greater* melatonin suppression (greater sensitivity) to evening phase delaying light compared with late and post-pubertal adolescents (Tanner 4 and 5), and these groups did not show a difference in melatonin suppression in response to morning phase advancing light exposure. A subsequent study[105] examined phase shifts in response to bright light exposure (80 minutes of intermittent bright light) delivered at various times across the 24-hour day in the laboratory to build a phase response curve (PRC) to bright light. The expectation was to find large phase delay shifts and small phase advance shifts because this would favor a delayed circadian system characteristic of older adolescents. Unexpectedly, however, phase delays and phase advances in older adolescents (14–17 years; Tanner 4 and 5) were similar in size[105] and did not differ from adults aged 30–45 years (Crowley & Eastman, unpublished). Taken together, these newer data suggest that light sensitivity as a function of pubertal status does not explain delayed circadian timing of older adolescents.

Two additional factors may be at play in the adolescent sleep and circadian timing delay. First, the maturational reduction in the rate of accumulation of "sleep pressure" across wakefulness[78,80] may "permit" teens to stay awake longer and therefore increase the opportunity for exposure to evening phase delaying light. Second, sleep restriction and the associated challenge of waking in the morning may lessen phase advancing morning light like adults.[106,107] Preliminary data[108] in adolescents (12.4–17.7 years) suggests that when sleep is shortened to 5.5 hours by staying awake late in room light (~100 lux) before and during 3 days of morning bright light, circadian phase can shift the wrong way (delay) or does not shift at all. When adolescents are given 10 hours of sleep opportunity, however, circadian phase shifted in the advance direction by ~2 hours as expected. Ongoing studies aim to tease apart the independent contributions of these common exposures—evening room light and sleep restriction—on the ability of the adolescent circadian system to phase advance to morning light.

Psychosocial Context

In addition to the sleep regulatory changes reviewed above, a number of psychosocial factors evolve as youngsters pass through adolescence. First, parent-set bedtimes become less common.[8,109,110] With less restriction over bedtime and greater evening alertness permitted by changes to sleep regulatory systems, many older adolescents stay awake later to study,[110,111] watch television or play video games,[112] and socialize.[110,113] Social interactions increasingly occur through use of technology.[114] A recent report indicates that 95% of American teens aged 13–17 years old have or have access to a cell phone and 97% use some sort of social media platform.[115] Access to media screens, such as television, video games, cell phones, and computers contributes to late bedtimes on school nights,[112,116] and more access to these screens is associated with fewer hours of sleep[116] and more disturbed sleep[116,117] on school nights. Studies indicate that light from media screens in the evening before bedtime may delay the circadian system and increase alertness,[118,119] though further work is needed. If so, such effects likely exacerbate the delayed circadian phase and heightened evening alertness that older adolescents already experience because of altered sleep regulation. On the other hand, a recent meta-analysis[120] of admittedly few studies of mostly adults showed mixed findings on the reduction of pre-bedtime short-wavelength light on sleep outcomes. Data also indicate that staying awake later on weekends to socialize or engage in other leisure activities and sleeping in on weekends may exacerbate the already delayed circadian system of teens.[101]

The combination of these biologic and psychosocial factors that favor (and perhaps exacerbate) late bedtimes are in direct conflict with the school schedule, particularly in communities with early school start times. As a consequence, school-night sleep is chronically restricted and many teens wake at an inappropriate time with respect to the circadian timing system. The negative consequences of short and ill-timed sleep are numerous, including sleepiness, depressed mood, immune and metabolic dysfunction, poor school performance, substance use, and driving accidents.[121] Education of school administrators, teachers, parents, and students about adolescent sleep needs remains critical, and targeted sleep interventions are needed to attenuate the risk of such poor outcomes.

Acknowledgments

We thank the National Institutes of Health for support of our research summarized in this chapter: MH52415, MH01358, MH45945, MH58879, HL71120, MH076969, MH079179, AA13252, MH078662, and HL105395. We also acknowledge our colleagues, fellows, students, staff, and participants who make important contributions to our research.

CLINICAL PEARLS

- Encourage parents to set a bedtime for their teenager.
- Encourage teens to avoid bright light and other stimulating activities in the evening before bedtime and to seek bright light (sunlight if possible) in the morning.
- Encourage teens to keep a consistent sleep-wake schedule across the week, including on weekends.
- As part of the medical community and a local community, be part of the discussion with school administrators, teachers, parents, and students about adolescent sleep needs and consequences of insufficient sleep in this age group.

References

1. Carskadon MA. Sleep in adolescents: the perfect storm. *Pediatr Clin North Am*. 2011;58(3):637–647.
2. Crowley SJ, Wolfson AR, Tarokh L, Carskadon MA. An update on adolescent sleep: New evidence informing the perfect storm model. *J Adolesc*. 2018;67:55–65.
3. Carskadon MA. Maturation of Processes regulating sleep in adolescents. In: Marcus CL, Carroll JL, Donnelly DF, Loughlin GM, eds. *Sleep in Children: Developmental Changes in Sleep Patterns*. 2nd ed. Informa Healthcare USA; 2008:95–114.
4. Crowley SJ, Acebo C, Carskadon MA. Sleep, circadian rhythms, and delayed phase in adolescence. *Sleep Med*. 2007;8(6):602–612.
5. Gradisar M, Gardner G, Dohnt H. Recent worldwide sleep patterns and problems during adolescence: a review and meta-analysis of age, region, and sleep. *Sleep Med*. 2011;12(2):110–118.
6. Wolfson AR, Carskadon MA. A survey of factors influencing high school start times. *NASSP Bulletin*. 2005;89(642):47–66.
7. Ziporyn TD, Owens JA, Wahlstrom KL, et al. Adolescent sleep health and school start times: setting the research agenda for California and beyond. A research summit summary. *Sleep Health*. 2022;8(1):11–22. https://doi.org/10.1016/j.sleh.2021.10.008.
8. Wolfson AR, Carskadon MA. Sleep schedules and daytime functioning in adolescents. *Child Dev*. 1998;69(4):875–887.
9. Olds T, Blunden S, Petkov J, Forchino F. The relationships between sex, age, geography and time in bed in adolescents: a meta-analysis of data from 23 countries. *Sleep Med Rev*. 2010;14(6):371–378.
10. Yang CK, Kim JK, Patel SR, Lee JH. Age-related changes in sleep-wake patterns among Korean teenagers. *Pediatrics*. 2005;115(suppl 1):250–256.
11. Kim SJ, Lee YJ, Cho SJ, Cho IH, Lim W. Relationship between weekend catch-up sleep and poor performance on attention tasks in Korean adolescents. *Arch Pediatr Adolesc Med*. 2011;165(9):806–812.
12. Galland BC, Short MA, Terrill P, et al. Establishing normal values for pediatric nighttime sleep measured by actigraphy: a systematic review and meta-analysis. *Sleep*. 2018;41(4).
13. Sadeh A, Dahl RE, Shahar G, Rosenblat-Stein S. Sleep and the transition to adolescence: a longitudinal study. *Sleep*. 2009;32(12):1602–1609.
14. Carskadon MA, Harvey K, Duke P, Anders TF, Litt IF, Dement WC. Pubertal changes in daytime sleepiness. *Sleep*. 1980;2(4):453–460.
15. Short MA, Weber N, Reynolds C, Coussens S, Carskadon MA. Estimating adolescent sleep need using dose-response modelling. *Sleep*. 2018:1–14.
16. Carskadon M, Mindell J, Drake C. Contemporary sleep patterns of adolescents in the USA: Results of the 2006 National Sleep Foundation Sleep in America poll. *J Sleep Res*. 2006;15(suppl 1):42.
17. Crowley SJ, Van Reen E, LeBourgeois MK, et al. A Longitudinal assessment of sleep timing, circadian phase, and phase angle of entrainment across human adolescence. *PLoS One*. 2014;9(11):e112199.
18. Burkart S, Parker H, Weaver RG, et al. Impact of the COVID-19 pandemic on elementary schoolers' physical activity, sleep, screen time and diet: a quasi-experimental interrupted time series study. *Pediatr Obes*. 2022;17(1):e12846.
19. Becker SP, Dvorsky MR, Breaux R, Cusick CN, Taylor KP, Langberg JM. Prospective examination of adolescent sleep patterns and behaviors before and during COVID-19. *Sleep*. 2021;44(8).
20. Meltzer LJ, Saletin JM, Honaker SM, et al. COVID-19 instructional approaches (in-person, online, hybrid), school start times, and sleep in over 5,000 U.S. adolescents. *Sleep*. 2021;44(12).

21. Borbely AA. A two process model of sleep regulation. *Hum Neurobiol*. 1982;1:195–204.

22. Achermann P, Dijk DJ, Brunner DP, Borbely AA. A model of human sleep homeostasis based on EEG slow-wave activity: quantitative comparison of data and simulations. *Brain Res Bull*. 1993;31(1-2):97–113.

23. Borbely AA, Achermann P. Sleep homeostasis and models of sleep regulation. *J Biol Rhythms*. 1999;14(6):557–568.

24. Borbely AA, Achermann P, Trachsel L, Tobler I. Sleep initiation and initial sleep intensity: interactions of homeostatic and circadian mechanisms. *J Biol Rhythms*. 1989;4(2):149–160.

25. Daan S, Beersma DG, Borbely AA. Timing of human sleep: recovery process gated by a circadian pacemaker. *Am J Physiol*. 1984;246(2 Pt 2):R161–83.

26. Edgar DM, Dement WC, Fuller CA. Effect of SCN lesions on sleep in squirrel monkeys: evidence for opponent processes in sleep-wake regulation. *J Neurosci*. 1993;13(3):1065–1079.

27. Dijk DJ, Czeisler CA. Contribution of the circadian pacemaker and the sleep homeostat to sleep propensity, sleep structure, electroencephalographic slow waves, and sleep spindle activity in humans. *J Neurosci*. 1995;15(5 Pt 1):3526–3538.

28. Borbely AA, Baumann F, Brandeis D, Strauch I, Lehmann D. Sleep deprivation: effect on sleep stages and EEG power density in man. *Electroencephalogr Clin Neurophysiol*. 1981;51: 483–493.

29. Dijk DJ, Brunner DP, Beersma DG, Borbely AA. Electroencephalogram power density and slow wave sleep as a function of prior waking and circadian phase. *Sleep*. 1990;13(5):430–440.

30. Moore RY. Circadian rhythms: Basic neurobiology and clinical applications. *Annu Rev Med*. 1997;48:253–266.

31. Lewy AJ, Sack RL. The dim light melatonin onset as a marker for circadian phase position. *Chronobiol Int*. 1989;6(1): 93–102.

32. Klerman H, St Hilaire MA, Kronauer RE, et al. Analysis method and experimental conditions affect computed circadian phase from melatonin data. *PLoS One*. 2012;7(4):e33836.

33. Klerman EB, Gershengorn HB, Duffy JF, Kronauer RE. Comparisons of the variability of three markers of the human circadian pacemaker. *J Biol Rhythms*. 2002;17(2):181–193.

34. Benloucif S, Guico MJ, Reid KJ, et al. Stability of circadian phase markers under regular sleep schedules. *Sleep*. 2003;26:A106.

35. Duffy JF, Cain SW, Chang AM, et al. Sex difference in the near-24-hour intrinsic period of the human circadian timing system. *Proc Natl Acad Sci USA*. 2011;108(suppl 3):15602–15608.

36. Eastman CI, Molina TA, Dziepak ME, Smith MR. Blacks (African Americans) have shorter free-running circadian periods than whites (Caucasian Americans). *Chronobiol Int*. 2012;29(8):1072–1077.

37. Duffy JF, Wright KP. Entrainment of the human circadian system by light. *J Biol Rhythms*. 2005;20(4):326–338.

38. Eastman CI, Tomaka VA, Crowley SJ. Sex and ancestry determine the free-running circadian period. *J Sleep Res*. 2017;26:547–550.

39. Aschoff J, Hoffmann K, Pohl H, Wever R. Re-entrainment of circadian rhythms after phase shifts of the zeitgeber. *Chronobiologia*. 1975;2:23–78.

40. Czeisler CA, Richardson GS, Zimmerman JC, Moore-Ede MC, Weitzman ED. Entrainment of human circadian rhythms by light-dark cycles: a reassessment. *Photochem Photobiol*. 1981;34:239–247.

41. Brainard GC, Hanifin JP, Greeson JM, et al. Action spectrum for melatonin regulation in humans: evidence for a novel circadian photoreceptor. *J Neurosci*. 2001;21:6405–6412.

42. Thapan K, Arendt J, Skene DJ. An action spectrum for melatonin suppression: evidence for a novel non-rod, non-cone photoreceptor system in humans. *J Physiol*. 2001;535:261–267.

43. Hannibal J, Hindersson P, Knudsen SM, Georg B, Fahrenkrug J. The photopigment melanopsin is exclusively present in pituitary adenylate cyclase-activating polypeptide-containing retinal ganglion cells of the retinohypothalamic tract. *J Neurosci*. 2002;22:RC191.

44. Provencio I, Rodriguez IR, Jiang G, Hayes WP, Moreira EF, Rollag MD. A novel human opsin in the inner retina. *J Neurosci*. 2000;20(2):600–605.

45. Gooley JJ, Lu J, Chou TC, Scammell TE, Saper CB. Melanopsin in cells of origin of the retinohypothalamic tract. *Nat Neurosci*. 2001;4(12):1165.

46. Berson DM, Dunn FA, Takao M. Phototransduction by retinal ganglion cells that set the circadian clock. *Science*. 2002;295(5557):1070–1073.

47. Wong KY, Dunn FA, Graham DM, Berson DM. Synaptic influences on rat ganglion-cell photoreceptors. *J Physiol*. 2007;582(Pt 1):279–296.

48. Guler AD, Ecker JL, Lall GS, et al. Melanopsin cells are the principal conduits for rod-cone input to non-image-forming vision. *Nature*. 2008;453(7191):102–105.

49. Moore-Ede MC, Sulzman FM, Fuller CA. *The Clocks That Time Us. Physiology of the Circadian Timing System*. Harvard University Press; 1982.

50. Minors DS, Waterhouse JM, Wirz-Justice A. A human phase-response curve to light. *Neurosci Lett*. 1991;133:36–40.

51. Revell VL, Eastman CI. How to trick Mother Nature into letting you fly around or stay up all night. *J Biol Rhythms*. 2005;20(4):353–365.

52. Khalsa SBS, Jewett ME, Cajochen C, Czeisler CA. A phase response curve to single bright light pulses in human subjects. *J Physiol*. 2003;549(3):945–952.

53. Czeisler CA, Kronauer RE, Allan JS, et al. Bright light induction of strong (type 0) resetting of the human circadian pacemaker. *Science*. 1989;244:1328–1333.

54. Kripke DF, Elliott JA, Youngstedt SD, Rex KM. Circadian phase response curves to light in older and young women and men. *J Circadian Rhythms*. 2007;5(1):4.

55. Revell VL, Molina TA, Eastman CI. Human phase response curve to intermittent blue light using a commercially available device. *J Physiol*. 2012;590(Pt 19):4859–4868.

56. Wright KP, Gronfier C, Duffy JF, Czeisler CA. Intrinsic period and light intensity determine the phase relationship between melatonin and sleep in humans. *J Biol Rhythms*. 2005;20:168–177.

57. Duffy JF, Rimmer DW, Czeisler CA. Association of intrinsic circadian period with morningness-eveningness, usual wake time, and circadian phase. *Behav Neurosci*. 2001;115:895–899.

58. Carskadon MA, Acebo C. Regulation of sleepiness in adolescents: Update, insights, and speculation. *Sleep*. 2002;25(6): 606–614.

59. Tarokh L, Carskadon MA. EEG delta power decline can begin before age 11: a reply to Campbell and Feinberg. *Sleep*. 2010;33(6):738.

60. Feinberg I, Campbell IG. The onset of the adolescent delta power decline occurs after age 11 years: a comment on Tarokh and Carskadon. *Sleep*. 2010;33(6):737. author reply 738.

61. Feinberg I. Schizophrenia: caused by a fault in programmed synaptic elimination during adolescence? *J Psychiatr Res.* 1982;17(4):319–334.

62. Feinberg I, Thode Jr. HC, Chugani HT, March JD. Gamma distribution model describes maturational curves for delta wave amplitude, cortical metabolic rate and synaptic density. *J Theor Biol.* 1990;142(2):149–161.

63. Matousek M, Petersen I. Automatic evaluation of EEG background activity by means of age-dependent EEG quotients. *Electroencephalogr Clin Neurophysiol.* 1973;35(6):603–612.

64. Gasser T, Jennen-Steinmetz C, Sroka L, Verleger R, Mocks J. Development of the EEG of school-age children and adolescents. II. Topography. *Electroencephalogr Clin Neurophysiol.* 1988;69(2):100–109.

65. Dustman RE, Shearer DE, Emmerson RY. Life-span changes in EEG spectral amplitude, amplitude variability and mean frequency. *Clin Neurophysiol.* 1999;110(8):1399–1409.

66. Campbell IG, Darchia N, Khaw WY, Higgins LM, Feinberg I. Sleep EEG evidence of sex differences in adolescent brain maturation. *Sleep.* 2005;28(5):637–643.

67. Tarokh L, Van Reen E, Lebourgeois M, Seifer R, Carskadon MA. Sleep EEG Provides evidence that cortical changes persist into late adolescence. *Sleep.* 2011;34(10):1385–1393.

68. Tarokh L, Carskadon MA. Developmental changes in the human sleep EEG during early adolescence. *Sleep.* 2010;33(6):801–809.

69. Jenni OG, Carskadon MA. Spectral analysis of the sleep electroencephalogram during adolescence. *Sleep.* 2004;27(4):774–783.

70. Gaudreau H, Carrier J, Montplaisir J. Age-related modifications of NREM sleep EEG: from childhood to middle age. *J Sleep Res.* 2001;10:165–172.

71. Feinberg I, Higgins LM, Khaw WY, Campbell IG. The adolescent decline of NREM delta, an indicator of brain maturation, is linked to age and sex but not to pubertal stage. *Am J Physiol Regul Integr Comp Physiol.* 2006;291(6):R1724–1729.

72. Williams RL, Karacan I, Hursch CJ, Davis CE. Sleep patterns of pubertal males. *Pediatr Res.* 1972;6(8):643–648.

73. Feinberg I, Koresko RL, Heller N. EEG sleep patterns as a function of normal and pathological aging in man. *J Psychiatr Res.* 1967;5(2):107–144.

74. Carskadon MA. The second decade. In: Guilleminault C, ed. *Sleep and Waking Disorders: Indications and Techniques.* Addison Wesley; 1982:99–125.

75. Karacan I, Anch M, Thornby JI, Okawa M, Williams RL. Longitudinal sleep patterns during pubertal growth: four-year follow up. *Pediatr Res.* 1975;9(11):842–846.

76. Kupfer DJ, Ulrich RF, Coble PA, et al. Application of automated REM and slow wave sleep analysis:II. Testing the assumptions of the two-process model of sleep regulation in normal and depressed subjects. *Psychiatry Research.* 1984;13:335–343.

77. Tarokh L, Carskadon MA, Achermann P. Dissipation of sleep pressure is stable across adolescence. *Neuroscience.* 2012;216:167–177.

78. Jenni OG, Achermann P, Carskadon MA. Homeostatic sleep regulation in adolescents. *Sleep.* 2005;28(11):1446–1454.

79. Campbell IG, Darchia N, Higgins LM, et al. Adolescent changes in homeostatic regulation of EEG activity in the delta and theta frequency bands during NREM sleep. *Sleep.* 2011;34(1):83–91.

80. Taylor DJ, Jenni OG, Acebo C, Carskadon MA. Sleep tendency during extended wakefulness: insights into adolescent sleep regulation and behavior. *J Sleep Res.* 2005;14(3):239–244.

81. Horne J, Ostberg O. A self-assessment questionnaire to determine morningness-eveningness in human circadian rhythms. *Int J Chronobiol.* 1976;4:97–110.

82. Smith CS, Reilly C, Midkiff K. Evaluation of three circadian rhythm questionnaires with suggestions for an improved measure of morningness. *J Applied Psychol.* 1989;74(5):728–738.

83. Carskadon MA, Vieira C, Acebo C. Association between puberty and delayed phase preference. *Sleep.* 1993;16(3):258–262.

84. Roenneberg T, Wirz-Justice A, Merrow M. Life between clocks: daily temporal patterns of human chronotypes. *J Biol Rhythms.* 2003;18(1):80–90.

85. Andrade MMM, Menna-Barreto L, Benedito-Silvo AA, Domenice S, Arnhold IJP. Sleep characteristics following change in adolescent maturity status. *Sleep Res.* 1993;22:521.

86. Randler C, Bilger S. Associations among sleep, chronotype, parental monitoring, and pubertal development among German adolescents. *J Psychol.* 2009;143(5):509–520.

87. Giannotti F, Cortesi F, Sebastiani T, Ottaviano S. Circadian preference, sleep and daytime behaviour in adolescence. *J Sleep Res.* 2002;11(3):191–199.

88. Kim S, Dueker GL, Hasher L, Goldstein D. Children's time of day preference: age, gender and ethnic differences. *Pers Individ Dif.* 2002;33(7):1083–1090.

89. Roenneberg T, Kuehnle T, Pramstaller PP, et al. A marker for the end of adolescence. *Curr Biol.* 2004;14(24):R1038–1039.

90. Roenneberg T, Kuehnle T, Juda M, et al. Epidemiology of the human circadian clock. *Sleep Med Rev.* 2007;11(6):429–438.

91. Fischer D, Lombardi DA, Marucci-Wellman H, Roenneberg T. Chronotypes in the US—Influence of age and sex. *PLoS One.* 2017;12(6):1–17.

92. Carskadon MA, Acebo C, Jenni OG. Regulation of adolescent sleep: Implications for behavior. *Ann NY Acad Sci.* 2004;1021:276–291.

93. Carskadon MA, Acebo C, Richardson GS, Tate BA, Seifer R. An approach to studying circadian rhythms of adolescent humans. *J Biol Rhythms.* 1997;12(3):278–289.

94. Hagenauer MH, Perryman JI, Lee TM, Carskadon MA. Adolescent changes in the homeostatic and circadian regulation of sleep. *Dev Neurosci.* 2009;31(4):276–284.

95. Melo PR, Goncalves BS, Menezes AA, Azevedo CV. Circadian activity rhythm in pre-pubertal and pubertal marmosets (*Callithrix jacchus*) living in family groups. *Physiol Behav.* 2016;155:242–249.

96. Carskadon MA, Acebo C. Intrinsic circadian period in adolescents versus adults from forced desynchrony. *Sleep.* 2005;28(abst suppl):A71.

97. Czeisler CA, Duffy JF, Shanahan TL, et al. Stability, precision, and near-24-hour period of the human circadian pacemaker. *Science.* 1999;284:2177–2181.

98. Wright KP, Hughes RJ, Kronauer RE, Dijk DJ, Czeisler CA. Intrinsic near-24-h pacemaker period determines limits of circadian entrainment to a weak synchronizer in humans. *PNAS.* 2001;98(24):14027–14032.

99. Crowley SJ, Eastman CI. Free-running circadian period in adolescents and adults. *J Sleep Res.* 2018:1–8.

100. Hagenauer MH, Lee TM. The neuroendocrine control of the circadian system: adolescent chronotype. *Front Neuroendocrinol.* 2012;33(3):211–229.

101. Crowley SJ, Carskadon MA. Modifications to weekend recovery sleep delay circadian phase in older adolescents. *Chronobiol Int.* 2010;27(7):1469–1492.

102. Sharkey KM, Carskadon MA, Figueiro MG, Zhu Y, Rea MS. Effects of an advanced sleep schedule and morning short wavelength light exposure on circadian phase in young adults with late sleep schedules. *Sleep Med*. 2011;12(7):685–692.

103. Weinert D, Kompauerova V. Light-induced phase and period reponses of circadian activity rhythms in laboratory mice of different age. *Zoology*. 1998;101:45–52.

104. Crowley SJ, Cain SW, Burns AC, Acebo C, Carskadon MA. Increased sensitivity of the circadian system to light in early/mid puberty. *J Clin Endocrinol Metab*. 2015;100(11):4067–4073.

105. Crowley SJ, Eastman CI. Human adolescent phase response curves to bright white light. *J Biol Rhythms*. 2017;32(4):334–344.

106. Burgess HJ, Eastman CI. Short nights attenuate light-induced circadian phase advances in humans. *J Clin Endocr Metab*. 2005;90(8):4437–4440.

107. Burgess HJ. Partial sleep deprivation reduces phase advances to light in humans. *J Biol Rhythms*. 2010;25(6):460–468.

108. Crowley SJ, Fournier CL, Eastman CI. Late bedtimes prevent circadian phase advances to morning bright light in adolescents. *Chronobiol Int*. 2018;35(12):1748–1752.

109. Carskadon MA. Patterns of sleep and sleepiness in adolescents. *Pediatrician*. 1990;17(1):5–12.

110. Loessl B, Valerius G, Kopasz M, Hornyak M, Riemann D, Voderholzer U. Are adolescents chronically sleep-deprived? An investigation of sleep habits of adolescents in the southwest of Germany. *Child Care Health Dev*. 2008;34(5):549–556.

111. Carskadon MA. Adolescent sleepiness: increased risk in a high-risk population. *Alcohol. Drugs and Driving*. 1989–1990;5/6(4/1):317–328.

112. Van den Bulck J. Television viewing, computer game playing, and internet use and self-reported time to bed and time out of bed in secondary-school children. *Sleep*. 2004;27(1):101–104.

113. Knutson KL, Lauderdale DS. Sociodemographic and behavioral predictors of bed time and wake time among US adolescents aged 15 to 17 years. *J Pediatr*. 2009;154(3):426–430. 430e1.

114. Valkenburg PM, Peter J. Online communication among adolescents: an integrated model of its attraction, opportunities, and risks. *J Adolesc Health*. 2011;48(2):121–127.

115. Anderson M, Jiang J. *Teens, social media & technology*. 2018: 2018.

116. Carter B, Rees P, Hale L, Bhattacharjee D, Paradkar MS. Association between portable screen-based media device access or use and sleep outcomes: a systematic review and meta-analysis. *JAMA Pediatr*. 2016;170(12):1202–1208.

117. Munezawa T, Kaneita Y, Osaki Y, et al. The association between use of mobile phones after lights out and sleep disturbances among Japanese adolescents: a nationwide cross-sectional survey. *Sleep*. 2011;34(8):1013–1020.

118. Cajochen C, Frey S, Anders D, et al. Evening exposure to a light-emitting diodes (LED)-backlit computer screen affects circadian physiology and cognitive performance. *J Appl Physiol*. 2011;110(5):1432–1438.

119. Chang AM, Aeschbach D, Duffy JF, Czeisler CA. Evening use of light-emitting eReaders negatively affects sleep, circadian timing, and next-morning alertness. *PNAS*. 2015;112(4):1232–1237.

120. Shechter A, Quispe KA, Mizhquiri Barbecho JS, Slater C, Falzon L. Interventions to reduce short-wavelength ("blue") light exposure at night and their effects on sleep: a systematic review and meta-analysis. *SLEEP Advances*. 2020;1(1).

121. Medeiros-Oliveira VC, Viana RS, Oliveira AC, Nascimento-Ferreira MV, De Moraes ACF. Are sleep time and quality associated with inflammation in children and adolescents? A systematic review. *Prev Med Rep*. 2023;35:102327. Published 2023 Jul 17. https://doi.org/10.1016/j.pmedr.2023.102327.

122. Tanner J. *Growth at Adolescence*. Oxford: Blackwell; 1962.

5

Pharmacology of Sleep in Children

Judith A. Owens and Vijayabharathi Ekambaram

CHAPTER HIGHLIGHTS

- Decision-making regarding medication for insomnia in the pediatric population should include review of the patient's clinical presentation, caregiver and patient preference and previous medication exposure, the properties of the available drug options and potential side effects.
- Pediatric providers should be involved in recommendations for melatonin use in children and counsel families about the relative pros and cons
- Medications for insomnia should be prescribed starting at the lower dosing range and for as short a time period as possible. There are some instances (e.g., for children with neurodevelopmental disorders such as autism) in which a more chronic course may be indicated, but clear expectations for treatment response should be discussed and drug holidays should be considered in these cases.

Introduction

This chapter will cover general principles of medication use for sleep disorders in children with a focus on prescription and over-the-counter (OTC) sedative/hypnotic medications for insomnia in children and adolescents; specific pharmacologic interventions for other sleep disorders (e.g., narcolepsy, restless legs syndrome [RLS]) are discussed in detail in those respective chapters. These general recommendations will be followed by a discussion of specific features of those sleep medications that have been identified as commonly used in pediatric settings.

It should be stated at the outset that behavioral interventions for pediatric insomnia (as is the case for insomnia in adults) are considered as the mainstay of treatment.[1] Thus pharmacotherapy should only be considered when behavior techniques are ineffective for a number of potential reasons and should always be used in combination with behavioral interventions. In addition, there is a relative lack of evidence-based literature related to efficacy, safety, and tolerability of medications used in treating children with insomnia. Recommendations for pharmacologic intervention for pediatric insomnia are derived mostly from adult data, case reports, or small case series in pediatric populations, as well as clinical experience. Very few published studies have documented the effectiveness of hypnotic/sedative use in children using randomized placebo-controlled clinical trials.[1-3] Furthermore, it should be noted that no medications are currently approved by the U.S. Food and Drug Administration (FDA) for use in treating insomnia in children under 18 years old, thus all use in clinical practice is considered "off-label."

However, despite the relative dearth of data, sedative/hypnotic medications and OTC sleep aids are prescribed frequently by practitioners. For example, in a national U.S. survey, about 88% of the child psychiatry practitioners recommended OTC medicines for the treatment of insomnia in a typical month.[4,5] Because many prescribing pediatric health care providers, including those in primary care and mental health settings as well as sleep medicine providers, may not be knowledgeable about or experienced with using these medications in children, there is a risk of inappropriate selection and overuse of as well as overdosing and underdosing. Therefore, a rational and systematic approach to pharmacotherapy based on the available evidence and clinical experience is critical to optimizing safety and efficacy when these medications are considered as part of the therapeutic approach.[3]

General Principles for Medication Use in Pediatric Insomnia

- Treatment strategies for insomnia should always be based on the systematic evaluation of possible etiologic factors, thus the decision to use hypnotic/sedative medications needs to be made after and in the context of a thorough clinical evaluation and diagnosis.
- As noted in the introduction, medication is very rarely a first choice or sole treatment for insomnia in children. In almost all cases, medication should be used in combination with nonpharmacologic behavioral management strategies. Although pharmacologic interventions may have a more rapid effect, nonpharmacologic treatments have been

shown to result in more sustained improvement[6,7] and avoidance of potential side effects associated with drugs.

- Existing unhealthy sleep practices should be addressed, and treatment recommendations must include the implementation of more appropriate sleep behaviors. Healthy sleep practices, commonly referred to as "good sleep hygiene," include modifiable daytime, bedtime, and within-sleep practices that positively impact sleep-wake transitions, psychophysiologic arousal, and the sleep environment. Although as a stand-alone intervention sleep hygiene measures are often not adequate to fully address insomnia symptoms, they are an integral part of the "treatment package."
- Psychoeducation for patients and families regarding the basics of sleep and sleep regulation is a critical component of appropriate medication management. For example, a child may have a bedtime that is inappropriately early from a developmental or circadian preference ("morningness-eveningness") standpoint or occurs during the so-called forbidden zone of increased circadian alertness immediately preceding the natural fall-asleep time. This situation may lead to sleep onset delay/bedtime refusal that is appropriately addressed with behavioral interventions and should not be treated with medication. Similarly, a late-day nap may reduce the sleep drive such that even large doses of medication are ineffective in facilitating sleep initiation at an appropriate bedtime. Clinicians can help parents understand the rationale for treatment recommendations by explaining that sleep is a biologic function influenced by multiple internal and external facilitating and inhibiting factors.
- Furthermore, it should be emphasized to caregivers that medication acts to facilitate rather than induce sleep.
- Clear, well-defined treatment goals must be established with the patient and caregivers. Specific agreed-upon treatment outcomes should be realistic, clearly defined, and measurable. Family and patient expectations in older children and adolescents regarding the potential impact of pharmacotherapy must be explicitly stated and appropriate. For example, the immediate goal of treatment should be to alleviate or improve rather than eliminate sleep problems.
- Potential modifications in dosage and timing should be reviewed ahead of time with the family. These include whether the medication is to be given on a nightly or an intermittent "as needed" basis, and if the latter case, what will be the criteria for administering the medication on any given night (e.g., sleep onset latency >45 minutes)? If middle-of-the-night dosing for night waking is to be employed, parameters governing this strategy should be clearly outlined (e.g., there must be at least a 4-hour remaining sleep opportunity after dosing). Caregivers and patients should be strongly cautioned against increasing medication dose without explicit medical input, especially for drugs with a narrow therapeutic index (e.g., clonidine).
- Any hypnotics, particularly those with high toxicity levels in overdose, should be used with extreme caution in patients with a history of depression and/or suicidal ideation because of the risk of non-accidental overdose.

- Adolescents in particular should be screened for alcohol and drug use before initiation of sleep medication, as many recreational substances may have additive effects when combined with sedatives/hypnotics. Urine/blood drug screening may be appropriate in some situations in which a history of substance use is unclear or potentially dangerous.
- Careful questioning and documentation of current use of any OTC sleep medications (including combination analgesics-hypnotics and "natural" preparations such as herbal and homeopathic remedies and supplements such as melatonin) are important to avoid overmedication and potential drug-drug interactions. In some cases, OTC sleep medications may not only interact with other prescription or OTC drugs but may exacerbate an underlying medical condition. Although generally viewed by parents as safe, the potential drug-drug interactions between most OTC and complementary/alternative therapies (i.e., herbal preparations) and supplements, and prescription sedative/hypnotics, as well as with other medications, is largely unknown and thus should be approached with caution.
- Similarly, clinical screening for use of OTC (i.e., caffeine) or prescription stimulants (such as psychostimulants) that may be causing or exacerbating insomnia symptoms or masking resultant daytime sleepiness is an important component for ensuring appropriate treatment with sedatives/hypnotics.
- Medication selection should be based on the clinician's judgment of the best possible match between the clinical circumstances (e.g., the type of sleep problem, patient and family characteristics, previous medication use) and the properties of currently available drugs (e.g., onset of action, safety, tolerability).
- The general properties of the available medications particularly onset and duration of action, should be appropriate for the presenting complaint. For example, for children with sleep-onset problems, a shorter-acting medication is generally desirable, whereas longer-acting medications should be considered for sleep maintenance problems.
- Consideration should be given to the timing of drug administration relative to the targeted time of sleep onset (e.g., within 30 minutes of "lights out") and to the "forbidden zone" phenomenon mentioned above. This period of heightened circadian-mediated alertness occurs in the evening immediately before sleep onset, making it more difficult to fall asleep during this 1- or 2-hour window. Because most hypnotic medications have their onset of action within 30 minutes of administration and peak within 1–2 hours, giving a sedative/hypnotic during that time window may be less effective (e.g., requiring a higher dose) and has the potential to induce dissociative phenomenon.[3] Timing and type of medication should also minimize "morning hangover" or persistent grogginess. In general, this means balancing likely effectiveness with choosing an agent with the shortest possible half-life.
- As with most psychotropic medications in children (especially those with clear evidence-based dosing ranges based on clinical trial results), dosing should be initiated at the

lowest level likely to be effective and increased as necessary based on treatment response and development of side effects. There should be clearly defined criteria for dose escalation with simultaneous monitoring for side effects. Close communication with the family with frequent follow-up visits is key to successful and safe management.

- On the other hand, it appears that some medications (e.g., zolpidem) are metabolized differently in younger children, and these data suggest that children may require higher doses than adults and anecdotally, a dose that is not adequate to induce sleep has been found to result in a "paradoxical" reaction in which the child becomes groggy and subsequently agitated and disinhibited. However, it should be noted that currently there are no label guidelines to this effect.
- Sedative/hypnotics should be used with caution when there is a potential for drug-drug interaction with concurrent medications (e.g., fluoxetine [a CYP2D6 and CYP2C19 inhibitor] and diphenhydramine).
- In general, abrupt discontinuation of medications, especially those that are being used on a nightly basis over a period of time, should be avoided. Drugs should be tapered gradually to reduce the possibility of rebound insomnia; this phenomenon appears especially prevalent at higher doses and with short/intermediate half-life drugs. In addition, other potential side effects may be avoided by a gradual weaning process; for example, medications that suppress REM sleep when abruptly discontinued may result in a "REM rebound" with an increase in vivid or disturbing dreams.
- It is essential to have a defined "exit strategy" at the time of initiation of sedative/hypnotic treatment. This includes consideration of caregiver/patient expectations regarding the duration of treatment and if, when, and how a trial off medication might be developed (e.g., during summer vacation).
- All medications prescribed for sleep problems should be closely monitored for the emergence of adverse effects. Some medications may also precipitate or exacerbate coexisting sleep problems. For example, immediate release alpha agonists such as clonidine may induce an increase in partial arousal parasomnias (e.g., sleepwalking) during the latter part of the night in susceptible children with a history of parasomnias.
- Insomnia in children commonly occurs with other primary sleep disorders (e.g., obstructive sleep apnea, RLS). Thus, the presence of both medically based and behaviorally based sleep disorders warrants attention. Also, the pharmacologic treatment of insomnia could exacerbate the coexisting sleep problems. For example, sedative/hypnotics with respiratory depressant properties (e.g., benzodiazepines [BZDs]) and medications that may cause significant weight gain (e.g., risperidone) should be avoided if the insomnia occurs in the presence of obstructive sleep apnea, and sedating selective serotonin reuptake inhibitors should be used with caution in the presence of insomnia, as they may increase symptoms of RLS.
- Patients, especially adolescents, should be cautioned to avoid hazardous activities (e.g., driving) after taking a hypnotic medication.

- Because some sleep medications are contraindicated in pregnancy, pregnancy screening should be carefully considered in sexually active females before initiating therapy, and the importance of contraception use during the course treatment should be discussed. This may warrant pregnancy testing in some situations.

Specific Medications Used for Pediatric Insomnia

The discussion in this chapter is focused mainly on three major categories of medications: (1) prescription drugs approved (in adults) by the U.S. Food and Drug Administration (FDA), (2) OTC drugs, and (3) off-label pediatric insomnia drugs. The clinical properties of selected medications are summarized in Table 5.1.

FDA-Approved Prescription Drugs (in Adults)

Benzodiazepine Receptor Agonists

BZDs act primarily through the somnogenic (sleep-inducing) neurotransmitter gamma-aminobutyric acid (GABA).[8] GABA's action on the events related to use such a drowning and central nervous system contributes to the anxiolytic, anticonvulsant, sedative, and muscle-relaxing effects of BZDs.[8,9] The shorter-acting BZDs are used in treating sleep-onset insomnia, and the longer-acting BZDs are used for sleep maintenance. BZD use in the pediatric population is limited because of their risk of addiction and potential side effect profile including morning hangover, daytime sleepiness, dizziness, headaches, anterograde amnesia (memory loss for events occurring between dosing and sleep onset), rebound insomnia, and withdrawal phenomena. In patients with suspected sleep-disordered breathing, BZDs should be used with caution because of their muscle relaxant properties. BZDs are also potent slow-wave sleep suppressants and, very importantly, have dependence/abuse potential.[9]

In general, in children, BZDs are used only for short-term insomnia or insomnia occurring in the context of comorbid conditions such as anxiety disorders, neurodevelopmental disorder, and seizure disorders, for which their other properties (e.g., anxiolytic, anticonvulsant, muscle relaxant) may be beneficial,[2] as well as for some parasomnias (e.g., refractory sleep terrors). Clonazepam is a relatively long-acting BZD that has been shown to be effective in the treatment of periodic limb movement disorder and parasomnias such as sleepwalking,[2,9] and may be considered in sleep maintenance insomnia especially in children with neurologic/neurodevelopmental conditions, with the caveat that a potential side effect is morning grogginess. The half-life of clonazepam ranges from 18 to 39 hours and reaches its maximum plasma concentration within 1 to 4 hours after oral administration. Clonazepam is also available as disintegrating tablets that are easily dissolvable when placed under the tongue.[3]

	Mechanism of Action	Available Strengths	Formulations	Common Side Effects	Comments
Benzodiazepine receptor agonists (BzDRA) Clonazepam (Klonopin)*	Bind to central GABA receptors	0.125 mg, 0.25 mg, 0.5 mg, 1 mg, 2 mg	Tablet, orally disintegrating tablet	Residual daytime sedation, rebound insomnia on discontinuation, psychomotor impairment, anterograde amnesia (dose dependent); respiratory impairment function	Also used to control partial arousal parasomnias (night terrors, sleepwalking)
Non-benzodiazepine receptor agonists (BzDRA) Zolpidem (Ambien)* Eszopiclone (Lunesta)*	Bind to α_1 subunits GABA receptors	5 mg, 10 mg (Zolpidem) 6.25 mg,12.5 mg (Zolpidem-CR) 1 mg, 2 mg, 3 mg (Lunesta)	Tablet, oral spray, sublingual tablet	Headache, retrograde amnesia; few residual next-day effects	Little clinical experience in children
Synthetic melatonin receptor agonist Ramelteon (Rozerem)*	Selective affinity MT_1, MT_2 receptors	8 mg	Tablet	Fatigue, headache, and dizziness; co-administration with fluvoxamne should be avoided; possible reduction in prolactin and testosterone levels	Avoid coadministration with fluvoxamine
Selective histamine receptor antagonist Doxepin (Silenor)*	Selective antagonism of the histamine H_1 receptor	3 mg, 6 mg	Tablet, capsule, oral liquid concentrate	Daytime somnolence and residual next-day effect	Used for sleep maintenance insomnia
Dual orexin receptor antagonists Suvorexant (Belsomra)*	Bind to OX1R and OX2R receptors and inhibit the activation of the arousal system	5 mg, 10 mg, 15 mg, 20 mg 5–10	Tablet	Daytime somnolence and abnormal dreams	Schedule IV drugs
Antihistamines Diphenhydramine (Benadryl) Cyproheptadine (Periactin) Hydroxyzine (Atarax)	Competitive histamine (H_1) receptor blocker in the central nervous system	12.5 mg, 25 mg (tablets); 12.5 mg/5 mL (liquid) (Benadryl) 4 mg, 2 mg/5 mL (Periactin); 25 mg, 50 mg (Atarax)	Tablet, capsule, syrup, injectable	Daytime drowsiness, GI (appetite loss, vomiting, constipation, dry mouth), paradoxical excitation	Weak soporifics; high-level parental/practitioner acceptance
Hormone analog Melatonin	Main effect suprachiasmatic nucleus; non-selective action at MT_1 and MT_2 receptors	1 mg, 2 mg, 3 mg, 5 mg (0.3–25)	Tablet; various strengths	Headache, nightmares, morning grogginess; possible exacerbation of comorbid autoimmune diseases	Used in children with developmental disabilities, autism, neurologic impairment, blindness; jet lag

Non-Benzodiazepine Receptor Agonists

Non-benzodiazepines are GABA-minergic drugs. Some are referred to as "Z-drugs," including zaleplon, zolpidem, and eszopiclone; they have similar pharmacology to BZDs but with different chemical structures.[9] They selectively bind and activate the α_1 subunits of the GABA-A receptor complex.[10]

TABLE 5.1	Clinical Properties of Selected Medications Used for Pediatric Insomnia—Cont'd				
Medications	Mechanism of Action	Available Strengths	Formulations	Common Side Effects	Comments
α-Agonists Clonidine IR Clonidine ER (Kapvay) Guanfacine IR (Tenex) Guanfacine ER (Intuniv)	α-Adrenergic receptor agonists; (guanfacine more selective) decrease NE release	0.025 mg, 0.1 mg (tablets); 0.05 mg/5mL (liquid); (clonidine IR) 0.1 mg; 0.2 mg (Kapvay) 1 mg, 2 mg, (Tenex); 1 mg, 2 mg, 3 mg, 4 mg (Intuniv)	Tablet, liquid, transdermal patch	Dry mouth, bradycardia, hypotension, rebound hypertension on discontinuation	Also used in daytime treatment of ADHD
Atypical antidepressants Trazodone	5-HT$_{2A/C}$ antagonist	50 mg, 100 mg, 150 mg (tablets); 10 mg/mL, 20 mg/mL (liquid)	Tablet, liquid	Dizziness, CNS overstimulation Cardiac arrhythmias, hypotension, priapism	May be used with comorbid depression

*Medications approved in adults by the U.S. Food and Drug Administration.
ADHD, Attention-deficit/hyperactivity disorder; CNS, central nervous system; GABA, gamma-aminobutyric acid; GI, gastrointestinal.

Zaleplon (ultrashort acting, 1–2 hours half-life) and zolpidem (short acting, 2–3 hours half-life) are primarily used for sleep initiation. Sublingual forms of zolpidem and zaleplon may be used for middle-of-the-night insomnia (if at least 5 hours remain before the desired wake time).[11] The intermediate–to–long acting forms (5–7 hours half-life) eszopiclone and zolpidem-CR are indicated for use in adults for sleep maintenance insomnia.[2,12]

Zaleplon has been reported to trigger sleepwalking in adolescents and may cause drowsiness, ataxia, dizziness, confusion, and slurred speech in excessive doses.[13] Zolpidem-induced complex sleep-related behaviors such as sleep eating, sleepwalking, and sleep driving have been documented extensively in adult studies; more recent reports of serious and life-threatening events related to use such a drowning and hypothermia have warranted an additional FDA "black box warning" for this class of drugs. Concerns have also been raised about its use in the pediatric population, and hallucinations have been reported in pediatric clinical trials.[2,14,15] Eszopiclone can cause an unpleasant metallic taste and headaches.[2,12]

Unlike BZDs, Z-drugs in their recommended doses do not typically cause rebound insomnia with abrupt discontinuation.[3] Longer-duration trials of Z-drugs in adults suggest continued hypnotic benefit at 6 months, without the development of tolerance.[12] The potential side effects of Z-drugs include headaches, dizziness, anterograde amnesia, confusion, and hallucinations.[13] Z-drugs are relatively contraindicated in patients with sleep apnea because they blunt the arousal response to hypoxemia.[2] Because the abuse/dependence potential is reported to be low, extended-release formulations do not have label limitations on duration of use.

Melatonin Receptor Agonists

Ramelteon is the only FDA-approved synthetic melatonin receptor agonist used in the treatment of insomnia in adults[16] and is believed to promote sleep largely through regulation of the circadian sleep-wake cycle rather than direct sedation per se.[16,17] Whereas clinical studies of ramelteon have shown an objective (PSG) reduction in sleep latency compared with placebo, subjective improvements are less consistently reported.[18] Ramelteon is rapidly absorbed and has a short elimination half-life (1–2.6 hours); its pharmacokinetics are altered by high-fat meals.[16]

Pediatric case series have documented ramelteon to be effective in the treatment of insomnia in children; it appears to be well tolerated in these reports and in clinical practice without significant daytime sedation.[17,19,20] Adult data also suggest there is little evidence of next-day impairment associated with the use of ramelteon.[16,19] The most frequently reported adverse events include fatigue, headache, and dizziness.[19] In contrast to GABA modulators, ramelteon has not shown potential for abuse, dependence, withdrawal, and rebound insomnia, and it is not a scheduled drug; this may be advantageous in clinical situations in which abuse potential is a concern.[16,17,20]

Selective Histamine Receptor Antagonists

The tricyclic antidepressant (TCA) doxepin (Silenor), at low doses (3–6 mg), is now FDA approved for sleep maintenance insomnia (not for sleep onset). At this low dose, doxepin exerts its sedative effect through selective antagonism of the alerting properties of the histamine H$_1$ receptor.[21] Half-life is 2–8 hours and elimination half-life is close to 24 hours.[21,22] Adult clinical studies have documented improvement in total sleep time, quality of sleep, and reduction in wake after sleep onset compared with placebo.[18] The common adverse effects reported include daytime somnolence and residual next-day effect largely with the 6-mg dose.[21]

Doxepin does not appear to have any abuse potential and is thus not a scheduled drug. Although it is available in a generic formulation as 10-mg capsules or 10-mg/mL oral liquid concentrate, this higher dosage has not been approved by the FDA for insomnia treatment.[18,21,22]

Dual Orexin Receptor Antagonists

Suvorexant, a dual orexin receptor antagonist, has a novel mechanism in that it blocks orexin receptors (OX1R and OX2R) and thus promotes sleep by reducing wakefulness and arousal.[23–25] Clinical studies of suvorexant have documented improvement in total sleep time and reduction in wake after sleep onset compared with placebo.[18] The most noticeable side effects reported in adult clinical trials are daytime somnolence and abnormal dreams; otherwise the medication appeared to be well tolerated.[23] However, because of its potential for addiction, it is classified as a schedule IV drug, and additionally, given its higher cost, it is not currently recommended as a first-line treatment for insomnia.[23]

A newer dual orexin receptor antagonist, lemborexant, was approved by the FDA on December 20, 2019.[24,26] Lemborexant has more OX2R inhibition, and it dissociates rapidly from orexin receptors compared with suvorexant; it is expected to have less risk of daytime sedation.[24,26]

Over-the-Counter (OTC) Drugs

Sedating Antihistamines

Antihistamines are often considered acceptable choices for families and health care providers because of their familiarity, low cost, and availability.[4] First-generation antihistamines (e.g., diphenhydramine, cyproheptadine, hydroxyzine) are histamine (H_1) receptor blockers in the central and peripheral nervous systems. They are lipid soluble, rapidly absorbed, and can easily pass through the blood-brain barrier, resulting in significant sedative and hypnotic effects compared with second- and third-generation antihistamines.[2,9]

Antihistamines are generally well tolerated in children, and their effects on sleep architecture appear to be minimal. However, a relatively rare but troublesome paradoxical excitation effect with disinhibited behavior may be observed. With regards to efficacy, one older randomized controlled trial in school-aged children documented subjective improvement in sleep latency and night waking.[27] However, another more recent pediatric study found that antihistamines were not more effective than placebo in reducing nighttime awakening in young children.[28]

Both diphenhydramine and cyproheptadine are available OTC, and hydroxyzine requires a prescription.[2,9,29]

The potential side effects include daytime drowsiness, confusion, and anticholinergic effects such as blurred vision,

dry mouth, constipation, and urinary retention. Tolerance may develop quickly with these medications and thus result in the need for dose escalation.[2,4,29]

Melatonin

Melatonin is a neurohormone that plays a significant role in the regulation of circadian sleep-wake cycles and core body temperature rhythms. Melatonin release by the pineal gland is mediated through the suprachiasmatic nucleus in the hypothalamus and its production is inhibited by exposure of the retina to light.[2,9] It promotes sleep through both chronobiotic (i.e., shifts the circadian sleep-wake cycle) and hypnotic (i.e., sedating) effects depending upon the dose and timing of administration. For example, a relatively larger hypnotic dose of melatonin (e.g., 3–5 mg) administered close to (30 minutes before) bedtime causes mild sedation and reduced sleep onset latency.[2] Alternatively, in children and adolescents with circadian phase delay, a smaller chronobiotic dose of melatonin (e.g., 0.3–0.5 mg) can be administered earlier in the evening (e.g., 1–2 hours before the desired bedtime) to advance sleep onset.

Exogenous melatonin is generally well tolerated, and there is considerable empirical evidence for the use of melatonin for sleep-onset insomnia in the pediatric population, specifically in children with autism.[30,31] However, only a handful of studies have documented reduction in sleep-onset latency in healthy children[32] and in children with attention-deficit/hyperactivity disorder (ADHD).[33,34] Melatonin is also clinically used in the correction of chronic or acute circadian rhythm disturbances in healthy children and adolescents (e.g., delayed sleep phase syndrome, jet lag) and in children with neurodevelopmental disorders (e.g., blindness, Rett syndrome).[35]

Exogenous synthetic melatonin is commercially available OTC in the United States in several different formulations, including liquid and "gummies"; it is considered a "dietary supplement" by the FDA and thus it is considered "safe until proven otherwise." Melatonin formulations may vary in strength, purity, and therefore potentially in safety and efficacy and concern have been raised regarding the actual content of melatonin in these commercial brands. One recent study analyzed a total of 31 commercial supplements by chromatography, documented actual melatonin content ranged from −83% to +478% of the labeled content; in addition, serotonin (5-hydroxytryptamine) was identified in over a quarter of the commercially available brands.[36] A recent study found similar variability in the "gummy" forms of melatonin; the actual melatonin content in 88% of samples tested did not meet label claim within +/-10% (required of OTC products).[37] In addition, an increase in calls to Poison Control Centers in the U.S. regarding melatonin increased by 530% between 2012–2021 530% between 2012–2021,[38] reflecting the substantial increase in the use of melatonin in the pediatric population.[39] Because of these variations, strong consideration should be given to using only "pharmaceutical-grade melatonin" that has a USP Verified Mark.

Melatonin has low and variable bioavailability due to extensive first-pass metabolism, and younger children appear to metabolize it more rapidly than older children.

The immediate-release melatonin has half-life close to 45 minutes, and it reaches its peak plasma concentration within 1 hour of administration.[25] Inhibitors (e.g., cimetidine and TCAs) and inducers (e.g., carbamazepine, omeprazole) of the enzyme that metabolizes melatonin (CYPA2) may impact concentration and efficacy/side effects. Commonly used doses of melatonin are 1 mg in infants, 2.5–3 mg in older children, and 5 mg in adolescents; use of melatonin in children with special needs have reported doses ranging from 0.5 to 10 mg, irrespective of age.

Melatonin is also available in controlled-release formulations with prolonged half-life of 3.5–4 hours, which may be used for sleep maintenance.[25] Whereas clinical trials of the controlled release melatonin minitablet (Circadin-CR) have yielded promising results in the European Union, use of extended-release preparations in the United States is limited by the lack of formulations that do not require swallowing a pill or capsule.

Melatonin generally has a low side effect profile and is considered generally safe even under conditions of long-term use.[40] However, prospective longitudinal studies are lacking, and a theoretical side effect of suppression of the hypothalamic-gonadal axis by melatonin has been proposed.[41] However, more recent studies have not found evidence of alterations in reproductive hormone levels in children on melatonin. Limited data also suggest that exogenous melatonin does not suppress endogenous melatonin levels. Because of its proinflammatory properties, melatonin should be used with caution in children with immune disorders or who are on immunosuppressants (e.g., corticosteroids).[2] Finally, the widespread increased use of melatonin in the pediatric population in the last decade, now marketed to "promote restful sleep" rather than solely to address sleep problems, has raised some alarms regarding inappropriate usage and potential long-term adverse effects.

Off-Label Drugs Used for Pediatric Insomnia

Alpha Agonists

Clonidine is a central and peripheral α-adrenergic agonist originally developed as an antihypertensive. Because of its highly sedating properties, it has generally been used in clinical practice for the treatment of sleep initiation insomnia in children with ADHD.[42] Despite its widespread use[4,5] in pediatric and psychiatry practice, the clinical data regarding safety and efficacy in children are largely limited to retrospective studies that appear to demonstrate subjective efficacy and a relatively low side effect profile.[43,44]

Due to its rapid absorption, it has an onset of action within 1 hour, and it reaches peak effects within 2–4 hours. Clonidine has minimal effects on sleep architecture, but may decrease both REM and slow-wave sleep. Thus its discontinuation can cause vivid dreams and increased sleepwalking/ sleep terrors (due to a rebound increase in REM and slow-wave sleep, respectively).[2,9]

Despite its relatively low adverse effect profile,[43] clonidine has a narrow therapeutic index, and there have been reports of overdose with this medication.[45] The potential side effects of clonidine include dry mouth, bradycardia, irritability, and hypotension, and abrupt discontinuation can cause rebound hypertension. Clonidine should be avoided in patients with diabetes and Raynaud's syndrome.[2,9]

Guanfacine, a selective α2A adrenergic receptor agonist, is associated with less sedation and cardiovascular side effects compared with clonidine, because of its α2A receptor selectivity.[2] Despite the lack of clinical studies in children, immediate-release guanfacine is frequently used for treating insomnia in pediatric and psychiatric practices. In a recent randomized, placebo-controlled trial of children with ADHD, extended-release guanfacine was associated with an increase in wake after sleep onset, and a decrease in total sleep time.[9,46]

Antidepressants

TCAs (amitriptyline, doxepin) and atypical antidepressants (trazodone, mirtazapine) are used for treating insomnia in both pediatric and adult populations, especially in mental health settings.[25] Despite their widespread use, there is a lack of methodologically studies in support of their use in insomnia. Therefore their use should generally be limited to clinical situations in which there are concurrent mood disorders with insomnia. The dosage of antidepressants for insomnia is typically less than the dosage used to treat mood disorders. Due to their anticholinergic effects, the majority of these antidepressants suppress REM sleep, and their abrupt withdrawal may lead to REM rebound and increased nightmares.[2]

Amitriptyline (dosing 10–25 mg) is one of the most sedating TCAs used for insomnia. The most commonly reported side effects include blurred vision, dry mouth, urinary retention, and orthostatic hypotension. Mirtazapine, an α_2-adrenergic, 5-HT antagonist has a high degree of sedation at low doses (e.g., 7.5 mg), and potential side effects include residual daytime sleepiness and weight gain.[2,25,47] Trazodone, a $5\text{-HT}_{2A/C}$ antagonist, is one of the most sedating antidepressants and appears to inhibit post-synaptic binding of serotonin and block histamine receptors.[47] It can cause "morning hangover" and has been associated with hypotension, arrhythmias, and serotonin syndrome; in the 50–150 mg dose range it has been associated with reports of priapism in males.[2,25]

Antipsychotics

Atypical antipsychotics (risperidone, olanzapine, quetiapine) are sometimes used for insomnia in children with underlying psychiatric and neurodevelopmental disorders. In general, they have effects on multiple neurotransmitters (muscarinic, histaminergic, serotoninergic) that promote sleep.[25,48] They vary in the degree of sedation, but most of these antipsychotics decrease sleep-onset latency, increase sleep continuity, and suppress REM sleep (in higher doses). However, their sedating effects may also interfere with daytime functioning, and their other significant side effects limit their use except in specialized circumstances when other medication choices have failed or are contraindicated.

Anticonvulsants

A number of antiepileptic drugs, including carbamazepine, phenobarbital, and valproic acid, are associated with increased daytime somnolence. Newer anticonvulsants have varying degrees of daytime sedation. For example, sedation rates with topiramate are 15–25% and 5–15% with gabapentin. Anticonvulsants typically cause dose-dependent sedation, although tolerance to this effect may develop.

Gabapentin, which has effects on dopamine, serotonin, and norepinephrine neurotransmitters, appears to increase slow-wave sleep, and has been shown to improve sleep maintenance and decrease RLS symptoms. In children with neurodevelopmental disorders, gabapentin (dosing range 5–15 mg/kg) has

shown promising results in improving refractory insomnia.[49] Potential improvements in pain control with gabapentin may have added benefit for some patients.

> **CLINICAL PEARLS**
> - Melatonin formulations available in the US are highly variable with regard to actual content compared to label claims.
> - USP certified "pharmaceutical grade" melatonin is strongly recommended.
> - Because there are currently no hypnotic medications approved for use in children, off-label use is primarily based on clinical experience.
> - Medication for childhood insomnia should always be combined with behavioral interventions.

Summary

In summary, clinicians working in pediatric settings need to evaluate all factors potentially contributing to the development and persistence of insomnia, including comorbid medical, psychiatric, and neurodevelopmental disorders; coexisting sleep disorders; caregiver behaviors; and patient practices interfering with sleep before considering sedative/hypnotic medication use. Behavior therapy should always be considered as the first modality of treatment; when behavior treatment is ineffective, pharmacologic management should

be considered in combination with behavior therapy, which is proven to have long-lasting patient outcomes. Overall, there is limited data in regard to medication use for pediatric insomnia. Selection of medication, when determined to be appropriate, should be based on pharmacokinetic and pharmacodynamic profiles of the individual drugs and the specific clinical circumstances (age, presence of comorbid medical or psychiatric conditions, concomitant medications, abuse potential, etc.).

References

1. Owens JA, Mindell JA. Pediatric insomnia. *Pediatr Clin North Am*. 2011;58(3):555–569.
2. Owens JA, Moturi S. Pharmacologic treatment of pediatric insomnia. *Child Adolesc Psychiatr Clin N Am*. 2009;18(4):1001–1016.
3. Pelayo R, Dubik M. Pediatric sleep pharmacology. *Semin Pediatr Neurol*. 2008;15(2):79–90.
4. Owens JA, Rosen CL, Mindell JA. Medication use in the treatment of pediatric insomnia: results of a survey of community-based pediatricians. *Pediatrics*. 2003;111(5 Pt 1):e628–35.
5. Owens JA, et al. Use of pharmacotherapy for insomnia in child psychiatry practice: a national survey. *Sleep Med*. 2010;11(7):692–700.
6. Mindell JA, et al. Behavioral treatment of bedtime problems and night wakings in infants and young children. *Sleep*. 2006;29(10):1263–1276.
7. Mindell JA, et al. Pharmacologic management of insomnia in children and adolescents: consensus statement. *Pediatrics*. 2006;117(6):e1223–1232.
8. Griffin CE 3rd, et al. Benzodiazepine pharmacology and central nervous system-mediated effects. *Ochsner J*. 2013;13(2):214–223.
9. Relia S, Ekambaram V. Pharmacological approach to sleep disturbances in autism spectrum disorders with psychiatric comorbidities: a literature review. *Med Sci (Basel)*. 2018;6(4).
10. Möhler H, Fritschy JM, Rudolph U. A new benzodiazepine pharmacology. *J Pharmacol Exp Ther*. 2002;300(1):2–8.
11. Zammit GK, et al. Sleep and residual sedation after administration of zaleplon, zolpidem, and placebo during experimental middle-of-the-night awakening. *J Clin Sleep Med*. 2006;2(4):417–423.
12. Walsh JK, et al. Nightly treatment of primary insomnia with eszopiclone for six months: effect on sleep, quality of life, and work limitations. *Sleep*. 2007;30(8):959–968.
13. Liskow B, Pikalov A. Zaleplon overdose associated with sleepwalking and complex behavior. *J Am Acad Child Adolesc Psychiatry*. 2004;43(8):927–928.
14. Blumer JL, et al. Potential pharmacokinetic basis for zolpidem dosing in children with sleep difficulties. *Clin Pharmacol Ther*. 2008;83(4):551–558.
15. Blumer JL, et al. Controlled clinical trial of zolpidem for the treatment of insomnia associated with attention-deficit/hyperactivity disorder in children 6 to 17 years of age. *Pediatrics*. 2009;123(5):e770–e776.
16. FDA. Highlights of Prescribing Information Rozerem (Ramelteon) Tablets. 2005. Accessed November 16, 2023. https://www.accessdata.fda.gov/drugsatfda_docs/label/2010/021782s011lbl.pdf
17. Stigler KA, Posey DJ, McDougle CJ. Ramelteon for insomnia in two youths with autistic disorder. *J Child Adolesc Psychopharmacol*. 2006;16(5):631–636.
18. Sateia MJ, et al. Clinical practice guideline for the pharmacologic treatment of chronic insomnia in adults: an American Academy of Sleep Medicine clinical practice guideline. *J Clin Sleep Med*. 2017;13(2):307–349.

19. Kawabe K, et al. The melatonin receptor agonist ramelteon effectively treats insomnia and behavioral symptoms in autistic disorder. *Case Rep Psychiatry*. 2014;2014:561071.

20. Miyamoto A, et al. [Treatment with ramelteon for sleep disturbance in severely disabled children and young adults]. *No To Hattatsu*. 2013;45(6):440–444.

21. Weber J, et al. Low-dose doxepin: in the treatment of insomnia. *CNS Drugs*. 2010;24(8):713–720.

22. Low-dose doxepin (Silenor) for insomnia. *Med Lett Drugs Ther*. 2010;52(1348):79-80.

23. Kawabe K, et al. Suvorexant for the treatment of insomnia in adolescents. *J Child Adolesc Psychopharmacol*. 2017;27(9):792–795.

24. Kishi T, et al. Lemborexant vs suvorexant for insomnia: a systematic review and network meta-analysis. *J Psychiatr Res*. 2020;128:68–74.

25. Dujardin S, Pijpers A, Pevernagie D. Prescription drugs used in insomnia. *Sleep Med Clin*. 2018;13(2):169–182.

26. Landry I, et al. Pharmacokinetics, pharmacodynamics, and safety of the dual orexin receptor antagonist lemborexant: findings from single-dose and multiple-ascending-dose phase 1 studies in healthy adults. *Clin Pharmacol Drug Dev*. 2021;10(2):153–165.

27. Russo RM, Gururaj VJ, Allen JE. The effectiveness of diphenhydramine HCl in pediatric sleep disorders. *J Clin Pharmacol*. 1976;16(5-6):284–288.

28. Merenstein D, et al. The trial of infant response to diphenhydramine: the TIRED study—a randomized, controlled, patient-oriented trial. *Arch Pediatr Adolesc Med*. 2006;160(7):707–712.

29. Daviss WB, Scott J. A chart review of cyproheptadine for stimulant-induced weight loss. *J Child Adolesc Psychopharmacol*. 2004;14(1):65–73.

30. Jan J, et al. Melatonin therapy of pediatric sleep disorders: recent advances, why it works, who are the candidates and how to treat. *Curr Pediatr Rev*. 2007;3:214–224.

31. Bendz LM, Scates AC. Melatonin treatment for insomnia in pediatric patients with attention-deficit/hyperactivity disorder. *Ann Pharmacother*. 2010;44(1):185–191.

32. van Geijlswijk IM, Korzilius HP, Smits MG. The use of exogenous melatonin in delayed sleep phase disorder: a meta-analysis. *Sleep*. 2010;33(12):1605–1614.

33. van der Heijden KB, et al. Prediction of melatonin efficacy by pretreatment dim light melatonin onset in children with idiopathic chronic sleep onset insomnia. *J Sleep Res*. 2005;14(2):187–194.

34. Van der Heijden KB, et al. Effect of melatonin on sleep, behavior, and cognition in ADHD and chronic sleep-onset insomnia. *J Am Acad Child Adolesc Psychiatry*. 2007;46(2):233–241.

35. Johnson KP, Malow BA. Sleep in children with autism spectrum disorders. *Curr Treat Options Neurol*. 2008;10(5):350–359.

36. Erland LA, Saxena PK. Melatonin natural health products and supplements: presence of serotonin and significant variability of melatonin content. *J Clin Sleep Med*. 2017;13(2):275–281.

37. Cohen PA, Avula B, Wang Y, Katragunta K, Khan I. Quantity of melatonin and CBD in melatonin gummies sold in the US. *JAMA*. 2023;329(16):1401–1402. https://doi.org/10.1001/jama.2023.2296.

38. Lelak K, Vohra V, Neuman MI, Toce MS, Sethuraman U Pediatric melatonin ingestions - United States, 2012-2021. *MMWR Morb Mortal Wkly Rep*. 2022;71(22):725–729. [published correction appears in MMWR Morb Mortal Wkly Rep. 2022 Jul 08;71(27):885]. https://doi.org/10.15585/mmwr.mm7122a1.

39. Hartstein LE, Garrison MM, Lewin D, Boergers J, LeBourgeois MK. Characteristics of melatonin use among US children and adolescents. *JAMA Pediatrics*. 2024;178(1):91–93. https://doi.org/10.1001/jamapediatrics.2023.4749.

40. Carr R, et al. Long-term effectiveness outcome of melatonin therapy in children with treatment-resistant circadian rhythm sleep disorders. *J Pineal Res*. 2007;43(4):351–359.

41. Luboshitzky R, et al. Increased nocturnal melatonin secretion in male patients with hypogonadotropic hypogonadism and delayed puberty. *J Clin Endocrinol Metab*. 1995;80(7):2144–2148.

42. Prince JB, et al. Clonidine for sleep disturbances associated with attention-deficit hyperactivity disorder: a systematic chart review of 62 cases. *J Am Acad Child Adolesc Psychiatry*. 1996;35(5):599–605.

43. Ingrassia A, Turk J. The use of clonidine for severe and intractable sleep problems in children with neurodevelopmental disorders—a case series. *Eur Child Adolesc Psychiatry*. 2005;14(1):34–40.

44. Xue M, et al. Autism spectrum disorders: concurrent clinical disorders. *J Child Neurol*. 2008;23(1):6–13.

45. Kappagoda C, et al. Clonidine overdose in childhood: implications of increased prescribing. *J Paediatr Child Health*. 1998;34(6):508–512.

46. Rugino TA. Effect on primary sleep disorders when children with ADHD are administered guanfacine extended release. *J Atten Disord*. 2018;22(1):14–24.

47. Younus M, Labellarte MJ. Insomnia in children: when are hypnotics indicated? *Paediatr Drugs*. 2002;4(6):391–403.

48. Keshavan MS, et al. Sleep quality and architecture in quetiapine, risperidone, or never-treated schizophrenia patients. *J Clin Psychopharmacol*. 2007;27(6):703–705.

49. Robinson AA, Malow BA. Gabapentin shows promise in treating refractory insomnia in children. *J Child Neurol*. 2013;28(12):1618–1621.

Key References

Feren S, Katyal A, Walsh J. Efficacy of hypnotic medications and other medications used for insomnia. *Sleep Med Clin*. 2006;1:387–397.

Jan J, Wasdell M, Reiter R, et al. Melatonin therapy of pediatric sleep disorders: recent advances, why it works, who are the candidates, and how to treat. *Curr Pediatr Rev*. 2007;3:214–224.

Malow B, Johnson K. Sleep in children with autism spectrum disorders. *J Child Neurol*. 2008;10:350–359.

Meolie AL, Rosen C, Kristo D, et al. Oral nonprescription treatment for insomnia: an evaluation of products with limited evidence. *J Clin Sleep Med*. 2005;1(2):173–187.

Mindell JA, Emslie G, Blumer J, et al. Pharmacologic management of insomnia in children and adolescents: consensus statement. *Pediatrics*. 2006;117(6):e1223–1232.

Owens JA, Babcock D, Blumer J, et al. The use of pharmacotherapy in the treatment of pediatric insomnia in primary care: rational approaches. A consensus meeting summary. *J Clin Sleep Med*. 2005;1(1):49–59.

Van der Heijden KB, Smits MG, Van Someren EJ, et al. Effect of melatonin on sleep, behavior, and cognition in ADHD and chronic sleep-onset insomnia. *J Am Acad Child Adolesc Psychiatry*. 2007;46(2):233–241.

Witek MW, Rojas V, Alonso C, et al. Review of benzodiazepine use in children and adolescents. *Psychiatr Q*. 2005;76(3):283–296.

Younus M, Labellarte MJ. Insomnia in children: when are hypnotics indicated? *Paediatr Drugs*. 2002;4(6):391–403.

Recommended Readings

Buysee D, Schweitzer P, Moul D. Clinical pharmacology of other drugs used as hypnotics. In: Kryger M, Roth T, Dement B, eds. *Principles and Practices of Sleep Medicine.* 4th ed. Elsevier Saunders; 2005:452–467.

Colle M, Rosenzweig P, Bianchetti G, et al. Nocturnal profile of growth hormone secretion during sleep induced by zolpidem: a double-blind study in young adults and children. *Horm Res.* 1991;35(1):30–34.

Meolie AL, et al. Oral nonprescription treatment for insomnia: an evaluation of products with limited evidence. *J Clin Sleep Med.* 2005;1(2):173–187.

Owens JA, et al. The use of pharmacotherapy in the treatment of pediatric insomnia in primary care: rational approaches. A consensus meeting summary. *J Clin Sleep Med.* 2005;1(1):49–59.

Satterlee W, Faries D. The effects of fluoxetine on symptoms of insomnia in depressed patients. *Psychopharmacol Bull.* 1995;31:227–237.

van Zyl LT, et al. L-tryptophan as treatment for pediatric non-rapid eye movement parasomnia. *J Child Adolesc Psychopharmacol.* 2018;28(6):395–401.

Walsh JK, Erman M, Erwin CW, et al. Subjective hypnotic efficacy of trazodone and zolpidem in DSM III-R primary insomnia. *Hum Psychopharm Clin.* 1998;13(3):191–198.

6

Promoting Healthy Sleep Practices

Allison Hayes Clarke, Brittany Nance, and Irina Trosman

CHAPTER HIGHLIGHTS

- Healthy sleep focuses on sufficient sleep time, safe sleep practices, and sleep hygiene.
- Primary care providers and school educators are gatekeepers to parental and child education on healthy sleep habits and sleep requirements.
- Education should be aimed at providing a safe sleep environment as recommended by the American Academy of Pediatrics guidelines for age-based sleep duration, and recommendations for sleep hygiene such as consistent bedtime, sleep routine, and avoidance of caffeine and electronics.
- Culture also plays a role in family sleep practices, so the provider must ensure that this is taken into account when providing recommendations, such as with bed sharing or bedtime routines.

Introduction

What do we mean by healthy sleep? How is that conceptualized? When we think about healthy sleep for children, we consider safety, sleep duration, timing, consistency, and factors that may disrupt sleep. Many biologic and cultural factors impact which sleep habits are considered healthy. Sleep duration is very important for children's well-being. Insufficient and poor quality sleep have been associated with significant physical and psychologic consequences including obesity, diabetes, injuries, depression, behavioral problems, and impairments in academic performance.[1-6]

The American Academy of Sleep Medicine (AASM) has recommended that children aged 6–12 years should regularly sleep 9–12 hours per 24 hours and teens aged 13–18 years should sleep 8–10 hours per 24 hours.[7] However, many U.S. children do not get an appropriate amount of sleep. For instance, one of the U.S. population-based reports based on self-reported sleep duration conducted by the Centers for Disease Control and Prevention (CDC) in 2016 suggested that approximately 58% of middle schoolers and 73% of high school students do not get the recommended amount of sleep each night.[7,8] Sleep duration was defined as <9 hours for students aged 6–12 years and <8 hours for those aged 13–18 years based on the previously published AASM

consensus statement.[7] Furthermore, parents often do not realize that their children are getting inadequate amounts of sleep[9,10] and may be unaware of the signs and potential consequences of poor sleep for their children.[11] Numerous factors impact insufficient sleep including increased use of screen time, mismatch between sleep schedules and school start times, overly scheduled evenings, caffeine consumption, and poor sleep habits. The reasons for sleep improvement with implementation of healthy sleep practices is still not completely understood. Some researchers speculate that healthy sleep practices enhance sleep regulation, synchronize the circadian clock, and create behavioral sleep conditioning.[10] Because better sleep education and sleep habits can have a significant impact on children's sleep duration and quality of life, health care providers should be engaged in early sleep health education and identification of knowledge gaps. This process should ideally start with prenatal parental education and continue throughout childhood.

Building Safe Sleep Practices

Bringing home a new baby is often an exciting, but scary time for new parents. Newborns and infants are growing and developing at a rapid pace, and their sleep is no different. Healthy sleep habits often start at the very beginning, with safe sleep practices in infancy.

Newborn safety has been researched extensively because of the risk of sudden infant death syndrome (SIDS) and other sleep-related deaths. Safety alerts from the Consumer Product Safety Commission (CPSC) in the 1990s raised concerns of bed-sharing and SIDS.[12-14] The American Academy of Pediatrics (AAP) recommendations are focused on a safe sleep environment with the goal to reduce the risk of all sleep-related infant deaths.[15] These recommendations include that infants should room-share for the first 6–12 months, sleeping on a firm surface in the supine position that is free from objects other than a fitted sheet. The AAP does not recommend bed-sharing or use of commercial devices that are not approved for sleep. At this time, an approved sleep device includes a "crib, bassinet, portable crib, or play yard that conforms to the safety standards of the Consumer Product Safety Commission (CPSC)."[15] See Table 6.1 for a complete list of recommendations.

Historically, many parents placed their newborns in their own bed. Bed-sharing refers to a sleeping arrangement in which an infant shares the same sleeping surface with another person. In contrast, co-sleeping refers to a sleeping arrangement in which a child is within arm's reach of their

TABLE 6.1 Summary of Recommendations with Strength of Recommendation[15]

A-Level Recommendations

Back to sleep for every sleep.

Use a firm sleep surface.

Breastfeeding is recommended.

Room-sharing with the infant on a separate sleep surface is recommended.

Keep soft objects and loose bedding away from the infant's sleep area.

Consider offering a pacifier at naptime and bedtime.

Avoid smoke exposure during pregnancy and after birth.

Avoid alcohol and illicit drug use during pregnancy and after birth.

Avoid overheating.

Pregnant women should seek and obtain regular prenatal care.

Infants should be immunized in accordance with AAP and CDC recommendations.

Do not use home cardiorespiratory monitors as a strategy to reduce the risk of SIDS.

Health care providers, staff in newborn nurseries and NICUs, and childcare providers should endorse and model the SIDS risk-reduction recommendations from birth.

Media and manufacturers should follow safe sleep guidelines in their messaging and advertising.

Continue the "Safe to Sleep" campaign, focusing on ways to reduce the risk of all sleep-related infant deaths, including SIDS, suffocation, and other unintentional deaths.

Pediatricians and other primary care providers should actively participate in this campaign.

B-Level Recommendations

Avoid the use of commercial devices that are inconsistent with safe sleep recommendations. Supervised, awake tummy time is recommended to facilitate development and to minimize development of positional plagiocephaly.

C-Level Recommendations

Continue research and surveillance on the risk factors, causes, and pathophysiologic mechanisms of SIDS and other sleep-related infant deaths, with the ultimate goal of eliminating these deaths entirely.

There is no evidence to recommend swaddling as a strategy to reduce the risk of SIDS.

Abbreviations: AAP, American Academy of Pediatrics; CDC, Centers for Disease Control and Prevention; SIDS, sudden infant death syndrome; NICU, neonatal intensive care unit.

mother, but not on the same sleeping surface. Thus, sleeping in the same room (i.e., room-sharing), but not in the same bed, is considered co-sleeping. Bed-sharing may make it easier to monitor an infant and keep it safe and breastfeed. Some parents love the idea of sleeping near their baby and others may have no other options due to socioeconomic factors. Bed-sharing is still prevalent in many unindustrialized cultures.[16] In the United States, room-sharing is recommended whereas bed-sharing is discouraged due to concerns of SIDS. Despite these recommendations, bed-sharing rates in the United States have risen over the past two decades.[17,18] It is more common among Black, Hispanic, and Asian infants than for non-Hispanic White infants. One study found rates of bed-sharing as high as 88%.[19] Possible reasons include breastfeeding, attachment and bonding facilitation, and cultural preferences. Acknowledging that parents do not always follow safe sleep recommendations, the AAP Task Force added bed-sharing modifications to their 2016 update and encouraged practitioners to have open conversations with caregivers about risk reduction.[15]

Understanding the family beliefs and the reasons for choosing a particular sleep environment should be taken into account. Parental education and review of AAP recommendations may improve parental understanding of infants' sleep safety. However, we can also try to provide support to the families who have to practice bed-sharing and adjust AAP recommendations to reduce the risk of a sudden unexpected infant death to the best of our ability. For instance, reviewing appropriate conditions such as breastfeeding, non-smoking, positioning infant supine on a firm mattress with no pillows or comforters, taking measures to make sure the infant cannot fall off the bed or get caught in bed gaps, temperature control, use of pacifier, and avoidance of alcohol exposure. During this time period, the child's primary care provider will serve as an important figure in providing parental guidance and education regarding safe sleep practices.

Adequate Sleep Duration

As children age, sleep duration becomes an important part of healthy sleep practices. Guidelines for sleep duration for each age group were developed by a panel of experts based on an extensive review of current research to date (Table 6.2).

TABLE 6.2 Sleep Duration Recommendations[7]

Age	Recommended Hours of Sleep
4–12 months	12–16 (including naps)
1–2 years	11–14 (including naps)
3–5 years	10–13 (including naps)
6–12 years	9–12
13–18 years	8–10

Adequate Duration

There are ranges of sleep recommended for each age as individual variability in sleep needs is influenced by many factors, including, but not limited to, genetic, medical, and environmental differences. Due to significant variability in duration and sleep patterns, no guidelines were provided for infants <4 months of age.[7] Research suggested that children and adolescents are getting significantly less sleep than recommended based on the previously mentioned guidelines.[7] The 2014 National Sleep Foundation, Sleep in America Poll, used a probability-based poll to sample 1,103 parents of children ages 6–17 aimed to represent the U.S. population. Parents reported their children ages 6–10 were receiving an average of 8.9 hours of sleep per night, well below the average number of hours recommended. The same is true across older children and adolescents, with parents estimating that 11- and 12-year-old children sleep an average of 8.2 hours per night, 13- to 14-year-olds sleep an average of 7.7 hours, and adolescents 15–17 sleep an average of 7.1 hours per night.[20] In particular, minority children are two to three times more likely to have inadequate sleep duration. Moreover, even though 97% of parents reported that they thought sleep was "very" or "extremely" important to their child's health/well-being, parents underestimated the number of hours of sleep their children needed each night with almost half of parents estimating their child or adolescent only needed 8 hours of sleep or less to function at their best.[20] One study, focusing on parental knowledge of sleep in youngsters between 3 months and 12 years of age, demonstrated large gaps in parental education regarding their children's sleep needs. In this study, more than half of parents believed that inadequate sleep increases the risk of being underweight and endorsed snoring as a sign of healthy sleep.[10]

Primary care providers and educators play an essential role in providing parental education; however, they may also lack both awareness and knowledge of the impact of sleep disturbances on the child's health. One study revealed the overall mean sleep knowledge test score of primary care physicians was 34%.[21]

Bedtime Routines and Sleep-Onset Associations

Bedtime routines have been defined as observable, predictable, and repetitive behaviors that occur daily in approximately the hour prior to the child falling asleep.[22,23] Use of a consistent, calming bedtime routine prior to sleep onset has been associated with numerous positive outcomes in children and their caregivers including, but not limited to, increased sleep duration among children, reduced nighttime awakenings, decreased bedtime resistance and sleep-onset latency, and improved perceptions of caregiver sleep.[23] Moreover, regular bedtime routines have been associated more broadly with child emotion and behavior regulation.

The goal of a healthy bedtime routine is to help children and adolescents transition from wakefulness to sleep. This is achieved by developing a routine that helps children to wind down, both because they associate their routine with the transition to sleep and because the activities aim to help children calm down and relax. Many activities may be included in a bedtime routine, such as taking a bath, brushing teeth, changing into pajamas, reading a book, singing a song, and sharing highlights from the day. The same routine does not work for all children and their families and it is important to learn which activities are most relaxing for each child. This is also important for children with autism spectrum disorders (ASDs). For example, some children with ASD or sensory disorders may be stimulated by bathing or taking a shower prior to bed. This may lead to greater difficulties falling asleep. Deep pressure, massage, rubbing on lotion, wearing weighted suspenders or vest, and/or swinging may be more appropriate and calming. The strategy can vary from child to child and may need to be adjusted according to the child's developmental stage and needs.[24] However, order and consistency among caregivers are very important.

There is a great variability in bedtime routine among families. Caregivers' work schedules, amount of homework, over-scheduling of activities, or late-ending social events or late evening extracurricular activities may culminate in delayed bedtime, shortened bedtime routine time (or absence of such), and subsequent shorter sleep time. Maladaptive bedtime routine activities may also include consumption of caffeine and activities that stimulate children, such as running or climbing, as well as, use of electronics prior to bedtime. These activities have been associated with poor and insufficient sleep as well as psychosocial and physical concerns.[23] In addition, caregiver presence at bedtime and related activities, such as feeding to sleep, have been associated with poor sleep continuity. Children learn to associate these caregivers or props with the ability to fall asleep. When they awaken in the middle of the night, they are unable to resume sleep unless their caregiver or sleep prop is present. In pediatric sleep medicine practice, children frequently present for evaluation of nocturnal awakenings. In fact, the frequency of night awakenings is one of the main factors by which parents judge the quality of their child's sleep.[25] During evaluation, it is not uncommon to uncover a history of sleep-onset association with bottle feeding or nursing, parental presence, rocking the child to sleep, or TV/screen time.

Advocates of reading to children demonstrated that daily reading aloud to or with children has positive impacts on early literacy skills, including language and cognitive development.[23] Bedtime routines that included reading, storytelling, or singing to children at bedtime at 3 years of age were associated with higher receptive vocabulary and overall language abilities at 5 years of age.[26] Additionally, having a language-based activity in the bedtime routine was associated with increased nighttime sleep duration in preschool-age children.[26] It is possible that this association may not be entirely related to the act of reading or singing itself, but rather, that parents who utilize language-based routines may engage in fewer maladaptive routines at bedtime (e.g., use of electronic devices).[23]

Contributing Factors

Definitions of healthy sleep habits are driven, at least in part, by cultural norms and expectations for parents and children. Many aspects of childhood sleep that are considered problematic by some are based on culture expectations for sleep behaviors. Factors that may be influenced by both biology and cultural expectations include, but are not limited to, sleep timing, duration, where and with whom we sleep, and sleep routines. How well an individual child's sleep behaviors, based on biology and development, match the cultural expectations for sleep determine whether or not a specific sleep behavior is considered problematic.[27] For instance, in some cultures, bed-sharing is the norm whereas other cultures pride themselves on teaching children to sleep independently. Although across cultures there is consensus that getting enough, and good quality, restorative sleep are important for health and development, the perception of healthy sleep practices may vary across the world.

Electronic devices have become commonplace in the lives of children and adolescents. It is estimated that, in the United States, children and adolescents are using some form of electronic device approximately 7 hours a day.[26,28] Results of the Sleep in America Poll[20] suggested that 72% of children and 89% of adolescents have at least 1 device in their bedroom. Moreover, many children and adolescents use their devices before and after bedtime, with one study estimating that 37% of adolescents texted after turning off the lights.[29] Research suggests that use of television and electronics contributes not only to reduced sleep duration, but also to poor sleep quality.[30] Watching television at bedtime has been associated with 30 minutes less total sleep time in children. Moreover, this television use has health consequences and has been associated with increased risk for obesity.[1,4,6,30]

Several ideas and theories have been proposed to explain the potential relationship between electronic media usage and sleep. These include that technology may interfere with sleep because sleep time is replaced by electronics use. Alternately, the alerting and arousing nature of electronics may interfere with drowsiness or the light emitted from the device may lead to delays in the body's natural circadian rhythm and may also cause activation in the moment. Moreover, use of electronic devices in bed or in the bedroom may reduce the association between bed and sleep.[31] The AAP issued new guidelines in 2016 that recommended limiting screen time to 1 hour a day of high-quality programs for kids 2–5 years of age and consistent limits on screen time for kids ages 6 and older.[32] However, despite AAP recommendations many children still are using screens for extended periods of time, especially during COVID-19 quarantine.

There are many other contributing factors that may disrupt healthy sleep including delayed phase sleep of adolescence, school start times, and chronic medical conditions. These topics, including expanded impact of technology on sleep, will be discussed in further chapters.

Thankfully, we know that brief parental education regarding healthy sleep habits can make a significant impact in parental knowledge and motivation to change sleep habits (Jones et al., 2013). Improvements in child sleep have been associated with parental functioning, including mood and stress management. This suggests the importance of establishing a consistent routine that allows them to feel empowered and helps the child to develop healthy sleep habits.[34]

CLINICAL PEARLS

- Research suggests that parents value sleep for their children, but lack knowledge about what this means and how to achieve healthy sleep practices.
- Health care providers can bridge this gap by providing education to families about safe sleep practices, average sleep duration as children grow, impacts of screen time on sleep, and the importance of limiting caffeine
- Establishing a sleep environment that is separate from daytime activities and routine that helps children to relax as transition to bed can reduce time to fall asleep and nocturnal awakenings and increase total sleep duration.
- Changes to sleep practices are best achieved when recommendations align with family values and goals and match the child's unique developmental needs.

Summary

Learning about healthy sleep habits should be an essential part of child and parental education. This can be delivered in the form of prenatal education including school-based educational programs, webinars, seminars, small class teachings, telephone follow-up after routine checkups with pediatric providers including nurses, booklets and sleep education websites, and direct discussion during well-child visits. This may have a significant impact on improving behaviors and psychologic health, as well as, healthy sleep practice in children.

In addition, sleep medicine education should be incorporated in training of primary care providers, school educators, and school curriculums. Primary care providers should start educating the families regarding healthy sleep habits during the very first visit and continue this process at every well-child visit. A number of questionnaires (i.e., Bedtime issues excessive daytime sleepiness night awakenings regularity and duration of sleep snoring [BEARS], Children's Sleep Habits Questionnaire, Sleep Disturbance Scale for Children, Sleep Self Report) are available to determine whether the child has sleep difficulties that may be at least partially related to poor sleep habits.

References

1. Chen X, Beydoun MA, Wang Y. Is sleep duration associated with childhood obesity? A systematic review and meta-analysis. *Obesity (Silver Spring)*. 2008;16(2):265–274. https://doi.org/10.1038/oby.2007.63.

2. Fitzgerald CT, Messias E, Buysse DJ. Teen sleep and suicidality: Results from the youth risk behavior surveys of 2007 and 2009. *J Clin Sleep Med*. 2011;7(4):351–356. https://doi.org/10.5664/JCSM.1188.

3. Lowry R, Eaton DK, Foti K, McKnight-Eily L, Perry G, Galuska DA. Association of sleep duration with obesity among US high school students. *J Obes*. 2012;2012:476914. https://doi.org/10.1155/2012/476914.

4. Magee L, Hale L. Longitudinal associations between sleep duration and subsequent weight gain: a systematic review. *Sleep Med Rev*. 2012;16(3):231–241. https://doi.org/10.1016/j.smrv.2011.05.005.

5. Owens J. Adolescent Sleep Working Group, Committee on Adolescence. Insufficient sleep in adolescents and young adults: An update on causes and consequences. *Pediatrics*. 2014;134(3):e921–e932. https://doi.org/10.1542/peds.2014-1696.

6. Patel SR, Hu FB. Short sleep duration and weight gain: A systematic review. *Obesity (Silver Spring)*. 2008;16(3):643–653. https://doi.org/10.1038/oby.2007.118.

7. Paruthi S, Brooks LJ, D'Ambrosio C, Hall WA, Kotagal S, Lloyd RM, Wise MS. Consensus Statement of the American Academy of Sleep Medicine on the Recommended Amount of Sleep for Healthy Children: Methodology and Discussion. *J Clin Sleep Med*. 2016;12(11):1549–1561. https://doi.org/10.5664/jcsm.6288.

8. Wheaton AG, Jones SE, Cooper AC, Croft JB. Short sleep duration among middle school and high school students – United States, 2015. *MMWR Morb Mortal Wkly Rep*. 2018;67(3):85–90. https://doi.org/10.15585/mmwr.mm6703a1.

9. Carskadon M, Mindell J, Drake C. Contemporary sleep patterns of adolescents in the USA: Results of the 2006 National Sleep Foundation Sleep in America poll. *J Sleep Res*. 2006;15:42.

10. Owens JA, Jones C. Parental knowledge of healthy sleep in young children: Results of a primary care clinic survey. *J Dev Behav Pediatr*. 2011;32(6):447–453. https://doi.org/10.1097/DBP.0b013e31821bd20b.

11. Owens J.A., Spirito A., McGuinn M., Nobile C. Sleep habits and sleep disturbance in elementary school-aged children. *J Dev Behav Pediatr*. 200;21(1), 27–36. doi:10.1097/00004703-200002000-00005

12. United States Consumer Product Safety Commission. CPSC warns against placing babies in adult beds; study finds 64 deaths each year from strangulation and suffocation. News from CPSC. Release #99-175; 1999a.

13. United States Consumer Product Safety Commission. Soft bedding may be hazardous to babies. Release #99-09; 1999b.

14. Nakamura S, Wind M, Danello MA. Review of hazards associated with children placed in adult beds. *Arch Pediatr Adolesc Med*. 1999;153(10):1019–1023. https://doi.org/10.1001/archpedi.153.10.1019.

15. SIDS and Other Sleep-Related Infant Deaths Updated 2016 Recommendations for a Safe Infant Sleeping Environment. *Pediatrics*. 2016;138(5): https://doi.org/10.1542/peds.2016-2938. e20162938.

16. Nelson EA, Taylor BJ, Jenik A, Vance J, Walmsley K, Pollard K, Nepomyashchaya V. International Child Care Practices Study: Infant sleeping environment. *Early Hum Dev*. 2001;62(1):43–55. https://doi.org/10.1016/s0378-3782(01)00116-5.

17. Colson ER, Willinger M, Rybin D, Heeren T, Smith LA, Lister G, Corwin MJ. Trends and factors associated with infant bed sharing, 1993–2010: The National Infant Sleep Position Study. *JAMA Pediatr*. 2013;167(11):1032–1037. https://doi.org/10.1001/jamapediatrics.2013.2560.

18. Willinger M, Ko CW, Hoffman HJ, Kessler RC, Corwin MJ. National Infant Sleep Position. Trends in infant bed sharing in the United States, 1993–2000: The National Infant Sleep Position study. *Arch Pediatr Adolesc Med*. 2003;157(1):43–49. https://doi.org/10.1001/archpedi.157.1.43.

19. Weimer SM, Dise TL, Evers PB, Ortiz MA, Welldaregay W, Steinmann WC. Prevalence, predictors, and attitudes toward cosleeping in an urban pediatric center. *Clin Pediatr (Phila)*. 2002;41(6):433–438. https://doi.org/10.1177/000992280204100609.

20. Appold K. Time for bed? America's kids aren't getting enough sleep: The national sleep foundation's 2014 poll found that children are getting less-than-recommended sleep, but parents can play a powerful role in establishing good sleep habits for their kids. *RT for Decision Makers in Respiratory Care*. 2014;27(5):24.

21. Papp KK, Penrod CE, Strohl KP. Knowledge and attitudes of primary care physicians toward sleep and sleep disorders. *Sleep Breath*. 2002;6(3):103–109. https://doi.org/10.1007/s11325-002-0103-3.

22. Mindell JA, Li AM, Sadeh A, Kwon R, Goh DY. Bedtime routines for young children: A dose-dependent association with sleep outcomes. *Sleep*. 2015;38(5):717–722. https://doi.org/10.5665/sleep.4662.

23. Mindell JA, Williamson AA. Benefits of a bedtime routine in young children: Sleep, development, and beyond. *Sleep Med Rev*. 2018;40:93–108. https://doi.org/10.1016/j.smrv.2017.10.007.

24. Malow BA, Adkins KW, Reynolds A, Weiss SK, Loh A, Fawkes D, Clemons T. Parent-based sleep education for children with autism spectrum disorders. *J Autism Dev Disord*. 2014;44(1):216–228. https://doi.org/10.1007/s10803-013-1866-z.

25. Palmstierna P, Sepa A, Ludvigsson J. Parent perceptions of child sleep: a study of 10,000 Swedish children. *Acta Paediatr*. 2008;97(12):1631–1639. https://doi.org/10.1111/j.1651-2227.2008.00967.x.

26. Hale L, Guan S. Screen time and sleep among school-aged children and adolescents: A systematic literature review. *Sleep Med Rev*. 2015;21:50–58. https://doi.org/10.1016/j.smrv.2014.07.007.

27. Jenni OG, O'Connor BB. Children's sleep: An interplay between culture and biology. *Pediatrics*. 2005;115(1 Suppl):204–216. https://doi.org/10.1542/peds.2004-0815B.

28. Council on Communications and Media, Strasburger VC Children, adolescents, obesity, and the media. *Pediatrics*. 2011;128(1):201–208. 10.1542/peds.2011–1066.

29. Adachi-Mejia AM, Edwards PM, Gilbert-Diamond D, Greenough GP, Olson AL. TXT me I'm only sleeping: Adolescents with mobile phones in their bedroom. *Fam Community Health*. 2014;37(4):252–257. https://doi.org/10.1097/FCH.0000000000000044.

30. Fuller C, Lehman E, Hicks S, Novick MB. Bedtime use of technology and associated sleep problems in children. *Glob Pediatr Health*. 2017;4 https://doi.org/10.1177/2333794X17736972.2333794X17736972.

31. Hysing M. Review: Recommendations for the assessment and management of sleep disorders in ADHD. *Evid Based Ment Health*. 2014;17(1):22. https://doi.org/10.1136/eb-2013-101560.

32. Council on Communications and Media Media and young minds. *Pediatrics*. 2016;138(5): https://doi.org/10.1542/peds.2016-2591. e20162591.

33. Jones CH, Owens JA, Pham B Can a brief educational intervention improve parents' knowledge of healthy children's sleep? A pilot-test. Health Educ J. 2013;72(5):601–610. https://doi.org/10.1177/0017896912464606

34. Mindell JA, Telofski LS, Wiegand B, Kurtz ES. A nightly bedtime routine: Impact on sleep in young children and maternal mood. *Sleep*. 2009;32(5):599–606. https://doi.org/10.1093/sleep/32.5.599.

PART II

Diagnosis

7

Taking a Sleep History

Stephen H. Sheldon

CHAPTER HIGHLIGHTS

- Clinical evaluation of the pediatric and adolescent patient is crucial for assessing and managing sleep and its disorders in the pediatric population.
- The clinical history is the main means of diagnosis and management.
- The process of developing a differential diagnosis in pediatric sleep medicine involves perceiving the patient situation, perceiving particular cues, and generating hypotheses.
- Historical details such as bedtime, sleep latency, habitual time of morning waking, sleep continuity, excessive daytime sleepiness, parasomnias, restless sleep, enuresis, and snoring are important factors to consider in the evaluation of sleep disorders in children.
- The physical examination must be comprehensive and include an extensive neuro-developmental evaluatio.

Introduction

Clinical evaluation is the most important part of the process of assessment and diagnosis of sleep and its disorders in the pediatric and adolescent patient. Next in importance comes the physical examination. Laboratory assessment may be valuable as well, though it is not always necessary. Careful and vigilant assessment and management of disordered sleep and alertness has the ability to foster appropriate physiologic development, promote sleep health, improve quality of life, improve performance, decrease accidents and injuries, facilitate recovery from other medical disorders, and prevent sequelae. Sleep-related symptoms are common in the pediatric patient. Comprehensive sleep history, physical examination with detailed examination of the head and neck, and judicious use of sleep-specific questionnaires guide decisions to diagnostic and therapeutic closure. This may also provide a guide to the decision to pursue additional diagnostic testing.[1] In adult-oriented care, information given by the patient should, when possible, be supplemented by a bed partner, family member, or roommate. Most often in the pediatric patient, the majority of historical information is provided by a parent and/or caretaker, with supplemental information provided by the patient. Therefore obtaining

a sleep history is frequently more difficult in evaluation of the pediatric patient, relying on secondhand information, often from a parent/caretaker who may have been asleep when the majority of nocturnal symptoms first appear.

Developing a Differential Diagnosis: Process of Solving Clinical Problems

Hypotheses form the basis of inquiry into patients' presenting problems. They are generated very early in the assessment, are then refined by completing the clinical history, and by performing a physical examination. The set of hypotheses is then further refined into an actual diagnosis or a list of possible (differential) diagnoses.[2] Laboratory testing may be needed when the history and physical examination alone do not lead to a final diagnosis.

Evaluation of the Clinical History

The abilities for establishing an appropriate initial hypothesis set and to subsequently test it by clinical inquiry require a wide knowledge base. Understanding of the pathophysiology, natural history, clinical manifestations, and patterns of symptom presentation for the various disorders is essential if one is to make an accurate diagnosis.

Sleep disturbances in children are common. When a sleepless child frequently disturbs parents during the night, parents will generally be quick to seek medical attention (especially when the child's sleep problems lead to symptoms of sleep deprivation in the parents). Similarly, profoundly sleepy children may reach the sleep professional early on (particularly if the child is falling asleep at inappropriate times such as during meals, while talking on the phone, or when opening presents at a birthday party). On the other hand, the child who is only mildly sleepy may not reach appropriate professional care until late in the course of the disorder because the symptoms of less than profound sleepiness are easy to miss. A youngster in a state of hypo-arousal may have symptoms considerably different than those of a sleepy adult. Thus, instead of overt sleepiness, sleepy children may present with hyperactivity, distractibility, attention difficulties, mood swings, increased frustration, and learning problems. These symptoms are too often inadequately addressed, usually with behavioral interventions with only limited consideration of the possibility of a sleep disorder. This is unfortunate, as screening for sleep problems generally does not take very long to perform.

In one study of 202 children who presented consecutively to a developmental and behavioral pediatric practice, parents and other primary caretakers were found to only infrequently report that the child under their care had a sleep problem, even when symptoms suggesting a sleep disorder were present.[3] Simply asking the parent the single question, "Does your child have a sleep problem?" is inadequate to determine the presence or absence of problematic sleep.

A sleep history obtained from a frustrated, sleepy parent can be vague and inaccurate, with the parent focusing, at times, on the wrong details. For example, parents often describe the child's sleep pattern only for the most severe or most recent night or period. A more accurate depiction of the sleep patterns across time can be obtained from a sleep diary, log, or chart. For this reason, the parent can be asked to maintain a sleep chart or log for a period of 2–4 weeks prior to the first visit (and then again during treatment). This item then becomes very helpful in identifying habitual sleep–wake cycle patterns and provides documentation of abnormalities occurring from night to night.[3] Maintaining a sleep log seems to improve observational skills of the child's caretaker, increases validity of observational data, and can be indirectly therapeutic. Parents might see on paper what actually happened most nights. Sleep disorder professionals might find review of such documents useful to clarify the actual pattern of what is happening and such review might well be the most accurate way of documenting progress.

It is important to begin with a screening process that might provide insight or cues to the practitioner that a problem requiring further consideration might be present. A structured approach to screening the history has been tested and validated.[4] An important first step is obtaining information regarding the typical/habitual sleep patterns and difficulties. A number of screening tools have been developed to assist the child health care practitioner in assessing for sleep-related disorders and have been comprehensively reviewed by Spruyt and Gozal.[5] These authors, however, concluded that very few of these tools fulfill all the necessary properties required, and only a few are standardized. None of the tools had any diagnostic power in and of themselves; thus making the diagnosis remains in the domain of the clinician. One questionnaire, the *BEARS* Screening Tool developed by Owens and Dalzell, had particular usefulness in the primary care setting as well as in the sleep medicine center.[6] It has questions regarding *b*edtime, *e*xcessive daytime sleepiness, *a*wakenings at night, *r*egularity/duration, and *s*noring, the answers to which suggest a series of possible diagnoses (Figs. 7.1–7.5).

Components of the Sleep History[1]

Before delving into the specifics of the sleep history it is useful to obtain details of the child's birth (obstetrical history of the mother, details of the pregnancy and delivery of the patient), whether congenital disorders were present; motor and cognitive development, school performance, medical history, orthodontic history, and relevant family medical history.

Obtaining the sleep history begins with a description of onset, severity, frequency, duration, and possible events surrounding the presenting sleep-related symptoms. This begins the process of hypotheses generation and testing these hypotheses by focused questioning with searching inquiry design. Inquiry design is dependent upon following appropriate problem-solving skills.

Associated *nocturnal symptoms* evolve from complaints including but not limited to sleep-related breathing disorders, sleep-related enuresis, nocturnal behaviors and motor activity (including description of behaviors), nighttime wakings, and other symptoms such as leg discomfort, restless sleep, hypnagogic and hypnopompic hallucination, nocturnal eating, and sleep paralysis. *Time of onset of symptoms* assists in a general assessment of the stage of sleep (or state transitions) within which symptoms occur or are most prevalent.

Daytime symptoms should also be assessed including but not limited to excessive daytime sleepiness, learning difficulties in school, hyperactivity, attention/concentration problems, mood disturbances, irritability, leg discomfort/growing pains, frequent morning headaches, difficulty moving in the morning, use of sleep aids (over the counter and prescription), utilization of other medications, and caffeine intake. *Assessment of the habitual sleep schedule* on school days, weekends, and holidays/vacations is very important in assessment of biologic rhythms and symptoms resulting from sleep deprivation. An evaluation of sleep health practices can provide important information regarding inappropriate sleep hygiene, unrealistic parental expectations, and environmental practices that may promote and/or unsuitably affect sleep. Finally, maintenance of a sleep diary or log can provide very useful longitudinal information, rather than cross-sectional data. Anecdotal data suggest parents will often describe what happened the night before presentation to the practitioner, or the worst night they have experienced. Yet, longitudinally, symptoms may deviate from these descriptions.

Bedtime

Knowledge of what parents believe is an appropriate bedtime and length of expected sleep can provide insight into the reasons for the problem sleep. For example, a 9-year-old child whose bedtime is 7:30 p.m. and whose scheduled waking is 7:00 a.m. most likely will be in bed too early (at a time when his or her circadian rhythm may not permit easy settling) and in bed too long (*inappropriate caretaker expectation*). On the other hand, knowledge that a child

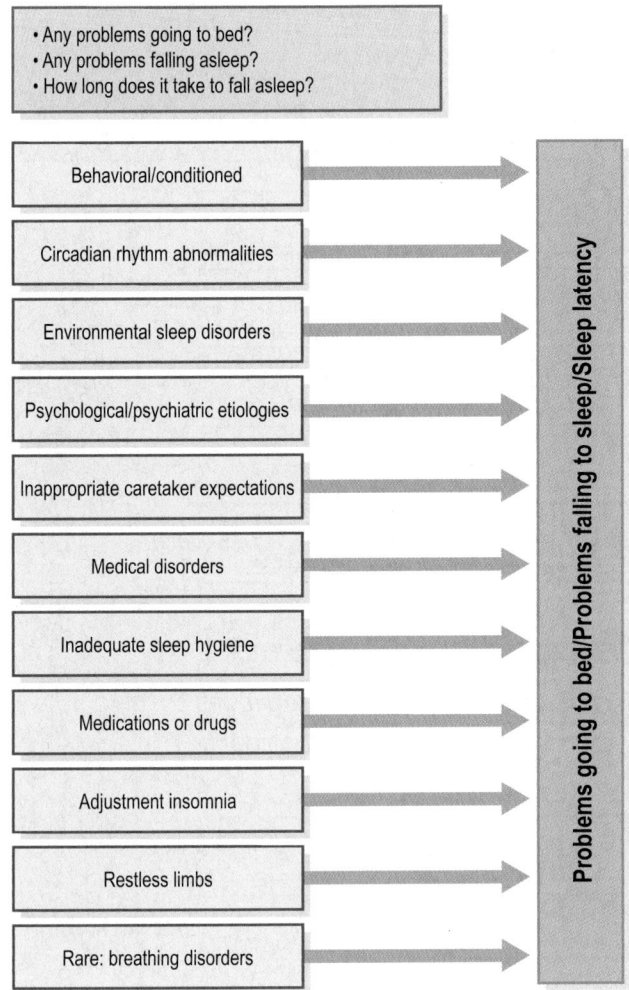

• **Fig. 7.1** Bedtime. (Adapted from Owens JA, Dalzell V. *Sleep Med.* 2005.)

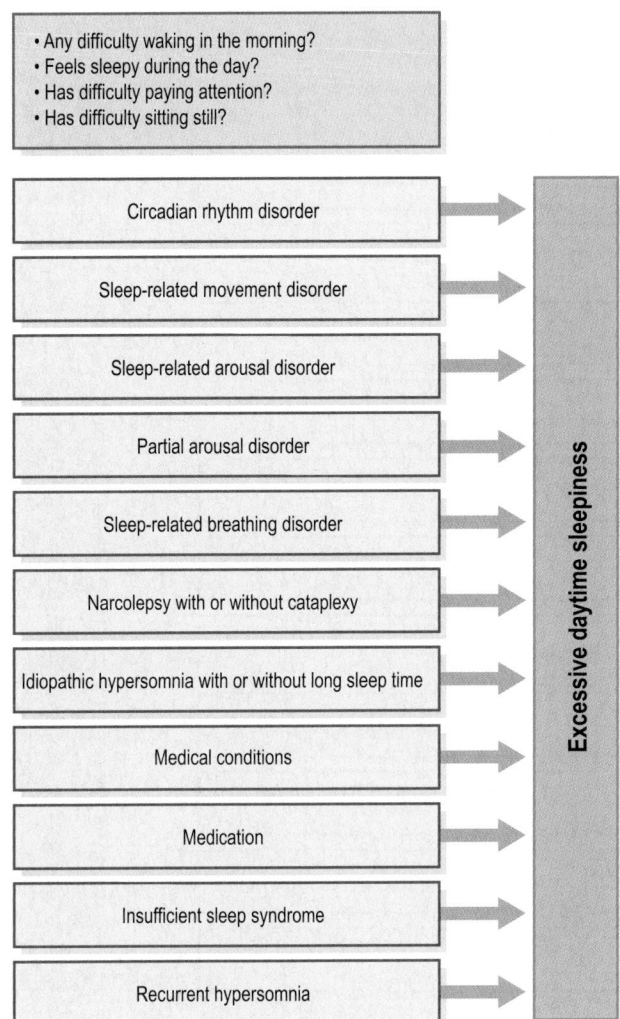

• **Fig. 7.2** Excessive daytime sleepiness. (Adapted from Owens JA, Dalzell V. *Sleep Med.* 2005.)

both falls asleep and wakes early (7:30 p.m. and 5:00 a.m.) suggests a circadian rhythm disorder might be present (*advanced sleep phase*). Similarly, a 2-year-old child whose bedtime is at 1:00 a.m. (because of the parents' work schedules) and who then wakes at 11:00 a.m. (and is difficult to wake earlier) may have a *delayed sleep phase* that, at least on weekdays when earlier wakings are necessary, can lead to a syndrome of *insufficient sleep* and profound daytime problems.

Sleep Latency

Sleep latency can provide information regarding the ease and speed of settling at night. This information, combined with the knowledge of habitual bedtime, can help in determination of the presence of behavioral, circadian, psychologic, and medical sleep-onset difficulties (*behavioral insomnia of childhood, sleep-onset association disorder, limit-setting sleep disorder, delayed or advanced sleep phase, anxiety-related sleep disorders, and restless limb syndrome*).

The history that the youngster can fall asleep easily and without difficulty when at the grandparent's house, or in the parents' bed, or on the sofa, or in front of the television strongly suggests a behavioral/conditioned etiology or anxiety rather than an organic cause for the sleeplessness because, when the cause of a child's sleeplessness is medically based, a child typically has difficulty falling asleep anywhere and under any circumstances. Also, when the cause is anxiety, the child usually has difficulty falling asleep in a room alone. Prolongation of the sleep latency must be assessed in conjunction with knowledge of bedtime for accurate interpretation. For example, a 4-hour sleep latency in a 9-year-old child has different meaning when the bedtime is 7:00 p.m. (which may be too early) than when it is 10:00 p.m.

Habitual Time of Morning Waking

Time of habitual morning waking helps determine total nocturnal sleep time and provides information as to circadian phase. Determination of whether morning waking

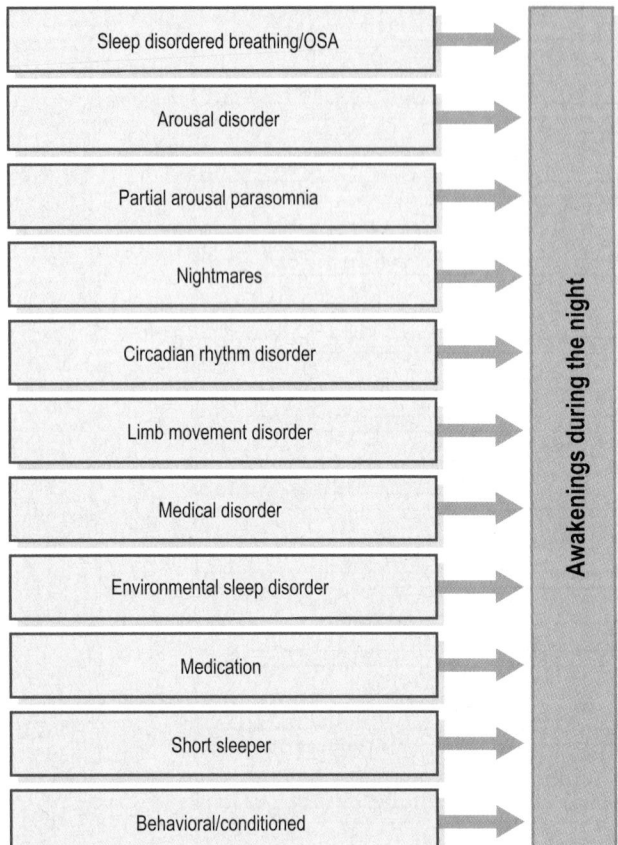

• **Fig. 7.3** Awakenings. OSA, obstructive sleep apnea. (Adapted from Owens JA, Dalzell V. *Sleep Med*. 2005.)

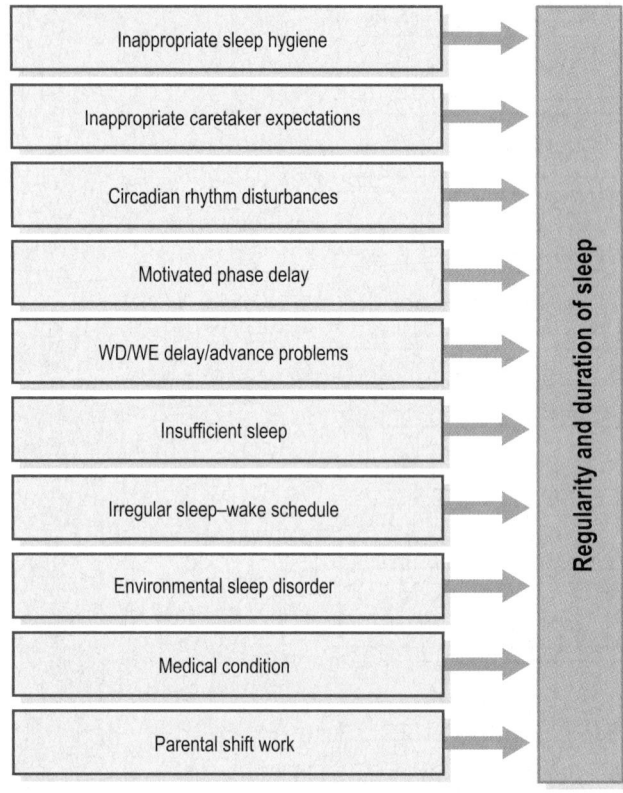

• **Fig. 7.4** Regularity and duration of sleep. WD, weekdays; WE, weekends. (Adapted from Owens JA, Dalzell V. *Sleep Med*. 2005.)

is spontaneous or induced is also important. The times of morning waking are also powerful contributors to circadian rhythm entrainment; if the times are inconsistent, *sleep–wake schedule abnormality* might be suggested.

It is important to determine the times of waking on weekends and holidays in addition to on weekdays (school days). Late sleep offset on weekends and holidays might suggest a *delayed sleep phase*. When wake-up times are variable, a *non–24-hour sleep–wake schedule* might be suspected, especially in a youngster with severe neurologic abnormalities.

Sleep Continuity

Sleep continuity problems may occur as isolated symptoms or in association with sleep-onset difficulties. Determination of timing, frequency, length, and characteristics of, and parental responses to, nocturnal wakings provides information regarding possible behavioral, circadian/schedule-related, and physiologic (medical) causes. Sleep-onset difficulties accompanied by sleep continuity

problems in the absence of physiologic abnormalities suggest the presence of *behavioral, schedule-related*, or *psychologic* etiologies that should be pursued by careful history. *Limit-setting problems* and insufficient parental tolerance are sometimes easy to detect when similar findings exist during the day. A history of wakings that are short only and whenever specific parental interventions are initiated (rocking, pacifier, feeding) may suggest (if not diagnose) the actual problem (*sleep-onset association disorders* or *excessive nocturnal feedings*).

Excessive Daytime Sleepiness

Determination of the presence of daytime sleepiness is vitally important. It can be difficult to determine the presence of excessive sleepiness in young infants, toddlers, and young children in whom daytime sleep is normal as expected. Total sleep times range from about 16–18 hours in the newborn to about 9–10 hours by late childhood. There is a gradual decline in total sleep time as the child matures.

By about 12 weeks of age (if not before) circadian rhythmicity of the sleep–wake cycle begins to be clear,

- Does the patient snore more than three nights per week?
- Are there pauses, snorts, gasps, or choking?
- Does the child breathe through her/his mouth?
- Does the child wake with headaches?
- Does the child wet the bed?
- Are there reported witnessed apneas?
- Is there sleep-related diaphoresis?
- Is/are there daytime sleepiness/hyperactivity/attention problems?
- Does the child wake with a dry mouth?

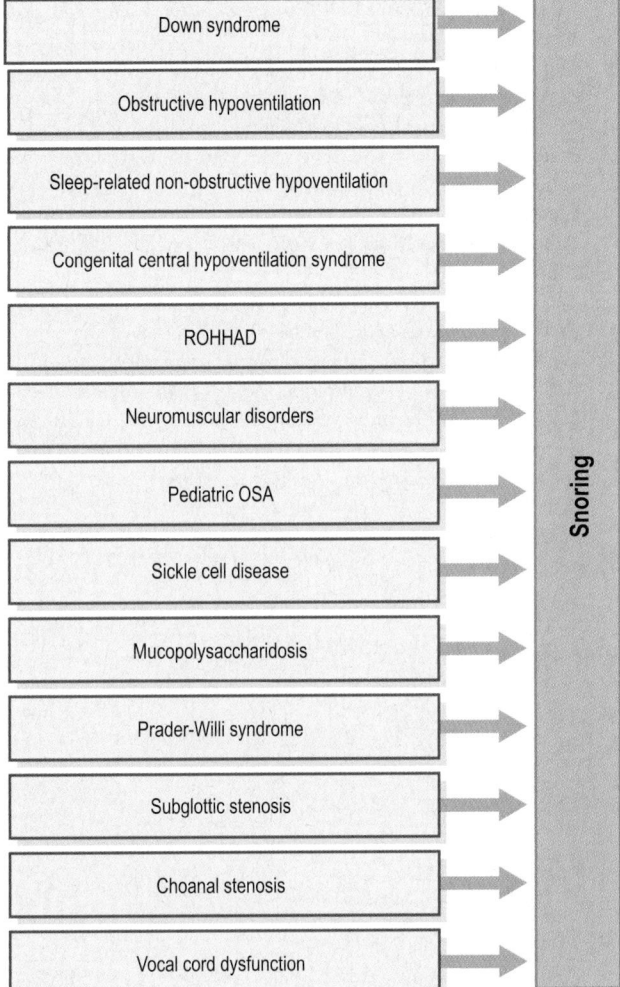

• **Fig. 7.5** Snoring. OSA, obstructive sleep apnea. ROHHAD, rapid-onset obesity with hypothalamic dysregulation, hypoventilation, and autonomic dysregulation. (Adapted from Owens JA, Dalzell V. *Sleep Med*. 2005.)

with the longest sleep period occurring at night and the longest wake period occurring during the day. At this age, daytime sleep occurs in about three to four discrete day-time naps. Naps consolidate at around 6 months into two briefer daytime sleep periods and, into the second year of life, into a single early afternoon sleep period. Daytime naps are typically given up by 3–5 years of age. There is a wide variation of normal, but youngsters habitually still napping at 6–7 years of age might be exhibiting symptoms of daytime sleepiness.

The Physical Examination

The physical examination needed depends on the medical history, the specifics of the sleep complaint, and the hypotheses generated during assessment. A healthy toddler who simply needs help giving up the pacifier at night may not need a full examination; a child with enuresis may require examination of the genitals, perineum, and spine; and a child with possible seizures or known neurologic abnormalities will require a more comprehensive and extensive neurodevelopmental evaluation. A complete discussion of the physical and developmental evaluation of children at various developmental levels may be found in several excellent resources.[7,8]

The most common areas requiring evaluation in children presenting with sleep complaints are those related to the airway because airway-related problems are often part of the differential diagnosis regardless of presenting complaint.[9–11]

These areas include:
- Habitus: For abnormal height, weight, and body mass index (obesity or failure to thrive).
- HEENT:
  1. For abnormal skull or facial features (craniosynostosis, facial asymmetry, midface hypoplasia, retrognathia, macroglossia, dental overjet, high arched and/or elongated palate).[12]
  2. For adenotonsillar and uvular enlargement and oropharyngeal crowding (modified Mallampati scale[13] [Table 7.1].
  3. For nasal obstruction (septal deviation, polyps, enlarged turbinates).
  4. For palatal abnormalities (high arching, presence of cleft).
  5. For thyroid enlargement.
- Chest and back: For chest or spine abnormalities (pectus excavatum, barrel-shaped, scoliosis).
- Neurologic: For abnormal tone (hypertonia, spasticity, hypotonia).

Other Assessments

Based on the clinical history and physical examination, other objective and/or laboratory assessments may be indicated. The role of polysomnography in diagnosis and management of pediatric sleep disorders is beyond the

 TABLE 7.1 **Modified Mallampati Scoring Criteria[13]**

Modified Mallampati Scoring:

- Class I: Soft palate, uvula, fauces, pillars visible
- Class II: Soft palate, uvula, fauces visible
- Class III: Soft palate, base of uvula visible
- Class IV: Only hard palate visible

scope of this chapter and is discussed elsewhere in this volume.

Depending upon the presenting complaint, physical examination, and synthesis of this information, a complete blood count (CBC), serum chemistry profile, serum iron and ferritin levels, and thyroid function testing may be appropriate. Neuroimaging with either magnetic resonance imaging (MRI) or computed tomography (CT) may be considered based on individual presentation, particularly in patients with preceding head trauma or children with abnormal neurologic examinations.[1]

CLINICAL PEARLS

- Clinical history is the most important part of the process of solving clinical problems.
- The ability to establish an initial hypothesis set and subsequent testing of these hypotheses requires a wide knowledge base.
- A structured approach to obtaining pertinent clinical information is essential to the diagnosis and management of sleep disorders in infants, children, and adolescents.

References

1. Shelgikar AV, Chervin R. Approach to and evaluation of sleep disorders. *Contin Minneap Minn*. 2013;19(1 *Sleep Disorders*):32–49. https://doi.org/10.1212/01.CON.0000427214.00092.0f.
2. Barrows HS, Tamblyn RM. *Problem-based learning: An approach to Medical Education*. Springer; 1980.
3. Ferber R. *Solve Your Child's Sleep Problems*. Simon & Schuster; 2006.
4. Sheldon SH, Ahart S, Levy HB. Sleep patterns in abused and neglected children. *Sleep Res*. 1991;20(333).
5. Spruyt K, Gozal D. Pediatric sleep questionnaires as diagnostic or epidemiological tools: A review of currently available instruments. *Sleep Med Rev*. 2011;15(1):19–32.
6. Owens JA, Dalzell V. Use of the "BEARS" sleep screening tool in a pediatric residents' continuity clinic: A pilot study. *Sleep Med*. 2005;6:63–69.
7. Kliegman R, St. Gemme III J. *Nelson Textbook of Pediatrics*. 21st ed. Elsevier; 2020.
8. Frankenberg WK, Thornton SM, Cohrs ME. *Pediatric Developmental Diagnosis*. Thieme-Stratton; 1981.
9. Epstein LJ, Kristo D, Strollo PJ. Clinical guideline for the evaluation, management and long-term care of obstructive sleep apnea in adults. *J Clin Sleep Med*. 2009;5(3):263–276.
10. Cataletto ME, Lipton AJ, Murphy TD. Childhood sleep apnea. Published online May 14, 2012. http://emedicine.medscape.com/article/1004104.
11. Chan J, Edman JC, Koltai PJ. Obstructive sleep apnea in children. *Am Fam Physician*. 2004;69(5):1147–1155.
12. Gozal D. Diagnostic approaches to respiratory abnormalities in craniofacial syndromes. *Semin Fetal Neonatal Med*. 2021;26(6):101292. https://doi.org/10.1016/j.siny.2021.101292.
13. Samsoon GL, Young J. Difficult tracheal intubation: A retrospective study. *Anaesthesia*. 1987;42:487–490.

8

Differential Diagnosis in Pediatric Sleep Medicine

Stephen H. Sheldon

CHAPTER HIGHLIGHTS

- There are various sleep disorders that can cause arousals/awakenings during sleep, including Nocturnal Eating/Drinking Syndrome, Disorders of Arousal From REM Sleep Nightmares, Sleep Paralysis, and REM Sleep Behavior Disorder/REM Sleep Without Atonia.
- Excessive daytime sleepiness in children can be caused by various sleep disorders, and it is important to assess the frequency and nature of nighttime awakenings.
- Insomnia is one of the most common presenting complaints in pediatric sleep medicine and can be caused by a variety of factors. Assessing problem sleeplessness involves asking questions about the duration of the problem, difficulties with bedtime and sleep onset, nighttime awakenings, and sleep quality in different environments.
- Clinical problem solving and establishing a comprehensive differential diagnosis are important in pediatric sleep medicine.

Differential Diagnosis

Recommendations for management of a child with sleep problems can be made only after an accurate diagnosis is established. Often symptoms are vague in the child, and parents seek medical advice only because the child's sleep problem is disrupting the parents' sleep. Difficulty functioning during the day can be the presenting symptom, and the child's sleep is frequently overlooked as a possible contributing or underlying factor. The child's health care practitioner may be faced with a dilemma: sorting out a confusing history.

Arriving at an appropriate sleep-related diagnosis involves a complex series of deductions. Generating an initial hypothesis set, testing these hypotheses by specific questioning of sleep-related symptoms, and gaining information from a physical examination are essential in the clinical reasoning process. A cornerstone to the process of appropriate clinical problem-solving and arriving at an accurate diagnosis is adequacy and completeness of the hypothesis set. Too little information about sleep disorders and the sleep–wake cycle is taught to medical professionals. This chapter is intended to be a quick reference for the busy practitioner. The practitioner may use this chapter to develop an appropriate hypothesis and subsequently a clear

and precise differential diagnosis that will include but not be limited to various sleep disorders that may affect daytime and nighttime functioning. Specific clinical facts that can be used to differentiate one sleep disorder from others are listed and briefly described. Comprehensive descriptions of each sleep-related disorder, diagnostic criteria, and suggestions for management are given elsewhere in this volume.

Not uncommonly, considerable overlap in disorder presentation exists. Problems that present with "problem sleeplessness" may also be associated with "excessive daytime sleepiness." Some disorders may be classified as partial arousals from sleep. At times, description of these sleep disorders is reiterated. However, presentation in different sections will be focused on the primary presenting complaint. Each diagnosis is covered more comprehensively in other chapters in this textbook.

Classification of disorders (Tables 8.1–8.5) have been adapted from the American Academy of Sleep Medicine, ICSD-3,[1] AASM Scoring Manual,[2] the BEARS screening tool,[3] and modified and updated from *Pediatric Sleep Medicine*, Appendix 3: Differential Diagnosis in Pediatric Sleep Medicine.[4]

Pediatric Insomnia (Problem Sleeplessness)

Insomnia is one of the most common presenting complaints presenting to the child health care practitioner. It may present as a disorder of initiating sleep, disorder of maintaining sleep, or both. As previously mentioned, there may be considerable overlap of symptoms and clear assessment of the child's sleep/wake patterns is essential in arriving at a diagnosis and appropriate management plan. Often there are a variety of causes and each must be addressed in order for adequate resolution to be possible. Insomnia that is present for less than 3 months is considered acute insomnia. If there is sudden onset of symptoms, this may be due to an identifiable stress or the precipitating event may be somewhat obscure. There may be family conflict or environmental issues that precipitate the symptoms. Sleeplessness is clearly a problem for the patient and the family. Chronic insomnia is defined as problem sleeplessness lasting more than 3 months and may be due to disorders that can range from conditioned (e.g.., sleep onset association disorder), inadequate sleep hygiene, inappropriate caretakers' expectations, to allergy, environmental issues, chronic pain syndromes, and Munchhausen's syndrome by proxy.

Assessing Problem Sleeplessness

Searching questions might include the following:

1. How long has the problem been present?
2. Does the child have problems going to bed and settling at a desired bedtime?
3. Does the child have difficulty falling to sleep once lights are turned out.
4. How long does it take for the child to fall to sleep?
5. Does the child wake at night? How long is the waking? How frequent are the wakings?
6. Does the child sleep well somewhere? Or, do they sleep poorly everywhere and under any circumstance?

 TABLE 8.1   **Diagnosis and Presentation of Insomnia/Sleeplessness**

Disorder	Principal Differentiating Considerations
Insomnia (Short-Term)	• Difficulty initiating and/or maintaining sleep has been present for a short time (less than 3 months). • Onset of the problem is sudden and may surround periods of acute stress, conflict, emotions, or environmental changes. Sleeplessness is clearly different from the child's normal sleep pattern. • There may be multiple manifestations including, but not limited to, bedtime struggles, problems falling to sleep or staying asleep, early morning waking, and/or problems falling to sleep at bedtime or after waking at night without parental intervention. • Daytime behavior and/or mood disorders may also be present. • A precipitating event may or may not be identified. • Stressors may, at times, be pleasant (e.g., holidays, birthdays, vacations).
Insomnia (Chronic)	• Difficulty initiating and/or maintaining sleep is present for 3 months or more. • Onset may be acute but persistent. • May have gradual onset.
Insomnia (Chronic) Inappropriate Sleep-Onset Associations	• Difficulty falling to sleep at a determined bedtime. Problems also center on nocturnal waking and/or an inability of the child to fall back to sleep. • Characteristic of this diagnosis is the ability of the child to rapidly return to sleep once the transitional object or behavior is provided. The child can fall to sleep easily somewhere and/or when certain conditions are present. • Children who sleep poorly and wake frequently during the night under *any* circumstances require further evaluation. • Problems also center on nocturnal waking and an inability of the child to fall back to sleep. • May be placed into bed already asleep. • Children require the same conditions for settling after a nighttime waking as they require to settle at the beginning of their nighttime sleep period.
Limit-Setting Sleep Disorder	• Child refuses to go to sleep at a time desired by the parents. • Parents give in to the child's protestations about sleep and limits are rarely set. • Daytime behavioral problems may be present. • Other parenting dysfunction might be identified. • Once sleep onset occurs, it is typically normal. • Once limits are set and enforced, sleep onset and maintenance problems typically improve.
Excessive Nocturnal Fluids	• Extremely frequent nighttime waking is noticed. • This disorder may be differentiated from sleep-onset association disorder by identifying that only a small volume of fluid is consumed, with the child rapidly returning to sleep once the feeding begins. • Most common during infancy. • Excessive fluids are ingested at night. • Differentiated from sleep-onset association disorder because the child will rapidly fall to sleep once feeding begins and not finish or complete the feeding.
Inadequate Sleep Hygiene	• There are irregular bedtimes, irregular times of morning sleep offset, and frequent napping. • Sleeping environment may be chaotic, cluttered, and used for other activities. • Settling at night may be difficult, and presenting complaints can vary.
Psychologic Disorders	• Comprehensive evaluation indicates the presence of a mood disorder, and the sleep complaint tends to increase in severity with the severity of the daytime symptoms. • Fears expressed during wakefulness may be present, and the child (and/or parent) may be able to identify the particular stressor. • Nightmares (anxiety dreams) often occur. Anxiety and fear seem to be generalized, with diurnal and nocturnal manifestations. • Primary anxiety may be present during the day. • Nocturnal fears may be elucidated from the history.
Environmental Sleep Disorders	• An identifiable environmental stimulus might be identified. • Clear temporal relationship to the onset of the sleep complaint with the environmental trigger is often identified. • Symptoms are related to the physical presence of the environmental stimulus, rather than a psychologic or emotional reaction. • Daytime symptoms may include excessive sleepiness from nocturnal sleep deprivation, attention-span problems, restlessness, poor school performance, lethargy, and malaise.

TABLE 8.1 Diagnosis and Presentation of Insomnia/Sleeplessness—Cont'd

Disorder	Principal Differentiating Considerations
Sleeplessness Associated With Allergy	<ul><li>Daytime symptoms of and manifestation of allergy are often identified but may not be considered to be part of the sleep complaint.</li><li>Daytime irritability; dermatologic lesions; wheezing, rhinorrhea, and other respiratory tract complaints; colicky abdominal pain (associated with food allergy); agitation; and lethargy may accompany the sleep complaints.</li><li>Food allergies may result in sleep complaints.</li><li>Sleeplessness due to allergy may be differentiated from sleep-disordered respiration by the absence of snoring or respiratory pauses during sleep, and the presence (as with food allergy) of other system involvement.</li><li>Nocturnal asthma, gastroesophageal reflux, and colic may be difficult to differentiate from food allergy and may require significant laboratory testing to eliminate these as causes of the sleep complaint (especially if allergic respiratory symptoms predominate).</li></ul>
Medication-Related Problem Sleeplessness	<ul><li>There is typically a history of medication use, particularly stimulant medicines.</li><li>Over-the-counter (OTC) medications (e.g., diphenhydramine) may produce a paradoxical response at bedtime.</li><li>Some OTC medications and some foods may contain caffeine that can disrupt sleep onset and/or maintenance.</li><li>Children, at any age, can have sleep onset and/or maintenance disrupted by medications.</li></ul>
Sleeplessness Associated with Respiratory Disorders	<ul><li>Snoring, restless sleep, gasping, or snoring can occur during wake-to-sleep transition, affecting sleep consolidation.</li><li>Central apneas may result in symptoms suggesting apparent life-threatening events.</li><li>Nocturnal and diurnal hypoventilation may be present.</li><li>There may be a history of primary pulmonary disease including, but not limited to, asthma, ciliary dyskinesia, and chronic obstructive pulmonary disease.</li><li>*Obstructive sleep apnea:* Sleep-onset difficulties are unusual but can occur when frequent occlusive and/or partially occlusive respiratory events prevent sleep consolidation. More frequently, nocturnal awakenings occur, often associated with very restless sleep.</li><li>*Central sleep apnea:* When symptoms are present, sleep maintenance insomnia is the typical complaint.</li><li>*Congenital central hypoventilation syndrome (CCHS):* Sleep onset is usually normal. Sleep maintenance problems exist with manifestations of arousals to lighter stages of sleep and awakening from sleep. Excessive daytime sleepiness may occur secondary to sleep fragmentation. Other morphologic and autonomic symptoms are typically present (see section of CCHS in the differential diagnosis of breathing disorders in children).</li><li>*Chronic pulmonary disorders and asthma:* Sleep disturbances are common and consist of difficulty in initiating sleep as well as maintenance insomnia. There are frequent awakenings, coughing, shortness of breath, and respiratory distress. Medications used in daytime management may exacerbate the sleep complaints. Daytime sleepiness may occur due to nocturnal sleep disruption and architectural fragmentation. Expiratory wheezing and/or nocturnal coughing may also be noted.</li><li>*Altitude-related respiratory abnormalities:* Acute onset (within 72 hours) of symptoms of sleeplessness after travel to elevations higher than 4000 m above sea level. Associated symptoms include headache, fatigue, and anorexia. Symptoms resolve after return to habitual altitude.</li></ul>
Sleeplessness Associated With Movement Disorders	<ul><li>There may be complaints of difficulty keeping limbs from moving after getting into bed.</li><li>Complaints may focus on presence of growing pains.</li><li>Kicking during sleep and very restless sleep may be present.</li><li>Rhythmic movements before sleep onset may be a principal complaint.<ul><li>*Restless leg (limb) syndrome:* Patients complain of disturbing feelings (aches, tingling, itching, or creeping sensations) in their limbs when they get into bed. Movement of the limbs seems to improve symptoms.</li><li>*Periodic limb movement disorder:* History may reveal frequent awakenings and unrefreshing sleep. Numerous partial arousals can occur. Sleep architecture and continuity can be significantly disrupted, and children may wake frequently at night complaining of limb "pains." There can be repetitive and stereotypic movements of one or both legs noted. Arms may also be involved. Parents may express concern about periodic jerking movements.</li><li>*Rhythmic movement disorder:* Rhythmic movements are seen before onset of sleep; but may also be identified during sleep. History may reveal rhythmic head banging, head rolling, body rocking, or head rocking. There are paroxysms of stereotypic, repetitive movements of large muscle groups. Episodes occur before sleep onset, and during light sleep, but may also be noted during slow-wave sleep. Similar rhythmic behaviors can occur during daytime naps and during wakefulness. Onset of symptoms is typically during the first 2 years of life. Episodes may occur frequently (almost nightly) or may be infrequent (less than once per week). Diurnal symptoms are unusual, and affected children are normal neurologically, behaviorally, and psychologically. If symptoms are severe (especially in patients with head banging), bruising and other physical injury may occur.</li></ul></li></ul>

(Continued)

TABLE 8.1 **Diagnosis and Presentation of Insomnia/Sleeplessness—Cont'd**

Disorder	Principal Differentiating Considerations

Sleeplessness Associated With Circadian Rhythm Disorders	• Complaints may focus on difficulty falling to sleep at a desired bedtime. Once asleep the child sleeps well and typically wakes late morning or afternoon.
	• Complaint may focus on excessive daytime sleepiness due to sleep restriction from difficulty falling to sleep at a desired time and early morning waking for school.
	• Complaint might focus on falling to sleep early in the evening easily but waking very early in the morning ready to start the day.
	• Complaints may center around days and nights being reversed.
	• Wake and sleep behaviors may be quite chaotic throughout the 24-hour light-dark cycle.
	• Caretakers' expectations require identification.
	  • *Delayed sleep phase syndrome:* Frequent presenting complaints are bedtime struggles and sleep-onset difficulties. Sleep onset may be delayed for hours. There are few, if any, complaints of nocturnal waking. Morning waking can be quite difficult. On weekends and vacations, the child may sleep into late morning or early afternoon hours.
	  • *Advanced sleep phase syndrome:* Problems center around early morning waking at a time significantly earlier than desired. Sleep onset is normal, but at an unusually early time. Sleep is otherwise normal and uninterrupted.
	  • *Non–24-hour sleep–wake disorder:* Sleep complaints are variable and changing due to a continuous delay in phase of the sleep–wake cycle. Patients can alternate from periods of extreme inability to sleep at night and severe sleepiness during the day, to a brief period where there are fewer sleep-related complaints.
	  • *Irregular sleep–wake schedule disorder:* Similar to the non–24-hour sleep–wake disorder, sleep and wake patterns are significantly variable, haphazard, and disorganized. No clear sleep–wake pattern can be discerned. Complaints may focus on sleeplessness, sleepiness, or both.

Inappropriate Caretakers' Expectations	• Expectations for sleep (including timing and duration) are inappropriate for the child's developmental level. • Just as an infant cannot walk like an adult, they cannot sleep like an adult until they are maturationally capable.
Munchausen's Syndrome by Proxy	• History, physical examination, and testing procedures are inconsistent. • Multiple medical personnel have been consulted. • Multiple treatments (often costly and invasive) have been reported to be unsuccessful. • Parent/caretaker may have a medical background and is typically well read regarding medical procedures. • Severe form of child abuse. • No objective evidence of a primary sleep-related disorder.
Infantile Colic	• Characteristically begins at about 2–3 weeks of age. • Paroxysms of crying occur in the later afternoon hours. • Spells occur for at least 3 days per week and last for 3 weeks or more. • No other medical reason for the crying paroxysms can be identified. • Most symptoms resolve by 4 months of age.
Sleep-Related Gastroesophageal Reflux Disorder	• Frequent episodes of spitting up and/or vomiting. • Failure to thrive may be present. • Snoring and/or stridulous respiration may be noted, particularly if there is pharyngeal reflux.
Chronic Pain Syndromes	• Symptoms of other chronic medical illness may be present (e.g., juvenile rheumatoid arthritis). • Acute or chronic otitis media or other infection may be present. • Complaints of difficulty falling to sleep due to pain or waking with pain may be present. • Principal symptoms may be related to the primary underlying medical condition.

Excessive Daytime Sleepiness (Problem Sleepiness)

Sleep disorders presenting with problem sleepiness are a heterogenous group that may have underlying functional and organic causes. A final common pathway is undesirable sleeping during times when the child should be awake, unavoidable sleep episodes (sleep attacks), an increased total sleep time during 24-hour periods, or problems waking alert and refreshed. Cognitive and/or performance problems may result. As with children presenting with problem sleeplessness, significant overlap in etiologies might exist. These sleep disorders may manifest sleepiness, sleeplessness, or both. Duplication of diagnoses and their description is unavoidable and have been included with modification to focus on the disorder when the presenting complaint is one of excessive sleepiness.

Symptoms of excessive sleepiness in children are variable and are often less clear than those of sleeplessness. Symptoms may be confusing on initial presentation. When extreme degrees of hypersomnolence are present, symptoms are usually obvious. Children are noted to fall to sleep at inappropriate times (e.g., during meals, at parties, while opening presents at Christmas, or on the playground). On the other hand, many sleepy children manifest behaviors that are paradoxical and may be mistaken for symptoms of other disorders or behavior problems. These symptoms may include, but are not limited to, the following:

hyperactivity
poor concentration
school difficulties
pathological shyness
fidgety behavior
habitual napping
habitual napping
and performance deficits

Additionally, there may be attention span problems
easy distractability, unusual aggressiveness
motor restlessness
Motor restlessness
rapid mood swings
decreased appetite
cognitive deficits
and difficulty reading

It is evident that these signs and symptoms may be shared with many childhood disorders. Evaluation should be considered incomplete if possible disorders of excessive somnolence are not comprehensively searched for and assessed. There may be specific overlap of diagnoses because symptoms may appear similar or not classic on initial presentation. Some disorders present with symptoms of problem sleepiness, problem sleeplessness, or both.

Assessing Problem Sleepiness

Searching questions and inquiry design might include the following questions:
1. Does the patient have difficulty waking in the morning?
2. Does the child feel sleepy during the day?
3. Does the child fall to sleep at odd times during the day?
4. Are there attention or concentration difficulties?
5. Are there learning issues?
6. Does the child have difficulty sitting still?

TABLE 8.2   Diagnosis and Presentation of Sleepiness

Disorder	Principal Differentiating Considerations
Problem Sleepiness Secondary to Behavioral and/or Psychophysiologic Disorders	This is a range of disorders that typically present with nocturnal symptoms. However, because of the presence of limited total sleep time, manifestations of problem sleepiness may occur and predominate.
Insufficient Sleep	<ul><li>Total daily sleep time is considerably shorter than age-appropriate norms.</li><li>Sleep restriction is typically volitional.</li><li>Total sleep time may be normal if children are allowed to wake spontaneously.</li><li>Daytime symptoms of sleepiness are often the presenting complaint.</li><li>Insufficient sleep may be the final common pathway for many disorders that result in excessive daytime sleepiness. Behavioral factors, circadian factors, and disorders of sleep stages and/or arousals from sleep all can be associated with insufficient sleep at night, causing symptoms of daytime fatigue, malaise, and sleepiness.</li><li>Presence of sleep restriction and short total sleep time for age differentiates these etiologies of problem daytime sleepiness from those with underlying central nervous system (CNS) or respiratory etiologies.</li><li>The disparity between the need for sleep and the amount of sleep actually obtained is significant.</li></ul>
Limit-Setting Sleep Disorder	<ul><li>Few, if any, limits on behavior are enforced at night.</li><li>Similar limits are not obligatory during the daytime.</li><li>Behavioral problems may be present.</li><li>Parents give in to the child's demands and rarely set limits on the child's behavior.</li></ul>
Inadequate Sleep Hygiene	<ul><li>Sleeping environment may not be conducive to sleep.</li><li>Schedules may not be appropriately set.</li><li>Children may be given too much autonomy over their bedtime and sleeping environment.</li></ul>
Mood Disorders	<ul><li>Complaints center on fatigue or malaise.</li><li>Inability to fall asleep at bedtime and early morning awakenings with an inability to fall back to sleep are common associated complaints.</li><li>Other daytime symptomatology of a mood disorder is typically present.</li><li>Bedtime struggles, early morning waking and inability to fall back to sleep may be present.</li></ul>
Environmental Sleep Disorder	<ul><li>Stimulating and/or uncomfortable environmental factors can be found.</li><li>Sleep returns to normal once the noxious environmental stimulus is removed.</li><li>A temporal relationship to the presence of the sleep-disturbing environmental factor might be identified.</li><li>Environmental factors disrupting the child's nocturnal sleep might initially go unrecognized.</li></ul>
Sleepiness Associated With CNS Etiologies	<ul><li>These diagnoses encompass a group of disorders with the primary cause originating from a CNS etiology. In children, profound sleepiness is usually easily identified. Children fall asleep at unusual and unexpected times. They may fall to sleep during a meal, while playing on a playground, at a party, or at other times when consolidated sleep would not be anticipated. Children very often fall to sleep during a car ride, but falling to sleep while talking to a friend on the telephone or at a birthday party is unusual. Symptoms might first be noticed by teachers because of frequent sleeping in class, difficulty in remembering tasks, and forgetfulness. Lesser degrees of sleepiness often result in paradoxical symptomatology. Principal symptoms might include but not be limited to hyperactivity, motor restlessness, attention-span problems, difficulty with concentration, school learning issues, moodiness, and forgetfulness.</li></ul>
Narcolepsy, Type 1	<ul><li>Positive family history of narcolepsy and cataplexy may be present.</li><li>Sleep attacks and unintentional sleep episodes are present.</li><li>Sleepiness may alternate with overactivity.</li><li>Cataplexy is present in Narcolepsy, Type 1, but may be overlooked or misinterpreted because symptoms may be partial and involve only muscles of the face or mouth. Eyelid fluttering, jaw drop, and/or apparent tongue thrusting may be manifestations of cataplexy. Generalized cataplexy may be described as partial epilepsy, *drop attacks*, or syncope.</li><li>Hypnagogic hallucinations may be misinterpreted as nightmares or anxiety-related sleep disorder.</li><li>Sleep paralysis may be described as refusal to wake rather than an inability to move at sleep offset.</li></ul>
Narcolepsy, Type 2	<ul><li>Symptoms are the same a Narcolepsy, Type 1 but cataplexy is notably absent.</li><li>Other narcoleptic symptoms may be identical.</li></ul>

TABLE 8.2 Diagnosis and Presentation of Sleepiness—Cont'd

Disorder	Principal Differentiating Considerations
Idiopathic Hypersomnia	• Naps and/or unintentional sleep episodes may be considerably long. • Naps are most often unrefreshing. • Cataplexy, hypnagogic hallucinations, and sleep paralysis are usually absent. • Autonomic dysfunction may be notable. • Associated symptoms might include migraine cephalgia, syncope, orthostatic hypotension, and Raynaud's phenomena. Syncope and orthostatic symptoms may be confused with cataplexy.
Post-traumatic Hypersomnia	• Complaints often focus on excessive daytime sleepiness and frequent daytime sleep episodes. • There is a history of head trauma. • Problem daytime sleepiness is different from the habitual pre-trauma sleep pattern. • Other post-trauma daytime symptoms are often present.
Kleine-Levin Syndrome (Recurrent Hypersomnia)	• Waxing and waning of symptoms. • Symptom-free periods are notable. • Behavioral symptoms are present during the symptomatic episodes. • Hypersomnolent phases may or may not be associated with binge eating and hypersexuality. • Onset is typically during the early adolescent years and typically in biological males. • Episodes last from a few days to a few weeks, spontaneously resolve, and may recur 2 to 12 times per year. • Social impairment during attacks is severe.
Munchausen Syndrome by Proxy	• Symptoms are factitious. • Multiple expensive and/or invasive medical interventions may have been conducted. • Multiple health care providers may be involved in the care of the youngster. • Symptoms are inconsistent with physical and/or laboratory findings.
Problem Sleepiness Associated With Circadian Rhythm Disturbances	
Long Sleeper	• Total sleep time is greater than expected for age. • Sleep is typically normal when allowed to sleep according to normal physiology. • Symptoms appear when sleep is restricted due to educational and social requirements. • At times there is a complaint of hypersomnia.
Delayed Sleep Phase Syndrome	• Sleep-onset difficulties are common, and principal complaints surround inability to fall asleep and problem sleeplessness. • Once asleep the child sleeps well. • If permitted to sleep without interruption, the child will sleep well into late morning or early afternoon. • Daytime symptoms of sleepiness are most significant during the morning hours. • When there are early morning responsibilities (e.g., school), parents frequently report difficulty waking the child, disorientation upon awakening, sluggishness, lassitude, crankiness, aggression, and/or an inability to perform required tasks. • Symptoms of excessive sleepiness are generally restricted to the morning hours.
Irregular Sleep–Wake Pattern	• Sleep episodes are erratic, disorganized, and unpredictable. • Total 24-hour sleep time may be normal. • Combination of problem sleepiness and problem sleeplessness is usually present. • Developmental and/or CNS abnormalities may be present.
Non–24-Hour Sleep–Wake Disorder	• Patients alternate between periods of profound daytime sleepiness and an inability to sleep at night and periods of relatively normal nocturnal sleep. • Prolonged periods of sleep may alternate with prolonged periods of wake. • May be seen in children with visual disabilities.
Sleepiness Due to Movement Disorders	
Periodic Limb Movement Disorder	• Complaints of non-refreshing sleep are common. • Kicking during sleep may be described. • Sleep is described as restless. • Growing pains or other limb pain complaints may be present.

(Continued)

TABLE 8.2	Diagnosis and Presentation of Sleepiness—Cont'd
Disorder	**Principal Differentiating Considerations**
Restless Leg Syndrome	• Complaints may center around an inability to fall to sleep because the child feels a compulsion to move arms or legs. • Typically associated with sleep onset difficulties. • The child may also complain of unusual feelings in the arms or legs, like ants are crawling about. • Some children may state their legs hurt or itch.
Sleepiness Due to Breathing Disorders	
Obstructive Sleep Apnea (OSA)	• Snoring is the principal symptom of pediatric OSA. • Sleep is often restless. • Frequent nocturnal waking may occur. • Sleep-related diaphoresis may occur. • Secondary sleep-related enuresis may be noted. • Paradoxical symptoms of hyperactivity, motor restlessness, and school performance difficulty may be present during the day. • The child may be overweight. • Adenotonsillar hypertrophy may be present. • High arch, elongated palate, and dental malocclusion may be noted.
Obesity-Hypoventilation Syndrome	• Profound problem daytime sleepiness, sleep attacks, and unintentional sleep episodes are often present. • Body mass index >95th percentile for age and sex. • Hypercapnia is present both during wake and sleep but seems to be worse during sleep and worst during REM sleep. • Obstructive sleep apnea may be present but not the principal cause of the persistent hypercapnia. • Systemic hypertension, pulmonary hypertension, and/or cor pulmonale may occur.
Congenital Central Hypoventilation Syndrome (CCHS)	• Hypoventilation is present both night and day. • Hypoxemia and hypercapnia typically are present but may be subtle because there can be little evidence of respiratory distress. • Most often diagnosed in infancy. • *PHOX2B* gene mutation is present. • Hirschsprung's disease is often associated with CCHS. • Other disorders of the autonomic nervous system are often present. • Neural crest tumors can be present. • Some patients present later in childhood, during adolescence, or young adulthood.

Arousals/Awakenings

As previously noted, many etiologies of disordered sleep in childhood can present with symptoms of sleeplessness, sleepiness, or both. At times, however, the presenting signs and symptoms may refer to neither decreased nor excessive sleep. Again, significant duplication and overlap exists. This section will focus on those entities that present most commonly as disorders of maintaining sleep, with symptoms of nocturnal waking, arousals, or partial arousals. Sleep disorders that have major presenting manifestations unrelated to sleepiness or sleeplessness will be described in greater detail.

Assessing Arousals and/or Wakings at Night

Waking at night may be troublesome for the entire family. Children may fully awaken or there may be a partial arousal. Partial arousals occur when a stimulus does not exceed the arousal threshold and there is "status dissociatus" or dissociative states. These partial arousals may have an endogenous or exogenous precipitating factor. Partial arousals display signs of overlapping states. Searching questions and inquiry design might include the following:

1. Does the child appear to wake frequently during the night? Is the child fully awake or seems to still be asleep (or disoriented)?
2. Does the child scream, yell, walk, cry, or talk during sleep?
3. Does the child fall back to sleep quickly or is it difficult for the child to return to sleep?
4. Does the child remember the arousal or waking?

 TABLE 8.3 **Arousals and Awakening**

Disorder	Principal Differentiating Considerations
Arousals Secondary to Psychophysiologic Etiologies Behavioral/Conditioned (Sleep-Onset Association Disorder)	• Problems may center on nocturnal waking and an inability of the child to fall back to sleep. • Characteristic of this diagnosis is the ability of the child to rapidly return to sleep once the transitional object or behavior is provided. • The child can fall to sleep easily somewhere and/or when certain conditions are present.
Disorders of Arousal From NREM Sleep	• Many symptoms are consistently associated with partial arousals from NREM sleep. Complaints may be varied and may change over time. Typically, there are recurrent paroxysms of incomplete awakening from sleep. Spells most often occur during the first third to first half of the major nocturnal sleep period. Inappropriate or complete lack of responsiveness to efforts of others to wake or redirect the child during the spell. It is not uncommon for redirection or intervention to increase the intensity of the paroxysm. • Spells can be associated with complex behaviors. Most episodes are brief, but some can last longer. Talking and shouting may occur during events, eyes are often open during a spell, the child is difficult to awaken, and if awakened there can be considerable disorientation or confusion. Most frequently, there is amnesia of the spell. Children may be surprised and occasionally concerned about behaviors exhibited during the night for which there is no recall. NREM partial arousals can occur after conditions that increase slow-wave sleep activity, such as during recovery from sleep deprivation, and can be exacerbated by fever and stress.
Sleepwalking, Agitated Sleepwalking, and Confusional Arousals	• Occurs during the first third to first half of the nocturnal sleep period. • Ambulation is most often quiet (but may be agitated). • Complex behaviors may be noted. • There is generally amnesia for the event. • Enuresis and urinary voiding at unusual places around the home is common. • There is typically no dream mentation. • Children most often rapidly return to sleep. • Exacerbating factors can include fever, sleep deprivation/restriction, medications, stress/anxiety, and/or bladder distension. • Somniloquy may occur during spells, and speech may or may not be incoherent. • Spells may be infrequent or may occur several times during a single sleep period. • Children may appear agitated during the spell and may occasionally run or thrash about. • Confusion and/or disorientation may appear to be profound.
Sleep Terrors	• Occur during the first third to first half of the night. • There is no displacement from the bed. • Spells have abrupt, sudden onset with a piercing, terrifying scream. • Spells are usually brief. • There is considerable agitation and autonomic discharge including, but not limited to, pupillary dilation, tachypnea, tachycardia, diaphoresis, and trembling. • Attempts to comfort the child may increase agitation. • There is amnesia for the event.

(Continued)

TABLE 8.3	Arousals and Awakening—Cont'd
Disorder	**Principal Differentiating Considerations**
Nocturnal Eating/Drinking Syndrome	• Dysfunctional eating and/or drinking occurs during and/or after an arousal from the major nocturnal sleep period. • Inappropriate weight gain may occur. • Amnesia for the event may or may not be present. • There is often an adverse effect on general health. • Unintentional injury to self or others may occur if a stovetop, oven, or microwave is turned on. • Spells can occur at any time during the night but do not occur during REM sleep.
Disorders of Arousal From REM Sleep	
Nightmares	• Arousal/awakening occurs during the second half or final third of the major sleep period (early morning hours). • Anxiety is related to disturbing dream mentation but is not intense. • There may be only mild autonomic discharge. • Waking may be prolonged with difficulty returning to sleep. • There is a clear and story-like dream report and memory of the awakening/arousal.
Sleep Paralysis	• Spells typically occur at morning sleep offset. • Although the child is awake and alert, they may not be able to open their eyes, move their arms or legs, or be able to talk. • Upon waking, the child may act frightened rather than resisting being awakened. • Sensation of inability to breathe may occur due to inhibition of accessory muscles of breathing. • Spells are typically brief. • Sleep paralysis may be isolated, familial (X-linked dominant), or a symptom of narcolepsy.
REM Sleep Behavior Disorder/REM Sleep Without Atonia	• There is significant sudden movement with swinging of the arms, kicking, or flailing of extremities. • Punching, kicking, and vocalizations are common. • Vivid dream recall is usually present. • Most occur during the second half or final third of the sleep period. • Injuries to self (and/or bedpartners) can occur.
Arousals/Awakenings Secondary to Medical Disorders	
Asthma	• A history of asthma may be elicited. • Symptoms of nocturnal wheezing and/or frequent nocturnal coughing might be present. • Nocturnal waking may be frequent. • There may be a significant history of allergy. • Past history of bronchodilator treatment may be elicited.
Epilepsy	• There may be a history of seizure disorder. • Other neurologic symptoms may be elicited. • History may be significant for abnormal electroencephalographic activity. • May occasionally present as an apparent life-threatening event, particularly if it occurs during sleep.
Other Sleep-Related Medical Disorders	• Symptoms principally related to the primary underlying medical condition may be present. • A history of chronic pain may be elicited. • There may be a history of chronic respiratory disorder. • Gastroesophageal reflux disease may be present. • Nightmares may be present. • A history of another chronic upper airway disorder may be present. • Other disorders might include, but are not limited to, abnormal swallowing syndrome, sleep-related laryngospasm, sleep choking syndrome, and terrifying hypnogogic hallucinations may also present with symptoms unrelated to sleepiness or sleeplessness.
Arousals and Waking Secondary to Sleep-Related Breathing Disorders	• A history of habitual snoring (≥3 nights per week) is present. • Snoring may be associated with respiratory pauses, snorts, gasps, or choking. • Restless sleep may be present. • There may be frequent nocturnal waking. • Sleep-related diaphoresis may be present. • Palate may be high, arched, and elongated. • Daytime sleepiness and/or hyperactivity may be present.

TABLE 8.3	Arousals and Awakening—Cont'd
Disorder	**Principal Differentiating Considerations**
Arousals and Waking Secondary to Acute and/or Chronic Pain Syndromes	• A history of a disorder associated with chronic pain may be present (e.g., juvenile rheumatoid arthritis, other chronic inflammatory disorders). • Acute infections including, but not limited to, acute suppurative otitis media may be present. • A history of chronic ear infections may be elicited. • There may be a history of chronic urinary and/or gastrointestinal complaints. • Migraine cephalgia may be present. • Non-refreshing sleep without significant daytime sleepiness may be the primary complaint. • Teething pain, posttraumatic pain, myalgia, cephalgia, orthopedic disorders, or any other disease associated with chronic pain may disrupt nocturnal sleep.
Nocturnal Leg Cramps	• Sudden abrupt waking from sleep occurs. • Waking is associated with clear cramping of a muscle or group of muscles. • Spells are episodic, not periodic. • No organic pathology can be found to account for the symptoms. • Rubbing, stretching, or massage of the affected limb may relieve the discomfort.
Arousals and/or Wakings Secondary to Circadian Rhythm Disorders	
Short Sleeper	• Total 24-hour sleep time is shorter than expected (<75% of age-appropriate norms) when compared with age-appropriate norms. • Nocturnal sleep is often shorter than expected. • Sleep is otherwise normal. • Children wake early in the morning refreshed and alert. • There is no significant daytime sleepiness.
Shiftwork by Proxy	• Parent(s)/caretaker(s) are involved in shift work. • Unusual sleep–wake schedules may be enforced for the children.
Advanced Sleep Phase	• Children fall to sleep easily in the late afternoon or very early evening. • Sleep is otherwise normal. • There is an early morning wake time. • Children wake refreshed and alert but at an undesirabley early time. • Total sleep time is consistent with age-appropriate norms. • Typically, there is no daytime sleepiness.
Irregular Sleep Phase	• Sleep and wake times are very haphazard and variable. • Total 24-hour sleep time is usually normal. • Long sleep periods and long wake periods are temporally unpredictable. • Sleep and wake bouts are unpredictable and scattered. • Neurocognitive difficulties and performance difficulties are often present. • No clear sleep–wake pattern can be discerned.

Regularity and Duration of Sleep

Every physiologic function exhibits rhythmic variation across the 24-hour day. Most notable is the sleep–wake cycle. Disorders of regularity and duration of sleep, therefore, are a group of clinical syndromes characterized by misalignment between the endogenous sleep–wake cycling and external/environmental phases. Typically, when asleep, sleep structure is normal. Disorders are related to the regularity and rhythm of sleep and wake when compared with the phase of required physiologic function. Like any other system, biologic rhythm systems may become dysfunctional. Symptoms may be clear or may be subtle. Children with disorders of the sleep–wake cycle may not complain of schedule problems. Symptoms may center on inability to initiate sleep, maintain sleep, or both. One of the most vital questions from which to assist in pursuing an appropriate inquiry design is, *"Does the child sleep well somewhere, under some conditions, and at some time during the day?"* The location and situation may not seem appropriate for sleep, but if the child sleeps well despite the location or situation, the likelihood that the problem is either behavioral, conditioned, or circadian misalignment is greater. If the child sleeps well under some circumstance the problem may relate to delayed sleep phase disorder, advanced sleep phase disorder, short sleeper, shift-work by proxy, inappropriate caretaker expectations, inappropriate sleep hygiene, environmental factors, or inappropriate sleep-onset associations. If the child sleeps poorly under all circumstances, non-24-hour sleep-wake disorder, irregular sleep-wake disorder, and chronic medical conditions should be considered.

Assessing Disorders of Sleep That Are Principally Associated With Sleep Timing, Regularity, and Duration

Searching Questions asked: Searching questions and inquiry design might include the following questions:
1. Has a regular sleep schedule been established for the child?
2. At what time does the child habitually get into bed?
3. At what time does the child habitually wake in the morning?
4. If appropriate, is there any difference in bedtime and/or wake time on school days compared to weekends and/or holidays?
5. What is the average total sleep time for every 24-hour cycle?

TABLE 8.4	Regularity and Duration of Sleep
Disorder	**Principal Differentiating Considerations**
Irregularity Related to Circadian Rhythm Disorders	
Delayed Sleep Phase	• Bedtime and sleep-onset time are much later than expected (bedtime struggles are common). • Sleep onset may be delayed for hours beyond the parents' desired bedtime for the child. • Daytime sleepiness likely occurs if early morning waking is required. • Sleeps late into morning or into afternoon when allowed to wake spontaneously (e.g., weekends, holidays). • Most alert in afternoon hours. • If allowed to sleep and wake spontaneously, sleep is normal and daytime performance is normal.
Advanced Sleep Phase	• The child falls to sleep much earlier than expected for age. • Sleep is generally normal and uninterrupted. • Very early morning waking to begin the day. • Wakes early alert and refreshed. • Daytime sleepiness is unusual with the only symptom being bedtime and consolidated sleep earlier than expected.
Non–24-Hour Sleep– Wake Syndrome	• Sleep complaints vary and change. • Patients periodically alternate from episodes of extreme sleeplessness with the sleep–wake cycle apparently reversed, with periods of relatively normal sleep. • Cycling may vary but seems to recur regularly throughout each month. • At times, wake periods may be prolonged (24–40 hours in length) and followed by prolonged sleep periods (14–24 hours in length). • May be present in sightless children.

TABLE 8.4 **Regularity and Duration of Sleep—Cont'd**

Irregular Sleep–Wake Syndrome	• Sleep pattern is variable and haphazard. • Complaints vary and often include sleepiness, sleeplessness, or both. • Total sleep time over a 24-hour period is usually within age-group norms, but long sleep periods and long wake periods are temporally unpredictable. • Parents might complain that their child "never sleeps." • Remainder of the day may also be chaotic and follow no regular schedule.
Irregularity Related to Behavioral/Conditioned Issues	
Inappropriate Sleep Hygiene	• Bedtime routines may be disrupted by arousing activities. • Sleep environment may be chaotic and filled with other activities such as eating, television, and computer games. • Sleep onset can be difficult, but the sleep complaint is variable and may be associated with irregular bedtimes and wake times. • In some children, excessive napping may disrupt nocturnal sleep.
Short Sleeper	• Total sleep time is substantially less than norms for age. • Sleep is otherwise normal and refreshing. • Sleep onset may be delayed. • Early morning wakings may occur. • Children typically wake refreshed and alert after a period of short nocturnal sleep. • No significant daytime sleepiness is present.
Inappropriate Caretaker Expectations	• There are clear expectations regarding the child's sleep–wake habits and cycling that are beyond the child's developmental level. • Bedtime may be too early in the evening for the child's age. • There can be a lack of understanding of normal developmental landmarks. • Expectations of a young infant to sleep through the night pay little attention to the developmental inability of the infant to consolidate sleep in a manner similar to an adult, just as the small infant cannot walk or talk like an older child or adult.
Irregularity of Sleep due to Medical Conditions	• A complex medical or neurologic condition is typically present. • Symptoms may be principally related to the primary underlying medical disorder. • Sleep–wake scheduling problems may take a variety of forms and can be quite irregular. • Virtually any medical condition may affect sleep in a variety of ways. • Sleep-related comorbidities may be present.

Sleep Breathing Disorders

Sleep-disordered breathing (SDB) is common and can be a serious cause of morbidity during childhood. This section is concerned with diagnosing the disorders of breathing during sleep in childhood. There is a wide range of symptoms, signs, and diagnoses that extend from simple snoring to obstructive sleep apnea syndrome (pediatric OSAS). There are also disorders that primarily present with sleep-related hypoventilation. Sleep-related hypoventilation syndrome may either be acquired or congenital. This section will assist in differentiating various forms of SDB in childhood. As previously stated, much overlap exists. Comprehensive discussion of each specific diagnosis may be found elsewhere in this text. Snoring is considered the most characteristic feature of pediatric OSA. If a child does snore more than 3 nights per week consideration should be given to assess for the presence of OSA. Additionally, complex sleep apnea, obesity hypoventilation, and medications/substance affect should also be considered. If SDB is suspected and the child does not habitually snore, OSA may still be present. Nevertheless, consideration should then be given to the possible presence of primary central sleep apnea, apnea of prematurity, apnea of infancy, central apnea with Cheynne-Stokes breathing, Congenital Central Hypoventilation Syndrome, and ROHHAD (Rapid-onset Obesity with Hypothalamic dysfunction, Hypoventilation, and Autonomic Dysregulation).

Assessing Disorders of Sleep With Sleep-Related Abnormalities of Breathing and Ventilation

Searching Questions asked: Searching questions that might be included in the inquiry design are as follows:

1. Does the child snore more than 3 nights per week?
2. Are there respiratory pauses, snorts, gasps, or choking?
3. Is there mouth breathing?
4. Frequent morning headaches?
5. Enuresis?
6. AWitnessed apnea?
7. Diaphoresis?
8. Restless sleep?
9. Neck hyper-extended during sleep?
10. Daytime sleepiness, over-activity, attention problems?
11. Morning dry mouth?
12. Poor school performance?

TABLE 8.5   Sleep Breathing Disorders

Disorder	Principal Differentiating Considerations
Primary Snoring	<ul><li>Snoring is present ≥3 nights per week.</li><li>No other nocturnal symptoms are reported.</li><li>Daytime symptoms are notably absent.</li><li>Diagnosis is principally based on polysomnography that shows the *absence of* apneas, hypopneas, periods of oxygen desaturation, hypercapnia, or electrocardiographic (ECG) changes.</li></ul>
Obstructive Sleep Apnea	<ul><li>Snoring is present ≥3 nights per week.</li><li>Other nocturnal symptoms are present, including, but not limited to, observed apneas; increased work of breathing; respiratory pauses, snorts, gasps, or choking; restless sleep; secondary enuresis; frequent nighttime waking; waking feeling unrefreshed.</li><li>Daytime symptoms are often present, including, but not limited to, hyperactivity, daytime sleepiness, learning difficulties, behavioral difficulties, and/or morning headaches.</li><li>Diagnosis is based on *polysomnographic evidence of the presence of* apneas, hypopneas, periods of oxygen desaturation, hypercapnia, and ECG changes (pediatric OSA).</li><li>Sleep fragmentation from frequent respiratory effort related arousals can also result in symptoms (formerly classified as upper airway resistance syndrome).</li></ul>

TABLE 8.5	Sleep Breathing Disorders—Cont'd

Disorder	Principal Differentiating Considerations
Sleep-Related Hypoxemia	<ul><li>Oxygen saturation falls to ≤90% for ≥5 consecutive minutes.</li><li>Principal etiology for the hypoxemia is not due to OSA or central sleep-disordered breathing.</li><li>Carbon dioxide levels are normal.</li><li>With primary pulmonary disease, underlying medical disorders or neurologic disorders or sleep-related hypoxemia may be present.</li><li>Hypoxemia is most likely due to the underlying medical/pulmonary/neurologic problem rather than OSA or central sleep apnea.</li></ul>
Obesity Hypoventilation Syndrome	<ul><li>BMI ≥95th percentile for age and gender.</li><li>Significant daytime sleepiness (sleep attacks and/or unintentional sleep episodes) are commonly present.</li><li>Sleep-related hypercapnia is notable.</li><li>Hypercapnia is commonly present during the daytime waking hours as well as during sleep.</li><li>OSA and its symptoms are often present.</li><li>Hypoventilation is not due to an underlying medical, pulmonary, or neurologic disorder.</li><li>Differentiated from obstructive hypoventilation by the *presence of* normal carbon dioxide levels during the day and/or the *absence of* compensated respiratory acidosis (chronically elevated serum bicarbonate levels).</li></ul>
Complex Sleep-Disordered Breathing	<ul><li>Pediatric OSA is present.</li><li>Central sleep apnea is also present.</li><li>Central sleep apnea persists once the obstructive component is resolved.</li><li>Medication that depresses respiratory function may also be contributing to or underlying both the obstructive and central components.</li></ul>
Sleep-Related Hypoventilation Due to a Medical Disorder	<ul><li>Carbon dioxide is elevated during sleep.</li><li>Hypercapnia is considered to be due to, but not limited to, primary pulmonary disease, neuromuscular disorder, or chest wall deformity.</li><li>Obstructive hypoventilation and/or obesity hypoventilation syndrome are notably absent.</li><li>Lower airway disease, primary pulmonary disease, chest wall abnormalities, and neurologic or neuromuscular disorders are usually present.</li><li>Hypercapnia is typically most severe in REM sleep.</li></ul>
Primary Central Sleep Apnea of Prematurity	<ul><li>The infant is <37 weeks of gestation.</li><li>Prolonged (≥20 seconds) apnea and/or cyanosis is seen.</li><li>Oxygen desaturations and/or bradycardic episodes are noted.</li><li>Excessive periodic breathing is present.</li><li>Resolves with maturation, most often by the time conceptional term (40 weeks' gestation) is reached.</li></ul>
Primary Central Sleep Apnea of Infancy	<ul><li>The infant is of *term gestation* (≥37 weeks).</li><li>Prolonged (≥20 seconds) apnea or cyanosis is seen.</li><li>Oxygen desaturations and/or bradycardic episodes are noted.</li><li>Excessive periodic breathing (>5% of the total sleep time) is present.</li><li>Transient central apneas are not uncommon in infants born at term. Etiology of central sleep apnea of infancy is unclear but may be related to delay in maturation of the central respiratory center. Some infants may present with an apparent life-threatening event. Infants with significant gastroesophageal reflux disorder may present with a cyanotic spell after eating. In neonates, reflux into the esophagus may be related to respiratory pause and bradycardia secondary to a vagal response. Exaggerated pulmonary stretch reflex (Hering-Breuer reflex) resulting in an expiratory apnea or hypopnea after an augmented breath (sigh) may also be present. The clinical significance of expiratory apneas and hypopneas in the newborn infant is unclear.</li></ul>

(Continued)

TABLE 8.5	Sleep Breathing Disorders—Cont'd	
Disorder	**Principal Differentiating Considerations**
Central Sleep Apnea With Cheyne-Stokes Breathing	• Central sleep apnea is present. • A pattern of apneustic breathing may be seen. • Waxing and waning of respiratory effort and flow is noted. • Periodic oxygen desaturations are commonly associated with respiratory pauses. • Is seen in children with abnormalities of the posterior fossa including, but not limited to, Chiari malformations and posterior fossa tumors.
Congenital Central Hypoventilation Syndrome (CCHS)	• Hypoventilation/hypercapnia is notably present during wakefulness and sleep. • *PHOX2B* gene mutation is present. • Hirschsprung's disease is common. • Other abnormalities of the autonomic nervous system can be identified including, but not limited to, hypotension, swallowing abnormalities, and decreased variability in heart rate. • Neural tumors (e.g., ganglioneuroma/ganglioneuroblastoma) may be present. • Respiration and ventilation is insensitive to hypoxemia and hypercapnia. • Late-onset central hypoventilation with hypothalamic dysfunction may occur.
ROHHAD(Rapid-Onset Obesity With Hypothalamic Dysfunction, Hypoventilation, and Autonomic Dysregulation)	• Sudden, unexplained, rapid onset of obesity is present (typically 10–20 kg within 6–12 months). • Hypoventilation is present (may be sleep related). • Hypoxemia during sleep and significant oxygen desaturation during wake may be noted. • Hypoventilation is deceptive and can be life-threatening because no respiratory distress or increased work of breathing is noted. • There is a blunted response to hypoxemia and hypercarbia. • Hypothalamic-mediated endocrinopathies are noted (precocious puberty, hypogonadism, hypothyroidism, growth hormone deficiency). • Tumors of neural origin may be present. • *PHOX2B* gene mutation is notably absent.

CLINICAL PEARLS

• Similar to all clinical problem-solving processes, appropriate clinical reasoning methods are used to evaluate pediatric sleep disorders.
• Arriving an appropriate sleep-related diagnosis involves a complex series of deductions.
• A cornerstone to the process of appropriate clinical problem-solving and arriving at an accurate diagnosis is adequacy and completeness of an initial hypothesis set.
• A broad knowledge base is required for clinical diagnostic accuracy involving signs and symptoms of a wide variety of sleep-related disorders.

References

1. American Academy of Sleep Medicine. *International Classification of Sleep Disorders*. 3rd ed. American Academy of Sleep Medicine; 2014.
2. Berry RB, Quan SF, Abreu AR, et al. for the American Academy of Sleep Medicine. *The AASM Manual for the Scoring of Sleep and Associated Events: Rules, Terminology and Technical Specifications.* Version 2.6. American Academy of Sleep Medicine; 2020.
3. Owens JA, Dalzell V. Use of the "BEARS" sleep screening tool in a pediatric residents' continuity clinic: a pilot study. *Sleep Med.* 2005;6:63–69.
4. Sheldon SH. Pediatric sleep medicine differential diagnosis, appendix 3. In: Sheldon SH, Spire JP, Levy HB, eds. *Pediatric Sleep Medicine*. WB Saunders; 1992:185–214.

PART III

Clinical Practice

The Insomnia (Disorders of Initiating and Maintaining Sleep)

9

Sleep and Colic

Anat Cohen Engler, Tamar Etzioni, and Giora Pillar

CHAPTER HIGHLIGHTS

- Infantile colic is a common syndrome characterized by excessive crying, mainly during evening and night hours, in an infant who is otherwise healthy. It is a benign, transient condition that usually resolves by the age of 6 months.
- The etiology and pathogenesis are not well understood. Most theories suggest a gastrointestinal (GI) disturbance or temperament and self-regulation issues.
- Parental reports suggest that infants with infantile colic have more sleeping problems, and shorter sleep duration. Nevertheless, objective studies that used polysomnography demonstrated that infants with or without colic had similar sleep duration and not substantially different sleep structure. This discrepancy may be due in part to differences in the infants' signaling behavior during nighttime and how they are perceived by their parents, rather than in their actual sleeping habits.
- The two nocturnal behaviors may have a common cause such as circadian disturbance, feeding method, and temperament.
- Melatonin has both sleep-promoting effects and a relaxing effect on the GI tract. Low levels of melatonin in early infancy may lead to both fragmented sleep and colic.

Terminology and Definitions

The most distinctive feature of infantile colic is excessive crying. Crying, especially in the evening, is a normal behavior of infants.[1] Recognizing which crying behavior should be considered excessive and requires further evaluation is a challenge for the clinician.

There is an extensive variety of definitions for excessive crying and colic. The most widely used is the one defined by Wessel in 1954, also known as "the rule of three": crying for more than 3 hours per day, for more than 3 days per week, and for longer than 3 weeks in an infant who is well-fed and is otherwise healthy.[2,3] Although widely acceptable, this definition is hard to apply as 3 weeks is a long time for parents to document and evaluate their infant's crying. It was also suggested that the 3-week cut-off is arbitrary. A more

practical definition, used in many studies, is the "modified Wessel criteria" requiring the infant to have fussed/cried for more than 3 hours a day on at least 3 days in any 1 week.[3–5]

Other definitions rely on different time frames as well as on parents' perception for what is considered "excessive." Reijneveld et al. demonstrated that different definitions apply to different groups of children.[6]

For the purposes of research, it is highly important to adhere to a unified definition in order for results to be comparable and for meta-analysis to be carried out. We recommend using the Wessel or modified Wessel criteria to keep unity between studies.

As for practical purpose, the Rome IV criteria suggested the following: (1) age less than 5 months when the symptoms start and stop; (2) recurrent and prolonged periods of crying, fussing, or irritability that start and stop without obvious cause and cannot be prevented or resolved by caregivers; and (3) no evidence of poor weight gain, fever, or illness.[5]

Another possibility is a percentile chart for "average" or "excessive" crying provided by Wolke et al. and based on a cross-country meta-analysis. As major differences were found between studies, this chart must be used only as a rough guide to recognize excessive crying.[3] Nevertheless, acute crying might be an obvious sign of a serious illness or even a life-threatening one, and must clearly not be ignored.

Properties and "Natural Course"

The typical colicky crying episodes are prolonged, practically unsoothable, and associated with a high-pitched cry. The episodes are sometimes accompanied by posture changes such as drawing up of the legs or clenched fists, flushing, and passing gas. Episodes are more common during evening and night hours.[7–9]

Besides differences in crying duration and intensity, it seems that the crying curve of the colicky infant resembles the one of the "average" infant. The overall duration of crying increases gradually until it peaks at about the age of 6–8 weeks, then declines until it reaches a plateau around the age of 3–4 months.[1,9]

Prevalence

The prevalence of infantile colic in the community is estimated to be 10–25%, depending on the definition used. Because there is a large variety of definitions and different considerations to babies' cries, it is hard to determine the exact prevalence rates.[3,6]

Pathogenesis

Although infantile colic is a well-known syndrome of excessive cry, the etiology and pathogenesis remain an enigma. Many theories exist, yet none is adequately evidence-based. It seems that infantile colic may be a shared presentation of different situations.

Most of the theories argue that a gastrointestinal (GI) disturbance and an associated abdominal pain cause the crying paroxysms. That belief is somewhat supported by clinical evidence and the infant's behavior during the bouts as described above. A machine learning–based algorithm found significant acoustic similarities between colicky cry and painful cry, which may suggest that the cry indeed originates in a painful stimulus.[10] Other theories suggest that the crying bouts may be related to temperament and regulation, or that the "excessive cry" simply represents the extreme end of the normal infantile crying behavior.[11] This section will describe the most accepted proposed causes of infantile colic.

Excessive Air Load in the Gastrointestinal Tract

Based on clinical observations that infants with colic tend to pass relatively large amounts of gas,[7] it is a common belief that excessive gas in the GI tract causes painful abdominal distention and subsequent crying bouts. Possible sources for excessive gas may be aerophagia and colonic bacterial fermentation of malabsorbed carbohydrates. This theory is somewhat supported by small studies,[12] though clinical trials with simethicone (a gas absorber) failed to prove symptomatic relieve in comparison with placebo when treating colicky infants.[13,14]

Dysmotility

Another common belief is that the origin of infants' crying is gut hyperperistalsis and intestinal smooth muscle spasm.[15] This theory is supported by evidence that antispasmodic agents, such as dicyclomine hydrochloride and cimetropium bromide, alleviate colic symptoms.[13,14] Transient dysregulation of the central nervous system was suggested as the reason for dysmotility, though no difference was found in the balance of autonomic nervous system between colicky and other infants.[16]

Altered Gut Microbiota

The role of intestinal microflora has been growing in importance. Different and less diverse gut-microflora, as well as lower counts of lactobacilli, were observed in colicky infants in comparison with healthy infants. The differences disappeared by the age of 3–4 months.[17,18]

Gut Hormones

The GI tract activity is highly regulated by different hormones. Some of them were suggested to play a role in the pathogenesis of infantile colic. Different studies found higher levels of motilin and ghrelin in colicky infants.[19] Motilin is speculated to promote gastric emptying, which increases small bowel peristalsis and decreases transit time. This can also relate to the dysmotility theory.

Infants with colic also seem to have higher levels of 5-hydroxy indoleacetic acid, a metabolite of serotonin,[20] and a delay in the development of melatonin circadian rhythm.[21] This supported the hypothesis that some features of colic might be caused by a serotonin–melatonin counterbalancing system involving the GI smooth muscles. Serotonin and melatonin have opposite effects on intestinal smooth muscle: serotonin causes contraction, whereas melatonin causes relaxation.[22] It was hypothesized that in some infants the balance between circulating serotonin concentrations and intestinal smooth muscle sensitivity to serotonin might lead to painful GI cramps in the evening when serotonin concentrations are highest.

Lack of melatonin in the first months of life may explain the lack of its needed relaxing effect.[21,23] However, some researchers believe there is no solid scientific evidence to support this hypothesis.[24]

Gastroesophageal Reflux

This was suggested to be related to the pathogenesis of infantile colic, though no convincing evidence exists. Apparently, this is a distinctive common GI pathology that may coexist with infantile colic.[25]

Food Allergy

Food allergy was also suggested to have a role in infantile colic. This assumption is mainly based on observational studies that demonstrated an improvement after applying a low-allergen diet. As evidence accumulates, this relation seems less clear.[26] Like gastroesophageal reflux, food allergy may also be a distinctive pathology that might mimic or coexist with infantile colic.

Infantile Migraine

Recent studies demonstrated an association between infantile colic and an increased risk for migraine headache in the future.[27,28] It is plausible that for some infants, infantile colic might be a migrainous phenomenon or that both phenomena share a common cause or predisposition.

Psychosocial Factors

Over the years, it was widely argued that excessive infant crying and feeding and sleep difficulties are problems of self-regulation.[11] It was also argued that the excessive crying is an early manifestation of a difficult temperament, and the colicky infant is often considered to be irritable and hypersensitive.[8] This assumption is almost impossible to examine in an unbiased longitudinal manner, thus evidence is conflicting.[8,29,30] Parental psychologic factors such as anxiety disorder, emotional stress, and depression were also found associated and predispose to infantile colic.[31,32]

Parental Smoking

Few studies indicated that exposure of the child to tobacco smoking by the mother during pregnancy and after delivery, and smoking by the father, were associated with excessive crying. Moreover, it was suggested that smoking is linked to increased plasma and intestinal motilin levels, and higher-than-average intestinal motilin and ghrelin levels seem to be related to elevated risk of infantile colic.[33]

Outcome and Prognosis

Infantile colic is a transient, self-limiting condition considered to have a favorable outcome, usually resolving by the age of 4–6 months.[8]

On psychologic grounds, several studies suggested that infants with colic are more emotional and are somewhat prone to negative moods and temper tantrums.[34,35] This was confronted by other studies, suggested that behavioral difficulties are associated only with unremitting excessive crying that lasts longer than 6 months, and therefore does not account as infantile colic.[36,37]

Despite the self-limiting nature and favorable outcome, infantile colic may have a serious impact on the parents. Other than preexisting maternal depression, mothers of infants with colic have a higher risk for developing consequential depression.[38]

Excessive crying is also associated with shaken baby syndrome and child abuse,[39,40] which emphasizes the need for a proper diagnosis and attention for this situation.

Diagnosis

Excessive infant crying is a very common situation, and the differential diagnosis is extremely broad. When excessive crying is prolonged, an organic disease is estimated to account for less than 5% of the cases.[41] Nevertheless, before making the diagnosis of infantile colic, an organic cause must be ruled out.

When faced with a crying infant, the importance of a thorough history and physical examination cannot be overemphasized. Situations that may cause similar symptoms such as gastroesophageal reflux, constipation, and cow milk protein allergy must be considered, as well as an acute illness or a neurologic or developmental problem.

- Parents should be asked about characteristics of the crying episodes such as duration, time of the day, and accompanying behavior.

• **BOX 9.1   Potential Causes for Prolonged Excessive Infantile Crying**

Gastrointestinal:
    Infantile colic
    Gastroesophageal reflux
    Rumination
    Feeding problems
    Constipation
    Milk protein allergy
Neurologic:
    Psychomotor retardation
    Communication problems
Difficulty breathing:
    Choanal atresia
    Laryngomalacia
    Congenital lung disease
Infection:
    Urinary tract infection
    Otitis media
Pain:
    Fracture
    Hernia
    Corneal abrasion
    Atopic dermatitis
Social problems:
    Neglect
    Abuse
    Inadequate relation with care giver
    Limit-setting sleep disorders

- Physical examination should be completed in a systematic head-to-toe manner with emphasis on the GI and neurologic systems. Signs of abuse or trauma must be sought as well.
- The infant's weight percentile should be considered.

Any finding suggestive of a specific pathology should be considered and evaluated appropriately. Box 9.1 lists potential causes for prolonged, excessive infantile cry. If the history and physical examination reveal no pathologic condition in an infant that gains weight properly, laboratory or radiographic examinations are usually not necessary. A recent retrospective cohort study found that the only useful laboratory examination when evaluating a crying infant with a normal history and physical examination is urine evaluation.[41]

Treatment

Once the diagnosis of infantile colic is made, the first step of management is reassuring of the parents, explaining that colic is a self-limiting condition and that the excessive crying does not reflect an underlying disease or bad parenting.[8] In addition, parents should be reassured that there is no negative prognosis for infantile colic.

As for interventional therapies, over the years many remedies have been proposed and studied as possible treatments for infantile colic. The main groups are pharmacologic, probiotics, dietary, and behavioral interventions based on the different possible etiologies/mechanisms. Unfortunately, because of lack of a standard definition and methodologic weaknesses in many of the clinical trials, the data do not deliver convincing evidence to support a specific treatment. Currently, it is still not clear which is the optimal treatment, and watchful waiting might just be the best medicine.

Probiotics

As mentioned above, infants with colic have distinctive gut microflora, with lower counts of lactobacilli among other differences. *Lactobacillus reuteri*, one of the few endogenous *Lactobacillus* species in the human GI tract, has been used safely for many years as a probiotic dietary supplement in adults, and there is evidence of safety after long-term dietary supplementation for newborn infants. One meta-analysis found *L. reuteri* had a clear benefit when given to breastfed infants, but no clear benefit was found for bottle-fed infants.[42] A recent systematic review and meta-analysis found that probiotics, especially *L. reuteri*, made little or no difference in the occurrence of infantile colic, but did seem to reduce daily crying time in the range of 25–65 minutes. There was no difference in the reporting of side effects in comparison to placebo.[13,43]

Dietary Interventions

Some trials suggested that dietary modification such as low-allergen diet (maternal for breastfed or formula for bottle-fed infants), may have some benefit.[44,45] Other studies regarding dietary interventions (e.g., partially hydrolyzed, high fiber, low-lactose formulas) are inconclusive. Unfortunately, all studies in that manner had a small number of participants and a high risk for bias, so a solid conclusion or recommendation is not possible based on current available data.[18,26]

Pharmacologic Interventions

Several pharmacologic agents were suggested and tested as treatment of infantile colic.
- Simethicone, a commonly used drug aimed to relieve gas-related symptoms, did not demonstrate conclusive benefit as a treatment for infantile colic.[13,14]
- Anticholinergic drugs were tested as possible therapies due to their antispasmodic effect.
- Dicyclomine has been proved to be an effective treatment for infantile colic; however, because of life-threatening side effects such as apnea, seizures and coma, the manufacturer has contraindicated the use of the drug in infants younger than 6 months and does not consider infantile colic as an indication for using the drug. Cimetropium bromide was found effective but had many side effects including sleepiness.[14,18]
- Proton pump inhibitors are sometimes prescribed for irritable infants as a treatment for suspected gastroesophageal reflux disease in the absence of clear clinical evidence. They were found ineffective in such situations.[13]

Considering all mentioned above, as for now, pharmacologic therapy is not recommended for infantile colic.[14]

Behavioral Interventions

Clinical trials examining the efficacy of behavioral interventions are problematic in nature. First, it is impossible to conduct a double-blind study, and bias may affect the results. Second, many of the examined interventions can cause overstimulation and therefore influence the results.

Parent training programs, which remain popular, seem to reduce infant crying time, though evidence is slim and the certainty of the evidence is low.[46]

Complementary and Alternative Medicine

Though popular, reported evidence regarding efficacy and safety are still lacking, small clinical trials regarding chiropractic, acupuncture, herbal, and massage therapies found some of these therapies, but not all, may have a minor alleviating effect.[47,48]

In conclusion, any combination of these approaches can be tried and individualized to each infant. If the diagnosis of infantile colic is correct, the most important approaches are parental reassurance and gaining time. As stated, the natural history is spontaneous alleviation by 6 months of age.

Infantile Colic and Sleep Problems

An association between infantile colic and sleep problems later on in life has previously been suggested by subjective parental testimonies.[34,49] This association was further explored, supported by some research and confounded by others.[35,37]

Such association is very difficult to explore for several reasons. First, as described above, there is a lack of a globally acceptable definition of colic. Results of different studies are incomparable, as different colic definitions were used. Second, most of the research used questionnaires to evaluate infants' sleep. This method was found unreliable,[50] especially as mothers of "quiet" infants tend to overestimate their child's sleeping time, whereas mothers of colicky infants tend to consider their child to be more difficult.[51]

Currently, no consensus is established. The two phenomena may influence each other and both may be affected by many factors, some of which may overlap. As the base of both phenomena is very complex and may be attributed to physiologic as well as psychologic factors, empiric isolation of each factor and a full understanding of the nature and relation of those behaviors may never be accomplished.

Infantile Colic and Sleep Problems Before the Age of Three Months

Some subjective studies supported the hypothesis that infants with colic tend to sleep less. This was ratified by subjective studies, but not corroborated by objective researches.

A very large population-based study was conducted by Crowcroft et al. Their results showed that colicky babies had significantly shorter periods of "longest continuous time asleep" and longer periods of "longest time awake" than other infants.[52] St. James-Roberts et al. found that colicky infants slept on average 77 minutes less than non-colicky infants at the age of 6 weeks; the clearest group differences were in the daytime.[53] White et al. found that colicky infants slept about 1.5–2 hours less in a course of the day when compared with infants without colic.[54] On the other hand, a recent longitudinal study found that most infants with prolonged colic at 5–6 weeks of age were settled at night at 12 weeks of age, and they "slept through the night" as soon as other infants.[55]

Those studies, although very important and informative, were based on parental reports alone.

Objective studies, which used polysomnography (PSG) to evaluate sleep, found that colicky infants have a similar total and nocturnal sleeping time and structure as other infants. These studies shed new light on the validity of observational diaries.

One study found that during late evening and night sleep, excessively and non-excessively crying infants had an equal total sleeping time, a normal nocturnal sleep structure, and similar sleep onset time.[56]

A more recent study used a 24-hour PSG to compare between two groups, colicky and non-colicky infants, according to modified Wessel criteria. The study found that colicky infants had the same total sleep time as non-colicky infants, though sleep structure was somewhat different. The total REM sleep time in a 24-hour period was equal between the two groups, but the excessively crying infants had relatively less REM sleep during the evening, and they "catch up" during the long night sleep, when they had a longer REM sleep compared with the control group.[57]

The studies described above used both PSG and diaries to assess infants' sleep time and compared the results. A clear discrepancy between diary reports and PSG results was revealed, as reported sleep time in the diary data for the control group was longer than the objectively observed sleep time. These findings suggest that research based on diary reports alone may be biased, and more objective studies are needed.

Infantile Colic and Sleep After the Age of Three Months

Another aspect studied is whether colicky infants have sleeping problems later on in life, after colic symptoms had subsided.

Some studies argued that formerly colicky infants had more sleep difficulties, especially restless sleep and multiple night awakenings.[49,58] A recent study that relied on parental estimation also found that severe infantile colic at the age of 3 months was associated with fragmented sleep and multiple night wakening, but not with sleep duration, at the age of 12 months.[59] Others have found no significant differences in reported sleeping patterns.[51]

Canivet et al. approached mothers of ex-colicky infants and infants who did not have colic when the children were

4 years old and asked them about their children's sleep-related behaviors in several ways: (1) whether they went to sleep easily, (2) whether they talked and cried in sleep, (3) whether they did not mind going to bed, (4) frequency of nightmares, and (5) being overtired. No differences were found in the two groups in any aspect.[35]

Bell et al. questioned parents of children aged 2–3 years whether they consider their child's daytime or nighttime sleep as problematic and whether their child had colic during infancy. No difference was found between parents of infants with or without colic. They suggested that former studies that found such a difference might had included infants whose excessive crying lasted for over 3 months, and therefore does not account as infantile colic.[37] Again, these are all subjective reports. Kirjavainen et al. in the same research described above, also examined 6-month-old infants. There was no difference in reported sleeping time. PSG showed more short awakenings (shorter than 5 minutes) in the control group, but other than that, the sleep was practically similar between the two groups.[56]

Explanations for a Possible Direct Relation

Few theories attempted to explain a possible direct relation between infantile colic and sleeping problems.

As crying and sleeping are mutually exclusive in nature, it is reasonable to think that crying bouts during sleeping hours may come at the expense of sleep itself. White et al. found that, in a group of colicky infants, there was an inverse relation between time spent crying and duration of sleep, though in non-colicky infants such a relationship did not exist. However, they also showed that when controlling for crying statistically, colicky infants still have a shorter nocturnal sleep time, though less dramatic than the original differences.[54]

The theory of excessive crying as a result of sleep deprivation was not supported by the aforementioned studies, which used PSG. The proportion of sleep stages, the number of stage shifts, the total sleep time, and the number of sleep apneas of excessively crying infants were similar to the known structure of normal sleep for their age.[56,57]

As described above, there is a difference between the sleeping time as reported by parents and the actual sleeping time that was objectively measured, meaning that at least part of the real difference may not be in the sleeping habits of the infants but rather at their behavior during waking hours or how they are perceived by their parents. It is possible that while awake, "non-colicky" infants stay quiet and soothe themselves back to sleep, making it hard to recognize their night wakening, in contrast to colicky infants who tend to cry or fuss. This ties in with the hypothesis that infant sleep–waking problems usually involve maintenance of signaling behaviors rather than a generalized disturbance.[55]

Another possible explanation is that parents of colicky infants are more stressed and more sensitive to their infant's night wakening and tend to describe their child as more difficult than they actually are. Furthermore, Kahn et al.

demonstrated that lower parental cry tolerance was associated with poorer intact sleep quality in a bidirectional manner through the first 6 months of life.[60]

Common Causes

The two nocturnal behaviors may not be dependent on each other but may have common escalating factors.

There are several potential such factors, which may influence both sleep and behavior and, when disturbed, result in both fragmented sleep and excessive crying/colic. Shinohara et al. used actigraphic sleep measures to explore the relation between excessive crying and sleep consolidation. They concluded that although excessive crying and proportion of active sleep decreased in parallel, the cause seems to be an influence of common causes rather than a direct relation.[61] The following is a brief discussion of such potential factors.

Circadian Disturbance

The circadian production of hormones such as cortisol and melatonin begins around the age of 6–8 weeks, and a mature day–night-related secretion pattern is established by the age of 3–4 months,[62] the same age that nocturnal crying bouts and fragmented nocturnal sleep resolves. A difference in the nature of both behaviors in some infants may, in part, be attributed to a difference in day–night rhythmicity development.

Colicky and non-colicky infants were found to have similar average salivary cortisol levels during a 24-hour period, though infants with colic had a less clearly defined daily rhythm of cortisol secretion.[21,54] Among infants with infantile colic, elevated cortisol was found to be associated with increased crying intensity (but not duration) and fragmented sleep, suggesting a common cause for both phenomena among some of the infants.[63]

Melatonin, "the dark hormone," has well-known sleep-promoting effects,[64,65] as well as a relaxing effect on intestinal smooth muscle.[22,24] As mentioned earlier, infants with infantile colic seem to have a delayed development of melatonin circadian rhythm.[21] Therefore, it is possible that an earlier maturation of circadian melatonin secretion might play a role in the resolution of infantile colic and the consolidation of nocturnal sleep.

Feeding Method

The influence of feeding method on excessive crying and nocturnal sleep has been sparsely studied, and the data set in this matter is slim. Different studies that investigated the influence of breastfeeding on infantile colic had contradictory results.[52,66,67] As for the relation between feeding method and sleep–wake patterns of the infant, there are consistent findings suggesting that breastfed infants are more easily aroused and have a more fragmented nocturnal sleep.[23,68] There are not enough supporting data about the differences in the overall length of nocturnal sleep to make a solid conclusion.[69]

In our recent research, we found that exclusively breastfed infants had significantly fewer colic attacks and a decreased attack intensity when compared with exclusively formula-fed infants. We found that the breastfed infants, although waking up more often, tend to have an overall longer nocturnal sleep than formula-fed ones, though these results were not statistically significant.[23]

We also confirmed, as had been previously described, that breast milk contains melatonin, whereas artificial formulas do not. Considering the aforementioned properties of melatonin, this provides a possible explanation to a common factor affecting both crying and nocturnal infantile sleep, as breastfed infants enjoy an extrinsic melatonin supplementation. More research in this area might be beneficial.

Cow Milk Protein Allergy

In the late 1980s, cow milk protein allergy was found to cause sleeping problems.[70] It is also believed to elicit colic symptoms, as described above. However, cow milk allergy is rare in comparison to both infant sleeping problems and infantile colic and therefore cannot indicate a common pathology.

Temperament and Problems of Self-Regulation

Infants with colic, using Wessel's criteria, are more likely to have a difficult temperament than non-colicky babies when the temperament assessment is performed at 4 months of age. Nonetheless, colic does not appear to be an expression of a permanently difficult temperament. As mentioned earlier, the complex interface of infant's crying behavior, sleeping habits, and temperament is almost impossible to explore in an unbiased manner, especially when relying on subjective parental reports. Taking that into consideration, some studies did suggest that infants with difficult temperament tend to briefer total sleep duration,[30] longer sleep latency, and more night wakefulness.[71] In a longitudinal study, difficult infant temperament at 4 months was not associated with sleeping problems at the age of 16 months.[29]

CLINICAL PEARLS

- The prevalence of infantile colic in the community is estimated to be 10-25% and is thought to be associated with a gastrointestinal disturbance leading to crying paroxysms.
- The overall duration of crying increases gradually until it peaks at about the age of 6–8 weeks, then declines until it plateaus at around 3–4 months of age.
- The limited available literature suggests that there are indeed notable associations between infantile colic and sleep disturbance. Sleep quality is worse at night in babies with infantile colic, however, overall sleep duration is similar to babies without infantile colic as a result of increased daytime sleep.
- Circadian disturbance, feeding problems, cow milk protein allergy, and self-regulation issues are among the influential factors that may play a role in the association with infantile colic and sleep.

References

1. St. James-Roberts I, Halil T. Infant crying patterns in the first year: normal community and clinical findings. *J Child Psychol Psychiatr.* 1991;32(6):951–968.

2. Wessel MA, Cobb JC, Jackson EB, et al. Paroxysmal fussing in infancy, sometimes called colic. *Pediatrics.* 1954;14(5):421–435.

3. Wolke D, Bilgin A, Samara M. Systematic review and meta-analysis: fussing and crying durations and prevalence of colic in infants. *J Pediatr.* 2017;1(185):55–61.

4. Barr RG, Rotman A, Yaremko J, Leduc D, Francoeur TE. The crying of infants with colic: a controlled empirical description. *Pediatrics.* 1992;90(1 Pt 1):14–21.

5. Benninga MA, Faure C, Hyman St PE, James Roberts I, Schechter NL, Nurko S. Childhood functional gastrointestinal disorders: neonate/toddler. *Gastroenterology.* 2016;150(6):1443–1455.e2.

6. Reijneveld SA, Brugman E, Hirasing RA. Excessive infant crying: the impact of varying definitions. *Pediatrics.* 2001; 108(4):893–897.

7. Barr RG. Colic and crying syndromes in infants. *Pediatrics.* 1998;102(5 suppl. E):1282–1286.

8. Savino F. Focus on infantile colic. *Acta Paediatr.* 2007;96(9): 1259–1264.

9. Brazelton TB. Crying in infancy. *Pediatrics.* 1962;29:579–588.

10. Parga JJ, et al. Defining and distinguishing infant behavioral states using acoustic cry analysis: is colic painful? *Pediatr Res.* 2020;87(3):576–580.

11. St. James-Roberts I, Alvarez M, Hovish K. Emergence of a developmental explanation for prolonged crying in 1- to 4-month-old infants: review of the evidence. *J Pediatr Gastroenterol Nutr.* 2013;57:S30–S35.

12. Infante D, Segarra O, Le Luyer B. Dietary treatment of colic caused by excess gas in infants: biochemical evidence. *World J Gastroenterol.* 2011;17(16):2104.

13. Ellwood J, Draper-Rodi J, Carnes D. Comparison of common interventions for the treatment of infantile colic: a systematic review of reviews and guidelines. *BMJ Open.* 2020;10(2):e035405.

14. Biagioli E, Tarasco V, Lingua C, Moja L, Savino F. Pain-relieving agents for infantile colic. *Cochrane Database Syst Rev.* 2016;9:CD009999.

15. Camilleri M, et al. What's new in functional and motility disorders in the lower GI tract? *Malta Med J.* 2017;29(2):3–13.

16. Kirjavainen J, Jahnukainen T, Huhtala V, et al. The balance of the autonomic nervous system is normal in colicky infants. *Acta Paediatr.* 2001;90(3):250–254.

17. deWeerth C, Fuentes S, Puylaert P, de Vos WM. Intestinal microbiota of infants with colic: development and specific signatures. *Pediatrics.* 2013;131(2):e550–e558.

18. Camilleri M, Park SY, Scarpato E, Staiano A. Exploring hypotheses and rationale for causes of infantile colic. *Neurogastroenterol Motil.* 2017;29(2):e12943.

19. Savino F, Grassino EC, Guidi C, et al. Ghrelin and motilin concentration in colicky infants. *Acta Paediatr.* 2006;95(6):738–741.

20. Kurtoglu S, Uzum K, Hallac IK, et al. 5 Hydroxy-3-indole acetic acid levels in infantile colic: is serotoninergic tonus responsible for this problem? *Acta Paediatr.* 1997;86:764–765.

21. İnce T, Akman H, Çimrin D, Aydın A. The role of melatonin and cortisol circadian rhythms in the pathogenesis of infantile colic. *World J Pediatr.* 2018;14(4):392–398.

22. Bubenik GA. Thirty four years since the discovery of gastrointestinal melatonin. *J Physiol Pharmacol.* 2008;59(suppl. 2):33–51.

23. Cohen-Engler A, Hadash A, Shehadeh N, et al. Breastfeeding may improve nocturnal sleep and reduce infantile colic: potential role of breast milk melatonin. *Eur J Pediatr.* 2012;171(4):729–732.

24. Bubenik GA. Gastrointestinal melatonin: localization, function, and clinical relevance. *Dig Dis Sci.* 2002;47(10):2336–2348.

25. Indrio F, et al. Gut motility alterations in neonates and young infants: relation to colic. *J Pediatr Gastroenterol Nutr.* 2013;57:S9–S11.

26. Gordon M, et al. Dietary modifications for infantile colic. *Cochrane Database Syst Rev.* 2018;10:CD011029.

27. Gelfand AA, Goadsby PJ, Allen IE. The relationship between migraine and infant colic: a systematic review and meta-analysis. *Cephalalgia.* 2015;35(1):63–72.

28. Sillanpää M, Saarinen M. Infantile colic associated with childhood migraine: a prospective cohort study. *Cephalalgia.* 2015;35(14):1246–1251.

29. Martini J, Petzoldt J, Knappe S, Garthus-Niegel S, Asselmann E, Wittchen HU. Infant, maternal, and familial predictors and correlates of regulatory problems in early infancy: the differential role of infant temperament and maternal anxiety and depression. *Early Hum Dev.* 2017;115:23–31.

30. Kaley F, Reid V, Flynn E. Investigating the biographic, social and temperamental correlates of young infants' sleeping, crying and feeding routines. *Infant Behav Dev.* 2012;35(3):596–605.

31. Petzoldt J, Wittchen HU, Wittich J, Einsle F, Höfler M, Martini J. Maternal anxiety disorders predict excessive infant crying: a prospective longitudinal study. *Arch Dis Child.* 2014;99(9):800–806.

32. van den Berg MP, van der Ende J, Crijnen AA, et al. Paternal depressive symptoms during pregnancy are related to excessive infant crying. *Pediatrics.* 2009;124(1):e96–e103.

33. Stroud LR, Paster RL, Goodwin MS, et al. Maternal smoking during pregnancy and neonatal behavior: a large-scale community study. *Pediatrics.* 2009;123(5):e842–e848.

34. Rautava P, Lehtonen L, Helenius H, et al. Infantile colic: child and family three years later. *Pediatrics.* 1995;96(1 Pt 1):43–47.

35. Canivet C, Jakobsson I, Hagander B. Infantile colic. Follow-up at four years of age: still more "emotional". *Acta Paediatr.* 2000;89(1):13–17.

36. Hemmi MH, Wolke D, Schneider S. Associations between problems with crying, sleeping and/or feeding in infancy and long-term behavioural outcomes in childhood: a meta-analysis. *Arch Dis Child.* 2011;96(7):622–629.

37. Bell G, Hiscock H, Tobin S, Cook F, Sung V. Behavioral outcomes of infant colic in toddlerhood: a longitudinal study. *J Pediatr.* 2018;201:154–159.

38. Petzoldt J. Systematic review on maternal depression versus anxiety in relation to excessive infant crying: it is all about the timing. *Arch Womens Ment Health.* 2018;21(1):15–30.

39. Lee C, Barr RG, Catherine N, Wicks A. Age-related incidence of publicly reported shaken baby syndrome cases: is crying a trigger for shaking? *J Dev Behav Pediatr.* 2007;28(4):288–293.

40. Reijneveld SA, van der Wal MF, Brugman E, Sing RA, Verloove-Vanhorick SP. Infant crying and abuse. *Lancet.* 2004;364(9442):1340–1342.

41. Freedman SB, Al-Harthy N, Thull-Freedman J. The crying infant: diagnosis testing and frequency of serious underlying disease. *Pediatrics.* 2009;123(3):841–848.

42. Sung V, et al. Lactobacillus reuteri to treat infant colic: a meta-analysis. *Pediatrics.* 2018;141(1):e20171811.

43. Ong TG, Gordon M, Banks SS, Thomas MR, Akobeng AK. Probiotics to prevent infantile colic. *Cochrane Database of Syst Rev.* 2019;3(3):CD012473.

44. Hill DJ, Roy N, Heine RG, et al. Effect of a low-allergen maternal diet on colic among breastfed infants: a randomized, controlled trial. *Pediatrics*. 2005;116(5):e709–715.

45. Lucassen PL, Assendelft WJ, Gubbels JW, van Eijk JT, Douwes AC. Infantile colic: crying time reduction with a whey hydrolysate: a double-blind, randomized, placebo-controlled trial. *Pediatrics*. 2000;106(6):1349–1354.

46. Gordon M, Gohil J, Banks SS. Parent training programmes for managing infantile colic. *Cochrane Database Syst Rev*. 2019;12(12):CD012459.

47. Savino F, Ceratto S, De Marco A, Cordero di Montezemolo L. Looking for new treatments of infantile colic. *Ital J Pediatr*. 2014;40(1):53.

48. Rosen LD, Bukutu C, Le C, Shamseer L, Vohra S. Complementary, holistic, and integrative medicine: colic. *Pediatr Rev*. 2007;28(10):381–385.

49. Weissbluth M, Davis AT, Poncher J. Night waking in 4- to 8-month-old infants. *J Pediatr*. 1984;104(3):477–480.

50. Sadeh A. Assessment of intervention for infant night waking: parental reports and activity-based home monitoring. *J Consult Clin Psychol*. 1994;62:63–68.

51. Lehtonen L, Korhonen T, Korvenranta H. Temperament and sleeping patterns in colicky infants during the first year of life. *J Dev Behav Pediatr*. 1994;15(6):416–420.

52. Crowcroft NS, Strachan DP. The social origins of infantile colic: questionnaire study covering 76,747 infants. *BMJ*. 1997;314(7090):1325–1328.

53. St. James-Roberts I, Conroy S, Hurry J. Links between infant crying and sleep-waking at six weeks of age. *Early Hum Dev*. 1997;48(1-2):143–152.

54. White BP, Gunnar MR, Larson MC, Donzella B, Barr RG. Behavioral and physiological responsivity, sleep, and patterns of daily cortisol production in infants with and without colic. *Child Dev*. 2000;71(4):862–877.

55. St. James-Roberts I, Peachey E. Distinguishing infant prolonged crying from sleep-waking problems. *Arch Dis Child*. 2011;96(4):340–344.

56. Kirjavainen J, Kirjavainen T, Huhtala V, et al. Infants with colic have a normal sleep structure at 2 and 7 months of age. *J Pediatr*. 2001;138(2):218–223.

57. Kirjavainen J, Lehtonen L, Kirjavainen T, et al. Sleep of excessively crying infants: a 24-hour ambulatory sleep polygraphy study. *Pediatrics*. 2004;114(3):592–600.

58. Savino F, Castagno E, Bretto R, Brondello C, Palumeri E, Oggero R. A prospective 10-year study on children who had severe infantile colic. *Acta Paediatr*. 2005;94:129–132.

59. Sette S, Baumgartner E, Ferri R, Bruni O. Predictors of sleep disturbances in the first year of life: a longitudinal study. *Sleep Med*. 2017;36:78–85.

60. Kahn M, Bauminger Y, Volkovich E, Meiri G, Sadeh A, Tikotzky L. Links between infant sleep and parental tolerance for infant crying: longitudinal assessment from pregnancy through six months postpartum. *Sleep Med*. 2018;50:72–78.

61. Shinohara H, Kodama H. Relationship between duration of crying/fussy behavior and actigraphic sleep measures in early infancy. *Early Hum Dev*. 2012;88(11):847–852.

62. Larson MC, White BP, Cochran A, et al. Dampening of the cortisol response to handling at 3 months in human infants and its relation to sleep, circadian cortisol activity, and behavioral distress. *Dev Psychobiol*. 1998;33(4):327–337.

63. Brand S, Furlano R, Sidler M, Schulz J, Holsboer-Trachsler E. "Oh, baby, please don't cry!": in infants suffering from infantile colic hypothalamic-pituitary-adrenocortical axis activity is related to poor sleep and increased crying intensity. *Neuropsychobiology*. 2011;64(1):15–23.

64. Doghramji K. Melatonin and its receptors: a new class of sleep-promoting agents. *J Clin Sleep Med*. 2007;3(suppl. 5):S17–S23.

65. Lavie P. Sleep-wake as a biological rhythm. *Annu Rev Psychol*. 2001;52:277–303.

66. Saavedra MA, da Costa JS, Garcias G, et al. Infantile colic incidence and associated risk factors: a cohort study. *J Pediatr (Rio J)*. 2003;79(2):115–122.

67. Lucassen PL, Assendelft WJ, van Eijk JT, et al. Systematic review of the occurrence of infantile colic in the community. *Arch Dis Child*. 2001;84(5):398–403.

68. Figueiredo B, Dias CC, Pinto TM, Field T. Exclusive breast-feeding at three months and infant sleep-wake behaviors at two weeks, three and six months. *Infant Behav Dev*. 2017;49:62–69.

69. Rosen LA. Infant sleep and feeding. *J Obstet Gynecol Neonatal Nurs*. 2008;37(6):706–714.

70. Kahn A, Mozin MJ, Rebuffat E, et al. Milk intolerance in children with persistent sleeplessness: a prospective double-blind crossover evaluation. *Pediatrics*. 1989;84(4):595–603.

71. Sorondo BM, Reeb-Sutherland BC. Associations between infant temperament, maternal stress, and infants' sleep across the first year of life. *Infant Behav Dev*. 2015;39:131–135.

10

Sleep and Gastroesophageal Reflux

Robert Troxler and Susan M. Harding

CHAPTER HIGHLIGHTS

- Gastroesophageal reflux (GER) is common in children, with 12% of infants having regurgitation and 5% of adolescents reporting heartburn.
- 2022 transient relaxations of the lower esophageal sphincter are responsible for most GER episodes that commonly occur during arousals from sleep.
- Weekly heartburn is reported in 5.2% and/or regurgitation is reported in 8.2% of U.S. adolescents.
- Sleep-related GER is associated with GER symptoms during sleep, arousals, obstructive sleep apnea, asthma, laryngospasm, hoarseness, and brief resolved unexplained events (BRUE).
- Diagnosis of sleep-related GER includes symptoms and esophageal pH and impedance monitoring.
- Treatment includes behavioral interventions, pharmacologic therapy (primarily proton pump inhibitors), and in carefully evaluated children, surgical fundoplication.

Introduction

Gastroesophageal reflux disease (GERD) is common in children of all ages and can significantly impact sleep. In infants, GERD is brought to the attention of the pediatrician in at 24% of 6-month-old visits. Regurgitation occurs in more than 66% of otherwise healthy infants and is one of the most common GI problems presenting to primary care offices.[1-3] Although recent guidelines regarding management of pediatric GERD have been published, further research is required to understand the impact of GERD on sleep in children.[4]

Gastroesophageal reflux (GER) is the retrograde passage of gastric contents into the esophagus. Regurgitation is a symptom of GER and is common in infants. The refluxate is acidic and contains digestive enzymes, such as pepsin and trypsin, that can injure the mucosal lining of the esophagus and upper airway. Intrinsic protective mechanisms exist to prevent or minimize this damage. Reflux becomes pathologic GERD when GER episodes result in troublesome symptoms or complications including vomiting, poor weight gain, heartburn, esophagitis, or extraesophageal symptoms.[5]

The impact of this common problem on sleep in pediatric patients will be explored in this chapter. To appreciate the implications of GERD on sleep, we will first review esophageal physiology during wakefulness and sleep.

Esophageal Physiology

The esophagus develops initially during the fourth week of gestation as a small outgrowth of the endoderm and later includes all three germ layers: the endoderm, mesoderm, and ectoderm. These layers give rise, respectively, to the epithelial lining; muscular layers, angioblast, and mesenchyme; and the neural components.[6]

The esophagus slowly increases its length so that at 20 weeks of gestation, esophageal length approximates 11 cm.[7] Esophageal length doubles during the first year of life.[6] Ultimately, the esophageal body in adults has a length of 18–22 cm, with the lower esophageal sphincter (LES) representing the distal 2–4 cm of the esophagus. The LES grows from a few millimeters in newborns and reaches its adult length during adolescence. In older children, the proximal 1.5–2 cm of the LES is encircled by the crural diaphragm and sits in the thoracic cavity, and the lower 2 cm resides in the abdominal cavity.[8]

The esophagus consists of three functionally distinct zones, including the upper esophageal sphincter (UES), the esophageal body, and the LES.[6]

The UES is an intraluminal high-pressure zone located between the pharynx and the cervical esophagus. The anterior wall includes the posterior surface of the cricoid cartilage, the arytenoid cartilage, and the interarytenoid muscles. The posterior wall includes the cricopharyngeus and thyropharyngeus muscles. The UES prevents refluxate from getting into the upper airway, and it prevents air from entering the esophagus during inspiration. The UES opens during belching, rumination, deglutition, regurgitation, and vomiting.[6]

The esophageal body begins at the edge of the cricopharyngeal muscle, and in adults, is comprised of striated skeletal muscle for the first 4–5 cm, followed by a transitional zone that contains both skeletal muscle and smooth muscle cells. Thus diseases affecting striated skeletal muscle can alter UES and proximal esophageal function. The distal 10–14 cm is comprised of smooth muscle cells.[6]

The LES is a high-pressure zone controlling the flow of materials between the esophagus and the stomach. The LES is comprised of an intrinsic muscular layer (intrinsic LES) and the extrinsic LES, which is the crural diaphragm. These two components of the LES are superimposed and linked together by the phrenoesophageal ligament. Both the intrinsic and extrinsic components of the LES contribute to LES competence. The LES is tonically contracted at rest and relaxes with esophageal distention and deglutination. The crural diaphragm portion of the LES creates spike-like increases in LES pressure during inspiration and relaxes with esophageal distention and vomiting.[8]

The esophagus accomplishes its role as a conduit to move food from the mouth to the stomach through peristalsis. The esophagus exhibits three different forms of peristalsis: primary peristalsis, secondary peristalsis, and deglutitive inhibition.[9]

Primary peristalsis is a reflex esophageal contraction that is initiated by swallowing and a contraction wave that moves from the pharynx to the stomach. This propulsive force is caused by the sequential contraction of the esophageal muscle layers. In children, the typical amplitude of the contraction ranges between 40 and 89 mm Hg, has a duration of 2.5–5 seconds, and a propagation velocity of 3.0 cm/sec.[10,11]

Secondary peristalsis occurs with esophageal luminal distention and is not associated with a swallow. It helps remove refluxate that was not cleared with primary peristalsis.[9]

Deglutitive inhibition results when a second swallow is initiated while a prior peristalsis is still occurring. This results in complete inhibition of the peristaltic contraction caused by the first swallow. With successive swallows, the esophagus remains in stasis until a final swallow produces a large "clearing wave" that sweeps the esophagus of its contents.[9]

The LES is constantly adapting to the changing pressure gradients between the stomach and the esophagus to maintain competency. During inspiration, the pressure gradient between the stomach and esophagus is 4–6 mm Hg and is countered by an LES pressure between 10 and 35 mm Hg. During the migrating motor complex of esophageal contractions, the LES vigorously contracts to prevent reflux of stomach contents into the esophagus. During inspiration, there is an increasingly negative intraesophageal pressure, while abdominal muscle contractions augment gastric pressure. Both of these situations increase the pressure gradient, predisposing to GER events. However, the contraction of the crural diaphragm during abdominal muscle contraction, vomiting, or straining helps to prevent reflux.[8] In addition to abdominal and intrathoracic pressures, the LES pressure is influenced by many other factors as listed in Table 10.1.[12]

During swallowing, the LES relaxes within 1–2 seconds of the primary peristaltic contraction and this relaxation lasts approximately 5–10 seconds. When the bolus arrives at

TABLE 10.1 Factors Influencing Lower Esophageal Pressure and Transient Lower Esophageal Sphincter Relaxation Frequency

	Increases LES pressure	Decreases LES pressure	Increases TLESR frequency	Decreases TLESR frequency
Eating behavior(s)			Calorically dense meals, large meals, later meal times	
Food(s)		Chocolate, coffee, ethanol, mint, peppermint	Carbonated beverages	
Hormone(s)	Gastrin, motilin, substance P	Cholecystokinin, gastric inhibitory polypeptide, glucagon, progesterone, secretin, vasoactive intestinal polypeptide	Cholecystokinin	
Medication(s)	Cisapride, domperidone, Metoclopramide, prostaglandin F2α	Barbituates, calcium channel blockers, diazepam, meperidine, morphine, nitrates, theophylline	Sumatriptan	Atropine, loxiglumide, morphine
Macronutrient(s)	Protein	Fat, carbohydrates	Fat	
Neural agent(s)	α-Adrenergic agonists, β-adrenergic antagonists, cholinergic agonists	α-Adrenergic antagonists, β-adrenergic agonists, cholinergic antagonists, serotonin	L-Arginine	Baclofen, cannabinoid receptor agonists, metabotropic glutamate receptor antagonists, L-NAME, serotonin

Abbreviations: *LES*, lower esophageal sphincter; *TLESR*: transient lower esophageal sphincter relaxation.

Adapted from Kahrilas PJ, Panolfino J. Esophageal motor function. In: Yamada Y, ed. *Textbook of Gastroenterology*. Blackwell Publishers; 2009:187–206; Newberry C, Lynch K. The role of diet in the development and management of gastroesophageal reflux disease: Why we feel the burn. *J Thorac Dis*. 2019;11(S12):S1594–S1601.

the LES, the LES pressure declines to gastric pressure, and the sphincter remains closed. Then, the intrabolus pressure forces the LES to open and the bolus enters the stomach. After 5–7 seconds, the LES rebounds to its original pressure and the LES undergoes an after-contraction, which ends the peristaltic contraction wave.[9]

Gas is vented from the stomach by belching where there is a transient lower esophageal sphincter relaxation (TLESR). TLESRs are abrupt declines in the LES pressure to gastric pressure that are not related to primary peristalsis, secondary peristalsis, or swallowing. There is also inhibition of the crural diaphragm with TLESRs.[13] TLESRs have a typical duration of 10–45 seconds. TLESRs occur up to six times per hour in normal adults and are more frequent immediately postprandially. They occur during arousals but not during stable sleep.[14] TLESRs are the most common reflux mechanisms. Although TLESRs do not generally result in severe GERD alone, TLESRs in addition to hiatal hernia, hypotensive LES, increased gastric pressure, or limited esophageal acid clearance results in esophageal injury.[15]

TLESRs can be triggered by gastric distention or vagal stimulation that occurs with endotracheal intubation. Gamma-aminobutyric acid (GABA) serves as an inhibitor of TLESRs.[8] Table 10.1 also reviews factors influencing TLESRs.[12]

LES pressures in children range between 10 and 40 mm Hg. LES pressures that are 5 mm Hg above the intragastric pressure are usually sufficient to prevent GER. LES motor patterns in infants and children are similar to those observed in adults.[8,16]

Mechanisms of Gastroesophageal Reflux

GER occurs when intraabdominal pressure exceeds intrathoracic pressure and the LES barrier. GER is prevented by normal LES and esophagogastric junction function. The intraabdominal portion of the esophagus is squeezed closed by abdominal pressure. In addition, the acuity of the angle where the esophagus enters the stomach (angle of His) serves as a component of the barrier at the gastroesophageal junction. A compromise in this region, as seen in hiatal hernia, predisposes to GER.[8,17]

The majority (81–100%) of GER episodes in infants, children, and adults are caused by TLESRs.[18] Omari and colleagues noted that 82% of GER episodes in premature infants and 91% of GER episodes in term infants occurred in association with TLESRs.[19,20] Kawahara and colleagues noted TLESRs in association with 58–69% of GER episodes in children being evaluated for GERD.[18]

Protective mechanisms limit damage to the esophagus and airway. Immediately after the refluxate enters the lower esophagus, the UES contracts to prevent entry into the pharynx. Secondary peristalsis also occurs, which helps clear the refluxate. Saliva, which contains bicarbonate, is then swallowed, neutralizing any adherent acidic remnants. Finally, mucosal glands in the esophagus produce mucus and bicarbonate, limiting esophageal mucosal damage.[9]

Airway protective mechanisms include the UES reflex, whose function depends on refluxate volume. Small refluxate volumes result in UES contraction, whereas large volumes stimulate a vagally mediated relaxation of the UES, allowing the refluxate to enter the pharynx. Simultaneously, this vagal response evokes a centrally meditated apnea with laryngeal closure to prevent aspiration. In older children, apnea is not provoked, but a coughing spell occurs in this situation.[21]

Impedance manometry and optical manometry have allowed for refinements and advances in the understanding of the pathogenesis and pathophysiology of GER. The pathophysiology of GER is multifactorial. Upstream factors such as impaired swallow function and xerostomia may limit delivery of acid-neutralizing saliva to the esophagus. Similarly, post-esophageal factors, such as acid hypersecretory state, delayed gastric emptying, or an acid pocket, may increase the frequency, availability or acidity of refluxate. There are also structural and hypomotility mechanisms that result in GER. Impaired esophageal clearance, esophagogastric junction dysfunction, and hiatal hernia all contribute to the development of GER.[17] Ultimately, GER is a failure of esophageal clearance and/or the esophagogastric junction barrier.

Esophageal Physiology During Sleep

Sleep and the circadian rhythm alter upper gastroesophageal function. Gastric acid secretion peaks between 8 p.m. and 1 a.m. Gastric myoelectric function is disrupted by sleep, resulting in delayed gastric emptying.[14] There is also delayed esophageal acid clearance during sleep. These factors predispose to GER during sleep.

The UES pressure decreases with sleep onset. Kahrilas and colleagues reported that UES pressure decreases from 40 ± 17 mm Hg during wakefulness to 20 ± 17 mm Hg during N1 sleep, and was lowest (8 ± 3 mm Hg) during N3 sleep.[22] The UES contractile reflex is altered during sleep, is triggered by smaller volumes of refluxate during REM sleep, and does not occur during N3 sleep. UES is influenced by position and is highest in the supine position and lowest in the left-lateral position.[23,24] The UES reflex is preempted by coughing and/or arousal. In contrast to the UES, the basal LES pressure does not vary during sleep and maintains a tonic contraction. Dysfunction at the UES contributes acid exposure to the airway and is associated with laryngopharyngeal, or extraesophageal, reflux.

The esophagus itself is impacted by the transition from wake to sleep. The frequency of TLESRs declines during sleep time. Almost all TLESRs occur during wakefulness or during brief arousals from sleep.[24]

Salivary secretion is not detectable during stable sleep.[14] In addition, swallowing frequency decreases by 50–80% during sleep time compared with wakefulness.[14] Similar to TLESRs, swallowing occurs during arousals and is almost nonexistent during stable sleep, thus, limiting primary peristalsis.[25] Esophageal acid clearance is also delayed during sleep. Orr and colleagues observed that 15 mL of 0.1 N HCl was cleared from the distal esophagus within 25 minutes during sleep, whereas it took only 6 minutes to clear when awake.[25] Sleep prolongs the latency to the first swallow if esophageal acid is present. Two different esophageal reflexes vary with sleep stage. The esophago-UES contraction reflex, which is triggered by esophageal distention, and secondary peristalsis, triggered by non–deglutition-associated local distention, remain in N2, decrease in rapid eye movement (REM) sleep, and disappear in slow-wave sleep.[24] This decrease in salivary secretion and diminished esophageal clearance of reflux in sleep results in prolonged contact of the esophageal mucosa with acidic refluxate.

Finally, during sleep, 40% of the refluxate reaches the proximal esophagus near the UES compared with <1% during wakefulness.[26] This, in addition to the lower UES pressure during sleep, may predispose to microaspiration of refluxate into the pharynx.

Despite the lack of some GERD-protective mechanisms during sleep, individual GER events are much less frequent during sleep than during wake. However, if GER occurs, the events are of a longer duration, and are more likely to result in esophagitis and Barrett's esophagus.[14]

Gastroesophageal Reflux Disease

GERD is a common pediatric illness and has protean manifestations.[27] A prospective Italian study documents that 12% of infants had regurgitation and 1% of children met criteria for GERD.[2] Among U.S. adolescents, aged 10–17 years, 5.2% reported heartburn and 8.2% reported acid regurgitation during the previous week.[1] GERD is also more frequent during early childhood when large fluid boluses are used for feeding.[28]

Certain special populations of pediatric patients are considered to be at an elevated risk for GERD and related complications. These populations include patients with a history of achalasia, esophageal atresia, chronic respiratory illnesses (bronchopulmonary dysplasia, idiopathic pulmonary fibrosis, cystic fibrosis), hiatal hernia, lung transplantation, obesity, neurologic impairment, or prematurity.[5]

Infants with GERD may present with regurgitation or vomiting associated with irritability, anorexia, feeding refusal, poor weight gain, dysphagia, painful swallowing, and back arching during feeding. Gastrointestinal (GI) bleeding, either hematemesis or hematochezia, may be a presenting symptom of GERD. GERD may also present with extraesophageal symptoms such as coughing, wheezing, choking, or upper respiratory symptoms.[5,29] GERD may also be associated with signs such as dental erosion, anemia, esophagitis, esophageal stricture, Barrett's esophagus, apnea spells, asthma, recurrent pneumonia due to aspiration, and recurrent otitis media.[4]

There are several concerning signs and symptoms that may be caused by GERD, or other etiologies, that must not be missed while evaluation for GERD is ongoing. These so called "red flags" include weight loss, lethargy, fever, excessive pain, dysuria, onset of vomiting after 6 months of age,

vomiting with increasing frequency after 12–18 months of age, or persistent forceful vomiting. Seizures, increasing head circumference, microcephaly or macrocephaly, nocturnal vomiting, or bulging fontanelle suggest intracranial etiologies. Other GI symptoms such as bilious emesis, hematemesis, chronic diarrhea, rectal bleeding, or abdominal distention also warrant further assessment.[4]

Adolescents and older children experience similar clinical presentations as adults with GERD. Typical complaints include heartburn, dyspepsia, sour burps, epigastric pain, and regurgitation. Gupta and colleagues described the presenting symptoms of GERD in pediatric patients. The most common symptoms included abdominal pain (70%), regurgitation (69%), and cough (69%). In patients between 1 and 36 months of age, symptoms of GERD included regurgitation (98%), irritability (41%), feeding problems (10%), failure to thrive (7%), and respiratory problems (18.6%). Toddlers and younger children (<6 years) more likely reported cough, anorexia/food refusal, and vomiting.[7] In a Finnish study examining children with GERD (mean age 6.7 years), the presenting symptoms included abdominal pain (63%), heartburn (34%), regurgitation (22%), vomiting (16%), retrosternal pain (18%), and respiratory symptoms (29%).[30] Adolescents with GERD reported esophageal symptoms (22.4%), regurgitation (21.4%), dysphagia (14.5%), shortness of breath (24.4%), wheezing (1.7%), and cough (17.9%).[31]

Extraesophageal manifestations of GERD are also present in children. El-Serag and colleagues compared 1,980 children with GERD (mean age 9.2 years) to a control group without GERD, examining the association of GERD with upper and lower respiratory disorders. They demonstrated that children with GERD were more likely to have sinusitis (4.2% vs. 1.4%), laryngitis (0.7% vs. 0.2%), asthma (13.2% vs. 6.8%), pneumonia (6.3% vs. 2.3%), and bronchiectasis (1.0% vs. 0.1%). After adjusting for age, gender, and ethnicity, GERD remained associated with all of these conditions.[32]

Differential Diagnosis of Gastroesophageal Reflux Disease

There are a myriad number of disorders that can present with findings similar to GERD. A complete review of all the illnesses that may mimic GERD is beyond the scope of this chapter. Conditions impacting the cardiac, endocrine, GI, neurologic, pulmonary, or renal systems may have similar signs and symptoms. In addition, infectious diseases, lead poisoning, or child neglect/abuse may present like GERD.[4] Specifically, eosinophilic esophagitis (EOE) is an entity that is easily mistaken for GERD. EOE presents with symptom constellations similar to GERD including esophageal dysfunction heartburn or dysphagia. Significant dysphagia, food impaction, and/or poor response to GERD therapy are symptoms that are common in EOE. Endoscopic biopsy specimens of the proximal and distal esophagus demonstrate >15 eosinophils/high power field.[33] Both entities demonstrate dilated intracellular spaces in addition to the clinical similarities.[34] New diagnostic modalities allow for the discrimination of these entities.[35]

Sleep-Related Gastroesophageal Reflux Disease

Sleep-related GERD may present with nocturnal awakenings with a sour taste in the mouth, burning discomfort in the chest, or nocturnal arousals. These arousals may disrupt sleep, leading to daytime sleepiness or insomnia.[14]

Few studies examine the epidemiology, severity, or range of clinical impact that is associated with sleep-related GERD in children.[27,36-43] In children, GERD during sleep is associated with increased sleep arousals, sleep fragmentation, and other sleep disturbances.[27] Kahn and colleagues evaluated 50 infants with occasional regurgitation and noted that 41 of 50 infants had proximal GER events, with 97 episodes occurring during sleep time. Reflux during sleep time occurred commonly during wakefulness (41%), or was associated with arousals. This study did not determine whether arousals led to the reflux or if the reflux led to the arousal from sleep.[36] A study by Sankaran and colleagues assessed 25 infants suspected of GER and brief resolved unexplained events (BRUE) with 24-hour impendence studies and 6-hour concurrent video-polysomnography. They described frequent acidic events that occurred more often in the awake state. Acid clearance time and proximal acid migration were higher in the awake state versus sleep. Sankaran and colleagues suggested that the sleep state appears to be protective of acid reflux in infants possibly due to greater chemosensory thresholds.[44] Machado and colleagues assessed 24 infants with simultaneous polysomnography and pH-impendence studies. Infants were found to have more non-acid GER episodes per hour during wake or wake after sleep onset compared with sleep (1.85 vs. 1.42 vs. 0.27, $p < 0.01$). There was no statistical difference between sleep states for acid GER. Of the 1,204 arousals recorded in the study, 13.7% occurred after a GER episode and 3.6% immediately preceded a GER episode. Thus non-acid GER appears to be a significant contributor to infant sleep disruption.[41]

Ghaem and colleagues examined 72 children with GERD and 3,102 controls, with a questionnaire, finding that children with GERD (aged 3–12 months) were less likely to have ever slept through the night by 12 months of age (20%) compared with the controls. Fifty percent of GERD children awakened and required parental attention more than three times nightly. These findings continued in children with GERD aged 12–24 months and 24–36 months, with only 8% and 4% sleeping through the night compared with 45% and 56% of controls. Sixty percent of 12–24 month-olds and 50% of 24–36 month-olds with GERD woke up more than three times nightly. Children with GERD had more awakenings and were less likely to sleep through the night.[37]

A prospective study in snoring, obese adolescents evaluated sleep via polysomnography and simultaneous multichannel intraluminal impedance and esophageal pH monitoring. In 13 subjects, a total of 113 reflux events were detected with 2.3 events per hour of wake after sleep onset and 0.6 events per hour of sleep ($p = 0.04$). In 38.5% of the subject's awakenings there was a significant association with reflux episodes.[42]

A prospective randomized controlled study in adolescents with GERD (ages 12–17 years) assessed the impact of 8 weeks of a proton pump inhibitor (PPI; esomeprazole) on quality of life (QoL) using the Quality of Life in Reflux and Dyspepsia Questionnaire. After 8 weeks of PPI, there was an improvement in the sleep dysfunction domains of the QoL instrument in the PPI-treated group. These findings suggested that GERD treatment may improve sleep in adolescents.[38] Another study by Orr found adult patients with reflux treated with rabeprazole (a PPI) demonstrated subjective improvements in sleep, but did not detect objective differences in their sleep.[45] Thus treatment of GERD may improve subjective sleep issues, but objective data are still lacking.

Obstructive Sleep Apnea

Both GERD and obstructive sleep apnea (OSA) share confounding variables and risk factors, including obesity.[14,15] In contrast to children, the relationship between OSA and GERD is better defined in adults. Wu and colleagues performed a meta-analysis that included 2,699 patients with OSA and GERD and determined there was a significant relationship between these two entities. There was a pooled odds ratio (OR) of 1.75 (95% confidence interval [CI] 1.18–2.59, $p < 0.05$) between OSA and GERD.[46] The relationship between sleep-related GERD and OSA was assessed by Wasilewska and colleagues with simultaneous esophageal pH monitoring and polysomnography in 24 children (ages 2–36 months) with sleep disturbances indicative of GERD and possible sleep-disordered breathing. Children with sleep-related GERD had a higher REM apnea-hypopnea index (AHI) (23.4 events per hour) compared with children without sleep-related GERD (AHI: 4.9 events per hour). These observations suggested that GERD is associated with more severe OSA during early childhood.[47]

Qubty and colleagues studied 139 infants between 0 and 17 months of age with OSA to determine comorbidities related to OSA. After excluding patients with central apnea greater than 50% of episodes, the most common comorbidity in their population was GERD with 68% of infants with OSA also having GERD. Prematurity (30%), genetic syndromes (30%), neuromuscular disease (34%), craniofacial disease (37%), and periodic limb movements of sleep (42%) were the other five most common comorbidities noted.[43] The impact of sleep-related GERD among children aged 6–12 years was assessed by Noronha and colleagues. Eighteen children with obstructive sleep apnea syndrome (OSAS) and tonsillar hypertrophy were evaluated with polysomnography with concomitant esophageal pH monitoring and the OSA-18 Questionnaire. The AHI was >1.0 for all patients and 41.1% of patients had esophageal pH values below 4 for more than 10% of sleep time. The esophageal pH values correlated with emotional distress and daytime problems on the OSA-18. A temporal correlation between individual GER events and apnea-hypopnea events was not apparent.[48]

Despite the linkage between these two conditions, the mechanisms by which GER and OSA are linked are not well understood. Several different prospective theories have been suggested. The first proposed mechanism suggests that inspiratory efforts increase due to obstruction of the upper airway leading to elevated negative pleural forces. These negative forces distend the esophagus and the LES. This, coupled with elevated abdominal pressures, push gastric contents into the esophagus.[15] Unfortunately, the observed physiology does not fully support this theory as the LES increases in pressure during obstructive periods to compensate for the negative pressure. Rather, most episodes of GER were due to TLESRs.[49]

A second postulated mechanism is that nocturnal GER results in sleep arousals that disrupt sleep and GER results in increased awakening and sleep deprivation. Although researchers have not detected a linear relationship between GER episodes and respiratory arousals on sleep studies while performing nocturnal polysomnography (NPSG) and pH-impendence monitoring, associations have been seen. Kim and colleagues assessed 216 adult patients with NPSG and esophagogastroduodenoscopy (EGD) and found that OSA was more severe in patients with patients with GERD (AHI 33.6 vs. 22.0, $p = 0.01$). Sleep efficiency was decreased in patients with endoscopically proven GERD (81.2% vs. 85.1%, $p = 0.02$).[50]

The final theorized mechanism is that GER results in pharyngeal edema that is more collapsible during apnea events.[15,51] There are limited studies assessing this proposed mechanism.

A recent study by Shepherd and colleagues suggested that obesity may be the connection between these two conditions. In this study, adult patients with obesity and OSA were compared with non-obese patients with OSA and a control of obese patients without OSA using NPSG, esophageal manometry, and pH-impedance monitoring. The authors described five key findings: the obese OSA group had more GER episodes than the non-obese OSA group, no difference in GER was seen between the two obese groups, the obese OSA group had more GER during the day than other groups, GER during sleep was four times greater for the obese groups (which were similar), and body mass index (BMI) was significantly associated with measures of GER severity. Together, these observations suggest that obesity plays a more important role in the pathogenesis of GER in OSA patients than degree of obstruction alone.[52]

Asthma, Laryngospasm, Hoarseness

Sleep-related GERD can trigger asthma and/or laryngospasm during sleep. There is an association between GERD and asthma but the direction of causality is not known, and may be bidirectional. Proposed mechanisms of interaction include microaspiration and a vagally mediated reflex

bronchoconstriction.[14] A systematic review assessed the association of pediatric asthma and GERD.[53] Twenty articles met the a priori inclusion criteria. Estimates of GERD prevalence in children with asthma ranged from 19.3% to 80.0%. Five studies compared 1,314 asthma patients with 2,434 controls. Based on these data, the average GERD prevalence in pediatric asthmatics was 22.0% compared with 4.8% in the controls. The pooled OR for having GERD in the asthma group was 5.6 (95% CI of 4.3–6.9).[53]

A prospective cohort of 1,037 New Zealanders was examined for GER symptoms and airway responsiveness at ages 11 years and 26 years. GER symptoms that were at least "moderately bothersome" were associated with asthma (OR 3.2, 95% CI 1.7–7.2), wheeze (OR 4.3, 95% CI 2.1–8.7), and nocturnal cough (OR 4.3, 95% CI 2.1 to 8.7) independent of BMI. Women with GER symptoms were more likely to have airflow obstruction. The direction of causality is not clear because patients with airway hyperresponsiveness at age 11 were more likely to report GER symptoms at age 26.[54]

The effect of GERD therapy on asthma outcomes shows conflicting data in children.[55,56] Khoshoo and colleagues described 44 pediatric asthmatics with GERD who were treated with omeprazole and metoclopramide, ranitidine, or fundoplication. Patients treated with omeprazole/metoclopramide or fundoplication had significantly fewer asthma exacerbations (0.33 and 0.66) over 6 months compared with patients on ranitidine (2.2).[55] Antithetically, Størdal and colleagues performed a randomized trial utilizing omeprazole or placebo for 12 weeks in 38 children with asthma and GERD (mean age 10.8 years). After 12 weeks, esophageal acid contact times decreased in the omeprazole group, but there were no differences in the asthma symptom score, lung function, or number of rescue beta-agonist uses between groups.[56] More information regarding the association between GERD and asthma in children is needed.

Sleep-related GERD may be associated with laryngeal findings as the acidic refluxate migrates into the larynx. Block and colleagues reported a retrospective review of 337 children (mean age 7.2 years) with hoarseness. Eighty-eight percent had laryngeal reflux and 30% had cough. Among the patients with cough and hoarseness (99 patients), 66% were found to have GERD. Also, 50% of patients who were treated for GERD utilizing a variety of behavioral and medical therapies had improvement or resolution of their hoarseness at 3 months, and 68% had resolution by 4.5 months.[57]

A recent review conducted by Chang and colleagues found limited data between pediatric cough and GERD.[58]

Brief Resolved Unexplained Events

A brief resolved unexplained event, formerly known as acute life-threatening events (ALTEs), is an event occurring in an infant younger than 1 year when the observer reports a sudden, brief, and now resolved episode of ≥1 of the following: (1) cyanosis or pallor; (2) absent, decreased, or irregular breathing; (3) marked change in tone (hyper- or hypotonia); and (4) altered level of responsiveness. A BRUE is diagnosed only when there is no explanation for a qualifying event after conducting an appropriate history and physical examination.[59]

Many disorders are implicated in BRUEs including seizures, infections, arrhythmias, and GERD.[59,60] In a systematic review of 2,912 publications including 643 infants with ALTEs, GERD was diagnosed in 227 (35%) infants, seizures in 83 (13%), lower respiratory tract infection in 58 (9%), and in 169 (26%) infants no diagnosis was made.[60] Despite the high prevalence of GERD, there is little data to support the role of GERD in ALTEs. Molloy and colleagues noted that there is rarely a temporal relationship between GERD events and apnea in premature infants.[61] Finally, Semeniuk and colleagues evaluated 264 patients aged 4–102 months with GERD and found 8 patients with symptoms of ALTEs. They described GERD as a causative factor of ALTEs in only 4.8% of their cohort.[62]

A retrospective observational study was performed with infants admitted to a single center for BRUE or OSA to determine the causes of OSA. This group of 82 patients (59 <12 months, and 23 between 12 and 24 months) was evaluated with NPSG, impedance-pH, and nasopharyngoscopy. In the younger group, 81% were admitted for BRUE and 19% for OSA and 50.8% of this group were found to have GERD. Laryngomalacia and GER were associated with elevated AHI in the younger group.[40]

Gastroesophageal Reflux Disease Diagnosis

For patients presenting with stereotypical features of sleep-related GERD, a thorough history and physical exam, that excludes other diagnoses, are sufficient to make the diagnosis. A comprehensive history for an infant suspected of GERD should include age of onset, detailed feeding history, pattern of vomiting, family medical history, growth trajectory, possible environmental triggers, previous interventions, and warning signs. Per the recent guidelines, in the absence of warning signs, diagnostic testing and/or therapies including acid suppression are *not* needed if there is no impact of the symptoms on feeding, growth, or acquisition of developmental milestones.[4]

Questions directed at the frequency of nighttime awakenings, substernal chest pain, indigestion, heartburn, nocturnal cough or choking, or chronic vomiting should lead to the diagnosis in most older children or adolescents.[28] Other patients may have only extraesophageal symptoms and present with excessive daytime sleepiness without an obvious historical cause, or waking up with laryngospasm, wheeze, or cough. Additionally, patients may note refluxate on their pillows.[14] However, historical findings do not discriminate patients with esophagitis.[28]

Diagnostic Interventions

Many diagnostic interventions have been used in the workup of children for GER and the recent European

Society of Pediatric Gastroenterology, Hepatology, and Nutrition (ESPGHAN) and North American Society for Pediatric Gastroenterology, Hepatology, and Nutrition (NASPGHAN) reviewed the literature supporting these practices. There was not enough evidence to support the routine use of barium contrast studies or ultrasonography in the diagnosis of GERD in infants and children, but these techniques could be used to exclude anatomical abnormalities.[4]

Endoscopy (EGD) has been used in the evaluation of patients for GERD; however, there is insufficient evidence to support EGD in the diagnosis of patients with GERD. The ESPGHAN/NASPGHAN working group recommends the use of EGD with biopsies to assess for complications of GERD or prior to escalation of therapy.[4]

Esophageal pH monitoring identifies acid GER episodes, and can be used in patients without typical GER symptoms. Esophageal pH monitoring is performed by placing a pH probe at a level corresponding to 87% of the nares-LES distance, based on published regression equations, by fluoroscopy or through manometric measurement of the LES location. Interpretation of the results involves calculating reflux index, which is the percentage of the recording time when esophageal pH falls below 4.0. The mean upper limit of normal is 12% in children up to 11 months, and 6% in children and adults.[28] The test is performed over 24 hours to increase the test's sensitivity and specificity, which approximates 90%. The reproducibility of the test ranges from 69–85%.[63] Additionally, esophageal pH monitoring can be integrated with polysomnography to allow unified visualization of the patient's sleep and esophageal pH.[14]

Esophageal electrical impedance monitoring allows for the detection of liquid and gas in the esophagus, regardless of pH. It is commonly combined with pH monitoring. pH-intraluminal impedance (pH-MII) monitoring has a high sensitivity compared with pH monitoring alone. Because a large number of GER events, especially post-prandial GER, are non-acidic, this technology allows for detection of more GER episodes. pH-MII allows for the detection and quantification of acidic, non-acidic liquids, and gas in the esophagus (Fig. 10.1). This technology is expensive, however, and requires a high degree of skill to interpret and has not been widely available to date. Jaimchariyatam and colleagues assessed adult patients with OSA and GERD with NPSG and esophageal pH-impedance monitoring and found that 44% of reflux events were acidic and 56% with non-acidic. The nocturnal reflux events were associated with preceding awakening and arousal (OR 3.71, $p < 0.001$ and OR 2.31, $p < 0.001$).[64] In addition, the clinical importance of non-acidic GER on pediatric sleep is unclear.[11] Recent studies in pediatrics have not demonstrated that pH-impedance monitoring alters clinical outcomes. pH-MII monitoring did not predict outcome of Nissen fundoplications nor predict risk of hospitalizations.[65,66] While pH-MII is not routinely recommended during diagnostic evaluation, there are scenarios that pH-MII may be useful.[4]

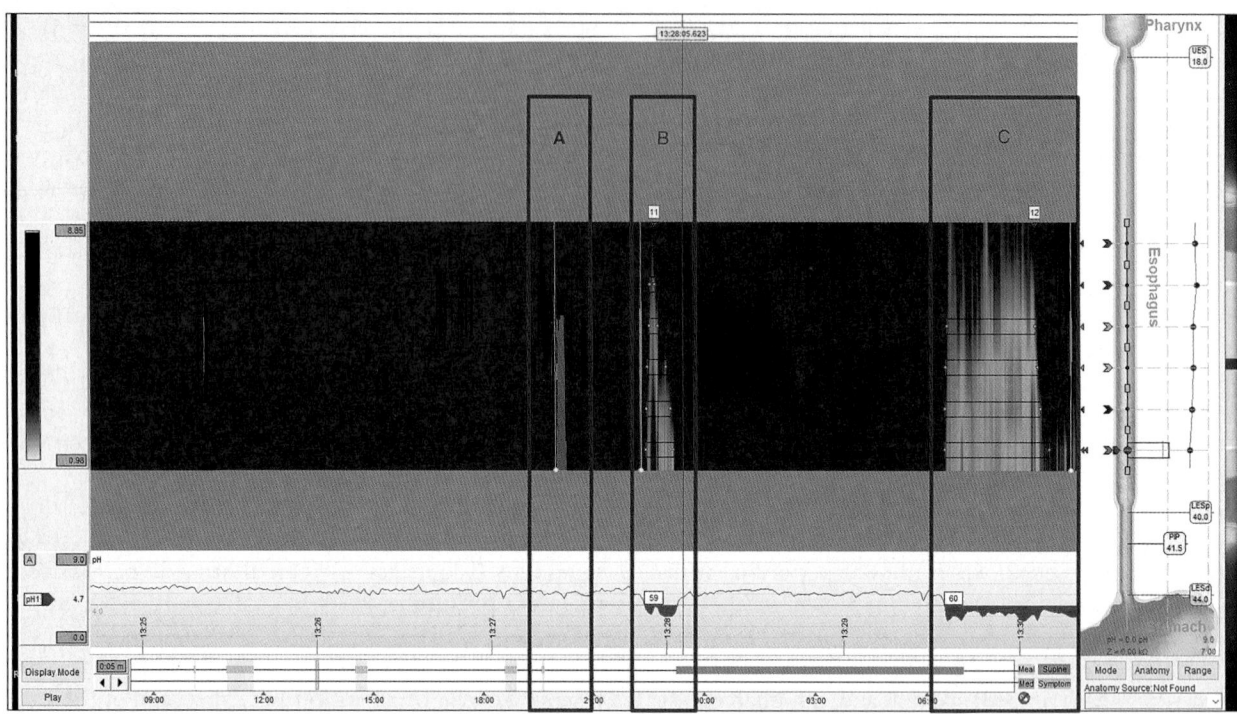

• **Fig. 10.1** pH-Intraluminal impedance monitoring (pH-MII) image demonstrating one episode of belching *(A)* and two episodes of acidic gastroesophageal reflux *(B, C)*. The data displayed are from the impedance monitoring port closest to the lower esophageal sphincter.

Gastroesophageal Reflux Disease Treatment

Management options for GERD include nonpharmacologic behavioral interventions, medical therapy, and surgical therapy. Appropriate treatment requires a thorough knowledge of chronotherapeutic principles to obtain optimal control of GERD.[28] Fig. 10.2 summarizes behavioral and medical therapy of GERD in children.[28]

Behavioral Interventions

Behavioral interventions during early childhood include formula thickening, modification of feeding regimens, positioning changes, and elevation of the head of the bed.[4] Milk thickening agents decrease visible regurgitation; however, these agents did not improve esophageal acid contact times, number of reflux episodes lasting greater than 5 minutes, or number of reflux episodes per hour.[67] Ummarino and colleagues compared a trial of thickened formula to family education/reassurance or magnesium alginate and simethicone. Thickening decreased median symptom scores over 8 weeks in all groups, but thickened feedings resulted in a 65.2% resolution of symptoms compared with 11.8% in the reassurance group ($p < 0.001$).[68] No definitive data demonstrated the superiority of any specific thickening agent.[4]

Feeding regimen modifications are helpful in the treatment of GER. These modifications include decreased feeding volumes with increased frequency of feedings, elimination of cow's milk protein, or transition to an extensively hydrolyzed or amino acid–based formula. Regurgitation may be the presenting complaint of patients with cow's milk protein allergy; therefore elimination of cow's milk protein may result in resolution of symptoms in patients who have an allergy to cow's milk protein, which presents similar to GERD.[69]

Positioning may also prevent GER episodes in infants. Tobin and colleagues studied 24 infants with GERD <5 months old with esophageal pH monitoring while being placed in different positions. Esophageal acid contact times were greatest in the supine position (15.3%) and lowest in the prone position (6.7%). There is conflicting data regarding the benefit of head-of-the-bed elevation by 30 degrees. The authors noted that the left decubitus position (esophageal acid contact time 7.7%) is a suitable alternative to prone positioning for the postural management of infants with symptomatic GERD.[70] Note that this recommendation is in contrast to the American Academy of Pediatrics recommendation that infants should sleep in the supine position. Supine positioning confers the lowest risk of sudden infant death syndrome (SIDS) and is the preferred position for infants to sleep.[71] A more recent study by Loots and colleagues described the left lateral decubitus position with head elevation at 30 degrees as associated with fewer GER events.[72] Due to the risk of SIDS, supine sleeping position is recommended as the safest sleep position for infants.

	Infants (Less than 12 months old)	Children (1-12 years old)	Adolescents (12-18 years old)
Behavioral Interventions	Formula Thickening Hydrolyzed protein formula for 2-4 weeks Prone or left-lateral decubitus positioning is best for GERD, but supine position recommended due to risk of SIDS	No evidence to support dietary restriction in children or adolescents Adult studies support limiting late night eating Weight loss if obese Avoid foods that decrease LES tone (peppermint, caffeine, chocolate, alcohol, high-fat meals)	

Medical Interventions

Acid Suppressive Therapy

Histamine-2 Receptor Antagonists

	Infants	Children	Adolescents
Cimetidine	10-20 mg/kg/day PO div Q6-12 hours	20-40 mg/kg/day PO div Q6H	1600 mg/day PO div Q6-12 hours
Famotidine	<3 mos: 0.5 mg/kg/day PO 3-12 mos: 1-2 mg/kg/day PO div BID	1-2 mg/kg/day div BID max 40 mg/day	20-40 mg PO BID
Nizatidine	>6 mos: 5-10 mg/kg/day PO div BID; Max 300 mg/day	5-10 mg/kg/day PO div BID Max: 300 mg /d	150 mg PO BID, max 300 mg per day
Ranitidine	As of April 1, 2020, withdrawn from United States Market due to contamination with probable carcinogen NMDA.		

Proton Pump Inhibitors

	Infants	Children	Adolescents
Esomeprazole	Not approved	1-11 yr: 10 mg PO QD	20-40 mg PO QD
Lansoprazole	Not approved	<30 kg: 15 mg PO QD >30 kg: 30 mg PO QD	15-30 mg PO QD
Omeprazole	Not approved	10-20 kg: 10 mg PO QD **or** 1 mg/kg/day PO div BID >20 kg: 20 mg PO QD	20 mg PO QD
Pantoprazole	Not approved	>5 yrs: 15-40 kg: 20 mg PO QD >40 kg: 40 mg PO QD	20-40 mg PO QD

Gastric Acid Buffers/ Barriers (Antacids, Alginate, Sucralfate)
Not recommended in chronic therapy as safe and convenient alternatives exist (H$_2$RAs and PPIs)

Prokinetic therapies

	Infants	Children	Adolescents
Baclofen*	Not approved	0.5 mg/kg/day 2-7 years: Max 40 mg/day 8-12 years: Max 60 mg/day	0.5 mg/kg/day Max 80 mg/day

* Consider prior to surgical intervention.

Bethanechol, erythromycin should not be used as first-line treatment.
Domperidone and metoclopramide should not be used the treatment of pediatric GERD.

• **Fig. 10.2** Summary of behavioral and medical therapies for treatment of gastroesophageal disease is pediatrics. GERD, gastroesophageal reflux disease; SIDS, sudden infant death syndrome; LES, lower esophageal sphincter; PO, by mouth; Q6, every 6 hours; BID, twice a day; QD, daily; NMDA, N-methyl-D-aspartate; H$_2$RA; histamine-2 receptor antagonist; PPI, protein pump inhibitor.

The efficacy of nonpharmacologic therapy in infant GERD was evaluated by Orenstein and colleagues. Caregivers of infants implemented a program utilizing GER feeding modifications, positioning, and tobacco smoke avoidance. Outcomes included the Infant Gastroesophageal Reflux Questionnaire-Revised. Among the 37 infants followed, GER scores improved in 59%, and 24% of patients no longer met diagnostic criteria for GERD after 2 weeks.[73]

Behavioral interventions during childhood and adolescence include weight management, dietary changes, sleep positional therapy, caffeine limitation, and smoking cessation. If possible, children should refrain from eating at least 3 hours before bedtime. In adults, sleep-related GERD episodes occur primarily during the first 2 hours of sleep time. There are minimal data examining behavioral therapy in children. Medications that can decrease LES pressure or increase the likelihood of GERD, include theophylline, anticholinergics, prostaglandins, calcium channel blockers, and alendronate.[14] Avoidance of these medications should be considered; however, there are no data in children examining the impact of these medications on GERD.

Pharmacologic Therapy

Pharmacologic treatment of GERD includes alginates, antacids, acid suppressive therapies, and prokinetic agents.

Alginates and Antacids

Alginates and antacids are designed to neutralize stomach acid and contain salts of sodium, potassium bicarbonate, aluminum, magnesium, or calcium. Antacids have major side effects and toxicities in children including milk-alkali syndrome. Although the British National Institute for Health Care Excellence guidelines have endorsed the use of alginates as an alternative therapy for thickening feeds in breastfed infants, the ESPGHAN/NASPGHAN guidelines do not recommend antacids/alginates for chronic treatment of children or infants with GERD.[4]

Acid Suppressive Therapy

There are two classes of acid suppressive therapy used in the treatment of GERD, histamine-2 receptor antagonists (H_2RAs) and PPIs. Both of these classes of medications are effective at increasing the pH of stomach contents and refluxate. There are limited data comparing the agents in pediatric populations, but rates of healing of erosive esophagitis are higher with PPI therapy.[28]

Histamine-2 Receptor Antagonists

H_2RAs inhibit the histamine-2 receptor of the gastric parietal cell and decrease gastric acid secretion. H_2RAs have a relatively quick onset of action and are useful for episodic symptom relief. Commonly used H_2RAs include famotidine, cimetidine, nizatidine, and ranitidine. Famotidine, one of the most commonly studied H_2RAs, has been shown to cause agitation and signs concerning for headaches in infants.[74] Other side effects include dizziness, constipation, anemia, and urticaria. Cimetidine has been associated

with gynecomastia, neutropenia, and thrombocytopenia, and reduces the hepatic metabolism of medications such as theophylline.[28] Tolerance to the H_2RA class of medications does develop in both children and adults. Thus H_2RAs are not ideal for chronic therapy for GERD in pediatric populations. ESPGHAN/NASPGHAN guidelines suggest that H_2RAs can be used in the treatment of reflux-related erosive esophagitis in infants and children if PPIs are not available or contraindicated.[4]

Proton Pump Inhibitors

PPIs inhibit the hydrogen-potassium ATPase channels that are the final step in gastric acid secretion. PPIs bind covalently with the cysteine residues of the hydrogen-potassium ATPase pump. PPIs are more effective at suppression of acidic secretions than the H_2RAs.[14,75] Commonly used PPIs include omeprazole, lansoprazole, pantoprazole, rabeprazole, and esomeprazole. There is some variation in the rates of activation and plasma half-life with the different PPIs; however, average half-life approximates 1–2 hours. Due to covalent bonding to the ATPase pump, the duration of action ranges from 15 hours for lansoprazole to 28 hours for omeprazole, and 46 hours for pantoprazole. PPIs are slow to achieve steady-state inhibition and generally require 3 days to achieve maximum impact. Children, ages 1–10 years, metabolize PPIs faster than adults and require a higher per kilogram dose compared with adults.[75] PPIs should be tapered and not discontinued abruptly as this would result in gastric acid hypersecretion.

The impact of treating GERD with PPIs on OSA in children has been studied by Wasilewska and colleagues in an evaluation with NPSG and 24-hour pH-metry. Thirty-seven children with OSA and GERD were evaluated with NPSG and pH-metry before and after 4–8 weeks of treatment with omeprazole. The AHI decreased from 13.08–8.22 per hour ($p < 0.01$) while on acid suppressive therapy.[76]

Minor side effects occur in 1–3% of patients on PPIs and include headache, diarrhea, abdominal pain, nausea, and rash. Major side effects are rare and include interstitial nephritis with omeprazole, hepatitis with omeprazole or lansoprazole, and visual disturbances with pantoprazole and omeprazole.[77]

There is a high frequency of nocturnal acid breakthrough among children on PPIs. Pfefferkorn and colleagues studied 18 children with esophagitis (mean age of 10.3 years) treated with 1.4 mg/kg of PPI divided twice daily and underwent esophageal pH testing after 3 weeks of therapy. They demonstrated that 89% of the patients had nocturnal acid breakthrough on the PPI.[78]

Finally, PPIs are most effective if they are administered as a single daily dose, 30 minutes before breakfast. This dosing corresponds with the timing of activation of stomach proton-potassium pumps after the overnight fast.[14] Infants require a higher dose (mg/kg) of PPI than older children due to more rapid metabolization and should be taken 30 minutes prior to the first meal of the day.[79]

Risks of Chronic Acid Suppression

Children taking H$_2$RAs or PPIs long term are at an increased risk of developing community-acquired pneumonia, acute gastroenteritis, and *Clostridium difficile* infection. These risks are thought to be conferred due to the medications limiting the gastric acid's ability to kill possible pathogenic microorganisms.[80] A prospective study of pediatric patients on acid suppressive therapies demonstrated increased gastric bacterial growth compared with untreated patients (46% vs. 18%, $p = 0.003$). There was elevated prevalence of *Staphylococcus, Streptococcus, Veillonella, Dermabacter,* and *Rothia* in the gastric fluid of patients on acid suppression therapies. There was a significant correlation between the abundance of *Corynebacterium* and *Propionibacterium* in gastric and lung fluid in patients on gastric suppressive medications ($p = 0.01$ and $p = 0.006$).[81] PPI use in 53,130 adults during the COVID-19 epidemic was independently associated with having a positive COVID-19 positive test. Taking once daily PPI increased COVID-19 positive tests twofold (adjusted odds ratio [aOR] 2.15; 95% CI, 1.9–2.44) and taking PPIs twice daily increased the risk by more than threefold (aOR 3.67; 95% CI, 2.93–4.60) after correcting for confounders. In this study, adults taking H$_2$RAs did not have an increased risk. Coronavirus appears to be easily destroyed when exposed to a gastric pH of less than 3, but survives in a more neutral pH.[82]

Based on the evidence available, infants and children with GERD who need pharmacotherapy should be treated with PPI as the first-line therapy for reflux-related erosive esophagitis. A 4- to 8-week course of H$_2$RAs or PPI is recommended as treatment for typical symptoms of GERD with follow-up assessment of treatment efficacy. Acid suppressive therapies are not recommended for infants with visible regurgitation who are otherwise healthy. Finally, extraesophageal symptoms should not be treated with acid suppressive medications except in the presence of typical GERD symptoms or with suggestive diagnostic testing.[4]

Prokinetics

There are several prokinetic medications that have been used in the treatment of GERD including baclofen, metoclopramide, domperidone, cisapride, and erythromycin. Baclofen is a muscle relaxant and antispasmodic that has been used in the treatment of GERD. In one randomized placebo-controlled trial in children with GERD, baclofen was demonstrated to decrease TLESRs and acid GER and increased the gastric emptying time.[83] Baclofen may be useful in treatment of GERD, but significant side effects have been noted in adult studies. These side effects range from drowsiness, dizziness, fatigue, and decreased seizure threshold. Given the limited data and the risk of side effects, baclofen could be considered prior to surgical intervention and after other medical therapies have failed.[4] Other prokinetic medications are not recommended in the treatment of children with GERD due to limited data and risk of significant side effects.

Referral to a Pediatric Gastroenterologist

For infants symptomatic with GERD without red flags for other conditions, an initial trial of feeding regimen alteration followed by elimination of cow's milk from breastfeeding mothers' diet and a transition to a protein hydrolysate formula or amino acid–based formula should be considered prior to referral to a pediatric gastroenterologist.[4]

For older children, medical therapy with a PPI should be initiated for 4–8 weeks and continued for another 4–8 weeks if improving. If GERD-related symptoms resolve, then the PPI should be stopped with plans for patient follow-up for evaluation of any recurrent symptoms. However, if the patient continues to have persistent GERD symptoms after 4–8 weeks of PPI therapy or is unable to tolerate weaning off the PPI therapy, then evaluation by a pediatric gastroenterologist should be considered.[4] Other indications for a pediatric gastroenterologist referral include "alarming" symptoms such as upper GI bleeding, persistence of failure to thrive, acute worsening of weight loss, or having difficulty swallowing or controlling secretions.[28]

Positive Airway Pressure

Continuous positive airway pressure (CPAP) is used for successful OSA treatment in children.[84] CPAP has also been shown to lead to improvements in GERD symptoms. Adult patients with good adherence to CPAP therapy demonstrate greater improvements in nocturnal acid reflux and daytime sleepiness.[85] In adults, CPAP controls OSA and decreases sleep-related GERD symptoms and esophageal acid contact times.[14] A recent study in adults found that CPAP use in patients with OSA and GERD and/or oropharyngeal reflux resulted in a decrease in oropharyngeal reflux events with a pH <6.0 (119.0 events without CPAP to 43.0 on CPAP, $p = 0.014$) and a decrease in esophageal reflex events with pH <4 from 4.5 to 0 events ($p = 0.017$).[86] CPAP increases esophageal, LES, and gastric pressures. The differential pressure between the esophagus and stomach (the so-called barrier pressure) increases with CPAP. Finally, CPAP causes a disproportionate increase in LES pressure compared with esophageal and gastric pressures. This increase may be due to reflex activation of the LES, or by the transmission of the CPAP pressure to the LES.[87] Despite this, there are scant data examining the effect of CPAP on sleep-related GERD in children. Animal model data demonstrate efficacy of PAP in neonatal models. Cantin and colleagues demonstrated that nasal CPAP with 6 cm H$_2$O had an inhibitory effect of GER in neonatal lambs.[88]

Surgical Therapies

Surgical interventions for GERD in pediatric patients are limited with options such as fundoplication, total esophagogastric dissociation, and radiofrequency ablation. Prior to any surgical intervention, a trial of transpyloric/jejunal feeding should be attempted.[4] In a study of 366 children with GERD and neurologic impairment there was no difference in rates of aspiration pneumonia or mortality between transpyloric feeding and fundoplication infants with neurologic disease.[89]

There are high rates of complication with transpyloric feedings including clogging (29%), dislodgement (66%), intussusception (20%), and perforation (2–3%).[4]

Surgical fundoplication involves wrapping a portion of the stomach around the LES to strengthen or tighten the LES. Published reports vary widely in the success of surgical interventions for GERD in children, with success rates ranging from 40% to 95%. Complication rates from open and laparoscopic reflux surgery are similar.[90] Complications of GERD surgery include splenectomy (0.2%), esophageal laceration (0.2%), infection, recurrent GERD (2.5–40%), small bowel obstruction, gastroparesis, and dumping syndrome. Long-term outcome studies of fundoplication show that 14% of children have GERD recurrence after Nissen fundoplication, and 20% have GERD recurrence in loose wrap procedures (i.e., <360-degree wrap).[28] The risks and benefits of fundoplication should be carefully assessed before consideration of surgery.[91]

Other surgical interventions, including total esophagogastric dissociation and radiofrequency ablation, do not have sufficient data to recommend these therapies as first-line surgical options for the treatment of GERD in children. Optimally, prior to considering surgical therapy, the child should be evaluated carefully by a pediatric gastroenterologist.

Future Directions

Novel diagnostics and therapeutics are currently being developed and evaluated. These diagnostics include novel impedance markers, mucosal impedance testing, salivary pepsin, and high-resolution manometry, which may result in increased sensitivity and accuracy in the diagnosis. Although new examinations and procedures, including electoral stimulation of the LES and magnetic sphincter augmentation, are approved by the U.S. Food and Drug Administration for adults, they are not yet recommended for children.[35,91] Minimal data exist evaluating sleep-related GERD in children. There is also a need for well-designed randomized trials evaluating the efficacy of GERD therapy in sleep-related GERD in children. Data emerging from adults cannot be extrapolated to children. Furthermore, pediatricians need to be educated that GERD does occur during sleep time and can adversely affect sleep and daytime functioning as well as potentially contribute to other comorbid disease states.

Conclusions

During sleep, there is significant alteration in the physiology of the gastroesophageal system that increases the likelihood of GER. Sleep-related GERD is associated with GER symptoms and alters sleep architecture. Sleep-related GERD can impact sleep, contribute to excessive daytime sleepiness, impair QoL, impact asthma severity, impact laryngitis, and is associated with OSA. There is still much research needed to assess the exact impact of sleep-related GERD on pediatric health and disease. Hopefully, future research will provide better methods of GERD identification, treatment, and prevention.

CLINICAL PEARLS

- Transient relaxations of the lower esophageal sphincter are responsible for most gastroesophageal reflux (GER) episodes that commonly occur during arousals from sleep.
- Weekly heartburn is reported in 5.2% and/or regurgitation is reported in 8.2% of U.S. adolescents.
- Sleep-related GER is associated with GER symptoms during sleep, arousals, obstructive sleep apnea, asthma, laryngospasm, hoarseness, and brief resolved unexplained events.
- Diagnosis of sleep-related GER includes symptoms and esophageal pH and impedance monitoring.
- Treatment includes behavioral interventions, pharmacologic therapy (primarily proton pump inhibitors), and in carefully evaluated children, surgical fundoplication.

References

1. Nelson SP, Chen EH, Syniar GM, Christoffel KK. Prevalence of symptoms of gastroesophageal reflux during childhood: A pediatric practice-based survey. Pediatric Practice Research Group. *Arch Pediatr Adolesc Med.* 2000;154(2):150–154. https://doi.org/10.1001/archpedi.154.2.150.

2. Campanozzi A, Boccia G, Pensabene L, et al. Prevalence and natural history of gastroesophageal reflux: Pediatric prospective survey. *Pediatrics.* 2009;123(3):779–783. https://doi.org/10.1542/peds.2007-3569.

3. Suwandhi E, Ton MN, Schwarz SM. Gastroesophageal reflux in infancy and childhood. *Pediatr Ann.* 2006;35(4):259–266.

4. Rosen R, Vandenplas Y, Singendonk M, et al. Pediatric Gastroesophageal Reflux Clinical Practice Guidelines. *J Pediatr Gastroenterol Nutr.* 2018;66(3):516–554. https://doi.org/10.1097/MPG.0000000000001889.

5. Lightdale JR, Gremse DA. Section on gastroenterology, hepatology, and nutrition. Gastroesophageal reflux: Management guidance for the pediatrician. *Pediatrics.* 2013;131(5):e1684–e1695. https://doi.org/10.1542/peds.2013-0421.

6. Skandalakis JE, Ellis H. Embryologic and anatomic basis of esophageal surgery. *Surg Clin of North Am.* 2000;80(1):85–155. https://doi.org/10.1016/S0039-6109(05)70399-6.

7. Gupta SK, Hassall E, Chiu Y-L, Amer F, Heyman MB. Presenting symptoms of nonerosive and erosive esophagitis in pediatric patients. *Dig Dis Sci.* 2006;51(5):858–863. https://doi.org/10.1007/s10620-006-9095-3.

8. Mittal RK, Balaban DH. The esophagogastric junction. *N Engl J Med.* 1997;336(13):1924–1932.

9. Diamant NE. Functional anatomy and physiology of swallowing and esophageal motility. In: Richter JE, Castell DO, eds. *The Esophagus.* 5 ed. Wiley-Blackwell; 2012:65–96.

10. Hillemeier AC, Grill BB, McCallum R, Gryboski J. Esophageal and gastric motor abnormalities in gastroesophageal reflux in infancy. *Gastroenterology.* 1983;84(4):741–746.

11. Mahony MJ, Migliavacca M, Spitz L, Milla PJ. Motor disorders of the oesophagus in gastro-oesophageal reflux. *Arch Dis Child*. 1988;63(11):1333–1338. https://doi.org/10.1136/adc.63.11.1333.

12. Kahrilas PJ, Panolfino J. Esophageal motor function. In: Yamada Y, ed. *Textbook of Gastroenterology*. Blackwell Publishers; 2009:187–206.

13. Mittal RK, Holloway RH, Penagini R, Blackshaw LA, Dent J. Transient lower esophageal sphincter relaxation. *Gastroenterology*. 1995;109(2):601–610. https://doi.org/10.1016/0016-5085(95)90351-8.

14. Harding SM. Gastroesophageal reflux during sleep. *Sleep Med Clin*. 2007;2(1):41–50. https://doi.org/10.1016/j.jsmc.2006.11.007.

15. Lim KG, Morganthaler TI, Katzka DA. Sleep and nocturnal gastroesophageal reflux. *Chest*. 2018;154(4):963–971. https://doi.org/10.1016/j.chest.2018.05.030.

16. Cucchiara S, Staiano A, Di Lorenzo C, et al. Esophageal motor abnormalities in children with gastroesophageal reflux and peptic esophagitis. *J Pediatr*. 1986;108(6):907–910. https://doi.org/10.1016/s0022-3476(86)80925-8.

17. Gyawali CP, Roman S, Bredenoord AJ, et al. Classification of esophageal motor findings in gastro-esophageal reflux disease: Conclusions from an international consensus group. *Neurogastroenterol Motil*. 2017;29(12):e13104–e13115. https://doi.org/10.1111/nmo.13104.

18. Kawahara H, Dent J, Davidson G. Mechanisms responsible for gastroesophageal reflux in children. *Gastroenterology*. 1997;113(2):399–408.

19. Omari TI, Barnett C, Snel A, et al. Mechanisms of gastroesophageal reflux in healthy premature infants. *J Pediatr*. 1998;133(5):650–654.

20. Omari TI, Barnett CP, Benninga MA, et al. Mechanisms of gastro-oesophageal reflux in preterm and term infants with reflux disease. *Gut*. 2002;51(4):475–479.

21. Oh JH, Michaudet C, Malaty J, et al. Relationship between sleep and acid gastro-oesophageal reflux in neonates. *J Sleep Res*. 2012;21(1):80–86. https://doi.org/10.1111/j.1365-2869.2011.00915.x.

22. Kahrilas PJ, Dodds WJ, Dent J, Haeberle B, Hogan WJ, Arndorfer RC. Effect of sleep, spontaneous gastroesophageal reflux, and a meal on upper esophageal sphincter pressure in normal human volunteers. *Gastroenterology*. 1987;92(2):466–471.

23. Eastwood PR, Katagiri S, Shepherd KL, Hillman DR. Modulation of upper and lower esophageal sphincter tone during sleep. *Sleep Med*. 2007;8(2):135–143. https://doi.org/10.1016/j.sleep.2006.08.016.

24. Bajaj JS, Bajaj S, Dua KS, et al. Influence of sleep stages on esophago-upper esophageal sphincter contractile reflex and secondary esophageal peristalsis. *Gastroenterology*. 2006;130(1):17–25. https://doi.org/10.1053/j.gastro.2005.10.003.

25. Orr WC, Johnson LF, Robinson MG. Effect of sleep on swallowing, esophageal peristalsis, and acid clearance. *Gastroenterology*. 1984;86(5 Pt 1):814–819.

26. Orr WC, Elsenbruch S, Harnish MJ, Johnson LF. Proximal migration of esophageal acid perfusions during waking and sleep. *Am J Gastroenterology*. 2000;95(1):37–42. https://doi.org/10.1111/j.1572-0241.2000.01669.x.

27. Sherman P.M., Hassall E., Fagundes-Neto U., et al. A global, evidence-based consensus on the definition of gastroesophageal reflux disease in the pediatric population. 2009;104(5):1278–1295. https://doi.org/10.1038/ajg.2009.129.

28. Vandenplas Y, Rudolph CD. Pediatric gastroesophageal reflux clinical practice guidelines: Joint recommendations of the North American Society for Pediatric Gastroenterology, Hepatology, and Nutrition (NASPGHAN) and the European Society for Pediatric Gastroenterology, Hepatology, and Nutrition (ESPGHAN). *J Pediatr Gastroenterol Nutr*. 2009;49(4):498–547.

29. Winter H.S. Gastroesophageal reflux in infants. http://www.uptodate.com. Accessed July 20, 2020.

30. Ashorn M, Ruuska T, Karikoski R, Laippala P. The natural course of gastroesophageal reflux disease in children. *Scand J Gastroenterol*. 2002;37(6):638–641.

31. Gunasekaran TS, Dahlberg M, Ramesh P, Namachivayam G. Prevalence and associated features of gastroesophageal reflux symptoms in a Caucasian-predominant adolescent school population. *Dig Dis Sci*. 2008;53(9):2373–2379. https://doi.org/10.1007/s10620-007-0150-5.

32. El-Serag HB, Gilger M, Kuebeler M, Rabeneck L. Extraesophageal associations of gastroesophageal reflux disease in children without neurologic defects. *Gastroenterology*. 2001;121(6):1294–1299. https://doi.org/10.1053/gast.2001.29545.

33. Liacouras CA, Furuta GT, Hirano I, et al. Eosinophilic esophagitis: Updated consensus recommendations for children and adults. *J Allergy Clin Immunol*. 2011;128(1):3–20.e6. https://doi.org/10.1016/j.jaci.2011.02.040.

34. Katzka DA, Ravi K, Geno DM, et al. Endoscopic mucosal impedance measurements correlate with eosinophilia and dilation of intercellular spaces in patients with eosinophilic esophagitis. *Clinical Gastroenterology and Hepatology*. 2015;13(7):1242–1248.e1. https://doi.org/10.1016/j.cgh.2014.12.032.

35. Naik RD, Evers L, Vaezi MF. Advances in the diagnosis and treatment of GERD: New tricks for an old disease. *Curr Treat Options Gastro*. 2019;17(1):1–17. https://doi.org/10.1007/s11938-019-00213-w.

36. Kahn A, Rebuffat E, Sottiaux M, Dufour D, Cadranel S, Reiterer F. Arousals induced by proximal esophageal reflux in infants. *Sleep*. 1991;14(1):39–42.

37. Ghaem M, Armstrong KL, Trocki O, Cleghorn GJ, Patrick MK, Shepherd RW. The sleep patterns of infants and young children with gastro-oesophageal reflux. *J Paediatr Child Health*. 1998;34(2):160–163.

38. Gunasekaran T, Tolia V, Colletti RB, et al. Effects of esomeprazole treatment for gastroesophageal reflux disease on quality of life in 12- to 17-year-old adolescents: An international health outcomes study. *BMC Gastroenterol*. 2009;9(1):673–676. https://doi.org/10.1186/1471-230X-9-84.

39. Kamal M, Tamana SK, Smithson L, et al. Phenotypes of sleep-disordered breathing symptoms to two years of age based on age of onset and duration of symptoms. *Sleep Med*. 2018;48:93–100. https://doi.org/10.1016/j.sleep.2018.04.008.

40. Nosetti L, Zaffanello M, De Bernardi F, et al. Age and upper airway obstruction: A challenge to the clinical approach in pediatric patients. *Int J Environ Res Public Health*. 2020;17(10):3531. https://doi.org/10.3390/ijerph17103531.

41. Machado R, Woodley FW, Skaggs B, Di Lorenzo C, Splaingard M, Mousa H. Gastroesophageal reflux causing sleep interruptions in infants. *J Pediatr Gastroenterol Nutr*. 2013;56(4):431–435. https://doi.org/10.1097/MPG.0b013e31827f02f2.

42. Machado RS, Woodley FW, Skaggs B, et al. Gastroesophageal reflux affects sleep quality in snoring obese children. *Pediatr Gastroenterol Hepatol Nutr*. 2016;19(1):12–18. https://doi.org/10.5223/pghn.2016.19.1.12.

43. Qubty WF, Mrelashvili A, Kotagal S, Lloyd RM. Comorbidities in infants with obstructive sleep apnea. *JCSM*. 2014;10(11):1213–1216. https://doi.org/10.5664/jcsm.4204.

44. Sankaran J, Qureshi AH, Woodley F, Splaingard M, Jadcherla S. Effect of severity of esophageal acidification on sleep vs wake periods in infants presenting with brief resolved unexplained events. *J Pediatr.* 2016;179(C):42–48.e1. https://doi.org/10.1016/j.jpeds.2016.08.066.

45. Orr WC, Goodrich S, Robert J. The effect of acid suppression on sleep patterns and sleep-related gastro-oesophageal reflux. *Alim Pharm Therap*. 2005;21(2):103–108. https://doi.org/10.1111/j.1365-2036.2005.02310.x.

46. Wu Z-H, Yang X-P, Niu X, Xiao X-Y, Chen X. The relationship between obstructive sleep apnea hypopnea syndrome and gastroesophageal reflux disease: A meta-analysis. *Sleep and Breathing*. 2019;23:389–397. https://doi.org/10.1007/s11325-018-1691-x.

47. Wasilewska J, Kaczmarski M. Sleep-related breathing disorders in small children with nocturnal acid gastro-oesophageal reflux. *Rocz Akad Med Bialymst*. 2004;49:98–102.

48. Noronha AC, de Bruin VMS, Nobre e Souza MA, et al. Gastroesophageal reflux and obstructive sleep apnea in childhood. *Int J Pediatr Otorhinolaryngol*. 2009;73(3):383–389. https://doi.org/10.1016/j.ijporl.2008.11.002.

49. Kuribayashi S, Massey BT, Hafeezullah M, et al. Upper esophageal sphincter and gastroesophageal junction pressure changes act to prevent gastroesophageal and esophagopharyngeal reflux during apneic episodes in patients with obstructive sleep apnea. *Chest*. 2010;137(4):769–776. https://doi.org/10.1378/chest.09-0913.

50. Kim Y, Lee YJ, Park JS, et al. Associations between obstructive sleep apnea severity and endoscopically proven gastroesophageal reflux disease. *Sleep and Breathing*. 2018;22:85–90. https://doi.org/10.1007/s11325-017-1533-2.

51. Dempsey JA, Veasey SC, Morgan BJ, O'Donnell CP. Pathophysiology of sleep apnea. *Physiol Rev*. 2010;90(1):47–112. https://doi.org/10.1152/physrev.00043.2008.

52. Shepherd K, Orr W. Mechanism of gastroesophageal reflux in obstructive sleep apnea: Airway obstruction or obesity? *JCSM*. 2016;12(01):87–94. https://doi.org/10.5664/jcsm.5402.

53. Thakkar K, Boatright RO, Gilger MA, El-Serag HB. Gastroesophageal reflux and asthma in children: A systematic review. *Pediatrics*. 2010;125(4):e925–e930. https://doi.org/10.1542/peds.2009-2382.

54. Hancox RJ, Poulton R, Taylor DR. Associations between respiratory symptoms, lung function, and gastro-oesophageal reflux symptoms in a population-based birth cohort. *Respiratory Reviews*. 2006;7:142.

55. Khoshoo V, Haydel R. Effect of antireflux treatment on asthma exacerbations in nonatopic children. *J Pediatr Gastroenterol Nutr*. 2020;44(3):331–335.

56. Størdal K. Acid suppression does not change respiratory symptoms in children with asthma and gastro-oesophageal reflux disease. *Arch Dis Child*. 2005;90(9):956–960. https://doi.org/10.1136/adc.2004.068890.

57. Block BB, Brodsky L. Hoarseness in children: The role of laryngopharyngeal reflux. *Int J Pediatr Otorhinolaryngol*. 2007;71(9):1361–1369. https://doi.org/10.1016/j.ijporl.2006.10.029.

58. Chang AB, Oppenheimer JJ, Kahrilas PJ, et al. Chronic cough and gastroesophageal reflux in children: CHEST guideline and expert panel report. *Chest*. 2019;156(1):131–140. https://doi.org/10.1016/j.chest.2019.03.035.

59. Tieder JS, Bonkowsky JL, Etzel RA, et al. Brief resolved unexplained events (formerly apparent life-threatening events) and evaluation of lower-risk infants. *Pediatrics*. 2016;137(5): https://doi.org/10.1542/peds.2016-0590. e20160590–e20160590.

60. McGovern MC. Causes of apparent life threatening events in infants: A systematic review. *Arch Dis Child*. 2004;89(11):1043–1048. https://doi.org/10.1136/adc.2003.031740.

61. Molloy EJ, Di Fiore JM, Martin RJ. Does gastroesophageal reflux cause apnea in preterm infants? *Neonatology*. 2005;87(4):254–261. https://doi.org/10.1159/000083958.

62. Semeniuk J, Kaczmarski M, Wasilewska J, Nowowiejska B. Is acid gastroesophageal reflux in children with ALTE etiopathogenetic factor of life threatening symptoms? *Adv Med Sci*. 2007;52:213–221.

63. Michail S. Gastroesophageal reflux. *Pediatr Rev*. 2007;28(3):101–110.

64. Jaimchariyatam N, Tantipornsinchai W, Desudchit T, Gonlachanvit S. Association between respiratory events and nocturnal gastroesophageal reflux events in patients with coexisting obstructive sleep apnea and gastroesophageal reflux disease. *Sleep Med*. 2016;22:33–38. https://doi.org/10.1016/j.sleep.2016.04.013.

65. Duncan DR, Amirault J, Johnston N, Mitchell P, Larson K, Rosen RL. Gastroesophageal reflux burden, even in children that aspirate, does not increase pediatric hospitalization. *J Pediatr Gastroenterol Nutr*. 2016;63(2):210–217. https://doi.org/10.1097/MPG.0000000000001092.

66. Rosen R, Levine P, Lewis J, Mitchell P, Nurko S. Reflux events detected by pH-MII do not determine fundoplication outcome. *J Pediatr Gastroenterol Nutr*. 2010;50(3):251–255. https://doi.org/10.1097/MPG.0b013e3181b643db.

67. Horvath A, Dziechciarz P, Szajewska H. The effect of thickened-feed interventions on gastroesophageal reflux in infants: Systematic review and meta-analysis of randomized, controlled trials. *Pediatrics*. 2008;122(6):e1268–e1277. https://doi.org/10.1542/peds.2008-1900.

68. Ummarino D, Miele E, Martinelli M, et al. Effect of magnesium alginate plus simethicone on gastroesophageal reflux in infants. *J Pediatr Gastroenterol Nutr*. 2015;60(2):230–235. https://doi.org/10.1097/MPG.0000000000000521.

69. Borrelli O, Mancini V, Thapar N, et al. Cow's milk challenge increases weakly acidic reflux in children with cow's milk allergy and gastroesophageal reflux disease. *J Pediatr*. 2012;161(3):476–481.e1. https://doi.org/10.1016/j.jpeds.2012.03.002.

70. Tobin JM, McCloud P, Cameron DJ. Posture and gastro-oesophageal reflux: A case for left lateral positioning. *Arch Dis Child*. 1997;76(3):254–258. https://doi.org/10.1136/adc.76.3.254.

71. Task Force on Sudden Infant Death Syndrome Moon RY. SIDS and other sleep-related infant deaths: Expansion of recommendations for a safe infant sleeping environment. *Pediatrics*. 2011;128(5):e1341–e1367. https://doi.org/10.1542/peds.2011-2285.

72. Loots C, Kritas S, van Wijk M, et al. Body positioning and medical therapy for infantile gastroesophageal reflux symptoms. *J Pediatr Gastroenterol Nutr*. 2014;59(2):237–243. https://doi.org/10.1097/MPG.0000000000000395.

73. Orenstein SR, McGowan JD. efficacy of conservative therapy as taught in the primary care setting for symptoms suggesting infant gastroesophageal reflux. *J Pediatr*. 2008;152(3):310–314. https://doi.org/10.1016/j.jpeds.2007.09.009. e311.

74. Orenstein SR, Shalaby TM, Devandry SN, et al. Famotidine for infant gastro-oesophageal reflux: A multi-centre, randomized,

placebo-controlled, withdrawal trial. *Alim Pharm Therap.* 2003;17(9):1097–1107. https://doi.org/10.1046/j.1365-2036.2003.01559.x.

75. Sachs G, Shin JM, Howden CW. Review article: The clinical pharmacology of proton pump inhibitors. *Alim Pharm Therap.* 2006;23(s2):2–8. https://doi.org/10.1111/j.1365-2036.2006.02943.x. Suppl 2.

76. Wasilewska J, Semeniuk J, Cudowska B, Klukowski M, Dębkowska K, Kaczmarski M. Respiratory response to proton pump inhibitor treatment in children with obstructive sleep apnea syndrome and gastroesophageal reflux disease. *Sleep Med.* 2012;13(7):824–830. https://doi.org/10.1016/j.sleep.2012.04.016.

77. Thomson ABR, Sauve MD, Kassam N, Kamitakahara H. Safety of the long-term use of proton pump inhibitors. *World J Gastroenterol.* 2010;16(19):2323–2330. https://doi.org/10.3748/wjg.v16.i19.2323.

78. Pfefferkorn MD, Croffie JM, Gupta SK, et al. Nocturnal acid breakthrough in children with reflux esophagitis taking proton pump inhibitors. *J Pediatr Gastroenterol Nutr.* 2006;42(2):160–165. https://doi.org/10.1097/01.mpg.0000189354.48043.4e.

79. Litalien C, Théorêt Y, Faure C. Pharmacokinetics of proton pump inhibitors in children. *Clin Pharmacokinet.* 2005;44(5):441–466. https://doi.org/10.2165/00003088-200544050-00001.

80. Canani RB. Therapy with gastric acidity inhibitors increases the risk of acute gastroenteritis and community-acquired pneumonia in children. *Pediatrics.* 2006;117(5):e817–e820. https://doi.org/10.1542/peds.2005-1655.

81. Rosen R, Amirault J, Liu H, et al. Changes in gastric and lung microflora with acid suppression: Acid suppression and bacterial growth. *JAMA Pediatr.* 2014;168(10):932–937. https://doi.org/10.1001/jamapediatrics.2014.696.

82. Almario CV, Chey WD, Spiegel B. Increased risk of COVID-19 among users of proton pump inhibitors. *Am J Gastroenterol.* 2020;115(10):1707–1715.

83. Omari TI, Benninga MA, Sansom L, Butler RN, Dent J, Davidson GP. Effect of baclofen on esophagogastric motility and gastroesophageal reflux in children with gastroesophageal reflux disease: A randomized controlled trial. *J Pediatr.* 2006;149(4):468–474.e2. https://doi.org/10.1016/j.jpeds.2006.05.029.

84. Waters KA, Everett FM, Bruderer JW, Sullivan CE. Obstructive sleep apnea: The use of nasal CPAP in 80 children. *Am J Respir Crit Care Med.* 1995;152(2):780–785. https://doi.org/10.1164/ajrccm.152.2.7633742.

85. Tamanna S, Campbell D, Warren R, Ullah MI. Effect of CPAP therapy on symptoms of nocturnal gastroesophageal reflux among patients with obstructive sleep apnea. *J Clin Sleep Med.* 2016;12(9):1257–1261. https://doi.org/10.5664/jcsm.6126.

86. Wang L, Han H, Wang G, et al. Relationship between reflux diseases and obstructive sleep apnea together with continuous positive airway pressure treatment efficacy analysis. *Sleep Med.* 2020;75:151–155.

87. Shepherd KL, Holloway RH, Hillman DR, Eastwood PR. The impact of continuous positive airway pressure on the lower esophageal sphincter. *Am J Physiol Gastrointest Liver Physiol.* 2007;292(5):G1200–G1205. https://doi.org/10.1152/ajpgi.00476.2006.

88. Cantin D, Djeddi D, Carrière V, et al. inhibitory effect of nasal intermittent positive pressure ventilation on gastroesophageal reflux. *PLoS ONE.* 2016;11(1):e0146742. https://doi.org/10.1371/journal.pone.0146742.

89. Srivastava R, Downey EC, O'Gorman M, et al. Impact of fundoplication versus gastrojejunal feeding tubes on mortality and in preventing aspiration pneumonia in young children with neurologic impairment who have gastroesophageal reflux disease. *Pediatrics.* 2009;123(1):338–345. https://doi.org/10.1542/peds.2007-1740.

90. Hassall E. Outcomes of fundoplication: Causes for concern, newer options. *Arch Dis Child.* 2005;90(10):1047–1052. https://doi.org/10.1136/adc.2004.069674.

91. Park S, Weg R, Enslin S, Kaul V. Ten things every gastroenterologist should know about antireflux surgery. *Clin Gastroenterol Hepatol.* 2020;18(9):1923–1929. https://doi.org/10.1016/j.cgh.2020.02.041.

11
Sleep and Pain

Valerie McLaughlin Crabtree, Kayla N. LaRosa, and Merrill S. Wise

CHAPTER HIGHLIGHTS

- The relationship between sleep and chronic pain is complex, multifactorial, and biopsychosocial in nature. The contribution of poor sleep to increased pain intensity and interference appears to be stronger than the contribution of pain to poor sleep. The relationship between sleep and pain is moderated by mood: with increasingly positive mood, the negative impact of poor sleep on reports of pain decreases.

- Evaluation of youth with pain and sleep issues begins with a thorough history of the pain, other medical and psychologic issues, and sleep. Because the perception of sleep quality and pain is subjective, it is essential to assess subjective reports of both.

- Youth with co-occurring pain and sleep disruption show benefit from hybrid models of cognitive-behavioral therapy that target the co-occurring symptoms. Improvements in sleep quality may influence pain perception indirectly by bolstering coping resources, thus limiting the degree that pain sensations interfere with the ability to engage in preferred activities.

- More research is needed to develop and evaluate pharmacologic treatment options for children with chronic pain and sleep issues.

Introduction

Chronic pain, described as pain occurring for 3 months or longer, is a relatively common condition and is estimated to occur in up to 83% of children and adolescents, depending on the type of pain. Headache is one of the most common complaints, and back pain is one of the least common.[1,2] When describing pain, it is important to consider the biopsychosocial aspects of the pain experience and the interference with daytime activities. The biopsychosocial approach to evaluating and managing pain includes a focus on multiple factors, including nociceptive, sociocultural, cognitive, behavioral, and emotional contributors to the pain experience.[3] Chronic pain is more common in girls than boys and in youth from lower socioeconomic status. As with many other biopsychosocial problems, rates of chronic pain increase with age across the pediatric developmental period.[1] It is important to note that chronic pain may be an entity itself (e.g., recurrent abdominal pain) or may be a direct result of another chronic condition (e.g., juvenile idiopathic arthritis[4]).

Many chronic pain conditions—including fibromyalgia, rheumatologic disorders, and other causes of musculoskeletal pain, functional abdominal pain, headaches and migraine, pain associated with cancer, sickle cell disease, complex regional pain syndrome, and spasticity-related pain in cerebral palsy—have been linked to disturbed sleep and daytime fatigue in children and adolescents. Over half of all children with chronic pain report disturbed sleep.[5–9] In systematic reviews, disturbance of sleep in children and adolescents with pain was demonstrated convincingly through self- and parent-reports, diary methodology, actigraphy, and polysomnography (PSG).[4,8] It is likely that chronic pain and related sleep disturbances in children also have a strong negative impact on the sleep and quality of life of parents and caregivers, although this has not been carefully investigated.[10]

This chapter will explore the consistent finding that sleep is disrupted in children and adolescents with pain, and we will examine this phenomenon from the perspective that a bidirectional relationship exists between pain and sleep. More studies support the impact of disrupted sleep on subsequent pain than support pain interfering with sleep.[4,8,11] Additionally, we will address mood as both a mediator and moderator of the relationship between pain and sleep, and on the functional impact of this relationship in youth. Daytime fatigue and reduced health-related quality of life are present in this population as well. Finally, we discuss pharmacologic and nonpharmacologic interventions designed to ameliorate sleep disturbances and, when possible, to diminish pain.

Chronic Pain

The most frequent sleep-related complaints in youth with chronic pain are difficulty initiating and maintaining sleep, shortened total sleep time, poor sleep quality, difficulty awakening in the morning, daytime sleepiness, and feeling unrested upon awakening.[4,8,11] Poor sleep in youth with chronic pain has a significant negative impact on physical, social, and emotional health-related quality of life through pathways such as activity limitation and functional disability.[12,13] For example, adolescents with poor sleep quality, poor sleep efficiency, and difficulty initiating and maintaining sleep have more limited daytime activities than adolescents with chronic pain who do not have poor sleep, even when controlling for pain and mood disturbances.[12] Further, in adolescents undergoing musculoskeletal surgery, poor sleep quality predicted the development of chronic pain but not acute pain.[14] These observations highlight the importance of understanding the role of disturbed sleep in pediatric pain patients instead of solely attributing daytime activity limitations and poor quality of life to chronic pain. In addition, poor sleep in children with juvenile idiopathic arthritis who have poor sleep were significantly more likely to have executive functioning difficulties. Poorer sleep predicted executive functioning difficulties irrespective of chronic pain group, indicating that disrupted sleep is likely a stronger driver of neurocognitive dysfunction than pain.[15] Furthermore, levels of sleep-related anxiety are reported to be higher in youth with chronic pain and are predictive of reports of insomnia.[9,15] This anxiety—likely reflecting intrusions of worry or

anxiety related to pain and/or functional limitations—also interferes with sleep onset and may lend itself to implementation of cognitive-behavioral interventions for insomnia.

Acute Pain

Most of the literature concerning sleep and pain is focused on the relationship between sleep disturbance and chronic pain, but acute pain is also associated with disrupted sleep. Post-surgical pain, acute injury, or relapsing and remitting pain associated with chronic conditions may negatively impact sleep, and painful occurrences are typically part of all children's lives on occasion.[16-18] In some cases, the psychologic impact of a traumatic event leading to the acute pain may contribute to sleep disturbance as well.[16] Similar to the relationship identified in chronic pain, more recent evidence has emerged that poor sleep quality and shorter sleep duration may be predictive of a higher likelihood of acute pain after surgery or an acute injury, whereas nighttime acute pain may be less predictive of nighttime sleep.[19,20] It is important to note that recent evidence supports the role of sleep deprivation in leading to a transition from acute to chronic pain in youth. Sleep deprivation is hypothesized to impact the sensory, psychologic, and social components of chronic pain development[21] (see Fig. 11.1).

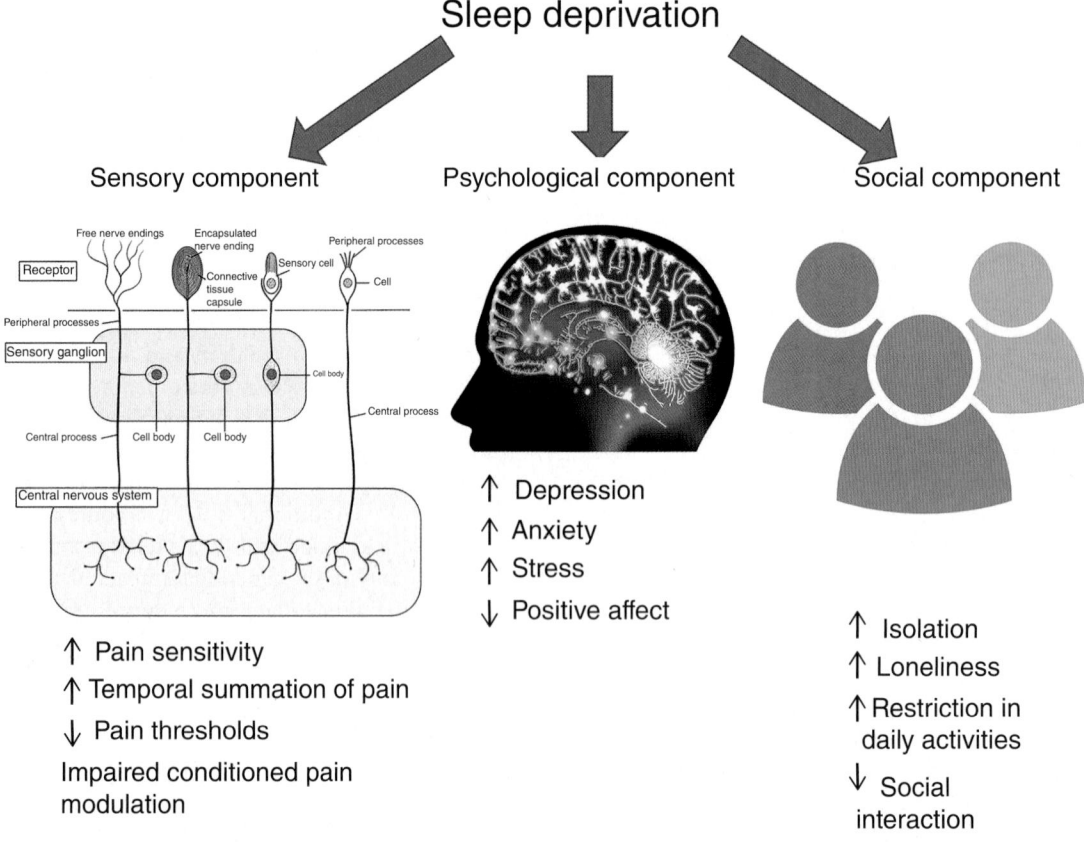

• **Fig. 11.1** Effects of sleep deprivation on sensory, psychologic, and social components involved in the transition to chronic pain. ↑ = Increased; ↓ = decreased. (Adapted from Andreucci A, Groenewald CB, Rathleff MS, Palermo TM. The role of sleep in the transition from acute to chronic musculoskeletal pain in youth-a narrative review. *Children (Basel)*. 2021;8(3):241.)

The potential role of sleep-disordered breathing in the experience of pain requires mention. Mental health disorders have not predicted the use of opioids in youth with acute pain episodes, but the presence of obstructive sleep apnea was predictive of opioid use, which may have been related to the increased likelihood of experiencing multiple pain episodes in children with obstructive sleep apnea (OSA).[22] Sleep-disordered breathing has been hypothesized to contribute to pain crises in youth with sickle cell disease, yet one study found that lower nadir oxygen saturation overnight, higher apnea-hypopnea indices, and higher oxygen desaturation index were not predictive of later vasoocclusive pain over a median of 4.9 years.[23]

Bidirectional Relationship of Pain and Sleep

More than 20 years ago, Lewin and Dahl[16] posited a theory in which sleep and pain have a bidirectional relationship. As such, pain may directly interfere with sleep whereby it inhibits sleep onset, induces nocturnal awakenings, and interferes with return to sleep. Conversely, a poor night's sleep is hypothesized to lead to increased experience of pain and decreased pain tolerance the next day. The role of potential mood dysregulation resulting from poor sleep is essential in Lewin and Dahl's model. More recently, Valrie and colleagues[8] conducted a systematic review of this bidirectional relationship between pain and sleep in youth with persistent pain. They expanded upon Lewin and Dahl's model by incorporating a broader biopsychosocial approach to conceptualizing pain and sleep in this population, whereby mood, physiology, and functional outcomes are incorporated into this complex relationship (see Fig. 11.2).

Importantly, poor sleep has been demonstrated to be predictive of reports of pain the next day. Furthermore, whereas daily variations in sleep have been shown to predict pain,

typical sleep quality had a greater influence on reports of pain.[24] Interestingly, whereas pain has been reported to be predictive of poor sleep quality the next evening in children with sickle cell disease,[25] this was not found in a sample of children with juvenile polyarticular arthritis[24] or in youth from a multidisciplinary pain clinic.[26] Although the relationship of sleep and pain was initially hypothesized as bidirectional, increasing evidence is highlighting the significant role of disrupted sleep on pain intensity and interference more than it is necessarily identifying a negative impact of pain on nighttime sleep.[11]

Recognizing the interrelated nature of pain and sleep in youth, Boggero and colleagues[27] evaluated the role of sleep in pain improvement after an intensive inpatient pain treatment. At the time of admission, whereas self-reports of insomnia symptoms were relatively high, actigraphic recordings of sleep did not demonstrate significantly impaired sleep quality. In youth with chronic pain admitted to the inpatient program, improvements were seen in both pain and self-reported sleep outcomes with reduced insomnia symptoms and excessive daytime sleepiness. Interestingly, youth who self-reported improved sleep outcomes were significantly more likely to have marked improvements in functional disability, pain severity, and coping.[27]

Methods of Sleep Assessment

Evaluation of the child with pain and sleep issues begins with a thorough history. In addition to ascertaining the child's duration, intensity, and quality of pain, a provider should take a thorough sleep history. Ideally, the clinician should possess a thorough understanding of normal development and sleep physiology in youth and should elicit the history directly from the child as often as possible, as well as obtain collateral report from the parent or caregiver. In addition to typical details, such as bedtime routines, habitual bed and rise times, and sleep duration, clinicians should ask about sleep quality, the degree of feeling refreshed upon awakening, possible sleep-related breathing problems, symptoms of restless legs syndrome and periodic limb movements, and parasomnias (sleepwalking, sleep talking, sleep terrors, and sleep bruxism). Obtaining a history of nap frequency and duration is also important, as is exploration of other manifestations of sleepiness during the day. Parents and caregivers should be asked their perceptions about the associations among pain, sleep quality, and daytime function, particularly if any temporal relationship is observed between pain, sleep, and pain interference with preferred activities. A thorough medication history is critical, especially because children with chronic or acute pain are likely to be taking several medications that can impact sleep and daytime alertness. Questions about mood, emotional regulation, and anxiety should also be included, particularly as they relate to both sleep and pain tolerance.

Both subjective and objective means of sleep assessment are important in youth with pain. Subjective measures range from single time point self-report questionnaires to daily

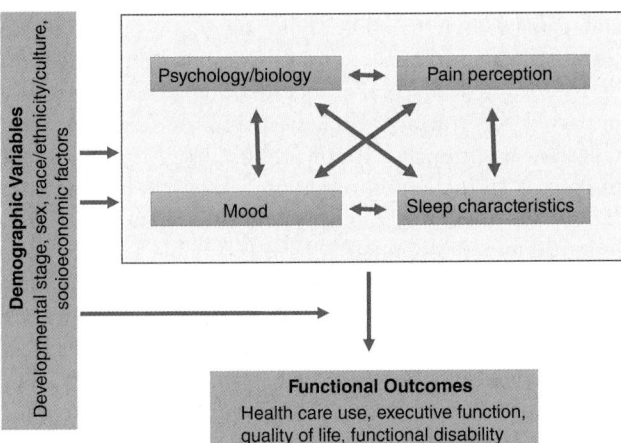

• **Fig. 11.2** A model of the pain-sleep relationship in pediatric persistent pain populations. (Adapted from Valrie CR, Bromberg MH, Palermo T, Schanberg LE. A systematic review of sleep in pediatric pain populations. *J Dev Behav Pediatr.* 2013;34(2):120–128.)

diary methods completed over multiple days. Depending on the developmental level of the child, measures can be completed by the child, the parent/caregiver, or (ideally) by both. Although parent reports are often relied upon in sleep research with youth, self-reports are also important to consider, particularly in older children. Descriptions of sleep have been found to be concordant between children and parents,[28,29] whereas adolescents and parents have been shown to have more discordant reports regarding sleep.[28]

Because interviews, questionnaires, and diaries are subjective, they are more appropriate to assess perception and awareness of sleep behaviors (night awakenings, resistance to sleeping alone, sleepwalking, night terrors, snoring, restless and disrupted sleep, and apneic pauses[30]). Objective data are important when there are concerns of non-behavioral sleep disturbances. The most used objective methods are actigraphy and PSG. Objective measurement periods can last from one night (PSG) to up to several weeks (actigraphy) and are best used to assess amount and timing of sleep (PSG or actigraphy) and stages of sleep, sleep quality, and causes of disrupted sleep (such as sleep apnea, periodic leg movements, parasomnias, or seizures [PSG][31]). PSG and actigraphy vary in terms of feasibility, impact on the child, duration, effort, cost, and reliability. Ideally, use of multiple measures is helpful, and findings can be viewed as complementary. Findings from each method should be closely integrated and interpreted within the context of the symptom(s) of concern.

Self-Report Questionnaires

Aspects of sleep to consider assessing via questionnaire include sleep patterns and habits, symptoms of disrupted sleep, and thoughts or beliefs about sleep. Most sleep questionnaires for children focus on sleep quality, sleep disruption, daytime sleepiness, and sleep duration. Some questionnaires also may assess sleep hygiene,[32] which is important in evaluating sleep among a population of youth with pain. Whereas objective measurement (i.e., actigraphy, PSG) is the gold standard for measuring sleep issues, subjective reports are important because of the benefit of minimal time and cost as well as permitting patient-reported outcomes. Two options for self-report measures are described, but other instruments may also be useful.

The Children's Report of Sleep Problems (CRSP)

The CRSP is a 60-item self-report questionnaire for children ages 8–18 years and features a parent proxy version. Sleep problems in a typical week are assessed through three modules: (1) Sleep Patterns, (2) the Sleep Hygiene Indices, and (3) the Sleep Disturbance Scale. The Sleep Patterns module features questions about bedtimes, wake times, sleep onset latency, night waking frequency and duration, nap sleep schedule variability, and subjective sleep quality, as well as the child's sleep during school, weekends, and holidays. The Sleep Hygiene Indices include a Caffeine Index, Activities the Hour Before Bed Index, Sleep Location, and Electronics Use at Sleep Onset subscales. Within the Sleep

Disturbance Scale, there are the following subscales: (1) Bedtime Fears/Worries, (2) Restless Legs, (3) Parasomnias, and (4) Insomnia. Raters indicate the frequency of sleep problems in a range from "never" to "always."

The CRSP features good internal consistency and relatively stable test-retest reliability in children and in adolescents. Day-to-day variability on this subscale was attributed to changes in the child's sleep location, which would be expected given frequent hospitalizations during treatment for children with cancer, who were included as an index clinical sample. The CRSP also demonstrated good agreement with actigraphy.[33,34]

PROMIS Sleep Disturbance and Sleep-Related Impairment

The Patient-Reported Outcomes Measurement Information System (PROMIS) pediatric sleep item banks include both self-report (ages 8–17) and parent-report (ages 5–17) forms. The full PROMIS pediatric sleep measure includes 28 items with 15 items contributing to the Sleep Disturbance item bank (i.e., sleep onset, disrupted sleep, and sleep quality) and 13 items contributing to the Sleep-Related Impairment item bank (i.e., wake time, excessive daytime sleepiness, and daytime function). Internal consistency and reliability are both high. Two short forms (4-item and 8-item) are also available based upon item response theory, providing high discrimination with ability to differentiate between those with and without sleep disturbance. Sixteen of the items within the total scale are also present in the adult PROMIS sleep banks, allowing for comparison across the developmental period.[35]

Self-Report Daily Diaries

Daily diaries can assist with the determination of directionality in the pain–sleep relationship. The sleep diary is completed upon awakening and gathers approximate bedtime, wake time, sleep quality, perceived number of night wakings, wake after sleep onset, and elements of sleep hygiene (location of sleep, medications taken, bedtime difficulties), and can be used in addition to actigraphy and PSG to document habitual sleep. Sleep diaries also allow the family to document atypical events that might have negatively impacted the youth's typical sleep routine (e.g., vacation, visitors). Additionally, youth and/or caregivers should be instructed to include information related to daytime pain experience, including intensity and interference with preferred activities. Sleep diaries have acceptable reliability and validity when child-completed daily sleep logs were compared against objective measures (actigraphy[36,37]) and are predictive of next-day pain in postoperative patients.[38] At least five weeknights of sleep diary are important to allow assessment of typical sleep.[39] Daily diaries have provided a unique methodology for elucidating the bidirectional relationship between pain and sleep in pediatric patients and often are useful in clinical practice for this purpose. However, difficulties with consistent sleep diary completion can lead to incomplete data and recall bias.

Actigraphy

An actigraph is a wristwatch-sized instrument usually worn on the non-dominant hand or ankle that measures movement over time through a piezoelectric or microelectromechanical accelerometer. These data are used as an indirect measure of sleep and wakefulness. Some models include an event button that can be pressed to signal bedtime and morning waking. The actigraph can be worn 24 hours a day for many days, and it captures data while the child sleeps in their normal environment. Actigraphy data can provide measures of total sleep duration, sleep onset latency, total time in bed, wake after sleep onset, and sleep efficiency (ratio of total sleep duration to total time spent in bed). Actigraphy provides unique data beyond what is available by sleep diary and/or PSG,[40] and it has been successfully used to measure the sleep patterns of children and adolescents experiencing a range of chronic pain conditions including migraine,[41] recurrent abdominal pain,[42] chronic musculoskeletal pain,[43] and sickle cell disease.[44]

Actigraphy has been beneficial in elucidating the bidirectional relationship between sleep and pain in youth. Fisher and colleagues[44] found that in youth with sickle cell disease, more daytime pain was associated with longer actigraph-documented wake after sleep onset and poorer sleep efficiency that night, whereas poorer sleep efficiency at night was associated with greater frequency and intensity of pain the next day. Further, worse actigraphically documented sleep was associated with greater pain in the postoperative period among youth.[45]

Nocturnal Polysomnography

Nocturnal PSG provides a comprehensive assessment of multiple physiologic parameters and is used primarily to assess individuals with suspected respiratory disturbance during sleep, or for characterization of certain movements or behaviors during sleep such as periodic limb movements and parasomnias. Children with habitual snoring, labored breathing, or witnessed apnea require PSG for evaluation of suspected OSA or other forms of sleep-related breathing disorders. Children on chronic steroids (prescribed for some forms of cancer or other painful conditions) may experience significant weight gain resulting in increased risk for OSA. Patients receiving chronic opioids can have altered sleep architecture, as well as elevated risk for sleep-related breathing problems. Both central sleep apnea and OSA and obstructive hypoventilation have been associated with opioid use.[46] An association has been found between children with both OSA and obesity and more rapid metabolism of intraoperative morphine in comparison to healthy weight controls.[47] Careful consideration must be given to prescribing opioids to pediatric patients with respect to impact on sleep.

Evidence-based practice parameters for respiratory indications for PSG in children provide clinical guidance regarding which children may benefit from PSG.[48]

Non-respiratory indications for PSG in this population include atypical or potentially injurious parasomnias and suspected periodic limb movement disorder (PLMD). PSG may be indicated when nocturnal seizures are being considered, particularly when there is uncertainty about whether seizures, respiratory disturbances during sleep, or parasomnias are occurring.[49]

Nocturnal PSG is a valid and reliable method for assessing sleep stage distribution and sleep architecture in children but, in the absence of clinical indications for respiratory or non-respiratory sleep disorders, the use of PSG to characterize sleep architecture in children with chronic pain is not likely to alter management or be cost-effective. From a research perspective, PSG (either in-laboratory or portable testing) may provide a useful method to investigate the important relationships between sleep and chronic pain in children. PSG findings in youth with chronic pain have shown mixed findings. Some studies have noted differences in chronic pain groups based on PSG parameters (such as increased N2 and decreased N3), whereas others have not.[50,51]

Comparing Subjective and Objective Measures

Subjective and objective assessment measures capture unique and complementary aspects of sleep; thus both methods have a place in pediatric sleep assessment. The different dimensions of sleep and sleep problems captured by subjective and objective measures also provide an explanation for discrepant research findings. Subjective reports reflect the child's or parents' actual perception of sleep. Objective measures, however, may be insensitive to the subtle causes of these perceived changes in sleep quality that contribute to the subjective experiences and are incapable of evaluating the importance of various domains of sleep to the individual. Because the perception of both sleep quality and pain are subjective, the role of obtaining patient-reported and caregiver-reported outcomes in studying the sleep of pediatric chronic pain patients is essential.

Role of Mood and Trauma

Because low mood has been shown to be associated with both poor sleep[52-57] and pain,[58,59] it is important to consider its role in the pain-sleep relationship. Mood has been found to serve as a mediator between the pain-sleep relationship. In children with sickle cell disease, those who had poor sleep were less likely to express pain the next day if they endorsed positive mood. For those with negative mood, a day with higher pain reports was associated with poorer sleep that night, and youth were then more likely to experience pain after a night of poor sleep.[25] A similar pattern has been demonstrated in children with juvenile polyarticular arthritis, such that a positive mood reduced the likelihood of poor sleep that would result in higher pain reports the next day.[24] In youth with other types of chronic pain, negative affect mediated the relationship been disrupted sleep and pain, but positive affect did not. This partial mediation was found related to negative affect predicting pain, whereas positive affect did not impact pain reports, and sleep quality predicted both positive and negative affect.[60]

Similarly, physical trauma can result in both psychologic trauma and painful conditions, and trauma exposure has been related to significantly disrupted sleep;[61-63] thus it is essential to consider the role of trauma in the pain-sleep relationship. A longitudinal study evaluating posttraumatic symptoms, sleep quality, and pain interference in youth with chronic pain demonstrated that baseline posttraumatic symptoms contributed to poor sleep quality, which led to greater pain interference 3 months later.[64] Similarly, in a sample of youth with chronic pain, although more posttraumatic stress symptoms were associated with reports of both pain intensity and interference, this relationship was partially mediated by reduced sleep quality.[65] This is an important model to consider when delivering interventions to improve this symptom cluster. Thus attention to both trauma symptoms and sleep may serve to prevent chronic pain interference on daytime functioning in youth.

Psychologic Interventions/Treatments

Cognitive-behavioral therapy (CBT) is a robust set of interventions that have demonstrated effectiveness for both pain and insomnia. CBT has demonstrated effectiveness on improving both pain and sleep in youth with headaches, fibromyalgia, and juvenile rheumatoid arthritis.[66-68] Critical elements included within CBT to address both pain and sleep included psychoeducation, identification of maladaptive thoughts accompanied by cognitive restructuring and thought stopping, self-assurance techniques, pleasant activity planning, activity pacing, problem-solving, sleep hygiene, stimulus control, sleep restriction, distraction techniques, and relaxation strategies (including deep breathing, visual imagery, and self-hypnosis). Inclusion of parent operant training can also be beneficial, as this provides the parent or caregiver with tools to reinforce healthy behaviors and avoid inadvertent reinforcement of pain-related behaviors.[68] Of particular importance to youth with chronic pain and problematic sleep, focusing on a hybrid CBT approach allows the clinician to tailor the CBT to elements of co-occurring symptoms, such as pain and sleep disturbance.[68] Improvements have been demonstrated in sleep habits, onset, and quality and in pain frequency, intensity, duration, interference, and catastrophizing.[66-68] Thus a growing body of literature demonstrates that CBT is likely to provide an effective set of interventions to improve the symptom cluster of chronic pain and sleep disruption in youth.

Although CBT has the most robust support for addressing pain and sleep disruption symptoms, eight sessions of mindfulness-based stress reduction (MBSR) in combination with music therapy improved both pain and sleep in youth with cancer.[69] Because this study used a combination of MBSR and music therapy, it is unclear which of the components are most important in alleviating cancer-related pain and sleep disturbance.

When measuring intervention outcomes, it is important to clearly assess sleep hygiene, scheduling, and perceived precipitating and perpetuating factors to poor sleep[70] in addition to obtaining a thorough pain history. A history of the patient's pain should assess not only pain severity but also pain interference, which captures how the pain sensation interferes with the youth's ability to engage in daily tasks and preferred activities. It is possible that improvements in sleep quality may not influence pain severity directly but rather improves pain interference and other pain-related outcomes indirectly by bolstering coping resources.[71]

Pharmacologic Interventions

Interventions directed at controlling pain during the major sleep period are likely to improve sleep quality and duration. There are few prospective studies designed to systematically evaluate pharmacologic interventions that address both chronic pain and sleep issues in children. In general, consideration should be given to combining pharmacologic and nonpharmacologic strategies to address both pain and sleep issues. The clinician should be aware of other sleep disorders that may be present, such as OSA and restless legs syndrome, before selecting a medication. Clear, well-defined treatment goals must be established as therapy is being started. As with other causes of insomnia, dosing of medication to address pain and sleep issues should be at the lowest level that is likely to be effective, followed by titration as necessary. Drug-drug interactions should be considered, and this includes certain over-the-counter agents that may affect sleep and wakefulness. Adolescents should be asked about recreational drug use, and drug screening may be indicated. Screening for pregnancy should be considered in adolescent girls, as some medications are contraindicated in pregnancy. Regardless of the medication selected, it is important to monitor closely for side effects including those that have an adverse impact on sleep or daytime alertness.

Benzodiazepine receptor agonists and non-benzodiazepine receptor agonists, which are commonly used to treat insomnia in adults, are not approved by the U.S. Food and Drug Administration (FDA) for use in children and thus are seldom used.[72] One exception is the use of clonazepam at bedtime for treatment of parasomnias that are frequent, disruptive, or potentially dangerous.

Tricyclic antidepressants, such as amitriptyline, have been used at bedtime for chronic pain and to help consolidation of sleep. Children with chronic pain plus restless legs syndrome or PLMD may benefit from gabapentin or pregabalin, or from other anticonvulsant medications such as carbamazepine or lamotrigine. Duloxetine (Cymbalta) is a newer selective serotonin and norepinephrine reuptake inhibitor with FDA approval in adults for treatment of diabetic peripheral neuropathic pain, fibromyalgia, chronic musculoskeletal pain, major depressive disorder, and generalized anxiety disorder (Eli Lilly and Company. Prescribing information. Indianapolis, IN 2011). However, use of duloxetine in children is off-label (not approved by the FDA), and the increased risk of suicidal thinking and behavior in children, adolescents, and young adults taking antidepressants for major depressive disorder and other psychiatric disorders limits use of this medication.

The effect of pregabalin on sleep and pain in adult participants with fibromyalgia was investigated in two studies, and findings were generally positive and associated with meaningful improvement in sleep and pain.[73,74] A randomized controlled trial of amitriptyline versus gabapentin for complex regional pain syndrome and neuropathic pain in children showed significant improvement in pain intensity scores and sleep.[75] A double-blind, crossover study of suvorexant in adult women with fibromyalgia showed improved sleep and reduced next-day pain sensitivity.[76] Generalization of these findings is limited by the disease model and the age group (usually adults). Nevertheless, it appears likely that certain medications have efficacy for controlling some forms of pain and improving sleep fragmentation.

The use of medical cannabis and related compounds in children with chronic pain is an emerging topic, but there are no medications in this category that are FDA approved for use in children for treatment of pain or sleep problems.[77] As this area of pharmacology evolves, clinical guidelines and evidence-based recommendations will be helpful.

Given the paucity of FDA-approved options in this area, much work is needed to develop and evaluate pharmacologic treatment options for children with chronic pain and sleep issues.[78]

Conclusion

A clear relationship between disrupted sleep and pain exists in children and adolescents with acute, episodic, and chronic pain. Whereas previously this was believed to be bidirectional, growing evidence indicates that disrupted sleep contributes to pain to a greater extent than pain contributes to poor sleep. This relationship appears to be moderated by mood and has an impact on daytime function including health-related quality of life. This chapter addresses the importance of fully assessing mood and sleep in pediatric patients with chronic pain as well as the utility of nonpharmacologic and pharmacologic methods of intervention in this patient population.

CLINICAL PEARLS

- A complex relationship between sleep and chronic pain is postulated in pediatric patients whereby the influence of poor sleep on pain intensity and interference is stronger than the contribution of pain to poor sleep.
- Negative mood moderates this relationship.
- Children and adolescents with co-occurring chronic pain and sleep disruptions benefit from cognitive-behavioral therapy that targets both symptoms.
- No medications are FDA-approved for improvement of sleep in children, and more research is needed to evaluate pharmacological treatment options for children with co-occurring chronic pain and sleep disruption.

References

1. King S, Chambers CT, Huguet A, et al. The epidemiology of chronic pain in children and adolescents revisited: a systematic review. *Pain*. 2011;152(12):2729–2738.
2. Treede RD, Rief W, Barke A, et al. A classification of chronic pain for ICD-11. *Pain*. 2015;156(6):1003–1007.
3. Liossi C, Howard RF. Pediatric chronic pain: biopsychosocial assessment and formulation. *Pediatrics*. 2016;138(5):e20160331.
4. Allen JM, Graef DM, Ehrentraut JH, Tynes BL, Crabtree VM. Sleep and pain in pediatric illness: a conceptual review. *CNS Neurosci Ther*. 2016;22(11):880–893.
5. Berrin SJ, Malcarne VL, Varni JW, et al. Pain, fatigue, and school functioning in children with cerebral palsy: a path-analytic model. *J Pediatr Psychol*. 2007;32(3):330–337.
6. Huntley ED, Campo JV, Dahl RE, Lewin DS. Sleep characteristics of youth with functional abdominal pain and a healthy comparison group. *J Pediatr Psychol*. 2007;32(8):938–949.
7. Long AC, Krishnamurthy V, Palermo TM. Sleep disturbances in school-age children with chronic pain. *J Pediatr Psychol*. 2008;33(3):258–268.
8. Valrie CR, Bromberg MH, Palermo T, Schanberg LE. A systematic review of sleep in pediatric pain populations. *J Dev Behav Pediatr*. 2013;34(2):120–128.
9. Palermo TM, Wilson AC, Lewandowski AS, Toliver-Sokol M, Murray CB. Behavioral and psychosocial factors associated with insomnia in adolescents with chronic pain. *Pain*. 2011;152(1):89–94.
10. Oh A, Koehler A, Yonker M, Troester M Sleep disorders and chronic pain syndromes in the pediatric population. *Semin Pediatr Neurol*. 2023;48:101085. https://doi.org/10.1016/j.spen.2023.101085.
11. Badawy SM, Law EF, Palermo TM. The interrelationship between sleep and chronic pain in adolescents. *Curr Opin Physiol*. 2019;11:25–28.
12. Palermo TM, Fonareva I, Janosy NR. Sleep quality and efficiency in adolescents with chronic pain: relationship with activity limitations and health-related quality of life. *Behav Sleep Med*. 2008;6(4):234–250.
13. Palermo TM, Kiska R. Subjective sleep disturbances in adolescents with chronic pain: relationship to daily functioning and quality of life. *J Pain*. 2005;6(3):201–207.
14. Rabbitts JA, Palermo TM, Zhou C, Meyyappan A, Chen L. Psychosocial predictors of acute and chronic pain in adolescents undergoing major musculoskeletal surgery. *J Pain*. 2020;21(11-12):1236–1246.
15. Ward TM, Ringold S, Metz J, et al. Sleep disturbances and neurobehavioral functioning in children with and without juvenile idiopathic arthritis. *Arthritis Care Res (Hoboken)*. 2011;63(7):1006–1012.
16. Lewin DS, Dahl RE. Importance of sleep in the management of pediatric pain. *J Dev Behav Pediatr*. 1999;20(4):244–252.
17. Ostojic K, Paget S, Kyriagis M, Morrow A. Acute and chronic pain in children and adolescents with cerebral palsy: prevalence, interference, and management. *Arch Phys Med Rehabil*. 2020;101(2):213–219.
18. Postier AC, Chambers C, Watson D, Schulz C, Friedrichsdorf SJ. A descriptive analysis of pediatric post-tonsillectomy pain and recovery outcomes over a 10-day recovery period from 2 randomized, controlled trials. *Pain Rep*. 2020;5(2):e819.
19. Lewandowski Holley A, Rabbitts J, Zhou C, Durkin L, Palermo TM. Temporal daily associations among sleep and pain in

treatment-seeking youth with acute musculoskeletal pain. *J Behav Med.* 2017;40(4):675–681.

20. Rabbitts JA, Groenewald CB, Tai GG, Palermo TM. Presurgical psychosocial predictors of acute postsurgical pain and quality of life in children undergoing major surgery. *J Pain.* 2015;16(3):226–234.

21. Andreucci A, Groenewald CB, Rathleff MS, Palermo TM. The role of sleep in the transition from acute to chronic musculoskeletal pain in youth—a narrative review. *Children (Basel).* 2021;8(3):241.

22. Zhang Y, Yang Y, Barnard M, Bentley JP, Ramachandran S. Opioid use for treatment of acute pain among children and adolescents enrolled in the Mississippi Medicaid program. *J Pharm Pract.* 20198971900198837767.

23. Willen SM, Rodeghier M, Rosen CL, DeBaun MR. Sleep disordered breathing does not predict acute severe pain episodes in children with sickle cell anemia. *Am J Hematol.* 2018;93(4):478–485.

24. Bromberg MH, Gil KM, Schanberg LE. Daily sleep quality and mood as predictors of pain in children with juvenile polyarticular arthritis. *Health Psychol.* 2012;31(2):202–209.

25. Valrie CR, Gil KM, Redding-Lallinger R, Daeschner C. Daily mood as a mediator or moderator of the pain-sleep relationship in children with sickle cell disease. *J Pediatr Psychol.* 2008;33(3):317–322.

26. Lewandowski AS, Palermo TM, De la Motte S, Fu R. Temporal daily associations between pain and sleep in adolescents with chronic pain versus healthy adolescents. *Pain.* 2010;151(1):220–225.

27. Boggero IA, Krietsch KN, Pickerill HM, et al. Improvements in sleep correlate with improvements in clinical outcomes among adolescents undergoing intensive interdisciplinary pain treatment. *Clin J Pain.* 2021;37(6):443–453.

28. Brimeyer C, Adams L, Zhu L, et al. Sleep complaints in survivors of pediatric brain tumors. *Support Care Cancer.* 2016;24(1):23–31.

29. Valrie CR, Gil KM, Redding-Lallinger R, Daeschner C. The influence of pain and stress on sleep in children with sickle cell disease. *Children's Health Care.* 2007;36(4):335–353.

30. Sadeh A. Commentary: comparing actigraphy and parental report as measures of children's sleep. *J Pediatr Psychol.* 2008;33(4):406–407.

31. Gregory AM, Sadeh A. Sleep, emotional and behavioral difficulties in children and adolescents. *Sleep Med Rev.* 2012;16(2):129–136.

32. Sen T, Spruyt K. Pediatric sleep tools: an updated literature review. *Front Psychiatry.* 2020;11:317.

33. Meltzer LJ, Avis KT, Biggs S, Reynolds AC, Crabtree VM, Bevans KB. The Children's Report of Sleep Patterns (CRSP): a self-report measure of sleep for school-aged children. *J Clin Sleep Med.* 2013;9(3):235–245.

34. Meltzer LJ, Brimeyer C, Russell K, et al. The Children's Report of Sleep Patterns: validity and reliability of the Sleep Hygiene Index and Sleep Disturbance Scale in adolescents. *Sleep Med.* 2014;15(12):1500–1507.

35. Forrest CB, Meltzer LJ, Marcus CL, et al. Development and validation of the PROMIS Pediatric Sleep Disturbance and Sleep-Related Impairment item banks. *Sleep.* 2018;41(6).

36. Gaina A, Sekine M, Chen X, Hamanishi S, Kagamimori S. Validity of child sleep diary questionnaire among junior high school children. *J Epidemiol.* 2004;14(1):1–4.

37. Sadeh A, Raviv A, Gruber R. Sleep patterns and sleep disruptions in school-age children. *Dev Psychol.* 2000;36(3):291–301.

38. Rabbitts JA, Zhou C, Narayanan A, Palermo TM. Longitudinal and temporal associations between daily pain and sleep patterns after major pediatric surgery. *J Pain.* 2017;18(6):656–663.

39. Short MA, Arora T, Gradisar M, Taheri S, Carskadon MA. How many sleep diary entries are needed to reliably estimate adolescent sleep? *Sleep.* 2017;40(3):zsx006.

40. Smith MT, McCrae CS, Cheung J, et al. Use of actigraphy for the evaluation of sleep disorders and circadian rhythm sleep-wake disorders: an American Academy of Sleep Medicine clinical practice guideline. *J Clin Sleep Med.* 2018;14(7):1231–1237.

41. Bruni O, Russo PM, Violani C, Guidetti V. Sleep and migraine: an actigraphic study. *Cephalalgia.* 2004;24(2):134–139.

42. Haim A, Pillar G, Pecht A, et al. Sleep patterns in children and adolescents with functional recurrent abdominal pain: objective versus subjective assessment. *Acta Paediatr.* 2004;93(5):677–680.

43. Tsai SY, Labyak SE, Richardson LP, et al. Actigraphic sleep and daytime naps in adolescent girls with chronic musculoskeletal pain. *J Pediatr Psychol.* 2008;33(3):307–311.

44. Fisher K, Laikin AM, Sharp KMH, Criddle CA, Palermo TM, Karlson CW. Temporal relationship between daily pain and actigraphy sleep patterns in pediatric sickle cell disease. *J Behav Med.* 2018;41(3):416–422.

45. Conrad N, Karlik J, Lewandowski Holley A, Wilson AC, Koh J. A Narrative review: actigraphy as an objective assessment of perioperative sleep and activity in pediatric patients. *Children (Basel).* 2017;4(4):26.

46. Rosen IM, Aurora RN, Kirsch DB, et al. Chronic opioid therapy and sleep: an American Academy of Sleep Medicine position statement. *J Clin Sleep Med.* 2019;15(11):1671–1673.

47. Dalesio NM, Lee CKK, Hendrix CW, et al. Effects of obstructive sleep apnea and obesity on morphine pharmacokinetics in children. *Anesth Analg.* 2020;131(3):876–884.

48. Aurora RN, Zak RS, Karippot A, et al. Practice parameters for the respiratory indications for polysomnography in children. *Sleep.* 2011;34(3):379–388.

49. Kotagal S, Nichols CD, Grigg-Damberger MM, et al. Non-respiratory indications for polysomnography and related procedures in children: an evidence-based review. *Sleep.* 2012;35(11):1451–1466.

50. de la Vega R, Miro J. The assessment of sleep in pediatric chronic pain sufferers. *Sleep Med Rev.* 2013;17(3):185–192.

51. Armoni Domany K, Nahman-Averbuch H, King CD, et al. Clinical presentation, diagnosis and polysomnographic findings in children with migraine referred to sleep clinics. *Sleep Med.* 2019;63:57–63.

52. Fitzgerald CT, Messias E, Buysse DJ. Teen sleep and suicidality: results from the youth risk behavior surveys of 2007 and 2009. *J Clin Sleep Med.* 2011;7(4):351–356.

53. Gruber R, Cassoff J, Frenette S, Wiebe S, Carrier J. Impact of sleep extension and restriction on children's emotional lability and impulsivity. *Pediatrics.* 2012;130(5):e1155–1161.

54. Lovato N, Gradisar M. A meta-analysis and model of the relationship between sleep and depression in adolescents: recommendations for future research and clinical practice. *Sleep Med Rev.* 2014;18(6):521–529.

55. Vriend JL, Davidson FD, Corkum PV, Rusak B, Chambers CT, McLaughlin EN. Manipulating sleep duration alters emotional functioning and cognitive performance in children. *J Pediatr Psychol.* 2013;38(10):1058–1069.

56. Winsler A, Deutsch A, Vorona RD, Payne PA, Szklo-Coxe M. Sleepless in Fairfax: the difference one more hour of sleep can make for teen hopelessness, suicidal ideation, and substance use. *J Youth Adolesc.* 2015;44(2):362–378.

57. Sivertsen B, Harvey AG, Reichborn-Kjennerud T, Torgersen L, Ystrom E, Hysing M. Later emotional and behavioral problems associated with sleep problems in toddlers: a longitudinal study. *JAMA Pediatr.* 2015;169(6):575–582. https://doi.org/10.1001/jamapediatrics.2015.0187.

58. Jonassaint CR, Jones VL, Leong S, Frierson GM. A systematic review of the association between depression and health care utilization in children and adults with sickle cell disease. *Br J Haematol.* 2016;174(1):136–147.

59. Soltani S, Kopala-Sibley DC, Noel M. The co-occurrence of pediatric chronic pain and depression: a narrative review and conceptualization of mutual maintenance. *Clin J Pain.* 2019;35(7):633–643.

60. Evans S, Djilas V, Seidman LC, Zeltzer LK, Tsao JCI. Sleep quality, affect, pain, and disability in children with chronic pain: is affect a mediator or moderator? *J Pain.* 2017;18(9):1087–1095.

61. Charuvastra A, Cloitre M. Safe enough to sleep: sleep disruptions associated with trauma, posttraumatic stress, and anxiety in children and adolescents. *Child Adolesc Psychiatr Clin N Am.* 2009;18(4):877–891.

62. Fellman V, Heppell PJ, Rao S. Afraid and awake: the interaction between trauma and sleep in children and adolescents. *Child Adolesc Psychiatr Clin N Am.* 2021;30(1):225–249.

63. Wamser-Nanney R, Chesher RE. Trauma characteristics and sleep impairment among trauma-exposed children. *Child Abuse Negl.* 2018;76:469–479.

64. Pavlova M, Kopala-Sibley DC, Nania C, et al. Sleep disturbance underlies the co-occurrence of trauma and pediatric chronic pain: a longitudinal examination. *Pain.* 2020;161(4):821–830.

65. Noel M, Vinall J, Tomfohr-Madsen L, Holley AL, Wilson AC, Palermo TM. Sleep mediates the association between PTSD symptoms and chronic pain in youth. *J Pain.* 2018;19(1):67–75.

66. Degotardi PJ, Klass ES, Rosenberg BS, Fox DG, Gallelli KA, Gottlieb BS. Development and evaluation of a cognitive-behavioral intervention for juvenile fibromyalgia. *J Pediatr Psychol.* 2006;31(7):714–723.

67. Klausen SH, Ronde G, Tornoe B, Bjerregaard L. Nonpharmacological interventions addressing pain, sleep, and quality of life in children and adolescents with primary headache: a systematic review. *J Pain Res.* 2019;12:3437–3459.

68. Law EF, Wan Tham S, Aaron RV, Dudeney J, Palermo TM. Hybrid cognitive-behavioral therapy intervention for adolescents with co-occurring migraine and insomnia: a single-arm pilot trial. *Headache.* 2018;58(7):1060–1073.

69. Liu H, Gao X, Hou Y. Effects of mindfulness-based stress reduction combined with music therapy on pain, anxiety, and sleep quality in patients with osteosarcoma. *Braz J Psychiatr.* 2019;41(6):540–545.

70. Spielman AJ, Caruso LS, Glovinsky PB. A behavioral perspective on insomnia treatment. *Psychiatr Clin North Am.* 1987;10(4):541–553.

71. Jungquist CR, O'Brien C, Matteson-Rusby S, et al. The efficacy of cognitive-behavioral therapy for insomnia in patients with chronic pain. *Sleep Med.* 2010;11(3):302–309.

72. Owens JA, Rosen CL, Mindell JA. Medication use in the treatment of pediatric insomnia: results of a survey of community-based pediatricians. *Pediatrics.* 2003;111(5 Pt 1):e628–635.

73. Roth T, Lankford DA, Bhadra P, Whalen E, Resnick EM. Effect of pregabalin on sleep in patients with fibromyalgia and sleep maintenance disturbance: a randomized, placebo-controlled, 2-way crossover polysomnography study. *Arthritis Care Res (Hoboken).* 2012;64(4):597–606.

74. Pauer L, Winkelmann A, Arsenault P, et al. An international, randomized, double-blind, placebo-controlled, phase III trial of pregabalin monotherapy in treatment of patients with fibromyalgia. *J Rheumatol.* 2011;38(12):2643–2652.

75. Brown S, Johnston B, Amaria K, et al. A randomized controlled trial of amitriptyline versus gabapentin for complex regional pain syndrome type I and neuropathic pain in children. *Scand J Pain.* 2016;13:156–163.

76. Roehrs T, Withrow D, Koshorek G, Verkler J, Bazan L, Roth T. Sleep and pain in humans with fibromyalgia and comorbid insomnia: double-blind, crossover study of suvorexant 20 mg versus placebo. *J Clin Sleep Med.* 2020;16(3):415–421.

77. U.S. Food and Drug Administration. FDA Regulation of Cannabis and Cannabis-Derived Products, Including Cannabidiol (CBD). Updated September 28, 2023. Accessed January 17, 2024. https://www.fda.gov/news-events/public-health-focus/fda-regulation-cannabis-and-cannabis-derived-products-including-cannabidiol-cbd.

78. Ciornei B, David VL, Popescu D, Boia ES. Pain management in pediatric burns: a review of the science behind It. *Glob Health Epidemiol Genom.* 2023;2023:9950870. Published 2023 Sep 15. https://doi.org/10.1155/2023/9950870.

12

Enuresis and Obstructive Sleep Apnea in Children

Oscar Sans Capdevila and Maria Eugenia Russi

CHAPTER HIGHLIGHTS

- Enuresis refers to the involuntary loss of urine during sleep that occurs at least twice a week in children older than 5 years of age (or the developmental equivalent) for at least 3 months.
- Enuretic episodes are considered frequent if they occur 4 or more times per week.
- Primary enuresis occurs in a child who has not been dry for at least 6 months, whereas secondary enuresis has an onset after a period of nocturnal dryness of at least 6 months.
- Enuresis classifies as monosymptomatic or non-monosymptomatic, with the latter correlating with daytime incontinence or other lower urinary tract symptoms like urgency.
- Daytime bladder control and coordination usually occurs by 4 years of age, however nighttime bladder control typically takes longer and is not expected until a child is 5–7 years old.
- Nocturnal enuresis is not a benign disorder; it has severe repercussions for the child and the family.
- The pathogenesis involves several possible mechanisms including nocturnal polyuria, detrusor overactivity, and an increased arousal threshold.

Abstract

Nocturnal enuresis (NE) is a common problem, affecting an estimated 5–7 million children in the United States and occurring more often in boys than in girls, with a 3:1 ratio.

According to the International Children's Continence Society, NE refers to the involuntary loss of urine after the age of 5 years, when most children are expected to have achieved full bladder control at night. It is classified as primary when the child has never achieved nighttime dryness, and secondary when NE occurs after a period of dryness of at least 6 months. To establish diagnosis of NE, a child 5–6 years old should have two or more bed-wetting episodes per month, and a child older than 6 years should have one or more wetting episode per month. To avoid confusion,
the International Children's Continence Society has defined enuresis as wetting that occurs at night, whereas they no longer refer to daytime incontinence as diurnal enuresis.[1]

Among the known risk factors to present NE, a significant correlation with obstructive sleep-disordered breathing (SDB) has emerged, in children and adults, over the last decade.[2,3] It seems clear that increased upper airway resistance during sleep manifested either as habitual snoring (HS) or documented obstructive sleep apnea (OSA) syndrome, increases the risk of enuresis. Most importantly, after successful treatment of the respiratory disorder during sleep, NE can be reduced or even eliminated. Thus, careful evaluation of SDB in enuretic patients is capital.

Epidemiology

The epidemiology of bedwetting is complicated by the variety of definitions used in studies. The prevalence of bedwetting decreases with age. The Avon Longitudinal Study found that infrequent bedwetting (defined in their study as bedwetting fewer than 2 nights per week) has a prevalence of 21% at 4 years and 6 months and 8% at 9 years and 7 months of age. NE (defined in their study as bedwetting more than 2 nights per week) has a prevalence of 8% at 4 years and 6 months and 1.5% at 9 years and 7 months of age.[4] An epidemiologic study in Hong Kong[5] defined bedwetting as 1 wet night over a 3-month period and reported a prevalence of 16.1% at 5 years, 10.1% at 7 years, and 2.2% at 19 years of age. The prevalence is greater for boys than girls at all ages.

Children tend to outgrow NE, with a spontaneous remission rate of about 14% annually among bedwetters (with 3% remaining enuretic as adults).[6]

NE is more common in boys. A quarter of school-aged children with NE have associated daytime symptoms (with or without wetting). Male sex and age younger than 9 years are considered major contributors to primary nocturnal enuresis (PNE) in children. It is well-known that boys have a great prevalence of NE compared with girls, by a 3:1 ratio (which tends to decline with age).[7]

Etiology

Important risk factors for PNE include family history, nocturnal polyuria, impaired sleep arousal, and nocturnal bladder dysfunction. NE has been linked to chromosomes 13, 12, 8 and 22, with a predominantly autosomal dominant inheritance.[8]

In two-thirds of children with NE, a disturbed circadian rhythm of antidiuretic hormone release and nocturnal polyuria have been found.[9] Defects in sleep arousal have also been associated with NE.[10] As many as a third of children with enuresis may have nocturnal detrusor overactivity, with reduced functional bladder capacity. These children have normal detrusor activity and a normal functional bladder capacity when they are awake, but a reduced functional bladder capacity with detrusor overactivity when they are asleep.[5]

Other risk factors for PNE include constipation,[11] developmental delay and other neurologic dysfunction,[12] attention-deficit/hyperactivity disorder,[13] upper airway obstruction,[14,15] and sleep apnea.[16]

Pathophysiology

Pathogenetic Heterogeneity

Enuresis is a clinically and pathogenetically heterogeneous disorder. Different groups of bedwetting children have different underlying defects and require different treatments to become dry.[17]

There are children who present nocturnal polyuria, with or without vasopressin deficiency. These children usually have no associated daytime bladder dysfunction[18] and wet their beds because nocturnal urine output exceeds the amount of urine that the bladder can accommodate, and they sleep too deeply to wake up when the bladder is full. Experts have chosen to call this subtype **diuresis-dependent enuresis**.[17]

There is a second group suffering from detrusor overactivity.[18,19] Many of these children have daytime symptoms such as urgency and/or incontinence, or are constipated,[11] and they wet their beds because of uninhibited detrusor contractions that fail to awaken the child from sleep. The term **detrusor-dependent enuresis** is used to define this subgroup.[17]

There are also children who exhibit signs of both diuresis and detrusor dependency to justify enuresis.[20]

Because neither nocturnal polyuria nor diminished functional bladder capacity adequately explains why children with NE do not wake up to void, the mechanism in patients with enuresis is thought to be multifactorial, with several different pathophysiologic mechanisms proposed.

Nocturnal Polyuria

The discovery by Nørgaard that many enuretic children have nocturnal polyuria demonstrated in a group of bedwetting children who lacked the physiologic nocturnal peak of vasopressin secretion and had a nocturnal urine production exceeding their functional bladder capacity.[21] This finding has since been repeated[22,23] and contradicted.[24] The possibility has also been put forward that polyuria is not necessarily always caused by vasopressin deficiency.[17]

Detrusor Overactivity

Support for the **detrusor overactivity** hypothesis is provided by the finding that children with enuresis go to the toilet more often than dry children, that they void smaller volumes, and that urgency symptoms are more common in this group.[18,19]

Sleep-Disordered Breathing

Significant correlation between enuresis and SDB has been established. HS is the most common clinical manifestation of SDB in children, a condition that ranges from primary snoring to severe OSA syndrome.[25] Studies on the epidemiology and symptoms of SDB have reported an increased frequency of enuresis in children with HS. Wang and colleagues reported that 46% of children with OSA diagnosed by polysomnography (PSG) had NE.[26]

In a European population questionnaire-based study, Kaditis and colleagues showed that 23.3% of children with NE were habitual snorers.[27] Similar results were found in a North American population-based study, in which 26.9% of habitual snorers presented enuresis with a predominant representation of males.[28]

In a questionnaire-based survey of a community sample of children in Greece, those children with HS reported more often the concurrent presence of PNE than those without HS.[15]

A recent cross-sectional study performed by Wada et al. was conducted on nearly 20,000 primary school children (5–12 years old) in Matsuyama, Japan. Associations between NE and the frequencies of snoring and unrefreshing sleep were evaluated using multivariate logistic and regression analyses.

Results of the study showed that although pathogenic mechanisms linking snoring and unrefreshing sleep to increased risk of NE are unknown, snoring, a surrogate reporter of SDB, is associated with increased urine production. Unrefreshing sleep may result from disrupted sleep, facilitating increased sleep pressure and elevated arousal thresholds. Thus, both SDB and unrefreshing sleep are potential independent risk factors of NE in school-aged children.[29]

Significant correlation between enuresis and OSA has been further supported by decreased frequency or complete resolution of NE after successful treatment of the breathing disorder during sleep. This will be discussed later in this chapter.

Deep Sleep With Reduced Arousability

Great controversy has existed for many years about whether enuresis reflects a sleep disorder. In fact, some studies based on surveys have found that children with NE are more subject to parasomnias (e.g., night terrors, sleepwalking) than children who do not wet the bed.[15]

Considering that most of patients with sleep apnea frequently complain about their awakenings to urinate but some of them do not fully awake to urinate and have enuresis, it is reasonable to think that there may be something abnormal with their arousal response. In that direction, several studies examine whether sleep characteristics may differ among children with and without enuresis, analyzing the "arousability" of these patients.[3,14,28,30,31] In most of them, normal polysomnographic findings were reported, failing to identify a specific "deep-sleep phenotype" that may explain the occurrence of enuresis in those children. However, when surveyed, parents consistently maintain that their children with NE are "deep sleepers," compared with their offspring who are not bedwetters.[15]

Regarding the location of the enuretic events within the sleep cycle, the voiding may occur during any sleep stage,[32] but it seems that children with severe, therapy-resistant enuresis preferably void during non-REM sleep.[33]

Increased Glomerular Filtration

It has been described that in obese adult patients, glomerular filtration rate is increased. Krieger and colleagues found in obese subjects with sleep apnea, higher fractional urinary flows, fractional sodium and chloride excretion, and a lower percentage of filtered sodium reabsorption, compared with normal subjects.[34] Interestingly enough, treatment with continuous positive airway pressure tended to normalize renal function in patients with OSA syndrome and was associated with reduced urinary output and sodium reabsorption. To our knowledge, no studies in children have been made to corroborate this hypothesis.

Natriuretic Peptides

One of the potential mechanisms accounting for the increased prevalence of enuresis in the context of SDB may be related to the release of both atrial (ANP) and brain natriuretic peptides (BNP) from cardiac myocytes after cardiac wall distension, as induced by the increased negative intrathoracic pressure swings that accompany the increased upper airway resistance in HS. Hence respiratory effort against a closed airway produces a rise in the negative intrathoracic pressure with the subsequent increase in the venous return and cardiac distension. In addition, the hypoxia associated with an apneic event may induce pulmonary vasoconstriction, causing right ventricular overload and atrial distension. All these mechanisms may explain the subsequent ANP release, enhancing urinary excretion.

According to that, Krieger and collaborators postulate that there is a correlation between ANP levels and the degree of negative intrathoracic pressure associated with apneas and hypoxemia. Release of this cardiac hormone (ANP) will in turn increase sodium and water excretion and will inhibit other hormones that regulate fluid homeostasis, such as vasopressin and the renin-angiotensin-aldosterone pathway.[34]

However, the role of ANP and BNP in that mechanism is somehow controversial. Patwardhan and colleagues showed in a community-based sample, lack of association of natriuretic peptides with OSA syndrome suggesting that undiagnosed OSA syndrome may not be associated with major alterations in left ventricular function, as reflected in morning natriuretic peptide levels.[35]

On the other hand, Kaditis and colleagues showed that in children with HS and apnea-hypopnea index (AHI) of at least 5 had a fourfold higher risk of nocturnal increase in BNP compared with subjects with AHI of 5 or fewer. Indeed, BNP was increased among snoring children and appeared to correlate with the severity of respiratory disturbance during sleep.[27]

Based on the cumulative evidence presented heretofore, it is possible that SDB may increase the frequency of enuresis in children though BNP-dependent mechanisms.

Pursuing that hypothesis, Sans and colleagues wanted to determine the prevalence of enuresis in young school-aged community children and assess whether the presence of HS would be associated with increased reports of enuretic symptoms; as well as to determine whether the degree of severity of SDB was accompanied by an increase in the frequency of enuresis, and whether higher morning BNP levels were present in SDB, particularly when enuresis is present.

Their findings support the notion that HS is associated with increased prevalence of NE, and that morning BNP levels are increased in enuretic children. However, the prevalence of enuresis does not appear to be modified by the severity of respiratory disturbance during sleep.

Taken together, they postulated that even mild increases in sleep pressure due to HS may raise the arousal threshold and promote enuresis, particularly among prone children, and those with elevated BNP levels. As a matter of fact, in children with a genetic propensity for enuresis, BNP levels tends to be enhanced by both HS and OSA syndrome, tipping the balance in favor of a pronounced enuretic symptomatology.[28]

The Three-Systems Model

This approach states that NE results from the interplay of three physiologic factors: defective sleep arousal, nocturnal polyuria, and bladder factors, such as lack of inhibition of bladder emptying during sleep, reduced bladder capacity, or bladder overactivity.[29,36] Of these three factors, the first two are also intimately associated with SDB.[29,36] HS, even with concurrent normal findings during PSG, can lead to not only abnormalities in behavior and cognition, as well as in cardiometabolic parameters, but can also increase the risk of NE,[28,37-39] whereas reciprocally, the presence of NE is associated with increased SDB risk. Thus, both SDB and unrefreshing sleep are potential independent risk factors of NE in school-aged children.

Secondary Nocturnal Enuresis

Risk factors for secondary NE include urinary tract infections (which may cause temporary detrusor and/or urethral instability), diabetes mellitus and diabetes insipidus, stress, sexual abuse, and other psychopathologic conditions, as well as some of the risk factors for PNE, such as constipation and upper-airway obstruction.[8]

Therapeutic Options in Children With Nocturnal Enuresis

The treatment of this common condition can be tailored according to the patient's underlying cause, and monitoring of treatment plays in a crucial role in a successful response. After identifying NE, it should ideally be treated early, preferably no later than age 6 years.[40] The treatment choice should be tailored to the patient's most likely underlying pathophysiology and coexisting disorders,[41] and it is essential to take into account that the patient's and family's motivation is a significant factor in the success of the intervention.[40] If the patient suffers from constipation, this problem should be treated first,[42] and any behavioral or psychologic comorbidities should be addressed as well because their presence negatively affects treatment adherence leading to lower success rates.[42] The initial approach is to try behavioral modifications, including restriction of fluid intake 2 hours before bedtime and of dairy 4 hours before bedtime (to avoid osmotic diuresis) and voiding before going to bed.[43] If the enuresis is infrequent and/or not distressing to the child or parents, treatment is not indicated.[44]

Only three therapies have stood the test of proper randomized, placebo-controlled trials. These are the **enuresis alarm, desmopressin**, and **imipramine treatment**.

Among these, **only the enuresis alarm and treatment with desmopressin** can presently be recommended for routine.[17]

The Enuresis Alarm

The alarm device consists of a urine detector, placed either in the child's underclothes or beneath the sheets, connected to an alarm clock that emits a strong wake-up signal. It works by the principle of waking the child from sleep at the moment of enuresis. Success rate is reported to be around 60–70%. Relapse after successful treatment occurs in 5–30% of children.[45]

Treatment With Desmopressin

Desmopressin is a synthetic vasopressin analog with antidiuretic action that has been used in enuretic children since the late 1970s. Side effects are rare and treatment is generally considered safe, provided that the patient does not consume large amounts of liquids while taking the drug.[46] Reported success rates have varied between 40% and 80%, but most children relapse after treatment, so the curative effect is low.[35,47,48]

Treatment of Sleep-Disordered Breathing

Weider and colleagues reported resolution or decreased frequency of PNE after relief of upper airway obstruction after adenotonsillectomy.[14] Similar results were reported by Leiberman and Basha and colleagues.[49,50] Interestingly enough, resolution of enuresis has been also reported in children with HS and nasal obstruction who received treatment with intranasal corticosteroids.

Appropriate treatment for SDB has been extensively explained in other chapters of this book.

Summary: Clinical Implications and Future Research

NE refers to the involuntary loss of urine after the age of 5 years, when children are expected to have achieved full bladder control at night. It is classified as primary when the child has never achieved nighttime dryness and secondary when bedwetting occurs after being dry for at least 6 months. The condition is considered primary in a child who has never been consistently dry during sleep for six months. Primary sleep enuresis is more common in boys than in girls by a 3:1 ratio.

As discussed before, enuresis is clinically and pathogenetically a heterogeneous disorder and, in this chapter, we want to emphasize the role of SDB in the disease. A link between HS and OSA syndrome has been established in children and adults. Several pathophysiologic mechanisms have been proposed to explain this association but, in the end, genetic predisposition to enuresis seems to be the most important factor even when compared with OSA syndrome severity. Effective treatment of upper airway resistance, even HS, may improve or resolve enuresis in those children.

Given all these considerations, careful evaluation of the presence of SDB (from HS to OSA syndrome) in enuretic patients is capital. Proper treatment can lead to resolution of the problem, thus improving the patient's self-esteem and quality of life.

Future Research: "The Central Hypothesis"

The mismatch between genotype and phenotype in enuresis led to the theory that enuresis, regardless of primary pathogenetic mechanism, may be ultimately caused by disturbances in a specific area in the brainstem.[32]

An inborn disturbance of the function of neuron groups in the upper pons may possibly give rise to the various subtypes of enuresis. The sympathetic branch of the autonomous nervous system is crucial for arousal from sleep[50] and urine storage (i.e., detrusor relaxation and urethral contraction)[51] and has an antidiuretic effect on the kidneys.[52] The parasympathetic system has largely opposite effects and is responsible for bladder emptying.[53]

The locus coeruleus (LC) is a pontine noradrenergic neuron group with pivotal roles both for arousal and for the autonomous nervous system, as the major noradrenergic nucleus of the central nervous system.[54] Arousal stimuli, such as bladder filling, exert their sleep-disrupting effects via the LC.[55] This theory has been corroborated by the findings that enuretic children have more nocturnal parasympathetic and less sympathetic activity than controls.[56,57] More studies are needed to further assess this "central hypothesis" approach for enuresis.

Electroencephalographic Recording and Evaluation of Arousal Dysfunction in Enuresis

Kawauchi and colleagues in 1998 published an elegant study based on changes in the structure of sleep spindles and delta waves on electroencephalography in patients with NE. The conclusions to their findings were that immaturity in the function of the thalamus and in the pons or in the lower tract might be the cause of the arousal dysfunction in patients with enuresis.[10]

When sleep structure (sleep architecture) is analyzed in enuretic patients by polysomnographic studies, little to no difference in sleep architecture of these enuretic patients versus controls has been found to account for the arousal dysfunction.

Assessing subtle electroencephalographic (EEG) changes during sleep (microstructure) provide more sensitivity that focus only on macrostructure. Cyclic alternating pattern (CAP) analysis may give a different perspective on what changes in sleep architecture occur in children with NE and may explain their lack of arousability.

In a recent study conducted by Soster et al., the sleep microstructure of 49 children (27 with enuresis) using CAP was analyzed. No differences in sex, age, and AHI in the patients with enuresis and the control patients were observed. The examination of sleep stage architecture in children with sleep enuresis showed a decrease in percentage of stage N3 sleep. CAP analysis showed an increase in CAP rate in stage N3 sleep and in phase A1 index during stage N3 sleep in the sleep enuresis group, but also a significant reduction of A2% and A3% and of phases A2 and A3 indexes, supporting the concept of decreased arousability in patients with sleep enuresis. The decrease of phase A2 and A3 indexes in these patients might reflect the impaired arousal threshold of children with sleep enuresis. Authors suggest that sleep fragmentation might result in a compensatory increase of slow-wave activity (indicated by the increase of CAP rate in stage N3 sleep) and may explain the higher arousal threshold (indicated by a decrease of phase A2 and A3 indexes) linked to an increased sleep pressure. These findings advocate the presence of a significant disruption of sleep microstructure (CAP) in children with sleep enuresis, supporting the hypothesis of a higher arousal threshold. The results of this study foster the view that CAP is a sensitive tool to analyze the non–rapid eye movement (NREM) sleep instability in sleep enuresis.[58]

Future studies integrating the evaluation of both autonomic and cortical arousals may be able to shed light on the concept of arousability in children with sleep enuresis using different methodologies of EEG analysis: spectral or NREM amplitude variability.

CLINICAL PEARLS

- Enuresis is very common in children and much more prevalent in adolescents than generally appreciated. Local urologic abnormalities account only for a 2–4% of the pediatric cases.
- Regarding the etiologies of enuresis, genetic, behavioral, psychological, size or abnormal reactivity of the bladder, lack of vasopresine release during sleep and delayed development have been suggested.
- Enuresis may be the sole manifestation of seizures and can accompany obstructive sleep apnea.
- Formal urologic evaluation is not indicated. Psychotherapy is only indicated if obvious psychopathology is present. Alarm (bell-and-pad device) is often effective. Tryciclic antidepressants are effective and may be employed only as a short-term treatment. Desmopressin (intranasally administered analogue) might be of benefit.
- Formal polysomnographic study with a full seizure montage is advised in patients with atypical histories or failure to respond to conventional therapy.

References

1. Vande Walle J, Rittig S, Bauer S, et al. American Academy of Pediatrics; European Society for Paediatric Urology; European Society for Paediatric Nephrology; International Children's Continence Society. Practical consensus guidelines for the management of enuresis. *Eur J Pediatr.* 2012;171(6):971–983.
2. Barone JG, Hanson C, DaJusta DG, Gioia K, England SJ, Schneider D. Nocturnal enuresis and overweight are associated with obstructive sleep apnea. *Pediatrics.* 2009;124(1): e53–e59.
3. Brooks LJ. Enuresis and sleep apnea. *Pediatrics.* 2005;116: 799–800.
4. Butler R, Heron J. An exploration of children's views of bedwetting at 9 years. *Child Care Health Dev.* 2008;34(1):65–70.
5. Yeung CK, Sreedhar B, Sihoe JD, Sit FK, Lau J. Differences in characteristics of nocturnal enuresis between children and adolescents: a critical appraisal from a large epidemiological study. *BJU Int.* 2006;97(5):1069–1073.
6. Bower WF, Moore KH, Shepherd RB, Adams RD. The epidemiology of childhood enuresis in Australia. *Br J Urol.* 1996;78(4):602–606.
7. Wille S. Nocturnal enuresis: sleep disturbance and behavioural patterns. *Acta Paediatr.* 1994;83:772–774.
8. Hunskaar S, Burgio K, Diokno A, Herzog AR, Hjälmås K, Lapitan MC. Epidemiology and natural history of urinary incontinence in women. *Urology.* 2003;62(4 Suppl 1): 16–23.
9. Rittig S, Knudsen UB, Nørgaard JP, Pedersen EB, Djurhuus JC. Abnormal diurnal rhythm of plasma vasopressin and urinary output in patients with enuresis. *Am J Physiol.* 1989;256(4 Pt 2): F664–F671.
10. Kawauchi A, Imada N, Tanaka Y, Minami M, Watanabe H, Shirakawa S. Changes in the structure of sleep spindles and delta waves on electroencephalography in patients with nocturnal enuresis. *Br J Urol.* 1998;81(Suppl 3):72–75.
11. Yazbeck S, Schick E, O'Regan S. Relevance of constipation to enuresis, urinary tract infection and reflux. A review. *Eur Urol.* 1987;13(5):318–321.
12. Järvelin MR. Developmental history and neurological findings in enuretic children. *Dev Med Child Neurol.* 1989;31(6): 728–736.
13. Duel BP, Steinberg-Epstein R, Hill M, Lerner M. A survey of voiding dysfunction in children with attention deficit-hyperactivity disorder. *J Urol.* 2003;170(4 Pt 2):1521–1523. discussion 1523-1524.
14. Weider DJ, Hauri PJ. Nocturnal enuresis in children with upper airway obstruction. *Int J Pediatr Otorhinolaryngol.* 1985;9(2):173–182.
15. Alexopoulos EI, Kostadima E, Pagonari I, Zintzaras E, Gourgoulianis K, Kaditis AG. Association between primary nocturnal enuresis and habitual snoring in children. *Urology.* 2006;68(2):406–409.
16. Brooks LJ, Topol HI. Enuresis in children with sleep apnea. *J Pediatr.* 2003;142:515–518.
17. Nevéus T. Sleep enuresis. *Handb Clin Neurol.* 2011;98:363–369.
18. Nevéus T, Hetta J, Cnattingius S, et al. Depth of sleep and sleep habits among enuretic and incontinent children. *Acta Paediatr.* 1999;88:748–752.
19. Yeung CK, Chiu HN, Sit FK. Bladder dysfunction in children with refractory monosymptomatic primary nocturnal enuresis. *J Urol.* 1999;162(3 Pt 2):1049–1055.
20. Nijman RJ. Role of antimuscarinics in the treatment of non-neurogenic daytime urinary incontinence in children. *J Urol.* 2004;63(3 Suppl 1):45–50.
21. Nørgaard JP, Pedersen EB, Djurhuus JC. Diurnal antidiuretic hormone levels in enuretics. *J Urol.* 1985;134:1029–1031.
22. Hunsballe JM, Hansen TK, Rittig S, et al. The efficacy of DDAVP is related to the circadian rhythm of urine output in patients with persisting nocturnal enuresis. *Clin Endocrinol.* 1998;49(6):793–801.
23. Vurgun N, Yiditodlu MR, Ypcan A, et al. Hypernatriuria and kaliuresis in enuretic children and the diurnal variation. *J Urol.* 1998;159(4):1333–1337.
24. Läckgren G, Nevéus T, Stenberg A. Diurnal plasma vasopressin and urinary output in adolescents with monosymptomatic nocturnal enuresis. *Acta Paediatr.* 1997;86(4):385–390.
25. Gozal D, O'Brien LM. Snoring and obstructive sleep apnoea in children: why should we treat? *Pediatr Respir Rev.* 2004;5:S371–S376.
26. Wang RC, Elkins TP, Keech D, Wauquier A, Hubbard D. Accuracy of clinical evaluation in pediatric obstructive sleep apnea. *Otolaryngol Head Neck Surg.* 1998;118:69–73.
27. Kaditis AG, Alexopoulos EI, Hatzi F, et al. Overnight change in brain natriuretic peptide levels in children with sleep disordered breathing. *Chest.* 2006;130:1377–1384.
28. Sans Capdevila O, McLaughlin Crabtree V, Kheirandish-Gozal L, Gozal D. Increased morning brain natriuretic peptide levels in children with nocturnal enuresis and sleep-disordered breathing: a community-based study. *Pediatrics.* 2008;121: e1208–e1214.
29. Wada H, Kimura M, Tajima T, et al. Nocturnal enuresis and sleep disordered breathing in primary school children: potential implications. *Pediatr Pulmonol.* 2018;53(11):1541–1548.
30. Cinar U, Vural C, Cakir B, Topuz E, Karaman MI, Turgut S. Nocturnal enuresis and upper airway obstruction. *Int J Pediatr Otorhinolaryngol.* 2001;59(2):115–118.
31. Umlauf MG, Chasens ER. Sleep disordered breathing and nocturnal polyuria: nocturia and enuresis. *Sleep Med Rev.* 2003;7(5):373–376.
32. Mikkelsen EJ, Rapoport JL. Enuresis: psychopathology, sleep stage, and drug response. *Urol Clin North Am.* 1980;7: 361–377.
33. Nevéus T, Stenberg A, Läckgren G, et al. Sleep of children with enuresis: a polysomnographic study. *Pediatrics.* 1996;106(6 Pt 1):1193–1197.
34. Krieger J, Petiau C, Sforza E, Delanoë C, Hecht MT, Chamouard V. Nocturnal pollakiuria is a symptom of obstructive sleep apnea. *Urol Int.* 1993;50(2):93–97.
35. Patwardhan AA, Larson MG, Levy D, et al. Obstructive sleep apnea and plasma natriuretic peptide levels in a community-based sample. *Sleep.* 2006;29(10):1301–1306.
36. Butler RJ, Robinson JC, Holland P, Doherty-Williams D. Investigating the three systems approach to complex childhood nocturnal enuresis—medical treatment interventions. *Scand J Urol Nephrol.* 2004;38:117–121.
37. Nevéus T. The role of sleep and arousal in nocturnal enuresis. *Acta Paediatr.* 2003;92:1118–1123.
38. Smith DL, Gozal D, Hunter SJ, Philby MF, Kaylegian J, Kheirandish-Gozal L. Impact of sleep disordered breathing on behavior among elementary school-aged children: a cross-sectional analysis of a large community-based sample. *Eur Respir J.* 2016;48:1631–1639.

39. Barnes ME, Huss EA, Garrod KN, et al. Impairments in attention in occasionally snoring children: an event-related potential study. *Dev Neuropsychol.* 2009;34:629–649.

40. Fagundes SN, Lebl AS, Azevedo Soster L, et al. Monosymptomatic nocturnal enuresis in pediatric patients: multidisciplinary assessment and effects of therapeutic intervention. *Pediatr Nephrol.* 2017;32(5):843–851.

41. Nevéus T. Pathogenesis of enuresis: Towards a new understanding. *Int J Urol.* 2017;24(3):174–182.

42. Franco I, von Gontard A, De Gennaro M. International Children's Continence Society. Evaluation and treatment of nonmonosymptomatic nocturnal enuresis: a standardization document from the International Children's Continence Society. *J Pediatr Urol.* 2013;9(2):234–243.

43. Graham KM, Levy JB. Enuresis. *Pediatr Rev.* 2009;30(5):165–172. quiz 173.

44. Gomez Rincon M, Leslie SW, Lotfollahzadeh S. *Nocturnal Enuresis.* StatPearls [Internet]. Treasure Island (FL): StatPearls Publishing; 2021.

45. Khalyfa A, Gharib SA, Kim J, et al. Peripheral blood leukocyte gene expression patterns and metabolic parameters in habitually snoring and non-snoring children with normal polysomnographic findings. *Sleep.* 2011;34:153–160.

46. Monda JM, Husmann DA. Primary nocturnal enuresis: a comparison among observation, imipramine, desmopressin acetate and bed-wetting alarm systems. *J Urol.* 1995;154(2 Pt 2):745–748.

47. Robson WL, Leung AK. Side effects and complications of treatment with desmopressin for enuresis. *J Natl Med Assoc.* 1994;86(10):775–778.

48. Glazener CM, Evans JH. Desmopressin for nocturnal enuresis. *Cochrane Database Syst Rev.* 2002(3):CD002112.

49. Basha S, Bialowas C, Ende K, Szeremeta W. Effectiveness of adenotonsillectomy in the resolution of nocturnal enuresis secondary to obstructive sleep apnea. *Laryngoscope.* 2005;115(6):1101–1103.

50. Leiberman A, Stiller-Timor L, Tarasiuk A, Tal A. The effect of adenotonsillectomy on children suffering from obstructive sleep apnea syndrome (OSAS): the Negev perspective. *Int J Pediatr Otorhinolaryngol.* 2006;70(10):1675–1682.

51. Bonnet MH, Arand DL. Heart rate variability: sleep stage, time of night, and arousal influences. *Electroencephalogr Clin Neurophysiol.* 1997;102(5):390–396.

52. de Groat WC, Booth AM. Physiology of the urinary bladder and urethra. *Ann Intern Med.* 1980;92(Pt 2):312–315.

53. Schrier RW, Liberman R, Ufferman RC. Mechanism of antidiuretic effect of beta-adrenergic stimulation. *J Clin Invest.* 1972;51:97.

54. Aston-Jones G, Rajkowski J, Cohen J. Locus coeruleus and regulation of behavioral flexibility and attention. *Prog Brain Res.* 2000;126:165–182.

55. Koyama Y, Imada N, Kayama Y, et al. How does the distention of urinary bladder cause arousal? *Psychiatry Clin Neurosci.* 1998;52(2):142–145.

56. Fujiwara J, Kimura S, Tsukayama H, et al. Evaluation of the autonomic nervous system function in children with primary monosymptomatic nocturnal enuresis power spectrum analysis of heart rate variability using 24-hour Holter electrocardiograms. *Scand J Urol Nephrol.* 2001;35(5):350–356.

57. Unalacak M, Aydin M, Ermis B, et al. Assessment of cardiac autonomic regulation in children with monosymptomatic nocturnal enuresis by analysis of heart rate variability. *Tohoku J Exp Med.* 2004;204:63–69.

58. Soster LA, Alves RC, Fagundes SN, et al. Non-REM sleep instability in children with primary monosymptomatic sleep enuresis. *J Clin Sleep Med.* 2017;13(10):1163–1170.

13

Bedtime Problems and Nightwakings

Melisa Moore and Jodi A. Mindell

CHAPTER HIGHLIGHTS

- Bedtime difficulties and frequent nightwakings are both common and persistent in young children, and such problems impact all areas of child functioning.
- Behavioral interventions (extinction, graduated extinction, positive routines, and social stories) have been shown to be highly effective and both preventative education and technology based interventions are promising.
- Rates of bedtime problems and frequent night wakings are higher in children with neurodevelopmental conditions, yet behavioral treatment remains the first line therapy.
- In addition to improving sleep, behavioral interventions also positively impact daytime behaviors, parent-child relationships, and parental well-being.

Introduction

In young children, bedtime difficulties and frequent nightwakings are both common and persistent, with 20–30% of children under the age of 3 years experiencing these sleep problems.[1–3] Furthermore, 84% of children with a sleep problem at ages 1–2 still have the same problem at age 3.[4] Studies have provided solid evidence that sleep problems affect emotional, cognitive, behavioral, and academic functioning in children,[4,5] and also are associated with important health concerns such as obesity.[6] Furthermore, sleep issues in children significantly impact daytime functioning and mental health of parents.[7,8]

Bedtime Problems

Bedtime problems occur in about 10–30% of preschoolers and toddlers.[1,3,9,10] Typical presentations include avoidance of bedtime (e.g., refusal to get into bed, stay in bed, or participate in the bedtime routine) and frequent requests after lights out (e.g., for drinks, hugs, or stories). Bedtime problems often begin as part of the emerging independence of toddlers, but they can continue or develop in preschoolers and school-aged children as well. Often children will test limits to determine boundaries and gain independence, both at night and during the day. In most cases these behaviors

are developmentally appropriate. However, at bedtime these behaviors may be more difficult for parents to address, and they can result in inconsistent bedtime routines or parental limits that change with the child's requests. When nighttime routines and appropriate rules are absent, inconsistent, or dependent upon the child's requests, bedtime problems may emerge.

Nightwakings

Frequent nightwakings are reported by 25–50% of parents[1,3,9,10] and are found to be most problematic in infants and toddlers aged 6 months to 3 years. The conditions under which the child learns to fall asleep (i.e., sleep associations) may directly impact the frequency of nightwakings, as may other behavioral factors and circadian issues; however, medical causes, such as reflux and obstructive sleep apnea, should also be considered. When sleep associations involve another person (typically a caregiver), it can be especially difficult for the child to return to sleep independently after normative nightwakings. Parental presence (e.g., rocking, feeding, or lying down with the child) has been shown to be one of the most common predictors of frequent nightwakings.[1] Although parents often perceive that their children with nightwakings have more frequent arousals than do other children, in fact such wakings are a normal part of sleep architecture and are experienced equally by children with and without reported nightwakings.[11] It is the child's signaling at times of waking—by crying, calling, or getting out of bed (because of difficulty returning to sleep independently)—that makes the parents aware of, and thus report as frequent, the nightwakings.

Children often have coexisting frequent nightwakings and bedtime problems. When bedtime problems lead to a long bedtime routine and increased time to sleep onset, caregivers may eventually do whatever it takes for everyone to get to sleep. Furthermore, inconsistent limit setting may facilitate the development of negative sleep associations. For example, a child may repeatedly prolong bedtime with demands (typically by calling out, crying, or having tantrums). If the caregiver eventually gives in to these demands, perhaps by lying down with the child or bringing them into the parental bed, these behaviors are reinforced. Thus, the sleep problem is related to both negative sleep onset associations and to a lack of appropriate limit setting.

Interventions

Interventions for bedtime problems and frequent nightwakings have been supported by a broad foundation of research. Mindell et al.,[12] found that 94% of 52 treatment studies for bedtime problems and frequent nightwakings of studies were efficacious, with over 80% of children demonstrating improvement; these improvements were maintained for 3–6 months. A similar review by Meltzer and Mindell[13] found significant small to large treatment effects with regard to sleep onset latency, number and duration of wakings, and sleep efficiency. Behavioral approaches for the treatment of bedtime problems and nightwakings are reviewed in the present chapter and include sleep hygiene, extinction, graduated extinction, positive routines and bedtime fading, parent education/prevention, social stories, and technology-based interventions incorporating these treatment modalities.

Positive Sleep Health

Sleep habit recommendations are typically a component of treatments for bedtime problems and frequent nightwakings. Any intervention to address childhood sleep problems should begin with an assessment, and if necessary, recommendations for improving overall sleep health. Positive sleep habits include having a consistent sleep schedule on weekdays and weekends that provides the opportunity for adequate sleep duration, a regular bedtime routine, and conditions that are conducive to falling asleep including having a dark, cool, and quiet environment. Several large-scale studies have found that absence of these sleep practices has a significant negative impact on bedtime and nighttime sleep behaviors.[12] Other important aspects of good sleep health include avoiding letting the child fall asleep while feeding but rather moving the feeding to the beginning of the routine, eliminating caffeine, and avoiding use of electronics 30–60 minutes before bedtime.

The evidence as to whether positive sleep health itself directly results in improvements in sleep is mixed. For example, one study[14] found that sleep hygiene alone significantly improved sleep in almost 20% of children with attention-deficit/hyperactivity disorder (ADHD) and insomnia. In contrast, another study found that although combined behavioral-educational intervention for new mothers resulted in significant improvement in maternal and infant sleep, teaching maternal sleep hygiene and providing basic information about infant sleep did not.[15] (Also see the "Education/Prevention" section.)

One specific aspect of children's sleep hygiene, a bedtime routine, has shown robust benefits in multiple areas of childhood functioning. A bedtime routine is a prescribed, consistent set of activities that occur immediately before bedtime, and may include several aspects of childhood health and well-being including nutrition (bedtime snack), hygiene (bath, brush teeth), communication (reading, singing), and physical contact (cuddling).[16] Although inclusion of a bedtime routine is often recommended to caregivers as part of well-child care or as a component of behavioral sleep interventions, the importance of the bedtime routine itself may be underappreciated.[16] For example, a 2009 study found that, compared with controls, a bedtime routine alone resulted in improvements in sleep onset latency, number of nightwakings, sleep continuity, problematic sleep behaviors, and maternal mood.[17] Another study demonstrated that a difference in sleep onset latency and nightwakings could be seen three nights after the introduction of a bedtime routine.[18] And one large-scale study of children birth to 6 years of age found a dose-dependent relationship between frequency of a bedtime routine and sleep outcomes, with each additional night per week of a bedtime routine associated with better sleep.[19]

Extinction

Standard extinction involves putting the child in the crib or bed at a consistent time and ignoring the child's negative behaviors (e.g., crying, yelling, tantrums), while monitoring for safety, until a specified wake time. Extinction is one of the earliest behavioral interventions developed and tested for bedtime problems and frequent nightwakings, and it has been well validated.[12] At least three randomized controlled trials (RCTs) provide empirical support for standard extinction. One RCT compared extinction to scheduled awakenings and to a control group. Based on parental reports it was found that the extinction group had fewer nightwakings than controls, and that the improvements seen occurred more quickly than in the scheduled awakenings group.[20] Extinction alone has also been compared with extinction combined with a medication (trimeprazine) or placebo.[21] Extinction was effective in all three groups—with improvements maintained at both 6 and 30 months—but the fastest response was in the extinction plus medication group.

Consistency is the key to success with extinction, yet most caregivers find their child's prolonged crying to be extremely stressful, thus the standard approach to extinction may not be a good solution for some parents. If parents respond to their child's yelling and crying after a period of time, the child's negative behavior is reinforced with attention and reward, increasing the likelihood of the behavior continuing. Parents should also be advised about the possibility of an initial or later *extinction burst* or brief worsening of negative behaviors. Although this is a normative part of the extinction process, parents may perceive this as evidence that the intervention is not working.

Graduated Extinction

Graduated extinction, like standard extinction, involves ignoring negative behaviors but for a specified duration or instituted in a stepwise manner. Graduated extinction may involve gradually moving the child into their own bedroom, moving the parent out of the child's bedroom (e.g., first sitting beside the bed, then in the doorway), checking at regular set or increasing intervals (5 minutes or first 5 minutes, then 10 minutes, then 15 minutes) and/ or providing brief reassurance and limited attention. The overall goal is to extinguish negative behaviors thereby increasing the independence of the child (e.g., move them into their bed/crib/room and allow them to develop their own soothing skills and positive sleep associations) and decreasing the child's reliance on a caregiver to help fall asleep at bedtime and return to sleep after normative nightwakings. Studies have found all such modifications of graduation extinction approaches to be efficacious.[11,12,22] In a clinical situation, the decision regarding the time between checks is usually based on parental comfort and acceptability, as well as on child temperament and the length of time the child will stay in bed (for toddlers).

A number of RCTs support the use of graduated extinction as an effective intervention for bedtime problems and frequent wakings. Gradisar and Jackson[23] compared graduated extinction to both bedtime fading and a sleep education control group. Both intervention groups had shorter sleep onset latency, fewer nightwakings, and less time awake after sleep onset than the control group. Additionally, they did not find adverse effects of the interventions at 12 months follow-up with regard to elevated stress response, parent-child interactions, or child emotional or behavioral functioning. Hiscock et al.,[24] compared graduated extinction, instituted at an 8-month well-child visit, to a control group. The intervention group demonstrated fewer sleep problems at both 10 and 12 months. Adams and Rickert[25] compared graduated extinction (ignoring the child for a set amount of time determined by the child's age and parent input) with positive bedtime routines. Both intervention groups were effective at reducing negative bedtime behaviors when compared with controls.

An RCT of 3- to 6-year-olds found the use of a bedtime pass to be an effective modification of graduated extinction. In this study, children were given a card (the bedtime pass), which could be traded in for a reasonable request (e.g., a visit from a caregiver or a drink of water).[26] After the bedtime pass was used, caregivers were instructed to ignore negative, attention-seeking behaviors from the child. Results demonstrated less frequent calling and crying out and shorter time to quieting in the intervention group compared with controls, and these improvements were maintained at three months. High parental satisfaction was noted.

Despite evidence that both graduated and standard extinction are effective, graduated extinction is almost always the recommended approach, as it is often perceived by parents and providers to be a "gentler" approach. Overall, graduated extinction interventions are typically the most widely used behavioral treatment for bedtime problems and nightwakings.

Positive Routines and Faded Bedtime

Positive routines with faded bedtime involves developing a short, enjoyable bedtime routine to be implemented at a time close to the time the child is currently falling asleep.

As soon as the child demonstrates negative behaviors, the enjoyable activity is stopped. Faded bedtime capitalizes on the idea of sleep restriction, which is used in the treatment of adult insomnia. A later bedtime should theoretically result in increased sleep pressure, which should facilitate a shorter sleep onset latency. In terms of the positive routines, the goal is for the child to develop an association between the positive bedtime routine and falling asleep quickly. Once this association is established, the child's bedtime is moved earlier in 15-minute increments. Unlike extinction, where the goal is to reduce negative behaviors, the goal of positive routines and faded bedtime is to increase sleep pressure and to reduce the physiologic and emotional arousal that accompanies bedtime conflict and for the child to develop or increase appropriate bedtime behaviors.[12]

At least three studies have found positive routines with faded bedtime to be effective in the treatment of bedtime problems and nightwakings.[25–27] One study of positive routines with faded bedtime that included a control group also had a group treated with graduated extinction. Before the later bedtime (in the positive routine group), the parent and child would complete 4–7 calm, pleasurable activities together; if the child began to have a tantrum, the parent was to end the activities and tell the child that it was time for bed; finally, the child's bedtime was gradually moved earlier until the desired time was reached. In this study, the positive routines with faded bedtime and the graduated extinction treatments were both significantly more effective than no treatment (the control group) but were not significantly different from each other. More recently, faded bedtime as a stand-alone intervention has been studied in preschool children in comparison with graduated extinction[23] (see previous section).

Social Stories

The use of social stories to visually and narratively present expectations around bedtime routines and sleep habits is common in children with neurodevelopmental conditions. One study investigated the use of a social story (the Sleep Fairy) in four typically developing children with the goal of reducing bedtime problems and frequent nightwakings.[28] The first pages of the book provided instructions for parents regarding setting clear expectations and providing contingent reinforcement. The rest of the story for children described a "sleep fairy" who would visit the child intermittently and secretly to see if they were asleep in their beds. If so, they would be given a small reinforcer. All four children, after 2 weeks of intervention, demonstrated decreased disruptive bedtime behaviors and no nightwakings. Parents were able to be consistent with the intervention (high-fidelity ratings) and also rated the intervention as highly acceptable. This approach is promising, as other approaches may be effective but not as tolerable for parents.

Education/Prevention

Parent education and prevention focuses on providing written or in-person information to prevent the development of bedtime problems and frequent nightwakings. Education typically involves provision of information about helping children develop self-soothing skills (including positive associations) and recommending positive sleep hygiene practices (including a consistent sleep schedule and a bedtime routine). Many educational programs advise putting children to bed awake and allowing them to return to sleep independently after normative nightwakings.[15] Multiple studies have been conducted showing that short preventative interventions (1–4 sessions) can improve infant sleep.[26,29–31] Cooney and colleagues used a two-session group parent education approach to teaching faded bedtime in preschool children. Improvements were found post-intervention in sleep onset latency, wake after sleep onset, and bedtime tantrums. These improvements were maintained at 2-year follow-up.[32] St. James-Roberts[30] and Adair[31] incorporated written sleep information into two routine well-child visits and found benefits in infant sleep. Wolfson et al.[33] randomly assigned first-time parents in child birthing classes to a sleep education group (2 classes before and 2 classes after childbirth) or to a control group. According to parent diaries, 72% of 3-week-old infants "slept through the night" compared with 48% in the control group. A study by Pinilla and Birch[34] found that by 8 weeks, 100% of infants in a parent education intervention slept through the night compared with 23% of controls.

A specific area of sleep prevention is the intersection of sleep and obesity. As early as the first 6 months of life, a link has been found between sleep duration and weight-for-length measures,[35] and it has been shown that total daily sleep duration of less than 12 hours during infancy is associated with overweight status in preschool-aged children.[36] Thus, there has been a call for clinicians and researchers to include sleep interventions in obesity-prevention efforts.[37] A pilot study from 2001[38] found that a behavioral intervention targeting feeding as well as sleep resulted in lower weight-for-length percentiles at 1 year of age, with increasing evidence supported by more recent RCTs that incorporate sleep recommendations.[39,40]

Technology

Though behavioral interventions have typically been conducted face-to-face, the use of technology in health care has increased dramatically over the past several years. Multiple studies have demonstrated improvements in sleep using app-based or computer-based interventions for young children. For example, Mindell designed an intervention based on responses to an expanded version of the Brief Infant Sleep Questionnaire (BISQ).[41] Parents were given information about how their child's sleep compared with a normative sample of same-aged children (*excellent, good,* or *disrupted*) along with customized, behaviorally based advice for how to improve their child's sleep. One week after the internet intervention, improvements were seen in latency to sleep onset, number and duration of nightwakings, and sleep continuity. Maternal confidence in managing their child's sleep, maternal sleep, and maternal mood were also significantly

improved. These improvements were maintained at 1 year post-intervention.[41,42]

Though most pediatric sleep practitioners have experience with telephone consultations or follow-up, a rapidly emerging area is video telemedicine, in part because of social distancing practices related to the COVID-19 pandemic. At least one center described a telemedicine approach (video visits) to child sleep problems before the COVID-19 pandemic,[43] and others have described their approaches during the pandemic.[44] It has been argued that the use of telemedicine, especially in urban settings, increases access to medical services.[45] It is likely that the research foundation for telemedicine in pediatric sleep will broaden in the near future as a result of the current increase in telemedicine interventions.

Treatment Implications

Although research clearly demonstrates that behavioral treatments for bedtime problems and nightwakings are effective at improving children's sleep, there are many who are resistant to behavioral interventions because of worries about harmful effects on other aspects of child development, such as the quality of the parent-child relationship. Concerns have been raised about the impact of behavioral sleep interventions on attachment, security, and mental health.[36] A review of secondary outcomes of behavioral sleep interventions did not find evidence to support iatrogenic effects.[8] Of 35 treatment studies that included a secondary outcome measure, no systematic negative effects were found on any measured child variable. Conversely, improvements were demonstrated in child mood, daytime behavior,[24,28,42,46–50] and temperament.[24,34] Several studies were also reviewed that focused on the impact of behavioral sleep interventions on the parent-child relationship.[42,48,49] Again, rather than demonstrating harmful effects, these studies found just the opposite. Young children with sleep disturbances initially scored lower (worse) on measures of attachment, security, and maternal bonding compared with good sleepers, and treatment gains improved security, attachment, and parent-child interactions.

Sleep Problems in Children With Neurodevelopmental Conditions

Although bedtime problems and frequent nightwakings are common in typically developing children, children with neurodevelopmental conditions such as autism spectrum disorders (ASDs) and ADHD are at an even higher risk for sleep problems. Over the past decade, there has been an increasing number of studies of sleep in children with neurodevelopmental conditions including ASDs and ADHD.

Autism Spectrum Disorders

Children with ASDs are at increased risk for bedtime problems and nightwakings compared with typically developing children, with 44–83% of children diagnosed with ASDs having a sleep problem based on actigraphy or parent report.[51–53] Sleep problems, prolonged nightwakings, and shorter sleep duration in children with ASDs have been shown to relate to more energetic, excited, and problematic daytime behaviors as well as to decreased social skills and increased stereotypic behaviors.[54]

It is the generally accepted standard of care that behavioral interventions are first-line treatment in treating sleep problems in children with ASDs.[55] Though behavioral interventions may be more challenging to implement and therefore may be offered less frequently than medications, parents of children with ASDs may prefer behavioral interventions to sleep medications.[56] Positive routines and faded bedtimes are behavioral sleep interventions that have been examined in at least two studies of children with ASDs and have been found to improve sleep.[57,58] Another study evaluated the efficacy of faded bedtime with response cost (i.e., negative consequences for inappropriate behaviors) combined with positive reinforcement in three children with ASD.[59] Sleep onset latency improved in all three cases during treatment and gains were maintained 12 weeks later. Daytime behavior, as measured by the Child Behavior Checklist (CBCL), a commonly used screening tool for externalizing and internalizing behaviors, improved, with scores moving from the borderline clinical range to the average range in two of the three children. Another study[60] of 20 children with ASDs (ages 3–10 years), whose parents attended a three-part workshop on the treatment of sleep issues, found significant improvements in hyperactivity, self-stimulatory behaviors, and repetitive behaviors in addition to significant improvements in sleep. For children with ASDs and/or ADHD, improvement in sleep problems has been shown to relate to improvements in parenting stress and mental health.[61]

ADHD

Children with ADHD have been reported to have more bedtime problems (e.g., longer time to sleep onset and bedtime resistance) than children without ADHD.[62,63] Behavioral sleep interventions have been shown to improve both sleep and symptoms of ADHD. For example, a two-session intervention providing recommendations for sleep hygiene and behavioral strategies for sleep problems found improvements in sleep, severity of ADHD symptoms, behavior, and quality of life at 3 and 6 months.[64] At least one case series[65] and one small study[14] have shown feasibility and parent satisfaction with behavioral sleep interventions. There has also been one recent RCT of a behavioral intervention for 27 children (aged 5–14 years) that found small changes in ADHD symptom scores from baseline to 5 months post-treatment after either a brief or extended treatment of sleep issues.[66] Early implementation of behavioral treatment may be critical as sleep disturbances can exacerbate symptoms of ADHD.[67]

CLINICAL PEARLS

- Ensuring positive sleep habits (sleep hygiene) is often the first step in any behavioral sleep treatment.
- A bedtime routine is critical.
- Behavioral approaches are the first line intervention for sleep problems in typically developing and neurodiverse children.
- Graduated extinction is the most common behavioral approach to bedtime problems and night wakings.

Summary

Overall, studies have found that bedtime problems and nightwakings are highly prevalent sleep disturbances in typically developing children, as well as in children with neurodevelopmental conditions such as ASD and ADHD. Behavioral interventions have been shown to be highly effective and include a number of different treatment techniques including extinction, graduated extinction, positive routines, and social stories. Preventive educational approaches are also effective, and technology-based interventions appear to be quite promising. Finally, not only do these behavioral interventions improve sleep disturbances, but they also appear to have a positive impact on secondary outcomes including daytime behaviors, parent-child relationships, and parental well-being.

References

1. Sadeh A, Mindell JA, Luedtke K, Wiegand B. Sleep and sleep ecology in the first 3 years: a web-based study. *J Sleep Res.* 2009;18(1):60–73.
2. Mindell JA, Kuhn B, Lewin DS, Meltzer LJ, Sadeh A, American Academy of Sleep Medicine. Behavioral treatment of bedtime problems and nightwakings in infants and young children. *Sleep.* 2006;29(10):1263–1276.
3. Williamson AA, Mindell JA, Hiscock H, Quach J. Child sleep behaviors and sleep problems from infancy to school-age. *Sleep Med.* 2019;63:5–8.
4. Kataria S, Swanson MS, Trevathan GE. Persistence of sleep disturbances in preschool children. *J Pediatr.* 1987;110(4):642–646.
5. Beebe DW. Cognitive, behavioral, and functional consequences of inadequate sleep in children and adolescents. *Pediatr Clin North Am.* 2011;58(3):649–665.
6. Hart CN, Carskadon MA, Considine RV, et al. Changes in children's sleep duration on food intake, weight, and leptin. *Pediatrics.* 2013;132(6):e1473–e1480.
7. Meltzer LJ, Mindell JA. Relationship between child sleep disturbances and maternal sleep, mood, and parenting stress: a pilot study. *J Fam Psychol.* 2007;21(1):67–73.

8. Moore M, Mindell JA. The impact of behavioral interventions for sleep problems on secondary outcomes in young children and their families. In: Wolfson A, Montgomery-Downs H, eds. *The Oxford Handbook of Infant, Child, and Adolescent Sleep and Behavior*. Oxford University Press; 2013.

9. Burnham MM, Goodlin-Jones BL, Gaylor EE, Anders TF. Nighttime sleep-wake patterns and self-soothing from birth to one year of age: a longitudinal intervention study. *J Child Psychol Psychiatry*. 2002;43(6):713–725.

10. Gaylor EE, Burnham MM, Goodlin-Jones BL, Anders TF. A longitudinal follow-up study of young children's sleep patterns using a developmental classification system. *Behav Sleep Med*. 2005;3(1):44–61.

11. Sadeh A. Assessment of intervention for infant nightwaking: parental reports and activity-based home monitoring. *J Consult Clin Psychol*. 1994;62(1):63–68.

12. Mindell JA, Kuhn BR, Lewin DS, Meltzer LJ, Sadeh A, American Academy of Sleep Medicine. Behavioral treatment of bedtime problems and nightwakings in infants and young children. *Sleep*. 2006;29(10):1263–1276. *Sleep*. 2006;29(10): 1263–1276.

13. Meltzer LJ, Mindell JA. Systematic review and meta-analysis of behavioral interventions for pediatric insomnia. *J Pediatr Psychol*. 2014;39(8):932–948.

14. Weiss MD, Wasdell MB, Bomben MM, Rea KJ, Freeman RD. Sleep hygiene and melatonin treatment for children and adolescents with ADHD and initial insomnia. *J Am Acad Child Adolesc Psychiatry*. 2006;45(5):512–519.

15. Stremler R, Hodnett E, Kenton L, et al. Effect of behavioural-educational intervention on sleep for primiparous women and their infants in early postpartum: multisite randomised controlled trial. *BMJ*. 2013;346:F1164.

16. Mindell JA, Williamson AA. Benefits of a bedtime routine in young children: sleep, development, and beyond. *Sleep Med Rev*. 2018;40:93–108.

17. Mindell JA, Telofski LS, Wiegand B, Kurtz ES. A nightly bedtime routine: impact on sleep in young children and maternal mood. *Sleep*. 2009;32(5):599–606.

18. Mindell JA, Leichman ES, Lee C, Williamson AA, Walters RM. Implementation of a nightly bedtime routine: how quickly do things improve? *Infant Behav Dev*. 2017;49:220–227.

19. Mindell JA, Li AM, Sadeh A, Kwon R, Goh DYT. Bedtime routines for young children: a dose-dependent association with sleep outcomes. *Sleep*. 2015;38(5):717–722.

20. Rickert VI, Johnson CM. Reducing nocturnal awakening and crying episodes in infants and young children: a comparison between scheduled awakenings and systematic ignoring. *Pediatrics*. 1988;81(2):203.

21. France KG, Blampied NM, Wilkinson P. Treatment of infant sleep disturbance by trimeprazine in combination with extinction. *J Dev Behav Pediatr*. 1991;12(5):308–314.

22. Blunden S. Behavioural treatments to encourage solo sleeping in pre-school children: an alternative to controlled crying. *J Child Health Care Prof Work Child Hosp Community*. 2011;15(2):107–117.

23. Gradisar M, Jackson K, Spurrier NJ, et al. Behavioral interventions for infant sleep problems: a randomized controlled trial. *Pediatrics*. 2016;137(6):e20151486.

24. Hiscock H, Bayer J, Gold L, Hampton A, Ukoumunne OC, Wake M. Improving infant sleep and maternal mental health: a cluster randomised trial. *Arch Dis Child*. 2007;92(11): 952–958.

25. Adams LA, Rickert VI. Reducing bedtime tantrums: comparison between positive routines and graduated extinction. *Pediatrics*. 1989;84(5):756.

26. Moore BA, Friman PC, Fruzzetti AE, MacAleese K. Brief report: evaluating the bedtime pass program for child resistance to bedtime—a randomized, controlled trial. *J Pediatr Psychol*. 2006;32(3):283–287.

27. Milan MA, Mitchell ZP, Berger MI, Pierson DF. Positive routines: a rapid alternative to extinction for elimination of bedtime tantrum behavior. *Child Behav Ther*. 1982;3(1):13–25.

28. Burke RV, Kuhn BR, Peterson JL. Brief report: a "storybook" ending to children's bedtime problems—the use of a rewarding social story to reduce bedtime resistance and frequent nightwaking. *J Pediatr Psychol*. 2004;29(5):389–396.

29. Kerr SM, Jowett SA, Smith LN. Preventing sleep problems in infants: a randomized controlled trial. *J Adv Nurs*. 1996;24(5):938–942.

30. St James-Roberts I, Gillham P. Use of a behavioural programme in the first 3 months to prevent infant crying and sleeping problems. *J Paediatr Child Health*. 2001;37(3):289–297.

31. Adair R, Bauchner H, Philipp B, Levenson S, Zuckerman B. Nightwaking during infancy: role of parental presence at bedtime. *Pediatrics*. 1991;87(4):500.

32. Cooney MR, Short MA, Gradisar M. An open trial of bedtime fading for sleep disturbances in preschool children: a parent group education approach. *Sleep Med*. 2018;46:98–106.

33. Wolfson A, Lacks P, Futterman A. Effects of parent training on infant sleeping patterns, parents' stress, and perceived parental competence. *J Consult Clin Psychol*. 1992;60(1):41–48.

34. Pinilla T, Birch LL. Help me make it through the night: behavioral entrainment breast-fed infants' sleep patterns. *Pediatrics*. 1993;91(2):436.

35. Sadeh A, Tikotzky L, Scher A. Parenting and infant sleep. *Sleep Med Rev*. 2010;14(2):89–96.

36. Taveras EM, Rifas-Shiman SL, Oken E, Gunderson EP, Gillman MW. Short sleep duration in infancy and risk of childhood overweight. *Arch Pediatr Adolesc Med*. 2008;162(4):305.

37. Paul IM, Hohman EE, Loken E, et al. Mother-infant room-sharing and sleep outcomes in the INSIGHT study. *Pediatrics*. 2017;140(1):e20170122.

38. Paul IM, Savage JS, Anzman SL, et al. Preventing obesity during infancy: a pilot study. *Obesity*. 2011;19(2):353–361.

39. Paul IM, Savage JS, Anzman-Frasca S, et al. Effect of a responsive parenting educational intervention on childhood weight outcomes at 3 years of age: the INSIGHT randomized clinical trial. *JAMA*. 2018;320(5):461.

40. Taylor BJ, Gray AR, Galland BC, et al. Targeting sleep, food, and activity in infants for obesity prevention: an RCT. *Pediatrics*. 2017;139(3):e20162037.

41. Mindell JA, Du Mond CE, Sadeh A, Telofski LS, Kulkarni N, Gunn E. Efficacy of an internet-based intervention for infant and toddler sleep disturbances. *Sleep*. 2011;34(4):451–458B.

42. Mindell JA, Du Mond CE, Sadeh A, Telofski LS, Kulkarni N, Gunn E. Long-term efficacy of an internet-based intervention for infant and toddler sleep disturbances: one year follow-up. *J Clin Sleep Med*. 2011;07(05):507–511.

43. Witmans MB, Dick B, Good J, et al. Delivery of pediatric sleep services via telehealth: the Alberta experience and lessons learned. *Behav Sleep Med*. 2008;6(4):207–219.

44. Paruthi S. Telemedicine in pediatric sleep. *Sleep Med Clin.* 2020;15(3):e1–e7.
45. Ronis SD, McConnochie KM, Wang H, Wood NE. Urban telemedicine enables equity in access to acute illness care. *Telemed E-Health.* 2017;23(2):105–112.
46. Richman N, Douglas J, Hunt H, Lansdown R, Levere R. Behavioural methods in the treatment of sleep disorders: a pilot study. *J Child Psychol Psychiatry.* 1985;26(4):581–590.
47. Seymour FW, Bayfield G, Brock P, During M. Management of night-waking in young children. *Aust J Fam Ther.* 1983; 4(4):217–223.
48. France KG. Behavior characteristics and security in sleep-disturbed infants treated with extinction. *J Pediatr Psychol.* 1992; 17(4):467–475.
49. Hiscock H, Bayer JK, Hampton A, Ukoumunne OC, Wake M. Long-term mother and child mental health effects of a population-based infant sleep intervention: cluster-randomized, controlled trial. *Pediatrics.* 2008;122(3):e621–e627.
50. Reid MJ, Walter AL, O'Leary SG. Treatment of young children's bedtime refusal and nighttime wakings: a comparison of "standard" and graduated ignoring procedures. *J Abnorm Child Psychol.* 1999;27(1):5–16.
51. Richdale AL, Schreck KA. Sleep problems in autism spectrum disorders: Prevalence, nature, & possible biopsychosocial aetiologies. *Sleep Med Rev.* 2009;13(6):403–411.
52. Richdale AL, Prior MR. The sleep/wake rhythm in children with autism. *Eur Child Adolesc Psychiatry.* 1995;4(3):175–186.
53. Wiggs L, Stores G. Sleep patterns and sleep disorders in children with autistic spectrum disorders: insights using parent report and actigraphy. *Dev Med Child Neurol.* 2004;46(6):372.
54. Schreck K. Sleep problems as possible predictors of intensified symptoms of autism. *Res Dev Disabil.* 2004;25(1):57–66.
55. Cuomo BM, Vaz S, Lee EAL, Thompson C, Rogerson JM, Falkmer T. Effectiveness of sleep-based interventions for children with autism spectrum disorder: a meta-synthesis. *Pharmacother J Hum Pharmacol Drug Ther.* 2017;37(5):555–578.
56. Wiggs L, Stores G. Behavioural treatment for sleep problems in children with severe learning disabilities and challenging daytime behaviour: effect on daytime behaviour. *J Child Psychol Psychiatry.* 1999;40(4):627–635.
57. Christodulu KV, Durand VM. Reducing bedtime disturbance and nightwaking using positive bedtime routines and sleep restriction. *Focus Autism Dev Disabil.* 2004;19(3):130–139.
58. Delemere E, Dounavi K. Parent-implemented bedtime fading and positive routines for children with autism spectrum disorders. *J Autism Dev Disord.* 2018;48(4):1002–1019.
59. Moon EC, Corkum P, Smith IM. Case study: a case-series evaluation of a behavioral sleep intervention for three children with autism and primary insomnia. *J Pediatr Psychol.* 2010;36(1):47–54.
60. Reed HE, McGrew SG, Artibee K, et al. Parent-based sleep education workshops in autism. *J Child Neurol.* 2009;24(8):936–945.
61. Martin CA, Papadopoulos N, Chellew T, Rinehart NJ, Sciberras E. Associations between parenting stress, parent mental health and child sleep problems for children with ADHD and ASD: Systematic review. *Res Dev Disabil.* 2019;93:103463.
62. Cortese S, Lecendreux M, Mouren M-C, Konofal E. ADHD and insomnia. *J Am Acad Child Adolesc Psychiatry.* 2006; 45(4):384–385.
63. Sadeh A, Pergamin L, Bar-Haim Y. Sleep in children with attention-deficit hyperactivity disorder: a meta-analysis of polysomnographic studies. *Sleep Med Rev.* 2006;10(6):381–398.
64. Hiscock H, Sciberras E, Mensah F, et al. Impact of a behavioural sleep intervention on symptoms and sleep in children with attention deficit hyperactivity disorder, and parental mental health: randomised controlled trial. *BMJ.* 2015;350:H68.
65. Mullane J, Corkum P. Case series: evaluation of a behavioral sleep intervention for three children with attention-deficit/hyperactivity disorder and dyssomnia. *J Atten Disord.* 2006;10(2):217–227.
66. Sciberras E, Fulton M, Efron D, Oberklaid F, Hiscock H. Managing sleep problems in school aged children with ADHD: A pilot randomised controlled trial. *Sleep Med.* 2011;12(9):932–935.
67. Dahl RE, Pelham WE, Wierson M. the role of sleep disturbances in attention deficit disorder symptoms: a case study. *J Pediatr Psychol.* 1991;16(2):229–239.

14

Attention Deficit, Hyperactivity, and Sleep Disorders

Grace Wang, Claire Bogan, Kristina Puzino Lenker, Susan Calhoun, James Luebbert, and Ronald D. Chervin

CHAPTER HIGHLIGHTS

- Daytime sequelae of sleep disorders can mimic and lead to a diagnosis of ADHD, sometimes for years, until the underlying cause is identified. Youth with ADHD are at higher risk for obstructive sleep apnea, restless legs syndrome, periodic limb movement disorder, delayed sleep-wake phase disorder, and insufficient sleep.
- Regulation of sleep and wakefulness appear to have shared neurochemical and neuroanatomical pathways with executive function.
- Psychotropic medications frequently used to treat ADHD and its behavioral and psychiatric co-morbidities can directly impact sleep and wakefulness.
- Comorbidities of ADHD, such as autism, oppositional defiant disorder, anxiety, and depression, may make sleep disturbances more challenging to manage, particularly with a chaotic psychosocial milieu.
- Behavioral sleep interventions are often important in efforts to address sleep disturbances in youth with ADHD.

Introduction

Sleep disturbances in children have long been associated with daytime impairment in the form of neurocognitive and behavioral deficits. In fact, dating back to 1892, Dr. William Osler, author of *Principles and Practices of Medicine*, observed that children with "loud and snorting" respirations with "prolonged pauses" demonstrated deficits in their cognitive functioning and development.[1] In 1976, Dr. Christian Guilleminault published a series of case studies describing children with obstructive sleep apnea (OSA) syndrome and its association with learning and attention problems.[2] International research efforts in the past several decades have illuminated additional important links between sleep problems and behavioral or neurocognitive deficits in children, with attention-deficit/hyperactivity disorder (ADHD) being one of the most well studied.

ADHD is a common, chronic neuropsychiatric disorder usually presenting in early childhood, with an estimated prevalence of ~7% in children.[3] Core symptoms include a functionally impairing level of inattention and distractibility, executive function deficits, increased behavioral and verbal impulsivity, and motor hyperactivity. The morbidity of ADHD symptomatology includes impaired academic performance, strained personal and professional relationships, and poor self-esteem and quality of life.[4] Moreover, ADHD is associated with depression, anxiety, and substance use disorders,[4,5] and has been identified as a major risk factor for accidents and suicide.[6]

The relationships between sleep, sleep and wake regulation, and ADHD symptomatology are complex. A thoughtful understanding and ability to identify various contributing factors is crucial to improve sleep, daytime functioning, and quality of life in these individuals.

Sleep Disturbances and Comorbidity of Neurocognitive and Behavioral Deficits

Sleep disturbances occur frequently in youth with ADHD (25–70%). Reported prevalence rates likely vary due to heterogeneity of study participants (e.g., ADHD subtype(s), presence of primary sleep disorders, psychiatric comorbidities, and medication status).[7,8]

Subjective Studies

Cortese et al., performed a 2009 meta-analysis of subjective (parent and teacher questionnaires on behavior and sleep) and objective studies (polysomnography [PSG], actigraphy). They compared sleep parameters in non-medicated youth with ADHD without anxiety or depression (722 pooled subjects) versus controls (628 pooled subjects). Subjective studies showed significantly more bedtime resistance, sleep-onset difficulties, night awakenings, difficulties with morning awakenings, sleep-disordered breathing (SDB), and daytime sleepiness in youth with ADHD.[9]

141

Objective Studies

In the Cortese meta-analysis, youth with ADHD, compared with those without ADHD, had a longer sleep-onset latency (actigraphy), decreased true sleep time (actigraphy), more stage shifts per hour of sleep (PSG), higher apnea-hypopnea index (AHI) (PSG), lower sleep efficiency (PSG), and reduced mean sleep latency (multiple sleep latency test [MSLT]).[9] In a 2006 meta-analysis by Sadeh et al., 333 youth with ADHD exhibited more periodic limb movements of sleep (PSG) than controls (231 subjects), though the effect size was small.[10] No other PSG parameters were significantly different between groups. Díaz-Román et al., completed a more recent[4] meta-analysis of PSG studies, and excluded children with primary sleep disorders in an effort to examine any distinctive sleep architecture of ADHD itself. Youth with ADHD spent more time in stage N1 sleep compared with controls. While not meeting statistical significance, those with ADHD also tended to have a prolonged sleep-onset latency.[4]

Unraveling the Complex Relationship Between Attention-Deficit/Hyperactivity Disorder and Sleep

The literature clearly supports an association between sleep disturbances and ADHD. However, among children with ADHD, subjective and objective measures of sleep show a high degree of variability among studies. These inconsistencies speak to the highly complex, multifaceted relationship between ADHD and sleep, and point to the possibility that children with ADHD are a heterogeneous population.

Increasingly, ADHD is conceptualized as a heterogenous syndrome that affects individuals across the entire 24-hour period. Over the past decade, research efforts sought to identify differences in sleep and wake patterns and prevalence of sleep problems among the ADHD "subtypes" (inattentive [ADHD-I], combined [ADHD-C], and hyperactive/impulsive [ADHD-HI]) with mixed results. However, one consistent finding that emerged was the report of greater daytime sleepiness in ADHD-I subjects.[11,12] Most recently, researchers have begun to conceptualize ADHD as distinct "phenotypes,"[13] each with a different mechanism of action mediating ADHD symptoms. They describe a hypo-arousal state resembling narcolepsy, delayed sleep-onset insomnia, SDB, restless legs syndrome (RLS)/periodic limb movements of sleep (PLMs), and epilepsy/sleep electroencephalogram (EEG) epileptiform discharges.[13,14]

OBJECTIVES

In this chapter, the following topics will be discussed to help unravel the complex relationship between attention-deficit/hyperactivity disorder (ADHD) and sleep.

- There is evidence that regulation of sleep, wakefulness, and executive function may have shared neurochemical and neuroanatomical underpinnings. Thus sleep disturbances in ADHD may be a manifestation of an inherent dysregulation of sleep and wakefulness that is associated with central nervous system dysfunction.
- Psychotropic medications frequently used to treat ADHD (and behavioral or psychiatric comorbidities) can have direct effects on sleep and wakefulness.
- Primary sleep disorders, such as obstructive sleep-disordered breathing (ranging from primary snoring to upper airway resistance syndrome to obstructive sleep apnea syndrome), restless legs syndrome and periodic limb movement disorder, and delayed sleep–wake phase disorder, may result in poor quality or insufficient sleep for age. Daytime sequelae of sleep disorders can mimic and lead to a diagnosis of ADHD, sometimes for years, until the underlying cause is identified.
- Comorbid sleep disturbances can exacerbate ADHD symptoms.
- Psychiatric and neurobehavioral conditions (e.g., anxiety, depression, conduct disorder, oppositional defiant disorder, and autism) are frequently comorbid with ADHD. These comorbidities may have a detrimental impact on nocturnal sleep, in terms of bedtime resistance, insomnia, poor quality sleep, and insufficient sleep duration, particularly when the family or psychosocial milieu is more chaotic.
- Screening and treatment for medical sleep disorders, and use of behavioral sleep interventions, are often important in efforts to address sleep disturbances in youth with ADHD.

Shared Neurobiology of Sleep and Wakefulness, and Regulation of Behavior and Executive Function

Similar neurochemical and neuroanatomical underpinnings have been identified in maintenance of the sleep and wake cycle, as well as regulation of higher order cognitive functions (e.g., executive function) and affect. The noradrenergic and dopaminergic systems, and derangements thereof, have been implicated in both ADHD and sleep and wake disturbances (Fig. 14.1). Dopamine (DA) neurons in the ventral tegmental area consolidate wakefulness and are also involved in sleep and wake regulation.[15] Interestingly, striatal DA receptors are abnormally few in medication-naïve subjects with ADHD.[16] In one study, parental reports showed 10% of youth with ADHD had sleep disturbances even before starting methylphenidate (MPH).[17] The locus coeruleus (LC), which is part of the reticular activating system, and which mediates noradrenergic transmission, is a key structure in regulation of arousal and the sleep and wake cycle. Suppression of LC norepinephrine (NE) neurotransmission elicits profound sedation.[18]

Indeed, psychostimulants like MPH are thought to improve ADHD core symptoms by increasing DA and NE in the frontal lobes and striatum.[19] The prefrontal cortex (PFC), for which two key receptors are DA D1 and α-2A adrenoreceptors (sensitive to noradrenaline and epinephrine), is central in mediation of both sleep and wakefulness and executive function (see Fig. 14.1). Executive function involves many higher order cognitive functions, including

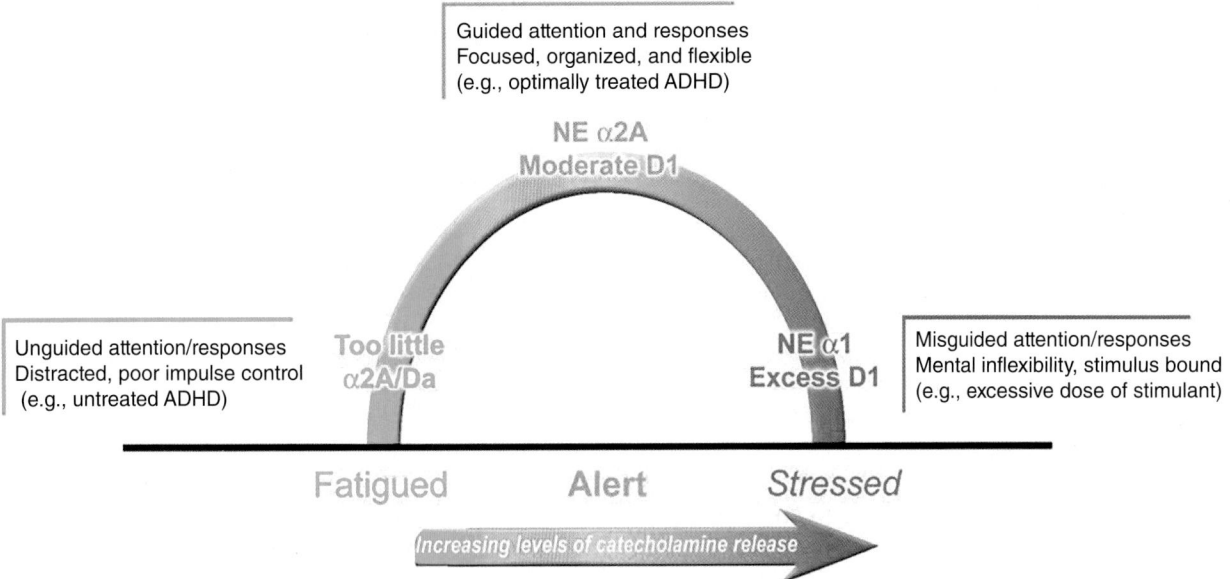

• **Fig. 14.1** Optimal prefrontal cortex (PFC) function and alertness require the proper neurochemical milieu. An optimal state of alertness and PFC function necessitates a moderate amount of the catecholamines, norepinephrine (NE) and dopamine (DA). There is an inverted U-dose–response relationship whereby inadequate NE and DA release is associated with fatigue and suboptimal PFC function (e.g., attention-deficit/hyperactivity disorder [ADHD] symptoms). Conversely, excessive NE and DA release is associated with a stressed state and mental inflexibility. Optimal PFC function is thus characterized by moderate noradrenergic stimulation of the postsynaptic α-2A receptors and moderate dopaminergic stimulation of the DA D1 receptors. Stimulants like methylphenidate are thought to improve ADHD core symptoms by increasing endogenous noradrenergic and dopaminergic stimulation of α-2A receptors and D1 receptors in the frontal lobes and striatum.[19] (From Arnsten AFT, Pliszka SR. Catecholamine influences on prefrontal cortical function: relevance to treatment of attention deficit/hyperactivity disorder and related disorders. *Pharmacol Biochem Behav.* 2011;99(2):211–216.)

organization and planning for the future, direction and maintenance of attention to a specific task at hand, and initiation and production of goal-oriented behavior[20] (Fig. 14.2). Further demonstrating shared neuroanatomical and neurochemical underpinnings between sleep and executive function, functional neuroimaging studies show similar decreased metabolic activity in the PFC in subjects with ADHD and in sleep-deprived subjects without ADHD. Drug-naïve youth with ADHD exhibited decreased cerebral regional blood flow in the orbitofrontal cortex, a PFC region involved in decision making.[21] In a study that subjected healthy subjects to 24 hours of sleep deprivation, significant decreases in regional cerebral metabolic rate for glucose were noted, predominantly in the PFC, thalamus, and posterior parietal cortex, with corresponding declines in cognitive performance and alertness.[22]

In conclusion, similar neurobiological underpinnings in sleep disturbances and ADHD (changes in noradrenergic and dopaminergic transmission, and PFC dysfunction) raise the possibilities that sleep disturbances could underlie ADHD in some cases, that ADHD could cause sleep disturbances in some cases, or that some third variable or process could cause both.

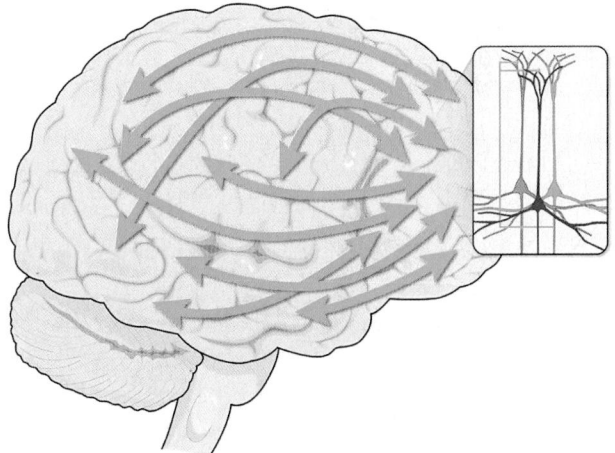

• **Fig. 14.2** Prefrontal cortex function and anatomy. Through extensive network connections with other brain regions, the prefrontal cortex plays a critical role in regulating attention, behavior, and emotion. The inattention, executive dysfunction, hyperactivity, and impulsivity seen in attention-deficit/hyperactivity disorder (ADHD) are thought to arise from abnormalities in the circuits involving the prefrontal cortex. (From Arnsten AFT, Pliszka SR. Catecholamine influences on prefrontal cortical function: relevance to treatment of attention deficit/hyperactivity disorder and related disorders. *Pharmacol Biochem Behav.* 2011;99(2):211–216.)

Psychotropic Medications Frequently Used in Treatment of Attention-Deficit/Hyperactivity Disorder and Effects on Sleep

Sleep disturbance in ADHD involves complex, multifactorial etiologies, and the use of stimulant medications in its treatment complicates research efforts. Table 14.1 has a summary of stimulant effects on sleep. Psychostimulants are first-line medications for treatment of ADHD core symptoms in youth, with U.S. Food and Drug Administration (FDA) approval for some agents in children as young as 3 years old.[23,24] Stimulants work by increasing synaptic availability of the monoamines DA and NE in the striatum and PFC, which are brain regions important for regulation of sleep and wakefulness, as well as executive function, behavior, and affect (see Fig. 14.1).[23] Increased DA and NE increases alertness and improves ADHD symptoms, but may also exacerbate sleep disturbances, if not iatrogenically introduce them.[25] In a meta-analysis, patients with ADHD, who were randomly assigned a stimulant and evaluated

TABLE 14.1 Stimulant Effects on Sleep: General Principles

Stimulant Effects on Sleep

- Stimulants work by increasing synaptic availability of the monoamines dopamine (DA) and norepinephrine (NE) in the striatum and prefrontal cortex (PFC), all brain regions important for regulation of sleep and wakefulness, as well as executive function, behavior, and affect.
- Increased DA and NE increases alertness and improves attention-deficit/hyperactivity disorder (ADHD) symptoms, but may also cause or exacerbate sleep disturbances.
- Common stimulant adverse effects on sleep include increased sleep-onset latency, decreased sleep efficiency, and shorter sleep duration.
- Stimulant adverse effects on sleep occur in a dose-dependent fashion. Higher doses result in increasingly shorter sleep duration and increased sleep-onset latency.[8]
- The severity of sleep disturbances associated with stimulants may attenuate with longer treatment duration.[26]
- If a child's stimulant regimen is thought to disturb sleep, clinicians should first consider adjusting the dose, timing, and formulation or choosing another agent, as opposed to prescribing a sleep aid. Being mindful of a medication's duration of action and the child's desired bedtime is important.
- Extended-release formulations of stimulants have fewer adverse side effects and result in decreased sleep-onset delay compared with immediate-release formulations, and the continuous therapeutic level of stimulant delivered may prevent rebound hyperactivity in the late afternoon and evening.
- If a child's bedtime resistance appears to be secondary to resumption of hyperactivity symptoms in the evening, then a late afternoon or early evening short-acting α-2 agonist like guanfacine or clonidine may be beneficial.

using objective sleep measures (PSG, actigraphy), exhibited overall longer sleep-onset latency, decreased sleep efficiency, and shorter sleep duration, regardless of the stimulant prescribed.[26] Another meta-analysis of six actigraphy studies in a patient with ADHD showed similar results with MPH compared with placebo.[27] The negative effects of stimulants on sleep occur in a dose-dependent fashion, such that higher doses result in increasingly shorter sleep duration and increased sleep-onset latency.[8] In fact, treatment-emergent insomnia was reported as a common stimulant adverse effect in ADHD.[23] However, the severity of sleep disturbances appears to attenuate with longer treatment duration.[26] Thus clinicians and families may choose to accept some degree of sleep disturbance (especially if adverse effects may diminish over time), in light of the psychosocial, developmental, and cognitive benefits conferred by stimulant treatment.

Although the *Diagnostic and Statistical Manual of Mental Disorders* (DSM) has not included sleep-related diagnostic criteria for ADHD since its third edition, and while there is no conclusive evidence to recommend screening with PSG, children with ADHD should be evaluated for symptoms of sleep disorders prior to initiating medication.[8,28,29] Treatment-emergent symptoms must be evaluated and monitored carefully.[17,26] Of note, the initial treatment approach involves behavioral and nonpharmacologic interventions.[8,24,30] Two recent randomized controlled trials (RCTs) showed that a brief behavioral intervention and group-based cognitive behavioral therapy (CBT) improved sleep in youth with ADHD treated with stimulants.[31,32] (For more information about behavioral sleep interventions in ADHD, see the section "Behavioral Management of Sleep Disturbances in Youth with Attention-Deficit/Hyperactivity Disorder.") If sleep disturbances persist despite conservative efforts, sleep medicine referral should be considered, and pharmacological management may be appropriate. Clinicians should first consider alternative medication trials and adjustments to dose and formulation before prescribing adjunctive sleep aids.[8] Treatment outcomes will differ depending on age, sex, and comorbidities, as well as medication dosage, formulation, duration, and previous trials.[8,28]

First, clinicians should consider a trial of an alternative stimulant, as stimulants have different pharmacodynamic and metabolic properties. Table 14.2 has a compilation of stimulant and nonstimulant medications commonly used in pediatric ADHD and clinical pearls for use in children with concurrent sleep disturbances. Therefore, there is no reliable way to predict individual patients' responses to any particular medication. Several recent studies suggest that lisdexamfetamine (a prodrug) compared with MPH better controls ADHD symptoms in youth, but may be associated with higher rates of insomnia.[8] If switching between stimulants does not produce the desired outcome, clinicians may consider monotherapy with a nonstimulant agent with the awareness that most studies show greater efficacy of stimulants compared with nonstimulants in treating ADHD core symptoms.[33,34] Atomoxetine (ATX) and extended-release (ER) formulations of clonidine and guanfacine have been widely studied and are approved by the FDA as monotherapies and as adjunctive therapies with stimulants for the treatment of ADHD in youth.[8,35] ATX acts as an NE reuptake inhibitor and may indirectly increase DA in the frontal lobes,[35,36] whereas clonidine and guanfacine act directly as α-2 adrenergic agonists at postsynaptic receptors in the PFC.[37] In a recent meta-analysis of double-blind RCTs for ATX in youth with ADHD, there was no increase in sleep-onset insomnia compared with placebo.[35] In a randomized, double-blind crossover study, twice-daily ATX compared with thrice-daily MPH showed significantly reduced sleep onset latency and better quality sleep as reported by both children and parents.[24,38] In contrast to stimulants, all of these nonstimulant medications are sedating and their most common adverse effects are fatigue, sedation, and hypersomnolence, which can lead to discontinuation.[8,37]

Next, clinicians should consider adjusting the timing and frequency of dosages or opt for changes in formulation to reduce sleep interference. Evening dosing of nonstimulant monotherapies can prevent hypersomnolence. ATX dosed in the evening is less associated with somnolence than morning dosing.[39] Studies indicate the somniferous effect of ER guanfacine is mild to moderate despite time of dosing, and the severity tends to decrease 2 weeks after initiation.[8,40–42] Although the activating effects of stimulants are known to interfere with sleep, studies and empirical observations also describe a paradoxical effect where, in some cases, effective treatment of hyperactivity with stimulants leads to improved sleep[26] (Fig. 14.3). One theory is that adherence with medication may have the indirect benefit of preventing bedtime resistance or sleep-onset delay caused by a "rebound effect" or withdrawal-emergent hyperactivity.[24,26] As a result, published guidelines have recommended an added dose of MPH 5 mg immediate release (IR) in the evening if a rebound effect is observed.[43,44] However, results of the previously mentioned meta-analysis by Kidwell et al., showed that decreased sleep efficiency linearly correlated with daily dose frequency of stimulant medication, so the choice of using this strategy to reduce bedtime overactivity should be carefully considered against the possibility of a dose-dependent detriment to sleep.[26] Perhaps counterintuitively, ER formulations of stimulants are shown to have fewer adverse effects and, similar to the previous theory, may even improve sleep due to continuous therapeutic levels of stimulant that prevent rebound hyperactivity.[26] Taken once daily, ER stimulants are effective for 8–12 hours and result in decreased sleep-onset delay compared with IR formulations taken two to three times per day.[26] In one study, osmotic-release oral delivery system MPH was associated with low incidence of insomnia, decreased nighttime awakenings, and increased stage 2 sleep.[8] Considering the pharmacokinetic profile of ER stimulants, clinicians may instruct caregivers not to give the medication any later than 10:00 a.m. to help ensure a normal bedtime.

Finally, if the earlier strategies are not successful, clinicians may choose to prescribe an adjunctive sleep aid. About one in five children with ADHD are prescribed sleep medications, though none are approved by the FDA for this specific indication.[8] In a recent systematic review, improvements in sleep-onset latency and total sleep duration were reported for melatonin, clonidine, and L-theanine (an amino acid), but not for guanfacine, zolpidem, or eszopiclone. However, the quality of evidence was moderate to low.[45] Melatonin is one of most widely used sleep aids in ADHD due to evidence that it can effectively advance delayed sleep–wake rhythms forward to decrease sleep-onset insomnia.[46] In youth with ADHD and chronic sleep-onset insomnia treated effectively with melatonin, 92% experienced a relapse of sleep-onset delay after discontinuation.[47] For this reason, as well as its tolerability and safety, patients tend to remain on this melatonin long term.[8,47] While the use of clonidine seems to be most efficacious as adjunctive therapy to stimulants,[37] it also has been studied and used empirically for decades as a safe and effective sleep aid for youth with ADHD.[8]

Conceptualizing Attention-Deficit/Hyperactivity Disorder and Its Inherent Heterogeneity

Advances in our understanding of ADHD have led to progressive conceptualization of ADHD as a "syndrome" with a constellation of symptoms stemming from heterogenous etiologies. For example, executive function deficits in one child may stem from the sleep fragmentation and recurrent, intermittent hypoxemia that accompany OSA. In another child, genesis of ADHD symptoms may be due to the chronic sleep deprivation that can accompany delayed sleep–wake phase disorder (DSWPD). The challenge to the practicing clinician is that these children may present in an identical fashion. Thus, while psychostimulants have traditionally been the mainstay of pharmacologic treatment for ADHD (as discussed in the last section), astute consideration of the underlying mechanism responsible for ADHD in any given child can lead to a different therapeutic direction (Table 14.3).

Literature supporting the association between ADHD symptomatology and sleep conditions (SDB, RLS/PLMs, DSWPD, insufficient sleep, and hypersomnolence) will be discussed in detail in the following section. Additionally, evidence for the link between ADHD and epilepsy/EEG interictal discharges will also be discussed.

Primary Sleep Disorders or Conditions Associated with Attention-Deficit/Hyperactivity Disorder

Primary sleep disorders can cause fragmented, poor quality, or insufficient sleep, and daytime sleepiness. Importantly, however, sleep disorders can also present with daytime neurobehavioral impairment that includes the inattention, hyperactivity, and impulsivity that characterize ADHD. Treatment of the underlying sleep disorder can improve, and possibly even resolve ADHD symptomatology, such that children may no longer meet DSM criteria after the SDB, insufficient sleep, or RLS are treated.

TABLE 14.2   **Stimulant and Nonstimulant Treatments for Attention-Deficit/Hyperactivity Disorder in Children and Effects on Sleep**

Common sleep-related side effects:
Sleep-onset insomnia, decreased sleep efficiency, shorter sleep duration, rebound phenomena, nightmares, anxiety.

Stimulants	Generic Name (Brand Name)	Mechanism of Action	Duration of Activity	Dosage Forms
Immediate Release (IR) Formulations	Methylphenidate (Ritalin)	Blocks reuptake of NE and DA into presynaptic neurons	3–4 hours	5, 10, and 20 mg tablets
	Methylphenidate (Methylin solution, Methylphenidate chewable)	Blocks reuptake of NE and DA into presynaptic neurons	3–4 hours	Methylin solution: 5 mg/mL, 10 mg/mL; Methylphenidate chewable (grape flavor): 2.5, 5, and 10 mg tablets
	Dexmethylphenidate (Focalin)	Blocks reuptake of NE and DA and increases release into extraneuronal space	3–5 hours	2.5, 5, and 10 mg tablets (2.5 mg Focalin equivalent to 5 mg Ritalin)
	D- & L-amphetamine sulfate (Evekeo, Evekeo ODT)	Blocks reuptake of NE and DA into presynaptic neurons	4–6 hours	Evekeo: 5, 10 mg tablets; Evekeo ODT: 5, 10, 15, and 20 mg orally disintegrating tablets)
	Dextroamphetamine sulfate (Zenzedi, ProCentra, generic [previously Dextrostat])	Promotes release of NE and DA from storage sites in presynaptic nerve terminals	4–6 hours	Zenzedi: 2.5, 5, 7.5, 10, 15, 20, 30 mg tablets; ProCentra: 5 mg/5 mL (bubblegum flavor); Generic: 5 and 10 mg tablets
	Mixed salts of amphetamine (Adderall)	Promotes release of NE and DA from storage sites in presynaptic nerve terminals; may also block reuptake	4–6 hours	5, 7.5, 10, 12.5, 15, 20, and 30 mg tablets
Extended/Sustained/ Delayed Release (ER) Formulations	Methylphenidate (Metadate ER)	Blocks reuptake of NE and DA into presynaptic neurons	3–8 hours variable	10 and 20 mg tablets (amount absorbed appears to vary)
	Methylphenidate (Concerta)	Osmotic controlled release (OROS) formulation; blocks reuptake of NE and DA into presynaptic neurons	12 hours	18, 27, 36, and 54 mg caplets
	Methylphenidate (Daytrana or generic)	Transdermal system Blocks reuptake of NE and DA into presynaptic neurons	12 hours (patch worn for 9 hours)	10 mg/9 hours (1.1 mg/hr), 15 mg/9 hours (1.6 mg/hr), 20 mg/9 hours (2.2 mg/hr), 30 mg/9 hours (3.3 mg/hr) transdermal patch
	Lisdexamfetamine (Vyvanse)	Prodrug that is converted to active component, dextroamphetamine Promotes release of NE and DA from storage sites in presynaptic nerve terminals; may also block reuptake	12 hours	Vyvanse: 10, 20, 30, 50, 60 and 70 mg tablets; Vyvanse Chewable: 10, 20, 30, 40, 50, and 60 mg chewable tablets (strawberry flavor)

Recommeded Starting Dose	FDA-Approved Maximum Dose for ADHD	FDA-Approved Indications for Children	Sleep Clinical Pearls
(5 mg twice daily before breakfast and lunch	60 mg/day (usually given in divided doses every 4 hours up to 3 times per day.)	Approved to treat ADHD in people aged 6 years and older	For children whose ADHD symptoms return to baseline in the evening and contribute to bedtime resistance, this may indicate inadequate evening ADHD medication coverage
(5 mg twice daily before breakfast and lunch)	60 mg/day (usually given in divided doses every 4 hours up to 3 times per day.)		Adding a low dose of IR stimulant may be beneficial on a case-by-case basis However, IR stimulants administered too close to bedtime may also exacerbate sleep-onset latency and contribute to bedtime resistance
(2.5 mg twice daily)	20 mg/day (maximum dose generally 10mg twice per day.)		Clinicians should make recommendations on the latest IR stimulant dosing time based on careful consideration of
(5 mg, 1–2 times per day)	5–40 mg/day (usually in 2 divided doses)		medication duration of activity, as well as the parents' preferred bedtime for the child
(3–5 years old: 2.5 my once daily; 6–17 years old: 5 mg once or twice daily)	40 mg/day (5-40 mg/day usually in 2 divided doses)	Approved to treat ADHD age 3 years and older	
(3–5 years old: 2.5 mg once daily; 6–17 years old: 5 mg once or twice daily)	40 mg/day (5-40 mg/day usually in 2 divided doses)		
(20 mg once daily)	60 mg/day	Approved to treat ADHD age 6 years and older	ER formulations provide continuous therapeutic levels of stimulant that can reduce rebound hyperactivity, as compared with IR formulations
(18 mg once daily)	6–12 Yrs: 54 mg; 13–17 Yrs.: 72 mg/day		Taken once daily, ER stimulants are effective for 8–12 hours and may result in less sleep-onset insomnia compared with IR formulations taken 2–3 times per day (25)
10 mg/9 hours (1.1 mg/hr)	30 mg/day		For some children, ER stimulants may worsen sleep-onset insomnia, oftentimes related to the timing of the single dose given earlier in the day
30 mg once daily	70 mg/day		Given the duration of action of ER stimulants, clinicians may instruct caregivers not to give the medication later than 10:00 a.m. to help ensure a normal bedtime; however, clinicians may need to individualize this cutoff time case by case

(Continued)

TABLE 14.2 **Stimulant and Nonstimulant Treatments for Attention-Deficit/Hyperactivity Disorder in Children and Effects on Sleep—Cont'd**

Common sleep-related side effects:
Sleep-onset insomnia, decreased sleep efficiency, shorter sleep duration, rebound phenomena, nightmares, anxiety.

Stimulants	Generic Name (Brand Name)	Mechanism of Action	Duration of Activity	Dosage Forms
Biphasic Formulations	Methylphenidate (Ritalin LA)	Spheroidal oral drug absorption systems (SODAS) of 50% IR and 50% delayed release. Blocks reuptake of NE and DA into presynaptic neurons	8 hours	20, 30, and 40 mg capsules; can be sprinkled
	Dexmethylphenidate (Focalin XR)	Blocks reuptake of NE and DA and increases release into extraneuronal space	12 hours	5, 10, 15, 20, 25, 30, 35, and 40 mg capsules
	Methylphenidate (Metadate CD)	30% IR and 70% delayed release. Blocks reuptake of NE and DA into presynaptic neurons	8 hours	20 mg capsule; can be sprinkled
	Mixed salts of amphetamine (Adderall-XR)	50% IR and 50% delayed release. Promotes release of NE and DA from storage sites in presynaptic nerve terminals; may also block reuptake	At least 8 hours (but appears to last much longer in certain patients)	5, 10, 15, 20, 25, and 30 mg capsules; can be sprinkled
	Dextroamphetamine (Dexedrine Spansule)	Promotes release of NE and DA from storage sites in presynaptic nerve terminals; may also block reuptake	8 hours	8.6, 17.3, 25.9 mg tablets (grape flavored)
	Methylphenidate (Cotempla XR-ODT)	Blocks reuptake of NE and DA into presynaptic neurons; dissolving tablet with 25% immediate-release microparticles and 75% extended-release	8 hours	5, 10, and 15 mg capsules
	Methylphenidate (Quillivant XR, Quillichew ER)	Quillivant XR: 20% of the dose is immediate-release and 80% extended-release; Quillichew: 30% of the dose is immediate-release and 70% extended-release	Quillivant XR: 12 hours; Quillichew ER: 8 hours	Quillivant XR: 10 mg/2 mL, 20 mg/4 mL, 30 mg/6 mL, 50 mg/10 mL oral suspension (banana flavored); Quillichew ER: 20, 30, and 40 mg chewable tablets (cherry flavored)

Recommeded Starting Dose	FDA-Approved Maximum Dose for ADHD	FDA-Approved Indications for Children	Sleep Clinical Pearls
20 mg once daily	60 mg/day	Approved to treat ADHD age 6 years and older	Bimodal formulations provide a mixed percentage of immediate and delayed release beads
			A clinical advantage of these formulations may be their rapid increase of drug levels in the morning delivered by IR beads, followed by one or two delayed release phases helping to maintain levels throughout the day
5 mg once daily	30 mg/day		
20 mg once daily	60 mg/day		The variety of pharmacokinetic profiles offered by these formulations provides clinicians with more options when individualizing medication regimens to meet a particular patient's needs
10 mg once daily	30 mg/day in children Recommended dose is 20 mg/day in adults		Sleep parameters may be affected similarly to ER formulations; therefore clinicians may instruct caregivers not to give the medication later than 10:00 a.m. (or determined on case-by-case basis) to help ensure a normal bedtime
5 mg once or twice daily	40 mg/day		
(17.3 mg once daily)	40 mg/day	Approved for 6 years and older	
20 mg once daily	60 mg/day	Approved for 6 years and older	

(Continued)

TABLE 14.2 Stimulant and Nonstimulant Treatments for Attention-Deficit/Hyperactivity Disorder in Children and Effects on Sleep—Cont'd

Nonstimulants	Generic Name (Brand Name)	Mechanism of Action	Duration of Activity	Dosage Forms
Common sleep-related side effects: Tiredness and sedation (often short-term or transient), depression, irritability, mood swings				
	Atomoxetine (Strattera)	Selectively inhibits the reuptake of NE with little to no activity at other neuronal reuptake pumps or receptor sites	5-hour plasma half-life but CNS effects appear to last much longer	10, 18, 25, 40, 60, and 80 mg capsules
	Guanfacine ER (Intuniv)	Selective α-2 agonist that preferentially binds postsynaptic α-2 adrenoreceptors in the PFC Reduces sympathetic outflow	Labeled for once-daily dosing	1, 2, 3, and 4 mg tablets
	Clonidine ER (Kapvay)	Postsynaptic α-2 agonist that stimulates receptors which may regulate subcortical activity in PFC Reduces sympathetic outflow	Labeled for twice-daily dosing	0.1 mg tablet

FDA, U.S. Food and Drug Administration; ADHD, attention-deficit/hyperactivity disorder; NE, norepinephrine; DA, dopamine; CNS, central nervous system; PFC, prefrontal cortex.
From Prince JB, Spencer TJ, Biederman J, Wilens TE. Pharmacotherapy of attention-deficit/hyperactivity disorder across the life span. In: Stern TA, Fava M, Wilens TE, Rosenbaum JF, eds. *Massachusetts General Hospital Comprehensive Clinical Psychiatry*. 2nd ed. Elsevier; 2016:538–551; Bangs, ME, Hazell P, Danckaerts M, Hoare P, Coghill DR, Wehmeier PM, Williams DW, Moore RJ, Levine L, Atomoxetine ADHD Odd Study Group. Atomoxetine for the treatment of attention-deficit/hyperactivity disorder and oppositional defiant disorder. *Pediatrics*, 2008;121(2), E314–E320. https://doi.org/10.1542/peds.2006-1880)

Recommended Starting Dose	FDA-Approved Maximum Dose for ADHD	FDA-Approved Indications for Children	Sleep Clinical Pearls
			Medications that reduce sympathetic tone (e.g., α agonists like guanfacine and clonidine) are sedating. Scheduling them close to bedtime can have the beneficial effect of decreasing sleep-onset latency. For children whose ADHD symptoms return to baseline in the evening and contribute to bedtime resistance, this may indicate inadequate evening ADHD medication coverage. Clinicians may consider scheduling an adjunctive dose of guanfacine or clonidine in the late afternoon or early evening, before trialing a low dose of IR stimulant, as the latter carries a higher risk of sleep interference. Atomoxetine monotherapy dosed in the evening is less associated with somnolence than morning dosing[39]
≤70 kg: 0.5 mg/kg for ≥3 days, then 1.2 mg/kg; >70 kg: 40 mg for ≥3 days, then 80 mg	Maximum of 1.4 mg/kg/day; not to exceed 100 mg per day	Approved to treat ADHD age 6 years and older. **Black box warning:** increased the risk of suicidal ideation in children or adolescents with ADHD (frequency of suicidal ideation in pediatric patients was 0.37%, with no suicides) (Bangs et al., 2008)	Atomoxetine monotherapy dosed in the evening is less associated with somnolence than morning dosing (Block et al., 2009).
1 mg daily or 0.05-0.08 mg/kg/day; may increase to 0.12 mg/kg/day	Not to exceed 4 mg per day	Approved to treat ADHD in youth 6–17 years old as monotherapy or as adjunctive treatment with stimulant	
0.1 mg at nighttime	0.1–0.2 mg given once or twice daily, not to exceed 0.4 mg daily		

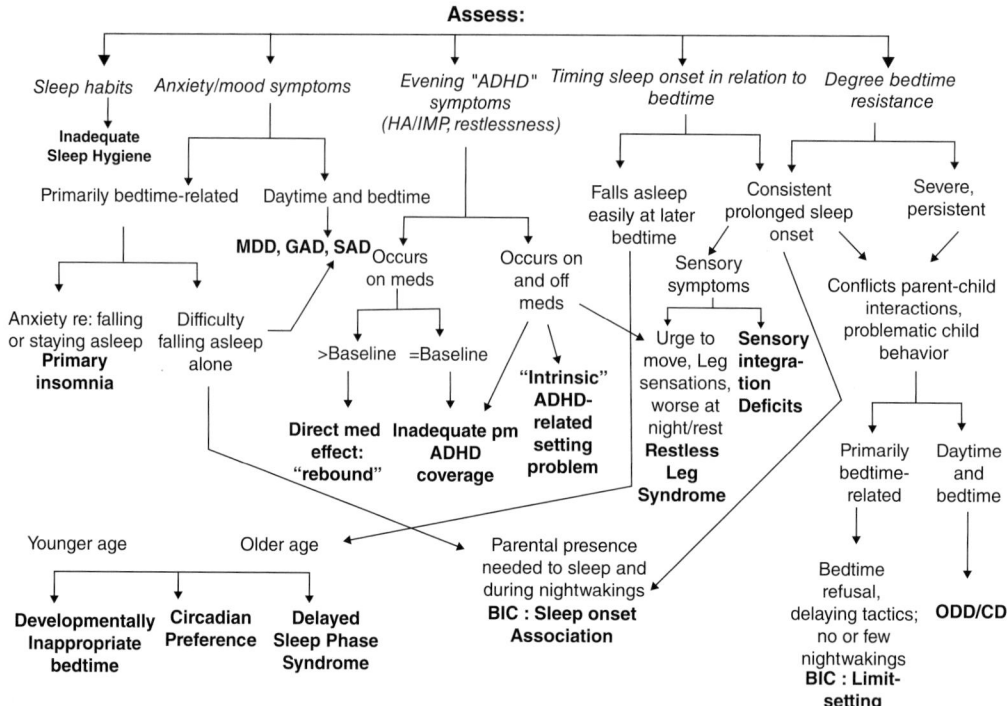

• **Fig. 14.3** Evaluation strategy for sleep-onset difficulties in children with attention-deficit/hyperactivity disorder (ADHD). Given the complexity of the relationship between ADHD and sleep, it is crucial to approach the patient's clinical presentation in a systematic manner. This algorithm addresses how to approach sleep-onset difficulties and bedtime resistance in children with ADHD. First, it is important to assess whether sleep hygiene is optimal and ensure that the child is not napping during the day or using sleep-disrupting products or medications (e.g., electronic devices, caffeine, psychostimulants) too close to bedtime. Additionally, it is important to assess whether the child's bedtime is age appropriate and whether there is enough homeostatic sleep drive at the attempted bedtime. If sleep hygiene is appropriate and bedtime is appropriate for age, then it is important to assess for medical, behavioral, and psychiatric conditions that can delay sleep. Medical conditions include restless legs syndrome, delayed sleep-phase disorder, nocturnal leg cramps, pain, etc. Behavioral and psychiatric conditions that can prolong sleep-onset latency include ADHD, oppositional defiant disorder (ODD), anxiety, and depression. Eliciting history from both the child and family is crucial. BIC, behavioral insomnia of childhood; CD, conduct disorder; GAD, generalized anxiety disorder; HA, hyperactivity; IMP, impulsivity; MDD, major depressive disorder; SAD, separation anxiety disorder. (From Owens JA. A clinical overview of sleep and attention-deficit/hyperactivity disorder in children and adolescents. *J Can Acad Child Adolesc Psychiatry*. 2009;18(2):92–102.)

TABLE 14.3	Evaluation and Management of Sleep Disturbances in Youth With Attention-Deficit/Hyperactivity Disorder: General Principles

- Sleep difficulties (e.g., bedtime resistance, night awakenings) in youth with attention-deficit hyperactivity disorder (ADHD) should involve a thorough and thoughtful evaluation of all medical contributing factors, such as obstructive sleep apnea, restless legs syndrome, periodic limb movements of sleep, and delayed sleep–wake phase disorder, as a first step. Please see the corresponding section in text on "Primary Sleep Disorders or Conditions Associated with Attention-Deficit Hyperactivity Disorder."
- Behavioral sleep problems (e.g., behavioral insomnia of childhood, sleep association, limit-setting, and combined types) should be addressed with behavioral sleep interventions and nonpharmacologic interventions before considering pharmacological management. These include setting an age-appropriate bedtime and creating a bedtime routine, optimizing sleep hygiene, and creating behavioral sleep plans with parental buy-in and positive reinforcement for the child. Please see the corresponding section in text on "Behavioral Management of Sleep Disturbances in Youth with Attention-Deficit Hyperactivity Disorder."
- If sleep-onset insomnia is thought to be secondary to a stimulant medication, clinicians should first consider alternative medication trials and adjustments to dose and formulation before prescribing adjunctive sleep aids.
- Medication treatments of sleep disturbances in ADHD should occur as a last step, only when all other conditions have been satisfied. Please see the corresponding section in text on "Psychotropic Medications Frequently Used in Treatment of Attention-Deficit Hyperactivity Disorder and Effects on Sleep."

Sleep-Disordered Breathing

Pediatric SDB encompasses a spectrum of pathology ranging from primary snoring to upper airway resistance syndrome to obstructive alveolar hypoventilation, and frank OSA.

Among the general pediatric population, the prevalence of OSA is in the range of 1–4%.[48] Habitual snoring is estimated at 5–12%.[48] An increased prevalence of SDB (25–57%) has been noted in youth with ADHD.[49] A robust literature supports the link between SDB and ADHD or ADHD

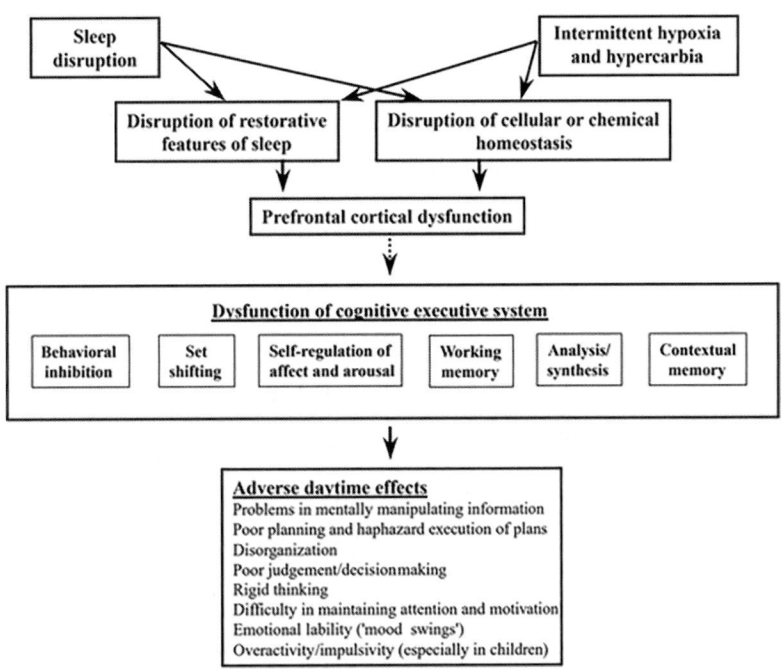

• **Fig. 14.4** Sleep fragmentation and intermittent gas exchange abnormalities associated with obstructive sleep apnea and effects on the prefrontal cortex. The sleep fragmentation and intermittent hypoxemia and hypercarbia associated with obstructive sleep apnea impair the normal restorative features of sleep and disrupt the homeostasis and viability of neurons and glia within particular brain regions, particularly the prefrontal cortex. Prefrontal cortex dysfunction ensues. Dysfunction of the prefrontal cortex leads to deficits in executive function, which manifests as difficulties with manipulation, analysis, and synthesis of information; memory impairment; and problems with regulation of behavior and affect. A child with obstructive sleep apnea may thus present with emotional lability, hyperactivity, impulsivity, difficulty sustaining attention and motivation, poor decision making, and poor execution of tasks requiring analysis and planning. (From Beebe DW, Gozal D. Obstructive sleep apnea and the prefrontal cortex: towards a comprehensive model linking nocturnal upper airway obstruction to daytime cognitive and behavioral deficits. *J Sleep Res*. 2002 Mar;11(1):1–16.)

symptomatology, related behavioral disorders including conduct disorder and oppositional defiant disorder, as well as other neurocognitive and neurobehavioral domains, including memory, mood, and academic achievement.[50]

SDB is associated with gas exchange abnormalities, including intermittent hypoxemia and hypercapnia (Fig. 14.4), increased oxidative stress and free radicals, and sleep fragmentation that in turn is associated with increased tumor necrosis factor (TNF)-α.[51] These processes also are associated with other inflammatory markers (e.g., C-reactive protein [CRP], interleukin [IL]-6, IL-8, etc.) that suggest systemic and local inflammation.[51] Consequences may include neuroinflammation, compromised integrity of the blood–brain barrier,[51] and neuronal apoptosis and neurologic dysfunction in certain areas of the brain, notably the PFC, which is required for executive function, and the hippocampus, which is important for learning and memory[49] (see Figs. 14.4–14.5). Intermittent hypoxemia in juvenile rats increased locomotor activity (a surrogate for behavioral hyperactivity) and impaired spatial learning.[52] Increased CRP levels were found in children with OSA; those with OSA and neurocognitive deficits had even higher CRP levels.[53] Degree of inflammation (CRP) has been noted in other studies to correlate with OSA severity (apnea/hypopnea index)[51] and to play a mediating role in the association of central obesity with OSA.[54] Of note, however, not all children with OSA exhibited neurocognitive deficits; thus

it is postulated that neurocognitive deficits are also influenced by genetic susceptibility and environmental factors. Treatment of SDB is associated with reduction in inflammation in children with OSA,[55] and, fortunately, significant improvement of cognitive deficits is possible if not guaranteed with SDB treatment (e.g., adenotonsillectomy [T&A] or continuous positive airway pressure [CPAP]).[51]

A meta-analysis in 2014 by Sedky et al., included 18 studies, comprising 1,113 children in the clinical group compared with 1,405 controls. Clinical subjects consisted of (1) children with SDB (874 subjects) who were evaluated for ADHD and (2) youth with ADHD (239 subjects) who were evaluated for SDB with PSG. The overall effect size assessing the relation between ADHD symptoms and SDB was 0.57, which is considered moderate. Of note, studies using a lower AHI cutoff (e.g., 1) had a higher effect size of 0.72; the authors hypothesized that mild OSA, compared with more severe forms, may be more closely related to ADHD symptoms. Age, gender, and body mass index (BMI) did not seem to moderate effect size.[49]

Whether a dose-dependent relationship exists between severity of SDB and severity of ADHD symptoms remains controversial. This question is complicated by how SDB severity is defined (e.g., AHI, severity of hypoxemia, degree of sleep fragmentation due to SDB, etc.). On the one hand, some evidence suggests that severity of hypoxemia correlates with executive function deficits.[56] Degree of sleep fragmentation secondary to respiratory events may also contribute to

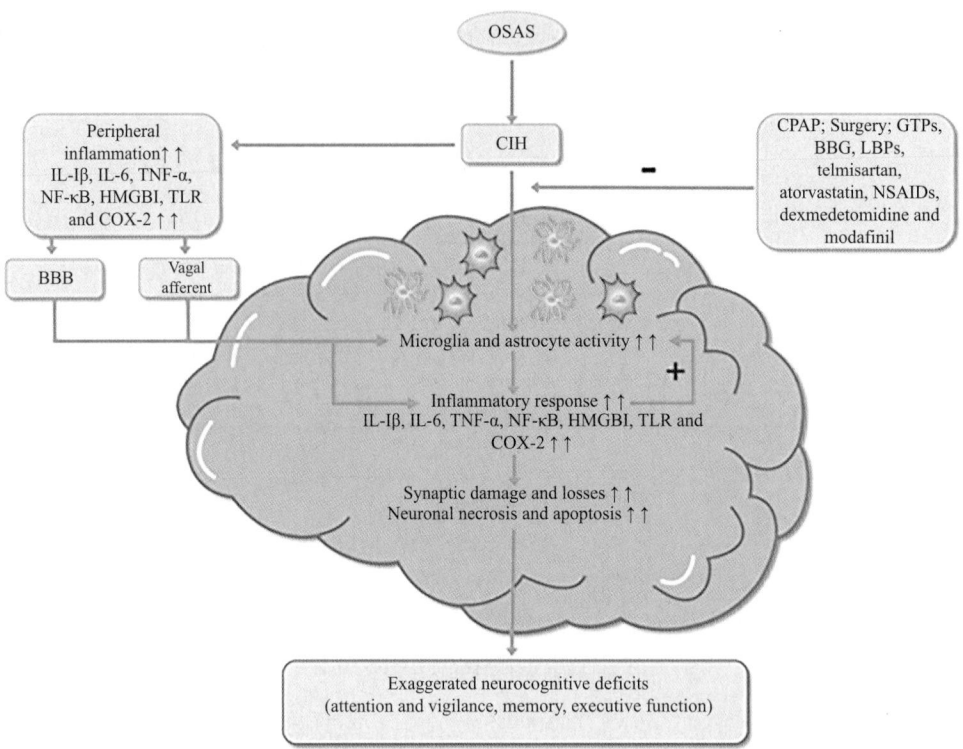

• **Fig. 14.5** Inflammation plays an important role in the cognitive dysfunction secondary to obstructive sleep apnea syndrome (OSAS). Chronic intermittent hypoxia (CIH) leads to peripheral inflammation, which contributes to central nervous system (CNS) inflammation by way of the blood–brain barrier (BBB) and vagal afferents. CNS inflammation results in proliferation of microglia and astrocytes, which induces release of inflammatory cytokines and propagating the neuroinflammatory response. This neuroinflammatory response leads to damage and loss of neuronal synapses, as well as necrosis and apoptosis of neurons. The loss of these critical components of the CNS results in neurocognitive deficits such as inattention, deficits in executive function, and impaired memory. Treatment of sleep-disordered breathing (SDB) is associated with reduction in inflammation in children with OSA,[55] and fortunately, significant improvement of cognitive deficits is possible if not guaranteed with SDB treatment (e.g., adenotonsillectomy or continuous positive airway pressure [CPAP]) (Liu et al., 2020). BBG, Brilliant Blue B; COX-2, cyclooxygenase-2; GTP, green tea catechin polyphenols; HMGB1, high mobility group box 1 protein; IL, interleukin; LBP, Llycium barbarum polysaccharides; NF-κβ, nuclear factor kappa beta; NSAID, nonsteroidal antiinflammatory drug; TLR, toll-like receptor; TNF-α, tumor necrosis factor-α. (From Liu X, Ma Y, Ouyang R, Zeng Z, Zhan Z, Lu H, et al. Inflammation and cognitive deficits in OSAS: The relationship between inflammation and neurocognitive dysfunction in obstructive sleep apnea syndrome. *J Neuroinflammation*. 2020 Aug 1;17(1):229.)

severity of attention deficits.[13] However, the AHI (the most commonly used objective measure of SDB severity) may not be a meaningful predictor of behavioral or cognitive deficits, including ADHD or its symptoms. For instance, Chervin et al., reported that the Pediatric Sleep Questionnaire – Sleep-Related Breathing Disorders (PSQ-SRBD) Scale predicted hyperactive behavior and its resolution 1 year after T&A for pediatric OSA, whereas polysomnographic findings did not.[57] Sleep laboratory–referred children found to have no OSA, as well as those confirmed to have OSA, both appear to have similarly elevated symptoms of ADHD.[58] Although children scheduled for T&A, compared with those scheduled for unrelated surgical care, had worse behavior and cognition at baseline, and no worse behavior or cognition 1 year after surgery, baseline polysomnographic results failed to show associations with baseline neurobehavioral measures or their improvement 1 year later.[59] A meta-analysis by Smith et al., found that snoring frequency, rather than

AHI, predicted poorer behavioral and cognitive functioning.[60] Similarly, Sedky et al., found a more robust effect size between ADHD and lower AHI (e.g., mild OSA), compared with higher AHI.[49] Considering the inverse, severe ADHD may not necessarily equate to higher risk for SDB. O'Brien et al., demonstrated an unexpectedly high prevalence of SDB symptoms in youth with "mild ADHD" symptoms, compared with youth with "significant ADHD" symptoms,[61] raising the question of whether mild ADHD and severe ADHD are clinically distinct entities.

The Sedky et al., meta-analysis also looked for differences in ADHD symptoms before and after T&A in the pediatric population.[49] A total of 529 youth with SDB were included, each with PSG pre-T&A and 1–13 months post-T&A. Hedges' *g* was 0.43, indicating a moderate degree of improvement in ADHD symptoms from before to after T&A.[49] When analyzed on an individual level, some children and adolescents with ADHD may no longer meet criteria for ADHD after T&A.

For instance, in one study, 28% of youth scheduled for T&A met DSM-5-TR criteria for ADHD. One year after T&A, 50% of those individuals no longer met DSM criteria for ADHD.[62] Similarly, in another study, ADHD scores normalized in 69% of 40 children who had undergone T&A 6 months prior.[63]

When behavioral and cognitive domains are separated, the literature currently supports improvement in subjective report of behavior and affect after T&A, but not necessarily in objectively measured tests of executive function. The Childhood Adenotonsillectomy Trial was a multicenter RCT conducted among 464 children with OSA to evaluate the effect of early T&A versus watchful waiting with supportive care (WWSC). Outcomes included measures of cognition, behavior, quality of life, and sleep (from full PSG).[64] Children 5–9 years of age with OSA were randomly assigned to either early T&A or WWSC. The primary outcome was the attention and executive-function score on the Developmental Neuropsychological Assessment (NEPSY), administered at baseline and 7 months later. No significant differences in attention and executive functioning were found between groups at the 7-month follow-up assessment. However, the early T&A group was associated with greater improvements in behavioral ratings by parents and teachers, better quality of life scores, and greater resolution of polysomnographic OSA parameters. Interestingly, 46% of children assigned to the WWSC experienced normalization of polysomnographic findings, suggesting that remission of OSA might be related to normal developmental trajectories such as widening or growth of the upper airway and other anatomical structures. Of note, the children's average baseline score for the attention and executive-function score (NEPSY) was close to the population mean of 100; additionally, children on medications for ADHD were excluded from the study. It is thus possible that the study population, with predominantly mild or mild to moderate OSA, also had relatively little ADHD symptomatology preintervention, which may have contributed to nonsignificant differences in executive function between the T&A and WWSC groups.

Restless Legs Syndrome and Periodic Leg Movements of Sleep/Periodic Limb Movement Disorder

Clinicians have long observed shared symptomatology in youth with ADHD and RLS, PLMs, and periodic limb movement disorder (PLMD). This has led to increased research efforts in recent years not only to characterize the nature of the comorbidity with ADHD, but to uncover shared pathophysiology that could lead to more effective treatment.

In the general pediatric population, the prevalence of RLS and PLMs in youth is 2–4% and 10%, respectively.[65,66] Youth with ADHD appear to have a higher overall prevalence of both RLS and PLMs compared with the general pediatric population, with a range of 7–52% for RLS[66-69] and 24–64% for PLMs.[66,70,71] Many studies have also explored the inverse of this bidirectional relationship. Approximately 25% of youth with RLS also experience ADHD symptomatology.[65,72,73] With regard to PLMs, approximately 45%

of youths with PLMs also had ADHD, though this percentage includes those with fewer PLMs than necessary to meet full diagnostic criteria for pediatric PLMD, which is a PLM index >5/hr of sleep.[68,70] This suggests that PLMs can cause clinically significant sleep fragmentation, resulting in daytime impairment. In a meta-analysis of 12 PSG studies, ADHD youth had significantly higher prevalence of PLMD and elevated PLMs compared with controls.[10] For instance, Silvestri et al., enrolled 55 children diagnosed with ADHD by DSM-5 criteria; the prevalence of PLMs was 40% and RLS was 26%.[74]

Possible Hypotheses Underlying the Comorbidity Among Attention-Deficit/Hyperactivity Disorder, Periodic Leg Movements of Sleep/Periodic Limb Movement Disorder, and Restless Legs Syndrome

Several hypotheses exist to describe the possible neurobiological mechanisms driving the comorbidity among ADHD, PLMs/PLMD, and RLS.

First, diurnal symptoms of inattentiveness, impulsivity, and hyperactivity may be the result of chronic sleep deprivation and fragmentation associated with PLMs and RLS. Second, the presence of PLMs or RLS in the setting of ADHD may correlate with unique subtypes or phenotypes of ADHD. Finally, the comorbidity of these disorders may result from dysfunction in a common biological substrate leading to the complex presentation of symptoms. Strong evidence supports the hypothesis that low serum ferritin levels, iron deficiency, and downstream dopaminergic dysfunction represent a common pathway linking ADHD, PLMs, PLMD, and RLS.[72]

Studies with objective sleep measures (e.g., PSG) demonstrate that PLMs/PLMD and RLS are associated with chronic sleep deprivation and poor quality sleep. Adolescents with PLMs demonstrated significant sleep fragmentation, manifested by increased wakefulness after sleep onset (WASO), increased N1 sleep, shorter total sleep time, and lower sleep efficiency.[65] Similarly, adolescents with comorbid ADHD and PLMs had increased N1 sleep, but unique to this age group was significantly increased sleep-onset latency and decreased N2 sleep (PSG).[65] The profound detriment to sleep experienced by adolescents with comorbid ADHD and PLMs in this study also correlated with clinically significant increases in internalizing (e.g., anxiety) and externalizing (e.g., impulsivity) behaviors compared with the general population, as well as to subjects with either ADHD or PLMs alone.[70] This suggests that children with co-occurring diagnoses of ADHD and PLMs may have higher behavioral and psychological symptom severity.

PLMs, PLMD, or RLS in the setting of ADHD may represent an ADHD phenotype with distinct neurobehavioral deficits and sleep parameters. In one study, subjects with the ADHD-H subtype, compared with those with ADHD-I, had significantly higher severity scores on the International RLS Rating Scale, opposition and hyperactivity scores on a standardized measure (SNAP-IV scales), and PLMs and periodic limb movements during wake (PLMW) indices.[74]

Role of Iron and Dopamine in Attention-Deficit/Hyperactivity Disorder

Interestingly, ADHD severity is correlated with positive family history of RLS, previous iron supplementation in infancy, and lower serum ferritin levels in youth with comorbid ADHD and RLS, compared with those solely with ADHD.[65,75] Additionally, children who were transiently iron deficient in infancy showed a significant increase of tibialis anterior electromyography (EMG) activity on PSG, suggesting that iron deficiency in early life can have persisting effects.[76] These findings point to the possibility that ADHD and RLS, PLMs, and PLMD share a common underlying pathophysiology of iron deficiency and dopaminergic hypofunction.[77] Iron is a cofactor for the hydroxylation of tyrosine in the rate-limiting step of DA biosynthesis; low iron stores in the brain cause synaptic dysfunction affecting dopaminergic transmission.[65,78] DA plays a prominent role in the pathophysiology of ADHD, and studies show that youth with ADHD have relatively low serum ferritin levels. Similarly, magnetic resonance imaging (MRI) studies show diminished iron stores in the thalami and striatum of ADHD subjects.[79]

Ferritin is a sensitive marker of iron deficiency, and serum ferritin levels >50 μ/L are considered optimal in patients vulnerable to RLS, whereas synthetic hypofunction of hemoglobin occurs <12 μg/L.[77] One study demonstrated that youth with ADHD had significantly lower serum ferritin levels than controls (mean levels of 21 μg/L vs. 46 μg/L, respectively), and subjects with both ADHD and RLS tended to have even lower ferritin levels than those with ADHD alone.[75] Though this finding did not reach statistical significance, it suggests a pathophysiologic association between comorbid ADHD and RLS. Konofal et al., later conducted a double-blind, placebo-controlled trial among 23 youth with ADHD, 19 of whom had low serum ferritin levels of <30 ng/mL. Subjects were randomized to 12 weeks of oral iron (ferrous sulfate) 80 mg daily or placebo. Subjects in the treatment group showed a significant improvement in the secondary end points including decreased mean scores on the Clinical Global Impression Severity Scale and the ADHD Rating Scale, as well as decreased scores on its hyperactive-impulsive and inattentive subscales. Notably, 14 subjects in the treatment group met criteria for possible RLS at baseline and only 2 met criteria at end point, demonstrating improvement in both ADHD and RLS symptoms with iron supplementation.[80]

Evening Chronotype and Delayed Sleep–Wake Phase Disorder

Youth with ADHD frequently present with difficulty falling asleep and bedtime resistance, with difficulty awakening for school and morning sleep inertia. Interestingly, this sleep-onset insomnia may have circadian underpinnings in a subset of ADHD individuals. A robust literature links ADHD and ADHD symptomatology with evening chronotype and DSWPD.[81] Chronic difficulty falling asleep at the desired time, in the context of DSWPD, leads to shorter nocturnal sleep periods and chronic sleep deprivation. Chronic sleep deprivation can manifest as daytime impairments in mood, behavior, and cognition, which are cardinal features of ADHD.

Individuals with evening chronotype are self-described "night owls"; chronotype can be influenced by physiologic, genetic, social, and environmental factors. Increased evening preference in subjects was associated with increased ADHD symptoms and poorer sustained attention on a continuous performance task.[82]

Individuals who meet diagnostic criteria for DSWPD demonstrate an even more exaggerated delay in the phase of the major sleep period in relation to the desired/socially acceptable sleep time (≥2 hours), with significant difficulty awakening at times required for obligations (e.g., school, work), sleep-onset difficulties, and nonrestorative sleep, all of which resolve when the individual sleeps on their preferred sleep–wake schedule. ADHD was associated with an increased prevalence of DSWPD, as well as later mid-sleep time on ad libitum sleep days.[83]

Physiologic Differences Between Youth With and Without Attention-Deficit/Hyperactivity Disorder

Although chronotype can also be influenced by social and environmental factors, physiologic differences between subjects with and without ADHD have emerged both in pediatric and adult populations, such as a later dim-light melatonin onset (DLMO).[83–85] A study of 110 medication-naïve children with ADHD found that 87 (79%) had sleep-onset insomnia. Children with versus without sleep-onset insomnia showed a phase delay as reflected by DLMO.[84] In a follow-up study, sleep hygiene did not seem to account for this difference.[86]

Differences in melatonin physiology and pineal function have been noted in ADHD subjects. Adults with ADHD and evening chronotype may have low pineal gland volumes.[87] In a study of 27 medication-free youth with ADHD compared with controls, there was an increase in daytime, nighttime, and 24-hour production of urinary 6-sulfatoxymelatonin, the main metabolite of melatonin.[88]

Further, differences in heart rate and heart rate variability have been identified in youth with ADHD, specifically increased heart rate in the afternoon and evening and diminished heart rate variability compared with controls, suggesting autonomic instability.[89,90] MPH treatment restores heart rate variability toward that seen in controls.[89]

Intervention Studies

Intervention studies are limited, though improvement in ADHD symptoms after treatment of the delayed sleep phase with melatonin or melatonin derivatives and bright light therapy (which advances the circadian phase) has been noted.

In one study involving 10 adult subjects with ADHD, 5 subjects received agomelatine for 4 weeks, in addition to their usual ADHD medication. Agomelatine is a selective agonist at melatonin MT_1 and MT_2 receptors and thereby induces a circadian phase advance. The patients on agomelatine experienced a reduction in ADHD symptoms on the Wender Utah Questionnaire.[91] When 29 adults with ADHD received 3 weeks of early morning light therapy during the fall or winter months, they experienced a significant circadian phase advance. This corresponded with a significant decrease in both subjective and objective measures of ADHD symptoms (improved inattention > hyperactivity) and improved mood (in those with seasonal depression as well as nonseasonal depression).[92]

Genetic and Environmental Factors in Evening Chronotype or Delayed Sleep–Wake Phase Disorder and Attention-Deficit/Hyperactivity Disorder

ADHD and evening chronotype or DSWPD may share genetic underpinnings. Loss of PER2 and BMAL1 molecular circadian rhythm (proteins that regulate the circadian clock) was reported in a small study of adults with ADHD.[93]

Environmental studies add a fascinating dimension to the story and suggest that ADHD and associated circadian rhythm disturbances may be due to insufficient bright light or visual tract abnormalities that prevent normal circadian entrainment. Natural daylight is the strongest zeitgeber for the circadian clock[94] and suppresses pineal gland production of melatonin. Geographically determined levels of solar irradiation are linked to distribution of chronotypes in populations; those living at higher latitudes with less solar irradiation are more frequently evening chronotypes.[95] Similarly, geographic areas associated with higher solar intensities are associated with lower prevalence of ADHD.[96] Interestingly, a higher level of self-reported photophobia is associated with ADHD.[97] Changes in the melanopsin photoreceptive system are postulated to play a role in circadian entrainment, as well as nonvisual responses to light, including photophobia.[98] As a whole, these observations suggest that absence or paucity of bright light, such as that due to geography, may be associated with higher prevalence of ADHD symptomatology. Additionally, some individuals may have abnormalities in the visual photoreceptive system that causes photophobia; thus this can lead to greater difficulty, or even inability, to achieve normal circadian entrainment with bright light.

Weakened Circadian Regulation of Sleep?

Some evidence also suggests that ADHD subjects may have a weakened circadian regulation of the sleep–wake cycle. In a study of 396 adults, social jetlag was associated with ADHD symptoms.[99]

Sleep Deprivation and Insufficient Sleep

Sleep deprivation and insufficient sleep are also implicated in neurobehavioral disturbances, including ADHD symptomatology and emotional dysregulation. Youth with ADHD frequently suffer from fragmented sleep, secondary to arousals from SDB and periodic limb movements of sleep, or insufficient sleep, for example, secondary to RLS, DSWPD, and behavioral insomnia. Adolescents with ADHD, compared with adolescents without ADHD, appear less likely to obtain sufficient sleep on school days and weekends (sleep diary, actigraphy), are more likely to fall asleep in class, and are more likely to have stayed up all night in the 2 weeks sampled.[100]

Brain regions affected by sleep deprivation include the PFC (executive function), basal ganglia (reward anticipation), and amygdala (emotional reactivity).[101] Functional MRI studies have demonstrated that sleep deprivation is associated with decrements in PFC function, with performance drops (e.g., arithmetic test).[102] Gruber et al., found that 1-hour sleep restriction led to deficits on a continuous performance test (CPT) in youth (ages 7–11) with ADHD as well as controls; deficits in youth with ADHD reached clinically significant levels of inattention on the CPT.[103] In another study, youth with ADHD were found to sleep less than the recommended number of hours for age (<9 hours) based on actigraphy and PSG; additionally, the sleep deprivation correlated negatively with Conners' ADHD ratings.[14]

Hypo-Arousal and Hypersomnolence

Youth with ADHD report increased daytime sleepiness on subjective measures.[9,104] More daytime sleepiness and inadvertent daytime dozing is primarily seen in children with ADHD-I, rather than ADHD-C and ADHD-H.[12,17]

Studies that have employed objective measures (e.g., MSLT) have shown conflicting results.[7] Some studies cited increased somnolence in medication-free youth with ADHD (without known primary sleep disorders), with reduced mean sleep latency.[105,106] and longer reaction time[106] compared with controls. Importantly, however, in the Golan et al., study (which demonstrated statistically significant differences in MSL in all five naps between ADHD youth and controls), 50% of the ADHD group had symptoms of SDB and 15% had periodic limb movements of sleep on PSG.[105] Other studies employing the MSLT did not show significant differences in MSL in youth with ADHD compared with controls.[107–109] Thus, the full nature of this relationship remains to be elucidated.

Given the high comorbidity of ADHD with primary sleep disorders, the excessive daytime sleepiness may be secondary to fragmented, poor quality sleep (e.g., due to SDB, PLMs) or insufficient sleep (e.g., secondary to sleep-onset insomnia with RLS and DSWPD). An inherent dysfunction of central nervous system mechanisms that promote wakefulness and arousal has been implicated in the pathogenesis of ADHD symptoms. It has been postulated that the motor hyperactivity seen in ADHD may actually be a compensatory mechanism to stay awake and alert.[106]

In terms of objective markers of sleepiness, researchers have also examined sleep microarchitecture, namely cyclic alternating pattern (CAP) analysis during non–rapid eye movement (NREM) sleep, which has also been employed in narcolepsy research.[110] The CAP may be a "code" for the physiological oscillating pattern seen during NREM sleep, which is hypothesized to be important for sleep building and maintenance.[111] Each CAP cycle is comprised of a transient arousal complex (phase A) that interrupts the slower theta/delta activities of NREM sleep (phase B). NREM sleep that shows the CAP is thought to represent a state of sustained arousal instability, as the individual fluctuates between a state of higher and lower arousal. As in other

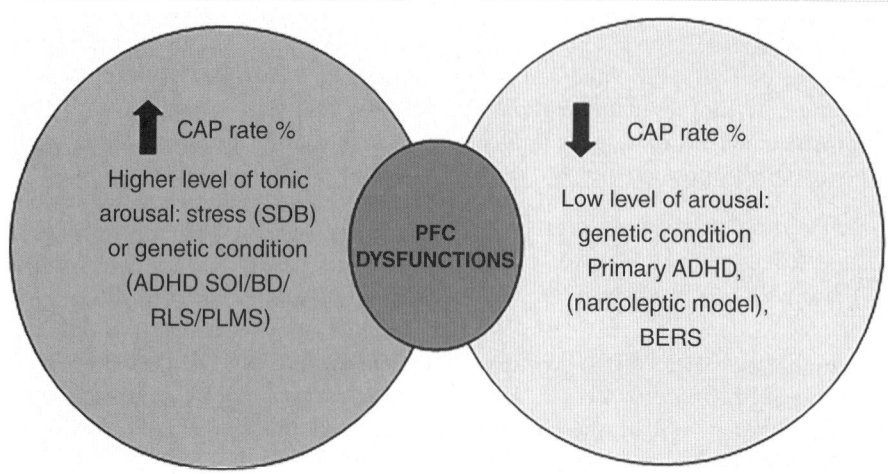

• **Fig. 14.6** Interaction between different levels of arousal during sleep and sleep-related attention-deficit/hyperactivity disorder (ADHD) phenotypes. Researchers have examined sleep microarchitecture in youth with ADHD, namely cyclic alternating pattern (CAP) analysis during non–rapid eye movement (NREM) sleep. CAP is an electroencephalogram (EEG) marker of unstable sleep. Differences in arousability during sleep may relate to different sleep-related ADHD phenotypes. As in other hypo-arousal conditions (e.g., narcolepsy, Prader-Willi syndrome), children who have the "primary" form of ADHD (described by Miano and colleagues as ADHD that cannot be explained by an underlying sleep disorder) appear to have lower total CAP rates, and lower CAP rates during stage N2 sleep compared with controls. Lower CAP rates may suggest excessive stability of NREM sleep, and therefore may characterize a state of "hypo-arousal" similar to that observed in narcolepsy. Conversely, higher levels of arousal and higher CAP rates are seen in primary sleep disorders that interrupt sleep (e.g., sleep-disordered breathing [SDB], periodic limb movements of sleep [PLMs]). BERS, benign epilepsy with rolandic spikes; BD, bipolar disorder; PFC, prefrontal cortex; RLS, restless legs syndrome; SOI, sleep-onset insomnia. (From Miano S, Parisi P, Villa MP. The sleep phenotypes of attention deficit hyperactivity disorder: the role of arousal during sleep and implications for treatment. *Med Hypotheses*. 2012 Aug;79(2):147–153.)

hypo-arousal conditions (e.g., narcolepsy, Prader-Willi syndrome), youth with ADHD have been found to have lower total CAP rates, and lower CAP rates during stage N2 sleep than controls,[112] though this result has not been consistent. The implications of this "excessive stability" in NREM sleep among youth with ADHD, and the relationship to executive function deficits, remain to be clarified (Fig. 14.6).

A recent meta-analysis examining sleep EEG microstructure in children and adolescents with ADHD found that slow-wave activity in individuals with ADHD was significantly higher in early childhood and declined in later childhood and adolescence compared with controls, with an inversion point around 10 years old. Another difference was total CAP rate and CAP A1 index in N2 sleep, with CAP A1 rate in NREM sleep significantly lower in ADHD patients than controls. The authors concluded that slow-wave activity and CAP A1 changes may be possible markers of altered cortical maturation in ADHD.[113]

Ictal and Interictal Epileptiform Discharges

A link between ADHD symptomatology and interictal epileptiform discharges (IEDs) during sleep (particularly centrotemporal and rolandic spikes) has been observed.[14] The reported prevalence for IEDs ranges from approximately 5%[114] to 50–60% in youth with ADHD without clinical seizures,[115] compared with 2–3% in youth without ADHD. Neuropsychological assessment in youth with benign epilepsy with centrotemporal or

rolandic spikes (BECRS) and IEDs during sleep revealed deficits in attention span, as well as other cognitive domains, including visuospatial short-term memory, verbal fluency, and academic performance; significant improvement in these domains was observed following remission of IEDs.[13]

In terms of epilepsy, population studies estimated a ADHD prevalence of approximately 12–17% in childhood epilepsy,[116] with predominance of ADHD–inattentive subtype.[116] Epilepsy appears to be more severe in individuals with comorbid ADHD.[117]

Stimulants may reduce seizure threshold in ADHD with comorbid epilepsy. Available data are limited on effects of antiepileptic medications, and other viable treatment options on ADHD symptomatology among children with IEDs.[13] Further research is required.

Behavioral Management of Sleep Disturbances in Youth with Attention-Deficit/Hyperactivity Disorder

Insomnia symptoms (difficulty initiating and maintaining sleep) are the most frequent parent-reported and self-reported sleep difficulties among youth with ADHD, and are often associated with bedtime resistance, delayed sleep onset, increased night awakenings, and shortened sleep duration. Fig. 14.3 has a systematic evaluation strategy for sleep-onset difficulties in children with ADHD.

Behavioral sleep interventions such as behavioral modification and cognitive behavioral therapy for insomnia (CBT-I) are recommended as the first-line approach, and preferred by parents, in the treatment of insomnia symptoms and chronic insomnia disorder in youth with ADHD.[118] Only after primary sleep disorders (e.g., OSA, RLS) have been identified and treated, and behavioral interventions maximized without adequate response, should initiation of pharmacotherapy be considered. Overall, findings on behavioral treatment of sleep difficulties among youth with ADHD are encouraging. However, unique challenges exist in the management of these children's sleep difficulties that require tailored treatment modalities and are the focus of this section.

Treatment Considerations

Psychiatric Comorbidities

Psychiatric comorbidities are common among children with ADHD, and the majority of youth with an ADHD diagnosis have at least one.[119] These comorbidities are often associated with sleep difficulties that may both result from and exacerbate comorbid psychiatric symptoms, making treatment of sleep difficulties in youth with ADHD more challenging. Specifically, up to 30% of children with ADHD have a comorbid anxiety disorder and 10–30% have a mood disorder.[120] Children with ADHD and comorbid anxiety or depression may be more vulnerable to the development of bedtime fears. They may ruminate and worry enough to delay sleep onset and require parental presence at night to initiate sleep.[121,122] Moreover, up to 78% of children with autism spectrum disorder meet criteria for comorbid ADHD, and frequently share similar common sleep challenges (i.e., difficulty with sleep initiation and maintenance, including delayed sleep onset, short sleep duration, multiple nighttime awakenings, and early morning awakening), which often persist into adulthood.[123] ADHD-related disruptive behavior disorders such as conduct disorder and oppositional defiant disorder may make affected youth particularly prone to developing bedtime conflicts, and in turn nighttime sleep disturbance including shorter sleep duration and lower sleep efficiency.[124]

Family Factors

Various familial factors may contribute to sleep difficulties in youth with ADHD, given the hereditary nature of ADHD, as well as the potential discord that it causes to the family system. In fact, data indicate that 25–30% of parents of children with ADHD have ADHD themselves, and their own ADHD symptoms might interfere with their ability to consistently implement a behavioral sleep plan.[30] Familial interactions and household environments, such as greater family conflict and disorganized and less structured family environments may also be associated with sleep difficulties.[125] In addition, parents of youth with ADHD are less likely to provide consistent and clear structure regarding household rules and bedtime routines, without which bedtime resistance may arise.

Furthermore, parental disagreement about how to handle bedtime problems and resistance can worsen the struggle, and thus should be an important point of discussion when plans for treatment are initiated. Clinicians should design a treatment plan to ensure buy-in from both parents to optimize success. Parents of children with ADHD, compared with other parents, may believe that their child's sleep problems are more intrinsic and less responsive to treatment.[126] Therefore, clinicians who address sleep difficulties in children with ADHD should work with parents to promote their own beliefs of effectiveness regarding interventions and to support families through frequent check-ins between follow-ups. This can help to ensure that the intervention is implemented accurately and consistently. Moreover, behavioral sleep interventions may need to be paired with treatment that addresses daytime behavior. Strategies may combine reinforcement charts, rewards, parent–child contracts, and other interventions.[127] Importantly, consistency from parents coupled with positive and immediate feedback to the child are key to successful implementation of behavioral sleep interventions.

Promotion of Sleep Hygiene

Children with ADHD tend to have poorer sleep hygiene than typically developing peers.[128,129] Therefore, clinicians may need to educate youth with ADHD and their families about good sleep hygiene practices that may have never been developed, or been developed and then abandoned due to resistance from the child (i.e., "the iPad is the only thing that calms my child down at night"). As youth with ADHD are constantly seeking parental attention and reinforcement for both positive and negative behaviors,[127] parents should be encouraged to attend consistently to positive behaviors (e.g., "I like the way you put your pajamas on"), instead of negative behaviors ("Shut off the video game and get to bed"). Furthermore, given that transitions between activities are often difficult, it can be helpful for parents to provide transition warnings prior to bedtime routine. Consistent sleep–wake scheduling and clearly defined bedtime routines (i.e., pictorial representation routines) are also important as they expose children to specific activities and cues, preparing them for and promoting appropriately timed and effective sleep, while encouraging successful transition between activities. Although implementation of good sleep hygiene practices is the foundation for behaviorally focused management of sleep difficulties, residual sleep disturbances may persist due to other factors (e.g., sleep disorders such as OSA and RLS and parents' unrealistic expectations about developmentally appropriate sleep behaviors).

Age

Adolescence itself presents a substantial risk for development of chronic insomnia disorder.[130] This risk[131] appears to be compounded by inherent qualities of ADHD (e.g., difficulty settling down, disorganized thoughts, and racing mind). Adolescents may benefit from different treatment modalities that encourage independent participation. One such treatment modality is CBT-I. This evidence-based therapy combines behavioral approaches (aimed at elimination of habits, behaviors and environmental disruptions that interfere with sleep) with cognitive techniques that examine, manage, and modify harmful sleep-related thoughts and beliefs.[132–134] In contrast to CBT-I, brief behavioral treatment of insomnia (BBT-I) is a concise, targeted therapy that focuses solely on behavioral techniques to optimize sleep–wake scheduling and strengthen healthy environmental cues to promote better sleep.[135,136]

Effectiveness of Behavioral Sleep Interventions

Although substantial evidence has demonstrated the effectiveness of behavioral treatment in typically developing children and adolescents with sleep difficulties,[137] less research has evaluated the effectiveness of behavioral sleep interventions in children with ADHD. However, recent systematic reviews of the literature support overall improvements in sleep behavior in young children with ADHD following behavioral sleep interventions.[30,138] Five RCTs[31,139–142] have been conducted with ADHD sample sizes ranging from 24 to 244, and one RCT compared individuals with ADHD to typically developing peers. The majority of the RCTs included telephone follow-up calls and assessment time points ranging from 5 weeks to 6 months. They demonstrated sleep improvements in terms of reduction in sleep-onset latency, increased sleep duration, and improvements in parent-reported sleep problems. Moreover, Cortese and colleagues[30] indicated empirical evidence for the efficacy of healthy sleep practices that included consistent bed and awakening time or targeting sleep duration: their data from a nonrandomized phase of an RCT demonstrated a decrease in sleep-onset delay in 21% of young children with ADHD.[143] Methodological differences across studies with various study designs and measures of assessment limit the ability to draw definitive conclusions about the effectiveness of behavioral sleep interventions in this specific population of children, and emphasize the need for further RCTs to demonstrate efficacy and optimize behavioral treatment strategies. Importantly, no RCTs have been conducted to support the effectiveness of CBT-I or BBT-I among adolescents with chronic insomnia disorder. Despite these methodological limitations to existing literature, promotion of good sleep hygiene and behavioral therapy remain the first-line treatment approach for youth with ADHD and comorbid sleep difficulties.

Future Directions

This chapter illustrates that a multitude of sleep problems and primary sleep disorders, such as SDB, insufficient sleep, RLS, and delayed sleep–wake phase disorder, can have consequential behavioral and neurocognitive consequences that can resemble ADHD or some would postulate, constitute one of the pathways to ADHD itself.

Further research into sleep-related ADHD phenotyping could lead to the identification of "predictors" of ADHD and help illuminate the natural history and prognosis of different ADHD phenotype trajectories. Biomarkers, such as decreased heart rate variability or dysregulation of melatonin secretion, and PSG analyses, such as those performed to identify CAPs, have generated interest in children with ADHD, and may prove helpful in early identification of risk for this adverse outcome, or in tracking treatment response. Similarly, because sleep disturbances in ADHD may represent an inherent, central nervous system dysregulation of sleep and wakefulness, future longitudinal studies are warranted to evaluate whether sleep disturbances in early childhood are a premorbid neurophysiological or behavioral sign of ADHD.

From a clinical standpoint, sleep-related ADHD phenotyping could spearhead the development of more targeted, patient-specific, and effective treatment options for youth with ADHD. For example, individuals with EEG indicating hypo-arousal would theoretically benefit from treatment with psychostimulants to increase NE and DA, thereby promoting arousal. Alternatively, children who suffer from insufficient or disturbed sleep, as seen in RLS and OSA, would benefit from treatment of their underlying sleep disorder. More precise therapies addressing the underlying pathophysiology of ADHD symptoms can hopefully minimize untoward adverse effects of ADHD treatment; for example, psychostimulants in children with ADHD and epilepsy can lower the seizure threshold.[144] Pragmatic trials to test the real-world effectiveness of sleep treatments are required to inform how best to sequence treatments and how best to target treatments to specific phenotypes in youth with ADHD.

Future studies will be needed to better define timing of any sleep-induced brain injury in relation to when phenotypic expression, such as ADHD symptomatology, can be observed. Some studies suggest that children with remote SDB symptoms, long since resolved, can nonetheless be at increased risk for development of ADHD symptoms.[144–146] If so, intervention to reverse the sleep-related brain injury may need to occur years before the neurocognitive or behavioral morbidity can be observed. It is also interesting to consider whether ADHD that stems from an "inherent" dysregulation of sleep and wakefulness in the central nervous system, as opposed to sleep disorders that are readily treatable such as SDB, is more likely to persist and require treatment.

One important question that remains to be answered definitively is whether sleep disturbances and SDB in particular actually cause ADHD. This is an important question because both ADHD and SDB are each so common in children. At least two studies, though not truly epidemiologic samples, estimated the population attributable risk percentage for habitual snoring (and any underlying SDB) and hyperactive behavior. One found that under the assumption that SDB can cause hyperactive behavior, and that the prevalence of habitual snoring or underlying SDB is about 8%, the proportion of children with hyperactive behavior whose problem would be eliminated by treatment of the SDB is 15%.[147] The other study estimated that the proportion of children whose hyperactive behavior would be eliminated by treatment of SDB is 25%.[148] With an estimated 70 million children in the United States alone with ADHD,[149] either figure would have enormous implications.

However, what neurobehavioral comorbidity is actually caused by SDB remains less than completely clear. The Childhood Adenotonsillectomy Trial (CHAT) study showed that children with OSA who were randomized to early T&A as opposed to watchful waiting for 7 months experienced clearly advantageous amelioration in behavior, a secondary outcome, but not executive function as the primary outcome.[64] Other nonrandomized studies have suggested improvement of both behavioral and cognitive functions,[59,150] but these trial designs cannot prove cause and effect. Additional data are needed to address this important question. The ongoing Pediatric Adenotonsillectomy Trial for Snoring (PATS) is an RCT that will show whether treatment for children with SDB symptoms, but little or no objective evidence for OSA, still benefit from early T&A more than they do from 12 months of watchful waiting.

These questions highlight the considerable work that remains to unravel the complex relationship between sleep and ADHD in youth. Moving forward, it is crucial that clinicians, researchers, families, and the greater community develop increased awareness that there are numerous sleep-related causes of ADHD that should be considered in the diagnosis and ongoing treatment of children with ADHD. A better understanding of these relationships will clarify mechanisms by which sleep problems may lead to ADHD (or vice versa), improve diagnostic accuracy, and increase patient-centeredness of therapeutic recommendations.

CLINICAL PEARLS

- Addressing the various medical, psychiatric, behavioral, and psychosocial factors contributing to each child's ADHD symptomatology is critical for treatment efficacy.
- Youth with ADHD have a significantly higher prevalence of obstructive sleep apnea, restless legs syndrome, periodic limb movement disorder, delayed sleep-wake phase disorder, and insufficient sleep than the general pediatric population, so it is prudent to screen for and treat these conditions. Treatment of the underlying sleep disorder(s) may alleviate or resolve ADHD symptoms.
- Difficulties with sleep onset in ADHD may be both physiologic (delayed melatonin secretion), as well as behavioral nature. Education on sleep hygiene, circadian phase advancement, and behavioral insomnia may be necessary.
- Careful attention should be given to the patient's medications, particularly stimulants, as they can directly impact wakefulness and sleep. Modifying formulation, dosage, duration of action, and timing may lead to the desired effect.

References

1. Osler W. *The Principles and Practice of Medicine*. Appleton and Co; 1892:335–339..
2. Guilleminault C, Eldridge FL, Simmons FB, Dement WC. Sleep apnea in eight children. *Pediatrics*. 1976;58(1):23–30.
3. Thomas R, Sanders S, Doust J, Beller E, Glasziou P. Prevalence of attention-deficit/hyperactivity disorder: A systematic review and meta-analysis. *Pediatrics*. 2015;135(4):e994–1001. https://doi.org/10.1542/peds.2014-3482.
4. Díaz-Román A, Hita-Yáñez E, Buela-Casal G. Sleep characteristics in children with attention deficit hyperactivity disorder: Systematic review and meta-analyses. *J Clin Sleep Med*. 2016;12(5):747–756. https://doi.org/10.5664/jcsm.5810.
5. Mulraney M, Giallo R, Lycett K, Mensah F, Sciberras E. The bidirectional relationship between sleep problems and internalizing and externalizing problems in children with ADHD: A prospective cohort study. *Sleep Med*. 2016;17:45–51. https://doi.org/10.1016/j.sleep.2015.09.019.
6. Manor I, Gutnik I, Ben-Dor DH, Apter A, Sever J, Tyano S, Zalsman G. Possible association between attention deficit hyperactivity disorder and attempted suicide in adolescents – A pilot study. *Eur Psychiatry*. 2010;25(3):146–150. https://doi.org/10.1016/j.eurpsy.2009.06.001.
7. Bioulac S, Micoulaud-Franchi JA, Philip P. Excessive daytime sleepiness in patients with ADHD–diagnostic and management strategies. *Curr Psychiatry Rep*. 2015;17(8):608. https://doi.org/10.1007/s11920-015-0608-7.
8. Tsai MH, Hsu JF, Huang YS. Sleep problems in children with attention deficit/hyperactivity disorder: Current status of knowledge and appropriate management. *Curr Psychiatry Rep*. 2016;18(8):76. https://doi.org/10.1007/s11920-016-0711-4.
9. Cortese S, Faraone SV, Konofal E, Lecendreux M. Sleep in children with attention-deficit/hyperactivity disorder: Meta-analysis of subjective and objective studies. *J Am Acad Child Adolesc Psychiatry*. 2009;48(9):894–908. https://doi.org/10.1097/CHI.0b013e3181ac09c9.
10. Sadeh A, Pergamin L, Bar-Haim Y. Sleep in children with attention-deficit hyperactivity disorder: A meta-analysis of polysomnographic studies. *Sleep Med Rev*. 2006;10(6):381–398. https://doi.org/10.1016/j.smrv.2006.03.004.
11. Chiang HL, Gau SSF, Ni HC, Chiu YN, Shang CY, Wu YY, Soong WT. Association between symptoms and subtypes of attention-deficit hyperactivity disorder and sleep problems/disorders. *J Sleep Res*. 2010;19(4):535–545. https://doi.org/10.1111/j.1365-2869.2010.00832.x.
12. Mayes SD, Calhoun SL, Bixler EO, Vgontzas AN, Mahr F, Hillwig-Garcia J, Parvin M. ADHD subtypes and comorbid anxiety, depression, and oppositional-defiant disorder: differences in sleep problems. *J Pediatr Psychol*. 2009;34(3):328–337. https://doi.org/10.1093/jpepsy/jsn083.
13. Miano S, Parisi P, Villa MP. The sleep phenotypes of attention deficit hyperactivity disorder: The role of arousal during sleep and implications for treatment. *Med Hypotheses*. 2012;79(2):147–153. https://doi.org/10.1016/j.mehy.2012.04.020.
14. Miano S, Amato N, Foderaro G, Pezzoli V, Ramelli GP, Toffolet L, Manconi M. Sleep phenotypes in attention deficit hyperactivity disorder. *Sleep Med*. 2019;60:123–131. https://doi.org/10.1016/j.sleep.2018.08.026.
15. Oishi Y, Lazarus M. The control of sleep and wakefulness by mesolimbic dopamine systems. *Neurosci Res*. 2017;118:66–73. https://doi.org/10.1016/j.neures.2017.04.008.

16. Fusar-Poli P, Rubia K, Rossi G, Sartori G, Balottin U. Striatal dopamine transporter alterations in ADHD: Pathophysiology or adaptation to psychostimulants? A meta-analysis. *Am J Psychiatry.* 2012;169(3):264–272. https://doi.org/10.1176/appi.ajp.2011.11060940.

17. Becker SP, Pfiffner LJ, Stein MA, Burns GL, McBurnett K. Sleep habits in children with attention-deficit/hyperactivity disorder predominantly inattentive type and associations with comorbid psychopathology symptoms. *Sleep Med.* 2017;21:151–159. https://doi.org/10.1016/j.sleep.2015.11.011.

18. Berridge CW, Schmeichel BE, España RA. Noradrenergic modulation of wakefulness/arousal. *Sleep Med Rev.* 2012;16(2):187–197. https://doi.org/10.1016/j.smrv.2011.12.003.

19. Rubia K, Alegria AA, Cubillo AI, Smith AB, Brammer MJ, Radua J. Effects of stimulants on brain function in attention-deficit/hyperactivity disorder: A systematic review and meta-analysis. *Biol Psychiatry.* 2014;76(8):616–628. https://doi.org/10.1016/j.biopsych.2013.10.016.

20. Horne JA. Human sleep, sleep loss and behaviour. Implications for the prefrontal cortex and psychiatric disorder. *Br J Psychiatry.* 1993;162:413–419. https://doi.org/10.1192/bjp.162.3.413.

21. Lee JS, Kim BN, Kang E, Lee DS, Kim YK, Chung JK, Cho SC. Regional cerebral blood flow in children with attention deficit hyperactivity disorder: Comparison before and after methylphenidate treatment. *Hum Brain Mapp.* 2005;24(3):157–164. https://doi.org/10.1002/hbm.20067.

22. Thomas M, Sing H, Belenky G, Holcomb H, Mayberg H, Dannals R, Redmond D. Neural basis of alertness and cognitive performance impairments during sleepiness. I. Effects of 24 h of sleep deprivation on waking human regional brain activity. *J Sleep Res.* 2000;9(4):335–352. https://doi.org/10.1046/j.1365-2869.2000.00225.x.

23. Faraone SV. The pharmacology of amphetamine and methylphenidate: Relevance to the neurobiology of attention-deficit/hyperactivity disorder and other psychiatric comorbidities. *Neurosci Biobehav Rev.* 2018;87:255–270. https://doi.org/10.1016/j.neubiorev.2018.02.001.

24. Konofal E, Lecendreux M, Cortese S. Sleep and ADHD. *Sleep Med.* 2010;11(7):652–658. https://doi.org/10.1016/j.sleep.2010.02.012.

25. Swanson J, Baler RD, Volkow ND. Understanding the effects of stimulant medications on cognition in individuals with attention-deficit hyperactivity disorder: A decade of progress. *Neuropsychopharmacology.* 2011;36(1):207–226. https://doi.org/10.1038/npp.2010.160.

26. Kidwell KM, Van Dyk TR, Lundahl A, Nelson TD. Stimulant medications and sleep for youth with ADHD: A meta-analysis. *Pediatrics.* 2015;136(6):1144–1153. https://doi.org/10.1542/peds.2015-1708.

27. De Crescenzo F, Armando M, Mazzone L, Ciliberto M, Sciannamea M, Figueroa C, Vicari S. The use of actigraphy in the monitoring of methylphenidate versus placebo in ADHD: A meta-analysis. *Atten Defic Hyperact Disord.* 2014;6(1):49–58. https://doi.org/10.1007/s12402-013-0122-x.

28. Becker SP. ADHD and sleep: Recent advances and future directions. *Curr Opin Psychol.* 2019;34:50–56. https://doi.org/10.1016/j.copsyc.2019.09.006.

29. Cortese S, Angriman M. Treatment of sleep disorders in youth with ADHD: What is the evidence from randomised controlled trials and how should the field move forward? *Expert Rev Neurother.* 2019;17(6):525–527. https://doi.org/10.1080/14737175.2017.1311789.

30. Cortese S, Brown TE, Corkum P, Gruber R, O'Brien LM, Stein M, Owens J. Assessment and management of sleep problems in youths with attention-deficit/hyperactivity disorder. *J Am Acad Child Adolesc Psychiatry.* 2013;52(8):784–796. https://doi.org/10.1016/j.jaac.2013.06.001.

31. Hiscock H, Sciberras E, Mensah F, Gerner B, Efron D, Khano S, Oberklaid F. Impact of a behavioural sleep intervention on symptoms and sleep in children with attention deficit hyperactivity disorder, and parental mental health: Randomised controlled trial. *BMJ.* 2015;350:h68. https://doi.org/10.1136/bmj.h68.

32. Vidal R, Castells J, Richarte V, Palomar G, García M, Nicolau R, Ramos-Quiroga JA. Group therapy for adolescents with attention-deficit/hyperactivity disorder: A randomized controlled trial. *J Am Acad Child Adolesc Psychiatry.* 2015;54(4):275–282. https://doi.org/10.1016/j.jaac.2014.12.016.

33. Faraone SV, Glatt SJ. A comparison of the efficacy of medications for adult attention-deficit/hyperactivity disorder using meta-analysis of effect sizes. *J Clin Psychiatry.* 2010;71(6):754–763. https://doi.org/10.4088/JCP.08m04902pur.

34. Hanwella R, Senanayake M, de Silva V. Comparative efficacy and acceptability of methylphenidate and atomoxetine in treatment of attention deficit hyperactivity disorder in children and adolescents: A meta-analysis. *BMC Psychiatry.* 2011;11:176. https://doi.org/10.1186/1471-244X-11-176.

35. Hvolby A. Associations of sleep disturbance with ADHD: Implications for treatment. *Atten Defic Hyperact Disord.* 2015;7(1):1–18. https://doi.org/10.1007/s12402-014-0151-0.

36. Bymaster FP, Katner JS, Nelson DL, Hemrick-Luecke SK, Threlkeld PG, Heiligenstein JH, Perry KW. Atomoxetine increases extracellular levels of norepinephrine and dopamine in prefrontal cortex of rat: A potential mechanism for efficacy in attention deficit/hyperactivity disorder. *Neuropsychopharmacology.* 2002;27(5):699–711. https://doi.org/10.1016/S0893-133X(02)00346-9.

37. Sallee F, Connor DF, Newcorn JH. A review of the rationale and clinical utilization of α2-adrenoceptor agonists for the treatment of attention-deficit/hyperactivity and related disorders. *J Child Adolesc Psychopharmacol.* 2013;23(5):308–319. https://doi.org/10.1089/cap.2013.0028.

38. Sangal RB, Owens J, Allen AJ, Sutton V, Schuh K, Kelsey D. Effects of atomoxetine and methylphenidate on sleep in children with ADHD. *Sleep.* 2006;29(12):1573–1585. https://doi.org/10.1093/sleep/29.12.1573.

39. Block SL, Kelsey D, Coury D, Lewis D, Quintana H, Sutton V, Sumner C. Once-daily atomoxetine for treating pediatric attention-deficit/hyperactivity disorder: Comparison of morning and evening dosing. *Clin Pediatr.* 2009;48(7):723–733. https://doi.org/10.1177/0009922809335321.

40. Sallee FR, McGough J, Wigal T, Donahue J, Lyne A, Biederman J, & SPD503 Study Group Guanfacine extended release in children and adolescents with attention-deficit/hyperactivity disorder: A placebo-controlled trial. *J Am Acad Child Adolesc Psychiatry.* 2009;48(2):155–165. https://doi.org/10.1097/CHI.0b013e318191769e.

41. Wilens TE, Bukstein O, Brams M, Cutler AJ, Childress A, Rugino T, Youcha S. A controlled trial of extended-release guanfacine and psychostimulants for attention-deficit/hyperactivity disorder. *J Am Acad Child Adolesc Psychiatry.* 2012;51(1):74–85.e2. https://doi.org/10.1016/j.jaac.2011.10.012.

42. Newcorn JH, Stein MA, Childress AC, Youcha S, White C, Enright G, Rubin J. Randomized, double-blind trial of guanfacine extended release in children with attention-deficit/

hyperactivity disorder: Morning or evening administration. *J Am Acad Child Adolesc. Psychiatry*. 2013;52(9):921–930. https://doi.org/10.1016/j.jaac.2013.06.006.

43. Cortese S, Holtmann M, Banaschewski T, Buitelaar J, Coghill D, Danckaerts M, European ADHD Guidelines Group Practitioner review: Current best practice in the management of adverse events during treatment with ADHD medications in children and adolescents. *J Child Psychol Psychiatry*. 2013;54(3):227–246. https://doi.org/10.1111/jcpp.12036.

44. Graham J, Banaschewski T, Buitelaar J, Coghill D, Danckaerts M, Dittmann RW, European Guidelines Group European guidelines on managing adverse effects of medication for ADHD. *Eur Child Adolesc Psychiatry*. 2011;20(1):17–37. https://doi.org/10.1007/s00787-010-0140-6.

45. Anand S, Tong H, Besag FMC, Chan EW, Cortese S, Wong ICK. Safety, tolerability and efficacy of drugs for treating behavioural insomnia in children with attention-deficit/hyperactivity disorder: A systematic review with methodological quality assessment. *Paediatr Drugs*. 2017;19(3):235–250. https://doi.org/10.1007/s40272-017-0224-6.

46. van Geijlswijk IM, Korzilius HPLM, Smits MG. The use of exogenous melatonin in delayed sleep phase disorder: A meta-analysis. *Sleep*. 2010;33(12):1605–1614. https://doi.org/10.1093/sleep/33.12.1605.

47. Hoebert M, van der Heijden KB, van Geijlswijk IM, Smits MG. Long-term follow-up of melatonin treatment in children with ADHD and chronic sleep onset insomnia. *J Pineal Res*. 2009;47(1):1–7. https://doi.org/10.1111/j.1600-079X.2009.00681.x.

48. Lumeng JC, Chervin RD. Epidemiology of pediatric obstructive sleep apnea. *Proc Am Thorac Soc*. 2008;5(2):242–252. https://doi.org/10.1513/pats.200708-135MG.

49. Sedky K, Bennett DS, Carvalho KS. Attention deficit hyperactivity disorder and sleep disordered breathing in pediatric populations: A meta-analysis. *Sleep Med Rev*. 2014;18(4):349–356. https://doi.org/10.1016/j.smrv.2013.12.003.

50. Owens JA. Sleep disorders and attention-deficit/hyperactivity disorder. *Curr Psychiatry Rep*. 2008;10(5):439–444. https://doi.org/10.1007/s11920-008-0070-x.

51. Liu X, Ma Y, Ouyang R, Zeng Z, Zhan Z, Lu H, Chen Y. The relationship between inflammation and neurocognitive dysfunction in obstructive sleep apnea syndrome. *J Neuroinflammation*. 2020;17(1):229. https://doi.org/10.1186/s12974-020-01905-2.

52. Row BW, Kheirandish L, Neville JJ, Gozal D. Impaired spatial learning and hyperactivity in developing rats exposed to intermittent hypoxia. *Pediatr Res*. 2002;52(3):449–453. https://doi.org/10.1203/00006450-200209000-00024.

53. Gozal D, Crabtree VM, Sans Capdevila O, Witcher LA, Kheirandish-Gozal L. C-reactive protein, obstructive sleep apnea, and cognitive dysfunction in school-aged children. *Am J Respir Crit Care Med*. 2007;176(2):188–193. https://doi.org/10.1164/rccm.200610-1519OC.

54. Gaines J, Vgontzas AN, Fernandez-Mendoza J, Calhoun SL, He F, Liao D, Bixler EO. Inflammation mediates the association between visceral adiposity and obstructive sleep apnea in adolescents. *Am J Physiol Endocrinol Metab*. 2016;311(5):E851–E858. https://doi.org/10.1152/ajpendo.00249.2016.

55. Ingram DG, Matthews CK. Effect of adenotonsillectomy on c-reactive protein levels in children with obstructive sleep apnea: A meta-analysis. *Sleep Med*. 2013;14(2):172–176. https://doi.org/10.1016/j.sleep.2012.11.011.

56. Kheirandish L, Gozal D. Neurocognitive dysfunction in children with sleep disorders. *Dev Sci*. 2006;9(4):388–399. https://doi.org/10.1111/j.1467-7687.2006.00504.x.

57. Chervin RD, Weatherly RA, Garetz SL, Ruzicka DL, Giordani BJ, Hodges EK, Guire KE. Pediatric sleep questionnaire: Prediction of sleep apnea and outcomes. *Arch Otolaryngol Head Neck Surg*. 2007;133(3):216–222. https://doi.org/10.1001/archotol.133.3.216. https://pubmed.ncbi.nlm.nih.gov/17372077/.

58. Chervin RD, Archbold KH. Hyperactivity and polysomnographic findings in children evaluated for sleep-disordered breathing. *Sleep*. 2001;24(3):313–320. https://doi.org/10.1093/sleep/24.3.313. https://pubmed.ncbi.nlm.nih.gov/11322714/.

59. Chervin RD, Ruzicka DL, Giordani BJ, Weatherly RA, Dillon JE, Hodges EK, Guire KE. Sleep-disordered breathing, behavior, and cognition in children before and after adenotonsillectomy. *Pediatrics*. 2006;117(4):e769–e778. https://doi.org/10.1542/peds.2005-1837. https://pubmed.ncbi.nlm.nih.gov/16585288/.

60. Smith DL, Gozal D, Hunter SJ, Kheirandish-Gozal L. Frequency of snoring, rather than apnea-hypopnea index, predicts both cognitive and behavioral problems in young children. *Sleep Med*. 2017;34:170–178. https://doi.org/10.1016/j.sleep.2017.02.028.

61. O'Brien LM, Mervis CB, Holbrook CR, Bruner JL, Klaus CJ, Rutherford J, Gozal D. Neurobehavioral implications of habitual snoring in children. *Pediatrics*. 2004;114(1):44–49. https://doi.org/10.1542/peds.114.1.44.

62. Dillon JE, Blunden S, Ruzicka DL, Guire KE, Champine D, Weatherly RA, Chervin RD. DSM-IV diagnoses and obstructive sleep apnea in children before and 1 year after adenotonsillectomy. *J Am Acad Child Adolesc Psychiatry*. 2007;46(11):1425–1436. https://doi.org/10.1097/chi.0b013e31814b8eb2.

63. Li HY, Huang YS, Chen NH, Fang TJ, Lee LA. Impact of adenotonsillectomy on behavior in children with sleep-disordered breathing. *Laryngoscope*. 2006;116(7):1142–1147. https://doi.org/10.1097/01.mlg.0000217542.84013.b5.

64. Marcus CL, Moore RH, Rosen CL, Giordani B, Garetz SL, Taylor HG, Childhood Adenotonsillectomy Trial (CHAT) A randomized trial of adenotonsillectomy for childhood sleep apnea. *New Eng J Med*. 2003;368(25):2366–2376. https://doi.org/10.1056/NEJMoa1215881. https://pubmed.ncbi.nlm.nih.gov/23692173/.

65. Angriman M, Cortese S, Bruni O. Somatic and neuropsychiatric comorbidities in pediatric restless legs syndrome: A systematic review of the literature. *Sleep Med Rev*. 2007;34:34–45. https://doi.org/10.1016/j.smrv.2016.06.008.

66. Picchietti D, Allen RP, Walters AS, Davidson JE, Myers A, Ferini-Strambi L. Restless legs syndrome: Prevalence and impact in children and adolescents–the Peds REST study. *Pediatrics*. 2007;120(2):253–266. https://doi.org/10.1542/peds.2006-2767.

67. de Weerd A, Aricò I, Silvestri R. Presenting symptoms in pediatric restless legs syndrome patients. *J Clin Sleep Med*. 2013;9(10):1077–1080. https://doi.org/10.5664/jcsm.3086.

68. Kwon S, Sohn Y, Jeong SH, Chung US, Seo H. Prevalence of restless legs syndrome and sleep problems in Korean children and adolescents with attention deficit hyperactivity disorder: A single institution study. *Korean J Pediatr*. 2014;57(7):317–322. https://doi.org/10.3345/kjp.2014.57.7.317.

69. Picchietti DL, England SJ, Walters AS, Willis K, Verrico T. Periodic limb movement disorder and restless legs

syndrome in children with attention-deficit hyperactivity disorder. *J Child Neurol.* 1998;13(12):588–594. https://doi.org/10.1177/088307389801301202.

70. Frye SS, Fernandez-Mendoza J, Calhoun SL, Vgontzas AN, Liao D, Bixler EO. Neurocognitive and behavioral significance of periodic limb movements during sleep in adolescents with attention-deficit/hyperactivity disorder. *Sleep.* 2018;41(10):zsy129. https://doi.org/10.1093/sleep/zsy129.

71. Picchietti DL, Underwood DJ, Farris WA, Walters AS, Shah MM, Dahl RE, Hening WA. Further studies on periodic limb movement disorder and restless legs syndrome in children with attention deficit hyperactivity disorder. *Mov Disord.* 1999;14(6):1000–1007.

72. Cortese S, Konofal E, Lecendreux M, Arnulf I, Mouren MC, Darra F, Dalla Bernardina B. Restless legs syndrome and attention-deficit/hyperactivity disorder: A review of the literature. *Sleep.* 2005;28(8):1007–1013. https://doi.org/10.1093/sleep/28.8.1007.

73. Pullen SJ, Wall CA, Angstman ER, Munitz GE, Kotagal S. Psychiatric comorbidity in children and adolescents with restless legs syndrome: A retrospective study. *J Clin Sleep Med.* 2011;7(6):587–596. https://doi.org/10.5664/jcsm.1456.

74. Silvestri R, Gagliano A, Aricò I, Calarese T, Cedro C, Bruni O, Bramanti P. Sleep disorders in children with attention-deficit/hyperactivity disorder (ADHD) recorded overnight by video-polysomnography. *Sleep Med.* 2009;10(10):1132–1138. https://doi.org/10.1016/j.sleep.2009.04.003.

75. Konofal E, Cortese S, Marchand M, Mouren MC, Arnulf I, Lecendreux M. Impact of restless legs syndrome and iron deficiency on attention-deficit/hyperactivity disorder in children. *Sleep Med.* 2007;8(7–8):711–715. https://doi.org/10.1016/j.sleep.2007.04.022.

76. Peirano P, Algarin C, Chamorro R, Manconi M, Lozoff B, Ferri R. Iron deficiency anemia in infancy exerts long-term effects on the tibialis anterior motor activity during sleep in childhood. *Sleep Med.* 2012;13(8):1006–1012. https://doi.org/10.1016/j.sleep.2012.05.011.

77. Picchietti MA, Picchietti DL. Advances in pediatric restless legs syndrome: Iron, genetics, diagnosis and treatment. *Sleep Med.* 2010;11(7):643–651. https://doi.org/10.1016/j.sleep.2009.11.014.

78. Didriksen M, Thørner LW, Erikstrup C, Pedersen OB, Paarup HM, Petersen M, Ullum H. Self-reported restless legs syndrome and involuntary leg movements during sleep are associated with symptoms of attention deficit hyperactivity disorder. *Sleep Med.* 2019;57:115–121. https://doi.org/10.1016/j.sleep.2019.01.039.

79. Wang Y, Huang L, Zhang L, Qu Y, Mu D. Iron status in attention-deficit/hyperactivity disorder: A systematic review and meta-analysis. *PLoS One.* 2017;12(1):e0169145. https://doi.org/10.1371/journal.pone.0169145.

80. Konofal E, Lecendreux M, Deron J, Marchand M, Cortese S, Zaïm M, Arnulf I. Effects of iron supplementation on attention deficit hyperactivity disorder in children. *Pediatr Neurol.* 2008;38(1):20–26. https://doi.org/10.1016/j.pediatrneurol.2007.08.014.

81. Coogan AN, McGowan NM. A systematic review of circadian function, chronotype and chronotherapy in attention deficit hyperactivity disorder. *Atten Defic Hyperact Disord.* 2017;9(3):129–147. https://doi.org/10.1007/s12402-016-0214-5.

82. Rybak YE, McNeely HE, Mackenzie BE, Jain UR, Levitan RD. Seasonality and circadian preference in adult attention-deficit/hyperactivity disorder: Clinical and neuropsychological correlates. *Compr Psychiatry.* 2007;48(6):562–571. https://doi.org/10.1016/j.comppsych.2007.05.008.

83. Bijlenga D, Van Someren EJW, Gruber R, Bron TI, Kruithof IF, Spanbroek ECA, Kooij JJS. Body temperature, activity and melatonin profiles in adults with attention-deficit/hyperactivity disorder and delayed sleep: A case-control study. *J Sleep Res.* 2013;22(6):607–616. https://doi.org/10.1111/jsr.12075.

84. Van der Heijden KB, Smits MG, Van Someren EJW, Gunning WB. Idiopathic chronic sleep onset insomnia in attention-deficit/hyperactivity disorder: A circadian rhythm sleep disorder. *Chronobiol Int.* 2005;22(3):559–570. https://doi.org/10.1081/CBI-200062410.

85. Van Veen MM, Kooij JJS, Boonstra AM, Gordijn MCM, Van Someren EJW. Delayed circadian rhythm in adults with attention-deficit/hyperactivity disorder and chronic sleep-onset insomnia. *Biol Psychiatry.* 2010;67(11):1091–1096. https://doi.org/10.1016/j.biopsych.2009.12.032.

86. van der Heijden KB, Smits MG, Gunning WB. Sleep hygiene and actigraphically evaluated sleep characteristics in children with ADHD and chronic sleep onset insomnia. *J Sleep Res.* 2006;15(1):55–62. https://doi.org/10.1111/j.1365-2869.2006.00491.x.

87. Bumb JM, Mier D, Noelte I, Schredl M, Kirsch P, Hennig O, Sobanski E. Associations of pineal volume, chronotype and symptom severity in adults with attention deficit hyperactivity disorder and healthy controls. *Eur Neuropsychopharmacol.* 2016;26(7):1119–1126. https://doi.org/10.1016/j.euroneuro.2016.03.016.

88. Büber A, Çakaloz B, Işıldar Y, Ünlü G, Bostancı HE, Aybek H, Herken H. Increased urinary 6-hydroxymelatoninsulfate levels in attention deficit hyperactivity disorder diagnosed children and adolescent. *Neurosci Lett.* 2016;617:195–200. https://doi.org/10.1016/j.neulet.2016.02.016.

89. Buchhorn R, Conzelmann A, Willaschek C, Störk D, Taurines R, Renner TJ. Heart rate variability and methylphenidate in children with ADHD. *Atten Defic Hyperact Disord.* 2012;4(2):85–91. https://doi.org/10.1007/s12402-012-0072-8.

90. Imeraj L, Antrop I, Roeyers H, Deschepper E, Bal S, Deboutte D. Diurnal variations in arousal: A naturalistic heart rate study in children with ADHD. *Eur Child Adolesc. Psychiatry.* 2011;20(8):381–392. https://doi.org/10.1007/s00787-011-0188-y.

91. Niederhofer H. Treating ADHD with agomelatine. *J Atten Disord.* 2012;16(4):346–348. https://doi.org/10.1177/1087054711417400.

92. Rybak YE, McNeely HE, Mackenzie BE, Jain UR, Levitan RD. An open trial of light therapy in adult attention-deficit/hyperactivity disorder. *J Clin Psychiatry.* 2006;67(10):1527–1535. https://doi.org/10.4088/jcp.v67n1006.

93. Baird AL, Coogan AN, Siddiqui A, Donev RM, Thome J. Adult attention-deficit hyperactivity disorder is associated with alterations in circadian rhythms at the behavioural, endocrine and molecular levels. *Mol Psychiatry.* 2012;17(10):988–995. https://doi.org/10.1038/mp.2011.149.

94. Wright KP, McHill AW, Birks BR, Griffin BR, Rusterholz T, Chinoy ED. Entrainment of the human circadian clock to the natural light-dark cycle. *Curr Biol.* 2013;23(16):1554–1558. https://doi.org/10.1016/j.cub.2013.06.039.

95. Leocadio-Miguel MA, Louzada FM, Duarte LL, Areas RP, Alam M, Freire MV, Pedrazzoli M. Latitudinal cline of chronotype. *Sci Rep.* 2017;7(1):5437. https://doi.org/10.1038/s41598-017-05797-w.

96. Arns M, van der Heijden KB, Arnold LE, Kenemans JL. Geographic variation in the prevalence of attention-deficit/hyperactivity disorder: The sunny perspective. *Biol Psychiatry*. 2013;74(8):585–590. https://doi.org/10.1016/j.biopsych.2013.02.010.

97. Kooij JJS, Bijlenga D. High prevalence of self-reported photophobia in adult ADHD. *Front Neurol*. 2014;5:256. https://doi.org/10.3389/fneur.2014.00256.

98. La Morgia C, Ross-Cisneros FN, Hannibal J, Montagna P, Sadun AA, Carelli V. Melanopsin-expressing retinal ganglion cells: Implications for human diseases. *Vision Res*. 2011;51(2):296–302. https://doi.org/10.1016/j.visres.2010.07.023.

99. McGowan NM, Voinescu BI, Coogan AN. Sleep quality, chronotype and social jetlag differentially associate with symptoms of attention deficit hyperactivity disorder in adults. *Chronobiol Int*. 2016;33(10):1433–1443. https://doi.org/10.1080/07420528.2016.1208214.

100. Becker SP, Langberg JM, Eadeh HM, Isaacson PA, Bourchtein E. Sleep and daytime sleepiness in adolescents with and without ADHD: Differences across ratings, daily diary, and actigraphy. *J Child Psychol Psychiatry*. 2019;60(9):1021–1031. https://doi.org/10.1111/jcpp.13061.

101. Maski KP, Kothare SV. Sleep deprivation and neurobehavioral functioning in children. *Int J Psychophysiol*. 2013;89(2):259–264. https://doi.org/10.1016/j.ijpsycho.2013.06.019.

102. Drummond SP, Brown GG, Stricker JL, Buxton RB, Wong EC, Gillin JC. Sleep deprivation-induced reduction in cortical functional response to serial subtraction. *Neuroreport*. 1999;10(18):3745–3748. https://doi.org/10.1097/00001756-199912160-00004.

103. Gruber R, Wiebe S, Montecalvo L, Brunetti B, Amsel R, Carrier J. Impact of sleep restriction on neurobehavioral functioning of children with attention deficit hyperactivity disorder. *Sleep*. 2011;34(3):315–323. https://doi.org/10.1093/sleep/34.3.315.

104. Bioulac S, Taillard J, Philip P, Sagaspe P. Excessive daytime sleepiness measurements in children with attention deficit hyperactivity disorder. *Front Psychiatry*. 2020;11(3). https://doi.org/10.3389/fpsyt.2020.00003.

105. Golan N, Shahar E, Ravid S, Pillar G. Sleep disorders and daytime sleepiness in children with attention-deficit/hyperactive disorder. *Sleep*. 2004;27(2):261–266. https://doi.org/10.1093/sleep/27.2.261.

106. Lecendreux M, Konofal E, Bouvard M, Falissard B, Mouren-Siméoni MC. Sleep and alertness in children with ADHD. *J Child Psychol Psychiatry*. 2000;41(6):803–812.

107. Palm L, Persson E, Bjerre I, Elmqvist D, Blennow G. Sleep and wakefulness in preadolescent children with deficits in attention, motor control and perception. *Acta Paediatr*. 1992;81(8):618–624. https://doi.org/10.1111/j.1651-2227.1992.tb12313.x.

108. Prihodova I, Paclt I, Kemlink D, Skibova J, Ptacek R, Nevsimalova S. Sleep disorders and daytime sleepiness in children with attention-deficit/hyperactivity disorder: A two-night polysomnographic study with a multiple sleep latency test. *Sleep Med*. 2010;11(9):922–928. https://doi.org/10.1016/j.sleep.2010.03.017.

109. Wiebe S, Carrier J, Frenette S, Gruber R. Sleep and sleepiness in children with attention deficit/hyperactivity disorder and controls. *J Sleep Res*. 2013;22(1):41–49. https://doi.org/10.1111/j.1365-2869.2012.01033.x.

110. Ferri R, Miano S, Bruni O, Vankova J, Nevsimalova S, Vandi S, Plazzi G. NREM sleep alterations in narcolepsy/cataplexy. *Clin Neurophysiol*. 2005;116(11):2675–2684. https://doi.org/10.1016/j.clinph.2005.08.004.

111. Terzano MG, Parrino L, Sherieri A, Chervin R, Chokroverty S, Guilleminault C, Walters A. Atlas, rules, and recording techniques for the scoring of cyclic alternating pattern (CAP) in human sleep. *Sleep Med*. 2001;2(6):537–553. https://doi.org/10.1016/s1389-9457(01)00149-6.

112. Miano S, Donfrancesco R, Bruni O, Ferri R, Galiffa S, Pagani J, Pia Villa M. NREM sleep instability is reduced in children with attention-deficit/hyperactivity disorder. *Sleep*. 2006;29(6):797–803. https://doi.org/10.1093/sleep/29.6.797.

113. Biancardi C, Sesso G, Masi G, Faraguna U, Sicca F. Sleep EEG microstructure in children and adolescents with attention deficit hyperactivity disorder: A systematic review and meta-analysis. *Sleep*. 2021;44(7):zsab006. https://doi.org/10.1093/sleep/zsab006.

114. Richer LP, Shevell MI, Rosenblatt BR. Epileptiform abnormalities in children with attention-deficit-hyperactivity disorder. *Pediatr Neurol*. 2002;26(2):125–129. https://doi.org/10.1016/s0887-8994(01)00370-8.

115. Silvestri R, Gagliano A, Calarese T, Aricò I, Cedro C, Condurso R, Tortorella G. Ictal and interictal EEG abnormalities in ADHD children recorded over night by video-polysomnography. *Epilepsy Res*. 2007;75(2–3):130–137. https://doi.org/10.1016/j.eplepsyres.2007.05.007.

116. Reilly CJ. Attention deficit hyperactivity disorder (ADHD) in childhood epilepsy. *Res Dev Disabil*. 2011;32(3):883–893. https://doi.org/10.1016/j.ridd.2011.01.019.

117. Davis SM, Katusic SK, Barbaresi WJ, Killian J, Weaver AL, Ottman R, Wirrell EC. Epilepsy in children with attention-deficit/hyperactivity disorder. *Pediatr Neurol*. 2010;42(5):325–330. https://doi.org/10.1016/j.pediatrneurol.2010.01.005.

118. Goodday A, Corkum P, Smith IM. Parental acceptance of treatments for insomnia in children with attention-deficit/hyperactivity disorder, autistic spectrum disorder, and their typically developing peers. *Children's Health Care*. 2014;43(1):54–71. https://doi.org/10.1080/02739615.2014.850879.

119. Spruyt K, Gozal D. Sleep disturbances in children with attention-deficit/hyperactivity disorder. *Expert Rev of Neurother*. 2011;11(4):565–577. https://doi.org/10.1586/ern.11.7.

120. Owens JA. A clinical overview of sleep and attention-deficit/hyperactivity disorder in children and adolescents. *J Can Acad Child Adolesc Psychiatry*. 2009;18(2):92–102.

121. Accardo JA, Marcus CL, Leonard MB, Shults J, Meltzer LJ, Elia J. Associations between psychiatric comorbidities and sleep disturbances in children with attention-deficit/hyperactivity disorder. *J Dev Behav Pediatr*. 2012;33(2):97–105. https://doi.org/10.1097/DBP.0b013e31823f6853.

122. Hansen BH, Skirbekk B, Oerbeck B, Richter J, Kristensen H. Comparison of sleep problem s in children with anxiety and attention deficit/hyperactivity disorders. *Eur Child Adolesc Psychiatry*. 2011;20(6):321–330. https://doi.org/10.1007/s00787-011-0179-z.

123. Thomas S, Lycett K, Papadopoulos N, Sciberras E, Rinehart N. Exploring behavioral sleep problems in children with ADHD and comorbid autism spectrum disorder. *J Atten Disord*. 2018;22(10):947–958. https://doi.org/10.1177/1087054715613439.

124. Aronen ET, Lampenius T, Fontell T, Simola P. Sleep in children with disruptive behavioral disorders. *Behav Sleep Med*. 2014;12(5):373–388. https://doi.org/10.1080/15402002.2013.821653.

125. Deault LC. A systematic review of parenting in relation to the development of comorbidities and functional impairments in children with attention-deficit/hyperactivity disorder (ADHD).

Child Psychiatry Hum Dev. 2010;41(2):168–192. https://doi.org/10.1007/s10578-009-0159-4.

126. Bessey M, Coulombe JA, Smith IM, Corkum P. Assessing parental sleep attitudes and beliefs in typically developing children and children with ADHD and ASD. *Children's Health Care.* 2013;42(2):116–133. https://doi.org/10.1080/0273961 5.2013.766096.

127. Barkley RA, Benton CM. *Your Defiant Child: Eight Steps to Better Behavior.* Guilford Press; 2013.

128. Martin CA, Hiscock H, Rinehart N, Heussler HS, Hyde C, Fuller-Tyszkiewicz M, Sciberras E. Associations between sleep hygiene and sleep problems in adolescents with ADHD: A cross-sectional study. *J Atten Disord.* 2020;24(4):545–554. https://doi.org/10.1177/1087054718762513.

129. van der Heijden KB, Stoffelsen RJ, Popma A, Swaab H. Sleep, chronotype, and sleep hygiene in children with attention-deficit/hyperactivity disorder, autism spectrum disorder, and controls. *Eur Child Adolesc Psychiatry.* 2018;27(1):99–111. https://doi.org/10.1007/s00787-017-1025-8.

130. Gradisar M, Gardner G, Dohnt H. Recent worldwide sleep patterns and problems during adolescence: A review and meta-analysis of age, region, and sleep. *Sleep Med.* 2011;12(2):110–118. https://doi.org/10.1016/j.sleep.2010.11.008.

131. Zhou ES, Owens J. Behavioral treatments for pediatric insomnia. *Curr Sleep Med Rep.* 2016;2(3):127–135. https://doi.org/10.1007/s40675-016-0053-0.

132. Edinger J. Overcoming Insomnia: A Cognitive Behavioral Therapy Approach. (C. Carney, trans.). Oxford University Press; 2018.

133. Morin C.M. Insomnia: A Clinical Guide to Assessment and Treatment. (C. A. Espie, trans.). Kluwer Academic/Plenum Publishers; 2013.

134. Perlis ML, Jungquist C, Smith MT, Posner D. *Cognitive Behavioral Treatment of Insomnia: A Session-by-Session Guide.* Springer Science & Business Media; 2015.

135. Gunn HE, Tutek J, Buysse DJ. Brief behavioral treatment of insomnia. *Sleep Med Clin.* 2019;14(2):235–243. https://doi.org/10.1016/j.jsmc.2019.02.003.

136. Troxel WM, Germain A, Buysse DJ. Clinical management of insomnia with brief behavioral treatment (BBTI). *Behav Sleep Med.* 2012;10(4):266–279. https://doi.org/10.1080/15402002.2011.607200.

137. Mindell JA, Kuhn B, Lewin DS, Meltzer LJ, Sadeh A, American Academy of Sleep Medicine. Behavioral treatment of bedtime problems and night wakings in infants and young children. *Sleep.* 2006;29(10):1263–1276. https://doi.org/10.1093/sleep/29.10.1263.

138. Rigney G, Ali NS, Corkum PV, Brown CA, Constantin E, Godbout R, Weiss SK. A systematic review to explore the feasibility of a behavioural sleep intervention for insomnia in children with neurodevelopmental disorders: A transdiagnostic approach. *Sleep Med Rev.* 2018;41:244–254. https://doi.org/10.1016/j.smrv.2018.03.008.

139. Corkum P, Lingley-Pottie P, Davidson F, McGrath P, Chambers CT, Mullane J, Weiss SK. Better nights/better days-distance intervention for insomnia in school-aged children with/without ADHD: A randomized controlled trial. *J Pediatr Psychol.* 2016;41(6):701–713. https://doi.org/10.1093/jpepsy/jsw031.

140. Keshavarzi Z, Bajoghli H, Mohamadi MR, Salmanian M, Kirov R, Gerber M, Brand S. In a randomized case-control trial with 10-years olds suffering from attention deficit/hyperactivity disorder (ADHD) sleep and psychological functioning improved during a 12-week sleep-training program. *World J Biol Psychiatry.* 2014;15(8):609–619. https://doi.org/10.3109/15622975.2014.922698.

141. Pelsser LM, Frankena K, Buitelaar JK, Rommelse NN. Effects of food on physical and sleep complaints in children with ADHD: A randomised controlled pilot study. *Eur J Pediatr.* 2010;169(9):1129–1138. https://doi.org/10.1007/s00431-010-1196-5.

142. Sciberras E, Mulraney M, Heussler H, Rinehart N, Schuster T, Gold L, Hiscock H. Does a brief, behavioural intervention, delivered by paediatricians or psychologists improve sleep problems for children with ADHD? Protocol for a cluster-randomised, translational trial. *BMJ Open.* 2017;7(4):e014158. https://doi.org/10.1136/bmjopen-2016-014158.

143. Weiss MD, Wasdell MB, Bomben MM, Rea KJ, Freeman RD. Sleep hygiene and melatonin treatment for children and adolescents with ADHD and initial insomnia. *J Am Acad Child Adolesc Psychiatry.* 2016;45(5):512–519. https://doi.org/10.1097/01.chi.0000205706.78818.ef.

144. Bonuck K, Freeman K, Chervin RD, Xu L. Sleep-disordered breathing in a population-based cohort: Behavioral outcomes at 4 and 7 years. *Pediatrics.* 2012;129(4):e857–e865. https://doi.org/10.1542/peds.2011-1402.

145. Beebe DW, Gozal D. Obstructive sleep apnea and the prefrontal cortex: Towards a comprehensive model linking nocturnal upper airway obstruction to daytime cognitive and behavioral deficits. *J Sleep Res.* 2002;11(1):1–16. https://doi.org/10.1046/j.1365-2869.2002.00289.x.

146. Chervin RD, Ruzicka DL, Archbold KH, Dillon JE. Snoring predicts hyperactivity four years later. *Sleep.* 2005;28(7):885–890. https://doi.org/10.1093/sleep/28.7.885.

147. Chervin RD, Archbold KH, Dillon JE, Panahi P, Pituch KJ, Dahl RE, Guilleminault C. Inattention, hyperactivity, and symptoms of sleep-disordered breathing. *Pediatrics.* 2012;109(3):449–456. https://doi.org/10.1542/peds.109.3.449. https://pubmed.ncbi.nlm.nih.gov/11875140.

148. Chervin RD, Dillon JE, Bassetti C, Ganoczy DA, Pituch KJ. Symptoms of sleep disorders, inattention, and hyperactivity in children. *Sleep.* 1997;20(12):1185–1192. https://doi.org/10.1093/sleep/20.12.1185. https://pubmed.ncbi.nlm.nih.gov/9493930/.

149. Forum on Child and Family Statistics. Child Population: Number of Children (in Millions) ages 0–17 in the United States by Age, 1950–2019 and Projected 2020–2050. Accessed [12/6/2020]. https://www.childstats.gov/americaschildren/tables/pop1.asp?fbclid=IwAR3MPAHMkiZkHSxlbf_IvtrsVCsrSkQnA9WNV2a6KjMRiaIeHsGZKs2B36A

150. Chervin RD, Ruzicka DL, Hoban TF, Fetterolf JL, Garetz SL, Guire KE, Giordani BJ. Esophageal pressures, polysomnography, and neurobehavioral outcomes of adenotonsillectomy in children. *Chest.* 2012;142(1):101–110. https://doi.org/10.1378/chest.11-2456. https://pubmed.ncbi.nlm.nih.gov/22302302/.

15

Sleep and Its Disturbances in Autism Spectrum Disorder

Paul Gringras

CHAPTER HIGHLIGHTS

- Children with Autism Spectrum Disorder (ASD) experience sleep challenges early in development and can sleep up to 45 minutes less than their typically developing peers daily.
- In addition to reduced nightly sleep duration, children with ASD also experience later bedtimes, earlier wake times, and more frequent awakenings.
- Learning challenges, anxiety, sensory concerns, melatonin deficiency, and epilepsy are among the ASD comorbidities associated with these sleep problems.
- Optimizing sleep, including melatonin supplementation, is ideal for improving the quality of life of the child with ASD.

Introduction

Families of young people with autism spectrum disorders (ASDs) often report that their children have problems falling asleep or staying asleep and that they don't seem to need as much sleep as their peers. These difficulties can arise in infancy, often before the child has a formal autism spectrum diagnosis. Although every day brings behavioral and learning challenges, poor sleep is often the final straw for these children's caregivers.

Epidemiologic studies in children with ASD show that these sleep difficulties start at a very young age and tend to persist.[1,2] Even when children with learning difficulties and medical comorbidities are excluded, an excess of sleep problems are still found in children with ASD.[2]

Given that the causes of ASD themselves are poorly understood, it comes as no surprise that the origins of sleep disorders in ASD are still unclear. Despite efforts by diagnostic systems to classify ASD as a single entity, the evidence is to the contrary. Indeed, the symptoms of ASD cluster in dimensions rather than into clear categories, and such an interpretation is likely to also provide an easier framework for exploring some of the associated sleep problems.[3]

A combination of epidemiologic and biologic studies is required to explore potential causal links and answer important questions, such as whether sleep problems appear as a secondary consequence of having an ASD; whether early and persistent sleep problems cause, or contribute to, the emergence of ASD; and whether ASD and its associated sleep problems share a common underlying pathophysiologic basis.

Autism is rarely the discrete entity described in many research studies. Comorbidity is the rule rather than the exception, and it is necessary to appreciate the often additive contributions of common comorbidities, such as attention-deficit/hyperactivity disorder (ADHD), learning difficulties, tics, and seizures, all of which have their own independent effects on sleep.

After discussing the prevalence and possible causes of sleep problems in ASD, an attempt will be made to review the various intervention modalities that are used in treating these sleep problems in children. This is an exciting and rapidly developing area that challenges researchers and clinicians, not just to establish what interventions can work, but also to determine how best to deliver them to large numbers of patients. Finally, we will look briefly beyond childhood at what is known about the long-term prognosis.

Epidemiology

In general, solid epidemiologic studies of sleep patterns, sleep behaviors, and sleep quality in patients with ASD are lacking. Studies have been small, lacked controls and have often used non-validated diagnostic tools.[4]

Two complementary research protocols that can be helpful are longitudinal cohort studies and controlled cross-sectional studies. The former have all the strengths of studying the temporal sequence of sleep problems in young people with ASD, and they can shed more light on possible directions of causality. However, they are often costly, retaining a cohort for years is difficult, and parameters studied are usually subjective. The latter are less expensive, they allow for the teasing out of possible confounders, and, if subjects are carefully matched, they permit the combination of objective and subjective measures.

Evidence from one of the longitudinal protocols comes from the Avon Longitudinal Study of Parents and Children

(ALSPAC), a prospective study of a cohort of over 14,000 children born in 1991–1992 in southwest England.[5] Parental reports of sleep duration were collected by questionnaires at eight time points from 6 months to 11 years, including from 86 children with an ASD diagnosis. Children with ASD slept for 15 to 45 minutes less each day compared with contemporary controls aged 30 months to 11 years old. The difference remained significant after adjusting for gender, epilepsy, high parity, and ethnicity. The difference in sleep duration mostly reflected changes in nighttime rather than daytime sleep duration. Nighttime sleep duration was shortened because of both later bedtimes and earlier waking times. Frequent wakings, defined as three or more times a night, were significantly more common in children with ASD from 30 months of age.

Another population-based cohort study assessed sleep problems at two age ranges (7–9 and 11–13 years).[2] A screening questionnaire was used to define autism spectrum problems and, in this group, the prevalence of chronic insomnia was more than 10 times that seen in controls; and, in the ASD children, the sleep problems were more persistent over time.

Evidence from a cross-sectional study comes from a study of children between 4 and 10 years of age randomly selected from a regional autism center.[4] This descriptive cross-sectional study compared both subjective and objective measures of sleep in an ASD cohort with those of typically developing (TD) controls. In this study, more than half of the families of the children with ASD (57.6%) voiced concerns about sleep problems, including the presence of long sleep latencies despite a bedtime routine, frequent night wakings, sleep terrors, and early risings. Only 12.5% of families of the TD cohort reported sleep concerns. Objective actigraphy measurements showed children with ASD took longer to fall asleep, were more active during the night, and had the longest nighttime duration of a wake episode. However, sleep efficiency, total sleep time, and the number of long wake episodes, as determined by actigraphy, were not statistically different between the ASD and TD cohorts.

Sleep Profiles and Sleep Architecture

Wiggs and Stores used sleep questionnaires, parental diaries, and actigraphy to describe the profile of sleep disturbance in children with ASD.[6] They found that the sleep disorders underlying the sleeplessness were most commonly behavioral, although sleep–wake cycle disorders and anxiety-related problems were also seen. They did not find that sleep patterns measured with actigraphy differed between those ASD children with or without reported sleeplessness. Similar findings were reported in studies by Malow[7] and Souders and colleagues,[4] who found the commonest sleep diagnoses were behavioral insomnia of childhood: sleep-onset type and insomnia due to ASD.

Importantly, Wiggs and Stores observed that some children with ASD woke at night without alerting their parents, which they termed "contented sleeplessness." This contented behavior contrasts with TD children who have sleep association disorder who signal or come into their parents' bedrooms. These important differences have contributed to the design of many of the current or proposed behavioral interventions discussed later in this chapter.

Sleep Architecture and Dreaming in ASD

A small, controlled study found that young adults with ASD have fewer recollections of dreaming than controls. Their dream content narratives after rapid eye movement (REM) sleep awakenings were shorter with fewer social and emotional experiences.[8] Spectral analysis of the same group showed distinctive slower alpha EEG patterns and asymmetries in the ASD group.[9]

Objective support for REM differences is inconsistent. One single-night polysomnography (PSG) study found REM sleep percentage was lower in children with ASD compared with both children with typical development and children with other developmental disorders.[10] Although interesting, the numbers of children were small and some of the differences found might relate to differences in mean age of the different groups of children. Additionally, a *first-night effect* might account for part of this finding and, in fact, one 2-night study did find that REM sleep percentage was lower on night 1 but not night 2.[11]

If REM differences in ASD are real, the potential implications are intriguing. REM sleep is greatest in the developing brain and may represent a protected time for neuroplasticity.[12] REM sleep is involved in memory consolidation and, according to several studies, normal cognitive function and processing of emotional memory.[13,14] An open label study successfully used donepezil to pharmacologically increase REM percentage in children, although this still lacks replication and the clinical impact of such an intervention is unknown.[15]

Causes of Sleep Problems in Children with ASD

Learning Difficulty and Anxiety

Children with ASD may present with varied language and cognitive phenotypes. Young people with high-functioning autism and Asperger's syndrome might have average or above-average cognitive abilities, in contrast to non-verbal children with profound learning difficulties. This level of cognitive impairment, although normally a strong predictor for sleep problems, seems less so in ASD where children across a wide range of cognitive abilities have been reported as having sleep problems at an equally high rate. It is tempting to speculate that, although sleep problems in general may be equally common among these groups, the specific nature of these problems is group dependent. A high rate of anxiety in many of the young people with Asperger's syndrome[16] is often encountered that exacerbates bedtime insomnia with perseverative rituals that further increase sleep latency.[17]

Sensory Issues

Hypersensitivities are well described in people with ASD.[18] Parents attest to the challenges of trimming nails, cutting hair, and even getting their children to wear clothes. The environmental nuances occurring at bedtime, with demands or needs around room and bed (e.g., special sheets, particular sounds, favorite pajamas) are often marked and problematic for families of children with ASD. The theory underlying the reasons for using weighted blankets and other weighted items for calming purposes on these youngsters is based on the idea of sensory integration, although as discussed in the interventions section, evidence of benefit from robust trials is lacking.

Genes, Neurobiologic Factors, and Melatonin

Although there have been many attempts to use putative genetic and biochemical findings from ASD studies to explain the sleep difficulties seen in children with ASD,[19] these attempts suffer from two fundamental problems: first, there is no evidence that ASD exists as a single disorder with a single cause; and second, the actual causal pathways that lead to ASD are poorly understood.

Although ASD was once thought to be caused by environmental factors, genetic factors are now considered to be more contributory to its pathogenesis. These include, for example, mutations in certain clock-related genes and in other genes that encode synaptic molecules associated with neuronal communication.[20] However, epigenetic mechanisms are also likely to be important, these mechanisms are affected by environmental factors (e.g., nutrition, drugs, and mental stress), and they control gene expression without changing DNA sequence.[21] For autism neurobiology, the reader is directed to a review by Budimirovic and Subramanian, although the field is constantly advancing.[22]

Perhaps the greatest efforts have centered on the hormone melatonin because of its known importance in sleep neurobiology and relevance also to ASD research. Abnormal platelet serotonin level remains one of the few consistent biochemical findings in children with autism.[23] Serotonin is a biochemical precursor to melatonin, and there has been considerable research into the components of this pathway. Genetic abnormalities have been reported in the two melatonin receptors,[24] and a variety of mutations have been described in acetylserotonin-o-methyltransferase (ASMT), one of the enzymes responsible for the synthesis of melatonin from serotonin.[24,25] However, the overall numbers of children in these studies whose ASD and sleep problems were associated with these specific ASMT mutations are very small and the findings have not been replicated in all genetic studies.[26]

Although the genetic findings still only explain a few case findings, there is other evidence that melatonin physiology is important in ASD. In one study by Leu and colleagues, the level of a melatonin metabolite was directly related to the amount of deep sleep in children with ASD.[27] The role of exogenous melatonin in treating the sleep of children with ASD is discussed later in the treatment section of this chapter.

Seizures

When a child (and particularly a very young child) presents initially with seizures, the focus of caretakers and clinicians is reducing the frequency and intensity of the seizures and investigating their causes. It is usually only later, when the seizures are under control, that a range of language, cognitive, social, behavioral, and sleep problems emerge or become recognized.[28] About 30% of children with autism also have epilepsy,[29] but it is still not known how often a shared underlying cause accounts for both disorders. However, seizures are often activated in sleep. So, when evaluating a child with autism who experiences unusual repetitive sleep-associated behaviors (or possible parasomnias), one should maintain a high index of suspicion of a possible underlying seizure disorder. Despite the technical challenges of studying these children (who may well be aversive to the investigations required), full electroencephalography (EEG) and PSG are often essential. For additional information on epilepsy and sleep, see also Chapter 44.

Comorbidities in ASD

Unfortunately, much of the sleep and ASD research has sought to study *pure* groups of children with ASD. Although this approach has certain advantages, it also reduces the generalizability to the real clinical situation where comorbidity of both medical and psychiatric conditions is the rule.[30]

When the prevalence of current comorbid DSM-IV disorders was carefully assessed in children and adolescents with ASD, 72% were diagnosed with at least one comorbid disorder.[30] Anxiety disorders (41%) and ADHD (31%) were the most common, but higher rates of obsessive–compulsive disorder, oppositional defiant disorder, and tic disorders were also present. Many of these disorders are themselves associated with sleep problems (see Chapters 15 and 46), and their frequency in children with ASD suggests they should not be ignored. Clinically, we have observed that there is often an additive effect, where the prolonged sleep latency and bedtime resistance commonly seen in children with ADHD[31] is exacerbated in ASD by an additional degree of cognitive rigidity and by a lack of empathy regarding the sleep of other family members.

Diagnostic Overshadowing—Diagnosing Other Sleep Disorders

Diagnostic overshadowing[32]—in the context of ASD with sleep problems—is the phenomenon of inadvertently over-focusing on the child's ASD (and assuming that the ASD itself is the cause of the child's insomnia) instead of remaining vigilant to other potential causes of the sleep disorders.

Obstructive sleep apnea (OSA) syndrome is common in the general pediatric population, and its peak incidence in preschool-aged children[33] occurs at a similar age to that when ASD is often first diagnosed.[34] However, there is no convincing epidemiologic evidence to suggest that OSA syndrome is more common in ASD, at least once one adjusts for confounders such as low muscle tone.[35]

Parents report an increased frequency of non–rapid eye movement (NREM) arousal disorders in children with ASD,[36] although robust studies are still lacking. Much of the time, simple clinical history combined with home video is sufficient to rule out much rarer nocturnal seizure disorders.[37]

In ASD, rhythmic movement disorder, such as head banging, can be severe, and it can be seen during the day—unrelated to sleep—as well as at night. The movements can persist to adulthood.[38] There is very little research on causes or treatments specific to ASD.

The diagnosis of restless leg syndrome in children with ASD is difficult because of the child's cognitive and language limitations. In some cases the finding of frequent arousing periodic limb movements (PLMs) on PSG can be very suggestive. Low long-term stores of iron (usually determined by low serum ferritin levels) can worsen such a disorder, and iron supplementation was shown to improve restless sleep in children with ASD in an open-label pilot study,[39] although the evidence for its use is better established in children with ADHD.

REM sleep behavior disorder (RBD) has been reported in one case series of children with ASD who were studied with PSG,[11] although a larger PSG study that excluded children on psychotropic medication did not document RBD or even periods of REM sleep without atonia.[7]

Treatment of Sleep Problems in ASD

Size of the Problem

Autism is certainly more common than was previously thought, and current estimates are of over 1 in 100 children being affected. As already discussed, over half of these children will have significant sleep problems. Although complex face-to-face multidisciplinary interventions may be effective, they are time-consuming and will fail to reach many youngsters suffering from a disorder this common. It is for this reason that booklet or web interventions are being proposed, and perhaps this is why behavioral interventions are often neglected in favor of perceived quicker pharmacologic options.

What and Who Are We Trying to Treat?

We need to differentiate those interventions designed to improve the sleep and quality of life of family members and other caretakers from those that demonstrably improve sleep quantity and quality for the child. Often there is an assumption that because parents report an improvement on a subjective sleep questionnaire, there is an actual improvement in the child's objective sleep parameters. In fact, this is rarely the case and, with the exception of sleep latency, parental questionnaires in interventional studies do not agree with objective findings on PSG or actigraphy.[40] This is, of course, not surprising as they are looking at different outcome measures, although both are clinically important.

Sleep disturbances in TD children are known to impact maternal sleep and daytime functioning with the extent of sleep disturbance significantly predicting maternal mood,

stress, and fatigue. There has not been enough research on health-related quality of life outcomes for parents and siblings in specific ASD groups. In part, this is because there is still debate about the best choice of outcome measures for children with autism and their carers.[41] Support groups have been shown to help the mental health and quality of life of mothers of children with ASD, but these have not focused on sleep issues alone.[42,43]

Measuring Sleep in Children With Autism

Investigating sleep, or any other medical disorder, can be more challenging in this group of children who may be disturbed by changes in the routine, the environment, or have sensory issues and poorly tolerate any monitoring.

Nevertheless, it is possible with careful planning, attention to the environment, and skilled physiologists to carry out the entire range of conventional sleep investigations, and it is important not to miss a diagnosis of OSA, PLM disorder, or even narcolepsy in a child with an ASD.

Sleep diaries are still the most commonly used subjective form of monitoring and whether paper based, or electronic, are easily completed and understood. The limitations are obvious, and exhausted parents can under- or overestimate night-wakings. For this reason actigraphy, when tolerated, has a growing acceptance and provides a more objective measure than parent report, and has gained popularity due to its ability to measure sleep–wake patterns for extended periods of time in the child's natural environment. In children with ASD, actigraphy can be particularly useful in an "*n* of 1" trial format. This term refers to a crossover design where the child acts as their own control, and periods off and on medication (and different doses of medication) are compared while monitoring sleep with actigraphy. Although PSG (with or without full EEG) is the gold standard for the diagnosis of many sleep disorders, it is expensive, only available at a few specialist centers, and a challenge in many children with ASD.

There is still a lack of agreement about what sleep measure matters the most, and in reality every situation is different. At times, the best choice of parameter will be quite simple; if, for example, the only problem is falling asleep, then sleep latency is the obvious treatment target.

Although night wakings are common in children with ASD, capturing them in a meaningful way is more difficult (e.g., there is a huge difference between 10 wakings between 10:30 p.m. and 11:30 p.m. and 10 wakings that occur every hour of the night).

Sleep fragmentation (or its converse, sleep efficiency) is sometimes used, but there is a lack of standardization on how it is defined, what is normal for a child with an ASD, and how much change matters.

The other common measure is total sleep time. A more recent related measure, "longest sleep period," shows promise as being responsive to change and correlates with changes in child's behaviors and parent's quality of life.[44] Table 15.1 summarizes potential treatment targets (based on sleep diaries or actigraphy).

TABLE 15.1 Suggested Clinical Goals for Treatment of Insomnia		
Measure (Units)	Clinical Goal (Significant Degree of Change)	Background Rationale
Sleep onset latency (minutes)	Aim for minimum 15 minutes' improvement and latency < 30 minutes	Parent focus group work and consensus[45]
Total sleep time (minutes)	Aim for a minimum of 45 minutes' improvement	Work by Sadeh on sleep restriction and extension in children[46]
Wake after sleep onset (minutes)	Huge variation: significant change 35 mins	Normative PSG[47]
Sleep efficiency (%)	Aim for >85%: significant change 6%	Normative PSG[47]
Longest sleep period	Aim for minimum 45 minutes' improvement	Based on 0.5 SD and HRQoL[44,47]

HRQoL, Health-related quality of life; *PSG*, polysomnogram; *SD*, standard deviations.
Reproduced from Leschziner G. *Oxford Handbook of Sleep Medicine.* Oxford University Press; forthcoming.

Interventions

Parent-Directed Behavioral Interventions

The basic principles of behavioral interventions for children and young people with ASD do not differ greatly from general principles of sleep environment normalization and appropriate *sleep hygiene* as discussed in Chapters 8 and 14. The most common treatments for many sleep insomnia type problems are behavioral sleep interventions (BSIs), which seek to provide parents with strategies they can implement to help their child "learn" healthy sleep behaviors and, if necessary, "unlearn" inappropriate sleep behaviors. BSIs can be delivered in a variety of modes including face-to-face[48], telephone[49], paper based,[45] and online/app based[50,51], making for the possibility of flexible and cost-effective interventions with wide reach. BSIs have well-demonstrated efficacy in randomized controlled trials (RCTs) for younger TD children, and older (up to 12 years of age) autism and ADHD populations[48,51,52].

Parent-directed behavioral sleep interventions should always the first line approach when treating insomnia in children with ASD, as with TD children. Exhausted parents may be reluctant to try such interventions, particularly if they have previously attempted with little success. However, they should be reassured that there is good evidence that they can be as effective as medications, but with more long-term benefits and without adverse effects.[53]

Environmental Interventions

The usual recommendations captured in "sleep hygiene" advice are equally important for children with NDD. A range of special environmental modifications for sleep in children with NDD are proposed and sometimes used, but often without robust evidence. Thus, weighted blankets when trialed were not found to improve BSIs in ASD.[54]

Less common solutions, such as "safe spaces," when carefully considered can provide a more contained safe bed, or bedroom, to start to allow parents to monitor their children safely from outside the child's room, and improve sleep associations to help the child learn to "self-soothe" without a parent's presence every night.

Pharmacologic Interventions in ASD

This section will primarily focus on melatonin; there is little robust evidence for the use of any other medications for sleep problems in ASD.

Melatonin

Melatonin is a hormone that is produced by the pineal gland in a circadian manner, and it is involved in the induction of sleep and in synchronization of the circadian system.

There is a wide variety of unlicensed fast-release, slow-release, and liquid preparations of melatonin. Many products rely on food-grade rather than pharmaceutical-grade melatonin, and some are expensive. A prolonged-release formulation of melatonin (Circadin) was licensed in the 2008 as a short-term treatment of insomnia in patients over 55 years of age. Many children are unable to swallow these tablets, and although they can be crushed (and thereby become immediate-release), the product license has limited children's access to a pharmaceutical-grade prolonged-release preparation. A prolonged-release melatonin minitablet (Slenyto) mimicking the endogenous release profile of the hormone at night has now been licensed in Europe by the Medicines and Healthcare products Regulatory Agency for children with autism. It was evaluated in a phase III multicenter randomized, placebo-controlled study of children with autism. The study began with a 13-week double-blind treatment period followed by an extended open-label period with continued efficacy and safety monitoring. Results included clinically significant improvement in caregivers' diary-reported sleep initiation and maintenance (sleep latency, total sleep time, longest sleep period).[3] Effects were maintained in the long term. The medication was well tolerated and no unexpected safety issues were reported. This study was the only Class 1 rated study in a recent practice guideline publication on the treatment for insomnia and disrupted sleep behavior in children and adolescents with ASD by the American Academy of Neurology.[55]

Secondary outcomes showed improvements in child's social functioning and behavior and in caregivers' well-being.

Lack of any head-to-head studies means that there are still no good data on whether, or when, immediate-release melatonin preparations should be used. There is additionally a number of melatonin analogs already produced or in development,[5] although they are virtually never used in the pediatric population. There is no evidence from equivalence studies of any superiority of these over melatonin itself.

Adverse Effects

In the more recent largest placebo-controlled studies to date involving children with learning difficulty, autism, and epilepsy,[45,56,57] and the most recent Neurim Slenyto[44] study, there were no excess adverse effects in the treatment group over that recorded for placebo, and in particular seizures were not worsened. A Cochrane Review found no worsening of seizure frequency in patients with epilepsy given melatonin.[58] There was no detectable impact on puberty in a paper by Malow and colleagues.[7]

Dose

The cut-off point between physiologic and pharmacologic doses in children is less than 500 µg. Physiologic doses of melatonin may result in very high receptor occupancy. The doses used in RCTs and published case series vary greatly, with between 500 µg and 5 mg being the most common doses although much lower and higher doses have been used. In one large RCT, 18% of children seemed to respond to a 500 mcg dose, but others seemed to require much higher doses (12 mg).[45] Increasing doses above 5 mg is likely to recruit direct sedative effects on melatonin, rather than just sleep phase–shifting properties. This might be necessary and helpful for some children with severe developmental disorders and brain injury.

Other Pharmacologic Options

The use of sedative antihistamines, chloral hydrate, clonidine, trazodone, gabapentin,[35,59,60] and occasionally atypical antipsychotic medications has been reported in case series and open-label studies as improving sleep of children with ASD. Such medications are often prescribed to also address behavioral and mood comorbidities in ASD, and carefully designed studies will be required to isolate which effects are specific to sleep.

Do Children With ASD Grow Out of Their Sleep Problems?

Well-meaning family members, friends, and professionals will often try to reassure an exhausted family that their sleepless child with ASD "will grow out of it." Unfortunately, there is no empirical evidence to suggest this is true. Anecdotally, parents whose children with ASD had reached young adulthood have told us that they simply gave up mentioning it, as "there seemed to be nothing more we could do." In addition, some young children with ASD eventually enter sheltered accommodation, where caretakers are awake at night anyway (so without having their own sleep disturbed), and the sleep problems of the youngsters under their care are less likely to be reported.

In an adult study with a clear control group, 20 adults with Asperger's syndrome (without medication) were compared with 10 healthy controls.[16] On subjective questionnaires and sleep diaries, the Asperger's subjects had more frequent difficulties falling asleep, longer sleep latencies, and more frequent early morning wakings than did the controls. In another non-controlled study, objective and subjective measures were used to investigate sleep in adolescents and young adults aged 15 to 25 years with autism and Asperger's syndrome.[61] This study found that although the sleep questionnaires completed by parents and caretakers revealed only a moderate degree of sleep problems, greater sleep disturbances were recorded with actigraphy.

This finding suggests that even though subjective complaints of sleep disturbances are less common in adolescents and young adults with autism (than they are in younger children), this may be due to the caretakers adapting to the sleep patterns rather than to an actual reduction in sleep disturbances. The adult studies discussed above focus on adults who would not have been exposed to many of the newer behavioral and pharmacologic interventions discussed in this chapter. Although the hope is that long-term improvements in sleep for people with ASD will be possible with current treatment options, this will require evidence from controlled trials with much longer follow-up periods than those used to date.

CLINICAL PEARLS

- Sleep difficulties may emerge in infancy and precede a formal diagnosis of ASD.
- Behavioral interventions are often effective, can be delivered online, and should precede pharmacologic treatments.
- Melatonin treatment is most effective when preceded by and then accompanied by a behavioral intervention.
- Melatonin primarily improves sleep-onset difficulties, has a smaller impact on total sleep duration, and is unlikely to improve nighttime waking.
- Doses of melatonin as low as 0.5 mg will be helpful for some children.
- A newly licensed preparation of prolonged-release melatonin did not cause an increase in early morning waking (described when immediate-release melatonin is used) and increased the longest sleep period.

References

1. Humphreys JS, Gringras P, Blair PS, et al. Sleep patterns in children with autistic spectrum disorders: a prospective cohort study. *Arch Dis Child.* 2014;99(2):114–118.
2. Sivertsen B, Posserud MB, Gillberg C, Lundervold AJ, Hysing M. Sleep problems in children with autism spectrum problems: a longitudinal population-based study. *Autism.* 2012;16(2):139–150.
3. Happé F, Ronald A. The "fractionable autism triad": a review of evidence from behavioural, genetic, cognitive and neural research. *Neuropsychol Rev.* 2008;18(4):287–304.

4. Souders MC, Mason TBA, Valladares O, et al. Sleep behaviors and sleep quality in children with autism spectrum disorders. *Sleep*. 2009;32(12):1566–1578.

5. Blair PS, Humphreys JS, Gringras P, et al. Childhood sleep duration and associated demographic characteristics in an English cohort. *Sleep*. 2012;35(3):353–360.

6. Wiggs L, Stores G. Sleep patterns and sleep disorders in children with autistic spectrum disorders: insights using parent report and actigraphy. *Dev Med Child Neurol*. 2004;46(6):372–380.

7. Malow BA, Marzec ML, McGrew SG, Wang L, Henderson LM, Stone WL. Characterizing sleep in children with autism spectrum disorders: a multidimensional approach. *Sleep*. 2006;29(12):1563–1571.

8. Daoust A-M, Lusignan F-A, Braun CMJ, Mottron L, Godbout R. Dream content analysis in persons with an autism spectrum disorder. *J Autism Dev Disord*. 2008;38(4):634–643.

9. Daoust A-M, Limoges E, Bolduc C, Mottron L, Godbout R. EEG spectral analysis of wakefulness and REM sleep in high functioning autistic spectrum disorders. *Clin Neurophysiol*. 2004;115(6):1368–1373.

10. Buckley AW, Rodriguez AJ, Jennison K, et al. Rapid eye movement sleep percentage in children with autism compared with children with developmental delay and typical development. *Arch Pediatr Adolesc Med*. 2010;164(11):1032–1037.

11. Thirumalai SS, Shubin RA, Robinson R. Rapid eye movement sleep behavior disorder in children with autism. *J Child Neurol*. 2002;1(3):173–178.

12. Hobson JA. REM sleep and dreaming: towards a theory of protoconsciousness. *Nat Rev. Neurosci*. 2009;10(11):803–813.

13. Stickgold R. Sleep-dependent memory consolidation. *Nature*. 2005;437(7063):1272–1278.

14. Maquet P. The role of sleep in learning and memory. *Science*. 2001;294(5544):1048–1052.

15. Buckley AW, Sassower K, Rodriguez AJ, et al. An open label trial of donepezil for enhancement of rapid eye movement sleep in young children with autism spectrum disorders. *J Child Adolesc Psychopharmacol*. 2011;21(4):353–357.

16. Tani P, Lindberg N, Nieminen-von Wendt T. Sleep in young adults with Asperger syndrome. *Neuropsychobiology*. 2004;50(2):147–152.

17. Gabriels RL, Cuccaro ML, Hill DE. Repetitive behaviors in autism: relationships with associated clinical features. *Res Dev Disabil*. 2005;26(2):169–181.

18. Lane AE, Dennis SJ, Geraghty ME. Brief report: further evidence of sensory subtypes in autism. *J Autism Dev Disord*. 2011;41(6):826–831.

19. Kotagal S, Broomall E. Sleep in children with autism spectrum disorder. *Pediatr Neurol*. 2012;47(4):242–251.

20. Bourgeron T. The possible interplay of synaptic and clock genes in autism spectrum disorders. *Cold Spring Harb Symp Quant Biol*. 2007;72:645–654.

21. Miyake K, Hirasawa T, Koide T, Kubota T. Epigenetics in autism and other neurodevelopmental diseases. *Adv Exp Med Biol*. 2012;724:91–98.

22. Budimirovic DB, Subramanian M. Neurobiology of autism and intellectual disability. Oxford Medicine Online. 2017. https://doi.org/10.1093/med/9780199937837.003.0052

23. Zafeiriou DI, Ververi A, Vargiami E. The serotonergic system: its role in pathogenesis and early developmental treatment of autism. *Curr Neuropharmacol*. 2009;7(2):150–157.

24. Jonsson L, Ljunggren E, Bremer A. Mutation screening of melatonin-related genes in patients with autism spectrum disorders. *BMC Med Genomics*. 2010;3:10.

25. Melke J, Botros HG, Chaste P. Abnormal melatonin synthesis in autism spectrum disorders. *Mol Psychiatry*. 2008;13(1):90–98.

26. Toma C, Rossi M, Sousa I. Is ASMT a susceptibility gene for autism spectrum disorders? a replication study in European populations. *Mol Psychiatry*. 2007;12(11):977–979.

27. Leu RM, Beyderman L, Botzolakis EJ. Relation of melatonin to sleep architecture in children with autism. *J Autism Dev Disord*. 2011;41(4):427–433.

28. Baca CB, Vickrey BG, Caplan R. Psychiatric and medical comorbidity and quality of life outcomes in childhood-onset epilepsy. *Pediatrics*. 2011;128(6):e1532–e1543.

29. Tuchman R, Cuccaro M. Epilepsy and autism: neurodevelopmental perspective. *Curr Neurol Neurosci Rep*. 2011;11(4):428–434.

30. Abdallah MW, Greaves-Lord K, Grove J. Psychiatric comorbidities in autism spectrum disorders: findings from a Danish historic birth cohort. *Eur Child Adolesc Psychiatry*. 2011;20(11-12):599–601.

31. Konofal E, Lecendreux M, Cortese S. Sleep and ADHD. *Sleep Med*. 2010;11(7):652–658.

32. Jopp DA, Keys CB. Diagnostic overshadowing reviewed and reconsidered. *Am J Ment Retard*. 2001;106(5):416–433.

33. Tauman R, Gozal D. Obstructive sleep apnea syndrome in children. *Expert Rev Respir Med*. 2011;5(3):425–440.

34. Fountain C, King MD, Bearman PS. Age of diagnosis for autism: individual and community factors across 10 birth cohorts. *J Epidemiol Community Health*. 2011;65(6):503–510.

35. Bruni O, Angriman M, Calisti F, et al. Practitioner review: treatment of chronic insomnia in children and adolescents with neurodevelopmental disabilities. *J Child Psychol Psychiatry*. 2018;59(5):489–508.

36. Goldman SE, Richdale AL, Clemons T. Parental sleep concerns in autism spectrum disorders: variations from childhood to adolescence. *J Autism Dev Disord*. 2012;42(4):531–538.

37. Kotagal S. Parasomnias in childhood. *Sleep Med Rev*. 2009;13(2):157–168.

38. Chisholm T, Morehouse RL. Adult headbanging: sleep studies and treatment. *Sleep*. 1996;19(4):343–346.

39. Dosman CF, Brian JA, Drmic IE. Children with autism: effect of iron supplementation on sleep and ferritin. *Pediatr Neurol*. 2007;36(3):152–158.

40. Sadeh A. The role and validity of actigraphy in sleep medicine: an update. *Sleep Med Rev*. 2011;15(4):259–267.

41. McConachie H, Livingstone N, Morris C, et al. Parents suggest which indicators of progress and outcomes should be measured in young children with autism spectrum disorder. *J Autism Dev Disord*. 2018;48(4):1041–1051.

42. Shu BC, Lung FW. The effect of support group on the mental health and quality of life for mothers with autistic children. *J Intellect Disabil Res*. 2005;49(Pt 1):47–53.

43. Hall HR. Families of children with autism: behaviors of children, community support and coping. *Issues Compr Pediatr Nurs*. 2012;35(2):111–132.

44. Gringras P, Nir R, Breddy J, Frydman-Marom A, Findling RL. Efficacy and safety of pediatric prolonged-release melatonin for insomnia in children with autism spectrum disorder. *J Am Acad Child Adolesc Psychiatry*. 2017;56(11):948–957.e4.

45. Gringras P, Gamble C, Jones A. Melatonin for sleep problems in children with neurodevelopmental disorders: randomised double masked placebo controlled trial. *BMJ*. 2012;345:e6664.

46. Sadeh A, Gruber R, Raviv A. The effects of sleep restriction and extension on school-age children: what a difference an hour makes. *Child Dev*. 2003;74(2):444–455.

47. Scholle S, Beyer U, Bernhard M, et al. Normative values of polysomnographic parameters in childhood and adolescence: quantitative sleep parameters. *Sleep Med.* 2011;12(6): 542–549.

48. Hiscock H, Sciberras E, Mensah F, et al. Impact of a behavioural sleep intervention on symptoms and sleep in children with attention deficit hyperactivity disorder, and parental mental health: randomised controlled trial. *BMJ.* 2015; 350:h68.

49. Stuttard L, Beresford B, Clarke S, Beecham J, Curtis J A preliminary investigation into the effectiveness of a group-delivered sleep management intervention for parents of children with intellectual disabilities. *J Intellect Disabil.* 2015;19(4):342–355.

50. Espie CA, Kyle SD, Williams C, et al. A randomized, placebo-controlled trial of online cognitive behavioral therapy for chronic insomnia disorder delivered via an automated media-rich web application. *Sleep.* 2012;35(6):769–781.

51. Mindell JA, Kuhn B, Lewin DS, Meltzer LJ, Sadeh A Behavioral treatment of bedtime problems and night wakings in infants and young children. *Sleep.* 2006;29(10):1263–1276.

52. Johnson SB, Riley AW, Granger DA, Riis J The science of early life toxic stress for pediatric practice and advocacy. *Pediatrics.* 2013;131(2):319–327.

53. Kirkpatrick B, Louw JS, Leader G. Efficacy of parent training incorporated in behavioral sleep interventions for children with autism spectrum disorder and/or intellectual disabilities: a systematic review. *Sleep Med.* 2019;53:141–152.

54. Gringras P, Green D, Wright B, et al. Weighted blankets and sleep in autistic children—a randomized controlled trial. *Pediatrics.* 2014;134(2):298–306.

55. Buckley AW, Hirtz D, Oskoui M, et al. Practice guideline: treatment for insomnia and disrupted sleep behavior in children and adolescents with autism spectrum disorder: Report of the Guideline Development, Dissemination, and Implementation Subcommittee of the American Academy of Neurology. *Neurology.* 2020;94(9):392–404.

56. Coppola G, Iervolino G, Mastrosimone M, La Torre G, Ruiu F, Pascotto A. Melatonin in wake-sleep disorders in children, adolescents and young adults with mental retardation with or without epilepsy: a double-blind, cross-over, placebo-controlled trial. *Brain Dev.* 2004;26(6):373–376.

57. Garstang J, Wallis M. Randomized controlled trial of melatonin for children with autistic spectrum disorders and sleep problems. *Child Care Health Dev.* 2006;32(5):585–589.

58. Brigo F, Igwe SC, Del Felice A. Melatonin as add-on treatment for epilepsy. *Cochrane Database Syst Rev.* 2016(8):CD006967.

59. Ming X, Gordon E, Kang N, Wagner GC. Use of clonidine in children with autism spectrum disorders. *Brain Dev.* 2008;30(7):454–460.

60. Robinson AA, Malow BA. Gabapentin shows promise in treating refractory insomnia in children. *J Child Neurol.* 2013;28(12):1618–1621.

61. Oyane NMF, Bjorvatn B. Sleep disturbances in adolescents and young adults with autism and Asperger syndrome. *Autism.* 2005;9(1):83–94.

16

Metabolic Syndrome and Obesity

W. Jerome Alonso and Craig Canapari

CHAPTER HIGHLIGHTS

- Sleep deprivation, sleep fragmentation and circadian misalignment have been demonstrated to contribute to the components of the Metabolic Syndrome (MetS).
- Insulin resistance, sympathetic activation, intermittent hypoxemia and an increased propensity for obesity appear to be central in the role of short sleep and obstructive sleep apnea on MetS.
- Interventions directed toward short sleep and obstructive sleep apnea have shown improvements in measures of glucose regulation, lipid metabolism, hypertension and obesity.

Introduction

Metabolic syndrome (MetS) was originally described in the adult population, with the observance of the tendency for the aggregation of cardiovascular risk factors, which have since been shown to be associated with increased risk for atherosclerotic cardiovascular disease (ASCVD)[1] and type 2 diabetes (T2DM).[2] A central factor in the pathogenesis of MetS appears to be insulin resistance;[3,4] but is not likely the sole unifying condition, with its absence being noted in some cases. Other mechanisms that have been thought to play a role in the relationship include the effect of obesity, increased inflammatory mediators, aggravated oxidative stress and endothelial dysfunction, and elevated cortisol levels. Defining the condition in the pediatric population is a greater challenge, and considerations should be made for determining scoring criteria across ages, taking into account physiologic changes in metabolism throughout the life cycle, and needing to define morphologic scores for truncal obesity. There is consensus for the following four main components: (1) abdominal obesity, (2) dyslipidemia, (3) hypertension, and (4) glucose dysregulation. Prevalence rates vary greatly among the criteria from 6–39% of the general population.[5] The diagnosis of the condition has also been shown to be unstable as children age.[6,7] Nonetheless, there is significant evidence that the presence of MetS and its component cardiovascular risk factors in childhood and adolescence are associated with markers for early and subclinical atherosclerosis[8] and increased risk of the development of T2DM and ASCVD.[9]

Obesity in Children

The significance of obesity in modern day society cannot be overstated, with recent evidence demonstrating 19.7% of U.S. children between the ages of 2 and 19 are obese, representing approximately 14.7 million children and adolescents, based on recent estimates between 2017–2020. The consequences of obesity are broad and far-reaching, with implications on physical health and psychosocial wellbeing. There are associations with hypertension,[10] insulin resistance and glucose dysregulation,[11–13] inflammatory markers,[14–16] elevated triglycerides and low high-density lipoprotein (HDL),[12] and vascular dysfunction.[17] There is also evidence of body image dissatisfaction, reduced quality of life, and lower self-esteem.[18] Recent interest has also been placed in the relationship between sleep fragmentation and deprivation on obesity.

A number of meta-analyses have been completed that have consistently shown an association between inadequate sleep and obesity.[19–21] In a meta-analysis by Deng and colleagues involving 33 studies (57,848 children and adolescents), short sleep was associated with a significant increase in risk of obesity for both nighttime short sleep (relative risk [RR] {1/4} 1.61, 95% confidence interval [CI] 1.38–1.89; $P < 0.001$) and 24-hour short sleep (RR {1/4} 1.22, 95% CI 1.10–1.35; $P < 0.001$) with a dose–response analysis showing significance in early childhood, preschool-age children, school-age children, and teenagers.[19] Experimental studies demonstrated an association among sleep deprivation, decreased leptin,[22,23] and elevated ghrelin;[24] these hormonal changes correlate with increased appetite and food intake.[25–27] Buxton and colleagues presented findings showing a reduction in resting metabolic rate with an extended sleep restriction coupled with a circadian disruption.[28] A study of twins demonstrated that chronic sleep curtailment magnifies the effect of genetic risk factors for obesity.[29] Brand and coworkers noted on a cross-sectional study in children and adolescents that sleeping more than 9 hours, and keeping screen time less than 4 hours, reduced the effect of genetic predisposition for obesity.[30] Behavioral correlates with insufficient sleep include maladaptive habits such as increased snacking[31] and general food intake.[32] A study of experimentally induced sleep curtailment in adolescents used functional magnetic resonance imaging (MRI)

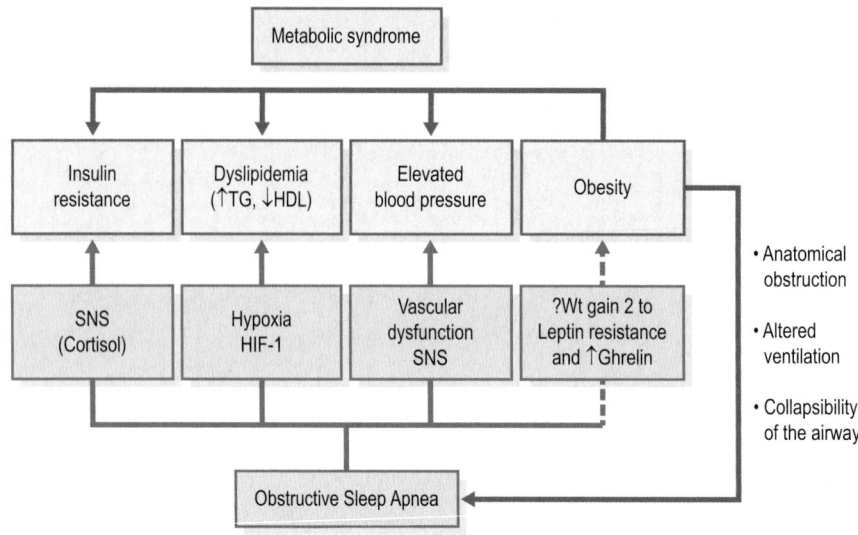

• **Fig. 16.1** Mechanistic contribution of obstructive sleep apnea (OSA) to metabolic syndrome. TG, triglycerides; HDL, high-density lipoprotein; SNS, sympathetic nervous system; HIF-1, hypoxia-inducible factor-1.

that showed a lack of increased neural inhibitory signaling with reduced sleep in both obese and non-obese subjects.[33] Contributory factors associated with both short sleep and obesity include increased availability of electronics, decreased parental supervision, later preferred sleep times and weekend bedtimes, early school times, and longer travel times.[34–36]

Obesity in the Context of Metabolic Syndrome

Obesity has been associated with elevations in blood pressure (BP),[10] insulin resistance and impaired glucose tolerance, inflammatory markers,[12] elevated triglycerides and low HDL,[12] and arterial wall stiffness and endothelial dysfunction.[17] Childhood obesity also confers an increased risk of future obesity and insulin resistance,[37] an increased risk of further weight gain over expected growth, and increased risk of the development of cardiovascular risk factors as young adults.[38] In particular, visceral fat has more adverse health outcomes compared with body mass index (BMI) or subcutaneous fat and offers an increase in the odds of developing MetS.[39] Although obesity has been demonstrated to have a larger role in the development of insulin resistance compared with obstructive sleep apnea (OSA),[40,41] there is evidence that OSA in the context of obesity may amplify the risk for insulin resistance and dyslipidemia.[40,42] Gozal and colleagues demonstrated an improvement in insulin resistance with adenotonsillectomy in the obese children alone, which supports an additive effect between OSA and obesity.[40] Fig. 16.1 describes a mechanistic model of the contribution of OSA and obesity to the MetS.

Obstructive Sleep Apnea and Obesity in Children

OSA is the sleep disorder most consistently associated with obesity. Epidemiologic characteristics in the general population suggest that 2% of school-age children[43] and 13% of preschool children are afflicted by the condition.[44] In contrast, 46–59% of obese children have OSA.[45–47] Contributing anatomic factors include adenotonsillar hypertrophy[48] and fat deposition in the lateral fat pads,[49] uvula,[50] and tongue.[51] There is also increased collapsibility of the upper airway with obesity in terms of the pharyngeal critical pressure of collapse (P_{crit}).[52] P_{crit} improves significantly with weight loss.[53] There is also increased work of breathing and lower oxygen reserves with truncal obesity.[54] Additionally, observational data suggest that OSA may predispose individuals to gain weight by derangement in adipocyte hormone functioning. Levels of the satiety hormone leptin are elevated in adults with obesity and OSA, and this has been postulated to be secondary to leptin resistance.[55–57] This relationship has also been demonstrated in children, with further elevations in leptin with increases in severity of hypoxemia independent of BMI Z-scores.[58] Leptin is reduced in children with MetS and OSA with initiation of continuous positive airway pressure (CPAP) therapy, suggesting a causal relationship.[59]

Sleep and the Components of Metabolic Syndrome

Sleep deprivation and sleep disruption have been observed to have associations with many of the parameters of MetS. A U-shaped association between sleep duration and MetS severity in adults was described in early cross-sectional data from the National Health and Nutrition Examination Survey (NHANES), with an almost equally high severity among those who slept <5 hours or >9 hours.[60] Subsequent studies in the pediatric population has shown variable findings, for either MetS or the individual components of the condition. Two studies have demonstrated an increased risk for MetS with short sleep duration.[61,62] OSA as a model of sleep fragmentation has also demonstrated a relationship with MetS. In the pediatric population, Redline and colleagues found a s6-fold increase in risk for MetS in obese adolescents who had sleep-disordered breathing (SDB).[63] A recent factor associated with components of MetS is circadian misalignment and later endogenous clock tendencies. A cross-sectional study in adults demonstrated that those with a socially imposed sleep time that had a discrepancy with their endogenous circadian rhythm showed lower HDL, higher triglycerides, higher plasma insulin, insulin resistance, and a higher waist circumference and BMI.[64]

Glucose Dysregulation

Glucose metabolism during sleep can be described as a series of homeostatic mechanisms that allow for maintenance of a stable blood glucose level during a period of fasting. A reduction of cerebral blood glucose consumption during sleep is a major factor in maintaining homeostasis during a sleep-related fast.[65] This may be related to a 30–40% reduction in brain utilization during slow-wave sleep (SWS).[66] Additional factors that may assist in glucose homeostasis include reduced peripheral utilization from decreased muscle tone and growth hormone–related insulin resistance. There is also evidence of an inhibition of insulin secretion that occurs with a rise in melatonin.[67] Leptin, an adipocyte satiety hormone, has also shown direct effects on insulin sensitivity and tissue glucose uptake; while having an inverse effect on hepatic gluconeogenesis.[68] Sleep disruption and fragmentation can exert its influence on these factors leading to derangement in glucose metabolism.

Dysregulation of glucose metabolism observed in insufficient sleep likely has contributions from a lack of a refractory period of the various stress hormones, a loss of a period of parasympathetic predominance, and the contribution of an increased tendency for obesity and its effects. These in turn can cause insulin resistance, glucose intolerance, and increased food intake. Elevated cortisol levels have been demonstrated in sleep deprivation in adults with associated insulin resistance.[69] However, markers of insulin insensitivity have been noted in healthy male adolescents with insufficient sleep despite normal levels of cortisol.[70] Sympathetic activity has also been shown to be elevated in sleep-deprived states, with associated inhibition of the secretion of leptin and insulin.[71] In a study of children between 8 and 11 years of age with 1 week of experimentally altered sleep duration, it was noted that there was a 134 kcal/day increase in food intake and increased measured weight in those with reduced sleep.[72] Obesity, which has been associated with short sleep as described earlier in the chapter, has long been known to be associated with glucose dysregulation, with mechanistic models relating to inflammation, adipocyte dysfunction, oxidative stress, endoplasmic reticulum stress, tissue aging, hypoxia, and change in genetic makeup.[73]

Inadequate sleep duration has been demonstrated in a number of meta-analyses in adult populations to have an independent association with incident T2DM.[74–76] In the pediatric population, a review from Dutil and Chaput found varied results, with 10 of 21 observational studies showing no association between sleep duration and markers of glucose dysregulation.[77] In two longitudinal studies, there was consistency in the association between inadequate sleep and insulin resistance, although only one showed a persistent association when controlling for BMI.[78] Experimental data from a randomized crossover study of 21 normal-weight male adolescents exposed to 3 nights of 4 hours per night sleep and 3 nights of 9 hours per night sleep showed increased insulin resistance in short sleepers as measured by the homeostasis model assessment of insulin resistance (HOMA-IR) index.[70] This was despite a similar amount of SWS. A prior SWS disruption trial in adults that utilized acoustic stimuli showed a 90% reduction of SWS over a 3-day period produced approximately a 25% reduction in insulin sensitivity without the expected compensatory rises in insulin secretion. Shaw and colleagues conducted a similar crossover study in prepubertal children that did not show any association between SWS disruption and fasting glucose, insulin levels, C-peptide levels, insulin sensitivity, or beta-cell responsiveness to a mixed meal.[79] Reduction in insulin sensitivity was only consistently observed in those with high insulin sensitivity, suggesting a resistance to the adverse effect of SWS disruption in this population, except for those with the least "metabolic reserve."

In the adult population, OSA has been demonstrated in large population-based studies like the Sleep Heart Health Study and the European Sleep Apnea Cohort to be associated with derangement in various aspects of glucose metabolism.[80–82] Sympathetic activation, activation of the hypothalamic-pituitary-adrenal axis, and oxidative stress relating to hypoxemia are all attributed factors affecting this relationship. Unfortunately, pediatric data are not as extensive and have had varying results. Fifteen studies have been identified examining the association between OSA and insulin resistance, with eight studies demonstrating a positive association between OSA and insulin resistance when using the HOMA-IR model.[63,83–89] The remaining seven studies failed to show an association after controlling for BMI.[90–95] A meta-analysis by Patinkin and colleagues involving eight of these studies, found a large and statistically significant elevation in insulin resistance among OSA subjects in compared with non-OSA subjects (g = 0.78, 95% CI 0.25–1.31; P = 0.02, I^2 = 87.8%).[96]

There have been several studies in adult populations investigating the effect of the treatment of OSA on measures of glucose dysfunction. Findings have differed in those with diabetes, prediabetes, and those without disorders of glucose metabolism. In patients without diabetes, some studies have found no significant effect of CPAP on glucose metabolism.[97–101] In patients with diabetes, several studies have examined the effect of treatment of OSA with CPAP on hemoglobin A1c (HbA1c). Results have been mixed, with some studies showing no effect, and others showing a modest benefit.[102–106] Findings are slightly more homogenous in the prediabetic population, with several studies showing improvement in insulin sensitivity and glucose tolerance.[107,108] In a population of prepubertal children, Gozal and colleagues published an interventional study with 62 children (37 obese and 25 non-obese) with SDB that underwent adenotonsillectomy that demonstrated an association between parameters of SDB and the insulin/glucose (I/G) ratio, and found a significant improvement in insulin resistance after treatment.[40] In an analysis of data from the Childhood Adenotonsillectomy Trial, a randomized control trial that included 464 children (ages 5–9.9) with OSA, adenotonsillectomy was not associated with a significant change in fasting blood glucose or fasting insulin with early surgical management versus watchful waiting.[109]

Circadian tendencies may also contribute to dysregulation of glucose metabolism. In adults, both later chronotypes and social jet lag have been associated with increased prediabetic risk.[110,111] In a case-control study of 18 adolescent subjects with diagnosed circadian rhythm disorders (10 with delayed sleep–wake phase; 6 with non–24-hour sleep–wake disorder; 1 irregular sleep–wake rhythm disorder; and 2 with hypersomnia), subjects were noted to have significantly higher levels of glucose on a 3-hour oral glucose tolerance test (OGTT) at the 30- and 120-minute measure, and increased serum insulin at the 120- and 150-minute recording.[112]

Dyslipidemia

Intermittent hypoxemia from SDB presents as the primary sleep-related mechanism affecting lipid metabolism, with evidence that the degree of hypoxemia significantly impacts degree of dyslipidemia.[113] Intermittent hypoxemia stimulates the production of hypoxia-inducible factor-1 in the liver, which in turn activates sterol regulatory element-binding protein-1 (SREBP-1) and stearoyl-CoA desaturase-1 (SCD).[114] SCD is an important gene controlled by SRBEP-1 that is instrumental in triglyceride and phospholipid biosynthesis.

Cross-sectional data from larger adult studies has demonstrated a tendency for a decrease in HDL cholesterol (HDL-C) and an increase in triglycerides with the presence of SDB.[115–118] However, this is inconsistent, with similar studies showing no significant association.[119–122] There have also been a number of studies in the pediatric population with similar conflicting findings, with three studies demonstrating an association between OSA and increased triglycerides,[84,87,88] and a number showing negative results. In a meta-analysis involving eight studies on the association of OSA on measures of dyslipidemia, Patinkin and colleagues found a small, but non-significant increase in triglycerides, a small and statistically elevated total cholesterol, and a significantly lower HDL-C.[96] Gozal and colleagues[40] examined the response on the lipid profile of children with OSA after having an adenotonsillectomy. The study involved 62 individuals (35 obese and 27 non-obese) and demonstrated

a significant reduction in total cholesterol and low-density lipoprotein (LDL) with reciprocal increases in HDL-C after a 6- to 12-month follow-up in both obese and non-obese children. In a retrospective study involving 24 obese children (11.8 ± 3.4 years) with OSA (17 were treated with CPAP and 5 underwent adenotonsillectomy), there was an associated improvement in total cholesterol from 179.8–168.9 mg/dL (−11 mg/dL, $P < 0.001$) and improvement in LDL from 117.7–103 mg/dL (−8.8 mg/dL, $P = 0.021$). In a cross-sectional, prospective, interventional, multicenter study of 113 obese children (11.3 ± 2.9 years),[123] patients were divided based on severity and received corresponding treatment as follows: (1) group 1, no polysomnographic evidence of OSA, respiratory disturbance index (RDI) <3 per hour who had no treatment administered; (2) group 2, mild OSA RDI ≥3 per hour, apnea-hypopnea index (AHI) <10 per hour, and/or obstructive hypoventilation without adenotonsillar hypertrophy who received dietary modification; (3) group 3, moderate to severe OSA with RDI ≥3 per hour and AHI >10 per hour, and/or obstructive hypoventilation with adenotonsillar hypertrophy who received adenotonsillectomy; and (4) group 4, moderate to severe OSA with RDI ≥3 per hour and AHI ≥10 per hour and/or presence of obstructive hypoventilation without adenotonsillar hypertrophy who received CPAP treatment. RDI and AHI were noted to be positively correlated with triglycerides in the surgically corrected group, with a negative correlation with HDL-C in the entire cohort and in the surgically resolved.

Hypertension

Elevated BP as a component of MetS has been demonstrated to have contribution from both insulin resistance[124] and obesity.[125] Hypertension has a strong association with SDB in adulthood with the condition being present in up to 50% of subjects with OSA.[126] However, data are conflicted in the pediatric population, with disagreement from three meta-analyses in regard to the presence of the association between SDB and hypertension in pediatric populations.[127–129] There has also been a lack of unifying evidence of the presence of an association between inadequate sleep and elevations in systolic or diastolic blood pressure.[78,130,131] The findings of elevated BP in a number of studies on short sleepers may be attributed to circadian misalignment, increased sympathetic activation, and increased renal sodium retention.[132]

The development of hypertension in the context of MetS is predominantly described as arising from the interaction between increased sympathetic nervous system (SNS) tone, insulin resistance, and derangement in vascular structure or function. As a parallel, SDB is also associated with a sympathetic predominance,[133] and associated insulin resistance, with evidence of reversibility with the treatment.[134,135] Hypoxemia, which is commonly seen in SDB, has been postulated to trigger vascular remodeling and an increase in inflammatory markers as seen in atherosclerosis.[136] Affectation of the renin-angiotensin-aldosterone system by hypoxemia in OSA has been postulated as well.[137] Sleep fragmentation also involved increased sympathetic activation.

The physiological profile of BP over a 24-hour period is characterized by a nighttime reduction described as the "nocturnal dipping" phenomena. This reduction in BP has been associated with an overall increase in markers of vagal tone and a decrease in sympathetic tone, even with the elimination of the effect of physical activity.[138] In comparison, wakefulness is characterized by BP variation being primarily reactive to the physical activity and posture,[139] whereas BP during sleep is controlled by posture and the transition into the stages of sleep.[138] Non–rapid eye movement (NREM) sleep is associated with an overall reduction in BP with an accompanying reduction in sympathetic tone, whereas rapid eye movement (REM) sleep is associated with bursts of sympathetic activation and an overall BP similar to wakefulness.[140] With partial sleep deprivation, there is an increase in mean BP during 24-hour BP monitoring, with the finding being more pronounced during nighttime sleep; this normalizes with subsequent sleep. There is also an increase in early morning BP surges with sleep deprivations.[141,142] Both sleep fragmentation and SWS deprivation attenuate nocturnal arterial BP dipping. However, subsequent day ambulatory BP is not significantly elevated.[143] Non-dipping of nocturnal systolic blood pressure (SysBP) and diastolic blood pressure (DiaBP) has been found in pediatric populations, as described by Ai and colleagues.[127]

A meta-analysis by Ai and colleagues, involving 3,081 participants from ages 3–17,[127] found both awake and nighttime SysBP were significantly higher in mild and moderate to severe OSA; DiaBP was elevated in awake and nighttime recordings in moderate to severe OSA, whereas mild OSA only showed increases in nighttime levels. Analysis of longitudinal data showed significantly higher SysBP in late adolescence or young adulthood in moderate to severe OSA, but not in mild OSA. Higher DiaBP was not evident in either moderate to severe OSA or mild OSA. The effect of surgical treatment of OSA in the pediatric population was examined by Kang and coworkers in a meta-analysis involving 12 studies of 1,193 children (mean age: 7.6; 54% boys).[144] Despite a significant reduction of the AHI by 9.4 events per hour (95% CI, −12.0 to −6.8), there was no evident improvement in postoperative office or 24-hour ambulatory SysBP or DiaBP after surgery. However, subgroup analysis showed a significant post-operative decrease in SysBP (−6.23 mm Hg, 95% CI, −7.78 to −4.67) and DiaBP (−7.93 mm Hg, 95% CI, −10.37 to −5.48) in children with hypertension.

Treatment of Obstructive Sleep Apnea in Obese Children

Adenotonsillectomy is considered to be first-line treatment of OSA in children. Unfortunately, it may be of limited benefit to children at risk for MetS. A meta-analysis from Friedman and colleagues has demonstrated only a 59.8% success rate in the treatment of OSA with adenotonsillectomy.[145] Furthermore, adenotonsillectomy is not as effective in the treatment of OSA in obese children; therefore it is likely to be less effective in the context of MetS.[40,146,147] Only a 12% cure rate (AHI <1) was demonstrated in a meta-analysis of adenotonsillectomy in obesity-related OSA.[148] As a result, the American Academy of Sleep Medicine supports repeat polysomnography after adenotonsillectomy in the context of obesity.[149] There is also evidence of the likelihood of weight gain over short-term follow-up post-adenotonsillectomy in both obese and non-obese children.[150]

CPAP is an alternative therapy with advantages for those who may be unresponsive to surgical management, those who are reluctant to pursue surgery, or special populations (i.e., trisomy 21 or complex OSA). In a retrospective chart review of 75 children (ages 7–17) divided among snorers, untreated OSA, and treated OSA, treated OSA was noted to have significant improvement in SysBP after 6 months of therapy.[151]

Naturally, weight loss is a critical goal in the treatment of obese children with OSA, as it reduces both OSA severity, secondary metabolic consequences, and cardiovascular risk. In a longitudinal study involving 62 obese/overweight (ages 7- to 18-year-olds) with OSA participating in a chronic care multidisciplinary overweight/obesity treatment clinic, there was significant improvement in AHI after an approximately 6.5-month follow-up (where 1 unit improvement in BMI standard deviation score was associated with a 55% improvement in AHI).[152] There is limited research on bariatric surgery in children. However, evidence from Kalra and coworkers showed resolution of OSA in a population of 10 morbidly obese adolescents (mean BMI = 60.8 ± 11.07) that underwent laparoscopic Roux-en-Y gastric after a mean weight loss of 58 kg (mean AHI at baseline vs. follow-up, 9.1 vs. 0.65).[45]

CLINICAL PEARLS

- Insulin resistance has shown a greater association with obstructive sleep apnea syndrome than with insufficient sleep; with likely contribution from the effect of intermittent hypoxemia, increased sympathetic tone, and behavioral tendencies that lean toward obesity.
- Intermittent hypoxemia from sleep-disordered breathing may exert its effect on stearoyl-CoA desaturase-1, leading to elevated triglycerides, low-density lipoprotein and lower high-density lipoprotein cholesterol.
- Treatment for obstructive sleep apnea in childhood has less consistent results and may be associated with further weight gain, but will likely benefit metabolic complications of obesity in the long term.
- Interventions targeting weight loss may allow for improvement in sleep duration and sleep-disordered breathing.

Summary

MetS is a collective of cardiovascular risk factors, including dysregulation of glucose metabolism, dyslipidemia, elevated BP, and truncal obesity, which may be worsened by sleep curtailment, sleep fragmentation, and circadian factors. OSA is a common disorder in obese children that may further predispose children to the downstream consequences of obesity. Studies implicate increased sympathetic activity, inflammation, intermittent hypoxemia, and the involvement of adipocytokines as mechanisms that cause MetS. Obesity holds a central role in contributing to the pathogenesis of the various components of MetS. There is evidence that short sleep increases the risk of being overweight in children. The rising rate of obesity must be taken seriously as a potential source of increased rates of both MetS and SDB.

References

1. Ford ES. Risks for all-cause mortality, cardiovascular disease, and diabetes associated with the metabolic syndrome: A summary of the evidence. *Diabetes Care*. 2005;28:1769–1778.
2. Ford ES, Li C, Sattar N. Metabolic syndrome and incident diabetes: Current state of the evidence. *Diabetes Care*. 2008;31:1898–1904.
3. Pladevall M, Singal B, Williams LK, Brotons C, Guyer H, Sadurni J, Falces C, Serrano-Rios M, Gabriel R, Shaw JE, Zimmet PZ, Haffner S. A single factor underlies the metabolic syndrome: A confirmatory factor analysis. *Diabetes Care*. 2006;29:113–122.
4. Kerr AG, Andersson DP, Rydén M, Arner P. Insulin resistance in adipocytes: Novel insights into the pathophysiology of metabolic syndrome. *Clin Nutr*. https://doi.org/10.1016/j.clnu.2023.12.012. Published online December 19, 2023.
5. Reinehr T, de Sousa G, Toschke AM, Andler W. Comparison of metabolic syndrome prevalence using eight different definitions: A critical approach. *Arch Dis Child*. 2007;92:1067–1072.
6. Goodman E, Daniels SR, Meigs JB, Dolan LM. Instability in the diagnosis of metabolic syndrome in adolescents. *Circulation*. 2007;115:2316–2322.
7. Gustafson JK, Yanoff LB, Easter BD, Brady SM, Keil MF, Roberts MD, Sebring NG, Han JC, Yanovski SZ, Hubbard VS, Yanovski JA. The stability of metabolic syndrome in children and adolescents. *J Clin Endocrinol Metab*. 2009;94:4828–4834.
8. Toledo-Corral CM, Ventura EE, Hodis HN, Weigensberg MJ, Lane CJ, Li Y, Goran MI. Persistence of the metabolic syndrome and its influence on carotid artery intima media thickness in overweight Latino children. *Atherosclerosis*. 2009;206:594–598.
9. Morrison JA, Friedman LA, Wang P, Glueck CJ. Metabolic syndrome in childhood predicts adult metabolic syndrome and type 2 diabetes mellitus 25 to 30 years later. *J Pediatr*. 2008;152:201–206.
10. Sorof JM, Lai D, Turner J, Poffenbarger T, Portman RJ. Overweight, ethnicity, and the prevalence of hypertension in school-aged children. *Pediatrics*. 2004;113:475–482.
11. Sinha R, Fisch G, Teague B, Tamborlane WV, Banyas B, Allen K, Savoye M, Rieger V, Taksali S, Barbetta G, Sherwin RS, Caprio S. Prevalence of impaired glucose tolerance among children and adolescents with marked obesity. *N Engl J Med*. 2002;346:802–810.
12. Steinberger J, Moorehead C, Katch V, Rocchini AP. Relationship between insulin resistance and abnormal lipid profile in obese adolescents. *J Pediatr*. 1995;126:690–695.
13. Arslanian S, Suprasongsin C. Insulin sensitivity, lipids, and body composition in childhood: is "syndrome X" present? *J Clin Endocrinol Metab*. 1996;81:1058–1062.
14. Cook DG, Mendall MA, Whincup PH, Carey IM, Ballam L, Morris JE, Miller GJ, Strachan DP. C-reactive protein concentration in children: Relationship to adiposity and other cardiovascular risk factors. *Atherosclerosis*. 2000;149:139–150.
15. Ford ES, National H, Nutrition Examination S. C-reactive protein concentration and cardiovascular disease risk factors in children: Findings from the National Health and Nutrition Examination Survey 1999–2000. *Circulation*. 2003;108:1053–1058.
16. Visser M, Bouter LM, McQuillan GM, Wener MH, Harris TB. Low-grade systemic inflammation in overweight children. *Pediatrics*. 2001;107:E13.
17. Tounian P, Aggoun Y, Dubern B, Varille V, Guy-Grand B, Sidi D, Girardet JP, Bonnet D. Presence of increased stiffness of the common carotid artery and endothelial dysfunction in severely obese children: A prospective study. *Lancet*. 2001;358:1400–1404.
18. Wardle J, Cooke L. The impact of obesity on psychological well-being. *Best Pract Res Clin Endocrinol Metab*. 2005;19:421–440.
19. Deng X, He M, He D, Zhu Y, Zhang Z, Niu W. Sleep duration and obesity in children and adolescents: Evidence from an updated and dose-response meta-analysis. *Sleep Med*. 2021;78:169–181.
20. Guo Y, Miller MA, Cappuccio FP. Short duration of sleep and incidence of overweight or obesity in Chinese children and adolescents: A systematic review and meta-analysis of prospective studies. *Nutr Metab Cardiovasc Dis*. 2021;31:363–371.
21. Miller MA, Kruisbrink M, Wallace J, Ji C, Cappuccio FP. Sleep duration and incidence of obesity in infants, children, and adolescents: A systematic review and meta-analysis of prospective studies. *Sleep*. 2018;41
22. Guilleminault C, Powell NB, Martinez S, Kushida C, Raffray T, Palombini L, Philip P. Preliminary observations on the effects of sleep time in a sleep restriction paradigm. *Sleep Med*. 2003;4:177–184.
23. Spiegel K, Leproult R, L'Hermite-Baleriaux M, Copinschi G, Penev PD, Van Cauter E. Leptin levels are dependent on sleep duration: Relationships with sympathovagal balance, carbohydrate regulation, cortisol, and thyrotropin. *J Clin Endocrinol Metab*. 2004;89:5762–5771.
24. Taheri S, Lin L, Austin D, Young T, Mignot E. Short sleep duration is associated with reduced leptin, elevated ghrelin, and increased body mass index. *PLoS Med*. 2004;1:e62.
25. Wren AM, Seal LJ, Cohen MA, Brynes AE, Frost GS, Murphy KG, Dhillo WS, Ghatei MA, Bloom SR. Ghrelin enhances appetite and increases food intake in humans. *J Clin Endocrinol Metab*. 2001;86:5992.
26. Levin F, Edholm T, Schmidt PT, Gryback P, Jacobsson H, Degerblad M, Hoybye C, Holst JJ, Rehfeld JF, Hellstrom PM, Naslund E. Ghrelin stimulates gastric emptying and

hunger in normal-weight humans. *J Clin Endocrinol Metab.* 2006;91:3296–3302.

27. Mars M, de Graaf C, de Groot CP, van Rossum CT, Kok FJ. Fasting leptin and appetite responses induced by a 4-day 65%-energy-restricted diet. *Int J Obes.* 2006;30:122–128.

28. Buxton OM, Cain SW, O'Connor SP, Porter JH, Duffy JF, Wang W, Czeisler CA, Shea SA. Adverse metabolic consequences in humans of prolonged sleep restriction combined with circadian disruption. *Sci Transl Med.* 2012;4 129ra143.

29. Watson NF, Harden KP, Buchwald D, Vitiello MV, Pack AI, Weigle DS, Goldberg J. Sleep duration and body mass index in twins: A gene-environment interaction. *Sleep.* 2012;35:597–603.

30. Brand C, Sehn AP, Todendi PF, de Moura Valim AR, Mattevi VS, Garcia-Hermoso A, Reis Gaya A, Reuter CP. The genetic predisposition to obesity has no influence on waist circumference when screen time and sleep duration are adequate in children and adolescents. *Eur J Sport Sci.* 2022;22:1757–1764.

31. Nedeltcheva AV, Kilkus JM, Imperial J, Kasza K, Schoeller DA, Penev PD. Sleep curtailment is accompanied by increased intake of calories from snacks. *Am J Clin Nutr.* 2009;89:126–133.

32. Brondel L, Romer MA, Nougues PM, Touyarou P, Davenne D. Acute partial sleep deprivation increases food intake in healthy men. *Am J Clin Nutr.* 2010;91:1550–1559.

33. Jensen CD, Duraccio KM, Barnett KA, et al. Sleep duration differentially affects brain activation in response to food images in adolescents with overweight/obesity compared to adolescents with normal weight. *Sleep.* 2019;42:1–11.

34. Chahal HS, St Fort N, Bero L. Availability, prices and affordability of essential medicines in Haiti. *J Glob Health.* 2013;3:020405.

35. Hayes JF, Balantekin KN, Altman M, Wilfley DE, Taylor CB, Williams J. Sleep patterns and quality are associated with severity of obesity and weight-related behaviors in adolescents with overweight and obesity. *Child Obes.* 2018;14:11–17.

36. Yeo SC, Jos AM, Erwin C, Lee SM, Lee XK, Lo JC, Chee MWL, Gooley JJ. Associations of sleep duration on school nights with self-rated health, overweight, and depression symptoms in adolescents: Problems and possible solutions. *Sleep Med.* 2019;60:96–108.

37. Steinberger J, Moran A, Hong CP, Jacobs Jr. DR, Sinaiko AR. Adiposity in childhood predicts obesity and insulin resistance in young adulthood. *J Pediatr.* 2001;138:469–473.

38. Sinaiko AR, Donahue RP, Jacobs Jr. DR, Prineas RJ. Relation of weight and rate of increase in weight during childhood and adolescence to body size, blood pressure, fasting insulin, and lipids in young adults. The Minneapolis Children's Blood Pressure Study. *Circulation.* 1999;99:1471–1476.

39. Taksali SE, Caprio S, Dziura J, Dufour S, Cali AM, Goodman TR, Papademetris X, Burgert TS, Pierpont BM, Savoye M, Shaw M, Seyal AA, Weiss R. High visceral and low abdominal subcutaneous fat stores in the obese adolescent: A determinant of an adverse metabolic phenotype. *Diabetes.* 2008;57:367–371.

40. Gozal D, Capdevila OS, Kheirandish-Gozal L. Metabolic alterations and systemic inflammation in obstructive sleep apnea among nonobese and obese prepubertal children. *Am J Respir Crit Care Med.* 2008;177:1142–1149.

41. Tauman R, O'Brien LM, Ivanenko A, Gozal D. Obesity rather than severity of sleep-disordered breathing as the major determinant of insulin resistance and altered lipidemia in snoring children. *Pediatrics.* 2005;116:e66–e73.

42. de la Eva RC, Baur LA Donaghue KC, Waters KA. Metabolic correlates with obstructive sleep apnea in obese subjects. *J Pediatr.* 2002;140:654–659.

43. Rosen CL, Larkin EK, Kirchner HL, Emancipator JL, Bivins SF, Surovec SA, Martin RJ, Redline S. Prevalence and risk factors for sleep-disordered breathing in 8- to 11-year-old children: Association with race and prematurity. *J Pediatr.* 2003;142:383–389.

44. Castronovo V, Zucconi M, Nosetti L, Marazzini C, Hensley M, Veglia F, Nespoli L, Ferini-Strambi L. Prevalence of habitual snoring and sleep-disordered breathing in preschool-aged children in an Italian community. *J Pediatr.* 2003;142:377–382.

45. Kalra M, Inge T, Garcia V, Daniels S, Lawson L, Curti R, Cohen A, Amin R. Obstructive sleep apnea in extremely overweight adolescents undergoing bariatric surgery. *Obes. Res.* 2005;13:1175–1179.

46. Marcus CL, Curtis S, Koerner CB, Joffe A, Serwint JR, Loughlin GM. Evaluation of pulmonary function and polysomnography in obese children and adolescents. *Pediatr Pulmonol.* 1996;21:176–183.

47. Silvestri JM, Weese-Mayer DE, Bass MT, Kenny AS, Hauptman SA, Pearsall SM. Polysomnography in obese children with a history of sleep-associated breathing disorders. *Pediatr Pulmonol.* 1993;16:124–129.

48. Gordon JE, Hughes MS, Shepherd K, Szymanski DA, Schoenecker PL, Parker L, Uong EC. Obstructive sleep apnoea syndrome in morbidly obese children with tibia vara. *J Bone Joint Surg Br.* 2006;88:100–103.

49. Mortimore IL, Marshall I, Wraith PK, Sellar RJ, Douglas NJ. Neck and total body fat deposition in nonobese and obese patients with sleep apnea compared with that in control subjects. *Am J Respir Crit Care Med.* 1998;157:280–283.

50. Stauffer JL, Buick MK, Bixler EO, Sharkey FE, Abt AB, Manders EK, Kales A, Cadieux RJ, Barry JD, Zwillich CW. Morphology of the uvula in obstructive sleep apnea. *Am Rev Respir Dis.* 1989;140:724–728.

51. Schwab RJ. Imaging for the snoring and sleep apnea patient. *Dent Clin North Am.* 2001;45:759–796.

52. Kirkness JP, Schwartz AR, Schneider H, Punjabi NM, Maly JJ, Laffan AM, McGinley BM, Magnuson T, Schweitzer M, Smith PL, Patil SP. Contribution of male sex, age, and obesity to mechanical instability of the upper airway during sleep. *J Appl Physiol.* 2008;104:1618–1624.

53. Schwartz AR, Gold AR, Schubert N, Stryzak A, Wise RA, Permutt S, Smith PL. Effect of weight loss on upper airway collapsibility in obstructive sleep apnea. *Am Rev Respir Dis.* 1991;144:494–498.

54. Arens R, Muzumdar H. Childhood obesity and obstructive sleep apnea syndrome. *J Appl Physiol.* 2010;108:436–444.

55. Harsch IA, Konturek PC, Koebnick C, Kuehnlein PP, Fuchs FS, Pour Schahin S, Wiest GH, Hahn EG, Lohmann T, Ficker JH. Leptin and ghrelin levels in patients with obstructive sleep apnoea: Effect of CPAP treatment. *Eur Respir. J.* 2003;22:251–257.

56. Ip MS, Lam KS, Ho C, Tsang KW, Lam W. Serum leptin and vascular risk factors in obstructive sleep apnea. *Chest.* 2000;118:580–586.

57. Vgontzas AN, Papanicolaou DA, Bixler EO, Hopper K, Lotsikas A, Lin HM, Kales A, Chrousos GP. Sleep apnea and daytime sleepiness and fatigue: Relation to visceral obesity, insulin resistance, and hypercytokinemia. *J Clin Endocrinol Metab.* 2000;85:1151–1158.

58. Tauman R, Serpero LD, Capdevila OS, O'Brien LM, Goldbart AD, Kheirandish-Gozal L, Gozal D. Adipokines in children with sleep disordered breathing. *Sleep*. 2007;30:443–449.

59. Nakra N, Bhargava S, Dzuira J, Caprio S, Bazzy-Asaad A. Sleep-disordered breathing in children with metabolic syndrome: The role of leptin and sympathetic nervous system activity and the effect of continuous positive airway pressure. *Pediatrics*. 2008;122:e634–e642.

60. Smiley A, King D, Bidulescu A. The Association between Sleep Duration and Metabolic Syndrome: The NHANES 2013/2014. *Nutrients*. 2019;11:2582.

61. Iglayreger HB, Peterson MD, Liu D, Parker CA, Woolford SJ, Sallinen Gafka BJ, Hassan F, Gordon PM. Sleep duration predicts cardiometabolic risk in obese adolescents. *J Pediatr*. 2014;164:1085–1090. e1081.

62. Hemati Z, Mozafarian N, Heshmat R, Ahadi Z, Motlagh ME, Ziaodini H, Taheri M, Aminaee T, Qorbani M, Kelishadi R. Association of sleep duration with metabolic syndrome and its components in children and adolescents; a propensity score-matched analysis: The CASPIAN-V study. *Diabetol Metab Syndr*. 2018;10:78.

63. Redline S, Storfer-Isser A, Rosen CL, Johnson NL, Kirchner HL, Emancipator J, Kibler AM. Association between metabolic syndrome and sleep-disordered breathing in adolescents. *Am J Respir Crit Care Med*. 2007;176:401–408.

64. Wong PM, Hasler BP, Kamarck TW, Muldoon MF, Manuck SB. Social jetlag, chronotype, and cardiometabolic risk. *J Clin Endocrinol Metab*. 2015;100:4612–4620.

65. Boyle PJ, Scott JC, Krentz AJ, Nagy RJ, Comstock E, Hoffman C. Diminished brain glucose metabolism is a significant determinant for falling rates of systemic glucose utilization during sleep in normal humans. *J Clin Invest*. 1994;93:529–535.

66. Maquet P. Functional neuroimaging of normal human sleep by positron emission tomography. *J Sleep Res*. 2000;9:207–231.

67. Peschke E. Melatonin, endocrine pancreas and diabetes. *J Pineal Res*. 2008;44:26–40.

68. da Silva AA, do Carmo JM, Hall JE. CNS Regulation of glucose homeostasis: Role of the leptin-melanocortin system. *Curr Diab Rep*. 2020;20:29.

69. Oster H, Challet E, Ott V, Arvat E, de Kloet ER, Dijk DJ, Lightman S, Vgontzas A, Van Cauter E. The functional and clinical significance of the 24-hour rhythm of circulating glucocorticoids. *Endocr Rev*. 2017;38:3–45.

70. Klingenberg L, Chaput JP, Holmback U, Visby T, Jennum P, Nikolic M, Astrup A, Sjodin A. Acute sleep restriction reduces insulin sensitivity in adolescent boys. *Sleep*. 2013;36:1085–1090.

71. Rayner DV, Trayhurn P. Regulation of leptin production: Sympathetic nervous system interactions. *J Mol Med (Berl)*. 2001;79:8–20.

72. Hart CN, Carskadon MA, Considine RV, Fava JL, Lawton J, Raynor HA, Jelalian E, Owens J, Wing R. Changes in children's sleep duration on food intake, weight, and leptin. *Pediatrics*. 2013;132:e1473–e1480.

73. Wondmkun YT. Obesity, Insulin resistance, and type 2 diabetes: Associations and therapeutic implications. *Diabetes Metab Syndr Obes*. 2020;13:3611–3616.

74. Cappuccio FP, D'Elia L, Strazzullo P, Miller MA. Quantity and quality of sleep and incidence of type 2 diabetes: A systematic review and meta-analysis. *Diabetes Care*. 2010;33:414–420.

75. Lee SWH, Ng KY, Chin WK. The impact of sleep amount and sleep quality on glycemic control in type 2 diabetes: A systematic review and meta-analysis. *Sleep Med Rev*. 2017;31:91–101.

76. Shan Z, Ma H, Xie M, Yan P, Guo Y, Bao W, Rong Y, Jackson CL, Hu FB, Liu L. Sleep duration and risk of type 2 diabetes: A meta-analysis of prospective studies. *Diabetes Care*. 2015;38:529–537.

77. Dutil C, Chaput JP. Inadequate sleep as a contributor to type 2 diabetes in children and adolescents. *Nutr Diabetes*. 2017;7:e266.

78. Hjorth MF, Chaput JP, Damsgaard CT, Dalskov SM, Andersen R, Astrup A, Michaelsen KF, Tetens I, Ritz C, Sjodin A. Low physical activity level and short sleep duration are associated with an increased cardio-metabolic risk profile: A longitudinal study in 8-11 year old Danish children. *PLoS One*. 2014;9:e104677.

79. Shaw ND, McHill AW, Schiavon M, Kangarloo T, Mankowski PW, Cobelli C, Klerman EB, Hall JE. Effect of slow wave sleep disruption on metabolic parameters in adolescents. *Sleep*. 2016;39:1591–1599.

80. Kent BD, Grote L, Ryan S, Pepin JL, Bonsignore MR, Tkacova R, Saaresranta T, Verbraecken J, Levy P, Hedner J, McNicholas WT. Diabetes mellitus prevalence and control in sleep-disordered breathing: The European Sleep Apnea Cohort (ESADA) study. *Chest*. 2014;146:982–990.

81. Seicean S, Kirchner HL, Gottlieb DJ, Punjabi NM, Resnick H, Sanders M, Budhiraja R, Singer M, Redline S. Sleep-disordered breathing and impaired glucose metabolism in normal-weight and overweight/obese individuals: The Sleep Heart Health Study. *Diabetes Care*. 2008;31:1001–1006.

82. Nagayoshi M, Punjabi NM, Selvin E, Pankow JS, Shahar E, Iso H, Folsom AR, Lutsey PL. Obstructive sleep apnea and incident type 2 diabetes. *Sleep Med*. 2016;25:156–161.

83. Bhatt SP, Guleria R, Kabra SK. Metabolic alterations and systemic inflammation in overweight/obese children with obstructive sleep apnea. *PLoS One*. 2021;16:e0252353.

84. Bhushan B, Ayub B, Loghmanee DA, Billings KR. Metabolic alterations in adolescents with obstructive sleep apnea. *Int J Pediatr Otorhinolaryngol*. 2015;79:2368–2373.

85. Bhushan B, Maddalozzo J, Sheldon SH, Haymond S, Rychlik K, Lales GC, Billings KR. Metabolic alterations in children with obstructive sleep apnea. *Int J Pediatr Otorhinolaryngol*. 2014;78:854–859.

86. Corgosinho FC, Ackel-D'Elia C, Tufik S, Damaso AR, de Piano A, Sanches de L, Campos RM, Silva PL, Carnier J, Tock L, Andersen ML, Moreira GA, Pradella-Hallinan M, Oyama LM, de Mello MT. Beneficial effects of a multifaceted 1-year lifestyle intervention on metabolic abnormalities in obese adolescents with and without sleep-disordered breathing. *Metab Syndr Relat Disord*. 2015;13:110–118.

87. Nandalike K, Agarwal C, Strauss T, Coupey SM, Isasi CR, Sin S, Arens R. Sleep and cardiometabolic function in obese adolescent girls with polycystic ovary syndrome. *Sleep Med*. 2012;13:1307–1312.

88. Watson SE, Li Z, Tu W, Jalou H, Brubaker JL, Gupta S, Huber JN, Carroll A, Hannon TS. Obstructive sleep apnoea in obese adolescents and cardiometabolic risk markers. *Pediatr Obes*. 2014;9:471–477.

89. Lesser DJ, Bhatia R, Tran WH, Oliveira F, Ortega R, Keens TG, Mittelman SD, Khoo MC, Davidson Ward SL. Sleep fragmentation and intermittent hypoxemia are associated with

decreased insulin sensitivity in obese adolescent Latino males. *Pediatr Res.* 2012;72:293–298.

90. Kelly A, Dougherty S, Cucchiara A, Marcus CL, Brooks LJ. Catecholamines, adiponectin, and insulin resistance as measured by HOMA in children with obstructive sleep apnea. *Sleep.* 2010;33:1185–1191.

91. Kalra M, Kumar S, Chakraborty R, et al. Association of obstructive sleep apnea with hyperinsulinemia in adolsecents with severe obesity. *Mineva Pneumol.* 2007;46:151–156.

92. Hannon TS, Lee S, Chakravorty S, Lin Y, Arslanian SA. Sleep-disordered breathing in obese adolescents is associated with visceral adiposity and markers of insulin resistance. *Int J Pediatr Obes.* 2011;6:157–160.

93. Koeck ES, Barefoot LC, Hamrick M, Owens JA, Qureshi FG, Nadler EP. Predicting sleep apnea in morbidly obese adolescents undergoing bariatric surgery. *Surg Endosc.* 2014;28:1146–1152.

94. Sundaram SS, Sokol RJ, Capocelli KE, Pan Z, Sullivan JS, Robbins K, Halbower AC. Obstructive sleep apnea and hypoxemia are associated with advanced liver histology in pediatric nonalcoholic fatty liver disease. *J Pediatr.* 2014;164:699–706. e691.

95. Van Hoorenbeeck K, Franckx H, Debode P, Aerts P, Ramet J, Van Gaal LF, Desager KN, De Backer WA, Verhulst SL. Metabolic disregulation in obese adolescents with sleep-disordered breathing before and after weight loss. *Obesity (Silver Spring).* 2013;21:1446–1450.

96. Patinkin ZW, Feinn R, Santos M. Metabolic consequences of obstructive sleep apnea in adolescents with obesity: A systematic literature review and meta-analysis. *Child Obes.* 2017;13:102–110.

97. Hoyos CM, Killick R, Yee BJ, Phillips CL, Grunstein RR, Liu PY. Cardiometabolic changes after continuous positive airway pressure for obstructive sleep apnoea: A randomised sham-controlled study. *Thorax.* 2012;67:1081–1089.

98. Kohler M, Stoewhas AC, Ayers L, Senn O, Bloch KE, Russi EW, Stradling JR. Effects of continuous positive airway pressure therapy withdrawal in patients with obstructive sleep apnea: A randomized controlled trial. *Am J Respir Crit Care Med.* 2011;184:1192–1199.

99. Salord N, Fortuna AM, Monasterio C, Gasa M, Perez A, Bonsignore MR, Vilarrasa N, Montserrat JM, Mayos M. A randomized controlled trial of continuous positive airway pressure on glucose tolerance in obese patients with obstructive sleep apnea. *Sleep.* 2016;39:35–41.

100. Lam JC, Lam B, Yao TJ, Lai AY, Ooi CG, Tam S, Lam KS, Ip MS. A randomised controlled trial of nasal continuous positive airway pressure on insulin sensitivity in obstructive sleep apnoea. *Eur Respir J.* 2010;35:138–145.

101. Chirinos JA, Gurubhagavatula I, Teff K, Rader DJ, Wadden TA, Townsend R, Foster GD, Maislin G, Saif H, Broderick P, Chittams J, Hanlon AL, Pack AI. CPAP, weight loss, or both for obstructive sleep apnea. *N Engl J Med.* 2014;370:2265–2275.

102. Myhill PC, Davis WA, Peters KE, Chubb SA, Hillman D, Davis TM. Effect of continuous positive airway pressure therapy on cardiovascular risk factors in patients with type 2 diabetes and obstructive sleep apnea. *J Clin. Endocrinol Metab.* 2012;97:4212–4218.

103. Shaw JE, Punjabi NM, Naughton MT, Willes L, Bergenstal RM, Cistulli PA, Fulcher GR, Richards GN, Zimmet PZ. The Effect of treatment of obstructive sleep apnea on glycemic control in type 2 diabetes. *Am J Respir Crit Care Med.* 2016;194:486–492.

104. West SD, Nicoll DJ, Wallace TM, Matthews DR, Stradling JR. Effect of CPAP on insulin resistance and HbA1c in men

with obstructive sleep apnoea and type 2 diabetes. *Thorax.* 2007;62:969–974.

105. Martinez-Ceron E, Barquiel B, Bezos AM, Casitas R, Galera R, Garcia-Benito C, Hernanz A, Alonso-Fernandez A, Garcia-Rio F. Effect of continuous positive airway pressure on glycemic control in patients with obstructive sleep apnea and type 2 diabetes. A randomized clinical trial. *Am J Respir Crit Care Med.* 2016;194:476–485.

106. Lam JCM, Lai AYK, Tam TCC, Yuen MMA, Lam KSL, Ip MSM. CPAP therapy for patients with sleep apnea and type 2 diabetes mellitus improves control of blood pressure. *Sleep Breath.* 2017;21:377–386.

107. Pamidi S, Wroblewski K, Stepien M, Sharif-Sidi K, Kilkus J, Whitmore H, Tasali E. Eight hours of nightly continuous positive airway pressure treatment of obstructive sleep apnea improves glucose metabolism in patients with prediabetes. A randomized controlled trial. *Am J Respir Crit Care Med.* 2015;192:96–105.

108. Weinstock TG, Wang X, Rueschman M, Ismail-Beigi F, Aylor J, Babineau DC, Mehra R, Redline S. A controlled trial of CPAP therapy on metabolic control in individuals with impaired glucose tolerance and sleep apnea. *Sleep.* 2012;35:617–625B.

109. Quante M, Wang R, Weng J, Rosen CL, Amin R, Garetz SL, Katz E, Paruthi S, Arens R, Muzumdar H, Marcus CL, Ellenberg S, Redline S. Childhood Adenotonsillectomy Trial (CHAT). The effect of adenotonsillectomy for childhood sleep apnea on cardiometabolic measures. *Sleep.* 2015;38:1395–1403.

110. Anothaisintawee T, Lertrattananon D, Thamakaison S, Knutson KL, Thakkinstian A, Reutrakul S. Later chronotype is associated with higher hemoglobin A1c in prediabetes patients. *Chronobiol Int.* 2017;34:393–402.

111. Koopman ADM, Rauh SP, van't Riet E, Groeneveld L, van der Heijden AA, Elders PJ, Dekker JM, Nijpels G, Beulens JW, Rutters F. The Association between Social Jetlag, the Metabolic Syndrome, and Type 2 Diabetes Mellitus in the General Population: The New Hoorn Study. *J Biol Rhythms.* 2017;32:359–368.

112. Tomoda A, Kawatani J, Joudoi T, Hamada A, Miike T. Metabolic dysfunction and circadian rhythm abnormalities in adolescents with sleep disturbance. *Neuroimage.* 2009;47(Suppl 2):T21–T26.

113. Savransky V, Jun J, Li J, Nanayakkara A, Fonti S, Moser AB, Steele KE, Schweitzer MA, Patil SP, Bhanot S, Schwartz AR, Polotsky VY. Dyslipidemia and atherosclerosis induced by chronic intermittent hypoxia are attenuated by deficiency of stearoyl coenzyme A desaturase. *Circ Res.* 2008;103:1173–1180.

114. Li J, Thorne LN, Punjabi NM, Sun CK, Schwartz AR, Smith PL, Marino RL, Rodriguez A, Hubbard WC, O'Donnell CP, Polotsky VY. Intermittent hypoxia induces hyperlipidemia in lean mice. *Circ Res.* 2005;97:698–706.

115. Newman AB, Nieto FJ, Guidry U, Lind BK, Redline S, Pickering TG, Quan SF, Sleep Heart Health Study Research G. Relation of sleep-disordered breathing to cardiovascular disease risk factors: The Sleep Heart Health Study. *Am J Epidemiol.* 2001;154:50–59.

116. Roche F, Sforza E, Pichot V, Maudoux D, Garcin A, Celle S, Picard-Kossovsky M, Gaspoz JM, Barthelemy JC, Group PS. Obstructive sleep apnoea/hypopnea influences high-density lipoprotein cholesterol in the elderly. *Sleep Med.* 2009;10:882–886.

117. Coughlin SR, Mawdsley L, Mugarza JA, Calverley PM, Wilding JP. Obstructive sleep apnoea is independently associated with

an increased prevalence of metabolic syndrome. *Eur Heart J.* 2004;25:735–741.

118. Czerniawska J, Bielen P, Plywaczewski R, Czystowska M, Korzybski D, Sliwinski P, Gorecka D. Metabolic abnormalities in obstructive sleep apnea patients. *Pneumonol Alergol Pol.* 2008;76:340–347.

119. Tan KC, Chow WS, Lam JC, Lam B, Wong WK, Tam S, Ip MS. HDL dysfunction in obstructive sleep apnea. *Atherosclerosis.* 2006;184:377–382.

120. Drager LF, Bortolotto LA, Lorenzi MC, Figueiredo AC, Krieger EM, Lorenzi-Filho G. Early signs of atherosclerosis in obstructive sleep apnea. *Am J Respir Crit Care Med.* 2005;172:613–618.

121. Drager LF, Bortolotto LA, Maki-Nunes C, Trombetta IC, Alves MJ, Fraga RF, Negrao CE, Krieger EM, Lorenzi-Filho G. The incremental role of obstructive sleep apnoea on markers of atherosclerosis in patients with metabolic syndrome. *Atherosclerosis.* 2010;208:490–495.

122. Kono M, Tatsumi K, Saibara T, Nakamura A, Tanabe N, Takiguchi Y, Kuriyama T. Obstructive sleep apnea syndrome is associated with some components of metabolic syndrome. *Chest.* 2007;131:1387–1392.

123. Alonso-Alvarez ML, Teran-Santos J, Gonzalez Martinez M, Cordero-Guevara JA, Jurado-Luque MJ, Corral-Penafiel J, Duran-Cantolla J, Ordax Carbajo E, MasaJimenez F, Kheirandish-Gozal L, Gozal D, Spanish Sleep N. Metabolic biomarkers in community obese children: Effect of obstructive sleep apnea and its treatment. *Sleep Med.* 2017;37:1–9.

124. Landsberg L. Hyperinsulinemia: Possible role in obesity-induced hypertension. *Hypertension.* 1992;19:I61–I66.

125. Sorof J, Daniels S. Obesity hypertension in children: A problem of epidemic proportions. *Hypertension.* 2002;40:441–447.

126. Shepard Jr. JW. Hypertension, cardiac arrhythmias, myocardial infarction, and stroke in relation to obstructive sleep apnea. *Clin Chest Med.* 1992;13:437–458.

127. Ai S, Li Z, Wang S, Chen S, Chan JW, Au CT, Bao Y, Li AM, Zhang J, Chan KC, Wing YK. Blood pressure and childhood obstructive sleep apnea: A systematic review and meta-analysis. *Sleep Med Rev.* 2022;65:101663.

128. Kwok KL, Ng DK, Chan CH. Cardiovascular changes in children with snoring and obstructive sleep apnoea. *Ann Acad Med Singap.* 2008;37:715–721.

129. Zintzaras E, Kaditis AG. Sleep-disordered breathing and blood pressure in children: A meta-analysis. *Arch Pediatr Adolesc Med.* 2007;161:172–178.

130. Cespedes EM, Rifas-Shiman SL, Redline S, Gillman MW, Pena MM, Taveras EM. Longitudinal associations of sleep curtailment with metabolic risk in mid-childhood. *Obesity (Silver Spring).* 2014;22:2586–2592.

131. Archbold KH, Vasquez MM, Goodwin JL, Quan SF. Effects of sleep patterns and obesity on increases in blood pressure in a 5-year period: Report from the Tucson Children's Assessment of Sleep Apnea Study. *J Pediatr.* 2012;161:26–30.

132. Gangwisch JE, Heymsfield SB, Boden-Albala B, Buijs RM, Kreier F, Pickering TG, Rundle AG, Zammit GK, Malaspina D. Short sleep duration as a risk factor for hypertension: Analyses of the first National Health and Nutrition Examination Survey. *Hypertension.* 2006;47:833–839.

133. Narkiewicz K, Somers VK. Cardiovascular variability characteristics in obstructive sleep apnea. *Auton Neurosci.* 2001;90:89–94.

134. Harsch IA, Schahin SP, Bruckner K, Radespiel-Troger M, Fuchs FS, Hahn EG, Konturek PC, Lohmann T, Ficker JH. The effect of continuous positive airway pressure treatment on insulin sensitivity in patients with obstructive sleep apnoea syndrome and type 2 diabetes. *Respiration.* 2004;71:252–259.

135. Harsch IA, Schahin SP, Radespiel-Troger M, Weintz O, Jahreiss H, Fuchs FS, Wiest GH, Hahn EG, Lohmann T, Konturek PC, Ficker JH. Continuous positive airway pressure treatment rapidly improves insulin sensitivity in patients with obstructive sleep apnea syndrome. *Am J Respir Crit Care Med.* 2004;169:156–162.

136. Lavie L. Obstructive sleep apnoea syndrome–an oxidative stress disorder. *Sleep Med Rev.* 2003;7:35–51.

137. Raff H, Roarty TP. Renin, ACTH, and aldosterone during acute hypercapnia and hypoxia in conscious rats. *Am J Physiol.* 1988;254:R431–R435.

138. Van de Borne P, Nguyen H, Biston P, Linkowski P, Degaute JP. Effects of wake and sleep stages on the 24-h autonomic control of blood pressure and heart rate in recumbent men. *Am J Physiol.* 1994;266:H548–554.

139. Kario K, Schwartz JE, Pickering TG. Ambulatory physical activity as a determinant of diurnal blood pressure variation. *Hypertension.* 1999;34:685–691.

140. Somers VK, Dyken ME, Mark AL, Abboud FM. Sympathetic-nerve activity during sleep in normal subjects. *N Engl J Med.* 1993;328:303–307.

141. Lusardi P, Zoppi A, Preti P, Pesce RM, Piazza E, Fogari R. Effects of insufficient sleep on blood pressure in hypertensive patients: A 24-h study. *Am J Hypertens.* 1999;12:63–68.

142. Tochikubo O, Ikeda A, Miyajima E, Ishii M. Effects of insufficient sleep on blood pressure monitored by a new multibiomedical recorder. *Hypertension.* 1996;27:1318–1324.

143. Sayk F, Teckentrup C, Becker C, Heutling D, Wellhoner P, Lehnert H, Dodt C. Effects of selective slow-wave sleep deprivation on nocturnal blood pressure dipping and daytime blood pressure regulation. *Am J Physiol Regul Integr Comp Physiol.* 2010;298:R191–R197.

144. Kang KT, Yeh TH, Ko JY, Lee CH, Lin MT, Hsu WC. Effect of sleep surgery on blood pressure in adults with obstructive sleep apnea: A systematic review and meta-analysis. *Sleep Med Rev.* 2022;62:101590.

145. Friedman M, Wilson M, Lin HC, Chang HW. Updated systematic review of tonsillectomy and adenoidectomy for treatment of pediatric obstructive sleep apnea/hypopnea syndrome. *Otolaryngol Head Neck Surg.* 2009;140:800–808.

146. Tauman R, Gulliver TE, Krishna J, Montgomery-Downs HE, O'Brien LM, Ivanenko A, Gozal D. Persistence of obstructive sleep apnea syndrome in children after adenotonsillectomy. *J Pediatr.* 2006;149:803–808.

147. Mitchell RB, Kelly J. Outcome of adenotonsillectomy for obstructive sleep apnea in obese and normal-weight children. *Otolaryngol Head Neck Surg.* 2007;137:43–48.

148. Costa DJ, Mitchell R. Adenotonsillectomy for obstructive sleep apnea in obese children: A meta-analysis. *Otolaryngol Head Neck Surg.* 2009;140:455–460.

149. Aurora RN, Zak RS, Karippot A, Lamm CI, Morgenthaler TI, Auerbach SH, Bista SR, Casey KR, Chowdhuri S, Kristo DA, Ramar K, American Academy of Sleep M. Practice parameters for the respiratory indications for polysomnography in children. *Sleep.* 2011;34:379–388.

150. Van M, Khan I, Hussain SS. Short-term weight gain after adenotonsillectomy in children with obstructive sleep apnoea: Systematic review. *J Laryngol Otol.* 2016;130:214–218.

151. DelRosso LM, King J, Ferri R. Systolic blood pressure elevation in children with obstructive sleep apnea is improved with positive airway pressure use. *J Pediatr.* 2018;195:102–107. e101.

152. Andersen IG, Holm JC, Homoe P. Impact of weight-loss management on children and adolescents with obesity and obstructive sleep apnea. *Int J Pediatr Otorhinolaryngol.* 2019;123:57–62.

SECTION II

The Hypersomnias

17

Narcolepsy

Suresh Kotagal

CHAPTER HIGHLIGHTS

- Childhood narcolepsy differs from that of adults from the standpoint of sleepiness and cataplexy being relatively subtle initially, hence, leading to the diagnosis being overlooked. There can be a lag of over 10 years between onset of symptoms and definitive diagnosis. Reduced levels of cerebrospinal fluid hypocretin (orexin) may enable diagnosis in preschool-age children, and in those who are receiving psychotropic medications.
- Childhood cataplexy is unique because it may manifest itself mainly in the form of transient facial weakness. Patients with cataplexy are generally positive for the histocompatibility antigen *DQB1*0602* and show low levels of cerebrospinal fluid hypocretin (orexin). Precocious puberty and obesity are also unique features of childhood narcolepsy–cataplexy.
- Key features of narcolepsy on polysomnography include nocturnal sleep-onset rapid eye movement (REM) periods, disturbed night sleep, REM sleep without atonia, and REM sleep behavior disorder.
- Comorbidities include behavioral disturbances, obesity, anxiety, and mood disturbances. Successful management of narcolepsy requires that comorbidities are managed concurrently. The evidence for pharmacotherapy of narcolepsy is not as robust as that in adults, but it is evolving.

Introduction

In 1880, Jean-Baptiste-Edouard Gélineau described narcolepsy as a pathologic condition that was characterized by recurrent, brief attacks of sleepiness.[1] He recognized that the disorder was accompanied by falls or *astasias*, which were subsequently termed cataplexy. Narcolepsy is a lifelong neurologic disorder of rapid eye movement (REM) sleep and homeostatic sleep–wake regulatory mechanisms in which there are attacks of *irresistible daytime sleepiness, cataplexy* (sudden loss of muscle control in the legs, trunk, face, or neck in response to emotional stimuli such as laughter, fright, anticipation of reward, or rage), *hypnagogic hallucinations* (vivid dreams at sleep onset), *sleep paralysis* (momentary inability to move at the time of sleep onset), and disturbed night sleep.[2] There are two forms of the disorder: narcolepsy with cataplexy (NT1) and narcolepsy without cataplexy (NT2). This chapter provides an overview of childhood narcolepsy.

Epidemiology

In a community-based survey from Olmsted County, Minnesota, the incidence of narcolepsy was estimated at 1.37 per 100,000 persons per year: 1.72 for men and 1.05 for women.[3] It was at its highest in the second decade of life, followed by a gradual decline thereafter. The prevalence was approximately 56 persons per 100,000 persons. In Japan, the prevalence has been estimated at 1 in 600,[4] and in Israel at 1 in 500,000.[5] Based on a survey of 20- to 60-year-olds, the prevalence of narcolepsy with cataplexy in Norway was estimated at 0.022%.[6] The exact prevalence rate of narcolepsy in childhood has been difficult to establish. Some epidemiologic studies had required the presence of cataplexy as a prerequisite for the diagnosis,[7] whereas others[8] have not made this stipulation. The lack of uniformity in clinical diagnostic criteria may explain variability in estimations of the prevalence of narcolepsy.[9] There is a slight male predominance for prevalence; in the Olmsted County study, the male:female ratio was 1.8:1.3. Narcolepsy has been recognized as early as 1 year of age, though most subjects are adolescents at the time of diagnosis. The increasing awareness of childhood narcolepsy in the lay press and scientific circles may alter the incidence and prevalence figures over the next few years. A seasonal variation in the incidence of narcolepsy was observed in China, with the lowest incidence in early winter and the highest incidence in spring.[10] The data from China also indicate an almost 3-fold increase in the incidence of narcolepsy following the 2009 H1N1 influenza pandemic, which suggested likely molecular mimicry and immune-mediated disturbance in the pathogenesis of this disorder.[10] Although narcolepsy is often diagnosed in the third and fourth decades, a meta-analysis of 235 subjects derived from three studies by Challamel and coworkers found that 34% of all subjects had onset of symptoms prior to the age of 15 years, 16% prior to the age of 10 years, and 4.5% prior to the age of 5 years (Fig. 17.1).[11] The use of cerebrospinal fluid (CSF) hypocretin (orexin) assay may facilitate early diagnosis, especially in preschool-age children in whom traditional sleep study criteria cannot

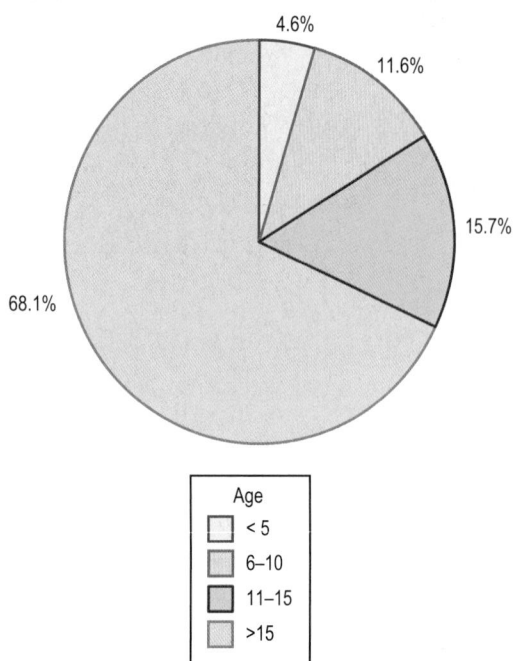

• **Fig. 17.1.** Age of onset of narcolepsy.[11]

be applied. A lag period of 10 years or more between the onset of symptoms and diagnosis has, however, been observed in adult subjects.[12,13] Cataplexy, the most reliable clinical feature of narcolepsy, may facilitate an earlier diagnosis of narcolepsy type 1. One the other hand, type 2 narcolepsy (without cataplexy), characterized mainly by sleepiness, may be more subtle and harder to recognize in its early stages.

Clinical Features

Preschool-Age Children

In their meta-analysis of 235 children, Challamel and coworkers found that 4.6% were <5 years at the time of diagnosis.[11] Sharp and D'Cruz have described a 12-month-old with hypersomnia who was subsequently confirmed to have narcolepsy.[14] In general, it is difficult to diagnose narcolepsy <4–5 years, because even unaffected children may take habitual daytime naps. Preschool-age children with narcolepsy may not be able to provide an accurate history of cataplexy, hypnagogic hallucinations, or sleep paralysis. The diagnosis may, however, be facilitated by documentation of cataplexy attacks on home cell phone in recorded video clips or on video-polysomnography (PSG), the latter showing skeletal muscle atonia and bursts of REMs coinciding with low-voltage, mixed-frequency activity on the electroencephalogram (EEG) during cataplexy attacks. The availability of CSF hypocretin (orexin) assay also facilitates the diagnosis of NT1 in preschool-age children (orexin levels are <110 pg/mL in NT1), but this does not apply to NT2, which is associated with hypocretin levels >110 pg/mL.

School-Age Children

Daytime sleepiness is an invariant and the most disabling feature. It appears as early as 5–6 years of age. There is a background of a constant, foggy feeling from drowsiness, superimposed on which are periods of more dramatic sleep attacks. Habitual afternoon napping is uncommon in healthy children older than age 5 or 6 years, and should raise a suspicion of narcolepsy. Several excellent sleep questionnaires are available for the initial assessment of sleepiness and longitudinal follow-up. The Pediatric Daytime Sleepiness Scale[15] and the Epworth Sleepiness Scale–Children and Adolescents[16] are two common sleep questionnaires. Naps in children with narcolepsy tend to be longer than those in adult patients (generally 30 to 90 minutes), and may not be consistently followed by a refreshed feeling.[16] The attacks of sleepiness are most likely to occur when the patient is carrying out monotonous or sedentary activities such as sitting in a classroom or reading a book. Sleepiness occurs regardless of the length of night sleep. The daytime sleepiness is frequently associated with automatic behavior of which the subject is unaware, and with impaired consolidation of memory, decreased concentration, executive dysfunction, and school-related learning problems. The irritability and mood swings that accompany sleepiness can mimic depression.[17,18] Children with daytime sleepiness may be mislabeled "lazy" and become the target of negative comments from their peers. Excessive sleepiness might also be overlooked by the parents until it starts adversely impacting mood, behavior, or academic performance. The behavioral changes are a consequence of impairment of function of the ventrolateral prefrontal cortex from sleepiness.[19]

Cataplexy, the second most common but most specific feature of narcolepsy, consists of a sudden loss of muscle tone in face, neck, back, or thigh muscles in response to emotional triggers such as laughter, fright, rage, excitement, surprise, or the anticipation of a reward. It is caused by the intrusion of the REM sleep–associated skeletal muscle atonia onto wakefulness.[20] Cataplexy is associated with hyperpolarization of spinal alpha motor neurons, with resultant atonia and areflexia due to active inhibition of skeletal muscle tone and a suppression of the monosynaptic H-reflex. A history of cataplexy may be difficult to elicit in young children. The author recalls a 6-year-old girl with proven narcolepsy who denied any episodic muscle weakness but would repeatedly fall down whenever she jumped on a trampoline. Consciousness remains intact during the cataplexy episodes, which can last 1–30 minutes. Respiration and cardiovascular function are unaffected. Challamel and coworkers found cataplexy in 80.5% of idiopathic narcolepsy and in 95% of symptomatic narcolepsy subjects.[11] Some of the unique features of childhood cataplexy include that it can be fairly subtle, and may be characterized often by transient facial weakness, with eyelid drooping, mouth falling open, and a slight head roll.[21]

Hypnagogic hallucinations are vivid dreams at sleep onset. They are vivid and sometimes frightening dreams upon awakening from sleep. *Sleep paralysis* is the momentary inability to move the body at sleep onset. These three phenomena at sleep onset/offset are related to intrusion of elements of REM sleep onto wakefulness.

Disturbed night sleep is common in narcolepsy. It is likely due to a decreased sleep homeostatic drive and altered non-REM (NREM)–REM sleep interaction.[22] Nocturnal arousals may be related to periodic or *aperiodic* limb movements. Periodic limb movements (PLMs) are rhythmic muscle contractions of 0.5–5 seconds' duration, with an inter-movement interval of 5–120 seconds, occurring in series of three or more, usually during stage N1 or N2. They may or may not be associated with evidence of cortical arousal on EEG. PLMs may be a marker for underlying restless legs syndrome.

Psychosocial problems in children with narcolepsy have been studied.[23] Compared with controls with hypersomnolence from other causes, children with narcolepsy show more behavioral difficulties, depressed mood, and impaired quality of life.

Obesity may develop at the onset of NT1, in association with hyperphagia and binge eating. It may be related to orexin deficiency, to the loss of the physiologic rise in leptin levels at night (leptin acts as an appetite suppressant), or to sedentary behavior and decreased basal metabolism. Weight gain at onset of NT1 is not related to prior use of anticholinergic medications, as it develops even before initiation of treatment with these drugs.[24] The weight gain may be accompanied by obstructive sleep apnea. *Precocious puberty* may also be seen in preteen boys and girls at onset of NT1.[25]

Infrequently, *REM sleep behavior disorder* (RBD) can be a presenting manifestation of narcolepsy.[26,27] It is characterized by motor dream enactment, typically in the form of flailing of arms and legs and yelling behavior during dreams. The PSG shows *REM sleep without atonia*, i.e., the persistence of muscle tone during REM sleep. The pathogenesis is decreased activity of the "REM off" neurons located in the sublaterodorsal region of the pons. Under physiologic conditions, these neurons, which are influenced by hypocretin, serve to inhibit muscle tone in REM sleep.[28]

Pathophysiology

The study of narcolepsy in humans has been advanced by its study in animals. Narcolepsy has been investigated in cats, miniature horses, quarter horses, Brahman bulls, and about 15 breeds of dogs. In animals, it shows a monogenic, autosomal recessive pattern of inheritance.[29] Cataplexy can be induced in cats by the injection of carbachol (an acetylcholine-like substance) into the pontine reticular formation.[30] Specifically, muscarinic type-2 receptors of acetylcholine have been implicated.[31] The food-elicited cataplexy test, used to study cataplexy in dogs, is based upon the supposition that the time taken for the consumption of food by narcoleptic animals whose eating is interrupted by cataplexy attacks is much longer than in animals without narcolepsy.

In 1999, Lin and coworkers demonstrated that canine narcolepsy is caused by a mutation in the hypocretin receptor-2 (orexin-2) gene.[32] Around the same time, Chemelli and colleagues established that a null mutation for the hypocretin-1 and hypocretin-2 peptides in mice produces aspects resembling human narcolepsy, including cataplexy.[33] The hypocretin-containing neurons are located primarily in the dorsolateral hypothalamus. They have widespread projections to the basal forebrain, amygdala, medial nuclei of the thalamus, periaqueductal gray matter, reticular formation, pedunculopontine nucleus, locus coeruleus, raphe nucleus, pontine tegmentum, and dorsal spinal cord.[20] Hypocretins 1 and 2 are peptides that are synthesized from preprohypocretin, and have corresponding receptors. Hypocretins stimulate food intake, increase the basal metabolic rate, and promote arousal.[33] The intravenous administration of hypocretin-1 (orexin A) in narcoleptic Doberman pinschers reduces cataplexy for up to 3 days, increases motor activity, promotes waking, and reduces sleep fragmentation in a dose-dependent manner.[34]

Histocompatibility Antigens and Human Narcolepsy

In 1984, an association between human narcolepsy and human leukocyte antigen (HLA) DR2 was reported in Japan by Juji and coworkers.[35] This association has been observed in other geographic regions of the world as well.[36–38] Consequently, an immunologic mechanism was suspected in the pathogenesis of human narcolepsy, but it was not definitively established. It was then demonstrated that the association with DR2 is only secondary, and that there is a stronger association of narcolepsy with the HLA DQ antigens, specifically *DQB1*0602* and *DQA1*0102*, which are present in 95–100% of patients.[39] This association is not specific for narcolepsy because it is also present in 12–38% of the general population.[39] In a study of 525 healthy subjects from the Wisconsin Sleep Cohort, Mignot and colleagues demonstrated that *DQB1*0602* positivity was linked to shorter REM latency, increased sleep efficiency, and decreased time spent in stage 1 NREM sleep.[40] Pelin and coworkers have demonstrated that homozygosity for these two haplotypes is associated with a 2- to 4-fold increase in the likelihood of developing narcolepsy over heterozygotes, but that the presence of these antigens does not influence the *severity* of the disease.[41]

Hypocretins and Human Narcolepsy

Unlike narcolepsy in dogs and mice, human narcolepsy–cataplexy is generally not associated with abnormalities in hypocretin receptors but rather with low to absent levels of CSF hypocretin-1 ligand.[42] In a postmortem study of human narcolepsy, Thannickal and colleagues found an 85–95% reduction in the number of hypocretin neurons in the hypothalamic region,[43] whereas melanin-concentrating hormone neurons, which are intermingled with the hypocretin neurons, remained unaffected, thus suggesting a targeted neurodegenerative process. Using a radioimmunoassay, Nishino and coworkers found that the mean CSF level of hypocretin-1 in healthy controls was 280.3 ± 33.0 pg/mL, and in neurologic controls it was 260.5 ± 37.1 pg/mL, whereas in those with narcolepsy, hypocretin-1 was either undetectable or <100 pg/mL.[44] The diagnostic sensitivity of low levels (<100 pg/mL) was 84.2%. Low to absent CSF hypocretin was found in 32 of 38 patients, who were all HLA *DQB1*0602* positive. HLA-negative narcolepsy patients had normal to high CSF hypocretin-1 levels. In another study, 92.3% of patients who were both *DQB1*0602* and cataplexy positive had undetectable CSF hypocretin-1 levels, whereas *DQB1*0602*-negative patients with cataplexy and *DQB1*0602*-negative patients without cataplexy had normal levels.[45] In a study of narcolepsy with cataplexy, narcolepsy without cataplexy and idiopathic hypersomnia, Kanbayashi and coworkers[46] found that all nine patients who were CSF hypocretin deficient were HLA *DQB1*0602* positive. In contrast, NT2 and idiopathic hypersomnia were associated with normal levels of CSF hypocretin (Fig. 17.2).

The CSF hypocretin (orexin) assay is most useful when an HLA *DQB1*0602*-positive patient with suspected NT1 is receiving central nervous system (CNS) antidepressants or stimulant drugs prior to formal diagnosis of narcolepsy, and discontinuation of these medications for obtaining a multiple sleep latency test (MSLT) is inconvenient or impractical. The CSF hypocretin (orexin) assay is also indicated when the suspected narcolepsy patient is <5 years old, which is below the recommended age range for the MSLT.

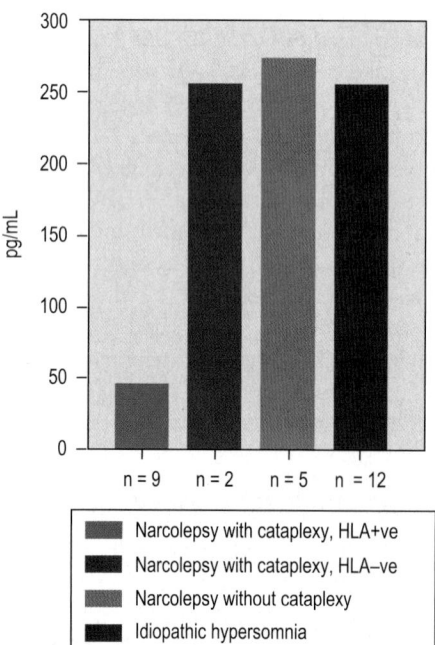

• **Fig. 17.2** Mean cerebrospinal fluid hypocretin-1 levels in various categories of hypersomnia. The narcolepsy-cataplexy group included three prepubertal children of ages 6, 7, and 10.[46] HLA, human leukocyte antigen.

The presence of HLA *DQB1*0602* is, per se, insufficient to precipitate narcolepsy. This is substantiated by the fact that *DQB1*0602*-positive monozygotic twins have been incompletely concordant for narcolepsy, with one of the pair developing narcolepsy–cataplexy at age 12 years and the other not until after having suffered emotional stress and sleep deprivation at the age of 45 years.[47] Human narcolepsy is therefore best explained on the basis of an interplay between genetic susceptibility and environmental factors. Major life events, such as a systemic illness, an injury, or bereavement, have been reported to occur in 82% of narcolepsy patients, compared with a 44% incidence in controls ($p < 0.001$).[48] A combination of genetic susceptibility and an acquired stress seems to trigger most cases of narcolepsy. In a study from China, subsequent to the 2009 H1N1 pandemic, there was a 3-fold increase in the incidence of narcolepsy.[10] Patients with *DQB1*0602* positivity may be more prone to develop NT1 after influenza infections or immunization.[49] In some patients, streptococcal infections are believed to trigger interaction between T-cell receptor and hypocretin cells via molecular mimicry[50] (see Fig. 17.2). The underlying cell-mediated immune derangement has been verified by the T-cell library method, a technique for detecting rare, antigen-specific T cells. Latorre and colleagues found that blood samples of NT1 and NT2 patients show the presence of hypocretin-reactive CD4+ and CD8+ T cells.[51] Cell-mediated immunity likely plays a key role in immune-mediated injury to the hypocretin system. Current pathophysiologic concepts are depicted in Fig. 17.3.

Monoamine Disturbances

Hypocretin deficiency leads to downregulation of arousal-mediating noradrenergic and dopaminergic pathways in the brainstem, and to relative upregulation of REM sleep-facilitating cholinergic pathways.[52] Montplaisir and coworkers measured serum and CSF levels of several biogenic amines and their metabolites,[53] such as dopamine (the metabolite is homovanillic acid), norepinephrine (the metabolite is 3-methoxy-4-hydroxyphenylethyleneglycol), epinephrine, and serotonin (the metabolite is 5-hydroxy indoleacetic acid), in patients with narcolepsy, in those with idiopathic hypersomnia, and in normal controls. Both narcolepsy and idiopathic hypersomnia patients had significantly decreased concentrations of dopamine and indoleacetic acid, a metabolite of tryptamine.[54] Dopamine and tryptamine are usually present in high concentrations in the basal ganglia. A relative deficiency of these compounds, probably mediated by downregulation of hypocretin, is likely involved in the development of sleepiness. Stimulants such as dextroamphetamine and methylphenidate, which are used in the treatment of hypersomnolence, tend to enhance dopamine release from presynaptic terminals. Activation of selective dopamine D2 receptor agonists also suppresses cataplexy.[54] This inhibition is believed to be indirectly mediated via activation of noradrenergic pathways.

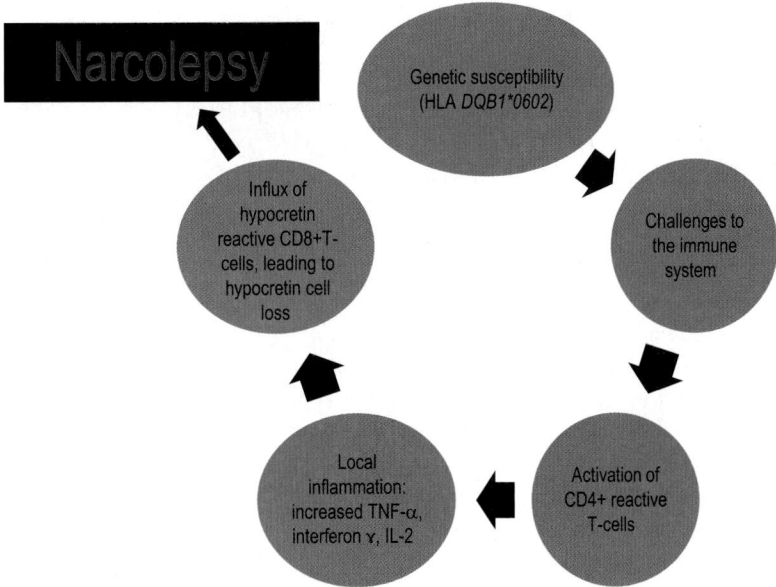

• Fig. 17.3 Presumed pathogenesis of narcolepsy.[52]. HLA, human leukocyte antigen; TNF, tumor necrosis factor; IL-2, interleukin-2.

Sleepiness in narcolepsy might also result from downregulation of histamine pathways in the brain.[55] The tuberomammillary region of the hypothalamus shows an increase in the number of histamine-producing cells, felt to be a compensatory reaction to the loss of hypocretin neurons. Histamine promotes wakefulness by activating the hypocretin pathways.

Secondary Narcolepsy

Although most narcolepsies are *idiopathic*, structural lesions of the hypothalamic region or brainstem may, on rare occasion, precipitate *secondary narcolepsy* in those who are biologically predisposed, likely due to disruption of the hypocretin pathways. Cerebellar hemangioblastomas, temporal lobe B-cell lymphomas, pituitary adenoma, third ventricular gliomas, craniopharyngiomas, head trauma, viral encephalitis, ischemic brainstem disturbances, sarcoidosis, and multiple sclerosis have been associated with narcolepsy.[56–65] Arii and colleagues described a hypothalamic tumor in a 16-year-old girl who manifested hypersomnolence, obesity, and low CSF hypocretin-1 levels, without cataplexy.[65] Although this patient did not meet the criteria for the diagnosis of narcolepsy, the report highlights the importance of hypocretins in the regulation of alertness, and its likely deficiency in cases of secondary narcolepsy.

Diagnosis

The diagnosis of narcolepsy is established on the basis of the history, combined with characteristic findings on the nocturnal PSG that is followed the next day by an MSLT, which is valid >5 years of age.[66] In preparation for the sleep studies, the patient should be withdrawn from all central nervous stimulants, hypnotics, antidepressants, and any other psychotropic agents for 2 weeks prior to the sleep studies, as these drugs may impact sleep architecture. In the case of drugs with a long half-life, such as fluoxetine, the drug-free interval may need to be 3–4 weeks. In preparation for the sleep studies, the patient should maintain a regular sleep–wake schedule, which can be verified by wrist actigraphy and sleep logs that are maintained for 1–2 weeks prior to the sleep studies.[67] A general physical examination should also be carried out to assess the Tanner stage of sexual development, as normal values for nocturnal total sleep time, daytime sleep latency, and daytime REM sleep latency are closely linked to the Tanner stages.[68]

During the PSG, multiple parameters of physiologic activity, such as the EEG (C3-A1, O2-A1 montage), eye movements, chin and leg electromyogram, nasal pressure, thoracic and abdominal respiratory effort, and oxygen saturation, are recorded simultaneously on a computerized sleep monitoring and analysis system.[69] The test helps exclude other sleep pathologies such as obstructive sleep apnea, PLM disorder, and idiopathic hypersomnia that can also lead to daytime sleepiness and mimic narcolepsy.

Patients with narcolepsy may exhibit a onset of REM sleep period, defined as occurring within 15 minutes of sleep onset (sleep-onset REM period [SOREMP]). This is a robust marker for narcolepsy. In a retrospective analysis of 148 children referred for evaluation of central hypersomnia disorders, a nocturnal SOREMP was found in approximately 54% of patients with NT1, compared with in only 2% of patients with other hypersomnias.[70] The specificity of a nocturnal SOREMP for diagnosis of NT1 was 97.3% (95% confidence interval [CI] 92.2–99.4), but the sensitivity was moderate at 54.8% (95% CI 38.7–78.2). Sleep efficiency is generally high (close to 90%), but there may be fragmentation of sleep due to increased non-specific arousals and PLMs. Another useful PSG clue to narcolepsy in adolescents is the presence of decreased nocturnal REM sleep latency (i.e., the time between sleep onset and the onset of the first 30-second epoch of REM sleep, but not necessarily as abbreviated as SOREMP). For example, in one study, the nocturnal REM sleep latency in narcoleptic subjects was <67 minutes (mean, 24.5 minutes; standard deviation [SD], 30; range, 0–66.5 minutes; $n = 8$) compared with a mean nocturnal REM sleep latency of 143.7 minutes in age-matched controls (range, 82.5–230.5; SD, 50.9 minutes; $P < 0.001$).[71] A similar conclusion was reached by Challamel and colleagues in their meta-analysis of 235 subjects[11] and in the pioneering work of Carskadon and coworkers.[72]

REM sleep without atonia or frank RBD are also important features of NT1.[73,74] They are likely related to loss of activation of REM "on" neurons that are located in the sublaterodorsal nucleus of the pons.[73–75]

Along with PSG, an MSLT is essential for the diagnosis of narcolepsy. It needs to be started 2 hours after the final morning awakening from PSG, and consists of 4–5 nap opportunities of 20-minute lengths at 2-hour intervals in a darkened, quiet room (e.g., at 1,000, 1,200, 1,400, and 1,600 hours).[66] While adults are required to sleep alone, young, preadolescent children may require parental presence in the sleep laboratory bedroom for reassurance. Eye movements, chin electromyogram, and EEG (generally C3-A2, O2-A1) are recorded. The MSLT quantifies the degree of sleepiness and helps assess the nature of the transition from wakefulness into sleep (i.e., wakefulness to NREM sleep, or wakefulness to REM sleep). The time interval between "lights out" and sleep onset is termed the *sleep latency;* a *mean sleep latency* is then derived from averaging all naps. A urine drug screen is obtained between the naps if the patient appears to be falling asleep very quickly and there is suspicion of drug-seeking behavior. A concerted effort should be made to ensure that the patient does not accidentally fall asleep between the naps. Typically, the mean sleep latency is shortened to less than 8 minutes in patients with narcolepsy, whereas in control children and adolescents it is between 14 and 18 minutes (Table 17.1).

In children without narcolepsy, the initial transition is from wakefulness into NREM sleep. In narcolepsy, however, the transition becomes from wakefulness into REM sleep. The characteristic feature of two or more SOREMPs may not be consistently present in the early stages of narcolepsy. Serial sleep studies may sometimes be needed to establish a definitive diagnosis (Fig. 17.4). Though the normative MSLT data established by Carskadon and colleagues[68] are widely used, it is conceivable that normal mean sleep latency in preadolescents is >20 minutes when there is in-home PSG followed by MSLT in the sleep laboratory.[76–78]

Serologic testing for the HLA *DQB1*0602* haplotype may be an adjunctive test, but it is not to be used to diagnose narcolepsy, as this haplotype is also present in 12–38%

TABLE 17.1	Normal Values for the Multiple Sleep Latency Test	
Stage of Development	Mean Sleep Latency (min)	Standard Deviation
Tanner stage I	18.8	1.8
Tanner stage II	18.3	2.1
Tanner stage III	16.5	2.8
Tanner stage IV	15.5	3.3
Tanner stage V	16.2	1.5
Older adolescents	15.8	3.5

Adapted from Carskadon MA. The second decade. In Guilleminault C, ed. *Sleeping and Waking Disorders: Indications and Techniques.* Addison-Wesley, 1982:99–125.

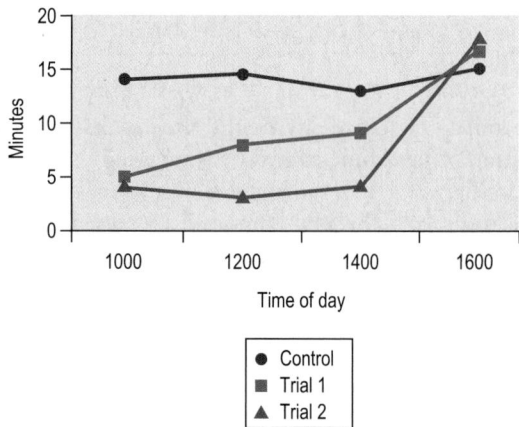

• **Fig. 17.4** Serial multiple sleep latency tests (MSLTs) in a 13-year-old child with evolving narcolepsy. MSLT trials 1 and 2 were carried out 9 months apart. They are compared with the MSLT findings of a healthy control. There is progressive decrease over time in the sleep latencies of the patient at 1,000, 1,200, and 1,400 hours along with an increase in the number of sleep-onset rapid eye movement periods. Sleep latencies in the final nap (1,600 hours) may be physiologically prolonged in children as a result of anticipation about going home, or the "last nap." *Reproduced from Kotagal S, Swink TD. Excessive daytime sleepiness in a 13-year old. Semin Pediatr Neurol. 1996;3:170–172.*

of the general population.[38] The CSF hypocretin (orexin) analysis is useful in establishing the diagnosis when psychotropic medications cannot be discontinued for safety reasons and for children <6–7 years of age because the MSLT is not valid in this age group.

Differential Diagnosis

By far, the most common disorder of excessive sleepiness in an adolescent is *insufficient nocturnal sleep.* To begin with, there is a physiologic shift in the sleep-onset time of most teenagers to between 10:30 p.m. and 11:00 p.m.[78] Also, the physiologic dim-light melatonin secretion starts to occur at a later time of the night, around 10:30 pm. The resultant physiologic delay in sleep onset is associated with a corresponding shift to a later morning wake up time. Linked to this physiologic phase delay, Carskadon and colleagues have documented SOREMPs during the MSLT of 12 of 25 healthy students.[79] Complicating the physiologic delay in sleep onset might be superimposed elements of *abnormal sleep hygiene* (such as use of caffeine, nicotine, illicit substances, late-night television viewing, phone calls, computer chats, video games, etc.). A circadian rhythm disturbance such as the *delayed sleep phase syndrome* might also delay sleep onset and be associated with insufficient night sleep and consequent daytime sleepiness.[80] The use of prescription drugs or over-the-counter sedatives such as antihistamines should also be considered as a possible cause of sleepiness. A high index of suspicion should be maintained for illicit drug use.

It is not uncommon for *obstructive hypoventilation* to present with obesity and sleepiness, and mimic narcolepsy.[81] The most common causes of childhood obstructive sleep apnea are adenotonsillar hypertrophy, neuromuscular disorders, and craniofacial anomalies such as Crouzon syndrome and Down syndrome. The *upper airway resistance syndrome* is an under-recognized type of obstructive sleep apnea leading to daytime sleepiness. It is characterized by habitual snoring, an increased number of breathing-related microarousals, and flow limitation on the nasal pressure tracing of the PSG.

Kleine-Levin syndrome, or *periodic hypersomnia*, is characterized by recurrent periods of sleepiness and behavioral disturbance.[82,83] It is common in adolescent males, who manifest 1- to 2-week periods of excessive sleepiness in association with amnesia and feelings of depersonalization. Though they have been dramatized, hyperphagia, anorexia, and hypersexual behavior tend to occur in only about half the patients. There may be a 2- to 10-pound weight gain during the sleepy periods, which may remits spontaneously, only to reappear a few weeks later. Anxiety may develop in the periods intervening in the sleepiness. No specific etiology has been found. The disorder subsides gradually over time. The nocturnal PSG shows decreased sleep efficiency and time spent in N3 sleep.[82,83] The MSLT may show moderate daytime sleepiness with a shortened mean sleep latency of 5–10 minutes, but fewer than two SOREMPs.

Idiopathic hypersomnia should also be considered in the differential diagnosis of narcolepsy. It is defined as a disorder associated with non-imperative sleepiness, long unrefreshing naps, difficulty reaching full awakening after sleep, and sleep drunkenness, as well as absence of SOREMPs during the MSLT.[84,85] Night sleep is quantitatively and qualitatively normal. The MSLT shows a short mean sleep latency, generally in the range of 5–10 minutes, but two or more SOREMPs, which would be suggestive of narcolepsy, are not seen.

Case Presentation

A 3-year-old girl was evaluated for a 6-week history of sleepiness and unsteadiness while standing and walking, leading to falls, occurring at least 8–10 times per day. The unsteadiness was intermittent, and was punctuated with long periods of stable balance and coordination. Her parents noticed that in addition to sleeping through the night, she began to take several long naps during the day, which was in excess of her prior napping habits. She remained afebrile. The brain magnetic resonance imaging scan, EEG, and serum ammonia, electrolytes, and thyroxine were normal. A lumbar puncture showed normal CSF cell count and differential, protein, and glucose. Video clips of the falls and muscle incoordination recorded by the father on his cell phone were reviewed, and they were suspicious for cataplexy. She possessed the histocompatibility antigen *DQB1*0602*. Consequently, 0.7 mL of the CSF that had been saved and frozen was sent for a hypocretin assay to Stanford University. The hypocretin level was low at 26 pg/mL (reference value is >110 pg/mL).[47] A diagnosis of narcolepsy–cataplexy (NT1) was established. Upon further questioning, the parents indicated that she had received a double dose of influenza A immunization approximately 4 weeks prior to onset of the symptoms. She was provided infusions of intravenous immunoglobulin G every 2 weeks for 3 months, without improvement in sleepiness or cataplexy. Symptomatic treatment was therefore started using a combination of methylphenidate 2.5 once a day and sodium oxybate (Xyrem) 2 g at night in two divided doses, with excellent results. Improvement has now been maintained for 11 years, though with uptitration in the dose to methylphenidate (Concerta) to 27 mg twice a day and sodium oxybate (Xyrem) to 4 g twice nightly. There have been no major side effects. She continues to do well academically and socially.

This case illustrates several aspects of narcolepsy–cataplexy. Cataplexy in preschool-age children may appear as episodes of abrupt muscle weakness that are not consistently associated with an emotional trigger such as laughter. Though not seen in the patient described earlier, transient facial and jaw muscle weakness may be the sole manifestation of cataplexy in preschool-age children. One needs to keep a high index of suspicion of narcolepsy in children who have abruptly developed new onset of sleepiness. Also, reviewing video clips recorded by the parents can be helpful, as exemplified by this case. The diagnosis in children below <5–6 years of age is problematic because the MSLT cannot be applied as it cannot distinguish physiologic napping from pathologic sleepiness. If cataplexy is present and the patient is positive for HLA *DQB1*0602*, there is a strong likelihood that CSF hypocretin will be low, thus assessing its levels becomes important. It is conceivable that in this patient, who was biologically predisposed to develop NT1 on the basis of the HLA *DQB1*0602*-positive status, the influenza immunization acted as a trigger for an immune-mediated degenerative process in the hypothalamus that led to reduced central nervous system hypocretin levels and precipitation of narcolepsy–cataplexy. The link between influenza immunization in North America and triggering of NT1 has, however, not been definitively established.

Management

General Measures

It is important to maintain regular sleeping and waking schedules. One to two planned naps during the day might help dissipate sleep pressure and daytime sleepiness. Regular exercise during the day might also enhance alertness and prevent excessive weight gain. Attention to comorbid obesity is important as it may predispose to sleep-disordered breathing. Psychiatric consultation should be arranged early in case of comorbid depression and anxiety. Because of the increased risk of accidents from sleepiness, patients should be cautioned against driving long distances and working near sharp, moving machinery.

Pharmacologic Therapy

The reader is referred to an upcoming evidence-based clinical practice guideline that is being published by the American Academy of Sleep Medicine.[86] Drugs commonly used for treatment are listed in Table 17.2. Except for sodium oxybate (Xyrem), which underwent a prospective, randomized, placebo-controlled study in children and was formally approved by the U.S. Food and Drug Administration, drug therapy for pediatric narcolepsy is on an "off-label" basis.

TABLE 17.2   Drugs Commonly Used in the Treatment of Narcolepsy

Symptom	Drug (trade name)	Dosage	Remarks
Daytime sleepiness	Modafinil (Provigil) Armodafinil (Nuvigil) Methylphenidate (Ritalin) methylphenidate (Ritalin SR) Methylphenidate (Concerta) Dextroamphetamine (Dexedrine) Amphetamine/ dextroamphetamine mixture (Adderall) Lisdexamfetamine (Vyvanse) Pitolisant (Wakix) Solriamfetol (Sunosi)	100–400 mg/day in 2 divided doses 50–500 mg/day in 2 divided doses 5–60 mg/day in 2 divided doses 18–54 mg/day in 2 divided doses up to age 12; up to 72 mg for those 12–18 years 10 –40 mg/day in 2 divided doses 10–40 mg/day in 2 doses 30–70 mg/day in 1–2 divided doses 8.9 mg once daily to a maximum of 35.6 mg/ once a day 75–150 mg/day in 1–2 doses	Side effects: headache, nervousness, anxiety, nausea, Stevens-Johnson syndrome, lowering efficacy of oral contraceptives Racemic enantiomer of modafinil; side effects are similar to modafinil Side effects common to all forms of methylphenidate: anorexia, weight loss, tremor, worsening of tics, insomnia, agitation, and headache Safety and efficacy not established <6 years Side effects common to amphetamines: anorexia, weight loss, tremor, worsening of tics, insomnia, agitation, headache; caution in heart disease or family history of sudden death Nausea, headache; QT interval prolongation; also effective against cataplexy Headache, insomnia; contraindicated with monoamine oxidase inhibitors
Cataplexy	Venlafaxine (Effexor) Clomipramine (Anafranil) Fluoxetine (Prozac) Sertraline (Zoloft) Sodium oxybate (Xyrem)	25–75 mg/day in 1–2 doses 25–75 mg/day in 1–2 doses 10–40 mg/day every morning 25–100 mg/day in 1–2 doses 3–9 g nightly in 2 divided doses, with first dose at bed onset, second dose 2.5–3 hours later	Common to venlafaxine and clomipramine: contraindicated with monoamine oxidase inhibitors; increased risk of suicidal thoughts Side effects common to sertraline and fluoxetine: nervousness, weight loss, dizziness, headache, constipation, xerostomia; increased risk of suicidal thoughts Side effects: worsening of depression, suicidal thoughts, sleepwalking, enuresis, worsening of sleep apnea, weight loss, tremor, constipation
Periodic limb movements/ restless legs syndrome	Elemental iron Clonazepam	3 mg/kg/day with orange juice 0.25–0.5 mg at bedtime	Side effects: constipation and abdominal discomfort Drowsiness

Note:
- The list of adverse effects/contraindications is not complete.
- Refer to package insert for details.
- All antidepressants are associated with a risk of increased suicidal ideation.
- Periodic follow-up is needed for all subjects to monitor for improvement and side effects.
- Patients may need a combination of drugs for optimum control of symptoms

The quality of evidence is generally low, with the literature composed mainly of small (<100 subjects), open-label design observational studies. It is not known whether, and to what extent, pharmacologic therapy improves the quality of life in childhood narcolepsy.

Daytime sleepiness is generally treated with stimulants such as methylphenidate (regular or extended-release formulations) or preparations of amphetamine.[87] The half-lives of amphetamine and methylphenidate are 10–12 hours and 3–4 hours, respectively. The side effects of these agents include loss of appetite, nervousness, tics, headache, and insomnia. Modafinil (Provigil), a drug whose mode of action is in part related to inhibition of dopamine active transporter, has also been reported to be effective in enhancing alertness and improving psychomotor performance in doses of 100–400 mg/day.[88] It works best if provided in two divided doses. The half-life is 3–4 hours. A racemic form, armodafinil, has a half-life of 10–14 hours and is now also widely utilized.[89] The potential side effects of modafinil and armodafinil include headache, nervousness, anxiety, and nausea. Stevens-Johnson syndrome is a rare but serious type of delayed hypersensitivity reaction with modafinil. It is characterized by a diffuse and progressive vasculitis that involves the skin (itchy, maculopapular rash), mucous membranes (oral ulceration), liver (elevated serum transaminases), and kidney (nephritis). It requires immediate discontinuation of modafinil/armodafinil, assessment for hepatic or renal involvement, and possible initiation of steroid therapy. Modafinil and armodafinil can decrease the potency of concurrently administered oral contraceptives.

Pitolisant is a wakefulness-promoting, histamine-3 receptor inverse antagonist/agonist. It is also effective against both sleepiness and cataplexy.[90] Absorption is not affected by food, the time to maximum concentration is around 3.5 hours, and it has an elimination half-life of about 20 hours. It is metabolized mainly by hepatic CYP2D6. Potential side effects include nausea, insomnia, and headache. In rare instances, the QT interval may be prolonged. Use in children is considered off-label. The dose in adults is 8.9 mg/day, which can be gradually titrated up if needed to 35.6 mg/day.

Solriamfetol is another recently introduced wakefulness-promoting agent, and is felt to work by inhibiting the reuptake of norepinephrine and dopamine.[91] The time-to-peak concentration is about 2 hours, which may be slightly delayed by food, and the half-life is around 7 hours. Over 90% of the drug is eliminated unchanged, hence, it is not recommended in patients with severe renal disease. Potential side effects include headache, nausea, anxiety, insomnia, and decreased weight. The dose is 75–150 mg/day in 1–2 doses.

Cataplexy is mediated in part by cholinergic pathways in the brainstem. Drugs with anticholinergic properties such as protriptyline and clomipramine were initially described as being effective for its control. Unfortunately, they are associated with significant side effects such as drowsiness, dryness of the mouth, and weight gain. Selective serotonin reuptake inhibitors such as fluoxetine may also be utilized to treat cataplexy, especially when there is coexisting depression.[92]

Gamma hydroxybutyrate (sodium oxybate; Xyrem) is an endogenous fatty acid with specific affinity for endogenous gamma-aminobutyric acid type B receptors.[93] It stabilizes nocturnal sleep, and has a modulating effect on GABAergic, dopaminergic, noradrenergic, and serotonergic neurons.[94] The drug is effective against both cataplexy and daytime sleepiness. The half-life is 30–60 minutes. It is typically provided in two divided doses, with the first dose at bedtime, and the second dose 2.5–3 hours after initial sleep onset. Adverse effects include dizziness, nausea, enuresis, exacerbation of sleep apnea, sleepwalking, somnolence, and weight loss.[95,96] Preexisting psychiatric conditions such as depression and anxiety may be worsened, so these conditions are relative contraindications for Xyrem use. There is a potential for abuse, and Xyrem should be avoided in patients who might pose a risk in this regard. Xyway is a calcium, magnesium, sodium, and potassium oxybate oral solution. The active ingredient is gamma hydroxybutyrate. It is effective against both daytime sleepiness and cataplexy, and may be indicated when there is a concern about avoiding extra sodium from Xyrem due to hypertension. Efficacy in children has not been studied, but is extrapolated from a previous pediatric study on Xyrem. It is provided as 4.5–9 g nightly in two divided doses, and is available through a centralized pharmacy. The prescription of both Xyrem and Xyway requires the prescriber and patient to undergo training through a Risk Evaluation and Mitigation Strategy (REMS) program. The medications are made available through a centralized pharmacy.

Due to the likelihood of immune dysfunction underlying narcolepsy, intravenous immunoglobulin G has been utilized early in the course of NT1, with variable, short-term results.[96] The lack of consistent improvement may be related to cell-mediated immunity, rather than humoral immunity, underlying the pathogenesis of narcolepsy.

Non-profit organizations such as *Wake Up Narcolepsy* and the *Narcolepsy Network* provide emotional support and advocacy for patients with narcolepsy and their families.

Future Directions

Further understanding of the role of T-cell dysfunction in the pathogenesis of narcolepsy might spur the development of therapies that specifically target this immune disturbance.[52] The small number of pediatric narcolepsy cases in individual medical centers has limited the launch of systematic, large-scale clinical investigations. The development of consortia-based treatment trials is being considered by several investigators. The high prevalence of anxiety disorders (odds ratio [OR] 4.56, 95% CI 1.99−10.44) and depression (OR 4.88, 95% CI 2.45−9.73) at the time of diagnosis of narcolepsy underscores the importance of providing early supportive psychologic/psychiatric services.[97] Unfortunately this has not happening consistently. Standards of care need to be developed that emphasize the management of comorbidities. The design of pharmacologic trials needs to include the assessment of patient preferences, cost of treatment, and the quality of life. Future treatments might also include selective agonists for hypocretin (orexin 2), administered via subcutaneous or intrathecal route.[98] Deep learning techniques of artificial intelligence (AI) may permit identifying transitions from wakefulness to REM sleep, or for assessing sleep state dissociation characteristic of narcolepsy.[99] When refined and applied to children in the ambulatory environment, this author hopes that AI techniques will facilitate early diagnosis of narcolepsy and facilitate timely intervention prior to the development of comorbidities.

CLINICAL PEARLS

- Preschool-age children may not be able to provide accurate information about their cataplexy. Reviewing video clips provided by parents may help document cataplexy.
- The manifestations of childhood sleepiness can at times be non-specific, in the form of inattentiveness, mood swings, and apathy. They represent dysfunction of the prefrontal cortex due to sleepiness.
- The measurement of cerebrospinal spinal fluid hypocretin (orexin) levels may enable a diagnosis of narcolepsy type 1. This test is useful in children <5–6 years of age for whom the multiple sleep latency test (MSLT) might be invalid, and when the patient is receiving medications that cannot be safely stopped for the MSLT, but which impact REM sleep, such as antidepressants.
- Obesity and precocious puberty may be evident at the onset of childhood narcolepsy–cataplexy symptoms.
- The spectrum of medications available to treat sleepiness and cataplexy is gradually increasing. Rational pharmacotherapy requires targeting the symptom(s) most bothersome to the patient.
- Comorbid anxiety and depression may be present at the onset of narcolepsy, and also require ongoing management.

References

1. Gélineau J. De la narcolepsie. *Gaz Hosp (Paris).* 1880;53:626–628.
2. American Academy of Sleep Medicine Central disorders of hypersomnolence. In: *The International Classification of Sleep Disorders – Third Edition (ICSD-3).* Online version. American Academy of Sleep Medicine; 2014.
3. Silber M, Krahn L, Olson E, et al. The epidemiology of narcolepsy in Olmsted County, Minnesota: A population-based study. *Sleep.* 2002;25:197–202.
4. Honda Y. Clinical features of narcolepsy: Japanese experience. In: Honda Y, Juji T, eds. *Narcolepsy.* Springer Verlag; 1988:2457.
5. Lavie P, Peled R. Narcolepsy is a rare disease in Israel. *Sleep.* 1987;10:608–609.
6. Heier MS, Evsiukova T, Wilson J, et al. Prevalence of narcolepsy with cataplexy in Norway. *Acta Neurol Scand.* 2009; 120(4):276–280.
7. Matsuki K, Honda Y, Juji T. Diagnostic criteria for narcolepsy and HLA-DR2 frequencies. *Tissue Antigens.* 1987;30:155–160.
8. Roffwarg HP. Sleep Disorders Classification Committee, Association of Sleep Disorders: Diagnostic classification of sleep and arousal disorders. *Sleep.* 1979;2:1–137.
9. Hublin C, Partinen M, Kaprio J, et al. Epidemiology of narcolepsy. *Sleep.* 1994;17(Suppl. 1):7–12.
10. Han F, Lin L, Warby SC, Faraco J, et al. Narcolepsy onset is seasonal and increased following the 2009 H1N1 pandemic in China. *Ann Neurol.* 2011;70(3):410–417.
11. Challamel MJ, Mazzola ME, Nevsimalova S, et al. Narcolepsy in children. *Sleep.* 1994;17S:17–20.
12. Overeem S, Reading P, Bassetti CLNarcolepsy. *Sleep Med Clin.* 2012;7(2):263–281.
13. Maski K, Steinhart E, Williams D, et al. Listening to the patient voice in narcolepsy: Diagnostic delay, disease burden, and treatment efficacy. *J Clin Sleep Med.* 2017;13:419.
14. Sharp SJ, D'Cruz OF. Narcolepsy in a 12-month-old boy. *J Child Neurol.* 2001;16:145–146.
15. Drake C, Nickel C, Burduvali E, Roth T, Jefferson C, Pietro B. The Pediatric Daytime Sleepiness Scale (PDSS): Sleep habits and school outcomes in middle-school children. *Sleep.* 2003;26(4):455–458.
16. Janssen KC, Phillipson S, O'Connor J, Johns MW. Validation of the Epworth Sleepiness Scale for Children and Adolescents using Rasch analysis. *Sleep Med.* 2017;33:30–35.
17. Kotagal S, Hartse KM, Walsh JK. Characteristics of narcolepsy in pre-teen aged children. *Pediatrics.* 1990;85:205–209.
18. Pearl PL, Efron L, Stein MA. Children, sleep, and behavior: A complex association. *Minerva Pediatr.* 2002;54:79–91.
19. Walker MP. Sleep, memory and emotion. *Prog Brain Res.* 2010;185:49–68.
20. Mahoney CE, Cogswell A, Coralink IJ, Scammell TE. The neurobiological basis of narcolepsy. *Nat Rev Neurosci.* 2019;20(2):83–93.
21. Pizza F, Antelmi E, Vandi S, et al. The distinguishing motor features of cataplexy: A study from video recorded attacks. *Sleep.* 2018;41(5). https://doi.org/10.1093/sleep/zsy026.
22. Maski K, Pizza F, Liu S, Steinhart E, et al. Defining disturbed night sleep and assessing its diagnostic utility for pediatric narcolepsy type 1. *Sleep.* 2020;13(6):686–690.
23. Stores G, Montgomery P, Wiggs L. The psychosocial problems of children with narcolepsy and those with excessive daytime sleepiness of uncertain origin. *Pediatrics.* 2006;118: e1116–e1123.
24. Kotagal S, Krahn LE, Slocumb N. A putative link between childhood narcolepsy and obesity. *Sleep Med.* 2004;5:147–150.
25. Poli F, Pizza F, Mignot E, et al. High prevalence of precocious puberty and obesity in childhood narcolepsy with cataplexy. *Sleep.* 2013;36:175–181.
26. Nevsimalova S, Prihodova I, Kemlink D, et al. REM sleep behavior disorder (RBD) can be one of the first symptoms of childhood narcolepsy. *Sleep Med.* 2007;7–8:784–786.
27. Lloyd R, Tippman-Peikert M, Slocumb N, et al. Characteristics of REM sleep behavior disorder in childhood. *J Clin Sleep Med.* 2012;8:127–131.
28. Peever J, Fuller PM. The biology of REM sleep. *Curr Biol.* 2017;27:R1237–R1248.
29. Tonokura M, Fujita K, Nishino S. Review of pathophysiology and clinical management of narcolepsy and dogs. *Vet Rec.* 2007;161(11):375–380.
30. Mitler MM, Dement WC. Cataplectic-like behavior in cats after microinjection of carbachol in the pontine reticular formation. *Brain Res.* 1974;68:335–343.
31. Reid MS, Tafti M, Geary JN, et al. Cholinergic mechanisms in cataplexy: I. Modulation of cataplexy via local drug administration into the paramedian pontine reticular formation. *Neuroscience.* 1994;59:511–522.

32. Lin L, Faraco J, Li R, et al. The sleep disorder, canine narcolepsy, is caused by a mutation in the hypocretin (orexin) receptor 2 gene. *Cell.* 1999;98:365–376.

33. Chemelli RM, Willie JT, Sinton CM, et al. Narcolepsy in orexin knock-out mice: Molecular genetics of sleep regulation. *Cell.* 1999;98:437–451.

34. John J, Wu M-F, Siegel JM. Systemic administration of hypocretin-1 reduces cataplexy and normalizes sleep and waking durations in narcoleptic dogs. *Sleep Res Online.* 2000; 3:23–28.

35. Juji T, Satake M, Honda Y, et al. HLA antigens in Japanese patients with narcolepsy. *Tissue Antigens.* 1984;24:316–319.

36. Billiard M, Seignalet J, Besset A, et al. HLA DR2 and narcolepsy. *Sleep.* 1986;9:149–152.

37. Langdon N, Lock C, Welsh K, et al. Immune factors in narcolepsy. *Sleep.* 1986;9:143–148.

38. Al Shareef SM, AlAnbay E, AlKhathlan MA, et al. HLA-DQB1*06:02 allele frequency and clinic-polysomnographic features in Saudi Arabian patients with narcolepsy. *Sleep Breath.* 2019;23(1):303–309.

39. Mignot E, Lin L, Rogers W, et al. Complex HLA-DR and -DQ interactions confer risk of narcolepsy-cataplexy in three ethnic groups. *Am J Hum Genet.* 2001;68:686–699.

40. Mignot E, Young T, Lin L, Fin L. Nocturnal sleep and daytime sleepiness in normal subjects with HLA-*DQB1*0602*. *Sleep.* 1999;22:347–352.

41. Pelin Z, Guilleminault C, Risch N, et al. HLA *DQB1*0602* homozygosity increases relative risk for narcolepsy but not disease severity in two ethnic groups. *Tissue Antigens.* 1998;51:96–100.

42. Nishino S, Ripley B, Overeem S, et al. Hypocretin (orexin) deficiency in human narcolepsy. *Lancet.* 2000;355:39–40.

43. Thannickal TC, Moore RY, Nienhuis R, et al. Reduced number of hypocretin neurons in human narcolepsy. *Neuron.* 2000;27:469–474.

44. Nishino S, Ripley B, Overeem S, et al. Low cerebrospinal fluid hypocretin (orexin) and altered energy homeostasis in human narcolepsy. *Ann Neurol.* 2001;50:381–388.

45. Krahn LE, Pankrantz VS, Oliver L, et al. Hypocretin (orexin) levels in cerebrospinal fluid of patients with narcolepsy: Relationship to cataplexy and *DQB1*0602*. *Sleep.* 2002;25:733–738.

46. Kanbayashi T, Inoue Y, Chiba S, et al. CSF hypocretin-1 (orexin-A) concentrations in narcolepsy with and without cataplexy and idiopathic hypersomnia. *J Sleep Res.* 2002;11:91–93.

47. Honda M, Honda Y, Uchida S, et al. Monozygotic twins incompletely concordant for narcolepsy. *Biol Psychiatry.* 2001;49:943–947.

48. Orellana C, Villemin E, Tafti M, et al. Life events in the year preceding the onset of narcolepsy. *Sleep.* 1994;17(Suppl. 1):50–53.

49. Dauvilliers Y, Montplaisir J, Cochen V, et al. Post-H1N1 narcolepsy-cataplexy. *Sleep.* 2010;33:1428–1430.

50. Kornum BR, Faraco J, Mignot E. Narcolepsy with hypocretin/orexin deficiency, infections, and autoimmunity of the brain. *Curr Opin Neurobiol.* 2011;21:897–903.

51. Latorre D, Kallweit U, Armentani E, et al. T-cells in patients with narcolepsy target self-antigens of hypocretin neurons. *Nature.* 2018;562(7725):63–68.

52. Mignot E, Taheri S, Nishino S. Sleeping with the hypothalamus: Emerging therapeutic targets for sleep disorders. *Nat Neurosci.* 2002;5(Suppl):1071–1075.

53. Montplaisir J, de Champlain J, Young SN, et al. Narcolepsy and idiopathic hypersomnia: Biogenic and related compounds in CSF. *Neurology.* 1982;32:1299–1302.

54. Nishino S, Arrigoni J, Valtier D, et al. Dopamine D2 mechanisms in canine narcolepsy. *J Neurosci.* 1991;11:2666–2671.

55. Valco PO, Gavrilov YV, Yamamoto M, et al. Increase of histaminergic tuberomammillary neurons in narcolepsy. *Ann Neurol.* 2013;74(6):794–804.

56. Autret A, Lucas F, Henry-Lebras F, et al. Symptomatic narcolepsies. *Sleep.* 1994;17S(Suppl. 1):21–24.

57. Madan R, Pitts J, Patterson MC, Lloyd R, Keating G, Kotagal S. Secondary narcolepsy in children. *J Child Neurol.* 2021;36(2):123–127.

58. Onofrj M, Curatola L, Ferracci F, et al. Narcolepsy associated with primary temporal lobe B-cell lymphoma in a HLA DR2 negative subject. *J Neurol Neurosurg Psychiatry.* 1992;55:852–853.

59. Schwartz WJ, Stakes JW, Hobson JA. Transient cataplexy after removal of craniopharyngoma. *Neurology.* 1984;34:1372–1375.

60. Lankford DA, Wellman JJ, Ohara C. Post-traumatic narcolepsy in mild to moderate closed head injury. *Sleep.* 1994;17S(Suppl. 1): 25–28.

61. Bonduelle C, Degos C. Symptomatic narcolepsies: A critical study. In: Guilleminault C, Dement WC, Passouant P, eds. *Narcolepsy.* Spectrum; 1976:312–332.

62. Rivera VM, Meyer JS, Hata T, et al. Narcolepsy following cerebral ischemia. *Ann Neurol.* 1986;19:505–508.

63. Schrader H, Gotlibsen OB. Multiple sclerosis and narcolepsy-cataplexy in a monozygotic twin. *Neurology.* 1980;30:105–108.

64. Kandt RS, Emerson RG, Singer HS, et al. Cataplexy in variant forms of Niemann–Pick disease. *Ann Neurol.* 1982;12:284–288.

65. Arii J, Kanbayashi T, Tanabe Y, et al. A hypersomnolent girl with decreased CSF hypocretin level after removal of a hypothalamic tumor. *Neurology.* 2001;56:1775–1776.

66. Kotagal S, Nichols CD, Grigg-Damberger MM, Marcus CL, Witmans MB, Kirk VG, D'Andrea LA, Hoban T. Non-respiratory indications for polysomnography and related procedures in children: An evidence-based review. *Sleep.* 2012;35(11):1451–1466.

67. Meltzer LJ, Montgomery-Downs HE, Insana SP, Walsh CM. The use of actigraphy for assessment in pediatric research. *Sleep Med Rev.* 2012;16(5):463–475.

68. Carskadon MA, Dement WC, Mitler MM, et al. Guidelines for the multiple. *sleep latency test (MSLT): A standard measure of sleepiness. Sleep.* 1986;9:519–524.

69. Kotagal S, Goulding PM. The laboratory assessment of daytime sleepiness in childhood. *J Clin Neurophysiol.* 1996;13:208–218.

70. Reiter J, Katz E, Scammell TE, Maski K. Usefulness of a nocturnal SOREMP for diagnosing narcolepsy with cataplexy in a pediatric population. *Sleep.* 2015;38(6):859–865.

71. Kotagal S. A developmental perspective on narcolepsy. In: Loughlin GM, Carroll JL, Marcus CL, eds. *Sleep and Breathing in Children.* Marcel Dekker; 2000:347–362.

72. Carskadon MA, Harvey K, Dement WC. Multiple sleep latency tests during the development of narcolepsy. *West J Med.* 1981;135:414–418.

73. Lloyd R, Tippman-Piekert M, Slocumb N, Kotagal S. Characteristics of REM sleep behavior disorder in childhood. *J Clin Sleep Med.* 2012;8(2):127–131.

74. Peever J, Fuller PM. The biology of REM sleep. *Curr Biol.* 2017:R1237–R1248.

75. Bin-Hasan S, Videnovic A, Maski K. Nocturnal REM sleep without atonia is a diagnostic biomarker of pediatric narcolepsy. *J Clin Sleep Med.* 2018;14(2):245–252.

76. Gozal D, Wang M, Pope DW. Objective sleepiness measures in pediatric obstructive sleep apnea. *Pediatrics.* 2001;108: 693–697.

77. Palm L, Persson E, Elmquist D, et al. Sleep and wakefulness in normal pre-adolescents. *Sleep*. 1989;12:299–308.

78. Carskadon MA. Factors influencing sleep patterns of adolescents. In: Carskadon MA, ed. *Adolescent Sleep Patterns: Biological, Social, and Psychological Perspectives*. Cambridge University Press; 2002:18–19.

79. Carskadon MA, Wolfson AR, Acebo C, et al. Adolescent sleep patterns, circadian timing, and sleepiness at a transition to early school days. *Sleep*. 1998;21:871–881.

80. Pavlova M. Circadian rhythm sleep-wake disorders. *Continuum (Minneap Minn)*. 2017;23:1051–1063. (4, *Sleep Neurology*).

81. Marcus CL, Brooks LJ, Draper KA, Gozal D, Halbower AC, Jones J, et al. Diagnosis and management of childhood obstructive sleep apnea syndrome. *Pediatrics*. 2012;130(3):e714–e755.

82. Gadoth N, Oksenberg A. Kleine Levin syndrome: An update and mini-review. *Brain Dev*. 2017;39(8):665–671.

83. Arnulf I. Kleine Levin syndrome. *Sleep Med Clin*. 2015;10(2):151–161.

84. Trotti LM. Idiopathic hypersomnia. *Sleep Med Clin*. 2017;12(3):331–344.

85. Leu-Semenescu S, Quera-Salva MA. Dauvilliers. French consensus. Idiopathic hypersomnia. Investigations and follow up. *Rev Neurol (Paris)*. 2017;173(1–2):32–37.

86. Maski K, Trotti LM, Kotagal S, Auger RR, Rowley JA, Hashmi SD, Watson NF. Treatment of central disorders of hypersomnolence. An American Academy of Sleep Medicine Clinical Practice Guideline. *J Clin Sleep Med*. 2021;17(9):1881–1893.

87. Wise MS, Arand DL, Auger RR, Brooks SN, Watson NF. Treatment of narcolepsy and other hypersomnias of central origin. *Sleep*. 2007;30:1712–1727.

88. Joo EY, Hong SB, Kim HJ, et al. The effect of modafinil on cortical excitability in patients with narcolepsy: A randomized, placebo-controlled, crossover study. *Sleep Med*. 2010;11:862–869.

89. Harsh JR, Hayduk R, Rosenberg R, et al. The efficacy and safety of armodafinil as treatment for adults with excessive sleepiness associated with narcolepsy. *Curr Med Res Opin*. 2006;22:761–774.

90. Dauvilliers Y, Bassetti C, Lammers GJ, et al. Pitolisant versus placebo or modafinil in patients with narcolepsy: A double-blind, randomised trial. *Lancet Neurol*. 2013;12:1068–1075.

91. Thorpy MJ, Shapiro C, Mayer G, et al. A randomized study of solriamfetol for excessive sleepiness in narcolepsy. *Ann Neurol*. 2019;85(3):359–370.

92. Dunlop BW, Crits-Christoph P, Evans DL, et al. Co-administration of modafinil and a selective serotonin reuptake inhibitor from the initiation of treatment of major depressive disorder with fatigue and sleepiness: A double-blind, placebo-controlled study. *J Clin Psychopharmacol*. 2007;27:614–619.

93. Koek W, France CP, Cheng K, Rice KC. GABA$_B$-positive receptor modulators: Enhancement of GABA$_B$ receptor agonist effects in vivo. *J Pharmacol Exp Ther*. 2010;335(1):163–171.

94. International Xyrem Study Group A double-blind, placebo-controlled study demonstrates sodium oxybate is effective for the treatment of excessive daytime sleepiness in narcolepsy. *J Clin Sleep Med*. 2005;1:391–397.

95. Mansukhani MP, Kotagal S. Sodium oxybate in the treatment of childhood narcolepsy-cataplexy: A retrospective study. *Sleep Med*. 2012;13:606–610.

96. Lecendreux M, Berthier J, Corny J, Bourdon O, Dossier C, Delclaux C. Intravenous Immunoglobulin Therapy in Pediatric Narcolepsy: A Nonrandomized, Open-Label, Controlled, Longitudinal Observational Study. *J Clin Sleep Med*. 2017;13:441–453.

97. Cohen A, Mandrekar St. J, Louis EK, Silber MH, Kotagal S. Comorbidities in a community sample of narcolepsy. *Sleep Med*. 2018;43:14–18.

98. Kaushik MK, Aritake K, Imanishi A, et al. Continuous intrathecal orexin delivery inhibits cataplexy in a murine model of narcolepsy. *Proc Natl Acad Sci U S A*. 2018;115(23):6046–6051.

99. Bandopadhyay A, Goldstein C. Clinical applications of artificial intelligence in sleep medicine: A sleep clinician's perspective. *Sleep Breath*. 2023;27:39–55.

18

Idiopathic Hypersomnia

Thuan Dang and Stephen H. Sheldon

CHAPTER HIGHLIGHTS

- Idiopathic hypersomnia (IH) can be difficult to differentiate from narcolepsy in children. As a result, it is a diagnosis of exclusion as it can be difficult to differentiate from the other disorders producing hypersomnolence.
- There can be a significant delay in diagnosis of IH as approximately two-thirds of patients develop symptoms before the age of 18, while the mean age of diagnosis was 30 years.
- Repeat PSG/MSLT testing may help quicken the path to diagnosis of IH.
- Behavioral therapy – including optimal sleep hygiene, patient safety, and scheduled naps – is the ideal initial treatment option.
- If stimulant medications are introduced, they should be used at the lowest doses tolerated and note closely for side effects such as delayed growth or excess anorexia.

Introduction

Excessive daytime sleepiness (EDS) in the pediatric and adolescent population is epidemic in our society. In the adolescent population, hypersomnolence manifests primarily as EDS. In part, symptoms are the result of school and lifestyle pressures. This is in combination with changes in circadian phase and total sleep time. In contrast, EDS manifesting as hypersomnolence is uncommon in young children. The primary manifestation of sleepiness in young children is hyperactivity. Young children respond to the symptom of sleepiness by increasing their motor activity to maintain alertness. However, even in this group, careful questioning does reveal symptoms of daytime sleepiness. The clinical definition of idiopathic hypersomnolence in childhood must consider this difference in the clinical response of children to the same "sleep pressure" manifested as EDS in adults.

Idiopathic hypersomnia (IH) is characterized by EDS and normal or long nocturnal sleep times, along with frequent and often prolonged naps. Both major sleep period and naps are typically unrefreshing.[1] Polysomnography (PSG) and the multiple sleep latency test (MSLT) demonstrate the absence of frequent periods of sleep onset with REM (SOREMP). The second edition of the *International Classification of Sleep Disorders: Diagnostic and Coding Manual* divides IH based

on nocturnal sleep time: idiopathic hypersomnia with long sleep time (ICD-10-CM G47.11) and idiopathic hypersomnia without long sleep time (ICD-10-CM G47.11). However, the third edition suggests that division of IH into these classifications lacks validity.[2] Table 18.1 contrasts the clinical criteria between these two diagnoses and narcolepsy without cataplexy (ICD-10-CM G47.419).[1] The key objective difference between narcolepsy and IH is SOREMP in two or more MSLT naps associated with narcolepsy.

Both disorders of IH are associated with difficult awakenings, sleep drunkenness, and unrefreshing primary sleep periods/naps.[1,3] Guilleminault and Pelayo have divided IH into three types based on etiology: those patients with a positive family history and positive HLA Cw2 antigen, a second type with history of viral infection, and a third group of those patients not included in the first two groups.[4] Bassetti and Aldrich divided their patients into three groups based on clinical symptoms.[3] The "classic idiopathic hypersomnia" group tended to have sleepiness that was not overwhelming, take unrefreshing naps of up to 4 hours, and have prolonged nighttime sleep and difficulty awakening. The second group, which they termed "narcoleptic type," presented with overwhelming EDS, took short refreshing naps, and awakened without sleepiness. Their third group was a "mixed group" with features of both syndromes.

Idiopathic hypersomnolence is a diagnosis of exclusion. A complete evaluation of other causes of hypersomnolence must be undertaken. The differential diagnosis of hypersomnolence is quite broad, ranging from mood disorders, to narcolepsy, to circadian rhythm disturbances or primary sleep disorders that cause EDS. Table 18.1 provides a framework based on etiology for further discussion of the differential diagnosis below.

Epidemiology

The incidence of diagnosis at major sleep centers varies from approximately 10% to 60% that of narcolepsy.[5,6] Anderson et al., in their series of 77 patients, noted that hypersomnia began at an age of 16.6 ± 9.4 years. Approximately two-thirds of patients developed symptoms before the age of 18. The mean age of diagnosis was 30 years.[5] In addition, Anderson et al. found 34% had a family history of

TABLE 18.1	Diagnostic Criteria		
	Narcolepsy Without Cataplexy	**Idiopathic Hypersomnia With Long Sleep Time**	**Idiopathic Hypersomnia Without Long Sleep Time**
	Complaint of EDS almost daily for >3 months	Complaint of EDS almost daily for >3 months	Complaint of EDS almost daily for >3 months
	Typical cataplexy not reported	Prolonged nocturnal sleep > 10 hr	Nocturnal sleep duration normal (6–10 hr)
	PSG demonstrates ≥6 hr sleep and no other cause for EDS	PSG demonstrates ≥6 hr sleep and no other cause for EDS	PSG demonstrates ≥6 hr sleep and no other cause for EDS
	Mean sleep latency < 8 min and ≥2 SOREMPs	Mean sleep latency < 8 min and <2 SOREMPs	Mean sleep latency < 8 min and <2 SOREMPs
	Hypersomnia not better explained by another sleep disorder, medical condition, behavioral problem, or substance abuse	Hypersomnia not better explained by another sleep disorder, medical condition, behavioral problem, or substance abuse	Hypersomnia not better explained by another sleep disorder, medical condition, behavioral problem, or substance abuse

EDS, Excessive daytime sleepiness; *PSG*, polysomnography; *SOREMP*, sleep onset with REM.
Based on American Academy of Sleep Medicine. *International Classification of Sleep Disorders. Diagnostic and Coding Manual*. 2nd ed. American Academy of Sleep Medicine; 2005.

similar symptoms, and, in eight cases, more than one family member was affected. Ali et al. in their series of 85 patients, found a familial incidence of 58%.[7]

Anderson found that 18% of IH patients were positive for the HLA *DQB1*0602* antigen compared with 98% of patients with narcolepsy.[5] The Cw2 antigen was observed in 10% of IH patients. A case report of three adolescent-onset cases of IH in a two-generation family raises the question of autosomal dominant inheritance.[8]

Children with central disorders of hypersomnia are vulnerable to sequelae related to learning; school performance; emotional functioning; engagement in curricular, extracurricular, and social activities; and quality of life. There is a complex relationship between neurobiologic features of IH, treatment, psychologic, sleep-related, and contextual factors across development.[9]

Pathophysiology

The underlying cause of the sleepiness in IH continues to be an active area of inquiry. Kanbayashi et al.[10] examined cerebrospinal fluid (CSF) levels of histamine in patients with IH, narcolepsy, obstructive sleep apnea (OSA) and normal neurologic controls. They found that low CSF histamine levels were mostly observed in non-medicated patients, and significant reductions compared with controls in histamine levels were observed only in non-medicated patients with hypocretin deficiency and with IH. In contrast, the levels in the medicated subjects with hypocretin deficiency and with IH did not differ significantly from those in control subjects. The authors also note that hypocretin-1 levels did not differ between medicated and non-medicated subjects in any of the hypersomnia categories.

Scammell and Mochizuki[11] note in an editorial in *Sleep* that reduced histamine signaling is an attractive

> **• BOX 18.1 Diagnostic Studies to Define Idiopathic Hypersomnia**
>
> - Sleep log
> - Polysomnography
> - Multiple sleep latency test/maintenance of wakefulness test
> - Actigraphy
> - Magnetic resonance imaging
> - Electroencephalography
> - Psychologic testing
> - Pediatric sleepiness scale

explanation for the sleepiness of IH. Parallel behavior between individuals with IH and mice with central histamine knockout (humans have great difficulty rousing from sleep in the morning, and mice lacking histamine exhibit a reduction in wake at the beginning of the usual active period).[12] Histamine H_3 receptors are inhibitory, exclusively located in the central nervous system (CNS).[10] H_3 receptor antagonists enhance central histaminergic neurotransmission specifically and are reported to enhance alertness in mouse models of narcolepsy. Kanbayashi's finding that low CSF histamine levels are observed in hypersomnia of central origin regardless of hypocretin-1 status suggests a wider role for this mechanism in the treatment of hypersomnia.[10]

Evaluation of Sleepiness in Children

Objective evaluation of sleepiness begins with a complete sleep history and physical examination to eliminate other causes of EDS (see Box 18.1). Sleep logs should be obtained to document sleep times, and actigraphy may be used to confirm the sleep log data. On the night before laboratory testing for daytime sleepiness, a polysomnogram should be obtained to confirm the absence of a primary sleep disorder. Hypersomnolence can be characterized quantitatively via the Multiple Sleep Latency Test (MSLT)[13] or Maintenance of Wakefulness Test (MWT).[14] Both tests measure the time to fall asleep during the daytime. The MSLT requires the patient to fall asleep, whereas the MWT requires the patient to stay awake. The mean adult sleep latency is 18.7 minutes. It is generally accepted that in the adult population the pathologic average sleep latency is 8 minutes or less as the result of the MSLT with an average sleep latency of 13.4 minutes.[15] Results from the MSLT and MWT often differ. Bonnet and Arand suggest that the MWT measures the sleep propensity and also the arousal system secondary to motivation and posture, whereas the MSLT is done supine and only measures sleep propensity.[16] Carskadon and Dement have demonstrated that sleep latency in children is age dependent.[17] Using Tanner stages to group children during adolescence, they observed a drop in average sleep latency on the MSLT of 20% between Tanner stages 1 and 3. This decreased sleep latency persisted in later adolescence (Tanner 4 and 5). In the same subjects, total sleep time and total rapid eye movement (REM) time remained constant but total slow-wave sleep (SWS) time deceased by 70%. Mean sleep latency of Tanner 1 and 2 children (mean age 12 years sleeping their habitual average of 9.1 hours) is 18 minutes. Compared with the college student (mean age 19 years, habitual sleep 7.1 hours) of less than 5.5 minutes. The definition of pathologic sleepiness in children must account for this age difference.

A number of pediatric sleepiness scales have been developed. Lewandowski et al. reviewed 21 measures and found that only six met "well-established" evidence-based assessment criteria.[18] Of these, only two—the Pediatric Daytime Sleepiness Scale[19] and the Sleep Disturbance Scale for Children[20]—assessed EDS. More recently, a modified pediatric Epworth Sleepiness Scale (ESS) has been developed and is titled the Epworth Sleepiness Scale for Children and Adolescents (ESS-CHAD).[21] It was concluded that the ESS-CHAD is a reliable and internally valid measure of daytime sleepiness in children between the ages of 6 and 16 years. Changes that were made to the adult-oriented ESS for pediatric patients did not affect the scale's capacity to measure daytime sleepiness. The EES-CHAD has also been shown to be sensitive and specific in children with craniopharyngioma.[22] Youngsters with craniopharyngioma are at high risk for EDS. This can be objective documented on MSLT, but patients frequently do not recognize or accurately report their sleepiness.

Clinical Presentation

Bassetti and Aldrich reviewed 42 cases of IH.[3] Onset of hypersomnolence was a mean age of 19±8 years (range 6–43 years). Onset was associated with insomnia in five, weight gain in two, viral illness in four, and minor head trauma in three. Forty-five percent of patients snored. Sixty percent took one or more involuntary naps during the day. Over half the subjects took naps of 30 minutes or longer, and

three-fourths reported the naps were unrefreshing. Over half of the patients had psychiatric problems. Polysomnographic recordings demonstrated short sleep latency of 6.6±5.7 minutes. Mean latency on the MSLT was 4.3±2.1 minutes. Five of 12 patients who underwent esophageal pressure monitoring were found to have upper airway resistance syndrome (UARS). None of these patients reported improved sleep with continuous positive airway pressure.

In their series of 77 patients with IH, Ali et al.[7] found that hypersomnia began at a mean ± SD age of 16.6 ± 9.4 years (range 0–46 years). Symptoms began before 18 years of age in 49 of 77 patients. Some patients and their families believed that the symptoms had been present from the first year of life, and, in 7 cases, worsening occurred over a period of several years. The mean age of diagnosis in this group was 30 years.[7] Precipitants were described by three subjects who reported a transient viral illness at the time of symptom onset, and one subject reported onset of symptoms over a day. The mean ESS score at initial presentation before treatment was 16.3±3.3 (range 11–24). In their study, Ali et al. noted that daytime somnolence interfered with work and social activities. The mean length of nighttime sleep reported was 9.2±1.8 hours, and this did not correlate with EES score.[7] There was no significant difference in MSLT between those with a long sleep time and those with a sleep time shorter than 10 hours. Seventy-six patients took nighttime sleep, and sleep drunkenness was not observed.[7]

Typically, symptoms begin during childhood including prolonged nighttime sleep, and awakening difficulties often precede the onset of daytime sleepiness. Roth reported continuous non-imperative sleepiness prolonged unrefreshing naps without dreaming and difficult arousal.[23] The risk of automobile accident or near-miss event was reported in 50% of 50 adult patients with IH over a 5-year period in Japan.[12]

Polysomnographic studies from Bassetti and Aldrich's 42 patients demonstrated a sleep efficiency of 93%, a mean of 20 total awakenings greater than 1 minute, 8% SWS, 18% REM sleep, automatic behaviors in 61%, and sleep paralysis in 40%.[3] Hours of sleep per day were 8.4±1.9, and time to activity in the morning was 42 minutes. Forza et al. studied 10 patients with IH;[24] all had onset before age 21. There was no statistical difference between IH patients and controls for total sleep time (TST) or sleep latency. Mean sleep latency was 9.1 minutes. IH patients demonstrated decreased SWS and increased REM sleep percentage with a sleep latency of 5.0 ±0.7 minutes.

Anderson et al.,[5] in their study of 77 IH patients, found a mean sleep latency of 11.5 minutes ± 8.2, increased mean SWS of 22.9% ± 8.7, and mean sleep efficiency of 94.3%. Ten patients had a sleep efficiency of less than 89%. REM sleep latency and percentages of light sleep and REM sleep were normal. Results from MSLT in this group of IH patients demonstrated that a mean sleep latency in patients with IH was 8.3±3.1 minutes, versus the narcolepsy group (4.1±2.6; $p < 0.001$). Comparison of the IH grouped by MSLT with sleep latency of at least 8 minutes or less than 8 minutes demonstrated no differences between these two groups in the duration of light sleep, SWS, REM sleep, sleep latency, sleep efficiency, REM sleep latency, body mass index, or untreated ESS.

Ali et al.[7] found the median nocturnal sleep latency was similar for males and females, but on MSLT, the mean sleep latency for males was lower than that for females. Thirteen patients had one SOREMP on either overnight polysomnography or MSLT, but none had two or more SOREMPs.

In a study of 75 patients with IH with and without long sleep time, Vernet and Arnulf[25] found that hypersomniacs had more fatigue, higher anxiety and depression scores, and more frequent hypnagogic hallucinations (24%), sleep paralysis (28%), sleep drunkenness (36%), and unrefreshing naps (46%) than controls. *DQB1*0602* genotype was similar, observed in 19% of controls and 24% of IH patients. Comparing the IH patients with long versus normal sleep time, those with long sleep time were younger, slimmer, and had more evening type characteristics and higher sleep efficiencies than those without long sleep time. MSLT latencies were normal (>8 minutes) in 71% of IH patients with long sleep time.[25]

Prevalence of EDS in children and adolescents was 29.2% in a recent study. It increased from 19.8% at Tanner stage 1 to 47.2% at Tanner stage 5.[26] EDS was significantly associated with short weekday time in bed, both long and short weekend time in bed, eveningness chronotype, insomnia symptoms, and sleep-disordered breathing symptoms.

Differential Diagnosis of Idiopathic Hypersomnolence

The differential diagnosis of idiopathic hypersomnolence includes those disorders that can produce EDS. A list based on etiology is seen in Box 18.2. History, physical examination,

• BOX 18.2 Differential Diagnosis of Hypersomnolence

- Neurologic disorders
  - Epilepsy and anticonvulsant therapy
  - Stroke
  - Tumor/increased intracranial pressure
  - Narcolepsy
- Primary sleep disorders
  - Insufficient sleep syndrome
  - Insomnia
  - Upper airway resistance syndrome
  - Obstructive sleep apnea syndrome
  - Restless legs syndrome
- Circadian disorders
  - Delayed phase syndrome
- Medical disorders
  - Infection: acute and chronic
  - Muscle diseases
  - Metabolic disorders
  - Prader–Willi syndrome
- Other disorders
  - Attention-deficit/hyperactivity disorder
  - Chronic fatigue syndrome/fibromyalgia
  - Kleine–Levin syndrome
  - Mood disorders
  - Drug dependence/abuse

polysomnography, and assessment of daytime sleep latency can usually exclude most of these diagnoses. Other chapters in this text cover most of these diagnoses, and this chapter will only touch on those that are outside of the primary sleep disorders.

It is often difficult to differentiate IH from narcolepsy, particularly in young children at presentation. Although symptoms may be present, classical MSLT findings may be absent, making definitive diagnosis difficult.[2] A repeat PSG/MSLT may be conducted 6–12 months later. Often the MSLT will show classical findings of narcolepsy at this time. Although not commonly performed, CSF hypocretin levels appear to be a definitive diagnostic test, provided it is interpreted within the clinical context.[27]

Primary Sleep Disorders

Whereas diagnostic criteria are well established for the primary sleep disorders in adults, normative data on which to base clinical decisions are only recently available for children. Thus, the reader must apply pediatric normative values when diagnosing sleep-disordered breathing[28] or restless legs syndrome/periodic leg movement disorder (RLS/PLMD).[29] Insufficient sleep syndrome is still the primary cause of daytime somnolence in most children. A number of studies have led to conflicting results with regards to school start times and daytime somnolence. Epstein et al. in Israel found decreased total sleep time and increased somnolence in fifth-grade pupils who started school at 7:10 a.m. versus 8 a.m.[30] A study in Maryland demonstrated no correlation of total sleep time with academic performance.[31]

UARS remains a diagnosis that must be excluded in this patient population. The use of esophageal pressure manometry is controversial, and consensus as to the usefulness of noninvasive measures, nasal pressure, and arterial tonometry has not been established in evaluation of upper airway resistance.

Neurologic Disorders

Narcolepsy remains the most difficult clinical syndrome to exclude in this group of disorders. It can present as young as 4 years of age and often cataplexy may not appear until later in life. However, the recent understanding that the absence of orexin/hypocretin as the pathophysiologic cause will facilitate accurate diagnosis of this patient group. CSF assay for the absence of orexin is becoming a routine clinical test.[32]

Heier et al. looked at CSF hypocretin-1 levels in patients with IH and those with narcolepsy with or without cataplexy. None of the patients with IH, narcolepsy without cataplexy, and those patients with HLA-negative narcolepsy with cataplexy had hypocretin levels less than 200,000 pg/mL. In contrast, 31 of 43 patients in the HLA-positive group had hypocretin levels less than 200,000 pg/mL.[33]

CNS lesions that produce increased intracranial pressure can be associated with hypersomnia. Poca et al. determined hypocretin levels in 26 patients with idiopathic intracranial hypertension and found no difference in these patients and their control group.[34] Subdural hematomas can produce an indolent syndrome of decreasing mental status and lethargy. Headache and vomiting are often associated with increased intracranial pressure. Epilepsy can produce a state in which the patient becomes lethargic and less responsive, the so-called petit-mal status or spike and wave stupor. During these periods, a pattern of the atypical continuous spike and wave discharges is observed on electroencephalography (EEG). Petit-mal status is often responsive to valproic acid with rapid return to normal state. Anticonvulsants also can produce sedation and EDS or paradoxical hyperactivity in children. Sedation appears to be common with carbamazepine, whereas hyperactivity is more common with phenobarbital.

Other Disorders

Attention-deficit/hyperactivity disorder (ADHD) is an active area of investigation as to its relationship to sleep disruption. Whereas both OSA syndrome and RLS/PLMD are associated with hyperactivity in children, ADHD is multifactorial in origin and sleep disorders that account for similar symptoms are noted in a significant fraction of children with ADHD.

Chronic fatigue/fibromyalgia syndrome is also a diagnosis of exclusion. Children often complain of diffuse muscle aches, and trigger points may be observed. The symptom is described as tiredness rather than true hypersomnia. Polysomnography may demonstrate an alpha–delta pattern on EEG.[35] Depression and UARS must be excluded in chronic fatigue patients as well.

Childhood mood disorders are commonly associated with sleep difficulties. Symptoms often manifest as insomnia, early morning awakenings, daytime sleepiness, or hypersomnia. Vgontzas et al. found increased sleep latency (54 minutes vs. 15 minutes), increased wake time after sleep onset (79 minutes vs. 56.8 minutes), and increased total wake time (134 minutes vs. 72 minutes) in patients with psychiatric etiologies for their hypersomnia compared with patients with IH. In patients with psychiatric disorders, REM sleep was decreased, compared with patients with IH.[36] Bipolar disorder may also present with hypersomnia during the depression phase of the illness. At times, there may be overlap with Kleine–Levin syndrome.

Circadian Disorders

Delayed-phase syndrome may also produce hypersomnolence. Affected children, however, report normal total sleep times in the presence of delayed sleep onset and morning hypersomnia. Non–24-hour sleep–wake cycles, as well as advanced sleep-phase syndrome, may also produce hypersomnolence. Sleep logs and/or actigraphy are often helpful in differentiating these problems.

Medical Disorders

Recovery from acute viral or bacterial illness often results in hypersomnolence. Hypersomnolence associated with fever and stiff neck should alert the examiner to possible meningitis. Stiff neck and other meningeal signs may be absent in children under 1 year of age. Lumbar puncture should always be performed if any question of meningitis exists. Kubota et al. report a case of acute disseminated encephalomyelitis associated with hypersomnolence as the major presenting feature and low hypocretin levels in the CSF.[37] Arii et al. describe hypersomnolence and low hypocretin levels in a child after removal of a hypothalamic tumor.[38]

Metabolic disorders may produce episodic mental status changes that produce sleepiness and altered mental status. Disorders of ammonia metabolism, lactate and pyruvate metabolism, and mitochondrial metabolism can be associated with episodic hypersomnia. Acute infection or other metabolic stress often precipitates these episodes. Muscle weakness can also be a source of hypersomnolence. In primary muscle disease, the dystrophies are often associated with decreased respiratory effort secondary to fatigue. Polysomnography demonstrates increasing REM-related central apnea as the first sign of weakness and need for nocturnal respiratory support.[39]

Prader–Willi syndrome is associated with obesity, craniofacial dysmorphism, hypotonia, hyperphasia, hypersomnia, and hypothalamic dysfunction. Manni et al. found sleep-onset REM periods in 5 of 10 children with Prader–Willi syndrome on MSLT.[40] None of the patients was Dr 15 or Dq 6 positive. Hypersomnia and SOREMPs could not be accounted for by sleep-disordered breathing alone; however, UARS was not excluded in these patients.

Treatment

The goal in IH is improvement in quality of life and improvement in symptoms of EDS. In untreated IH patients older than 20 years, Ozaki et al.[41] found decreased subscale scores in seven of nine domains of the SF-36 compared with normal. The changes did correlate with ESS scores in domains of autonomy, in controlling one's own job schedule, experience of divorce or break-up with a partner due to symptoms, experience of being forced to relocate or being dismissed due to symptoms, and perception of support of others. Treatment improved ESS scores. They concluded that the decrease of health-related quality of life could be attributed to psychologic, social, and environmental factors, such as lifestyle or social support rather than subjective sleepiness.[41] Comparing patients with IH and narcolepsy without cataplexy, Dauvilliers et al. found similar results of the Beck Depression Scale and SF-36 in both groups. These results contrasted with the narcolepsy with cataplexy group, who demonstrated higher mean scores and increased percentage with a score greater than 7 (31.8% vs. 18.1% in the IH group) on the Beck inventory.[42]

Treatment of IH is focused on symptom control, as the primary etiology remains unknown. The goal of therapy is to allow the patient to enjoy normal alert functioning and restful nocturnal sleep.

The approach to therapy is sleep hygiene, appropriate use of stimulant medication, and safety for the patient.

TABLE 18.2	Stimulants Used for Treatment of Idiopathic Hypersomnolence		
Name	Duration of Action (hr)	Contraindications	Special Considerations
Methylphenidate	4–6	Increased risk of cardiac arrhythmias	
Time release preps	8–12		Longer action
Dexmethylphenidate	4–6		Isomer of parent compound
Dextroamphetamines	4–6		
Time spans	6–12		
Mixed salts	4–6		
Extended release preps	8–12		Longer duration of action
Modafinil	6–8		Non-amphetamine drugs
Armodafinil	6–8		
Pemoline	12	High risk of liver disease	Rarely used

Sleep hygiene measures should include scheduled naps and regular sleep periods of 8–10 hours nightly. Medications, drugs, or alcohol that promote sleepiness should be avoided. Stimulant medication should be used at the lowest effective doses tolerated. Growth problems secondary to anorexia can be a limiting factor for stimulant use in some children. In addition, a balanced plan of stimulant use must be maintained so as not to interfere with nighttime sleep. The newer, longer-acting stimulants (Table 18.2) have been beneficial in management, keeping medicine out of the school setting and decreasing the need for late afternoon dosing. The American Academy of Child and Adolescent Psychiatry has produced a practice parameter for stimulant use in children, adolescents, and adults.[43] In 2007, the American Academy of Sleep Medicine produced a practice parameter for the treatment of narcolepsy and other hypersomnias of central origin.[44] They concluded, "Treatment of hypersomnia of central origin with methylphenidate or modafinil in children between the ages of 6 and 15 appears to be relatively safe." They recommend regular follow-up of patients to monitor response to treatment and side effects and to enhance the patient's adaptation to the disorder.[44]

A number of retrospective studies examined modafinil versus methylphenidate. Ali et al.[7] followed 85 patients for a median duration of 2.4 years. In their group, 65% of patients demonstrated a "complete response" to pharmacotherapy. Methylphenidate was more commonly used as a first-line agent before December 1998, but after its approval modafinil became the more commonly used first drug. At the last visit, 92% of patients were on monotherapy and 51% on methylphenidate versus 32% on modafinil. No difference in the response rate between the two drugs was demonstrated.[7] Adult dosing in this study was 367.4 ± 140.9 mg for modafinil and 50.9 ± 27.3 mg for methylphenidate.[7] Lavault et al.[45] reviewed response to therapy with modafinil in 104 patients with IH (59 with long sleep time compared with patients with narcolepsy with cataplexy). They found similar response to modafinil in both patient populations. Improvement in ESS scores was greater in the IH group without long sleep time compared with those with long sleep time. Loss of efficacy and habituation were rare. Adult doses of modafinil in this study ranged from 50 to 600 mg.[45] In 66 patients with IH, Anderson et al. found that 11 had spontaneous remission. No clinical characteristics could be identified to differentiate the spontaneous remitters.[5] In this study, 24 of 39 patients treated with modafinil had a 4-point or greater reduction in ESS.[5]

Summary

IH remains a diagnosis of exclusion, and at times it can be difficult to differentiate from the other disorders producing hypersomnolence (see Table 18.1). Continued research is necessary to better characterize this disorder in children. Treatment should be symptomatic; naps, improved sleep hygiene, and stimulants should be used in concert to improve quality of life in affected children. Although no dosing studies are available for children, both modafinil and methylphenidate appear to be safe and effective treatments. The role of histamine in the etiology of IH in children requires further exploration and may lead to future treatment in hypersomnias of central origin.

CLINICAL PEARLS

- Idiopathic hypersomnia is a diagnosis of exclusion.
- Narcolepsy without cataplexy can be distinguished by sleep-onset REM periods.
- Inadequate sleep hygiene is the most common cause of daytime sleepiness in adolescents and adults.
- Use of actigraphy may be helpful to distinguish the disorder from the consequences of inadequate sleep.

References

1. American Academy of Sleep Medicine. *International Classification of Sleep Disorders. Diagnostic and Coding Manual.* 2nd ed. American Academy of Sleep Medicine; 2005.
2. American Academy of Sleep Medicine. *International Classification of Sleep Disorders. Diagnostic and Coding Manual,* 3rd ed. American Academy of Sleep Medicine; 2014.
3. Bassetti C, Aldrich MS. Idiopathic hypersomnia: a series of 42 patients. *Brain.* 1997;120:1423–1435.
4. Guilleminault C, Pelayo R. Idiopathic central nervous system hypersomnia. In: Kryger MH, Roth T, Dement WC, eds. *Practice and Principles of Sleep Medicine.* 3rd ed. W.B. Saunders; 2000:687–692.
5. Anderson KN, Pilsworth S, Sharples LD, et al. Idiopathic hypersomnia: a study of 77 cases. *Sleep.* 2007;30(10):1274–1281.
6. Han F, Lin L, Li J, et al. Presentations of primary hypersomnia in Chinese children. *Sleep.* 2011;34(5):627–632.
7. Ali M, Auger RR, Slocumb NL, et al. Idiopathic hypersomnia: clinical features and response to treatment. *J Clin Sleep Med.* 2009;5(6):562–568.
8. Janackova S, Motte J, Bakchine S, et al. Idiopathic hypersomnia: a report of three adolescent-onset cases in a two-generation family. *J Child Neurol.* 2011;26(4):522–525.
9. Graef DM, Byars KC, Simakajornboon N, Dye TJ. Topical review: a biopsychosocial framework for pediatric narcolepsy and idiopathic hypersomnia. *J Ped Psychology.* 2020;45(1):34–39.
10. Kanbayashi T, Kodama T, Kondo H, et al. CSF histamine contents in narcolepsy, idiopathic hypersomnia and obstructive sleep apnea syndrome. *Sleep.* 2009;32(2):181–187.
11. Scammell TE, Mochizuki T. Is low histamine a fundamental cause of sleepiness in narcolepsy and idiopathic hypersomnia? *Sleep.* 2009;32(2):133–134.
12. Parmentier R, Ohtsu H, Djebbara-Hannas Z, et al. Anatomical, physiological, and pharmacological characteristics of histidine decarboxylase knock-out mice: evidence for the role of brain histamine in behavioral and sleep-wake control. *J Neurosci.* 2002;22:7695–7711.
13. Carskadon MA, Dement WC, Mitler MM, et al. Guidelines for the multiple sleep latency test (MSLT): a standard measure of sleepiness. *Sleep.* 1986;9:519–524.
14. Mitler MM, Gujavarti KS, Browman CP. Maintenance of wakefulness test: a polysomnographic technique for evaluation of treatment efficacy in patients with excessive somnolence. *Electroencephalogr Clin Neurophysiol.* 1982;53:658–661.
15. Mitler MM, Carskadon MA, Hirshkowitz M. Evaluating sleepiness. In: Kryger MH, Roth T, Dement WC, eds. *Practice and Principles of Sleep Medicine.* 3rd ed. W.B. Saunders; 2000.
16. Bonnet MH, Arand DL. Arousal components which differentiate the MWT from the MSLT. *Sleep.* 2001;24:441–447.
17. Carskadon MA, Dement WC. Sleepiness in the normal adolescent. In: Guilleminault C, ed. *Sleep and Its Disorders in Children.* Raven Press; 1987:53–66.
18. Lewandowski AS, Toliver-Sokol M, Palermo TM. Evidence-based review of subjective pediatric sleep measures. *J Pediatr Psychol.* 2011;36(7):780–793.
19. Drake C, Nickel C, Burduvali E, et al. The Pediatric Daytime Sleepiness Scale (PDSS): sleep habits and school outcomes in middle-school children. *Sleep.* 2003;26(4):455–458.
20. Bruni O, Ottaviano S, Guidetti V, et al. The Sleep Disturbance Scale for Children (SDSC). Construction and validation of an instrument to evaluate sleep disturbances in childhood and adolescence. *J Sleep Res.* 1996;5(4):251–261.
21. Janssen KC, Phillipson S, O'Connor J, Johns MW. Validation of the Epworth Sleepiness Scale for children and adolescents using Rasch analysis. *Sleep Med.* 2017;33:30–35.
22. Crabtree VM, Klages KL, Sykes A, et al. Sensitivity and specificity of the Modified Epworth Sleepiness Scale in children with craniopharyngioma. *J Clin Sleep Med.* 2019;15(10):1487–1493.
23. Roth B. *Narcolepsy and Hypersomnia.* Karger; 1980.
24. Forza E, Gaudreau H, Petit D, et al. Homeostatic sleep regulation in patients with idiopathic hypersomnia. *Clin Neurophysiol.* 2000;111:277–282.
25. Vernet C, Arnulf I. Idiopathic hypersomnia with and without long sleep time: a controlled series of 75 patients. *Sleep.* 2009;32(6):753–759.
26. Liu Y, Zhang J, Li SX, Chan NY, et al. Excessive daytime sleepiness among children and adolescents: prevalence, correlates, and pubertal effects. *Sleep Med.* 2018;53:1–8.
27. Mignot E, Lammers GJ, Okun RB, et al. The role of cerebrospinal fluid hypocretin measurement in the diagnosis of narcolepsy and other hypersomnias. *Arch Neurol.* 2002;59(10):1553–1562.
28. Goodwin JL, Enright PL, Morgan WJ, et al. Correlates of obstructive sleep apnea in 6–12 year old children. The Tucson Children Assessment of Sleep Apnea Study (TUCASA). *Sleep.* 200225 abstract supplement:A80.
29. Kohrman MH, Kerr SL, Schumacher S. Effect of sleep disordered breathing on periodic leg movements of sleep in children. *Sleep.* 1997:20.
30. Epstein R, Chillag N, Lavie P. Starting times of school: effects on daytime functioning of fifth grade children in Israel. *Sleep.* 1998;21:250256.
31. King J, Gould B, Eliasson A. Association of sleep and academic performance. *Sleep Breath.* 2002:4548.
32. Nishino S, Ripley B, Overeem S, et al. Hypocretin (orexin) deficiency in human narcolepsy. *Lancet.* 2000;355:3940.
33. Heier MS, Evsiukova T, Vilming S, et al. CSF hypocretin-1 levels and clinical profiles in narcolepsy and idiopathic CNS hypersomnia in Norway. *Sleep.* 2007;30(8):969973.
34. Poca MA, Galard R, Serrano E, et al. Normal hypocretin-1 (orexin A) levels in cerebrospinal fluid in patients with idiopathic intracranial hypertension. *Acta Neurochir Suppl.* 2012;114:221225.
35. Whelton CL, Salit I, Moldofsky H. Sleep, Epstein–Barr virus infection, musculoskeletal pain and depressive symptoms in chronic fatigue syndrome. *J Rheumatol.* 1992;19:939943.
36. Vgontzas AN, Bixler EO, Kales A, et al. Differences in nocturnal and daytime sleep between primary and psychiatric hypersomnia: diagnostic and treatment implications. *Psychosomatic Med.* 2000;62:220226.
37. Kubota H, Kanbayashi T, Tanabe Y, et al. A case of acute disseminated encephalomyelitis presenting hypersomnia with

decreased hypocretin level in cerebrospinal fluid. *J Child Neuro.* 2002;17:537539.

38. Arii J, Kanbayashi T, Tababe Y, et al. A hypersomnolent girl with decreased CSF hypocretin level after removal of a hypothalamic tumor. *Neurology.* 2001;56:17751776.

39. Kerr SL, Kohrman MH. Polysomnogram in Duchenne muscular dystrophy. *J Child Neurol.* 1994;9:332334.

40. Manni R, Politini L, Nobili L, et al. Hypersomnia in the Prader–Willi syndrome: clinical-electrophysiological features and underlying factors. *Clin Neurophysiol.* 2001;112:800805.

41. Ozaki A, Inoue Y, Nakajima T, et al. Health-related quality of life among drug-naïve patients with narcolepsy with cataplexy, narcolepsy without cataplexy, and idiopathic hypersomnia without long sleep time. *J Clin Sleep Med.* 2008;4(6):572578.

42. Dauvilliers Y, Paquereau J, Bastuji H, et al. Psychological health in central hypersomnias: the French Harmony study. *J Neurol Neurosurg Psychiatry.* 2009;80:636641.

43. Greenhill LL, Plixzka S, Dulcan MK. Work Group on Quality Issues. Practice parameter for the use of stimulant medications in the treatment of children, adolescents, and adults. *J Am Acad Child Adolesc Psychiatry.* 2002;4126S49S.

44. Kapur VK, Brown T, Swick TJ, et al. Standards of Practice Committee of the AASM. Practice parameters for the treatment of narcolepsy and other hypersomnias of central origin. *Sleep.* 2007;30(12):17051711.

45. Lavault S., Dauvilliers Y., Drouot X., et al. Benefit and risk of modafinil in idiopathic hypersomnia vs. narcolepsy with cataplexy. Sleep Med. 2011;12:550556.

19

Kleine-Levin Syndrome and Recurrent Hypersomnias

Stephen H. Sheldon and Brittany Nance

CHAPTER HIGHLIGHTS

- Kleine-Levin syndrome is an uncommon disorder occurring most often in males (but can occur in females) during middle adolescence.
- It is characterized by recurrent hypersomnia with cognitive abnormalities, altered perception, eating disorder, and disinhibited behavior, with return to normalcy during asymptomatic periods
- Underlying etiology is unclear and the exact pathophysiological mechanism is still to be determined.
- Treatment may include lithium therapy, but is generally aimed at symptomatology, and therapeutic response varies.
- Most often, there is spontaneous resolution of symptoms without noted sequelae.

Introduction

Kleine-Levin syndrome (KLS) is an unusual disorder of recurrent episodes of excessive sleepiness and prolonged total sleep time. It generally presents in late adolescence, but its etiology remains largely unknown. There are multiple hypotheses that include functional imaging demonstrating hypoperfusion, autoimmune correlation, genetics, and precipitating events such as infections, head trauma, alcohol, sleep deprivation, and/or stress.[1] KLS is considered to be extremely rare with an estimated prevalence of 1–2 per million (male to female ratio of 2:1).[2]

Clinical Characteristics

Hypersomnia is the characteristic symptom of KLS.[3] Sleepiness is profound and, during spells, patients may sleep continuously for more than 20 hours. Hypersomnia may last from several days to several weeks, recurring at least one time in an 18-month period, and presenting with one, but not all, of the following: "cognitive abnormalities, altered perception, eating disorder (hyperphagia or anorexia), and disinhibited behavior such as hypersexuality" (Box 19.1).[4]

Recurrent episodes of hypersomnia may be brief and last less than 1 week or may be prolonged and last up to 30 days with normal physical examination. Characteristic of KLS is recurrence of episodes of hypersomnia and behavioral abnormalities. During asymptomatic periods there is a return to normal alertness, behavior, and cognitive function.[4] There are few studies looking at long-term sequelae; however, there is growing concern regarding long-term cognitive deficits including verbal retrieval and speed of processing, as well as impairment of working memory and visuospatial processing.[5,6]

It is thought that KLS is a relapsing-remitting disorder with average duration of approximately 14 years from diagnosis; however, it may persist in some patients.[5] Due to this, patients often develop anxiety surrounding recurrence of episodes.

Menstruation-associated hypersomnia has been reported in female patients. Recurrent periods of hypersomnolence occur and are coupled to menses. Occasionally, mental disturbances also occur, and also occur with the menstrual cycle.[7] There are several reports that have found that treatment with oral contraceptive pills is successful for the management of menstruation-associated hypersomnia.[8,9]

Etiology

The cause of recurrent hypersomnia is unknown, but likely multifactorial. A possible viral etiology may be present in some cases. In other cases, there may be a suggestion of a local encephalitis in the region of the diencephalon.[10-12] Because many patients report a history of preceding infection, a post-infectious, autoimmune mechanism has also been suggested.[6] Recently, a case report of a pediatric patient with post-infectious KLS was found to have anti-N-methyl-D-aspartate (NMDA) type glutamate receptor antibody levels in his cerebrospinal fluid (CSF).[13] Patients with anti-NMDA encephalitis have been reported to have significant sleep-related disturbances including hypersomnia with hyperphagia and hypersexuality in the post-recovery period.[14] Ortega-Albas and colleagues have suggested

• **BOX 19.1**   **Diagnostic Criteria for Kleine-Levin Syndrome (ICSD-3-TR, 2023)[4]**

Criteria A–E must be met
A. The patient experiences at least two recurrent episodes of excessive sleepiness and sleep duration, each persisting 2 days to 5 weeks.
B. Episodes recur usually more than once a year and at least every 18 months.
C. The patient has normal alertness, cognitive function, behavior, and mood between episodes.
D. The patient must demonstrate at least one of the following during an episode:
   1. Cognitive dysfunction
   2. Altered perception
   3. Eating disorder (anorexia or hyperphagia)
   4. Disinhibited behavior (such as hypersexuality)
E. The hypersomnolence and related symptoms are not better explained by another sleep disorder; medical, neurologic, or psychiatric disorder (especially bipolar disorder); or use of drugs or medications.

that the excitatory and inhibitory symptoms of KLS may be explained by disruptions in the glutamate/gamma-aminobutyric acid (Glu-GABA) system and there is some speculation that gamma-hydroxybutyrate (GHB) may trigger KLS, which would further strengthen the hypothesis for the role of Glu-GABA disruption in KLS.[15,16] It is difficult to diagnostically test this hypothesis, and benzodiazepines, which are known GABA agonists, have not shown significant impact on KLS symptoms. However, there have been multiple reports of GABA antagonists providing effectiveness in reduction of at least subjective KLS symptoms with clarithromycin[17,18] and flumazenil.[19] Recurrent transient episodes of unresponsiveness and clearly identified stage 2 sleep pattern with the presence of sleep spindles has also been reported due to bilateral paramedian thalamic infarctions.[20] Although the exact cause of recurrent hypersomnia and other manifestations is still unclear, the symptoms of hypersomnolence, excessive and compulsive eating, hypersexuality, recurrence, and absence of any identifiable abnormalities between spells is suggestive of a functional abnormality at the level of the diencephalon. The hypothalamus may also be involved. Indeed, identical symptoms have been reported in patients with tumors of the hypothalamus or third ventricle and in patients with epidemic encephalitis. Most literature and case reports suggest that this recurrent hypersomnia is caused by dysfunction of the hypothalamus and midbrain limbic system. Neuroimaging has been used to evaluate brain function in KLS.[21] More recently, fluorodeoxyglucose positron emission tomography/computed tomography (FDG PET/CT) has shown marked symmetric hypometabolism in the thalamus and hypothalamus as well as mild homogeneous decreased glucose metabolism in the cortex in the symptomatic phase of KLS. When asymptomatic much less severe hypometabolism in the thalamus and hypothalamus was identified.[22] Recently, there have been studies demonstrating single-photon emission computerized tomography (SPECT) may be of use due to frontotemporal hypoperfusion. Vigren and coworkers found that during a symptomatic period 48% patients studied had frontal and/or temporal hypoperfusion on SPECT.[23] Another study, comparing asymptomatic and symptomatic KLS with control group utilizing SPECT found evidence of hypoperfusion in the frontotemporal region, but specifically cited increased hypoperfusion in the right dorsomedial prefrontal cortex and right temporoparietal junction with persistence of hypoperfusion in the asymptomatic period.[24] There is also evidence that brainstem dysfunction may also be involved. Recurrent hypersomnia associated with decreased blood flow in the thalamus on SPECT has also been reported.[25] During the remission period, there were no abnormal data in these tests.

Neuroendocrine function in patients with KLS has been assessed; however, only a limited number of subjects have been investigated and most literature consists of case reports. Investigation is complicated by the inability to predict timing of episodes, lack of a prodromal period, and relatively rapid recovery once symptoms begin. Nonetheless, some abnormal laboratory data reported include a paradoxical growth hormone response to thyroid-releasing hormone stimulation,[26] a blunted cortisol response to insulin-induced hypoglycemia,[27,28] and an absent thyroid-stimulating hormone response to thyroid-releasing hormone.[27] These findings suggest a possible dysfunction within the hypothalamic-pituitary axis. However, other basal and post-stimulation values of hormones are usually normal and laboratory values are normal during the asymptomatic periods between spells.

Studies of nocturnal or 24-hour secretory patterns of pituitary hormones have been conducted in a limited number of patients. Normal secretory pattern of growth hormone was reported in one patient, but the sampling at 4-hour intervals was sparse.[29] Normal 24-hour patterns of melatonin, prolactin, and cortisol secretion have been reported.[30] Gadoth and colleagues found an increased nocturnal prolactin secretory pattern and an abnormally flat nocturnal luteinizing hormone secretory pattern, whereas follicle-stimulating hormone and thyroid-stimulating hormone secretory patterns were normal.[26] Chesson and coworkers compared 24-hour secretions in the symptomatic and the asymptomatic period and found that values obtained during nocturnal sleep showed a significantly decreased growth hormone, but increased prolactin and thyroid-stimulating hormone, in a direction that supports the hypothesis that dopamine tone is reduced during the symptomatic period in KLS.[31] However, Mayer and colleagues found only minor hormonal changes in five patients.[32] Altogether, these data suggest some functional disturbance in the hypothalamic-pituitary axis in KLS, but the disturbance may be in response to the sleep-related and behavioral changes rather than a cause. An observation supporting a diencephalic dysfunction is the occurrence of dysautonomic features in some patients.[33]

Recurrent hypersomnia may occur with space-occupying lesions of the central nervous system (CNS), idiopathic recurring stupor, and certain psychologic/psychiatric conditions. Tumors in the region of the third ventricle, such as cysts, astrocytomas, and/or craniopharyngiomas, may be responsible for intermittent obstruction of the third ventricle leading to headache, vomiting, sensory disturbances, and intermittent impairment of alertness. Less frequently, tumors in other CNS locations may result in hypersomnia. Tumors in the middle fossa may disrupt the suprachiasmatic nucleus and an irregular sleep–wake pattern or a free-running state might occur. If a free running state occurs, hypersomnia may alternate with sleeplessness at a regular interval as the pacemaker cycles at its inherent rhythm. Recurrent hypersomnia may also develop after encephalitis or head trauma. Periodic hypersomnia has also been reported in a patient with a Rathke's cleft cyst.[34]

Major recurrent depression and bipolar affective disorder can be associated with excessive sleepiness.[35] Patients with psychogenic recurrent hypersomnia complain of extreme sleepiness and fatigue and may spend many hours in bed. Continuous night-and-day polygraphic recording often fails to demonstrate increased total sleep time despite the complaint of sleepiness.[36]

There may be genetic or familial predisposition as well. LMOD3 variants have been found in some families with KLS,[37] and in those with birthing difficulties, TRANK1 variants have also been noted.[38]

Evaluation

The diagnosis of KLS is typically based on clinical features. Laboratory evaluations are occasionally useful, because the diagnosis may be one of exclusion of other similar pathology. Complete blood count (CBC), platelet count, electrolytes, renal and liver function tests, calcium, phosphorus, serum protein electrophoresis, immunoglobulins, antinuclear antibodies, rheumatoid factor, and serum titers for herpes simplex, Epstein-Barr virus, cytomegalovirus, varicella-zoster, mumps, and measles have all been found to be normal in patients with KLS both during episodes and between episodes. CSF evaluation with cultures for bacteria, mycobacterium, virus, and fungi have also been shown to be negative.

Routine electroencephalogram (EEG) obtained during attacks may show generalized slowing of background activity or may be unremarkable. Magnetic resonance imaging (MRI) is normal during and between spells of hypersomnia.[31] Prolonged polysomnographic monitoring may reveal the increased total sleep time. During symptomatic periods, the multiple sleep latency test (MSLT) can reveal abnormal sleep latencies and sleep-onset rapid eye movement (REM) periods (SOREMPs). Therefore, it has been suggested the MSLT may be useful in diagnosis, especially when the polysomnography and MSLT are performed no earlier than the second night after the onset of hypersomnolence.[39] During asymptomatic periods polysomnography and MSLT are both normal.[40]

Lin and colleagues demonstrated a possible disruption in circadian rhythm during symptomatic episodes of KLS in which case actigraphy may play a role during episodes of hypersomnia.[41] There is no current diagnostic testing to confirm diagnosis; therefore it requires the exclusion of other disorders, which may be difficult. This commonly includes the exclusion of psychiatric disorders such as bipolar disorder, or other sleep-related hypersomnias such as narcolepsy.

Treatment

Interventions are focused on terminating the hypersomnia episode. Amphetamines and methylphenidate, and modafinil have been utilized in both treatment and prevention.[42] However, stimulant therapy has been shown to not be very effective and increases agitation during the symptomatic phase of KLS.[2] Antiepileptic drugs such as valproic acid, carbamazepine, phenytoin, lamotrigine, and gabapentin have been effective in preventing symptoms in some patients.[43] If Glu-GABA disruption is considered there may be a role for clarithromycin, which is recommended in the treatment of idiopathic hypersomnia,[44] or GABAergics such as amantadine and sodium oxybate to target excitatory symptoms, corticosteroids to target long-term inhibitory symptoms, and lithium to stabilize symptoms.[15] Although new guidelines suggest only lithium as treatment for KLS, no other treatment has been formally recommended or suggested, including intravenous (IV) corticosteroids.[44] Generally, the effectiveness of maintaining wakefulness, treating symptoms, and prevention of recurrences using a variety of therapeutic approaches does not seem effective.

CLINICAL PEARLS

- Kleine-Levin syndrome (KLS) is a rare disorder characterized by recurrent episodes of excessive sleepiness, prolonged total sleep time, and uncharacteristic behavior; separated by extended periods of normal sleep and behavior.
- Exact cause of KLS is unknown, but is believed to be multifactorial, with possible viral, autoimmune, and genetic factors playing a role.
- During episodes of hypersomnia, patients may sleep continuously for more than 20 hours and experience cognitive abnormalities, altered perception, eating disorders, and disinhibited behavior.
- Treatment for KLS is focused on managing symptoms. However, the effectiveness of these treatments is limited.
- Most patients with KLS experience spontaneous resolution of symptoms without any long-term sequelae.

References

1. Habra O, Heinzer R, Haba-Rubio J, Rossetti AO. Prevalence and mimics of Kleine-Levin syndrome: A survey in French-speaking Switzerland. *J Clin Sleep Med.* 2016;12(8):1083–1087.

https://doi.org/10.5664/jcsm.6040. [published Online First: Epub Date].

2. Dauvilliers Y, Barateau L. Narcolepsy and other central hypersomnias. *Continuum (Minneap Minn)*. 2017;23(4, Sleep Neurology):989–1004. 10.1212/CON.0000000000000492 [published Online First: Epub Date].

3. Dye TJ Idiopathic hypersomnia and Kleine-Levin Syndrome: Primary disorders of hypersomnolence beyond narcolepsy. Semin Pediatr Neurol. 2023;48:101082. https://doi.org/10.1016/j.spen.2023.101082.

4. American Academy of Sleep Medicine. *The International Classification of Sleep Disorders. Third Edition*. American Academy of Sleep Medicine; 2023. 3–TR ed.

5. Uguccioni G, Lavault S, Chaumereuil C, Golmard JL, Gagnon JF, Arnulf I. Long-term cognitive impairment in Kleine-Levin syndrome. *Sleep*. 2016;39(2):429–438. https://doi.org/10.5665/sleep.5458. [published Online First: Epub Date].

6. Miglis MG, Guilleminault C. Kleine-Levin syndrome. *Curr Neurol Neurosci Rep*. 2016;16(6):60. https://doi.org/10.1007/s11910-016-0653-6. [published Online First: Epub Date].

7. Billiard M, Guilleminault C, Dement WC. A menstruation-linked periodic hypersomnia. Kleine-Levin syndrome or new clinical entity? *Neurology*. 1975;25(5):436–443. https://doi.org/10.1212/wnl.25.5.436. [published Online First: Epub Date].

8. Sachs C, Persson HE, Hagenfeldt K. Menstruation-related periodic hypersomnia: A case study with successful treatment. *Neurology*. 1982;32(12):1376–1379. https://doi.org/10.1212/wnl.32.12.1376. [published Online First: Epub Date].

9. Suau GM, Cabrera V, Romaguera J. Menstruation-related hypersomnia treated with hormonal contraception: Case report and review of literature. *P R Health Sci J*. 2016;35(1):40–42.

10. Kesler A, Gadoth N, Vainstein G, Peled R, Lavie P. Kleine Levin syndrome (KLS) in young females. *Sleep*. 2000;23(4):563–567.

11. Carpenter S, Yassa R, Ochs R. A pathologic basis for Kleine-Levin syndrome. *Arch Neurol*. 1982;39(1):25–28. https://doi.org/10.1001/archneur.1982.00510130027005. [published Online First: Epub Date].

12. Fenzi F, Simonati A, Crosato F, Ghersini L, Rizzuto N. Clinical features of Kleine-Levin syndrome with localized encephalitis. *Neuropediatrics*. 1993;24(5):292–295. https://doi.org/10.1055/s-2008-1071559. [published Online First: Epub Date].

13. Tani M, Konishi Y, Nishida T, Takahashi Y, Kusaka T. A case of Kleine-Levin syndrome with positive anti-NMDA-type glutamate receptor antibodies. *Pediatr Int*. 2020;62(3):409–410. https://doi.org/10.1111/ped.14088. [published Online First: Epub Date].

14. Arino H, Munoz-Lopetegi A, Martinez-Hernandez E, et al. Sleep disorders in anti-NMDAR encephalitis. *Neurology*. 2020;95(6):e671–e684. https://doi.org/10.1212/WNL.0000000000009987. [published Online First: Epub Date].

15. Ortega-Albas JJ, Lopez R, Martinez A, Carratala S, Echeverria I, Ortega P. Kleine-Levin syndrome, GABA, and glutamate. *J Clin Sleep Med*. 2021;17(3):609–610. https://doi.org/10.5664/jcsm.9058. [published Online First: Epub Date].

16. Vaillant G, Martin M, Groos E, Larabi IA, Alvarez JC, Arnulf I. A strange New Year's Eve: Triggers in Kleine-Levin syndrome. *J Clin Sleep Med*. 2021;17(2):329–332. https://doi.org/10.5664/jcsm.8858. [published Online First: Epub Date].

17. Trotti LM, Bliwise DL, Rye DB. Further experience using clarithromycin in patients with Kleine-Levin syndrome. *J Clin Sleep*

Med. 2014;10(4):457–458. https://doi.org/10.5664/jcsm.3634. [published Online First: Epub Date].

18. Rezvanian E, Watson NF. Kleine-levin syndrome treated with clarithromycin. *J Clin Sleep Med*. 2013;9(11):1211–1212. https://doi.org/10.5664/jcsm.3176. [published Online First: Epub Date].

19. Trotti LM, Saini P, Koola C, LaBarbera V, Bliwise DL, Rye DB. Flumazenil for the treatment of refractory hypersomnolence: Clinical experience with 153 patients. *J Clin Sleep Med*. 2016;12(10):1389–1394. https://doi.org/10.5664/jcsm.6196. [published Online First: Epub Date].

20. Bjornstad B, Goodman SH, Sirven JI, Dodick DW. Paroxysmal sleep as a presenting symptom of bilateral paramedian thalamic infarctions. *Mayo Clin Proc*. 2003;78(3):347–349. https://doi.org/10.4065/78.3.347. [published Online First: Epub Date].

21. Engstrom M, Latini F, Landtblom AM. Neuroimaging in the Kleine-Levin Syndrome. *Curr Neurol Neurosci Rep*. 2018;18(9):58. https://doi.org/10.1007/s11910-018-0866-y. [published Online First: Epub Date].

22. Xie H, Guo J, Liu H, Song W. Do the symptoms of Kleine-Levin syndrome correlate with the hypometabolism of the thalamus on FDG PET? *Clin Nucl Med*. 2016;41(3):255–256. https://doi.org/10.1097/RLU.0000000000001043. [published Online First: Epub Date].

23. Vigren P, Engstrom M, Landtblom AM. SPECT in the Kleine-Levin syndrome, a possible diagnostic and prognostic aid? *Front Neurol*. 2014;5:178. https://doi.org/10.3389/fneur.2014.00178. [published Online First: Epub Date].

24. Kas A, Lavault S, Habert MO, Arnulf I. Feeling unreal: A functional imaging study in patients with Kleine-Levin syndrome. *Brain*. 2014;137(Pt 7):2077–2087. https://doi.org/10.1093/brain/awu112. [published Online First: Epub Date].

25. Nose I, Ookawa T, Tanaka J, et al. Decreased blood flow of the left thalamus during somnolent episodes in a case of recurrent hypersomnia. *Psychiatry Clin Neurosci*. 2002;56(3):277–278. https://doi.org/10.1046/j.1440-1819.2002.00979.x. [published Online First: Epub Date].

26. Gadoth N, Dickerman Z, Bechar M, Laron Z, Lavie P. Episodic hormone secretion during sleep in Kleine-Levin syndrome: Evidence for hypothalamic dysfunction. *Brain Dev*. 1987;9(3):309–315. https://doi.org/10.1016/s0387-7604(87)80051-7. [published Online First: Epub Date].

27. Koerber RK, Torkelson R, Haven G, Donaldson J, Cohen SM, Case M. Increased cerebrospinal fluid 5-hydroxytryptamine and 5-hydroxyindoleacetic acid in Kleine-Levin syndrome. *Neurology*. 1984;34(12):1597–1600. https://doi.org/10.1212/wnl.34.12.1597. [published Online First: Epub Date].

28. Fernandez JM, Lara I, Gila L, O'Neill of Tyrone A Tovar J, Gimeno A. Disturbed hypothalamic-pituitary axis in idiopathic recurring hypersomnia syndrome. *Acta Neurol Scand*. 1990;82(6):361–363. https://doi.org/10.1111/j.1600-0404.1990.tb03317.x. [published Online First: Epub Date].

29. Gilligan BS. Periodic megaphagia and hypersomnia–an example of the Kleine-Levin syndrome in an adolescent girl. *Proc Aust Assoc Neurol*. 1973;9:67–72.

30. Thompson C, Obrecht R, Franey C, Arendt J, Checkley SA. Neuroendocrine rhythms in a patient with the Kleine-Levin syndrome. *Br J Psychiatry*. 1985;147:440–443. https://doi.org/10.1192/bjp.147.4.440. [published Online First: Epub Date].

31. Chesson Jr. AL, Levine SN, Kong LS, Lee SC. Neuroendocrine evaluation in Kleine-Levin syndrome: Evidence of reduced

dopaminergic tone during periods of hypersomnolence. *Sleep*. 1991;14(3):226–232.

32. Mayer G, Leonhard E, Krieg J, Meier-Ewert K. Endocrinological and polysomnographic findings in Kleine-Levin syndrome: No evidence for hypothalamic and circadian dysfunction. *Sleep*. 1998;21(3):278–284. https://doi.org/10.1093/sleep/21.3.278. [published Online First: Epub Date].

33. Hegarty A, Merriam AE. Autonomic events in Kleine-Levin syndrome. *Am J Psychiatry*. 1990;147(7):951–952. https://doi.org/10.1176/ajp.147.7.951. [published Online First: Epub Date].

34. Autret A, Lucas B, Mondon K, et al. Sleep and brain lesions: A critical review of the literature and additional new cases. *Neurophysiol Clin*. 2001;31(6):356–375. https://doi.org/10.1016/s0987-7053(01)00282-9. [published Online First: Epub Date].

35. Jeffries JJ, Lefebvre A. Depression and mania associated with Kleine-Levin-Critchley syndrome. *Can Psychiatr Assoc J*. 1973;18(5):439–444. https://doi.org/10.1177/070674377301800516. [published Online First: Epub Date].

36. Billiard M, Cadilhac J. [Recurrent hypersomnia]. *Rev Neurol (Paris)*. 1988;144(4):249–258.

37. Al Shareef SM, Basit S, Li S, et al. Kleine-Levin syndrome is associated with LMOD3 variants. *J Sleep Res*. 2019;28(3):e12718. https://doi.org/10.1111/jsr.12718. [published Online First: Epub Date].

38. Ambati A, Hillary R, Leu-Semenescu S, et al. Kleine-Levin syndrome is associated with birth difficulties and genetic variants in the TRANK1 gene loci. *Proc Natl Acad Sci U S A*. 2021;118(12):e2005753118. doi: 10.1073/pnas.2005753118 [published Online First: Epub Date].

39. Rosenow F, Kotagal P, Cohen BH, Green C, Wyllie E. Multiple sleep latency test and polysomnography in diagnosing Kleine-Levin syndrome and periodic hypersomnia. *J Clin Neurophysiol*. 2000;17(5):519–522. https://doi.org/10.1097/00004691-200009000-00012. [published Online First: Epub Date].

40. Huang YS, Lin YH, Guilleminault C. Polysomnography in Kleine-Levin syndrome. *Neurology*. 2008;70(10):795–801. https://doi.org/10.1212/01.wnl.0000304133.00875.2b. [published Online First: Epub Date].

41. Lin C, Chin WC, Huang YS, et al. Different circadian rest-active rhythms in Kleine-Levin syndrome: A prospective and case-control study. *Sleep*. 2021;44(9):zsab096. https://doi.org/10.1093/sleep/zsab096. [published Online First: Epub Date].

42. Huang YS, Lakkis C, Guilleminault C. Kleine-Levin syndrome: Current status. *Med Clin North Am*. 2010;94(3):557–562. https://doi.org/10.1016/j.mcna.2010.02.011. [published Online First: Epub Date].

43. Itokawa K, Fukui M, Ninomiya M, et al. Gabapentin for Kleine-Levin syndrome. *Intern Med*. 2009;48(13):1183–1185. https://doi.org/10.2169/internalmedicine.48.2204. [published Online First: Epub Date].

44. Maski K, Trotti LM, Kotagal S, Auger RR, Rowley JA, Hashmi SD, Watson NF. Treatment of central disorders of hypersomnolence: An American Academy of Sleep Medicine clinical practice guideline. *J Clin Sleep Med*. 2021;17(9):1881–1893.

20

Posttraumatic and Post-Neurosurgical Hypersomnia

Stephen H. Sheldon and Thuan Dang

CHAPTER HIGHLIGHTS

- Children who suffer significant head injury frequently experience significant sleep disturbances. Closed-head trauma is the most common event resulting in posttraumatic hypersomnia.
- Symptoms resulting from closed-head injury depend on the location of injury within sleep-regulating brain areas. Areas of the brain expected to be involved are those most commonly related to maintaining wakefulness, including but not limited to the brainstem reticular formation, posterior hypothalamus, and the region of the third ventricle.
- In the hypersomnolent patient, polysomnography and multiple sleep latency testing should be considered to determine the nature of the posttraumatic nocturnal sleep disturbances as well as rule out coexisting pathologies such as obstructive sleep apnea syndrome and periodic limb movement disorder. This may not always be possible in patients with severe traumatic brain injury.
- Evaluation of depression and anxiety that could present as attention-deficit/hyperactivity disorder in posttraumatic hypersomnolent patients is recommended when evaluating for sleep disturbances.
- No specific medications are approved for posttraumatic hyposomnolence, and further studies identifying prevalence and treatment are needed.

For children with posttraumatic and post-neurosurgical hypersomnia the best-fitting diagnosis within the *International Classification of Sleep Disorders* (ICSD), Third Edition, is hypersomnia due to a medical condition.[1] Diagnostic criteria require excessive sleepiness for a duration of more than 3 months, although it may be more pragmatic to make this clinical diagnosis earlier. References cited in the ICSD are more applicable for adults. There is no clear distinction made for posttraumatic hypersomnia in children. Children who suffer significant head injury frequently experience significant sleep disturbances, particularly when the injury is severe enough to result in major loss of consciousness. Nonetheless, sleep disturbances may follow minor

trauma in which a brief loss of consciousness occurs. In all instances, sleep patterns after the injury vary notably from the pretrauma sleep habits.

Closed-head trauma is the most common event resulting in posttraumatic hypersomnia. Similar symptoms may occur after neurosurgical procedures and other brain traumas. It appears that the cause is less important than the location. Symptomatically, there is a variable period of initial coma that evolves into a posttraumatic hypersomnolence and excessive daytime sleepiness with or without sleep attacks or unintentional sleep episodes. Nocturnal sleep may or may not be prolonged compared with the preinjury period. When total sleep time within each 24-hour day is increased, the term "posttraumatic hypersomnia" is fitting. Associated symptoms are typically due to daytime sleepiness (e.g., concentration difficulties, amnesia of recent events, fatigue, and occasional visual problems). Patients typically complain of unrefreshing sleep and long total sleep time. Chronic headache and minor neurologic signs of traumatic brain injury (TBI) may also be present.

Every year in the United States, approximately 56,800 people die and more than 2.87 million seek medical care for TBIs. Of these deaths, 2,529 deaths are among children. Approximately 5.3 million Americans live with brain injury–associated long-term disabilities, such as seizure disorders and cognitive and psychosocial impairments.[2] TBI is a leading cause of morbidity and mortality in children. Each year, over a 250,000 children seek emergency care because of head trauma. In 2014, an estimated 812,000 children (age 17 or younger) were treated in U.S. emergency departments for concussion or TBI. Fortunately, the majority of children (90%) suffer only from minor injuries. Nevertheless, 37,000 children require hospitalization, and up to 2,529 children per year do not survive their sustained injuries.[3] The Centers for Disease Control and Prevention (CDC) in the United States reports TBI-related death rates for the different age groups as follows: 5.7/100,000 (0–4 years), 3.1/100,000 (5–9 years), and 4.8/100,000 (10–14 years). This rate increases approximately 5-fold (24.3/100,000) for patients between 15 and 19 years. Pediatric TBI is most commonly caused by falls and non-accidental injury in younger children, and road traffic accidents (as pedestrians or passengers) in older children and adolescents.[4]

Head trauma has been reported to increase the likelihood of sleep-disordered breathing.[5] A polysomnogram may be necessary to exclude this etiology for the hypersomnia. The mechanism by which head trauma may result in sleep-disordered breathing is not clear. It is hypothesized that a whiplash type of injury may damage the pharyngeal nerves, which would alter some of the airway reflexes. Performing a polysomnogram may not be clinically possible in a child after a head injury. Empiric use of positive airway pressure (PAP) therapy should be used very cautiously because basilar skull fractures are a contraindication to PAP due to potential pneumocephaly.

Ideally, quantification of hypersomnia with a multiple sleep latency test (MSLT), may be helpful, especially to distinguish true sleepiness from fatigue or depression. However, in the presence of severe trauma, conducting and interpreting an MSLT may not be possible. The ICSD specifically states that a clinical complaint of excessive sleepiness is "far more important" than a short sleep latency on an MSLT.[1]

A key question asked by patients and family members when addressing posttraumatic or post-neurosurgical hypersomnia is how long will the condition last and will it spontaneously resolve with time. To evaluate the prevalence and natural history of sleepiness following TBI, Watson and colleagues undertook a prospective cohort study of 514 young men and adolescents with TBI. The TBI group was compared with 132 non-cranial trauma controls, and 102 trauma-free controls. Subjects were evaluated at 1 month and 1 year after injury. Sleepiness was measured subjectively with a self-administered questionnaire from which the following four questions were asked: (1) I am sleeping or dozing most of the time – day or night, (2) I sit around half asleep, (3) I sleep or nap more during the day, and (4) I sleep longer during the night. At the 1-month time point more than half of the TBI subjects reported sleepiness (55%). Of interest, 41% of non-cranial trauma controls also reported sleepiness, as did only 3% of trauma-free controls. The TBI group was not only more likely to report being sleepy, but the severity of the sleepiness was also greater as a greater percentage of subjects with TBI endorsed each of the four sleepiness items than did both the trauma controls and trauma-free controls at 1 month. One year following injury, 27% of TBI subjects, 23% of non-cranial trauma controls, and 1% of trauma-free controls reported sleepiness.[2]

In this study, patients with TBI were sleepier than non-cranial trauma controls at 1 month but not 1 year after injury. The cause of the residual sleepiness is unclear. One important factor in predicting persistent sleepiness is the severity of trauma. The brain injury of the majority of patients in this study was considered mild. To better understand the role of severity, the brain-injured subjects were divided into injury-severity groups based on time to follow commands (TFC) after the injury. The subgroup that was able to follow commands less than 24 hours after injury was less sleepy at the 1-month measurement than the 7- to 13-day and 14-day or longer TFC groups. At 1 year, the non-cranial trauma control group and the ≤24-hour TFC group were less sleepy than the 14-day or longer TFC group. Overall sleepiness improved in many patients in this study, with the TBI group more likely to improve than the non-cranial trauma group. Sleepiness improved in 84–100% of TBI patients compared with 78% of the non-cranial trauma control group. However, about a quarter of TBI subjects remained sleepy 1 year after injury. In addition, patients with more severe brain injuries were unable to participate in the study and the authors felt this could have resulted in an underestimation of the true extent of sleepiness in the TBI group.[2]

It is of interest that significant and persistent hypersomnia was present in the non-brain trauma group even though the sleepiness was not as severe as the TBI group. No details about the type of trauma in the former group are provided.[2] This raises the question of the cause of the hypersomnia. We can speculate that perhaps adolescents' and young adults' whiplash-type injuries were included in the non-brain trauma group which, as mentioned earlier, can develop sleep-disordered breathing. Non-brain trauma victims may have poor sleep for other reasons that can lead to daytime hypersomnia. For example, chronic pain and insomnia may develop in this population.

Symptoms resulting from closed-head injury depend on the location of injury within sleep-regulating brain areas. Areas of the brain expected to be involved are those most commonly related to maintaining wakefulness, including but not limited to the brainstem reticular formation, posterior hypothalamus, and the region of the third ventricle. Shearing forces along the direction of main fiber pathways can lead to microhemorrhages in these areas. High cervical cord trauma has also been known to cause sleepiness and unintentional sleep episodes.[6,7] Whiplash injury may result in hypersomnia, with consequent sleep-disordered breathing. In these cases, the hypersomnolence appears to be secondary to the respiratory abnormality.[5] Contrecoup injuries commonly occur at the base of the skull and may result in organic posttraumatic sleepiness. These types of injury occur in areas of bony irregularities (especially the sphenoid ridges), with consequent damage to the inferior frontal and anterior temporal regions, including the basal forebrain.[8] Injury to the posterolateral hypothalamus provides a potential physiologic explanation for post-injury sleepiness. Levels of hypocretin, an alerting neuropeptide, have been shown to be lower in patients with acute moderate to severe TBI.[9,10] Thus, trauma-induced transient reductions in hypocretin may be an unappreciated cause for hypersomnia. This would be consistent with case reports of posttraumatic narcolepsy and cataplexy.[11] Injury of the ascending reticular activating system following mild TBI was reported in two cases that suggest injury to the ascending reticular activating system is a pathogenetic mechanism of fatigue and hypersomnia in patients with TBI.[12] Hypersomnia and insomnia are not the only sleep symptoms that can develop after a TBI.

Rodrigues and Silva have reported a patient with aggressive body movements during rapid eye movement (REM) sleep and periodic limb movements after a TBI consistent with REM sleep-behavior disorder.[13]

A multicenter prospective study was performed on sleep disturbances in children with TBI by Tham and colleagues.[14] This study followed 729 children for 24 months following a TBI and compared them to 197 children with orthopedic injury (OI), who served as controls. Sleep disturbance was assessed using only one question from a standardized questionnaire completed by the parents. Specifically, "How often did he/she have a problem with trouble sleeping in the last 4 weeks?" Response options include "never" = 0, "almost never" = 1, "sometimes" = 2, "often" = 3, and "almost always" = 4. Additional data were collected to determine functional outcomes in the areas of adaptive behavior skills and activity participation. Parental reports of preinjury sleep disturbances were compared with reports of post-injury changes at 3, 12, and 24 months. The average age of the patients was 9 years. Both cohorts (children with TBI and OI) displayed increased sleep disturbances after injury. However, children with TBI experienced higher severity and more prolonged duration of sleep disturbances compared with children with OI. Risk factors for disturbed sleep included mild TBI, psychosocial problems, and frequent pain. Sleep disturbances emerged as significant predictors of poorer functional outcomes in children with moderate or severe TBI. The authors found that using a multivariate model with demographic and psychosocial factors, mild TBI was a significant predictive factor for sleep disturbances in their cohort. The authors proposed as an explanation that persons with mild TBI may have increased recognition of post-injury impairments; therefore they may be more likely to report sleep disturbances as an injury complication. In children with mild TBI, sleep disturbances may also be a symptom of increased awareness of post-injury changes subsequently reported by parents and caregivers. The other important predictors of sleep disturbances in the TBI cohort were frequent pain and the presence of psychosocial problems.

An important distinction between children and adults with TBI is that the neurosystem is maturing but not yet completely developed. The timing of the injury relative to the child's age and maturation needs to be considered. Crowe and colleagues studied participants injured across various stages of childhood to examine the influence of age on recovery and see if it fits an early vulnerability or critical developmental periods model. A total of 181 children with TBI were categorized into four age-at-injury groups: infant, preschool, middle childhood, and late childhood. They were evaluated at least 2 years post-TBI with neurocognitive testing (IQ). The study found that overall, the middle childhood group had lower IQ scores across all domains. The authors concluded that contrary to expectations, children injured in middle childhood demonstrated the poorest outcomes, which may coincide with a critical period of brain and cognitive development.[15]

A consistent finding in the literature is that children with more severe TBI have a greater likelihood of neurocognitive deficits than children with mild TBI. Longitudinal data with 10-year post-injury follow-up confirm this.[16–19] Children with mild TBI tend not to exhibit long-lasting impairment. However, some children even with relatively mild trauma can have persistent cognitive problems. Babikian and colleagues studied predictors of these persistent problems. They found that preinjury variables such as parental education, premorbid behavior and/or learning problems, and school achievement predicted cognitive impairments in children with otherwise mild TBI.[20] Given this information, it might be expected that children with prior subacute sleep disturbances are more likely to report sleep problems with mild TBI than children who otherwise slept well preinjury.

In evaluating a child with sleep disturbances after a TBI, the possibility of confounding depression should be considered. Max and colleagues prospectively studied 177 children with TBI and measured emergence of new-onset depression symptoms 6 months after TBI. The population studied was predominantly male with a mean age of 10 years. The authors found an incidence of 11% of "novel definite/subclinical depressive disorders." Among these children, they further identified subsets of children with non-anxious depression and anxious depression. Emergence of depressive disorder was significantly associated with older age at the time of injury, family history of anxiety disorder, left inferior frontal gyrus (IFG) lesions, and right frontal white matter lesions.[21]

Children with TBI have been described as having symptoms consistent with attention-deficit/hyperactivity disorder (ADHD).[22] A prospective study of 82 children with TBI with a mean age of 5 found that, compared with a control group of children with orthopedic injuries, severe TBI was associated with significantly greater anxiety problems. In addition, over time, children who sustained a severe TBI at an earlier age had significantly higher levels of parent-reported symptoms of ADHD and anxiety.[23] Unfortunately, sleep disorders were not specifically evaluated in the methods described.

In the hypersomnolent patient, polysomnography and MSLT should be considered to determine the nature of the posttraumatic nocturnal sleep disturbances as well as rule out coexisting pathologies such as obstructive sleep apnea syndrome and periodic limb movement disorder. Comprehensive treatment of hypersomnia in this population will require evaluating the underlying cause of hypersomnia. In children with TBI who have lost consciousness or are recovering from coma it may seem obvious that the hypersomnia is due to the brain injury. However, a careful history must always be taken, and the presence or absence of prior sleep disturbances should be determined. Other causes of hypersomnolence should also be considered in the evaluation of the patient with suspected posttraumatic hypersomnia. Hydrocephalus, subdural hematoma, meningitis, encephalitis, and seizure disorders should be considered as contributing to sleep disturbances.[24] Physical examination can reveal the possibility of minor focal neurologic signs, especially those of brainstem origin. Daytime fatigue may be due to insomnia. The possibility of a medication effect should also be considered. When comprehensive nocturnal polysomnography reveals the presence of sleep-disordered breathing after head trauma, the sleep-related breathing disorders must first be managed before determining the extent to which each comorbid condition contributes to the hypersomnolence. The recognition that head trauma can be a precipitating factor to syndromes leading to excessive daytime sleepiness is important, and a comprehensive evaluation of all patients who exhibit excessive sleepiness after head trauma is needed.

Galland and colleagues conducted a systematic literature review on interventions for sleep problems in children with TBI and found very little evidence-based data in this population.[25] They did describe a case report of a 6-year-old boy with a traumatic right-sided hemorrhage in the basal ganglia with pathological crying and poor sleep. The crying decreased and the sleep improved with the use of citalopram.[26]

Given the description of ADHD complaints in children with TBI, it is not surprising that the use of stimulants in children with TBI has been described and reviewed.[27–30] No specific trials of stimulants for hypersomnia in children with TBI were located. In adults, modafinil for hypersomnia associated with TBI has been reported with mixed results.[30] The use of modafinil in children has been discouraged due to cutaneous adverse reactions.[31] Methylphenidate has been studied in children with TBI predominantly to treat cognitive and behavioral difficulties.[27,28,32–34] A small randomized trial by Williams and colleagues failed to find a significant improvement of cognitive function in children with TBI using methylphenidate. These children only received 4 days of treatment.[33] In a treatment trial by Mahalick and colleagues using methylphenidate in children with TBI, a significant improvement in attention and concentration on neuropsychologic tests was found. In this placebo-controlled trial, methylphenidate was given for 14 days.[34] In a study of survivors of childhood brain tumors with hypersomnia, the most common medications prescribed were modafinil and methylphenidate. Nineteen of 36 patients (53%) reported complete resolution of daytime sleepiness, 16 (44%) reported partial improvement, and 1 (3%) reported only mild to no improvement. School function as measured by school grades could not be determined in 9 patients, improved in 25, and was reported as unchanged in 5.[35] Clearly, further research is needed before the use of stimulants in this pediatric population can unequivocally be recommended. A behavioral approach to sleep disorders, especially if insomnia is present, may be a better alternative.

In the absence of sufficient evidence-based research to standardize the treatment of children with posttraumatic and post-neurosurgical hypersomnia, patients are forced to rely on available resources and variable regional sleep medicine expertise. Fortunately, newer techniques such as brain tissue oxygenation monitoring are being applied to children after TBI to maximize neurologic outcome.[36] More recent information allows us to anticipate, for patients and families, the possible likelihood of recovery and of persistent symptoms. Given the ongoing neurocognitive development of children, we cannot continue to merely extrapolate medical decisions based on studies in adults. TBIs are among the most common and tragic events that can befall an otherwise healthy child. We need further research, specifically treatment intervention trials, for a wide age range of children to develop appropriate management protocols.

CLINICAL PEARLS

- Children who suffer significant head trauma frequently experience significant sleep disturbances after the injury, particularly when the trauma is severe enough to result in major loss of consciousness, although sleep disturbances may also follow minor trauma with only a brief loss of consciousness.
- Head trauma has been reported to increase the likelihood of sleep-disordered breathing.
- In the presence of severe trauma, conducting and interpreting a multiple sleep latency test may not be possible.
- Confounding depression and anxiety should be considered in a child with sleep disturbances after a traumatic brain injury.
- No specific medication trials for posttraumatic hypersomnia are available; however, stimulants for cognitive deficits in this population have been reported to have mixed results.

References

1. American Academy of Sleep Medicine. *International Classification of Sleep Disorders*. 3rd ed TR. American Academy of Sleep Medicine; 2023.
2. Watson NF, Dikmen S, Machamer J, et al. Hypersomnia following traumatic brain injury. *J Clin Sleep Med*. 2007;3:363–368.
3. Pinto PS, Poretti A, Meoded A, et al. The unique features of traumatic brain injury in children. Review of the characteristics of the pediatric skull and brain, mechanisms of trauma, patterns of injury, complications and their imaging findings – part 1. *J Neuroimaging*. 2012;22:e1–e17.
4. Pinto PS, Meoded A, Poretti A, et al. The unique features of traumatic brain injury in children. Review of the characteristics of the pediatric skull and brain, mechanisms of trauma, patterns of injury, complications, and their imaging findings – part 2. *J Neuroimaging*. 2012;22:e18–e41.
5. Guilleminault C, Yuen KM, Gulevich MG, et al. Hypersomnia after head-neck trauma: A medicolegal dilemma. *Neurology*. 2000;54:653–659.
6. Adey W, Porter RW. EEG patterns after high cervical lesions in man. *Arch Neurol*. 1968;19:377–383.
7. Hall CS. Sleep attacks: Apparent relationship to atlantoaxial dislocation. *Arch Neurol*. 1975;32:58–59.
8. Ommaya AK, Grubb Jr RL, Naumann RA. Coup and contrecoup injury: Observations on the mechanics of visible brain injuries in the rhesus monkey. *J Neurosurg*. 1971;35:503–516.

9. Baumann CR, Bassetti CL, Valko PO, et al. Loss of hypocretin (orexin) neurons with traumatic brain injury. *Ann Neurol.* 2009;66:555–559.

10. Baumann CR, Stocker R, Imhof HG, et al. Hypocretin-1 (orexin A) deficiency in acute traumatic brain injury. *Neurology.* 2005;65:147–149.

11. Lankford DA, Wellman JJ, O'Hara C. Posttraumatic narcolepsy in mild to moderate closed head injury. *Sleep.* 1994;17:S25–S28.

12. Jang SH, Kwon HG. Injury of the ascending reticular activating system in patients with fatigue and hypersmonia following mild traumatic brain injury: Two case reports. *Medicine.* 2016;95(6):e2628.

13. Rodrigues RN, Silva AA. [Excessive daytime sleepiness after traumatic brain injury: Association with periodic limb movements and REM behavior disorder: Case report]. *Arq Neuropsiquiatr.* 2002;60:656–660.

14. Tham SW, Palermo TM, Vavilala MS, et al. The longitudinal course, risk factors, and impact of sleep disturbances in children with traumatic brain injury. *J Neurotrauma.* 2012;29:154–161.

15. Crowe LM, Catroppa C, Babl FE, et al. Timing of traumatic brain injury in childhood and intellectual outcome. *J Pediatr Psychol.* 2012;37:745–754.

16. Catroppa C, Godfrey C, Rosenfeld JV, et al. Functional recovery ten years after pediatric traumatic brain injury: Outcomes and predictors. *J Neurotrauma.* 2012;29:2539–2547.

17. Anderson V, Godfrey C, Rosenfeld JV, et al. 10 years outcome from childhood traumatic brain injury. *Int J Dev Neurosci.* 2012;30:217–224.

18. Anderson V, Godfrey C, Rosenfeld JV, et al. Predictors of cognitive function and recovery 10 years after traumatic brain injury in young children. *Pediatrics.* 2012;129:e254–e261.

19. Anderson V, Catroppa C, Godfrey C, et al. Intellectual ability 10 years after traumatic brain injury in infancy and childhood: What predicts outcome? *J Neurotrauma.* 2012;29:143–153.

20. Babikian T, McArthur D, Asarnow RF. Predictors of 1-month and 1-year neurocognitive functioning from the UCLA longitudinal mild, uncomplicated, pediatric traumatic brain injury study. *J Int Neuropsychol Soc.* 2012:1–10.

21. Max JE, Keatley E, Wilde EA, et al. Depression in children and adolescents in the first 6 months after traumatic brain injury. *Int J Dev Neurosci.* 2012;30:239–245.

22. Levin H, Hanten G, Max J, et al. Symptoms of attention-deficit/hyperactivity disorder following traumatic brain injury in children. *J Dev Behavioral Pediatr.* 2007;28:108–118.

23. Karver CL, Wade SL, Cassedy A, et al. Age at injury and long-term behavior problems after traumatic brain injury in young children. *Rehabil Psychol.* 2012;57:256–265.

24. Grigg-Damberger M. Neurologic disorders masquerading as pediatric sleep problems. *Pediatr Clin North Am.* 2004;51:89–115.

25. Galland BC, Elder DE, Taylor BJ. Interventions with a sleep outcome for children with cerebral palsy or a post-traumatic brain injury: A systematic review. *Sleep Med Rev.* 2012;16:561–573.

26. Andersen G, Stylsvig M, Sunde N. Citalopram treatment of traumatic brain damage in a 6-year-old boy. *J Neurotrauma.* 1999;16:341–344.

27. Jin C, Schachar R. Methylphenidate treatment of attention-deficit/hyperactivity disorder secondary to traumatic brain injury: A critical appraisal of treatment studies. *CNS Spectr.* 2004;9:217–226.

28. Nicholls E, Hildenbrand AK, Aggarwal R, et al. The use of stimulant medication to treat neurocognitive deficits in patients with pediatric cancer, traumatic brain injury, and sickle cell disease: A review. *Postgrad Med.* 2012;124:78–90.

29. Castriotta RJ, Murthy JN. Sleep disorders in patients with traumatic brain injury: A review. *CNS Drugs.* 2011;25:175–185.

30. Castriotta RJ, Atanasov S, Wilde MC, et al. Treatment of sleep disorders after traumatic brain injury. *J Clin Sleep Med.* 2009;5:137–144.

31. Kumar R. Approved and investigational uses of modafinil: An evidence-based review. *Drugs.* 2008;68:1803–1839.

32. Hornyak JE, Nelson VS, Hurvitz EA. The use of methylphenidate in paediatric traumatic brain injury. *Pediatr Rehabil.* 1997;1:15–17.

33. Williams SE, Ris MD, Ayyangar R, et al. Recovery in pediatric brain injury: Is psychostimulant medication beneficial? *J Head Trauma Rehabil.* 1998;13:73–81.

34. Mahalick DM, Carmel PW, Greenberg JP, et al. Psychopharmacologic treatment of acquired attention disorders in children with brain injury. *Pediatr Neurosurg.* 1998;29: 121–126.

35. Khan RB, Merchant TE, Sadighi ZS, et al. Prevalence, risk factors, and response to treatment for hypersomnia of central origin in survivors of childhood brain tumors. *J Neurooncol.* 2018;136(2):379–384.

36. Stippler M, Ortiz V, Adelson PD, et al. Brain tissue oxygen monitoring after severe traumatic brain injury in children: Relationship to outcome and association with other clinical parameters. *J Neurosurg Pediatr.* 2012;10:383–391.

21

Medication-Related Hypersomnia

MARY ANNE TABLIZO, ROCHELLE YOUNG, and MANISHA WITMANS

CHAPTER HIGHLIGHTS

- Hypersomnia in children may be from a primary sleep disorder such as narcolepsy, secondary to a medical or psychiatric condition, or related to medications that affect the sleep–wake state.
- The sedating side effects of some medications are often used off-label to help children initiate and/or maintain sleep; however, there are limited data on the use of sedative and hypnotic agents for use in the pediatric population.
- Because of the paucity of studies available regarding the use of hypnotic agents in the pediatric population, there is very sparse data on recommended doses, safety profile, and efficacy available for the majority of these medications.

Introduction

Many commonly used medications and substances in children can affect the sleep–wake state. This chapter aims to provide an overview of medications that cause excessive sleepiness or hypersomnia in children, whether this is an intended effect or unintended consequence of their use and/or misuse for treatment of sleep disorders or other health problems.

Hypersomnia

In the International Classification of Sleep Disorders (ICSD-3), conditions that manifest as hypersomnia are in the category of Central Disorders of Hypersomnolence. Among the well-described conditions causing hypersomnia are narcolepsy with and without cataplexy, idiopathic hypersomnia, Kleine-Levin syndrome, and hypersomnia due to medical disorders, medications or substances, and hypersomnia associated with psychiatric disorders.[1] Hypersomnia presents as inability to stay awake during a time that an individual should be alert. The sleepiness is out of proportion for age, gender, and developmental stage. The clinical complaints include excessive sleepiness, irrepressible sleep, non-refreshing sleep, and falling asleep during the day. Excessive sleepiness may be associated with increased sleep need beyond the recommended duration for age, need for nap beyond age-appropriate norms, or difficulty waking

after an adequate sleep period.[1] What makes hypersomnia challenging to recognize in children is that they may not present clinically the same way as adults. Manifestations of sleepiness in children may present as hyperactivity, motor restlessness, mood and emotional regulation difficulties, and poor academic performance. It is often only identified in children when it interferes with academic performance or when abnormal behavior is observed.

Hypersomnia in children can occur in the context of medication use intended for treatment of medical and psychiatric conditions that affect sleep–wake regulation and cause excessive sleepiness as an adverse effect. Several drugs are known to have sleep-promoting effects in children and are used off-label as sleep aids. In addition to sedatives and hypnotics, different classes of medication may have side effects of sleepiness when used for different pharmacologic indications other than sleep. These drug classes include anticonvulsants, antihistamines, antidepressants, antipsychotics, cardiovascular drugs, opioid analgesics and several other medications that are not commonly used in pediatric population. Hypersomnia may also be observed from other medication side effects such as sleep interruptions from motor restlessness and with the abrupt cessation of chronic stimulant use or abuse.

Sleep–Wake Continuum: Anatomy and Its Substrates

Sleep and wake states are generated by specific neurotransmitters in specific neuronal systems that together have widespread projections in the brain. Medications may exert their effects along various pathways to inhibit or enhance sleep.

Wakefulness and alertness are maintained by neurons in the ascending reticular formation in the brainstem. These neurons send projections to the thalamocortical pathways via two routes, the dorsal pathway in the posterior thalamus, and the ventral pathway in the basal forebrain. Neurons superolateral to the mammillary body of the posterior hypothalamus is a key wake-promoting region that has direct anatomical connections with other wake-promoting structures including brainstem nuclei of the ascending activating system, the basal forebrain, and the cerebral cortex. In contrast, sleep is promoted by inhibiting wake-promoting regions. The well-studied sleep-promoting region is the anterior hypothalamus, specifically the intermediate nucleus/ventrolateral preoptic area and adjacent median preoptic nucleus.[2,3]

Previous studies showed that acetylcholine is important for vigilance and cortical activation. Locus coeruleus neurons using norepinephrine project diffusely to the forebrain and brainstem to maintain cortical activation. Further studies suggest that norepinephrine and adrenergic receptors are important for stimulating and maintaining activating processes, whereas dopaminergic nuclei in the midbrain ventral tegmental areas are important in stimulating behavioral arousal. The posterior thalamic neurons have histamine, which has been long assumed to play a role in vigilance and have widespread projections to areas of the hypothalamus and cortex. Orexin (hypocretin) also has widespread projections across the forebrain and cortex is involved in maintaining wakefulness. Serotonergic neurons from the raphe nuclei are also important in maintaining wakefulness.

Medications may cause sleepiness, by either promoting sleep-activating neurons (gamma-aminobutyric acid [GABA]), or inhibiting the wake-promoting regions (antihistamines, anticholinergic, 5-HT$_2$ antagonist, α-1 antagonist, dopamine antagonist).[4] Adenosine is another neurotransmitter involved in sleep–wake regulation in the homeostatic process and may promote sleep through anticholinergic activity in the basal forebrain and brainstem. Melatonin, a circadian regulating hormone, is also a sleep promoting neuromodulator.[4,5]

Recent advances in genetics research including the mapping of the human genome and gene sequencing has led to the growth of pharmacogenetics to help determine medication effects on an individual's neurotransmitters and their regulation. These evaluations enable genetic factors involved in the modulation of therapeutic and adverse responses to pharmacotherapy to further our understanding of the implications of the administration of pharmacologic agents. This information can be used for personalized medicine approaches in determining the effects of medications including patients with sleep disorders.[6]

Abuse or Misuse of Prescription and Over-the-Counter Medications Contributing to Hypersomnia

The use of medications has climbed steadily over the years in all fields of medicine, particularly in sleep medicine, either to promote wakefulness or sleepiness, depending on the presenting problem. Our collective desire to manipulate and regulate sleep–wake cycles is rampant across society, children and adolescents are no exception, either because of parental and societal expectations or their own in meeting all their social and personal demands. Strategic and direct marketing to consumers and prescribers has contributed to the widespread use of pharmacologic agents to manipulate and treat sleep. Compounding this problem is that medications are

no longer available just to those with prescribing authority. Internet access has enhanced the spread of drug information as well as the distribution of medications, fueling the phenomenon. There is an increasing expenditure in prescription drugs over the years that proves increasing need and use of medications.[7,8] The misperception, particularly in adolescents, that medications prescribed by physicians and dispensed by pharmacists are safer than illicit drugs has resulted in a widespread epidemic of misuse of both prescription and over-the-counter (OTC) medications.[9] This has resulted in the intentional abuse of prescribed and OTC medications to affect mood, performance, and sleep–wake state. A wide variety of classes of medications that contain the potential for abuse includes sedatives, opioids and derivatives, stimulants, and tranquilizers and muscle relaxants, as well as other centrally acting agents.

The intake of prescription drugs for non-medical use is increasing among teenagers.[10–12] The National Survey on Drug Use and Health revealed in 2018 that approximately 1 in 5 Americans aged 12 and older used an illicit drug in the past year, with prescription pain relievers being the most commonly used category of drugs, after marijuana. The majority of these medications are obtained from friends or relatives (51.3%), 37.6% from physicians, and 6.5% from strangers; 0.6% reported obtaining the drug some other way. Non-medicinal use of psychotherapeutics occurred in 3.5 million children 12 and older. The types of medications used non-medicinally included pain relievers (1.9 million), tranquilizers (1.2 million), stimulants (1 million), and sedatives/hypnotics (251,000).[13] Most recently, a global estimate by the United Nations (UN) is based on available data from 130 countries in 2016: 13.8 million young people (mostly students) aged 15–16 years used cannabis at least once in the previous 12 months. A high prevalence of cannabis use was reported in West and Central Europe (20%) and North America (18%).[14] These data suggest that use of psychoactive substance for non-medicinal purposes is common among youth.

A particular abuse of medications in adolescents that warrants special consideration is the use of OTC medication used for cough and cold preparations. Factors that promote the likelihood of abuse include the ease of accessibility, as most of these medications are widely available in homes, are relatively inexpensive, and decreased perception of potential harm because they are legal. The abuse of these drugs is strongly associated with abuse of alcohol and other illicit substances. Previous data showed adolescents abuse prescription medication and cough medication to "get high."[15] Many adolescents obtain these medications from their peers, their social network of friends, relatives, or physicians. These medications may be used as sleep aids or alerting agents used as study aids. There is also less social stigma for use of these medications rather than street drugs.[16]

Since the legalization of marijuana across various states, there have been increased reports of unintentional ingestion of marijuana in children <6 years of age. Following 2009, when marijuana became legalized with more relaxed enforcement laws nationally, there was a mean annual increase of

27% per year, rising to 742 ingestions per year or 2.98 ingestions per 100,000 population, respectively, in 2017. More than 70% of all cases occurred in states with legalized marijuana. Of all pediatric patients, 54.6% received some form of hospital-based care, of which 7.5% required critical care. The prevalence rate of reported drowsiness was 38% in this study.[16]

For the clinician, the challenge lies in trying to differentiate not only if the complaint of hypersomnia is a result of the complex interplay of development, sociocultural influence on sleep–wake regulation and a possible sleep disorder, but also being able to differentiate iatrogenic causes of sleepiness that may further compound the presenting complaint. Use of stimulant medication or caffeine, either in the form of energy drinks or excessive use of other forms of caffeine, as a countermeasure, may mask the true sleepiness that is present for the given adolescent. For patients on anticonvulsant medications, either as a mood stabilizer or for their epilepsy, teasing apart the true sleepiness versus the sleepiness resulting from medications, neurologic condition, or even psychiatric disorder can be quite challenging.

Medications That Result in Sleepiness as Either an Intended or Unintended Consequence

Many different classes of medications can induce sleepiness. These drugs are intended for different pharmacologic indications including sedation to promote sleep for patients with insomnia and, in some cases, somnolence is an adverse effect of the medication. The sedating side effects of some of these medications are often used off-label to help adults and children initiate and maintain sleep. There are limited available data for their safety and efficacy specifically for the pediatric population. Most of the information available on these medications are obtained from adult studies and effects on children may not be the same. The data on medication-related sleep architecture changes are also mostly obtained from adults. The following medications can cause hypersomnia. The medications are presented alphabetically according to their drug class and pharmacologic properties and indications.

Anticonvulsants

Anticonvulsant medications suppress seizure activity but can also cause unwanted central nervous system (CNS) effects. Medications used in the treatment of epilepsy have been found to be sedating, thus challenging the clinician to distinguish sleepiness related to epilepsy from sleepiness due to drug therapy. The neurochemical basis for sleepiness is dependent on the class of medication.

Barbiturates are one of the oldest class of medications used as anticonvulsants. While barbiturates can cause wide spectrum of CNS depression, phenobarbital is one of the barbiturates that is used as anticonvulsants at low doses can cause hypnosis.[17] Phenobarbital is used as an antiepileptic drug in the neonatal and pediatric population. It causes sedation especially during initiation therapy, but tolerance can develop when given long term. Sedation is absent at lower concentrations during long-term therapy, but it may be seen when therapy is initiated or when the dosage is increased.[18] Anticonvulsants that act on $GABA_A$ receptors such as phenobarbital, tiagabine, and vigabatrin generally cause significant sleepiness.

Levetiracetam is another anticonvulsant drug (ACD) approved by the U.S. Food and Drug Administration (FDA) for use in infants and children. The mechanism for its anti-seizure activity is unclear. Although it appears to be well tolerated in children, drowsiness is a common reported adverse effect.[17] Topiramate has an FDA approval for focal, generalized tonic-clonic (GTC) seizures and Lennox-Gastaut syndrome as an initial monotherapy for children >10 years old and adjunctive therapy for as young as 2 years of age.[17] It can cause sleepiness by GABA increase and sodium blockade as two of several proposed mechanisms of action.[3] Carbamazepine and phenytoin are used as ACD in children and drowsiness is a frequent untoward reported effect.[17] The mechanism for sedation in carbamazepine and phenytoin appears to be mediated by slowing the rate of recovery of voltage-activated Na^+ channels from inactivation.[17,19] Valproate (Depakote) is also reported to cause sleepiness by acting on both GABA synthesis and sodium channel blockade. These medications may be used to induce and optimize the sleep period due to their sedating properties.[18,19]

Gabapentin is a centrally acting GABA agonist with high lipid solubility that can cross the blood–brain barrier (BBB) and is used as an anticonvulsant.[17] Because of its sedating effect, gabapentin is used off-label in children for the treatment of insomnia in patients with neurologic conditions. It is also used for children with restless legs syndrome (RLS). The data on its use for insomnia and RLS in children are limited. The residual excessive daytime sleepiness resulting from gabapentin may interfere with daytime functioning.[19,20]

Polysomnographic (PSG) studies of established antiepileptic drugs in general decrease sleep latency and increase total sleep time (TST). Levetiracetam, gabapentin, pregabalin, and tiagabine increase slow-wave sleep (SWS).[20]

Antidepressants

Dependent upon the specific antidepressant agent chosen, medications in this category can be either activating or sedating. Sleep-enhancing antidepressants may result in hypersomnia even at clinically therapeutic doses.[20] The antidepressants commonly prescribed as sleep aids in the United States include the tricyclic antidepressants (TCAs; doxepin, trimipramine, amitriptyline), trazodone, and mirtazapine. Of these, doxepin is the only FDA-approved antidepressant for insomnia in adults but not in children.[20]

Although they are classified as antidepressants, most of these drugs have other pediatric pharmacologic indications such as for anxiety, obsessive compulsive disorder, and treatment of enuresis, just to name a few.

Atypical Antidepressants

Mirtazapine (Remeron) is an atypical antidepressant that is highly sedating. This medication has widespread effects on norepinephrine, histamine, alpha-adrenergic systems, and serotonin. The sedating effect is through a 5-HT_{2A}, H_1 and 5-HT_{2C} receptor antagonist mechanism. There is decrease in sedation with increasing dose, which is suggested to be due to alpha-2 antagonism at higher doses.[20] Mirtazapine is widely used to treat adults and even older children with depression and insomnia, but its FDA approval is for depression in patients 18 years and older.[21] One study showed efficacy with use of mirtazapine for anxiety in children 5–17 years old with autism spectrum disorder.[22]

Trazodone is an antidepressant known to have sedating and hypnotic effects. It enhances sleep by acting at the 5-HT_{2A} and H_1 antagonist. Although safety and efficacy have not been established in children and adolescents, it has been widely used in children and adolescents with depression for its hypnotic properties. In addition to its notable side effect of residual daytime sleepiness, incidence of priapism has been reported in adults. PSG studies indicate that trazodone decreases sleep latency, may improve sleep continuity, and increases SWS, but it does not affect rapid eye movement (REM) sleep.[20]

Serotonin-Norepinephrine Reuptake Inhibitors

Duloxetine is a serotonin-norepinephrine reuptake inhibitors classified as antidepressants. The efficacy of duloxetine is not well established for treatment of depression in the pediatric population, but it has an FDA approval for the treatment of generalized anxiety disorder in children aged 7 years and older.[23] A systematic review of the efficacy, safety, and tolerability of duloxetine showed somnolence as one of the major adverse effects.[24] Duloxetine has mild 5-HT_{2A}/ and 5-HT_{2c} antagonism. Due to its serotonergic property, it is also associated with motor restlessness and may exacerbate preexisting RLS and periodic limb movements that can cause daytime sleepiness.

Selective Serotonin Reuptake Inhibitors

Selective serotonin reuptake inhibitors (SSRIs) are effective and widely used in children and adolescents for the treatment of depressive disorder.[25] Fluoxetine has been approved for treatment of depression for children ≥8 years old and escitalopram for ≥12 years old. There are other FDA-approved indications for pediatric use of SSRIs such as for obsessive-compulsive disorder (sertraline ≥6 years old, fluoxetine ≥7 years old, and fluvoxamine ≥8 years old) and as an adjunctive treatment for cataplexy in type I narcolepsy.

Despite being placed in one category, each drug in this class has different activity, indications, and adverse effects depending on their chemical structure. Sedation is an unlikely side effect for SSRI but is reported in some. Specifically, fluvoxamine, and citalopram tend to cause drowsiness and are used for patients with insomnia and underlying depression. Citalopram has mild H_1 and 5-HT_{2c} antagonism. Fluvoxamine is proposed to cause drowsiness

by modulating calcium release, inhibit sodium channel, and inhibit melatonin degradation.[20] Interestingly, insomnia is also reported as an untoward effect of citalopram and fluvoxamine in some patients. Fluoxetine and sertraline generally can cause sleep-onset delay, but fluoxetine is also reported to induce sedation as the dose is increased. Studies on healthy adults and patients with depressive disorder suggest that SSRIs tend to decrease sleep time, decrease REM sleep, suppress SWS, and increase awakenings.[26] SSRIs are also associated with motor restlessness and may exacerbate preexisting RLS and periodic limb movements. Daytime sleepiness maybe related to sleep disruption from motor restlessness and sleep architecture changes attributed to the use of SSRIs.[26]

Tricyclic Antidepressants

TCAs have both serotonergic and noradrenergic effects and are indicated for major depressive disorder. Depending on the chemical structure, each of the tricyclics have secondary effects and use. TCAs have an additional anticholinergic and central H_1 receptor blockade that can cause sedation. Tertiary amine TCAs, such as doxepin, have the most potent H_1 receptor antagonist property among the tricyclics and is commonly used for maintenance insomnia in adults with depression. Trimipramine is another TCA that has antihistaminergic properties that can cause sedation. Amitriptyline has the most anticholinergic property. Because of their sedating effects, they are also prescribed as sleep aids.[27] In general, these drugs decrease sleep latency, increase TST, and decrease REM sleep while increasing phasic eye movements during REM. Drugs with less affinity for H_1 receptors (e.g., nortriptyline, desipramine) that are more adrenergic are less sedating and may promote insomnia in some patients.[28]

For pediatric patients with depressive disorder, tricyclics are not commonly used because of lack of studies on their efficacy and unfavorable side effects.[29] Amitriptyline is approved for use as an antidepressant for children >12 years of age. Imipramine is used in the pediatric population for treatment of nocturnal enuresis. Amitriptyline is used for chronic migraines in children and teens to improve sleep and treat chronic pain. It is also used for nocturnal enuresis but not FDA approved for this disorder.[28]

Antihistamines

Allergy Medications

Antihistamines are used for treatment of hypersensitivity reactions that present as rhinitis, urticaria, conjunctivitis, and atopic diseases. They are available both as prescription and OTC preparations. The central properties of these classes are also used for suppressing motion sickness and for sedation. Antihistamines are often used as sleep aids, off-label in children due to their sedating properties, especially at higher doses. First-generation antihistamines (diphenhydramine, chlorpheniramine, hydroxyzine, doxylamine) cross the BBB and bind to histamine type 1 receptors in the brain and are the most sedating in this medication class.[30] The effects may be augmented when used in conjunction with sedative hypnotics, or narcotic agents. These agents are generally regarded as less harmful because they are readily available and widely used. Their effects, however, can be profound and they do have addictive potential. Diphenhydramine is a commonly available antihistamine drug that is often used off-label for sedation and as a hypnotic for children. Diphenhydramine is commonly used for allergy and atopic disorders, and many do not appreciate the potential harmful effects of the medications, including the risk for dependence. Some abuse this medication for its potential euphoric effects. Additionally, diphenhydramine, along with other antihistamines, has anticholinergic effects, especially at higher doses or prolonged use. It is often used as a hypnotic, even in young children; however, the somnolent effect can be inconsistent, ranging from a paradoxical excitation to noted somnolence and sedation. Chlorpheniramine and brompheniramine are also sedating first-generation antihistamines that are marketed for allergies and commonly formulated in cold products. The FDA has recommended that the use of OTC children's cough and cold medicines that contain mixtures of antihistamines and decongestants should not be given in children <2 years of age due to various side effects that can be fatal. The FDA also has a public advisory that the non-prescription products are not to be used for sedation in children.

Doxylamine is a first-generation antihistamine formulated for allergy and cold relief for both adults and children. Doxylamine and diphenhydramine are marketed as a non-prescription sleep aid. The long elimination T1/2 of these antihistamines (9–10 hours) make residual daytime sleepiness in the morning a common complaint.[18] It is associated with rebound insomnia after prolonged use.

Hydroxyzine is a centrally acting H_1 histamine receptor antagonist that is used for sedation, as an anxiolytic, and for pruritus in atopic disorders. Off-label, this agent is used for sedation even in children with insomnia. This medication, like other sedating antihistamines, can result in daytime sleepiness.

The newer generation antihistamines (cetirizine, levocetirizine, desloratadine, loratadine, fexofenadine) are hydrophilic and do not cross the BBB, hence, they are much more selective, enabling treatment of atopy with less associated sedation. Cetirizine has higher incidence of drowsiness than most other second-generation antihistamines despite negligible penetration into the brain.[30]

Appetite Stimulant

Cyproheptadine is a type of antihistamine with anticholinergic and antiserotonergic properties used to stimulate appetite, treat allergies and drug-induced serotonin syndrome, and used off-label to prevent migraine attacks in older children and adolescents. Its sedating property is due to antihistaminergic and anticholinergic effects. Like diphenhydramine, it can penetrate the BBB. It should be used with caution in infants and children as it may cause CNS depression.[30]

Antiemetic

Antihistamines that are primarily used for motion sickness such as dimenhydrinate and meclizine can cause drowsiness. They are antihistamines for nausea and are also used for their sedative properties. The effects are similar to those of diphenhydramine. Dimenhydrinate is an H_1 histamine receptor antagonist and interacts with other neurotransmitters, either directly or indirectly. It can also interact with other neurotransmitters including acetylcholine, serotonin, norepinephrine, dopamine, opioids, or adenosine.[30] Although it is available over the counter, and appears to be benign, this drug also has abuse potential and does result in hypersomnia.

Promethazine is another antihistamine that has prominent sedating effect and is mainly used for nausea, vomiting, motion sickness, surgical anesthesia, and as hypnotic pre- and post-operative adjunct. Promethazine has also significant anticholinergic property.[30]

Antihypertensives

Alpha-2 Agonists

Centrally acting alpha-2 adrenergic agonists such as clonidine and guanfacine, are used primarily as antihypertensive in adults. Clonidine and guanfacine have been used off-label for insomnia in children because of their sedating effects. Clonidine is one of the commonly used off-label medications for insomnia in children. It has FDA approval for use in children with attention-deficit/hyperactivity disorder (ADHD) from 6 to 17 years of age. Because of this, it commonly helps with insomnia in children with ADHD. Data regarding its use for insomnia are mostly anecdotal with limited data in terms of efficacy. It is generally well tolerated with minimal side effects such as daytime drowsiness. It decreases sleep latency and increases SWS that can make patients prone to have parasomnias.[31] Among the other off-label uses of clonidine in children include constitutional growth delay in children, Tourette's syndrome, mania, psychosis, and RLS.[18]

Guanfacine is a more selective alpha-2 adrenergic receptor agonist that is also used off-label for insomnia but is less sedating than clonidine. Guanfacine has FDA approval for children with ADHD in children aged 6–17 years old. It has a longer half-life than clonidine, which can help with sleep maintenance, but it has higher potential for daytime somnolence.

Alpha-1 Adrenergic Blockers

Prazosin is an alpha-1 adrenergic receptor antagonist that acts on the post-synaptic alpha-1 adrenergic receptor. Prazosin helps facilitate sleep and is used as a sedative in addition to treatment for post-traumatic disorder (PTSD) sleep disturbance and nightmares in adults. Case reports and case series reported improvement in PTSD-related nightmares and sleep disorders in the pediatric group, but this has not been systematically evaluated.[32]

Antipsychotic Agents

In treatment of acute psychosis, sedation may be helpful, but the daytime sleepiness may interfere with the patient's cognitive function and daily function for chronic use. Antipsychotic medications with concomitant antihistaminergic and anticholinergic properties are the most sedating. The sedating effect of antipsychotics agents can be determined based on their degree of H_1 receptor antagonism.[33,34]

First-Generation Antipsychotics

The antipsychotic agents are classified into two groups. The first-generation agents, also known as *typical antipsychotics*, are dopamine receptor antagonists (chlorpromazine, thioridazine, haloperidol, loxapine). This group also has noradrenergic, cholinergic, and histaminergic blocking action. Chlorpromazine and thioridazine are the most sedating drugs in the first-generation antipsychotic group due to their high H_1 and $5\text{-}HT_{2A}$ antagonism.[34] The first-generation antipsychotics have limitations due to significant side effects such as extrapyramidal symptoms.[33]

Second-Generation Antipsychotics

The second-generation group, also known as *atypical antipsychotic* agents, are serotonin-dopamine antagonists (aripiprazole, asenapine, olanzapine, risperidone, quetiapine). Second-generation groups have lesser side effects with lower risk of extrapyramidal symptoms; hence they are more commonly used antipsychotics.[33]

Aripiprazole, asenapine, risperidone, and quetiapine have FDA approval for acute treatment of bipolar disorder in children >10 years old. Olanzapine is indicated for both bipolar and schizophrenia for children >13 years old. Risperidone and aripiprazole are also used (with FDA approval) for patients >6 years old for treatment of irritability associated with autism. Ziprasidone, quetiapine, and olanzapine are commonly used and have been studied for behavioral problems in autism but have not been approved by the FDA for this indication.

Because of their sedating properties, atypical antipsychotic agents such as olanzapine, quetiapine, and risperidone have been used off-label for treatment of insomnia in children with concomitant behavioral and psychiatric issues. Olanzapine promotes sleep by blocking H_1 and serotonin ($5\text{-}HT_{2C}$) receptors.[34] Quetiapine has been widely used off-label for its sedating property in children and adolescents because it is an adrenergic antagonist with potent antihistamine properties.[34] Lurasidone is an atypical second-generation antipsychotic agent approved for use in pediatric patients (10–17 years of age) for bipolar depression and long-term symptom control of schizophrenia for patients 13–17 years old. Like other antipsychotic agents, it may impair judgment and can result in daytime sleepiness.[35]

In one study on antipsychotic medication use in adolescents, of 327 patients, sedation was a reason for discontinuation with quetiapine (13%) followed by olanzapine (7.3%), risperidone (4.2%), and aripiprazole (2%). All these medications affected sleep patterns with a decrease in insomnia but with daytime tranquilizing effects, especially in adolescents.[36]

Dopamine Agonists

As the precursor of dopamine, dopaminergic agents are used to treat dystonic disorders. They are used for the treatment of RLS and periodic limb movement disorder in adults. Patients with RLS are found to have decreased dopamine receptor expression and mild dopaminergic hypofunction. Data on the use of dopaminergic medications (carbidopa/levodopa, pramipexole, ropinirole) in children with RLS and periodic limb movement disorder is scarce and are mostly based on retrospective review and case series.[37]

Dopamine does not cross the BBB; levodopa is used because it does cross the BBB and is converted to dopamine in the brain. Commonly, levodopa is formulated with DOPA decarboxylase inhibitor, which prevents the peripheral conversion of levodopa to dopamine to prevent untoward side effects. In addition, the enzymatic breakdown enables the medication to be used at lower doses centrally to produce effective outcomes. The lack of receptor subtype selectivity causing increased adverse effects is the main therapeutic limitation of the use of dopaminergic agonists. Carbidopa has been used in dystonia associated with cerebral palsy and certain metabolic disorders. Excessive daytime sleepiness and sudden onset of sleep can occur with this agent, so it should be used with caution.[5]

Opioids and Morphine Derivatives

As the management of chronic pain has garnered more attention and awareness, there has been a steady increase in use of prescription pain medications, including OTC remedies. The neurobiology of pain is complex and involves both central and peripheral mechanisms. Simply, pain disrupts sleep while sleep deprivation may increase pain sensitivity.[38] Opioid peptides may be involved in the modulation of various biologic processes including sleep with somnolence as a common side effect.[39] In patients in pain, therapeutic doses of morphine decrease or eliminate pain intensity and at the same time can produce drowsiness, changes in mood, and mental clouding. The side effects may be more pronounced as the dose is increased including respiratory depression.[18]

Opioids and their derivatives are the most commonly abused prescription medications, resulting in social programs and dispensary interventions to stave off the epidemic. In 2015, about 9.7% of 12th graders reported misuse of Vicodin (an opiate narcotic) in a national survey, whereas up to 18% of 11th graders used opiates without a prescription.[40,41] The 2018 National Survey on Drug Use and Health reported that approximately 2.8% of adolescents between the ages of 12 and 17 misused opioids. In 2018, 1.9 million young adults between the ages of 18 and 25 misused opioids.[42]

Opioids bind to receptors across various regions in the brain, and, at high doses, can cause sleepiness and respiratory depression. Morphine congeners such as codeine and hydrocodone are also used as antitussives because of their central actions.[43] Long-term use of opioids and its derivatives can lead to physical dependence, tolerance, and addiction. Combination of opioids in addition to other sedating agents such as alcohol, antihistamines, or sedatives can result in life-threatening respiratory depression, coma, and death.

Sleep medicine has also embraced the use of opioids and its derivatives as an alternative treatment for RLS or Willis-Ekbom disease in adults.

Sedative-Hypnotics

Sedatives are drugs that decrease activity, relax and calm the recipient by depressing the CNS, and produce sleepiness, whereas hypnotics are drugs that are used to induce drowsiness, prolong or improve the quality of sleep, or produce partial anesthesia. These agents bind to GABA moieties at the benzodiazepine (BZD) receptor. GABA is a major inhibitory neurotransmitter in the brain. The sleep-promoting GABAergic neurons inhibit wake-promoting circuitry.[44]

Barbiturate

Barbiturates are used as ACDs and were also once used extensively as sedatives and hypnotics. Barbiturates enhance the binding of GABA to $GABA_A$ receptors. They potentiate GABA-induced Cl^- currents by prolonging bursts of channel opening. Barbiturates have been used in children for sleep induction and as anticonvulsants and anesthetics. Phenobarbital was introduced as a sedative and hypnotic in 1912. Since then, many commercially available barbiturate analogs have been introduced. Barbiturates decrease sleep latency, increase TST, decrease number of awakenings, increase N2 sleep, decrease REM sleep, and decrease N3 or SWS. After repetitive use, tolerance can develop and the effect on total sleep may decrease. Barbiturates are now seldom prescribed as sedatives and hypnotics because newer sedatives have a much safer pharmacologic profile. Barbiturates can cause significant CNS depression compared with BZDs, with the risk of fatal overdose leading to respiratory depression.[18] Significant drowsiness the following day is a common reported adverse effect.[45]

Benzodiazepines

Although BZDs are classified as sedative/hypnotics, they have limited use as hypnotics in children because of safety concerns. They are also used in pediatric groups as anxiolytics, anticonvulsants, and muscle relaxants. BZDs reduce the neuronal excitability of the sleep–wake centers resulting in sleepiness. The receptor complex of GABA agonists includes a group of ligand-gated ion channels, the mechanism of which is at the BZD binding sites on $GABA_A$ receptor and its

associated chloride channel. Each of these compounds displays unique aspects pertaining to their individual receptor subtype involved in binding that results in different patterns of effects. As such, GABA agonists with a shorter half-life, such as midazolam, tend to be used in practice as amnestics for invasive procedures, whereas BZDs with longer half-lives are being prescribed as sleep aids; however, effects can last the following waking hours and may cause daytime sleepiness. Memory impairment and rebound insomnia are reported on short-acting BZDs (triazolam and midazolam). Poor daytime function is often seen in long-acting BZDs such as diazepam and flurazepam.[46] BZDs can affect sleep architecture by decreasing alpha waves, increase in low-voltage fast activity, decrease sleep latency, and decrease number of awakenings. The TST is increased despite a decrease in SWS and decreased time spent in REM.[20] BZDs increase TST by increasing sleep stage 2, decrease duration of sleep stage 1, increase the number of cycles of REM, and decrease body movement. The effects on the sleep architecture decline after chronic nocturnal use. When discontinued, there is a rebound increase in the amount of REM.[18] There is an increased risk of habituation, which limits its use in children.

Chloral hydrate

Chloral hydrate was once widely used for sedating children for procedures and as a hypnotic agent. However, small clinical trials and observational studies showed that it was not as effective compared with other sedative agents due to delayed onset of action, sustained duration, and significant adverse effects.[47] Notable effects of this class of medication include reduced anxiety, anterograde amnesia, sedation, and memory impairment. Respiratory depression can occur when combined with other sedatives and hypnotics. Chloral hydrate is no longer available in the United States.

Melatonin

Melatonin is a hormone that may have a hypnotic effect given as a supplement to endogenous melatonin secreted by the pineal gland. It is used in adults and children for sleep-onset insomnia, delayed sleep phase disorder, and jet lag.[18] It is commonly used for treatment of insomnia in children with comorbidities such as developmental delay, ADHD, and autism spectrum disorder. It is also used anecdotally for treatment of parasomnia.[48] Common complaints from patients are daytime somnolence. Melatonin is discussed more extensively in another part of this book.

Nonbenzodiazepine Receptor Agonists

Non-BZD receptor agonists, commonly referred to as Z compounds, include zolpidem, zaleplon, zopiclone, and eszopiclone. Their therapeutic effect as hypnotics is due to agonist effects at the BZD site of the $GABA_A$ receptor. This group of drugs acts selectively on one of the GABA type A receptor subtypes. Z compounds are marketed to have less potential for dependence and side effects compared to BZDs because of this selectivity. Zolpidem is effective in shortening sleep latency and prolonging sleep time in patients with insomnia due to its longer half-life (about 2 hours), which can cover 8 hours of sleep especially if given as extended release. Compared with zaleplon (half-life 1 hour), which has a shorter half-life, late night administration of zolpidem is associated with morning sedation due to its longer half-life. There is less REM sleep suppression with zolpidem and zaleplon compared with BZDs.[18] Eszopiclone is an S isomer of zopiclone and has a peak concentration of 1 hour and half-life of 6 hours. This drug is used to help initiate sleep and sleep maintenance if given at least 4 more hours before time of arising to avoid residual daytime sedation. This medication is FDA approved for adults without limit of duration of administration based on previous data showing no tolerance for at least 6 months.[18] These drugs are classified as schedule IV in the United States, indicating potential for abuse similar to concerns with BZDs. There is limited data on the use of non-BZDs in children and are not FDA approved for use in pediatric population.[49]

Orexin Receptor Antagonist

Suvorexant is an FDA-approved orexin receptor antagonist that is available for treatment of insomnia in adults. It works by selectively blocking the binding of neuropeptides orexin A and B to receptors OX1R and OX2R (promotes wakefulness) with primary adverse effect of daytime somnolence.[50] The most common side effect of suvorexant usage reported during clinical trials is daytime sleepiness in adults. One study in adolescents also showed excessive sleepiness noted as an adverse effect.[51] Lemborexant is an FDA-approved (12/2019) orexin receptor antagonist indicated for sleep-onset and sleep-maintenance insomnia. It has a 17- to 19-hour half-life, with residual sleepiness as the most common adverse reaction reported. The safety and efficacy in the pediatric population have not been established.[52]

Ramelteon (Melatonin Receptor Agonist)

Ramelteon is a synthetic melatonin receptor that acts on melatonin receptors MT1 and MT2 causing sleepiness. Ramelteon has been shown to reduce sleep latency and is indicated for treatment of both transient and chronic insomnia. Ramelteon is useful in chronic insomnia, with no tolerance reported even after 6 months of drug administration.[53] There was no evidence of rebound insomnia or withdrawal effects when ramelteon was discontinued. Drowsiness is one of the reported adverse effects in small number of patients.[18] There is limited literature on the use of ramelteon in children other than from several case reports of its successful use. In one case report, ramelteon effectively treated night terror and sleepwalking in an 11-year-old with ADHD. This was presumed to be secondary to reduced slow-wave dysregulation.[54] It was also reported to be effective for delayed sleep–wake phase disorder in a 15-year-old patient.[55] Some studies also suggest ramelteon is effective

when used for sleep disturbance in the pediatric population with autism and cerebral palsy.[56] Additional studies are needed.

Other Medications That Can Cause Daytime Sleepiness

Atomoxetine

This is a non-stimulant indicated for treatment of ADHD in patients ≥6 years old. It inhibits presynaptic norepinephrine reuptake, resulting in increased synaptic norepinephrine and dopamine.[57] Somnolence was one of the adverse reactions (8%) reported in clinical trials in children and adolescents. PSG study in ADHD showed increased REM latency.[18]

Dextromethorphan

This hydrobromide is chemically related to codeine. It used to be classified as a synthetic opioid, until recently when the sigma 1 receptor is not considered an opioid receptor anymore. It is a common ingredient in OTC cough and cold remedies in the United States.[58,59] The use of this medication at higher doses, referred to as "sheeting," is where upward of 8–16 tablets are consumed at once, has been reported.[14,60] High doses can result in effects similar to that of phencyclidine or ketamine. As dextromethorphan is converted to dextrorphan, it can cause dissociative effects by antagonizing the N-methyl-D-aspartate (NMDA) receptor.[61] Although dextromethorphan use has decreased since 2006, it is still a significant concern. In 2015, the Monitoring the Future survey found that 3.1% of students in 8th to12th grade reported OTC cough medicine abuse.[61] In addition, many cough syrup preparations contain additional significant active ingredients such as antihistamine, decongestant, and analgesic. Intoxication with this medication presenting to the emergency room can be associated with sleepiness in up to 24% of cases.[59] At high doses, the effects can be profound and life-threatening.

Baclofen and Tizanidine

These are skeletal muscle relaxants often used in children with spasticity and contracture. Baclofen has sedating effects because it is a GABA derivative, and it is $GABA_B$ receptor agonist. It has been shown to improve TST and sleep efficiency and decrease wake after sleep onset.[62,63] Hypersomnia is a potential side effect but its prevalence has not been documented in the literature. Tizanidine can cause sedation because of its effect on the alpha-2 adrenergic receptor and has been used in children with cerebral palsy.[64]

Complementary Alternative Medications

Complementary alternative medication (CAM) use has increased substantially over the past decade. In sleep medicine, many of these agents are used as sleep aids and are discussed in the associated relevant chapters. The use of CAM in children is commonly reported in children whose parents also used CAM. Adolescents aged 12–17 years, children with multiple health conditions, and those whose families either delayed or did not use conventional medical care because of cost were also more likely to use CAM, suggesting that CAM use may be more common than reported in the literature.[65] There are few reports of Valerian for use in sleep disorders in children. Hypersomnia is not commonly reported as a concerning side effect when taking CAM therapies.[66]

Cannabinoids

Marijuana, also known as cannabis, is a psychoactive drug that is obtained from the cannabis plant. As legalization of marijuana becomes more commonplace, there is no topic more controversial than the use of marijuana in clinical practice. Within the United States, there are an estimated 55 million recent active users, defined as 1–2 users within the previous year, and 35 million regular users, defined as 1–2 users per month.[67] It appears that cannabis has a staggering rising trend of use, for both medical and recreational use. According to a California survey from 2013–2015, use of marijuana for 11th grade students was 38% versus 8% for 7th grade students. In addition, 12% reported weekly use.[67,68] The main active ingredient in cannabis is delta-9-tetrahydrocannabinol (THC), which affects the brain because of its psychoactive properties. It can cause sedation by increasing adenosine. The other active compound being evaluated extensively for medical purposes in cannabis is cannabidiol (CBD). CBD is a non-intoxicating phytocannabinoid that has shown analgesic, antiinflammatory, anticonvulsant, and anxiolytic activities without the psychoactive effect of THC.[17] The psychotropic effects likely are due to activation of CB1 receptors in the CNS by inhibiting arousal, whereas CB2 receptors in the periphery affect immune cells, and are thought to play a role in inflammation and immune response and are associated with causing alertness. There appears to be antagonistic effects of THC and CBD on each other with respect to the sleep–wake cycle, therefore the proportion and the concentration of the compounds determine the sedative versus alerting properties. Marijuana appears to improve sleep with certain conditions including PTSD, multiple sclerosis (MS), and chronic pain. Overall marijuana appears to help with faster sleep onset, decreased nighttime arousals, and improved overall sleep quality.[69] Marijuana has also been used as a coping mechanism for those with sleep disturbances as it is often self-administered for pain, anxiety, and insomnia.[70]

CBD has an FDA approval for treatment of certain types of seizures associated with Lennox-Gastaut syndrome or Dravet syndrome for young children.[70–72] Although clinical studies are lacking, observational studies report improvement in behavior and sleep in pediatric patients with autistic spectrum disorder. Somnolence is a commonly reported adverse effect for its use especially with higher doses of CBD.

Evaluating Hypersomnia Resulting From Medications: Considerations for the Clinician

Pharmacologic treatments required in the management of medical conditions in children and adolescents may result in a clinical presentation of hypersomnia. In addition, medications used for the treatment of disorders of sleepiness and/or sleeplessness may confound the clinical picture, leaving the sleep specialist with the challenge of evaluating the role of medication in relation to sleep–wake regulation. A thorough review of prescribed medications, OTC medication, dosage, frequency, and timing should be undertaken. It is important to consider the medications in view of the circadian factors that may enhance or inhibit the effect of medication.

Adolescents should specifically be asked about the use of prescription, non-prescription, or OTC medications; complementary alternative substances; and illicit drug use in a nonthreatening/nonjudgmental manner. Given the high prevalence of abuse of some of these agents among adolescents, additional history about associated mood problems, learning disabilities, and sleep disorders should be sought. Management of the abuse of these medications is beyond the scope of this chapter. Adolescents and their parents should be cautioned about the safety profile of medications, encouraged to not share medications, and warned about signs suggesting abuse, such as frequent prescription refills or altered behavior and academic performance at school. Pharmacists should equally be vigilant in questioning refills and in storing the medications appropriately behind the counter. Internet shopping for medications should be banned for children <18 years of age, with strict legislation.

CLINICAL PEARLS

- The possibility of hypersomnia associated with medication use must be explored and assessed in children and adolescents presenting with excessive sleepiness.
- Medications used to treat different medical conditions including sleep disorders may result in sleepiness being an intended/unintended consequence; therefore one should consider both nighttime and daytime effects on sleep when prescribing medication.
- Hypersomnia in adolescents should prompt the clinician to inquire about what pharmacologic or nonpharmacologic agents are being used that can affect the sleep–wake continuum.

Summary

Sleep–wake regulation is a complex process with the potential to be further confounded by the use of prescription or non-prescription drugs. Resulting hypersomnia must be evaluated by the clinician in the context of the social, medical, and physical parameters of the patient, with particular diligence applied to the adolescent. With the large number of medications available that may result in a presentation of hypersomnia, it is the role of medical personnel to remain diligent in their assessment of the sleepy patient. Ultimately, it is imperative for the clinician to be aware of the different classes of medications, their associated effects, and the trends of use of these medications by children and adolescents.

References

1. Silber M, Arnulf I, Kotagal S, Scammell T, Overrem S. Central disorders of hypersomnolence. In: Sateia M, ed. *International Classification of Sleep Disorders.* 3rd ed. American Academy of Sleep Medicine; 2014:143–182.
2. Saper CB, Scammell T, Lu J. Hypothalamic regulation of sleep and circadian rhythms. *Nature.* 2005;437:1257–1263.
3. Boes AD, Fischer D, Geerling JC, Bruss J, Saper CB, Fox M. Connectivity of sleep and wake promoting regions of the human hypothalamus observed during wakefulness. *Sleep.* September 2018;41(9):zsy108.
4. Holst SC, Landolt HP. Sleep-wake neurochemistry. *Sleep Med Clin.* 2018;13:137–146.
5. Torterolo P, Monti JM, Vanini G. Neurochemistry and pharmacology of sleep. In: Murillo-Rodriguez E, ed. *The Behavioral, Molecular, Pharmacological, and Clinical Basis of the Sleep-Wake Cycle.* Elsevier; 2019:45–83.
6. Cavallari LH, Mosley S. Johnson J. Pharmacogenetics. In: Wecker L, Taylor DA, Theobald RJ, eds. *Brody's Human Pharmacology: Mechanism-Based Therapeutics.* 6th ed. Elsevier; 2019:39–46.
7. Office of the National Drug Control Policy (ONDCP). Teens and Prescription Drugs: An Analysis of Recent Trends on the Emerging Drug Threat. Executive Office of the President; 2007.
8. Schumock GT, Stubbings J, Hoffman JM, Wiest MD, Suda KJ, Rim MH, Tadrous M, Tichy EM, Cuellar S, Clark JS, Matusiak LM, Hunkler RJ, Vermeulen LC. National trends in prescription drug expenditures and projections for 2019. *Am J Health Syst Pharm.* July 2019 18;76(15):1105–1121. https://doi.org/10.1093/ajhp/zxz109.PMID:31199861.
9. Substance Abuse and Mental Health Services Administration.. *Results from the 2010 National Survey on Drug Use and Health: Summary of National Findings, NSDUH Series H-41, HHS Publication No. (SMA) 11-4658.* Substance Abuse and Mental Health Services Administration; 2011.
10. Gonzales R, Brecht ML, Mooney L, et al. Prescription and over the counter drug treatment admissions to the California Public Treatment System. *J Subst Abuse Treat.* 2011;40:224–229.
11. Kann L, McManus T, Harris WA, et al. Youth Risk Behavior Surveillance – United States, 2015. *MMWR Surveill Summ.* 2016;65(6):1–174. https://www.cdc.gov/healthyyouth/data/yrbs/pdf/2015/ss6506_updated.pdf.
12. Levine D. "Pharming": The abuse of prescription and over-the counter drugs in teens. *Curr Opin Pediatr.* 2007;19:270–274.
13. Substance Abuse and Mental Health Services Administration. Key substance use and mental health indicators in the United States: Results from the 2018 National Survey on Drug Use and Health (HHS Publication No. PEP19-5068, NSDUH Series H-54). Center for Behavioral Health Statistics and Quality, Substance Abuse and Mental Health Services Administration; 2019. https://www.samhsa.gov/data/

14. UNODC.. *United Nations office on drugs and crime.* World Drug Report; 2017.
15. Bryner JK, Wang UK, Hiu JW, et al. Dextromethorphan abuse in adolescence: An increasing trend: 1999–2004. *Arch Pediatr Adolsec Med.* 2006;160:1217–1222.
16. Leubitz A, Spiller H, Jolliff H, Casavant M. Prevalence and clinical characteristics of unintentional ingestion of marijuana in children younger than 6 years in states with and without legalized marijuana laws. *Pediatr Emerg Care.* 2021;37(12):e969–e973. https://doi.org/10.1097/PEC.0000000000001841.
17. Metcalf CS, Smith MD, Wilcox KS. Pharmacotherapy of the epilepsies (Chapter 20). In: Brunton LL, Knollmann BC, eds. *Goodman & Gilman's The Pharmacological Basis of Therapeutics.* 14th ed. McGraw-Hill; 2022.
18. Mihic SJ, Mayfield J. Hypnotics and sedatives (Chapter 22). In: Brunton LL, Knollmann BC, eds. *Goodman & Gilman's The Pharmacological Basis of Therapeutics.* 14th ed. McGraw-Hill; 2022:1–27.
19. Lu J, Greco MA. Sleep circuitry and the hypnotic mechanism of GABA drugs. *J Clin Sleep Med.* 2006;2(2):S19–S26.
20. Schweitzer PK, Malhotra RK. Clinical pharmacology of drugs that affect sleep and wake (Chapter 53). In: Meir H, Kryger MD, eds. *Principles and Practice of Sleep Medicine.* 7th ed. Elsevier; 2022:519–547.
21. Weston C. Antidepressant drugs (Chapter 7). In: Bowers RT, Weston C, Mast RC, Jackson JC, eds. *Green's Child and Adolescent Clinical Psychopharmacology.* 6th ed. Lippincott Williams and Wilkins; 2018.
22. McDougle CJ, Thom RP, Ravichandran CT, Palumbo ML, Politte LC, Mulitte JE, Keary CJ, Erickson CA, Stigler KA, Mathieu-Frasier L, Posey DJ. A randomized double blind, placebo-controlled pilot trial of mirtazapine for anxiety in children and adolescents with ASD. *Neuropsychoparhmacolgy.* 2022;47(6):1263–1270.
23. Emslie GJ, Prakash A, Zhang Q, Pangalio BA, Bangs ME, March JS. A double blind efficacy and safety study of Duloxetine in children with major depressive disorder. *J Child Adolesc Psychopharmacol.* May 2014;24(4):170–179.
24. Rodrigues-Amorim D, Olivares JM, Spuch C, Rivera-Baltanas R. A systematic review of efficacy, safety, and tolerability of duloxetine. *Front Psychiatry.* 2020;11:554899.
25. Garland E.J., Kutcher S., Virani A., Elbe D. Update on the use of SSRIs and SNRIs with children and adolescents in clinical practice. *J Can Acad Child Adolesc Psychiatry.* 25(1):4–10.
26. Fabre V, Krystal AD, Bonnavion P. Serotonin and sleep (chapter 53). In: Meir H, Kryger MD, eds. *Principles and Practice of Sleep Medicine.* 7th ed. Elsevier; 2022:497–505.
27. Hazell P, Mirzaie M. Tricyclic drugs for depression in children and adolescents. *Cochrane Database Syst Rev.* 2013;2013(6):CD002317.
28. Hirsch M, Birnbaum R. Tricyclic and tetracyclic drugs: Pharmacology, administration and side effects. *UpToDate.* 2020

29. Tsapakis EM, Joldani F, Tando L, Baldessastus RJ. Efficacy of antidepressant in juvenile depression: Meta analysis. *Br J Psychiatry*. 2008;193(1):10.

30. Zuraw BL, Christiansen SC. Histamine, bradykinin, and their antagonists. In: Brunton LL, Knollmann BC, eds.*Goodman & Gilman's The Pharmacological Basis of Therapeutics*. 14th ed. McGraw-Hill; 2022.

31. Prince JB, Wilens TE, Biederman J, et al. Clonidine for sleep disturbances associated with attention-deficit hyperactivity disorder: A systematic chart review of 62 cases. *J Am Acad Child Adolesc Psychiatry*. 1996;35:599.

32. Ferrafiat V, Soleimani M, Chaumette B, et al. Use of prazosin for pediatric post-traumatic stress disorder with nightmares and/or sleep disorder: Case series of 18 patients prospectively assessed. *Front Psychiatry*. 2020;11:724.

33. Chokhawala K, Stevens L.*Antipsychotic medications. StatPearls [Internet]*. StatPearls Publishing; 2023.

34. Meyer J. Pharmacotherapy of psychosis and mania. (Chapter 19). In: Brunton LL, Knollmann BC, eds.*Goodman & Gilman's The Pharmacological Basis of Therapeutics*. 14th ed. McGraw-Hill; 2022.

35. Sunovion Pharmaceuticals Inc. Latuda® (lurasidone hydrochloride) tablets prescribing information. Sunovion Pharmaceuticals, 2010.

36. Al-Dhaher Z, Kapoor S, Saito E, Krakower S, David L, Ake T, Kane JM, Correll CU, Carbon M. Activating and tranquilizing effects of first-time treatment with aripiprazole, olanzapine, quetiapine, and risperidone in youth. *J Child Adolesc Psychopharmacol*. 2016;5:458–470.

37. Dye TJ, Gurbani N, Simakajornboon N. How does one choose the correct pharmacotherapy for a pediatric patient with restless legs syndrome and periodic limb movement disorder?: Expert Guidance. *Exp Opin Pharmacother*. 2019;20(13):1535–1538.

38. Schug S, Garrett W, Gillespie G. Opioid and non-opioid analgesics. *Best Pract Res Clin Anaesthesiol*. 2003;17:91–110.

39. Inturrisi C. Clinical pharmacology of opioids for pain. *Clin J Pain*. 2002;18:S3–S13.

40. Johnson LD, O'Malley PM, Bachman JG, et al. Monitoring the future national results on adolescent drug use: Overview of key findings. *National Institute on Drug Abuse*. 2009:7583–7587.

41. Austin G., Hanson T., Polik J., Zheng C. Highlight: 15th Biennial California Student Survey Drug, Alcohol and Tobacco Use 2013–2015. California Attorney General's Office.

42. Substance Abuse and Mental Health Services Administration. (2019). Key substance use and mental health indicators in the United States: Results from the 2018 National Survey on Drug Use and Health (HHS Publication No. PEP19-5068, NSDUH Series H-54). Center for Behavioral Health Statistics and Quality, Substance Abuse and Mental Health Services Administration; 2019. https://www.samhsa.gov/data/

43. Jutkiewicz EM, Traynor JR. Opioid analgesics (Chapter 23). In: Brunton LL, Knollmann BC, eds.*Goodman & Gilman's The Pharmacological Basis of Therapeutics*. 14th ed. McGraw-Hill; 2022.

44. Wisden W, Yu X, Franks NP. GABA receptors and the pharmacology of sleep. *Handb Exp Pharmacol*. 2019;253:280–283.

45. Nishino S, Sakai N, Mishima K, Mignot E, Dement C. Sedatives– hypnotics (Chapter 43). In: Schatzberg AF, Nemeroff CB, eds.*Textbook of Psychopharmacology*. 5th ed. American Psychiatric Association; 2017.

46. Monti JM. General Principle of treatment of sleep dysfunction and pharmacology of drugs used in sleep disorders (Chapter 55). In: Chokroverty S, ed.*Sleep Disorders Medicine*. Springer; 2017:190–1198.

47. Macias CG, Chumpitazi CE. Sedation and anesthesia for CT: Emerging issues for providing high-quality care. *Pediatr Radiol*. 2011;41(Suppl 2):517.

48. Ozcan O, Donmez YE. Melatonin treatment for childhood sleep terror. *J Child Adolesc Psychopharmacol*. 2014;24(9):528–529.

49. Sangal RB, Blumer JL, Lankford DA, et al. Eszopiclone for insomnia associated with attention-deficit/hyperactivity disorder. *Pediatrics*. 2014;134:e1095.

50. Dujardin S, Pijpers A, Pevernagie D. Prescription drugs used in insomnia. *Sleep Med Clin*. 2020;15(2):133–145.

51. Kawabe K, Horiuchi F, Ochi M, Nishimoto K, Ueno S, Oka Y. Suvorexant for the treatment of insomnia in adolescents. *J Child Adolesc Psychopharmacol*. 2017;27:792–795.

52. Scott L.J. Lemborexant: First approval. drugs. 2020 Mar;80(4):425–432. http://doi.org/10.1007/s40265-020-01276-1.PMID: 32096020.

53. Sateia MJ, Buysse DJ, Krystal AD, Neubauer DN, Heald JL. Clinical Practice Guideline for the Pharmacologic Treatment of Chronic Insomnia in Adults: An American Academy of Sleep Medicine Clinical Practice Guideline. *J Clin Sleep Med*. February 2017;13(2):307–309.

54. Sasayama D, Washizuka S, Honda H. Effective treatment of night terrors and sleepwalking with ramelteon. *J Child Adolesc Psychopharmacol*. 2016;26(10):948.

55. Takeshima M, Shimizu T, Ishikawa H, Kanbayashi T. Ramelteon for delayed sleep-wake phase disorder: A case report. *Clin Psychopharmacol Neurosci*. February 2020;18(1):167–169.

56. Miyamoto A, Fukuda I, Tanaka H, et al. Treatment with ramelteon for sleep disturbance in severely disabled children and young adults. [Japanese]. *No To Hattatsu*. 2013;45(6):440–444.

57. Bushe CJ, Savill NC. Systematic review of atomoxetine data in childhood and adolescent attention-deficit hyperactivity disorder 2009–2011: Focus on clinical efficacy and safety. *JPsychopharmacol*. 2014;28(3):204–211.

58. Windhab LG, Gastberger S, Hulka LM, Baumgartner MR, Soyka M, Muller TJ, Seifritz E, Mutschler J. Dextromethorphan abuse among opioid-dependent patients. *Clin Neuropharmacol*. 2020;43(5):127.

59. Lessenger JE, Feinberg SD. Abuse of prescription and over the counter medications. *J Am Board Fam Med*. 2008;21:45–54.

60. Spangler DC, Loyd CM, Skor EE. Dextromethorphan: A case study on addressing abuse of a safe and effective drug. *Subst Abuse Treat Prev Policy*. 2016;11(1):22. https://doi.org/10.1186/s13011-016-0067-0.

61. Schwartz RH. Adolescent abuse of dextromethorphan. *Clin Pediatr (Phil)*. 2005;44:565–568.

62. Raad S, Wilkerson M, Jones K, Orr W. The effect of baclofen on objective and subjective sleep measures in a model of transient insomnia. *Sleep Med*. 2020;72:130–134.

63. Mohon RT, Sawyer K, Pickett K, et al. Sleep-related breathing disorders associated with intrathecal baclofen therapy to treat patients with cerebral palsy. A cohort study and discussion. *Neurorehabilitation*. 2021;48(4):481–491.

64. Tanaka H, Fukuda I, Miyamoto A, et al. Effects of tizanidine for refractory sleep disturbances in disabled children with spastic quadriplegia. *No To Hattatsu*. 2003;36(6):455–460.

65. Davis MP, Darden PM. Use of complementary and alternative medicine by children in the United States. *Arch Pediatr Adolesc Med*. 2003;157(4):393–396.

66. Italia S, Wolfenstentter S, Teuner C. Patterns of complementary and alternative Medicine (CAM) use in children: A systematic review. *Eur J Pediatr.* 2014;173(11):1413–1428.

67. Black E, Hocum B, Black K. Ethics and science, cannabinoids and healthcare. *Primary Care Rep.* January 2018;24(1).

68. National Academies of Sciences, Engineering, and Medicine.. *The health effects of cannabis and cannabinoids: The current state of evidence and recommendations for research.* The National Academies Press; 2017. https://doi.org/10.17226/24625.

69. Kuhathasan N, Dufort A, MacKillop J, Gottschalk R, Minuzzi L, Frey BN. The use of cannabinoids for sleep: A critical review on clinical trials. *Exp Clin Psychopharmacol.* 2019 Aug;27(4):383–401. https://doi.org/10.1037/pha0000285.

70. Babson KA, Bonn-Miller MO. Sleep disturbances: Implications for cannabis use, cannabis use cessation, and cannabis use treatment. *Curr Addict Rep.* 2014;1:109–114. https://doi.org/10.1007/s40429-014-0016-9.

71. Hadland SE, Knight JR, Harris SK. Medicinal marijuana: Review of the science and implication for developmental behavioral pediatric practice. *Dev Behav Pediatr.* 2015;36:115.

72. Epidiolex (cannabidiol) oral solution. Accessdata.fda.gov. Revised 2021. ID: 4942762.

SECTION III

Sleep & Breathing Disorders

22

Normal Respiratory Physiology During Sleep in Infants and Children

John L. Carroll

CHAPTER HIGHLIGHTS

- Thoracic cage & chest wall mechanics, rib cage motion and dynamic lung volume physiology play a significant role in a full understanding of pediatric respiratory development and pediatric sleep disordered breathing.
- Central apneas occur normally in newborns and to a lesser extent, in children. Obstructive apneas are less common in newborns and children.
- Factors such as respiratory frequency, tidal volume, and periodic breathing play a significant role in normal pediatric ventilation and are frequently compromised in pediatric sleep-disordered breathing.

Introduction

The diaphragm, chest wall muscles and upper airway muscles are under continuous, dynamic central nervous system (CNS) control by neurons that are, in turn, heavily modulated by states of wakefulness, non–rapid eye movement (NREM) and rapid eye movement (REM) sleep. Neural control of breathing consists not only of phasic activity driving rhythmic breathing movements, but also tonic modulation of muscle activity to maintain optimum thoracic cage configuration, lung volumes, and upper airway patency. Central drive to respiratory muscles is modulated by sensory information from a complex system of mechanosensors and chemosensors, the input of which may be gated by sleep state. The central respiratory pattern generator (CPG) itself is comprised of a highly complex network of interacting neuronal groups that exhibit oscillatory firing behavior resulting from their reciprocal, cyclical interactions. The CPG is subject to modulation by wakefulness and sleep states not only via mechanoreceptor and chemoreceptor inputs, but also via inputs from other neurons in the brainstem, hypothalamus, and cortex. Given the extent to which normal breathing is dependent on real-time neural modulation, the profound effects of sleep on breathing pattern and ventilation are a key component of normal respiratory physiology and play an important role in sleep-disordered breathing (SDB).

All aspects of the human respiratory system, including structural, mechanical, and neural control, undergo profound maturational changes during growth and development. Breathing begins before birth, with fetal breathing movements in utero, and respiratory system maturation continues throughout childhood, with different developmental time frames for individual components, as body size increases ~20-fold from infancy to late adolescence. Concurrent maturation of the nervous system, including the effect of wakefulness and sleep state on respiratory control, imposes another layer of important functional changes during growth and development. Thus respiratory system physiology and the effects of sleep on breathing vary throughout life, from infancy through elderly adulthood, and these changes are highly relevant to sleep medicine.

As pointed out by previous authors, several factors frustrate attempts to summarize the normal effects of sleep on breathing during postnatal development.[1] Although numerous articles explore respiratory system mechanics and respiratory control maturation in sleeping children, there are many fewer that explore the effects of sleep, per se, on breathing. Another frustration is the heavily skewed focus on infants, especially preterm infants, whereas large gaps exist in the literature on sleep and breathing in older children and adolescents. Studies that span the entire developmental age range, from infancy through late adolescence, are rare. The methods used to assess the sleep state in these studies vary from full polysomnography to simple observation, often relying on indirect indicators of sleep state. Finally, there is enormous variation in the methods and techniques used to assess respiratory system function, which have evolved over time and vary between studies. In this chapter we will selectively highlight important effects of sleep on normal respiratory physiology during childhood.

Thoracic Cage and Pulmonary Mechanics

The mammalian respiratory system consists of a gas exchanger (the lungs), which are cyclically inflated and deflated by a pump (the diaphragm; rib cage; and intercostal, accessory and abdominal muscles), via a single partially collapsible intake manifold (the nose, mouth, and upper airway). The ability of the respiratory pump to achieve adequate gas exchange depends, in part, on resistive and elastic loads imposed and the real-time response of the system. Although the rib cage is commonly thought of as a "structural" element of the respiratory system, the muscular components are all under continuous neural modulation and subject to further modulation by sleep state.

Chest Wall Mechanics

Rib cage geometry in infants and children differs markedly from that of adults. Openshaw and colleagues, using chest radiographs and computed tomography (CT) scans from individuals 1 month to 31 years of age, found that the dome of the diaphragm and head of the sternum were higher in children, relative to thoracic vertebrae.[2] The ribs of infants and young children were more horizontal (less downward slope) compared with older children and adults and downward slope of the ribs increased with age. These changes occurred primarily between infancy and 2–3 years. The cross-sectional shape of the thorax also changed, being more rounded in infancy and becoming more ovoid (adult pattern) by about 3 years of age.[2]

Compliance of an expandable structure (e.g., lung or chest wall) is defined as the change in volume for a given change in pressure. In infancy, chest wall compliance is several fold higher than lung compliance and is even higher, relative to lung compliance, in preterm infants.[3–6] With age, chest wall compliance decreases relative to lung compliance; thus the chest wall becomes stiffer with age while lung compliance changes little. Chest wall compliance becomes approximately equal to lung compliance, as in adults, by the second year of life due to bone ossification and increased muscle mass.[4,7]

The high chest wall compliance of the neonate has clinical relevance. Passive (relaxed) resting lung volume (V_r) is determined by the balance between the outward recoil of the chest wall and the inward recoil of the lungs. Fig. 22.1 shows the static volume pressure curves of the lung (L) and chest wall (CW) typical of a newborn and an adult.[8] Note that lung compliance is quite similar at both ages, whereas the chest wall is much less stiff (more compliant) in the newborn (see Fig. 22.1, left). When the chest wall is highly compliant, the inward recoil of the lungs (L) is less opposed, resulting in a lower resting lung volume (see Fig. 22.1, left). As the lungs are the major reservoir for oxygen, low resting lung volume predisposes infants to rapidly developing hypoxemia and atelectasis.[9,10]

Paradoxical Inward Rib Cage Motion

In normal infants, without lung disease or upper airway obstruction, the highly compliant infant chest wall leads to the well-known phenomenon of "paradoxical inward rib cage motion" (PIRCM), also called thoracoabdominal asynchrony or "paradoxing" (informal). Multiple studies show that the rib cage of otherwise normal infants collapses during the inspiratory descent of the diaphragm and is associated with deflation of the rib cage, independent of upper airway obstruction.[11–14] The degree of thoracoabdominal asynchrony is significantly greater in preterm versus full-term infants.

PIRCM is more likely to occur during REM sleep due to lower chest wall muscle tone and increased chest wall compliance. Even in full-term normal infants, PIRCM occurs during REM sleep and is associated with a lower and more variable PaO_2.[15] In mature, healthy, full-term infants with PIRCM during REM sleep, thoracic gas volume (TGV) was 31% reduced compared with TGV during NREM sleep.[14] Such a large decrease in TGV during REM sleep markedly increases the probability of hypoxia with brief respiratory events, especially given that REM is the predominant sleep stage in infants and O_2 stores (primarily the lungs) are low relative to metabolic rate.[9,10]

At what age do normal infants stop exhibiting PIRCM during childhood? This is a key question for sleep medicine

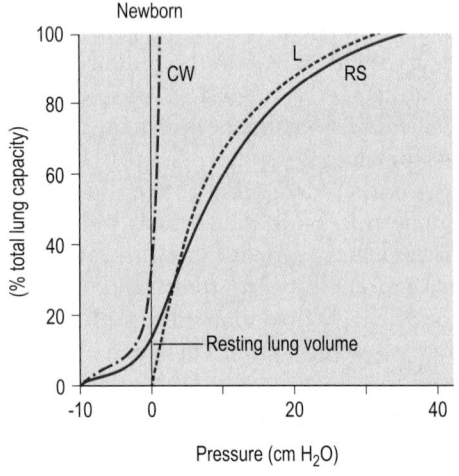
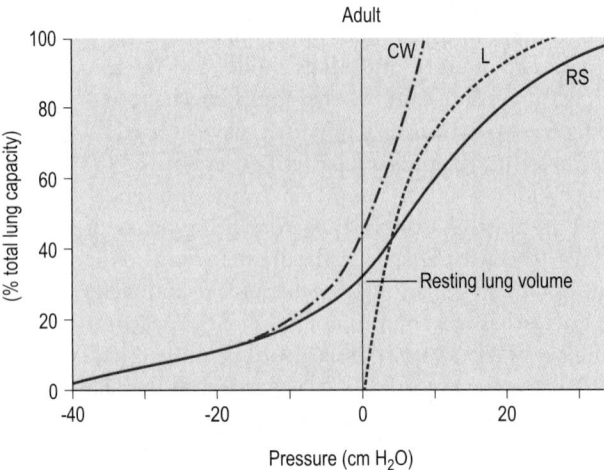

• **Fig. 22.1** Pressure volume curves of the respiratory system. The *solid line* represents the compliance of the respiratory system. The chest wall *(CW; dash-dot line)* is highly compliant in the newborn compared with the adult, whereas lung (L) compliance *(dashed line)* changes little with age.[8] RS, respiratory system.

specialists, as PIRCM is considered a sign of increased upper airway resistance or obstruction in older children and adults. Gaultier and colleagues studied healthy infants between 7 and 31 months of age using polysomnography and diaphragmatic electromyography (EMG) during a daytime nap. The duration of PIRCM during sleep decreased as postnatal age increased.[16] By 3 years of age, PIRCM is "rare or absent" in normal children[11,17] and does not occur during REM sleep in normal adolescents.[18] Therefore finding PIRCM in a child older than 3 years of age (with normal neuromuscular function) should raise suspicion for increased upper airway resistance or obstruction. However, it is important to note that the amount of measured "paradoxical breathing" (PIRCM) may depend heavily on the technology used to detect it. In a study of 55 normal children 2–9 years of age without SDB, PIRCM was detected in 40% of 30-second sleep epochs when piezo technology was used versus only 1.5% of epochs when respiratory inductance plethysmography (RIP) was used to detect thoracoabdominal motion.[19]

Dynamic Maintenance of End-Expiratory Lung Volume

Inhibition of respiratory muscle tone at any age results in a decrease in lung volume.[20–23] In other words, lung volume is maintained, in part, by respiratory muscle activity. In full-term infants, during tidal breathing in NREM sleep, end-expiratory lung volume (EELV) is maintained above the passive relaxed lung volume (V_r).[24] This is accomplished by multiple mechanisms including expiratory "braking" using muscles of the upper airway, and postinspiratory inspiratory activity (PIIA) of the diaphragm, such that the next breath begins before the end of the previous expiration.[24–26]

The strategy of maintaining EELV above V_r is sleep state dependent. Several studies of EELV in full-term infants were performed during behavioral NREM sleep but did not study the effects of sleep per se. When sleep state was studied, TGV was found to be greater in NREM sleep compared with REM sleep in full-term infants, suggesting that EELV was better maintained in NREM sleep.[14] Preterm infants also maintain EELV above passive V_r, also with clear sleep state dependency. Preterm infants at approximately 32-weeks' gestational age were studied during the first week of life during REM and NREM sleep. In NREM sleep, a shortened expiratory time (Te) and diaphragmatic braking resulted in maintenance of EELV above V_r. In contrast, during REM sleep, Te was longer and expiratory braking was reduced such that EELV approached V_r.[26]

The dynamically maintained EELV, which helps maintain SpO_2 in infants, may be lost during apnea. Preterm infants approximately 29 weeks' gestational age were studied during central apnea using intercostal muscle and diaphragm surface EMG activity as well as anteroposterior (AP) diameter of the rib cage and abdomen (as a measure of EELV).[22] During apnea, decreased activity of the respiratory muscles correlated with loss of EELV. The apnea-related drop in

EELV was greater during NREM sleep, suggesting that EELV was better maintained during NREM compared with REM sleep.[22] Thus infants are able to compensate for the "mechanical disadvantage" of their highly compliant chest wall by maintaining EELV above passive V_r during sleep, although they do this less effectively during REM sleep. This has important clinical implications, given the importance of lung O_2 stores in infants for maintaining normal SpO_2. The loss of EELV in infants during apnea increases the likelihood and speed of O_2 desaturation.

How long does the active maintenance of EELV above V_r persist during infancy? In healthy infants and children aged 1 month to 8 years, studied using RIP-derived tidal breathing flow-volume loops to assess breathing strategy, the flow-volume pattern during expiration was "interrupted" up to 6 months of age, consistent with dynamic maintenance of an elevated EELV during this period.[27] Between 6 and 12 months expiratory flow-volume patterns were a mixture of "interrupted" and "uninterrupted," indicating a transitional period. After 1 year of age, expiratory flow-volume patterns were "uninterrupted," consistent with relaxed or passive EELV.[27] Thus the transition from dynamic maintenance of elevated EELV to the mature, adult-like, passive or relaxed EELV occurs during the second half of the first year of life.

Relative Contribution of Rib Cage and Abdomen to Tidal Volume

Postnatal developmental changes in chest wall compliance and active maintenance of EELV predict that the relative contributions of the rib cage and abdomen to tidal volume (V_T), and the effects of sleep, are likely to change with maturation. In studies of normal supine adults, the average rib cage contribution to V_T fell by 25–32% during REM sleep compared with waking, consistent with the normal skeletal muscle atonia that occurs during REM sleep.[23,28] Similarly, in healthy, term infants, the rib cage contribution to V_T was found to be lower in REM versus NREM sleep.[29] As anticipated based on normal maturation of chest wall compliance, the contribution of the rib cage to V_T during NREM and REM sleep (measured using RIP) increases during infancy between 1 and 26 months of age.[30,31]

Response to Mechanical Loading of the Respiratory System During Sleep

Elastic and resistive loads on the respiratory system are intrinsic to the normal lungs, chest wall, and upper airway. In adults, nasal and upper airway resistance increase during normal sleep, although with considerable individual variation.[32–34] Numerous disorders impose additional loading on the respiratory system, including lung disease and sleep-related upper airway obstruction, and the normal respiratory system responds with load compensation strategies that vary with type of load, age, position, and sleep state.

An added load is typically defined as anything that requires increased respiratory muscle effort to maintain minute ventilation (V_E). The ability of the system to compensate for increased loading can be studied using externally imposed elastic or resistive loads. Unfortunately, although most of the available studies in children have been performed *during* sleep, few have examined the effects of sleep per se on the respiratory system response to loading. In addition, it is difficult to compare studies due to the variety of methodologies used. Nevertheless, these studies have relevance in the context of SDB, which imposes abnormal mechanical loads on the respiratory system. The key points highlighted here are (1) developmental changes in compensation for resistive loading and (2) how load compensation is affected by sleep.

Resistive Loading

Examples of natural resistive loads include nasal obstruction, upper airway obstruction, bronchospasm, and laryngospasm. Experimental resistive loading, typically accomplished by having a subject breathe through a known resistance, can be inspiratory only, expiratory only, or both. Awake, normal adults are able to compensate for added resistive loads and maintain V_E and V_T.[35,36] This compensatory ability depends on the adequacy of the respiratory control system response as well as chest wall stability and respiratory muscle strength.[35,37] During REM and NREM sleep in normal adults, progressive addition of inspiratory resistive loads decreases V_E, largely due to inadequate prolongation of inspiratory time (Ti) in the presence of increased inspiratory resistance.[36]

The much greater compliance of the chest wall during infancy, especially in preterm infants, predicts that infants may not cope well with inspiratory resistive loading. Before adding increased inspiratory resistance, preterm and full-term infants during NREM sleep exhibited similar baseline lung resistance and compliance, although the preterm infants exhibited greater asynchrony compared with full-term.[37] When presented with an inspiratory resistive load, full-term infants were able to maintain V_E and V_T with little effect on thoracoabdominal synchrony. In contrast, identical inspiratory loading in preterm infants resulted in decreased V_T and V_E as well as increased chest wall asynchrony, suggesting that the preterm infant is less able to compensate due to chest wall instability.[37]

Resistive loading alters vagally mediated reflexes that modify mechanical and neural inspiratory duration. For example, in a study of full-term, 2- to 3-day-old infants during NREM sleep, application of increasing inspiratory resistive loads (to a single breath) resulted in progressive prolongation of Ti, shortening of Te and decreasing V_T.[38] These changes were also reflected in "neural" V_T, Ti, and Te as measured by EMG.[38] In the same group of infants (during NREM sleep), increasing expiratory resistive loading was associated with progressive decrements in V_E and prolongation of (neural and mechanical) Te, with little effect on Ti.[39] In summary, both inspiratory and expiratory resistive loading decrease minute ventilation in infants, but effects on breathing pattern differ.

In addition, the effects of mechanical loading on respiratory timing in infants tend to be more pronounced with resistive loads versus elastic loads.[38–40] Unfortunately, although studies were often performed during sleep, the effects of sleep per se were typically not examined.

Very few studies have reported the effects of respiratory mechanical loading in older normal children. Marcus and coworkers studied the effects of inspiratory resistive loading in normal children ~9 years of age.[41] When presented with a flow-resistive load for 3 minutes during sleep, in both REM and NREM sleep, there was an immediate fall in V_T and V_E, which was proportional to the magnitude of the resistance and associated with a small increase in the ratio of Ti to total breath time (Ttot) due to shortening of Te.[41] A similar study of inspiratory resistive loading during NREM sleep in normal young adults (mean age 20.5 years) also reported a marked drop in V_T (and V_E), proportional to the magnitude of the resistive load.[42] This was associated with significant prolongation of Ti and increase of Ti/Ttot, with no change in respiratory rate.[42]

Elastic Loading

Examples of natural respiratory elastic loads include atelectasis, pulmonary edema, pulmonary fibrosis (lung), and obesity or abdominal distension (chest wall). Although there are multiple ways to experimentally impose an elastic load on the respiratory system, a common approach is to have the subject breathe from a closed-volume reservoir (elastic load varies with the size of the reservoir). In normal adults, during wakefulness, application of an inspiratory elastic load is compensated immediately such that V_T and V_E are preserved.[43] However, during NREM sleep, sustained inspiratory elastic loading caused a sustained drop in V_T and V_E until they were restored by increasing PCO_2.[43] Thus, during NREM sleep in adults, compensatory responses to elastic loading only occur when respiratory effort is increased by chemical stimuli.

In full-term quietly sleeping infants, application of an elastic load during inspiration caused a marked fall in V_T and prolongation of Ti, with little effect on Te.[38] Application of an elastic load during expiration in the same-age infants also caused a marked drop in V_T and prolongation of Ti, with little effect on Ti.[39] Similarly, in preterm infants ~31 weeks' gestational age and ~8 days' postnatal age, addition of external elastic loads caused a marked drop in V_T and prolongation of Ti and Te, the magnitude of which increased progressively with the magnitude of the elastic load.[40]

When application of respiratory elastic loading during sleep is prolonged in term and preterm infants, V_T initially drops but progressively increases during subsequent breaths indicating a compensatory response.[13] In both term and preterm infants, load compensation was more effective during NREM sleep. During REM sleep elastic loading increased rib cage distortion, which limited the ability to compensate.[13] Increased respiratory elastic load occurs in numerous clinical conditions, including hyperinflation, obesity, and neuromuscular disorders, and compensatory responses may be blunted by sleep, especially REM sleep.

Complete Airway Occlusion: Effects on Breathing During Sleep

Although review of the extensive literature on the Hering-Breuer (HB) and other lung-inflation reflexes is beyond the scope of this chapter, several points about the respiratory timing effects of total airway occlusion in children will be highlighted here. In 1868, Breuer and Hering described the role of the pulmonary slowly adapting stretch receptors (fibers carried in the vagus nerves) in determining the rate, depth, and timing of tidal breathing.[44] The HB reflexes are classically elicited in several ways; occlusion of the airway at the beginning of inspiration prolongs Ti, whereas airway occlusion at end inspiration prolongs Te. The HB reflexes can be elicited in normal, unsedated adults, but volumes larger than the normal tidal volume range are required and evidence for the persistence of HB reflexes beyond infancy is controversial.[45] In spite of multiple early studies suggesting that the HB reflexes participate in controlling tidal breathing during infancy, their role during postnatal development remains controversial.[38,39,46,47]

In full-term infants 2–3 days of age, during NREM sleep, total occlusion of the airway during inspiration (for a single breath) resulted in marked prolongation of mechanical and neural (EMG) Ti, as expected due to removal of vagally mediated feedback from pulmonary slowly adapting stretch receptors, without effect on Te.[38] In the same group of infants, total airway occlusion during expiration (for a single breath) led to marked prolongation of Te, without effect on Ti.[39] Beyond the newborn period, prolongation of Te by end-inspiratory occlusion persisted throughout the first year, although the magnitude of the Te prolongation decreased with age.[48,49]

Studies in preterm infants indicate that reflex effects of inspiratory airway occlusion on timing depend on gestational age at birth and chronologic age. In one study of preterm infants, ~30 weeks' gestational age and ~8 days old, the prolongation of Ti was similar to that seen in term infants.[50] Closer examination of the effects of maturity and age yielded different results. Preterm infants born at 27–32 weeks' gestational age and studied within the first 3–4 days exhibited wide variation in the response to inspiratory occlusion.[51] Ti was prolonged in some and shortened in others, whereas the overall magnitude of prolongation was much less than the ~30% prolongation of Ti observed in full-term infants.[51] In the same group of infants, the response to inspiratory occlusion was still immature at 7–10 days, but was similar to the full-term response by 14 days. In preterm infants born at 33–36 weeks' gestational age, the Ti prolongation with inspiratory occlusion was mature by 7–10 days, suggesting that the rapidity of maturation depends on the degree of maturity at birth.[51]

Sleep may profoundly affect HB reflexes in infants. In a study of preterm infants 30–36 weeks' "postconceptual age" (sic), using observational sleep staging, occlusion of a normal tidal breath at end inspiration resulted in an average Te prolongation of 87% in NREM sleep compared with 419% in REM sleep.[47] However, another study, using single-breath inspiratory occlusions in term newborns, found increased HB activity in NREM compared with REM sleep.[52]

Caution should be exercised in the interpretation of studies using mechanical loading or total airway occlusion. As noted previously, most studies only study infants during NREM sleep. Many studies only examined the effects of occlusion for brief durations, even a single breath or parts of a breath. Reflex effects during longer occlusions may lead to increasing compensatory adaptations over time. In addition, these methods may evoke other reflex effects from face masks used and some authors have suggested that the upper airway negative pressure and other reflexes may contribute, potentially confounding interpretation.[53]

Maintenance of Upper Airway Patency During Sleep in Normal Children

The pharyngeal airway, extending from the nasal choanae to the epiglottis, is a collapsible tube composed of muscle and soft tissues, without support from bony structures except for the posterior pharyngeal wall.[54] Pharyngeal patency depends on mechanical factors (muscle mass, connective tissue, submucosal fat, mucosal edema, perfusion, position, etc.) as well as activity of the muscles that compose and surround the airway.[54,55] The pharyngeal muscles may act to stiffen the airway soft tissues, making them less deformable by intraluminal negative pressure, or actively dilate the airway and change its caliber.[54]

The pharyngeal airway is bounded by the posterior pharyngeal wall, anchored at the top by the palatal muscles (musculus uvulae, palatoglossus, palatopharyngeus, tensor veli palatini, and levator veli palatini), at the bottom by the hyoid muscles (thyrohyoid, mylohyoid, stylohyoid, geniohyoid, and sternohyoid), and anteriorly by the genioglossus muscle.[54,56] The activity of these muscle groups is largely responsible for the maintenance of airway patency during sleep. It is important to note that, although most studies to date have focused on the genioglossus muscle, innervated by the hypoglossal nerve (cranial nerve [CN] XII), upper airway tone is influenced by input from other motoneuron groups including the motor vagus (CN X), glossopharyngeal (CN IX), facial (CN VII), and motor trigeminal (CN V).[55] In addition, motoneurons of the cervical ventral horn may contribute to airway patency via their influence on neck and jaw position as well as lung volume.[55] As these muscles are modulated by state, sleep may profoundly affect pharyngeal patency and reflex responses (e.g., to negative pressure).

A full review of normal upper airway structure, physiology, and its development is beyond the scope of this chapter. The reader is referred to several excellent reviews of upper airway structural development during childhood.[57–63] Here we review what is known about the physiology of upper airway collapsibility in infants and children, how it can be measured, how airway patency is affected by sleep, and the effects of puberty and age.

Critical Closing Pressure, P_{crit}

The human upper airway behaves as a Starling resistor, modeled as a tube with rigid segments on either end and a collapsible segment in a sealed box in between (representing the collapsible pharynx and surrounding tissue mass).[64] The patency of the collapsible segment is determined by the mechanical factors noted earlier and by the activity of upper airway muscles. P_{crit}, the *critical closing pressure* of the collapsible segment, is the pharyngeal lumenal pressure when collapse occurs (Fig. 22.2). In this model, the upstream (nasal) and downstream (hypopharyngeal/tracheal) segments have defined resistances and fixed diameters.

During inspiration, diaphragm contraction and thoracic cage expansion lower pressure in the downstream segment, creating a pressure gradient for inspiratory airflow. The degree of inspiratory airflow limitation (if any) depends on the pressure gradient between the upstream segment (P_{us}) and P_{crit} and is independent of downstream pressure (P_{ds}). P_{us} at the nares is atmospheric pressure (zero cm H_2O, reference) and P_{crit}, in normals, and is typically less than -10 cm H_2O. Therefore, although there is a small pressure drop across the upstream segment, in normal subjects upstream pressure remains sufficiently greater than the pressure in the collapsible segment such that inspiratory airflow is unimpeded (see Fig. 22.2, top).[64,65]

Any condition that increases P_{crit} (upper airway dilator muscle hypotonia, sedation, anesthesia, obesity, edema) may reduce the difference between P_{us} and P_{crit}, with resulting inspiratory airflow limitation (see Fig. 22.2, middle). When P_{crit} exceeds P_{us}, complete obstruction occurs (see Fig. 22.2, bottom).[54,55,64,65] In simple terms, when pharyngeal critical closing pressure is positive to atmospheric pressure, complete airway collapse occurs during inspiration, and upstream (nasal) positive pressure (greater than P_{crit}) is required to restore pharyngeal patency (e.g., nasal continuous positive airway pressure [CPAP]). In normal infants, children, and adults, P_{crit} is negative during wakefulness and sleep, usually less than -10 cm H_2O, and the pharyngeal airway is always patent, with no inspiratory airflow limitation.

Variations in P_{crit} during wakefulness and sleep are due largely to its dependence on upper airway dilator muscle activity. During normal breathing, airway patency is heavily influenced by state-dependent activity of the upper airway dilator muscles. In addition, upper airway dilator muscles are activated by negative pressure in the airway, sensed by negative pressure receptors primarily in the larynx.[54,66] Finally, the negative pressure reflex and respiratory drive to the upper airway dilator muscles are strongly influenced by the levels of chemical respiratory drive (PaO_2 and $PaCO_2$) from the peripheral and central chemoreceptors.[67-71] All of these factors combine to make P_{crit} dynamic, varying with position, sleep state, levels of chemical stimuli, and other factors that affect pharyngeal deformability.

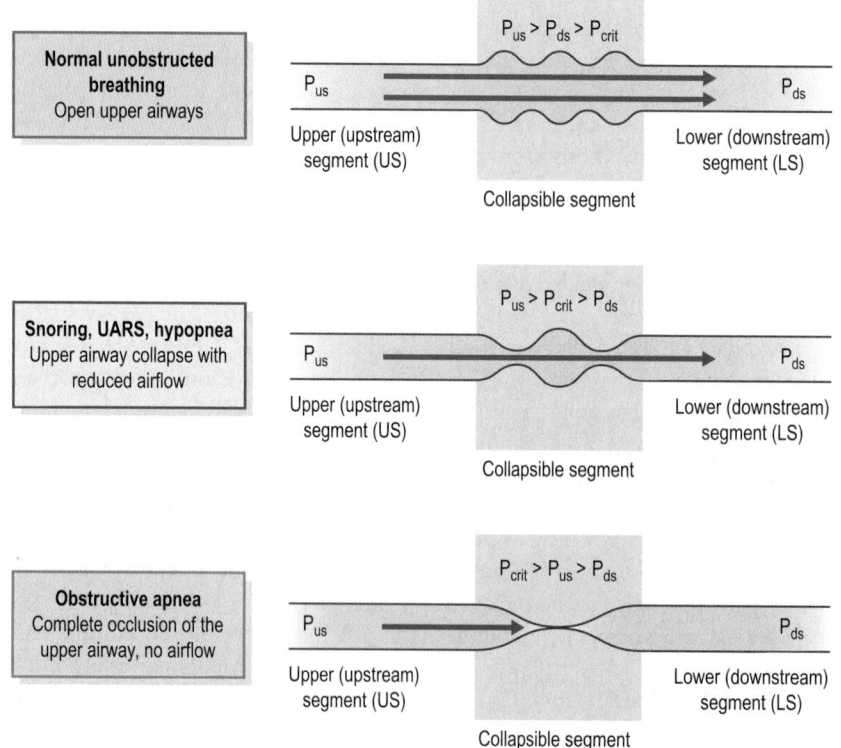

• **Fig. 22.2** The upper airway modeled as a Starling resistor; airflow through a tube with rigid upstream (nasal airway) and downstream (hypopharyngeal airway) segments, and a collapsible segment in a sealed box in between (pharyngeal airway). The upstream and downstream segments have defined resistances and fixed diameters. The patency of the collapsible segment depends on the pressure exerted by the surrounding tissues (P_{crit}). See text for explanation.[65] P_{ds}, pressure downstream; P_{us}, pressure upstream; UARS, upper airway resistance syndrome.

Measurement of Upper Airway Collapsibility

Upper airway collapsibility can be well characterized by two values: (1) the slope of the linear relationship between maximal inspiratory flow (*y*-axis) and upstream (nasal) pressure (*x*-axis) and (2) P_{crit}, the *x*-axis intercept (zero flow). The relationship between upper airway maximal inspiratory flow (V_{Imax}) and nasal pressure (P_N) may be termed V_{Imax}/P_N and is also termed "S_{PF}" (slope of the pressure-flow relationship) in the pediatric literature.[72] P_{crit} and V_{Imax}/P_N can be determined experimentally in individual subjects to obtain numerical measures of upper airway collapsibility. Their classical laboratory measurement yields values that "characterize" upper airway collapsibility during sleep for a particular sleep stage and specific method of measurement, in an individual subject. P_{crit} and V_{Imax}/P_N are typically measured during slow-wave sleep (SWS) and are difficult to measure during wakefulness or REM sleep.

In humans, P_{crit} of the upper airway is typically measured during tidal breathing, using a nasal mask attached to source of negative or positive pressure. A pneumotachograph is used to measure inspiratory airflow and P_N is measured at the mask.[73,74] In normal subjects there is no inspiratory flow limitation when nasal pressure is zero (atmospheric pressure), so negative pressure is applied via the nasal mask and made more negative in steps to produce a V_{Imax} versus P_N relationship, as shown in Fig. 22.3. When maximal inspiratory airflow (for tidal breaths at a given pressure) is plotted versus nasal mask pressure, a linear relationship is obtained and extrapolated to zero flow. The slope of the V_{Imax}/P_N relationship (S_{PF} in the literature) represents the collapsibility of the upper airway and the *x*-axis (zero flow) intercept represents P_{crit} (see Fig. 22.3). This approach has been used to characterize upper airway collapsibility in numerous studies of normal children[75] and adults.[73,74] In children with SDB,

when airflow limitation or obstructive apnea are already present at baseline (nasal mask pressure = 0), a linear pressure–flow relationship can be obtained in a similar manner by applying positive pressure via nasal mask, increasing in steps until airflow limitation is abolished.

Dynamic Upper Airway Negative Pressure Reflexes: Activated Versus Hypotonic P_{crit}

In normal children during neuromuscular paralysis P_{crit} is about −7.5 cm H_2O,[77] much higher than the P_{crit} of normal children during sleep, which is about −25 cm H_2O using the "activated" method of measurement (see later).[72,78,79] Loads imposed on the upper airway that generate negative pressure in the pharynx and larynx cause reflex activation of upper airway dilator muscles to stiffen and/or alter the caliber of the airway.[54] This has very important implications for the measurement of the V_{Imax}/P_N relationship and P_{crit}. When upper airway collapsibility is measured in the classical way, by progressively stepping down nasal (mask) pressure, the upper airway dilator muscles are reflexively activated as nasal pressure is decreased (made more negative). Fig. 22.4 shows a normal subject, in stage 2 NREM sleep, starting from a nasal mask holding pressure of 5 cm H_2O.[80] Fig. 22.4, left, shows the "activated" approach, in which P_N is decreased 1–2 cm H_2O every 10 minutes, without returning to baseline holding pressure. This results in recruitment of compensatory upper airway dilator muscle activity as evidenced by the marked genioglossus muscle EMG activity (see Fig. 22.4). The P_{crit} and V_{Imax}/P_N relationship measured using the activated approach include the effects of anatomical factors as well as compensatory activation of dilator muscle activity; thus the term activated P_{crit}.[72,81]

The "hypotonic" method of measuring the V_{Imax}/P_N relationship and P_{crit} was developed to avoid the effects of upper airway dilator muscle recruitment during the measurement. This method, shown in Fig. 22.4, right, also starts from a holding pressure but decreases P_N for only five breaths and then returns to baseline holding pressure. In the example shown in Fig. 22.4, right, nasal mask pressure was lowered without activation of compensatory upper airway dilator muscle activity, as indicated by the absence of genioglossus muscle activation (EMG_{GG}).[80] The hypotonic approach characterizes upper airway collapsibility without the effects of compensatory dilator muscle activity; therefore it reflects mainly anatomic factors contributing to obstruction.[72,81,82]

When both the activated and hypotonic methods of upper airway pressure-flow measurement are used in the same individual, important additional information is gained. Differences in P_{crit} and the slope of V_{Imax}/P_N, measured using the activated and hypotonic methods, reflect the magnitude of compensatory upper airway dilator muscle responses. As illustrated in Fig. 22.5, use of the hypotonic method results in a higher (less negative) P_{crit} and steeper slope of the V_{Imax}/P_N relationship, compared with the activated method. In sharp contrast, the activated method applied to the same child results in a much flatter slope of the V_{Imax}/P_N relationship and P_{crit} is shifted far to the left (more negative, less

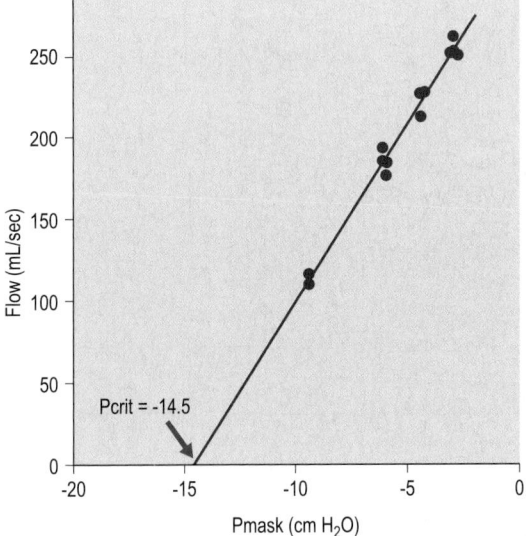

• **Fig. 22.3** Typical measurement of pharyngeal critical closing pressure in a normal subject. The slope of the pressure-flow relationship (in mL/s/cm H_2O) represents airway conductance and the *x*-axis intercept (zero flow) represents critical closing pressure (P_{crit}).[76]

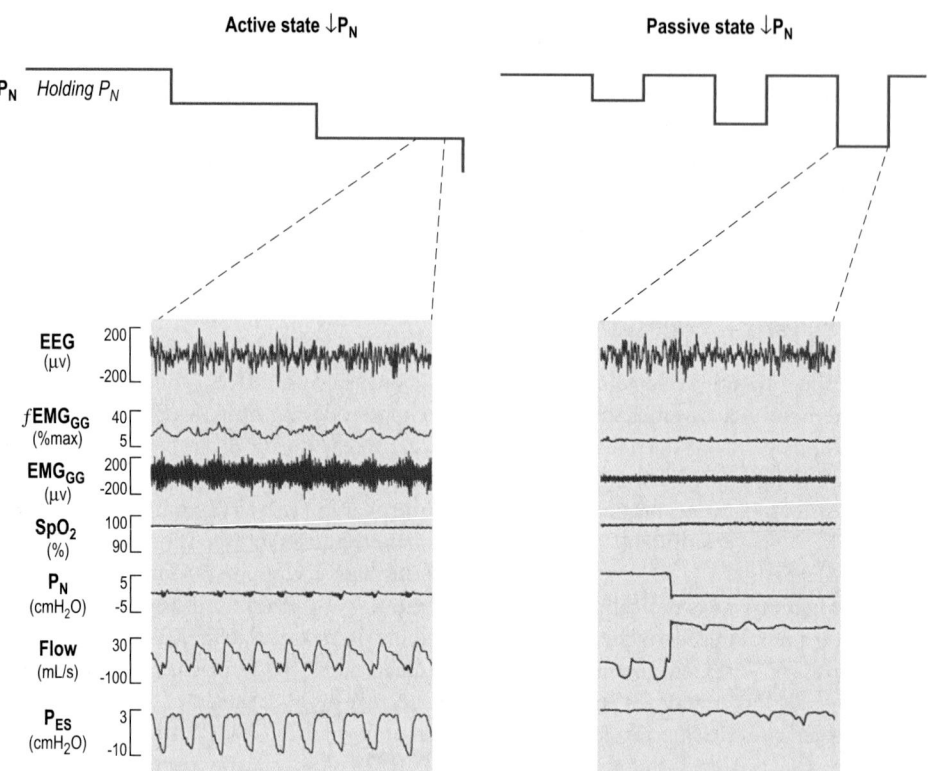

• **Fig. 22.4** Comparison of the two methods of measuring upper airway collapsibility in a control subject. *Left:* "Activated" method. *Left upper:* From holding pressure of 5 cm H_2O during stage 2 non–rapid eye movement (NREM) sleep, nasal mask *(P_N)* pressure is lowered in steps about every 10 minutes. *Left lower:* At −3 cm H_2O nasal pressure, inspiratory flow limitation occurs and compensatory dilator muscle activity *(EMG_GG)* is markedly increased. *Right:* "Hypotonic" method. *Right upper:* Starting from the same holding pressure (5 cm H_2O) in stage 2 NREM sleep, nasal mask pressure is lowered intermittently for five breaths only and then returned to the baseline holding pressure. *Right lower:* At −3 cm H_2O, in sharp contrast to the activated method *(left)*, there is no compensatory upper airway dilator muscle activation.[80] EEG, electroencephalography; P_{ES}, esophageal pressure.

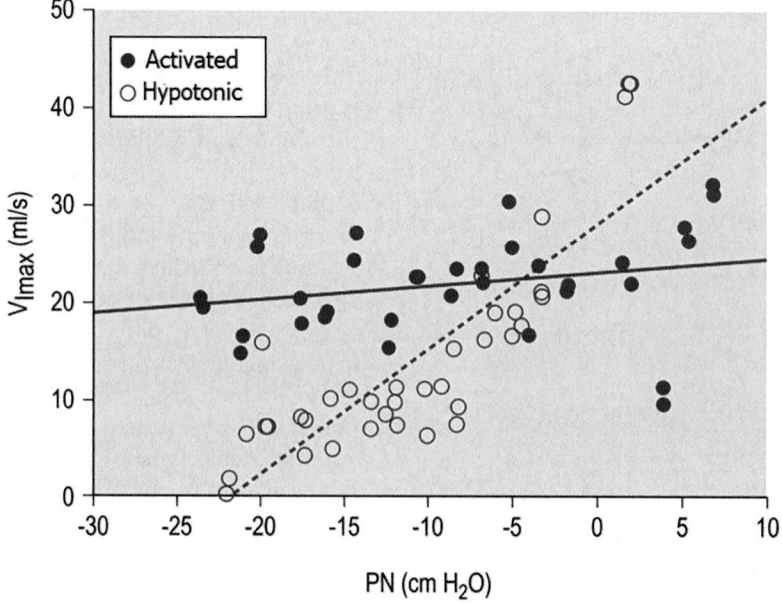

• **Fig. 22.5** Example of "activated" versus "hypotonic" method of measuring upper airway pressure-flow relationships in a child. With the activated method compensatory muscle responses decreased airway collapsibility. With the hypotonic technique, compensatory dilator muscle responses are not activated; resulting in a higher P_{crit} and steeper slope (S_{PF}).[72]

collapsible airway; see Fig. 22.5).[72] Thus, when the activated method was used, upper airway dilator muscle recruitment preserved V_{Imax} in spite of increasingly negative P_N, indicating strong dynamic regulation of airway patency.

P_{crit} and the slope of the V_{Imax}/P_N relationship have been studied extensively in normal adults and children and in subjects with SDB, before and after airway surgery, pre and post weight loss, before and after puberty, and a variety of other conditions. Both measures of upper airway collapsibility correlate strongly with apnea-hypopnea index (AHI) in subjects with SDB and improve with interventions that reduce AHI.

Upper Airway Collapsibility in Normal Children: Effects of Age

Early studies, using the activated method to determine P_{crit} and the slope of V_{Imax}/P_N, revealed a striking difference between normal adults and children. In adults, the V_{Imax}/P_N relationship was relatively steep and P_{crit} was approximately -5 to -30 cm H_2O.[83] In sharp contrast, the slope of the V_{Imax}/P_N relationship in normal children was nearly flat, making it difficult to obtain a P_{crit} value by extrapolation to zero flow. This indicated that normal children have a remarkable ability to maintain upper airway patency despite increasingly negative pressure in the airway lumen. The slope of the V_{Imax}/P_N relationship averaged ~8.5 mL/s/cm H_2O in children compared with ~30 mL/s/cm H_2O in adults.[83]

Later studies covered a larger age range and used both the activated and the hypotonic methods for determining upper airway collapsibility. In adults, the V_{Imax}/P_N relationship is steeper than in children, indicating that the adult airway is more collapsible compared with infants and children (Fig. 22.6).[72] Fig. 22.6, right, shows that the method used (activated vs. "hypotonic") had little effect on the slope or on P_{crit} in adults. Other studies in normal adults suggest that P_{crit} is slightly left-shifted (more negative) by 5–10 cm H_2O, with little change in slope, using the activated versus hypotonic approach.[80,84]

The V_{Imax}/P_N relationship in infants is relatively flat, P_{crit} is much more negative compared with adult values and neither are affected by the activated versus hypotonic method (see Fig. 22.6, left). This indicates that the infant upper airway is far less collapsible compared with the adult airway, in spite of being narrower.[72] The lack of difference between the activated and hypotonic approaches in infants (see Fig. 22.6, left) should not be interpreted as a lack of compensatory upper airway muscle activity during infancy. Indeed, the infant airway is heavily dependent upon dilator muscle activity.[85] The reason that the activated versus hypotonic V_{Imax}/P_N curves are about the same in infants is likely due to very rapid activation of compensatory responses, within one to two breaths of negative pressure application, such that *both curves* reflect activated upper airway dilator muscles.[86,87] In other words, the activated versus hypotonic approach does not work for infants, as a way to separate activated versus hypotonic responses, because the timing of their compensatory responses to negative pressure is so rapid.[72]

Upper airway collapsibility in school-aged children is strongly influenced by compensatory dilator muscle responses to negative pressure, as indicated by the large difference between the activated versus hypotonic approach to V_{Imax}/P_N and P_{crit} measurement (see Fig. 22.5; see Fig. 22.6, middle).[72,79] Adolescents also exhibit a marked difference, between an activated and hypotonic measurement approach, in the slope of the upper airway V_{Imax}/P_N relationship and P_{crit}, which increases with age.[88] The increase in adolescent upper airway collapsibility with age, approaching adult values by late adolescence, is independent of Tanner stage.[89] Normal, nonsnoring obese adolescents exhibit normal, vigorous upper airway neuromotor responses to negative pressure loading (using the activated and hypotonic methods) that are nearly identical to those of lean controls.[88]

In summary, with increasing age, from infancy through adolescence, P_{crit} becomes less negative and the slope of the V_{Imax}/P_N relationship becomes steeper. Thus, compared with adults, the upper airway of infants and children is relatively resistant to collapse, largely due to highly effective compensatory neuromotor responses to negative pressure during sleep. This may explain, in part, why children have less obstructive SDB and snore less than adults, despite having a smaller, narrower upper airway. Indeed, defective upper airway neuromotor responses to loading are believed to be a major factor in the pathophysiology of obstructive SDB in children.[90,91]

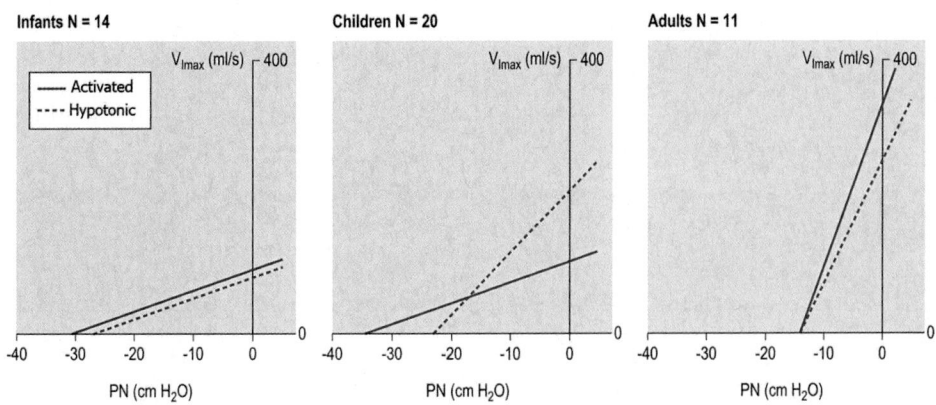

• **Fig. 22.6** Median V_{Imax}/P_N relationships for normal infants (*left*), children (*middle*), and adults (*right*) using the "activated" and "hypotonic" methods. See text for explanation.[72]

Effects of Sleep Stage on Maintenance of Upper Airway Patency

It is well known that obstructive SDB usually occurs during REM sleep in children,[92] possibly related to decreased upper airway dilator muscle activity,[93–95] decreased sensitivity of upper airway reflexes to chemical stimuli,[69] or other factors. Unfortunately, little is known about the physiology of upper airway collapsibility during REM sleep. The earliest studies in this area found that arousal tends to occur with negative pressure or occlusion challenges during REM sleep; therefore studies are typically performed only during stage 2 NREM sleep.[75] Therefore most data on effects of wakefulness, REM, and NREM sleep on upper airway physiology have been performed using nonchallenge protocols, typically by measuring genioglossus muscle EMG during sleep.

In normal, nonsnoring, asymptomatic children studied using EMG_{GG} during polysomnography, tonic EMG_{GG} activity was highest during wakefulness, decreased to 65% of wakefulness level during NREM sleep, and further decreased to about half of wakefulness level during REM sleep.[93] In normal children, no phasic EMG_{GG} activity was observed during sleep.[93] A recent study in adults with SDB, using hypotonic P_{crit}, found that P_{crit} was more negative (airway less collapsible) in SWS (deeper) compared with stage 2 NREM (lighter) sleep. The same study found that P_{crit} was higher (airway more collapsible) in REM sleep compared with both NREM stage 2 and SWS.[96] This confirms that P_{crit} varies with sleep state and, as anticipated, upper airway collapsibility (as measured by P_{crit}) is increased during REM sleep.

Dynamic Neuromotor Responses to Upper Airway Negative Pressure Loading

Dynamic upper airway responses have been studied in normal children (approximately 9–16 years of age) using negative pressure challenges (via nasal mask) during polysomnography, while recording EMG_{GG}.[97] As illustrated in Fig. 22.7, the upper airway neuromotor responses to negative pressure may develop quite rapidly. In this example, phasic EMG_{GG} activity can be observed even on breath 1 of the negative pressure challenge (see Fig. 22.7). As EMG_{GG} activity increases progressively breath by breath, inspiratory flow limitation decreases until flow limitation is abolished by breath 5 (see Fig. 22.7). These rapid-onset EMG_{GG} responses to negative pressure were highly variable between individuals.[97] In another study, adolescents exposed during NREM sleep to progressive stepping down of nasal pressure showed greater activation of EMG_{GG} using the activated method compared with the hypotonic approach. Normal, nonsnoring obese adolescents showed much greater activation of EMG_{GG} during sleep compared with lean controls, suggesting that they maintain upper airway patency during sleep via increased compensatory upper airway neuromotor activity compared with lean controls.[88]

Effects of Chemical Stimuli on Upper Airway Collapsibility

The effect of chemical stimuli on the upper airway muscles is a complex topic, beyond the scope of this chapter. Suffice it to say that both hypoxia and hypercapnia increase the activity of some (but not all) of the upper airway dilator muscles.[54,98,99] In humans, although stimulation of the upper airway muscles by CO_2 in adults is greatly reduced during sleep (compared with wakefulness), this response appears to be preserved during sleep in children.[72] The main effect of increased PCO_2, studied in normal school-aged children during NREM sleep, using the activated approach for measuring upper airway collapsibility, was an increase in inspiratory flow at a given nasal pressure. This effect was greatest for mild negative nasal pressures and diminished with increasingly negative P_N.[72]

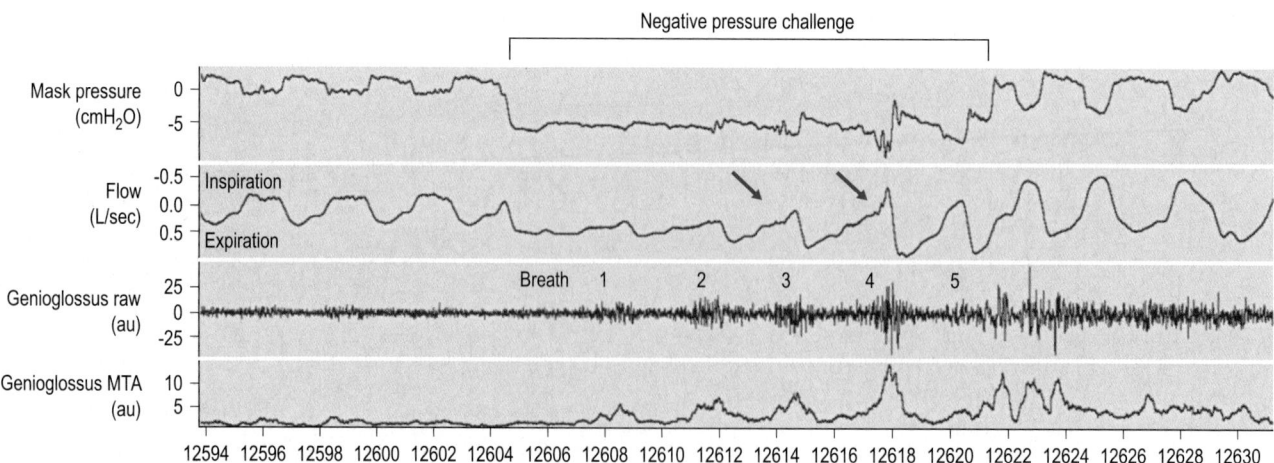

• **Fig. 22.7** Dynamic, breath-by-breath response to negative pressure challenge in a normal child. See text for explanation. MTA, moving time average.[97]

Ventilation During Sleep in Normal Children

Respiratory Frequency

Breathing pattern becomes more regular with age. Parmelee studied a group of premature infants from 30 weeks' gestation and a group of term infants. In preterm infants, regular breathing occurs only 10% of the time at 36 weeks' gestation and 30% of the time in infants at 40 weeks' gestation.[100] For both premature and term infants, breathing became more regular over the 8-month period studied. In general, respiratory rate is lower during sleep than during wakefulness.[101–103] There is a general consensus that the respiratory rate,[52,104–108] and particularly the variability of respiratory frequency,[104] is higher in REM sleep compared with NREM sleep. This may be related to the markedly increased excitation observed in medullary respiratory neurons during REM sleep.[109] Breathing frequency is not different between sexes,[110–112] at least in the first weeks of life. However, the range of respiratory frequencies is quite large, ranging from ~30 to near 70 breaths/min for infants in the first 2 weeks.[31,108,110–112] In addition to variability in recording methodologies and time-of-day of recordings, ambient temperature and even the type of feeding[113] may have influenced the measurement and contributed to the large range of observations.

A large meta-analysis compiled normal heart rate (143,346 children) and respiratory rate data (3,881 children) from 69 studies across the age range from 0 to 18 years.[114] Respiratory rate was highest in the first several weeks of life, declined steadily during the first year, showed accelerated decline between 1 and 2 years, and then continued to decline slowly until 18 years of age (Fig. 22.8). Similarly, normal heart rate is highest during the first month of life and declines across all of childhood through 18 years of age.[114] A recent study of normal awake and sleeping respiratory rate from birth through 18 years used an optical probe such that respiratory rate could be measured without artifacts in an observer's presence.[101] The results (560 awake and 103 sleeping children) confirmed and extended data from previous studies and provided normal respiratory rate centiles across the entire childhood age range.[100]

Multiple other studies have confirmed the general trend of respiratory rate decreasing with age throughout childhood,[31,101,103,114–117] an increase in regular breathing,[100] and a smaller difference in respiratory frequency between NREM and REM sleep.[100] For instance, in one longitudinal study respiratory frequency declined from 41 breaths/min at 1 month of age to 31 breaths/min at 5–6 months for both sleep states,[113] but others have found the decrease in respiratory rate is primarily in REM sleep.[118] In another study, which examined 57 normal infants, respiratory frequency was higher in 2–5 weeks, and 6–10 weeks compared with newborns, or 11- to 18-week-old infants.[107] Beyond 1 month of age, males breathe more rapidly than females, suggesting a slower maturation of the respiratory control system in males.[119]

In older children between 9 and 13 years, respiratory rate is highest in wakefulness and stage 1 sleep and lowest in stage 2 sleep.[120] Although average respiratory rate is the same in males and females, the variance of rate is higher in males.[116,120] In a study of adolescents, respiratory rate decreased in going from wakefulness to NREM sleep and increased during REM sleep[18]; in another, respiratory frequency was not different between NREM and REM sleep.[121]

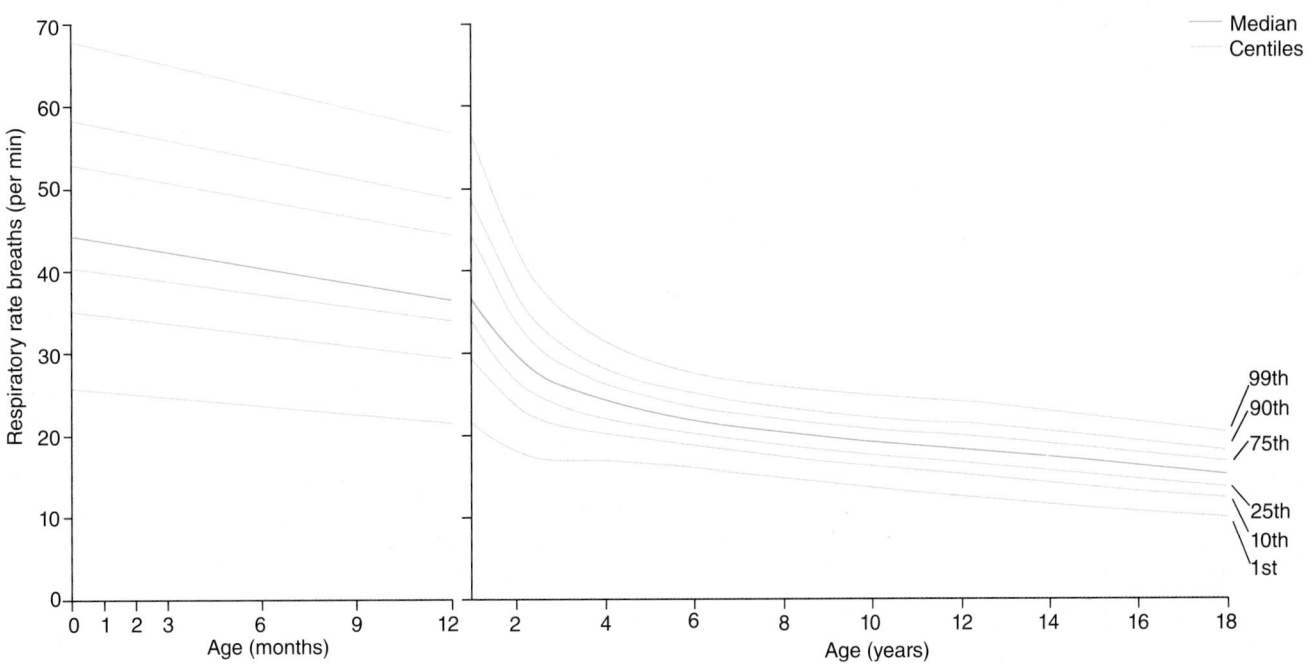

• **Fig. 22.8** Respiratory rate in normal children from birth to 18 years of age.[114]

Tidal Volume

In preterm infants ~31 weeks' gestational age, studied at ~3 weeks of age, average tidal volume during sleep was 6.7–7.0 mL/kg during sleep and did not differ between REM and NREM sleep.[122] Average tidal volume for term infants during the first week of life is about 4.6–4.9 mL/kg.[105,123] In contrast to respiratory frequency, generally no significant difference was observed in tidal volume between REM and NREM sleep in babies[52,104,105] or only a slight decrease in tidal volume was observed.[105] This is perhaps surprising because the chest wall and abdominal wall are more synchronous in NREM sleep, but during REM sleep abdominal wall and chest wall are asynchronous, and tidal volume is negatively correlated with the phase shift between the two.

In older babies at 2 months of age, using barometric plethysmography, V_T was greater in NREM sleep than REM sleep.[116] In adolescents, tidal volume was not significantly changed between wakefulness, NREM sleep, and REM sleep.[18]

Minute Ventilation

As expected for an increase in breathing frequency and little or no change in V_T, minute ventilation is generally increased in REM sleep compared with NREM sleep,[52,104,105,122] but this was not found uniformly in all studies.[106,116] This is perhaps surprising because of the thoracoabdominal asynchrony in REM sleep, but an increase in minute ventilation is even observed in preterm infants in which the chest wall is most compliant.[122] As expected from the greater variability of respiratory frequency in REM sleep, minute ventilation also showed higher variability in REM sleep.[104]

In adolescents, minute ventilation decreased by 8% in going from wakefulness to NREM sleep and increased by 4% in going from NREM to REM sleep.[18] In another study of older children, minute ventilation was not different between NREM and REM sleep.[121] In adults, data from numerous studies indicate that V_E falls about 15–18% in NREM and REM sleep, due largely to a decrease in V_T without a change in respiratory rate, although variability is higher between studies.[124] Some of the variation between studies may be due to measurement of respiratory rate during tonic versus phasic REM sleep.

Duty Cycle

In newborn babies during NREM sleep, there is a positive correlation between V_T and Ttot, between Ti and Te, and between V_T and Ti.[105] However, Ti/Ttot does not vary with sleep state,[116] but the variability of Ti/Ttot was increased in REM sleep.[106] With age, there is a general increase in most duty cycle parameters, such as V_T, V_{TOT}, Ti, Te, V_T/Ti, and V_T/Ttot.[116] At greater than 2 months of age, V_T/Ttot was smaller in NREM sleep.[116] In adolescents, the Ti/Ttot was not significantly different among sleep states.[18]

Sighs

Sighs or augmented breaths are spontaneous deep breaths several times larger than regular tidal breaths. Some sighs appear to be a "breath on top of a breath," which is characterized by a biphasic respiratory pattern, which is a long inspiratory duration with an abrupt change in inspiratory flow rate halfway through the inspiratory phase.[125] These intermittent deep breaths are believed to serve an important function in re-expanding collapsed lung segments. Sighs are common in the newborn period, particularly during REM sleep, and are associated with periodic breathing, which occurs in about half the subjects and is unrelated to sleep stage.[126] The frequency of sighs decreases with postnatal age.[125,127] It is unclear whether they are more numerous in NREM sleep: one study concluded that they are,[128] whereas another concluded that they are not.[127] Retarded expiratory flow, possibly due to postinspiratory inspiratory diaphragmatic activity, is also mostly encountered in NREM sleep.[128] Spontaneous sighs appear to increase the probability of a subsequent apnea along with oscillatory respiratory efforts.[129]

Normal Apnea

Apneas are common in the newborn period,[102,130,131] decrease in frequency with age,[108,132] and are often associated with body movements.[126] They are especially prevalent in preterm newborns,[130,133] they occur more often in REM than NREM sleep,[107,112,113,134–138] and last longer in REM sleep.[113] Apnea also appeared to occur more commonly in breastfed infants[113] and may occur more in females than males beyond 1 month of age.[113,119,136]

Apnea durations of 6–10 seconds are especially common during infancy, are generally considered to be normal,[102,126,139] and are more likely to occur during REM sleep.[108] Most apneas are central apneas and obstructive or mixed apneas are infrequent in the newborn period,[135] but increase between 3 and 6 weeks and then diminish by 3 months.[132] Their incidence is affected by sleep position, and are more common in the prone position.[140] Others have found that in young infants obstructive apneas are more common than central apneas.[138] In a study of 88 full-term healthy infants between 12 and 18 months of age, apnea density (minutes of apnea per 100 minutes of quiet time) remained constant at 0.5 and did not differ across ages or between sexes.[141]

Apneas become less common at older ages[135] and cannot be reliably predicted from recordings from the first week of life.[102] By 1 year of age, no apneas >20 seconds were observed in a population of infants.[134] A recent study found no central apnea >11 seconds in a large group (562 subjects) of healthy infants 1 year of age.[142] Here the time and duration of recording may play a role because greater recording times are associated with an increase in apnea index, perhaps due to the influence of circadian rhythms.[143] Again, there appears to be a prevalence of central apneas over obstructive apneas in children 2–9 years with an apnea index of 0.08/hr for central apneas and 0.01/hr for obstructive apneas.[19]

In normal children 9–13 years of age, apnea lasting 5 seconds or longer was observed in all subjects, ranging from 3 to 40 per night, with an average of about 18 per night.[120] Some of these central pauses lasted up to 25 seconds and were most prevalent in stage 1 and REM sleep compared with stages 2–4.[120] In children 1–18 years old, the prevalence of central apneas lasting longer than 10 seconds was 30%.[144] No mixed apneas were observed in any normal children or adolescents.[144]

In contrast to obstructive apnea, central apnea lasting >10 seconds occurs in normal children and is slightly more common in NREM sleep compared with REM sleep.[144] Often central apnea was not associated with significant O_2 desaturation, which was observed with only 19% of central apneas.[145] The lowest O_2 desaturation observed was 88%. There was no apparent difference between children demonstrating apneas and those that did not. Both groups spent the same amount of time in REM sleep (18% of total sleep time).

In a study of normal children age 1–18 years, 18% had obstructive apneas, but they were rare, averaging only 0.1 obstructive apneas per sleep hour, never longer than 10 seconds duration and not correlated with age.[144] In normal children 1–15 years of age, central apneas were much more common compared with obstructive apneas (89% incidence).[145] Obstructive apneas were observed in only 4% of normal children and were not associated with a specific sleep stage.[145] Of those normal children exhibiting obstructive apneas, the apnea index was about 0.37–0.56.[144,145] Compared with normal children, obstructive apneas in adults are more common and increase with advancing age.[146]

The physiologic and clinical importance of normal apnea pauses is uncertain. Analysis of event recording in infants (about 6–7 months of age) demonstrates that of 1,306 apneic events lasting longer than 15 seconds, only 14.9% were associated with bradycardia.[147] Follow-up on patients that demonstrated prolonged apneas, some exceeding 25 seconds, indicated that none had subsequent life-threatening events.[147] In older children (9–13 years), apneas lasting greater than 5 seconds also occurred frequently.[120] These pauses were most frequent in stage 1 and REM sleep compared with stages 2–4[120] and most occurred in association with sigh or movement.[18] Another study in adolescents recorded 5.5 central apneas lasting longer than 10 seconds per night,[18] but these were not associated with an O_2 desaturation below 90%.[144]

Over multiple studies, the overall apnea index is near 1,[145,148] which is considerably less than that observed in adults.[146] This underscores the conclusion that normative data developed in adults do not apply to the pediatric population,[149] although it may apply to adolescents in some cases.[150]

Periodic Breathing

Periodic breathing, characterized by periodic respiratory pauses, is common in the newborn period, especially in preterm infants.[100] As with apnea, periodic breathing is more common in REM sleep compared with NREM sleep.[151] The incidence of periodic breathing appears to decrease over the first 3 months of life.[112,135]

O$_2$ Saturation

Numerous studies over the last three decades have provided a wealth of reference data for normal O_2 saturation in infants and children, measured using pulse oximetry. The Collaborative Home Infant Monitoring Evaluation (CHIME) study reported O_2 saturation data for normal infants 2–25 weeks of age.[152] Average baseline O_2 saturation was >95% as anticipated, but brief apnea events and brief decreases in O_2 saturation were also observed (about four per hour) and are part of normal oxygenation and breathing pattern.[152] A large recent study of normal Canadian infants during sleep at 1 year of age reported a median O_2 saturation of 97% and an O_2 desaturation (≥3% drop) index of 6.7 per hour, but time with an O_2 saturation <92% was only 0.1% of the time.[142]

Terrill and colleagues recently reported a novel way to summarize large amounts of normal O_2 saturation data using SpO_2 cumulative-frequency, desaturation-depth versus incidence and desaturation-duration versus incidence plots.[153] The authors applied this method to normal infants 2 weeks to 2 years of age. The resulting SpO_2 cumulative frequency reference curves showed that median O_2 saturation ranged between 98% and 99% over the first 2 years and was no different between NREM and REM sleep.[154] In addition to summarizing large amounts of normal SpO_2 data, this approach can be used to describe O_2 saturation phenotypes that characterize particular disorders associated with sleep-related O_2 desaturation.

Control of Ventilation During Sleep

Ventilatory Response to Hypoxia

The hypoxic ventilatory response normalized to weight decreases with age, from $-0.035\,L\cdot kg^{-1}\cdot min^{-1}\cdot SaO_2^{-1}$ in children to $-0.024\,L\cdot kg^{-1}\cdot min^{-1}\cdot SaO_2^{-1}$ in adults, similar to the age-dependent decrease in hypercapnic ventilatory response.[155] This may serve an important purpose in promoting respiratory stability as high levels of peripheral chemoreceptor responsiveness are correlated with respiratory instabilities, particularly apnea and oscillatory breathing patterns.[156,157] This is consistent with an age-dependent decrease in peripheral chemoreceptor drive to breath, which continues at least through 28 years.[158]

In adult men, the hypoxic ventilatory response decreased to two-thirds waking value in NREM sleep and to one-third waking value in REM sleep,[159] although another study found similar values in NREM sleep and wakefulness.[160] The response appears to be state dependent. Stimulation of breathing with 15% O_2 caused a biphasic response in wakefulness and REM but a sustained increase in NREM sleep.[161]

Ventilatory Response to Hyperoxia

In premature infants, the response to reducing peripheral chemoreceptor input by breathing 100% O_2 caused ventilation to drop by 28% in wakefulness, 39% in REM sleep, and 37% in NREM sleep and often caused an apnea lasting 8–11 seconds.[161] In older infants, the drop in minute ventilation in response to a step increase in inspired O_2 is similar in REM and NREM sleep, primarily due to a decrease in V_T compared with frequency (F).[104]

Ventilatory Response to Hypercapnia

The absolute ventilatory response to hypercapnia during wakefulness increases with the weight of the subject over the period of 4–49 years, but when normalized to body weight, the ventilatory response decreases with age.[155,162] The normalized ventilatory response in children was $0.056\,L\cdot kg^{-1}\cdot min^{-1}\cdot torr\ P_{ET}CO_2^{-1}$ and in adults was $0.032\,L\cdot kg^{-1}\cdot min^{-1}\cdot torr\ P_{ET}CO_2^{-1}$. The ventilatory response to CO_2 is generally linear; thus it may be extrapolated to the point where ventilation is zero, the CO_2 threshold. The CO_2 threshold was also lower in children compared with adults, 36 versus 40 torr. When normalized to weight, there are no significant ventilatory differences between males and females, except for a slightly lower CO_2 threshold in females.[155] The decrease in hypercapnic ventilatory response is paralleled by a decrease in airway occlusion pressure ($P_{0.1}$) during hypercapnic stimulation, a measure of ventilatory drive, which also decreases with age.[163]

Control of $PaCO_2$ appears to be sleep-stage dependent. End-tidal CO_2 for older children (1–15 years) exceeds 45 mm Hg about 1.6–2% of total sleep time.[145] $P_{ET}CO_2$ was >50 mm Hg for 0.3% total sleep time,[145] similar to the conclusion of Brouillette, who considered 45 mm Hg to be the upper limit of normal.[164] This is less than earlier values of Marcus et al.,[144] which included >45 mm Hg approximately 7% of the time and >50 mm Hg 0.5% of the time. Despite the hypoventilation, as indicated by CO_2 values, desaturation events (lower than 92%) are very rare in the normal population and may represent the most accurate parameter to determine whether respiratory pathology exists.[144,165] Although different in sleep, the ventilatory response to CO_2 was the same in both NREM and REM sleep.[122]

Normal Arousal from Sleep

Arousal from sleep represents an important defense response against an ongoing respiratory challenge. Spontaneous arousals are a normal part of REM and NREM sleep.[166] For instance, in preterm and term infants, arousals (as defined by behavior) not associated with apnea occurred at a rate of 0.23/min.[167] The frequency increased to 0.59/min in sleep periods with apnea and was significantly higher during long apneic periods, during mixed versus central apnea and during severe versus mild apnea.[167] The arousal frequency may be influenced by sleep position. In healthy term infants, during REM sleep the prone position is associated with significantly fewer arousals compared with supine; however, the rate of arousal is the same (prone vs. supine) in NREM sleep.[168] Overall, the rate of arousals is lower in the prone compared with supine positions at 3 months of age.[169] Normal values for arousal index on polysomnography are higher in infants compared with older children. Two studies of healthy infants, one <30 days of age, the other <45 days of age living at high-altitude, reported normal arousal indices of 14.7/hr and 19/hr, respectively.[170,171] In contrast, healthy children 1.1–1.7 years of age have an average arousal index of 8.5/hr, indicating a normal decrease with age.[172]

Despite their association with apnea termination, arousal may not be essential because most apneic events appear to terminate without arousals, at least in younger infants.[167] In older (prepubertal) children during NREM sleep, termination of obstructive apnea events was associated with electroencephalography (EEG) arousal in only 12%, with movement in the rest.[173] Here, movement occurred in the absence of EEG changes. In comparison, all REM sleep apneas were terminated with a movement.[173] Thus arousal as defined by EEG changes do not appear to be a prerequisite for apnea termination.

Hypercarbia is a strong stimulus for arousal and probably plays a critical role in apnea termination. In a group of normal infants aged 7.3 weeks, the arousal threshold to increased CO_2 was 48.4 torr.[174] An even lower arousal threshold, 40.1 torr, was reported for 1–25 months of age.[175] This CO_2 threshold is only slightly greater than the normal resting level of CO_2. Similarly, in children 9 weeks of age, raising CO_2 to 60 torr by adding CO_2 to the inspired air caused arousal in all children.[176] In older children at 4.4 years of age, every child aroused when CO_2 was increased to 60 torr.[177] Although most of the ventilatory drive due to CO_2 is due to central chemoreceptors, arousal from sleep due to increased CO_2 appears to be dependent on peripheral chemoreceptors, at least in experimental models where it may be reduced by carotid sinus nerve section or hyperoxia.[178,179]

Compared with hypercarbia, hypoxia appears to be a weaker stimulus for arousal. In normal infants, arousal was observed 70% of the time when FiO_2 was decreased to 0.15.[174] In another study, an FiO_2 of 0.15 caused arousal in only 32% of the trials.[180] In infants 9 weeks of age, hypoxia (80 torr) failed to cause arousal in most cases, and in a group of infants averaging 12 weeks of age, hypoxia (80 torr) caused arousal in only 8 of 18 infants.[176] Arousal to hypoxia appears to occur more frequently in the older infant. In infants 1–25 months (average age 8 months) arousal to hypoxia (78 torr) occurred in all instances.[175] Position also has a significant influence. Hypoxia-induced arousal threshold is higher in the prone position compared with the supine position.[181]

There is limited information on the state dependence of hypoxia-induced arousal from sleep in humans. In normal term infants, the level of PaO_2 is significantly lower and more variable in REM sleep compared with NREM sleep.[15] However, the frequency of arousal during hypoxia is higher in REM compared with NREM sleep for infants studied at 2–5 weeks, 2–3 months, and 5–6 months.[182–184] This difference may be related to the rate of O_2 desaturation in the two states because no difference in level of O_2 saturation at the time of arousal was observed between the sleep states.[185]

The rate of desaturation may also be important. In lambs, where the rate of desaturation could be experimentally controlled, arousal from NREM sleep occurred at an SaO_2 of 80–83%[186]; however, during REM sleep arousal occurred between 44% and 76% SaO_2 with the lower value associated with the most rapid development of hypoxia.[186] Similar results were found in other laboratories in which the SaO_2 at arousal was lower in REM than NREM sleep[187] and significantly reduced by carotid nerve denervation.[188]

State-related differences in arousal threshold have been observed for other stimuli. Arousal threshold in response to a nasal air jet is significantly higher (i.e., stronger jet pressure required) in NREM sleep compared with REM sleep at 2–3 weeks and at 2–3 months,[189] but the difference is absent in the premature infant.[190] This is similar to the higher threshold for arousal from air-jet stimulation in the prone position during both NREM and REM sleep,[191,192] but this may be dependent on age because it was not observed at 2–3 weeks or 5–6 months postterm.[192]

In conclusion, arousal serves an important function in the termination of some apneic events but does not appear to be involved in the majority of cases. Increases in CO_2 in particular can initiate arousal but decreases in SaO_2 may also evoke arousal. In general, the threshold for arousal is higher in NREM sleep compared with REM sleep.

Summary

With respect to normal respiratory physiology during sleep, infancy is a time of rapid CNS, neural respiratory control, respiratory system structural and mechanical maturation, and developmental plasticity and vulnerability. Rib cage geometry, which differs markedly in infants compared with that of adults, becomes more adult-like by about 3 years of age. The high chest wall compliance of the newborn decreases with age and becomes approximately equal to lung compliance, as in adults, by the second year of life, resulting in higher resting lung volume. Concurrently, the contribution of the rib cage to tidal volume during sleep increases over the first 26 months of life. PIRCM (thoracoabdominal asynchrony), so commonly observed in term newborns and even more so in preterm newborns, decreases with age over the first 2–3 years of life. PIRCM after age 3 is abnormal and can be reliably used as a sign of abnormal physiology (e.g., increased upper airway resistance). The dynamic maintenance of EELV greater than passive V_r, characteristic of the newborn and infants up to ~6 months of life, transitions to passive or relaxed EELV by about 1 year of age. Mechanical loading of the respiratory system reveals infant vulnerability, especially in preterm newborns due, in part, to their high chest wall compliance. Infancy is also a time of respiratory control immaturity and instability, frequent central apnea, and period breathing, all of which resolve or decline with maturation.

Childhood, between infancy and adolescence, continues to be a time of rapid growth and maturation of neural respiratory control continues across childhood. Ventilatory drive decreases with age. Ventilatory responses to both hypoxia and hypercapnia (adjusted for body weight) decrease with age. Although the upper airway is smaller in young children and increases in size throughout childhood, the upper airway is much less collapsible in infants and children compared with adults. This is due to robust, dynamic, reflex regulation of upper airway collapsibility, likely mediated by negative pressure reflexes that persist throughout childhood and into adolescence, but are greatly reduced in adults. Central apnea continues to occur normally in children but is less frequent than in the newborn. Obstructive apnea is uncommon in infants and children, but becomes more common in adults and continues to increase with age throughout the entire life span into elderly adulthood.

Adolescence is a time of physiologic transition as children literally become adults over a 6- to 7-year time period. Thus there may be very large differences in normal respiratory physiology between a 13- and 18-year-old. The upper airway, for example, is "child-like" in early adolescence and collapsibility (e.g., as characterized by V_{Imax}/P_N and P_{crit}) progressively increases during adolescence to "adult-like" values by late-adolescence.

Understanding normal respiratory physiology during sleep is essential to advance understanding of sleep-related breathing disorders, as well as understanding the effects of sleep on pulmonary and respiratory system disorders. A deep understanding of normal respiratory physiology during sleep is also clinically useful and greatly strengthens mechanistic insights into sleep-related breathing disorders. Together, the studies reviewed in this chapter constitute an impressive wealth of important knowledge and paint a relatively clear picture of normal respiratory physiology maturation. However, as noted in the introduction, there are still major gaps and inconsistencies, in part due to the enormous variation in and lack of standardization of definitions, experimental approaches, methodologies, etc. The increasing number of mechanistic studies and life-spanning studies from infancy to late adolescence are, perhaps, promising signs.

CLINICAL PEARLS

- A clear understanding of typical respiratory physiology during the pediatric stage of life is necessary to adequately assess sleep-related breathing disorders.
- The period from infancy through adolescence is a time of rapid growth and development of the central nervous system, neural respiratory control, and mechanical respiratory ventilation.
- In infancy, thoracoabdominal asynchrony, which is common in newborns and preterm babies due to immature rib cage geometry, resolves over the first three years of life in normal development.
- During childhood, central apneas and ventilatory drive along with ventilatory responses to hypoxia and hypercapnia decrease with age.
- Finally, during adolescence, the upper and lower airway progressively become more 'adult-like' becoming less narrow and more collapsible amongst other factors.

References

1. Gaultier C. Respiratory adaptation during sleep from the neonatal period to adolescence. In: Guilleminault C, ed. *Sleep and Its Disorders in Children*. Raven, Press; 1987:97.
2. Openshaw P, Edwards S, Helms P. Changes in rib cage geometry during childhood. *Thorax*. 1984;39:624–627.
3. Gerhardt T, Bancalari E. Chestwall compliance in full-term and premature infants. *Acta Paediatr Scand*. 1980;69:359–364.
4. Papastamelos C, Panitch HB, England SE, Allen JL. Developmental changes in chest wall compliance in infancy and early childhood. *J Appl Physiol*. 1995;78:179–184.
5. Richards CC, Bachman L. Lung and chest wall compliance of apneic paralyzed infants. *J Clin Invest*. 1961;40:273–278.
6. Davis GM, Coates AL, Papageorgiou A, Bureau MA. Direct measurement of static chest wall compliance in animal and human neonates. *J Appl Physiol*. 1988;65:1093–1098.
7. Allen J, Gripp KW. Development of the thoracic cage. In: Haddad GG, Abman SH, Chernick V, eds. *Chernick-Mellins Basic Mechanisms of Pediatric Respiratory Disease*. 2nd ed. BC Decker; 2002:124–138.
8. Agostoni E, Mead J. Statics of the respiratory system. In: Fenn WO, Rahn H, eds. *Handbook of Physiology*. American Physiological Society; 1964:401.
9. Cherniack NS, Longobardo GS. Oxygen and carbon dioxide gas stores of the body. *Physiol Rev*. 1970;50:196–243.
10. Cook CD, Cherry RB, O'Brien D, Karlberg P, Smith CA. Studies of respiratory physiology in the newborn infant. I. Observations on normal premature and full-term infants. *J Clin Invest*. 1955;34:975–982.
11. Kohyama J, Sakuma H, Shiiki T, Shimohira M, Hasegawa T. Quantitative analysis of paradoxical inward rib cage movement during sleep in children. *Psychiatry Clin Neurosci*. 2000;54:328–329.
12. Henderson-Smart DJ, Read DJ. Depression of respiratory muscles and defective responses to nasal obstruction during active sleep in the newborn. *Aust Paediatr J*. 1976;12:261–266.
13. Knill R, Andrews W, Bryan AC, Bryan MH. Respiratory load compensation in infants. *J Appl Physiol*. 1976;40:357–361.
14. Henderson-Smart DJ, Read DJ. Reduced lung volume during behavioral active sleep in the newborn. *J Appl Physiol*. 1979;46:1081–1085.
15. Martin RJ, Okken A, Rubin D. Arterial oxygen tension during active and quiet sleep in the normal neonate. *J Pediatr*. 1979;94:271–274.
16. Gaultier C, Praud JP, Canet E, Delaperche MF, D'Allest AM. Paradoxical inward rib cage motion during rapid eye movement sleep in infants and young children. *J Dev Physiol*. 1987;9:391–397.
17. Gaultier C. Cardiorespiratory adaptation during sleep in infants and children. *Pediatr Pulmonol*. 1995;19:105–117.
18. Tabachnik E, Muller NL, Bryan AC, Levison H. Changes in ventilation and chest wall mechanics during sleep in normal adolescents. *J Appl Physiol*. 1981;51:557–564.
19. Traeger N, Schultz B, Pollock AN, Mason T, Marcus CL, Arens R. Polysomnographic values in children 2-9 years old: Additional data and review of the literature. *Pediatr Pulmonol*. 2005;40:22–30.
20. Muller N, Volgyesi G, Becker L, Bryan MH, Bryan AC. Diaphragmatic muscle tone. *J Appl Physiol*. 1979;47:279–284.
21. Muller NL, Bryan AC. Chest wall mechanics and respiratory muscles in infants. *Pediatr Clin North Am*. 1979;26:503–516.
22. Lopes J, Muller NL, Bryan MH, Bryan AC. Importance of inspiratory muscle tone in maintenance of FRC in the newborn. *J Appl Physiol*. 1981;51:830–834.
23. Tusiewicz K, Moldofsky H, Bryan AC, Bryan MH. Mechanics of the rib cage and diaphragm during sleep. *J Appl Physiol*. 1977;43:600–602.
24. Kosch PC, Stark AR. Dynamic maintenance of end-expiratory lung volume in full-term infants. *J Appl Physiol*. 1984;57:1126–1133.
25. Kosch PC, Hutchinson AA, Wozniak JA, Carlo WA, Stark AR. Posterior cricoarytenoid and diaphragm activities during tidal breathing in neonates. *J Appl Physiol*. 1988;64:1968–1978.
26. Stark AR, Cohlan BA, Waggener TB, Frantz 3rd ID, Kosch PC. Regulation of end-expiratory lung volume during sleep in premature infants. *J Appl Physiol*. 1987;62:1117–1123.
27. Colin AA, Wohl ME, Mead J, Ratjen FA, Glass G, Stark AR. Transition from dynamically maintained to relaxed end-expiratory volume in human infants. *J Appl Physiol*. 1989;67:2107–2111.
28. Stradling JR, Chadwick GA, Frew AJ. Changes in ventilation and its components in normal subjects during sleep. *Thorax*. 1985;40:364–370.
29. Hershenson MB, Stark AR, Mead J. Action of the inspiratory muscles of the rib cage during breathing in newborns. *Am Rev Respir Dis*. 1989;139:1207–1212.
30. Hershenson MB, Colin AA, Wohl ME, Stark AR. Changes in the contribution of the rib cage to tidal breathing during infancy. *Am Rev Respir Dis*. 1990;141:922–925.
31. Balasubramaniam SL, Wang Y, Ryan L, Hossain J, Rahman T, Shaffer TH. Age-related ranges of respiratory inductance plethysmography (RIP) reference values for infants and children. *Paediatr Respir Rev*. 2019;29:60–67.
32. Wiegand L, Zwillich CW, White DP. Collapsibility of the human upper airway during normal sleep. *J Appl Physiol*. 1989;66:1800–1808.
33. Hudgel DW, Martin RJ, Johnson B, Hill P. Mechanics of the respiratory system and breathing pattern during sleep in normal humans. *J Appl Physiol*. 1984;56:133–137.
34. Hudgel DW, Robertson DW. Nasal resistance during wakefulness and sleep in normal man. *Acta Otolaryngol*. 1984;98:130–135.

35. Freedman S, Campbell EJ. The ability of normal subjects to tolerate added inspiratory loads. *Respir Physiol.* 1970;10:213–235.

36. Wiegand L, Zwillich CW, White DP. Sleep and the ventilatory response to resistive loading in normal men. *J Appl Physiol.* 1988;64:1186–1195.

37. Deoras KS, Greenspan JS, Wolfson MR, Keklikian EN, Shaffer TH, Allen JL. Effects of inspiratory resistive loading on chest wall motion and ventilation: Differences between preterm and full-term infants. *Pediatr Res.* 1992;32:589–594.

38. Kosch PC, Davenport PW, Wozniak JA, Stark AR. Reflex control of inspiratory duration in newborn infants. *J Appl Physiol.* 1986;60:2007–2014.

39. Kosch PC, Davenport PW, Wozniak JA, Stark AR. Reflex control of expiratory duration in newborn infants. *J Appl Physiol.* 1985;58:575–581.

40. Boychuk RB, Seshia MM, Rigatto H. The immediate ventilatory response to added inspiratory elastic and resistive loads in preterm infants. *Pediatr Res.* 1977;11:276–279.

41. Marcus CL, Moreira GA, Bamford O, Lutz J. Response to inspiratory resistive loading during sleep in normal children and children with obstructive apnea. *J Appl Physiol.* 1999;87:1448–1454.

42. Pillar G, Schnall RP, Peled N, Oliven A, Lavie P. Impaired respiratory response to resistive loading during sleep in healthy offspring of patients with obstructive sleep apnea. *Am J Respir Crit Care Med.* 1997;155:1602–1608.

43. Wilson PA, Skatrud JB, Dempsey JA. Effects of slow wave sleep on ventilatory compensation to inspiratory elastic loading. *Respir Physiol.* 1984;55:103–120.

44. Schelegle ES. Functional morphology and physiology of slowly adapting pulmonary stretch receptors. *Anat Rec A Discov Mol Cell Evol Biol.* 2003;270:11–16.

45. Hamilton RD, Winning AJ, Horner RL, Guz A. The effect of lung inflation on breathing in man during wakefulness and sleep. *Respir Physiol.* 1988;73:145–154.

46. Trippenbach T. Pulmonary reflexes and control of breathing during development. *Biol Neonate.* 1994;65:205–210.

47. Hand IL, Noble L, Wilks M, Towler E, Kim M, Yoon JJ. Hering-Breuer reflex and sleep state in the preterm infant. *Pediatr Pulmonol.* 2004;37:61–64.

48. Rabbette PS, Fletcher ME, Dezateux CA, Soriano-Brucher H, Stocks J. Hering-Breuer reflex and respiratory system compliance in the first year of life: A longitudinal study. *J Appl Physiol.* 1994;76:650–656.

49. Rabbette PS, Costeloe KL, Stocks J. Persistence of the Hering-Breuer reflex beyond the neonatal period. *J Appl Physiol.* 1991;71:474–480.

50. Gerhardt T, Bancalari E. Apnea of prematurity: II. Respiratory reflexes. *Pediatrics.* 1984;74:63–66.

51. Thach BT, Frantz 3rd HW ID, Adler SM, Taeusch 3rd HW Jr. Maturation of reflexes influencing inspiratory duration in human infants. *J Appl Physiol.* 1978;45:203–211.

52. Finer NN, Abroms IF, Taeusch HW Jr. Ventilation and sleep states in newborn infants. *J Pediatr.* 1976;89:100–108.

53. Mathew OP. Apnea of prematurity: Pathogenesis and management strategies. *J Perinatol.* 2011;31:302–310.

54. Jordan AS, White DP. Pharyngeal motor control and the pathogenesis of obstructive sleep apnea. *Respir Physiol Neurobiol.* 2008;160:1–7.

55. Dempsey JA, Veasey SC, Morgan BJ, O'Donnell CP. Pathophysiology of sleep apnea. *Physiol Rev.* 2010;90:47–112.

56. Horner RL. Motor control of the pharyngeal musculature and implications for the pathogenesis of obstructive sleep apnea. *Sleep.* 1996;19:827–853.

57. Arens R, Muzumdar H. Childhood obesity and obstructive sleep apnea syndrome. *J Appl Physiol (1985).* 2010;108:436–444.

58. Katz ES, Mitchell RB, D'Ambrosio CM. Obstructive sleep apnea in infants. *Am J Respir Crit Care Med.* 2012;185:805–816.

59. Katz ES, D'Ambrosio CM. Pathophysiology of pediatric obstructive sleep apnea. *Proc Am Thorac Soc.* 2008;5:253–262.

60. Fleck RJ, Shott SR, Mahmoud M, Ishman SL, Amin RS, Donnelly LF. Magnetic resonance imaging of obstructive sleep apnea in children. *Pediatr Radiol.* 2018;48:1223–1233.

61. Arens R, Marcus CL. Pathophysiology of upper airway obstruction: A developmental perspective. *Sleep.* 2004;27:997–1019.

62. Pohunek P. Development, structure and function of the upper airways. *Paediatric Resp Rev.* 2004;5:2–8.

63. Praud JP, Reix P. Upper airways and neonatal respiration. *Respir Physiol Neurobiol.* 2005;149:131–141.

64. Gold AR, Schwartz AR. The pharyngeal critical pressure. The whys and hows of using nasal continuous positive airway pressure diagnostically. *Chest.* 1996;110:1077–1088.

65. Kirkness JP, Krishnan V, Patil SP, Schneider H. Upper airway obstruction in snoring and upper airway resistance syndrome. In: Randerath WJ, Sanner BM, Somers VK, eds.*Sleep Apnea.* Karger; 2006:79–89.

66. Chamberlin NL, Eikermann M, Fassbender P, White DP, Malhotra A. Genioglossus premotoneurons and the negative pressure reflex in rats. *J Physiol.* 2007;579:515–526.

67. Gauda EB, Carroll JL, McColley S, Smith PL. Effect of oxygenation on breath-by-breath response of the genioglossus muscle during occlusion. *J Appl Physiol.* 1991;71:1231–1236.

68. Pillar G, Malhotra A, Fogel RB, et al. Upper airway muscle responsiveness to rising PCO(2) during NREM sleep. *J Appl Physiol.* 2000;89:1275–1282.

69. Horner RL, Liu X, Gill H, Nolan P, Liu H, Sood S. Effects of sleep-wake state on the genioglossus vs. diaphragm muscle response to CO(2) in rats. *J Appl Physiol.* 2002;92:878–887.

70. Lo YL, Jordan AS, Malhotra A, et al. Genioglossal muscle response to CO_2 stimulation during NREM sleep. *Sleep.* 2006;29:470–477.

71. Weiner D, Mitra J, Salamone J, Cherniack NS. Effect of chemical stimuli on nerves supplying upper airway muscles. *J Appl Physiol.* 1982;52:530–536.

72. Marcus CL, Fernandes Do Prado LB, Lutz J, et al. Developmental changes in upper airway dynamics. *J Appl Physiol.* 2004;97:98–108.

73. Smith PL, Wise RA, Gold AR, Schwartz AR, Permutt S. Upper airway pressure-flow relationships in obstructive sleep apnea. *J Appl Physiol.* 1988;64:789–795.

74. Schwartz AR, Smith PL, Wise RA, Gold AR, Permutt S. Induction of upper airway occlusion in sleeping individuals with subatmospheric nasal pressure. *J Appl Physiol.* 1988;64:535–542.

75. Marcus CL, McColley SA, Carroll JL, Loughlin GM, Smith PL, Schwartz AR. Upper airway collapsibility in children with obstructive sleep apnea syndrome. *J Appl Physiol.* 1994;77:918–924.

76. Litman RS, McDonough JM, Marcus CL, Schwartz AR, Ward DS. Upper airway collapsibility in anesthetized children. *Anesth Analg.* 2006;102:750–754.

77. Isono S, Shimada A, Utsugi M, Konno A, Nishino T. Comparison of static mechanical properties of the passive pharynx between

normal children and children with sleep-disordered breathing. *Am J Respir Crit Care Med.* 1998;157:1204–1212.

78. Schultz HD, Del Rio R, Ding Y, Marcus NJ. Role of neurotransmitter gases in the control of the carotid body in heart failure. *Respir Physiol Neurobiol.* 2012;184:197–203.

79. Marcus CL, Katz ES, Lutz J, Black CA, Galster P, Carson KA. Upper airway dynamic responses in children with the obstructive sleep apnea syndrome. *Pediatr Res.* 2005;57:99–107.

80. McGinley BM, Schwartz AR, Schneider H, Kirkness JP, Smith PL, Patil SP. Upper airway neuromuscular compensation during sleep is defective in obstructive sleep apnea. *J Appl Physiol.* 2008;105:197–205.

81. Marcus CL, Keenan BT, Huang J, et al. The obstructive sleep apnoea syndrome in adolescents. *Thorax.* 2017;72:720–728.

82. Schwab RJ, Kim C, Bagchi S, et al. Understanding the anatomic basis for obstructive sleep apnea syndrome in adolescents. *Am J Respir Crit Care Med.* 2015;191:1295–1309.

83. Marcus CL, Lutz J, Hamer A, Smith PL, Schwartz A. Developmental changes in response to subatmospheric pressure loading of the upper airway. *J Appl Physiol.* 1999;87:626–633.

84. Patil SP, Schneider H, Marx JJ, Gladmon E, Schwartz AR, Smith PL. Neuromechanical control of upper airway patency during sleep. *J Appl Physiol.* 2007;102:547–556.

85. Wilson SL, Thach BT, Brouillette RT, Abu-Osba YK. Upper airway patency in the human infant: Influence of airway pressure and posture. *J Appl Physiol.* 1980;48:500–504.

86. Carlo WA, Miller MJ, Martin RJ. Differential response of respiratory muscles to airway occlusion in infants. *J Appl Physiol.* 1985;59:847–852.

87. Gauda EB, Miller MJ, Carlo WA, Difiore JM, Johnsen DC, Martin RJ. Genioglossus response to airway occlusion in apneic versus nonapneic infants. *Pediatr Res.* 1987;22:683–687.

88. Huang J, Pinto SJ, Yuan H, et al. Upper airway collapsibility and genioglossus activity in adolescents during sleep. *Sleep.* 2012;35:1345–1352.

89. Bandla P, Huang J, Karamessinis L, et al. Puberty and upper airway dynamics during sleep. *Sleep.* 2008;31:534–541.

90. Carrera HL, McDonough JM, Gallagher PR, et al. Upper airway collapsibility during wakefulness in children with sleep disordered breathing, as determined by the negative expiratory pressure technique. *Sleep.* 2011;34:717–724.

91. Gozal D, Burnside MM. Increased upper airway collapsibility in children with obstructive sleep apnea during wakefulness. *Am J Respir Crit Care Med.* 2004;169:163–167.

92. Goh DY, Galster P, Marcus CL. Sleep architecture and respiratory disturbances in children with obstructive sleep apnea. *Am J Respir Crit Care Med.* 2000;162:682–686.

93. Katz ES, White DP. Genioglossus activity during sleep in normal control subjects and children with obstructive sleep apnea. *Am J Respir Crit Care Med.* 2004;170:553–560.

94. Schwartz AR, O'Donnell CP, Baron J, et al. The hypotonic upper airway in obstructive sleep apnea: Role of structures and neuromuscular activity. *Am J Respir Crit Care Med.* 1998;157:1051–1057.

95. Horner RL. Emerging principles and neural substrates underlying tonic sleep-state-dependent influences on respiratory motor activity. *Philos Trans R Soc Lond B Biol Sci.* 2009;364:2553–2564.

96. Carberry JC, Jordan AS, White DP, Wellman A, Eckert DJ. Upper airway collapsibility (P_{crit}) and pharyngeal dilator muscle activity are sleep stage dependent. *Sleep.* 2016;39:511–521.

97. Katz ES, Marcus CL, White DP. Influence of airway pressure on genioglossus activity during sleep in normal children. *Am J Respir Crit Care Med.* 2006;173:902–909.

98. Onal E, Lopata M, O'Connor TD. Diaphragmatic and genioglossal electromyogram responses to isocapnic hypoxia in humans. *Am Rev Respir Dis.* 1981;124:215–217.

99. Onal E, Lopata M, O'Connor TD. Diaphragmatic and genioglossal electromyogram responses to CO_2 rebreathing in humans. *J Appl Physiol.* 1981;50:1052–1055.

100. Parmelee AH, Stern E, Harris MA. Maturation of respiration in prematures and young infants. *Neuropadiatrie.* 1972;3:294–304.

101. Herbert A, Pearn J, Wilson S. Normal percentiles for respiratory rate in children-reference ranges determined from an optical sensor. *Children (Basel).* 2020:7.

102. Hoppenbrouwers T, Hodgman JE, Arakawa K, Harper R, Sterman MB. Respiration during the first six months of life in normal infants. III. Computer identification of breathing pauses. *Pediatr Res.* 1980;14(11):1230–1233.

103. Rusconi F, Castagneto M, Gagliardi L, et al. Reference values for respiratory rate in the first 3 years of life. *Pediatrics.* 1994;94:350–355.

104. Bolton DP, Herman S. Ventilation and sleep state in the newborn. *J Physiol.* 1974;240:67–77.

105. Hathorn MK. The rate and depth of breathing in new-born infants in different sleep states. *J Physiol.* 1974;243:101–113.

106. Andersson D, Gennser G, Johnson P. Phase characteristics of breathing movements in healthy newborns. *J Dev Physiol.* 1983;5:289–298.

107. Curzi-Dascalova L, Gaudebout C, Dreyfus-Brisac C. Respiratory frequencies of sleeping infants during the first months of life: Correlations between values in different sleep states. *Early Hum Dev.* 1981;5:39–54.

108. Adamson TM, Cranage S, Maloney JE, Wilkinson MH, Wilson FE, Yu VY. The maturation of respiratory patterns in normal full term infants during the first six postnatal months. II: Sleep states and apnoea. *Aust Paediatr J.* 1981;17:257–261.

109. Orem JM, Lovering AT, Vidruk EH. Excitation of medullary respiratory neurons in REM sleep. *Sleep.* 2005;28:801–807.

110. Curzi-Dascalova L, Lebrun F, Korn G. Respiratory frequency according to sleep states and age in normal premature infants: A comparison with full term infants. *Pediatr Res.* 1983;17:152–156.

111. Haddad GG, Lai TL, Mellins RB. Determination of ventilatory pattern in REM sleep in normal infants. *J Appl Physiol.* 1982;53:52–56.

112. Hoppenbrouwers T, Harper RM, Hodgman JE, Sterman MB, McGinty DJ. Polygraphic studies on normal infants during the first six months of life. II. Respiratory rate and variability as a function of state. *Pediatr Res.* 1978;12:120–125.

113. Steinschneider A, Weinstein S. Sleep respiratory instability in term neonates under hyperthermic conditions: Age, sex, type of feeding, and rapid eye movements. *Pediatr Res.* 1983;17:35–41.

114. Fleming S, Thompson M, Stevens R, et al. Normal ranges of heart rate and respiratory rate in children from birth to 18 years of age: A systematic review of observational studies. *Lancet.* 2011;377:1011–1018.

115. O'Leary F, Hayen A, Lockie F, Peat J. Defining normal ranges and centiles for heart and respiratory rates in infants and children: A cross-sectional study of patients attending an Australian tertiary hospital paediatric emergency department. *Arch Dis Child.* 2015;100:733–737.

116. Haddad GG, Epstein RA, Epstein MA, Leistner HL, Marino PA, Mellins RB. Maturation of ventilation and ventilatory pattern in normal sleeping infants. *J Appl Physiol.* 1979;46:998–1002.

117. Scholle S, Wiater A, Scholle HC. Normative values of polysomnographic parameters in childhood and adolescence: Cardiorespiratory parameters. *Sleep Med.* 2011;12:988–996.

118. Carse EA, Wilkinson AR, Whyte PL, Henderson-Smart DJ, Johnson P. Oxygen and carbon dioxide tensions, breathing and heart rate in normal infants during the first six months of life. *J Dev Physiol.* 1981;3:85–100.

119. Hoppenbrouwers T, Hodgman JE, Harper RM, Sterman MB. Respiration during the first six months of life in normal infants: IV. Gender differences. *Early Hum Dev.* 1980;4:167–177.

120. Carskadon MA, Harvey K, Dement WC, Guilleminault C, Simmons FB, Anders TF. Respiration during sleep in children. *West J Med.* 1978;128:477–481.

121. Huang J, Colrain IM, Panitch HB, et al. Effect of sleep stage on breathing in children with central hypoventilation. *J Appl Physiol.* 2008;105:44–53.

122. Davi M, Sankaran K, Maccallum M, Cates D, Rigatto H. Effect of sleep state on chest distortion and on the ventilatory response to CO_2 in neonates. *Pediatr Res.* 1979;13:982–986.

123. Cross KW. The respiratory rate and ventilation in the newborn baby. *J Physiol.* 1949;109:459–474.

124. Krieger J, Maglasiu N, Sforza E, Kurtz D. Breathing during sleep in normal middle-aged subjects. *Sleep.* 1990;13:143–154.

125. Thach BT, Taeusch HW Jr. Sighing in newborn human infants: Role of inflation-augmenting reflex. *J Appl Physiol.* 1976;41:502–507.

126. Ellingson RJ, Peters JF, Nelson B. Respiratory pauses and apnea during daytime sleep in normal infants during the first year of life: Longitudinal observations. *Electroencephalogr Clin Neurophysiol.* 1982;53:48–59.

127. Curzi-Dascalova L, Plassart E. Respiratory and motor events in sleeping infants: Their correlation with thoracico-abdominal respiratory relationships. *Early Hum Dev.* 1978;2:39–50.

128. Radvanyi-Bouvet MF, Monset-Couchard M, Morel-Kahn F, Vicente G, Dreyfus-Brisac C. Expiratory patterns during sleep in normal full-term and premature neonates. *Biol Neonate.* 1982;41:74–84.

129. Fleming PJ, Goncalves AL, Levine MR, Woollard S. The development of stability of respiration in human infants: Changes in ventilatory responses to spontaneous sighs. *J Physiol.* 1984;347:1–16.

130. Southall DP, Richards J, Brown DJ, Johnston PG, de Swiet M, Shinebourne EA. 24-hour tape recordings of ECG and respiration in the newborn infant with findings related to sudden death and unexplained brain damage in infancy. *Arch Dis Child.* 1980;55:7–16.

131. Hoppenbrouwers T, Hodgman JE, Harper RM, Hofmann E, Sterman MB, McGinty DJ. Polygraphic studies of normal infants during the first six months of life: III. Incidence of apnea and periodic breathing. *Pediatrics.* 1977;60:418–425.

132. Guilleminault C, Ariagno R, Korobkin R, et al. Mixed and obstructive sleep apnea and near miss for sudden infant death syndrome: 2. Comparison of near miss and normal control infants by age. *Pediatrics.* 1979;64:882–891.

133. Gabriel M, Albani M, Schulte FJ. Apneic spells and sleep states in preterm infants. *Pediatrics.* 1976;57:142–147.

134. Gould JB, Lee AF, James O, Sander L, Teager H, Fineberg N. The sleep state characteristics of apnea during infancy. *Pediatrics.* 1977;59:182–194.

135. Flores-Guevara R, Plouin P, Curzi-Dascalova L, et al. Sleep apneas in normal neonates and infants during the first 3 months of life. *Neuropediatrics.* 1982;13(Suppl):21–28.

136. Waite SP, Thoman EB. Periodic apnea in the full-term infant: Individual consistency, sex differences, and state specificity. *Pediatrics.* 1982;70:79–86.

137. Rigatto H. Breathing and sleep in preterm infants. In: Loughlin GMCJ, Marcus CL, eds.*Sleep and Breathing in Children: A Developmental Approach.* Dekker; 2000:495–523.

138. Vecchierini MF, Curzi-Dascalova L, Trang-Pham H, Bloch J, Gaultier C. Patterns of EEG frequency, movement, heart rate, and oxygenation after isolated short apneas in infants. *Pediatr Res.* 2001;49:220–226.

139. Stein IM, White A, Kennedy JL Jr, Merisalo RL, Chernoff H, Gould JB. Apnea recordings of healthy infants at 40, 44, and 52 weeks postconception. *Pediatrics.* 1979;63:724–730.

140. Fernandes do Prado LB, Li X, Thompson R, Marcus CL. Body position and obstructive sleep apnea in children. *Sleep.* 2002;25:66–71.

141. Kelly DH, Riordan L, Smith MJ. Apnea and periodic breathing in healthy full-term infants, 12-18 months of age. *Pediatr Pulmonol.* 1992;13:169–171.

142. Vezina K, Mariasine J, Young R, et al. Cardiorespiratory monitoring data during sleep in healthy Canadian infants. *Ann Am Thorac Soc.* 2020;17:1238–1246.

143. Hoppenbrouwers T, Jensen D, Hodgman J, Harper R, Sterman M. Respiration during the first six months of life in normal infants: II. The emergence of a circadian pattern. *Neuropadiatrie.* 1979;10:264–280.

144. Marcus CL, Omlin KJ, Basinki DJ, et al. Normal polysomnographic values for children and adolescents. *Am Rev Respir Dis.* 1992;146:1235–1239.

145. Uliel S, Tauman R, Greenfeld M, Sivan Y. Normal polysomnographic respiratory values in children and adolescents. *Chest.* 2004;125:872–878.

146. Berry RB, Block AJ. Positive nasal airway pressure eliminates snoring as well as obstructive sleep apnea. *Chest.* 1984;85:15–20.

147. Weese-Mayer DE, Morrow AS, Conway LP, Brouillette RT, Silvestri JM. Assessing clinical significance of apnea exceeding fifteen seconds with event recording. *J Pediatr.* 1990;117:568–574.

148. Acebo C, Millman RP, Rosenberg C, Cavallo A, Carskadon MA. Sleep, breathing, and cephalometrics in older children and young adults. Part I – Normative values. *Chest.* 1996;109:664–672.

149. Rosen CL, D'Andrea L, Haddad GG. Adult criteria for obstructive sleep apnea do not identify children with serious obstruction. *Am Rev Respir Dis.* 1992;146:1231–1234.

150. Accardo JA, Shults J, Leonard MB, Traylor J, Marcus CL. Differences in overnight polysomnography scores using the adult and pediatric criteria for respiratory events in adolescents. *Sleep.* 2010;33:1333–1339.

151. Fenner A, Schalk U, Hoenicke H, Wendenburg A, Roehling T. Periodic breathing in premature and neonatal babies: Incidence, breathing pattern, respiratory gas tensions, response to changes in the composition of ambient air. *Pediatr Res.* 1973;7:174–183.

152. Hunt CE, Corwin MJ, Weese-Mayer DE, et al. Longitudinal assessment of hemoglobin oxygen saturation in preterm and term infants in the first six months of life. *J Pediatr.* 2011;159:377–383.e1.

153. Terrill PI, Dakin C, Edwards BA, Wilson SJ, MacLean JE. A graphical method for comparing nocturnal oxygen saturation profiles in individuals and populations: Application to healthy infants and preterm neonates. *Pediatr Pulmonol.* 2018;53:645–655.

154. Terrill PI, Dakin C, Hughes I, Yuill M, Parsley C. Nocturnal oxygen saturation profiles of healthy term infants. *Arch Dis Child.* 2015;100:18–23.

155. Marcus CL, Glomb WB, Basinski DJ, Davidson SL, Keens TG. Developmental pattern of hypercapnic and hypoxic ventilatory responses from childhood to adulthood. *J Appl Physiol.* 1994;76:314–320.

156. Nock ML, Difiore JM, Arko MK, Martin RJ. Relationship of the ventilatory response to hypoxia with neonatal apnea in preterm infants. *J Pediatr.* 2004;144:291–295.

157. Al-Matary A, Kutbi I, Qurashi M, et al. Increased peripheral chemoreceptor activity may be critical in destabilizing breathing in neonates. *Semin Perinatol.* 2004;28:264–272.

158. Springer C, Cooper DM, Wasserman K. Evidence that maturation of the peripheral chemoreceptors is not complete in childhood. *Respir Physiol.* 1988;74:55–64.

159. Douglas NJ, White DP, Weil JV, et al. Hypoxic ventilatory response decreases during sleep in normal men. *Am Rev Respir Dis.* 1982;125:286–289.

160. Hedemark LL, Kronenberg RS. Ventilatory and heart rate responses to hypoxia and hypercapnia during sleep in adults. *J Appl Physiol.* 1982;53:307–312.

161. Rigatto H, Kalapesi Z, Leahy FN, Durand M, MacCallum M, Cates D. Ventilatory response to 100% and 15% O2 during wakefulness and sleep in preterm infants. *Early Hum Dev.* 1982;7:1–10.

162. Avery ME, Chernick V, Dutton RE, Permutt S. Ventilatory response to inspired carbon dioxide in infants and adults. *J Appl Physiol.* 1963;18:895–903.

163. Gaultier C, Perret L, Boule M, Buvry A, Girard F. Occlusion pressure and breathing pattern in healthy children. *Respir Physiol.* 1981;46:71–80.

164. Brouillette RT, Weese-Mayer DE, Hunt CE. Breathing control disorders in infants and children. *Hosp Pract (Off Ed).* 1990;25:82–85. 8, 93–96 passim.

165. Chipps BE, Mak H, Schuberth KC, Talamo JH, Menkes HA, Scherr MS. Nocturnal oxygen saturation in normal and asthmatic children. *Pediatrics.* 1980;65:1157–1160.

166. Thach BT, Lijowska A. Arousals in infants. *Sleep.* 1996;19:S271–S273.

167. Thoppil CK, Belan MA, Cowen CP, Mathew OP. Behavioral arousal in newborn infants and its association with termination of apnea. *J Appl Physiol.* 1991;70:2479–2484.

168. Kato I, Scaillet S, Groswasser J, et al. Spontaneous arousability in prone and supine position in healthy infants. *Sleep.* 2006;29:785–790.

169. Kahn A, Groswasser J, Sottiaux M, Rebuffat E, Franco P, Dramaix M. Prone or supine body position and sleep characteristics in infants. *Pediatrics.* 1993;91:1112–1125.

170. Duenas-Meza E, Bazurto-Zapata MA, Gozal D, Gonzalez-Garcia M, Duran-Cantolla J, Torres-Duque CA. Overnight polysomnographic characteristics and oxygen saturation of healthy infants, 1 to 18 Months of age, born and residing at high altitude (2,640 meters). *Chest.* 2015;148:120–127.

171. Daftary AS, Jalou HE, Shively L, Slaven JE, Davis SD. Polysomnography reference values in healthy newborns. *J Clin Sleep Med.* 2019;15:437–443.

172. Scholle S, Wiater A, Scholle HC. Normative values of polysomnographic parameters in childhood and adolescence: Arousal events. *Sleep Med.* 2012;13:243–251.

173. Praud JP, D'Allest AM, Nedelcoux H, Curzi-Dascalova L, Guilleminault C, Gaultier C. Sleep-related abdominal muscle behavior during partial or complete obstructed breathing in prepubertal children. *Pediatr Res.* 1989;26:347–350.

174. McCulloch K, Brouillette RT, Guzzetta AJ, Hunt CE. Arousal responses in near-miss sudden infant death syndrome and in normal infants. *J Pediatr.* 1982;101:911–917.

175. van der Hal AL, Rodriguez AM, Sargent CW, Platzker AC, Keens TG. Hypoxic and hypercapneic arousal responses and prediction of subsequent apnea in apnea of infancy. *Pediatrics.* 1985;75:848–854.

176. Ward SL, Bautista DB, Woo MS, et al. Responses to hypoxia and hypercapnia in infants of substance-abusing mothers. *J Pediatr.* 1992;121:704–709.

177. Marcus CL, Bautista DB, Amihyia A, Ward SL, Keens TG. Hypercapneic arousal responses in children with congenital central hypoventilation syndrome. *Pediatrics.* 1991;88:993–998.

178. Fewell JE, Kondo CS, Dascalu V, Filyk SC. Influence of carotid-denervation on the arousal and cardiopulmonary responses to alveolar hypercapnia in lambs. *J Dev Physiol.* 1989;12:193–199.

179. Baker SB, Fewell JE. Effects of hyperoxia on the arousal response to upper airway obstruction in lambs. *Pediatr Res.* 1987;21:116–120.

180. Milerad J, Hertzberg T, Wennergren G, Lagercrantz H. Respiratory and arousal responses to hypoxia in apnoeic infants reinvestigated. *Eur J Pediatr.* 1989;148:565–570.

181. Martin RJ, Herrell N, Rubin D, Fanaroff A. Effect of supine and prone positions on arterial oxygen tension in the preterm infant. *Pediatrics.* 1979;63:528–531.

182. Parslow PM, Cranage SM, Adamson TM, Harding R, Horne RS. Arousal and ventilatory responses to hypoxia in sleeping infants: Effects of maternal smoking. *Respir Physiol Neurobiol.* 2004;140:77–87.

183. Verbeek MM, Richardson HL, Parslow PM, Walker AM, Harding R, Horne RS. Arousal and ventilatory responses to mild hypoxia in sleeping preterm infants. *J Sleep Res.* 2008;17:344–353.

184. Parslow PM, Harding R, Cranage SM, Adamson TM, Horne RS. Arousal responses to somatosensory and mild hypoxic stimuli are depressed during quiet sleep in healthy term infants. *Sleep.* 2003;26:739–744.

185. Horne RS, Parslow PM, Harding R. Postnatal development of ventilatory and arousal responses to hypoxia in human infants. *Respir Physiol Neurobiol.* 2005;149:257–271.

186. Fewell JE, Baker SB. Arousal from sleep during rapidly developing hypoxemia in lambs. *Pediatr Res.* 1987;22:471–477.

187. Davidson TL, Fewell JE. Arousal response from sleep to tracheal obstruction in lambs during postnatal maturation. *Pediatr Res.* 1994;36:501–505.

188. Fewell JE, Taylor BJ, Kondo CS, Dascalu V, Filyk SC. Influence of carotid denervation on the arousal and cardiopulmonary responses to upper airway obstruction in lambs. *Pediatr Res.* 1990;28:374–378.

189. Read PA, Horne RS, Cranage SM, Walker AM, Walker DW, Adamson TM. Dynamic changes in arousal threshold during sleep in the human infant. *Pediatr Res.* 1998;43:697–703.

190. Horne RS, Sly DJ, Cranage SM, Chau B, Adamson TM. Effects of prematurity on arousal from sleep in the newborn infant. *Pediatr Res.* 2000;47:468–474.

191. Horne RS, Ferens D, Watts AM, et al. The prone sleeping position impairs arousability in term infants. *J Pediatr.* 2001;138:811–816.

192. Horne RS, Bandopadhayay P, Vitkovic J, Cranage SM, Adamson TM. Effects of age and sleeping position on arousal from sleep in preterm infants. *Sleep.* 2002;25:746–750.

23

Apnea of Prematurity

Christian F. Poets

CHAPTER HIGHLIGHTS

- Apnea of prematurity is a misnomer, as only intermittent hypoxia has been shown to be associated with impaired outcome (e.g., death or disability).
- Hypoxic ventilatory depression and the proximity between the apneic and eupneic CO_2 threshold are key to understanding its pathophysiology.
- Treatment should be incremental, starting with prone, head-elevated positioning and caffeine administration, followed by nasal continuous positive airway pressure and synchronized nasal ventilation.

Introduction

Apnea of prematurity (AOP) affects almost every extremely low gestational age neonate (ELGAN) and also many more mature infants. Its pathophysiology, however, is incompletely understood. This chapter reviews observational studies better to understand the pathophysiology of AOP. Of the three components contributing to AOP (apnea, bradycardia, and intermittent hypoxemia [IH]), we will focus on the latter as it is most relevant to the long-term outcome of an infant. Based on these data, current strategies to treat or prevent AOP/IH will be reviewed.

Pathophysiology

The Role of Upper Airway Obstruction

Traditionally, apnea is divided into central, obstructive, and mixed. Many apparently "central" apneas, however, involve a loss of airway tone that results in intermittent airway obstruction,[1] whereas active glottic closure, similar to that preventing outflow of lung water during in utero apnea,[2] has also been observed in AOP, potentially preserving lung volume during apnea also *ex utero*. Airway obstruction may also prolong initially short respiratory pauses.[3] Thus the narrow upper airways of preterm infants seem to be actively kept open via a respiratory center input, and whether an apnea will appear as central or obstructive simply depends on which component of this input is activated first (diaphragm or upper airway).

Relationship Between Apnea, Bradycardia, and Desaturation

Apnea, bradycardia, and desaturation during AOP are closely temporally related. According to own data on 80 preterm infants, 83% of bradycardias (heart rate [HR] less than two-thirds of baseline) were accompanied by an apnea (≥ 4 sec), 86% by a fall in pulse oximeter saturation (SpO_2) to less than or equal to 80%, and 79% by both apnea and desaturation.[4] The interval between apnea and bradycardia was extremely short (median, 4.8 sec), as was that between bradycardia and desaturation (median, 4.2 sec). This was predominantly because the interval between the onset of apnea and that of desaturation, corrected for the time it takes for the blood to travel from the lung to the pulse oximeter sensor site, was only 0.8 seconds, suggesting an extremely low functional residual capacity (FRC) in these infants (Fig. 23.1).[4]

These observations support the concept that hypoxemia causes bradycardia (e.g., via stimulation of peripheral chemoreceptors),[5] the occurrence of which is facilitated by the absence of the pulmonary inflation reflex during apnea. The latter would also explain why, despite a similar severity of the accompanying hypoxemia, bradycardia is more common with central than with mixed or obstructive apnea.[6]

Changes in Lung Volume, Apnea, and Desaturation

Why is the interval between apnea and desaturation onset so short? This may again be related to a reduced FRC. In preterm infants, relaxation volume is only 10–15% of total lung capacity and thus very close to residual volume, predisposing them to the development of peripheral airway closure.[7] To compensate for this disadvantage, these infants actively maintain their end-expiratory lung volume above relaxation volume, which is one reason for their high respiratory rate.[8] In fact, lung volume is 20% lower after an apnea than after a sigh; that is, apnea results in a loss of FRC, which is restored with the resumption of breathing after apnea[9] or by a sigh.[10] This suggests that one of the main functions of sighs in preterm infants is to reverse falls in lung volume caused by apneas.[10,11]

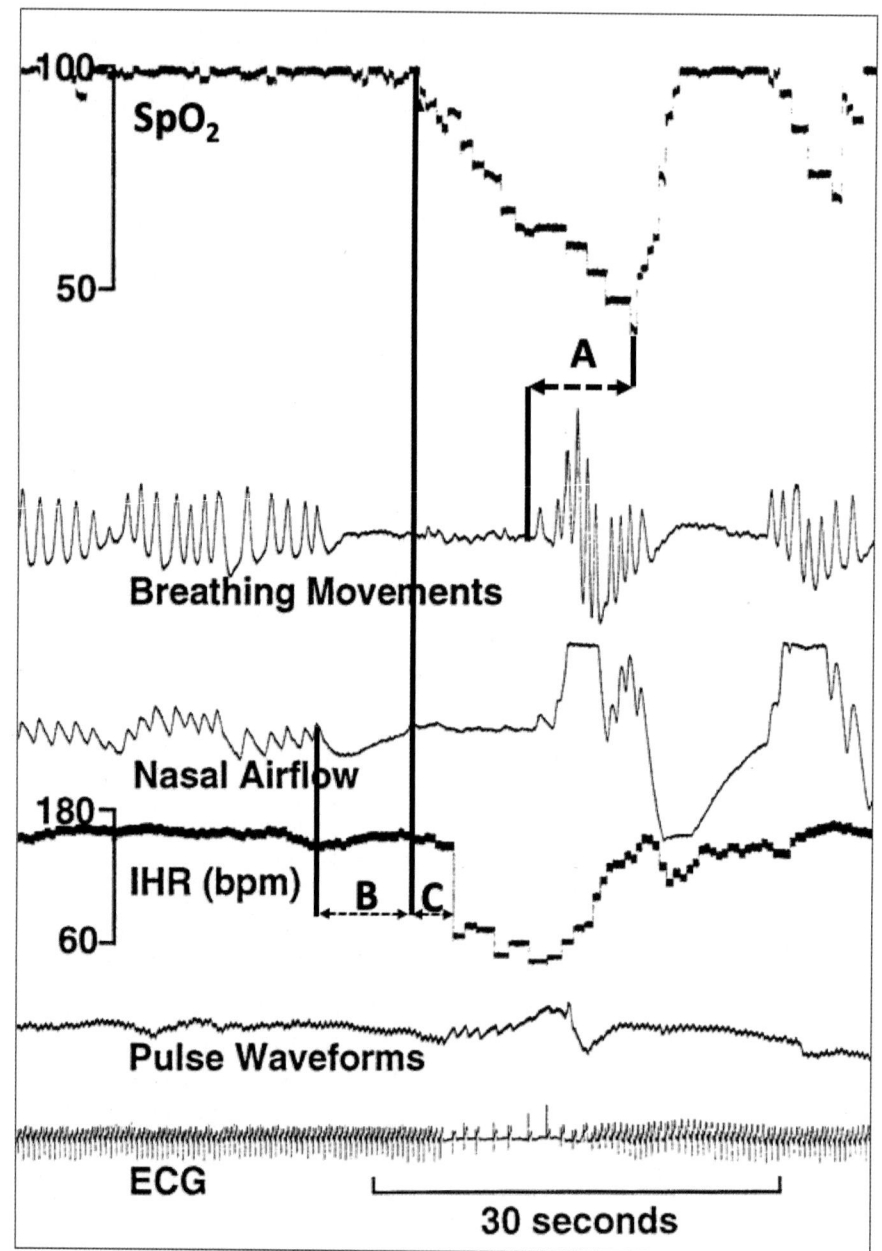

• **Fig. 23.1** Example for the close temporal relationship between apnea, bradycardia, and desaturation. The delay caused by the time it takes for the blood to travel from the lung to the pulse oximeter sensor attached to the foot can be estimated from the delay between the first breath after an apnea and the onset of the recovery in SpO_2 (A). This must be subtracted from the interval between the onset of apnea and that of desaturation (B) and from the interval between the onset of bradycardia and that of desaturation (C). Abbreviations: ECG, Electrocardiogram; IHR, Instantaneous Heart Rate. Modified from Poets CF. Pathophysiology of apnea of prematurity: implications from observational studies. In: Mathew OP. *Respiratory Control and Its Disorders* in the Newborn. Marcel Dekker, Inc.; 2003:295-316.)

During periodic apnea, SpO_2 falls twice as fast as during isolated apnea.[12] Although a reduced mixed venous O_2 saturation after a prior fall in SpO_2 may also contribute to this, another reason is a progressive fall in lung volume during the repeated apneas, resulting in peripheral airway closure. The complex interrelations of the factors influencing the speed of the fall in SpO_2 during AOP have been modeled mathematically.[13]

A loss in lung volume may also be decisive for the development of hypoxemia after abdominal muscle contractions in ELGANs, being involved in 80% of their desaturations to less than 75% SpO_2 in one study, and being associated with an average decrease in resting lung volume by 69% of tidal volume.[14]

A potential consequence of this reduction in lung volume is a (further) inhibition of respiration via activation of the Hering-Breuer deflation reflex. In term infants, this vagally mediated reflex terminates expiration while initiating inspiration. In preterm infants, however, induction of this reflex via chest compression resulted in a shortening of inspiratory time and a tendency to have short apneas (2–5 sec).[15] The same may occur if lung volume falls spontaneously (e.g., during apnea).

Conversely, an increase in lung volume apparently stabilizes breathing by reducing loop gain (i.e., the sensitivity of the negative feedback loop of the chemoreflex control of the respiratory system), whereas a reduced lung volume will increase the instability of the respiratory control system, as evident during periodic breathing.[16]

These considerations provide a theoretical basis for the effectiveness of strategies like the application of continuous positive airway pressure (CPAP) in reducing the frequency and/or severity of AOP in preterm infants.

The Role of Feeding and Gastroesophageal Reflux

Symptoms of AOP often increase in relation to feeding. We studied the effect of bottle feeding, as compared with slow (1-hr) and bolus (10-min) gavage feeding, on AOP and found 3 times more desaturations to less than or equal to 80% with bottle than with bolus gavage feeding, but no further reduction with slow gavage feeding. There were always significantly more desaturations in the hour feeds were given than during the following 2 hours, but the effect of feeding method persisted throughout these 3-hr feeding intervals. Interestingly, there was no significant effect of feeding technique on the frequency of apnea or bradycardia (Fig. 23.2).[17]

Thus bottle feeding may confer a significantly increased risk of episodic desaturation, which may be quite long-lasting. It is puzzling, however, that slow gavage feeding offered no advantage over bolus gavage feeding. Might gastroesophageal reflux (GER), occurring with either feeding method, be an explanation for this?

With the multiple intraluminal impedance (MII) technique, GER can be detected, independent of acidity, via changes in impedance caused by a liquid bolus inside the esophagus. We recorded MII, together with cardiorespiratory (CR) signals, in 19 infants with AOP.[18] MII signals were analyzed, independent of CR signals, for reflux episodes. CR signals were analyzed for apneas (≥4 sec), desaturations to less than or equal to 80%, and bradycardias to less than or equal to 100 bpm. A temporal relationship between GER and a CR event was considered present if both commenced within 20 seconds of each other. We found a high rate of both apnea and GER, but apnea frequency within 20 seconds of a reflux episode was not significantly different

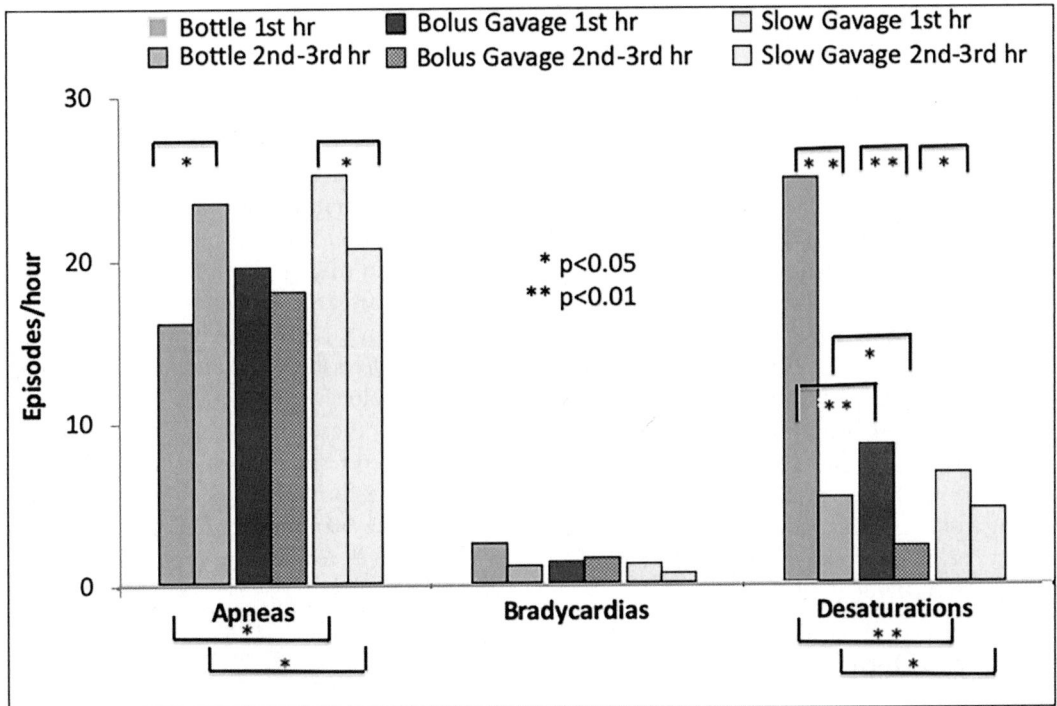

• **Fig. 23.2** Apnea, bradycardia, and desaturation rates during the hour feedings were given compared with the following 2 hours in 30 preterm infants studied at 34 (SD 1.4) weeks' gestational age.

from that during reflux-free epochs (mean, 0.19/min vs. 0.25/min); the same was true for desaturations and brady-cardias. Also, GER occurred similarly often *before* as *after* an apnea. Only in the few apneas (3.5%) that were associated with GER reaching the pharyngeal level, significantly more (45 vs. 26) occurred *after* rather than *before* GER. Thus although both CR events and GER were common, they did not, with few exceptions, appear to be temporally related. Similar results have since been reported by others,[19,20] and a recent randomized controlled trial (RCT) on metoclo-pramide involving 466 preterm infants also found no effect of this common antireflux drug on episodes of cyanosis or apnea.[21] Thus giving antireflux medications to infants to treat their AOP is likely futile.

Chest Wall Distortion, Anatomic Dead Space, and Diaphragmatic Fatigue

Chest wall distortion, clinically apparent as paradoxical breathing, is common in infants and is especially visible in preterm infants. It has been suggested that this distor-tion increases the volume displacement of the diaphragm during inspiration.[22] In longitudinal studies, Heldt showed that the minute volume displacement of the diaphragm was almost twice as large as pulmonary ventilation at 29–30 weeks' gestational age (GA) and fell to approximately 90% of pulmonary ventilation at 36 weeks' GA. Concomitantly, diaphragmatic work was almost halved.[23] The author specu-lated that this additional workload may represent not only a significant calorie expenditure in these infants, but con-tributes to the development of diaphragmatic fatigue and apnea. Further contributing is that, because of neonates' rel-atively large head size, anatomic dead space is approximately 45% of tidal volume in neonates but only 25% in adults.[24]

Circumstantial evidence that muscle fatigue may indeed be involved in neonatal apnea stems from the time course of apnea in term and preterm infants. AOP becomes more problematic (and prevalent) toward the end of the first and during the second week of life,[25] whereas chemore-ceptor resetting, which otherwise might also explain this phenomenon, is essentially complete within approximately 24–48 hours after birth. A mechanism through which labored breathing may produce apnea in preterm infants is the intercostal-phrenic inhibitory reflex. This may be elic-ited both by rib cage distortion[26] and respiratory loading[27] and is known to inhibit respiratory effort in infants.

Thus it is conceivable that similar to the obstructive sleep apnea syndrome in adults, where an increased work of breathing resulting from upper airway obstruction may lead to an increased rate of central apneas, the same mechanism may also play a role in AOP.

Hypoxic Ventilatory Depression

Fetal breathing is diminished if oxygen supply via the pla-centa is reduced.[28] For the fetus, respiratory movements are a waste of energy under these circumstances. This behavior,

however, although counterproductive ex utero, continues after preterm birth,[29] switching to a mature hypoxic ventila-tory response only at approximately 36 weeks' postconceptual age (PCA). This correlates well with the natural course of AOP.[30] While the classic hypoxic response is biphasic, consisting of an initial increase followed by a decrease in ventilation,[30,31] ELGANs show an immediate reduction in minute ventilation during hypoxia, which is due mainly to a fall in respiratory rate.[32]

The clinical relevance of this maturational phenomenon was demonstrated in a substudy of the Surfactant Positive Airway Pressure and Pulse Oximetry Trial (SUPPORT), one of the five large multicenter studies comparing the effects of a higher (91–95% SpO_2) vs. a lower (85–89%) target range for SpO_2 in ELGANs. By recording desatura-tion rates until 36 weeks' PCA in infants randomized in their center, the authors found significantly (2–3 times) more desaturations to less than or equal to 80% for at least 10 seconds in the first 11 days of life and again between 8 weeks of age, and reaching 36 weeks' PCA in those infants who had been randomized to the lower SpO_2 target group.[33] This observation is best explained by the effects seemingly small decreases in baseline SpO_2 have on hypoxic ventila-tory depression.[34]

As mentioned earlier, an important question is which molecular mechanisms are responsible for this hypoxic ventilatory depression. This is yet unknown, but one can-didate is the creatine-phosphocreatine (PCr) system. In the absence of oxidative phosphorylation, provision of phos-phate for the generation of adenosine triphosphate (ATP) relies predominantly on the PCr pool, before anaerobic glycolysis, with increased production of lactate and H^+, is activated. This is particularly relevant to tissues with a high energy metabolism, such as the central nervous system. A fall in intracellular ATP is an important trigger for hypox-emia-induced neuronal damage, and maintenance of ATP levels is therefore of fundamental importance for neuronal protection from hypoxemic insult.[35] The neonatal brain is relatively deficient in creatine, and it is tempting to specu-late that the much earlier onset of the hypoxic ventilatory depression in this age group is related to a decreased avail-ability of PCr in the neonatal brainstem.

Brainstem slices from pups of creatine-fed mice (2 g/kg/day) did indeed show higher phosphocreatine contents and significantly less hypoxic ventilatory depression (−14% vs. −41%) than those from non-supplemented control ani-mals. This corresponded to nearly constant cerebral ATP levels in the former versus a 54% decrease in the latter animals after 30 minutes of anoxia.[36] Also, measurements of the maximal respiratory amplitudes in such pups during hypoxia showed an increase by 51%, compared with 22% in control animals.[37] An RCT of creatine supplementation (200 mg/kg/day) to preterm infants with AOP, however, starting at around 2 weeks of age and being administered for 14 days, showed no effect at all on AOP,[38] although this could have been due to an insufficient dose and/or dura-tion of treatment. This issue deserves further study.

Relevance of the pCO_2 Apneic Threshold

Respiratory drive also depends on CO_2. A baseline concentration of partial pressure of carbon dioxide (pCO_2) is essential for breathing to occur; conversely, if pCO_2 falls considerably below its eupneic baseline, apnea sets in. The pCO_2 value at which this occurs is called the apnea-hypopnea threshold; it is approximately 3.5 Torr below eupneic pCO_2 in healthy adults.[39] The closer this eupneic pCO_2 is to apneic threshold pCO_2, the more unstable breathing gets, as minor behavioral changes in ventilation would be sufficient to propel the pCO_2 to below threshold, inducing apnea. The spontaneous pre-apneic threshold in term and preterm neonates is only 1–1.3 mm Hg below eupneic values, potentially destabilizing respiration in neonates compared with older subjects.[39] The logical clinical consequence of these findings, namely CO_2 inhalation as a treatment for AOP, has indeed been shown to be effective, but less so than methylxanthine treatment.[40] As a proof of concept, however, the latter study confirmed the relevance of the CO_2 apneic threshold in eliciting apnea in preterm infants.

Influence of the Thermal Environment

There are several case studies suggesting that overheating causes apnea in infants,[41,42] but for ethical reasons only few studies tested the opposite (i.e., whether cold stress stimulates breathing). One study, performed in three preterm infants, showed that apnea was more likely to occur during a *decrease* rather than an *increase* in incubator temperature.[43] Tourneux et al., measured energy expenditure and apnea rate in 22 preterm infants at thermoneutrality (32.5°C) and at ambient temperatures 2°C below and above this level. Apneas were less frequent and shorter in duration with cold exposure (during which oxygen consumption increased), but there was no association between body temperature and apnea rate.[44] Thus, the likelihood of apnea to occur seems to be inversely related to metabolic drive, although not necessarily to ambient temperature.

Termination of Apnea

As important as the question of what *causes* an apnea is that of what *terminates* it. In adults, recovery from apnea is usually associated with arousal from sleep, probably via activation of peripheral chemoreceptors. In preterm infants, the situation is more complex as here, motor activity may *precede* the onset of apnea and continues during apnea (i.e., apnea occurs *after* arousal rather than resulting in it).[45] In contrast, when looking for signs of behavioral arousal in sleep-related apneas, this seemed more likely to occur with longer (>15 sec) compared with shorter (5–15 sec) apneas, with those that were associated with hypoxemia (SpO_2 < 80%) or bradycardia (HR < 100/min), and with mixed compared with central apneas.[45] Thus several factors may affect the occurrence of arousal during apneas in preterm infants: sleep state, severity of hypoxemia/hypercapnia,

airway afferent input, and sleep fragmentation/habituation resulting from previous apneic episodes. Whatever the precise mechanism, it seems that chemoreceptor activation, but not cortical arousal, is required for apnea termination.

Relevance

Until recently, very little was known about if and when the triad of apnea, bradycardia, and desaturation in preterm infants, better known as AOP, becomes potentially harmful. Recently, the author reported on a secondary analysis of SpO_2 and pulse rate data recorded for the first 10 weeks in 1,035 participants in the Canadian Oxygen Trial (COT), another trial comparing 91–95% vs 85–89% target SpO_2 in ELGANs and their association with 18-month outcomes. This analysis helped to assess the long-term effects of these events by revealing the following associations[46,47]:

- Mean percentages of recorded time with IH (SpO_2 <80% for ≥10 sec) for the least and most affected 10% of infants were at 0.4% and 13.5%, respectively, whereas %time spent bradycardic (HR <80/min without IH) was rarer at 0.1% and 0.3%, respectively.
- Having been in the highest decile for %time with IH events lasting at least 1 minute was associated with 3.4-fold increased odds of developing the primary outcome of death beyond 36 weeks or disability at 18 months, with this association becoming non-significant for shorter events.
- Odds ratios for secondary outcomes of COT (motor impairment, cognitive or language delay, and severe retinopathy of prematurity) were 3-fold to 5-fold increased after prolonged hypoxemia.
- Bradycardia, in the absence of concomitant hypoxemia, did not significantly add to the risk of adverse outcome.
- The severity of IH, expressed as the area under the curve, and the rate with which IH events occurred, added little prognostic value compared with the simpler-to-determine %time below 80% SpO_2.
- Associations between hypoxemic exposure and adverse outcomes were stronger at later postnatal ages (i.e., at 8–10 weeks), and for infants assigned to a target range of 91–95% compared with a target range of 85–89% SpO_2.
- More recently, another post hoc analysis of the COT data also showed an association between the risk of developing severe bronchopulmonary dysplasia (BPD) and IH, which increased from 5% for infants in the lowest decile for IH exposure to 77% for those in the highest decile.

Investigators from the above-mentioned SUPPORT group reported a similar analysis, but they had recorded the SpO_2 only during the first 3 postnatal days and could associate these data only with 90-day survival, not with other outcomes. Survival was at 47.4% for infants born small for gestational age (SGA) who had fewer than 15 episodes/day with SpO_2 less than 80% for 20–60 seconds, but at 77.6% for SGA infants with fewer than 15 such episodes/day. A similar, albeit smaller effect size was seen for longer IH events (1–5 min), but again only for SGA infants. No increased mortality was seen in infants with frequent IH but normal birth weight.[48] These data thus confirm an association between IH events occurring shortly after birth and mortality, albeit only for SGA infants. Interestingly, SGA did not increase IH-related mortality in the COT study.

More recently, the above group looked at associations between IH and BPD in a group of SUPPORT participants from their own center and, similar to the COT study data, found that this diagnosis was associated with an increased number per day of IH events between postnatal days 7 and 28 and a longer cumulative duration of IH.[49]

Given these associations of long-term outcomes with IH, but not with bradycardia, it seems prudent to focus on the avoidance of IH, particularly of episodes lasting for 1 minute or longer, if we want to reduce adverse sequelae of AOP as the main cause of IH in extremely preterm infants.

Treatment

For space constraints, this review will focus on interventions for AOP that have already been proven beneficial, except for doxapram (see later).

Prone Head-Elevated Positioning

In the prone position, the chest wall is stabilized and thoracoabdominal asynchrony reduced. Although some individual studies showed less apnea in the prone position in preterm infants,[50,51] a Cochrane analysis found no such effect.[52] A small study, however, showed that a 15-degree head-elevated tilt prone position was associated with a 49% reduction in desaturations to less than 85%.[53] Two subsequent studies reinvestigated the issue and found only a slight (−13%) reduction in the frequency of desaturation/bradycardia compared with the horizontal position; one found also no advantage for the so-called three-stair position (a variation of the head-up tilt position based on the Kinesthetics Infant Handling concept).[54,55] This much less clear advantage of the head-up tilt position may be because infants in the earlier study[53] had received no other treatment for AOP, whereas in the more recent studies all had received caffeine and most CPAP. The prone, head-up tilt position may therefore be considered mainly a first-line intervention for AOP, because it offers little additional effect in infants already treated with caffeine or CPAP.

Continuous Positive Airway Pressure and Synchronized Nasal Ventilation

CPAP has been shown to reduce extubation failure in preterm infants, despite the fact that most systems currently available do *not* reduce work of breathing. CPAP can be applied via a nasopharyngeal tube, nasal prongs, or masks. Reintubation rates are 40% lower with prongs (relative risk [RR] 0.59 [0.41–0.85]; number needed to treat [NNT] 5) than with the nasopharyngeal tube.[56] A meta-analysis comparing CPAP failure rates with prongs versus masks found

an even lower rate of CPAP failure with the latter facial interfaces (RR 0.72 [0.53–0.97]).[57] Thus masks are the preferred means of applying CPAP to the infant.

In recent years, applying a flow (1–10 L/min) of heated humidified gas via high-flow nasal cannula (HHFNC) has become quite popular for preventing IH in preterm infants. Effectiveness of this intervention is probably related to the fact that, similar to CPAP, it generates a distending pressure in the airways of 4–5 cm H_2O.[58] In a multicenter study, 52 of 152 infants randomized to HHFNC, but only 39 of 151 infants randomized to CPAP, had shown an increase in FiO_2 of greater than 0.2, a pH less than 7.2, a pCO_2 greater than 60 mm Hg or greater than 1 apnea/24 hours with bag ventilation or greater than 6 with stimulation within 7 days after extubation (34.2% vs. 25.8%; risk difference 8.4%; 95% CI 1.9–18.7).[59] The study was aimed at non-inferiority of HHFNC versus conventional CPAP. Also, the current meta-analysis on the topic shows no significant differences in the rate of therapy failure between HHFNC and conventional nasal CPAP systems.[60] Thus HHFNC probably can be used as an alternative to CPAP for the prevention of IH.

An extension to CPAP is nasal intermittent positive pressure ventilation (N-IPPV), which has a higher effectiveness than CPAP in preventing extubation failure (RR 0.21 [0.10–0.45]; NNT 3), but only if the IPPV is synchronized with the infant's breathing efforts.[61] Synchronization with the infant's breathing efforts is important because of the above-mentioned glottic closure often occurring during apparently central apneas. Typically, an inspiratory pressure of 15–20 cm H_2O, applied at a rate of 10–20/min, is combined with a CPAP level of 5–6 cm H_2O. There is concern that this might result in gastric distension, but this has not been confirmed in meta-analysis. When we compared nonsynchronized N-IPPV with nasal CPAP delivered via a variable flow device that reduces work of breathing (Infant Flow, EME, Brighton, UK), the rate of bradycardia and desaturation was 50% lower with the latter device than with either CPAP applied through a standard ventilator or N-IPPV.[62] Similar results have been reported by others.[63] Nasal CPAP may also be combined with nasal high-frequency oscillatory ventilation. In a crossover trial enrolling 42 infants, both the number of desaturations to less than 80% SpO_2 and the duration of time spent below this level were significantly reduced.[64] Thus, use of a technique that reduces work of breathing, synchronized N-IPPV or applies nasal high-frequency oscillatory ventilation may improve success rates for nasal ventilatory support in reducing IH events.

Caffeine

Methylxanthines increase chemoreceptor sensitivity and respiratory drive and can also improve diaphragmatic function. Of the substances available, caffeine has a wider therapeutic range and fewer side effects than theophylline. In the large, randomized Caffeine for Apnea of Prematurity (CAP) trial, caffeine (or placebo) was started during the first 10 days of life in infants of 500–1250 g birth weight until no longer considered necessary for AOP treatment. Mechanical ventilation, CPAP, and oxygen administration could all be discontinued 7–10 days earlier in infants treated with caffeine. Most important, however, are the data on the primary outcome (i.e., death or disability) at 18 months' corrected age. These showed that caffeine was associated with a 23% reduction in this outcome (odds ratio [OR] 0.77; 95% CI 0.64–0.93). This benefit was particularly strong for cerebral palsy: 4.4% vs. 7.3% of infants had this outcome (RR 0.58; 0.39–0.87).[65] Somewhat unexpected, and not primary end points, were the findings of a 40% lower risk of BPD (36% vs. 47%; OR 0.6; 95% CI 0.5–0.8), a 30% lower risk of developing a symptomatic patent ductus arteriosus (OR 0.7; 0.5–0.8), and a 40% reduction in the risk of developing stage 4 or 5 retinopathy of prematurity (ROP) or requiring treatment for ROP (5% vs. 8%; OR 0.6; 0.4–0.9) in the caffeine group.[66] A 5-year follow-up to this study showed that the preventive effect of caffeine on motor impairment persists even into middle childhood.[67] Even at an 11-year follow-up of this cohort, caffeine therapy, compared with placebo, was still associated with a reduced risk of motor impairment (OR 0.66 [0.48–0.90]; $p = 0.009$).[68] Regarding other long-term (side) effects, sleep studies performed in 201 former CAP participants at age 5–12 years showed no difference in sleep disorders in subjects treated with neonatal caffeine compared with placebo.[69]

In subgroup analyses, the effect of caffeine on the primary outcome was found to be restricted to infants requiring respiratory support at randomization; that is, caffeine had no effect on death or disability in infants *not* requiring CPAP or IPPV.[70] Interestingly, the reduced duration of the need for ventilatory support was only evident in those who were randomized within their first 3 days of life.

Because of the above data, and because at least 90% of infants less than 1,250 g birth weight are considered candidates for caffeine administration, the latter may be considered within the first 3 days of age in any infant less than 1,250 g who requires respiratory support and has developed or is likely to develop AOP (i.e., is very immature and still being ventilated). It is important, however, also to consider when to discontinue caffeine treatment. Here, CAP study infants received caffeine up to a median GA of 34 weeks. It is possible, however, that a longer duration of treatment will be even more beneficial, particularly given that the more mature brain is less tolerant to the detrimental effects of intermittent hypoxia, and caffeine still reduces rates of IH at 35–36 weeks' GA.[71,72] A longer duration of treatment, however, may equally well be detrimental. This must therefore be tested in a further RCT.

In the CAP study, a loading dose of 10 mg/kg caffeine base (intravenous [IV] or orally) and a maintenance dose of 2.5–5 mg/kg once daily were used. Subgroup analysis, however, revealed that the reduction in death or disability was more pronounced in infants receiving an average dose of greater than 3.5 mg/kg/day than it was in infants receiving caffeine at a lower dose.[73]

Another RCT compared a loading dose of 40 mg/kg caffeine base (maintenance dose 10 mg/kg/day) with a "conventional" 10/2.5 mg/kg regimen in 234 infants born at a mean GA of 27 weeks. Infants in the high-dose group had only half the risk of failing extubation within 48 hours of caffeine loading or to require reintubation and mechanical ventilation or doxapram within 7 days of caffeine loading (15.0% vs. 29.8%; RR 0.51 [0.31–0.85]).[74] The study was underpowered, however, for assessing effects on neurodevelopment. A recent RCT in infants less than 30 weeks' GA investigating high-dose versus standard-dose caffeine was stopped prematurely because of a much higher incidence (36% vs. 10%) of intracerebellar hemorrhage in the high-dose compared with the standard-dose group;[75] such high doses should thus not be used in infants less than 30 weeks' GA. In more mature infants (mean GA, 35.7 weeks), however, a daily dose of 10 mg/kg was apparently well tolerated, although resulting in a mean salivary caffeine concentration of 71 μg/mL.[72]

Doxapram

Doxapram stimulates peripheral chemoreceptors at low and central ones at high doses and also has direct effects on respiratory rhythm generation in the pre-Bötzinger complex and its related motor output centers.[76] It shows a clear dose-response curve, with a 50% reduction in apnea rate occurring in 47%, 65%, 82%, and 89% of infants at doses of 0.5, 1.5, 2.0, and 2.5 mg/kg/hr, respectively.[77] Most studies used a continuous IV infusion, although some suggest that the IV solution may also be given orally at twice the dose with good effect (enteral absorption is approximately 50%).[78] Short-term side effects become quite common at doses above 1.5 mg/kg/hr and include irritability, myoclonus, elevated blood pressure, and gastric residuals. Of concern is the fact that the long-term effects of doxapram are unknown. This is particularly worrying given that in a study on factors associated with poor development in extremely low birth weight infants, the only difference found was that infants with a mental development index (MDI) less than 70 had received a mean cumulative doxapram dose of 2,233 mg, compared with 615 mg in matched controls without developmental delay ($p < 0.01$).[79] Although such a retrospective analysis cannot distinguish whether this reflects sequelae of IH/severe AOP (for which doxapram had been ordered) or a direct drug effect, it clearly raises concern. In the CAP trial,[65] infants in the placebo group had not only been more likely to develop cerebral palsy, but had also been three times more likely to receive doxapram.

The yet largest cohort study on long-term effects of doxapram analyzed 2-year follow-up data in 142 doxapram-treated infants born at less than 1,250 g or less than 30 weeks' GA and 284 controls and found a significantly *lower* risk of the combined outcome of death or neurodevelopmental delay in the doxapram group after adjusting for confounders (OR 0.54 [0.37–0.78]).[80] Given these conflicting data in the absence of safe alternatives, doxapram is used in the author's institution on an individual basis in selected infants with frequent IH despite synchronized N-IPPV plus caffeine, but no such approach may be possible in other parts of the world where doxapram is only available with benzyl alcohol as a preservative.[81]

Summary

In summary, treatment for AOP may follow an incremental approach, starting with infant care procedures such as prone positioning, followed by caffeine and CPAP/N-IPPV/noninvasive high frequency oscillation ventilation (N-HFOV) (Table 23.1). We urgently need data on the efficacy and side effects of pharmacologic treatments such as doxapram, or new treatment modalities that may be based on the pathophysiology of this condition as summarized above.

CLINICAL PEARLS

- Apnea of prematurity is a misnomer, as only intermittent hypoxia, not apnea, has been shown to be associated with impaired outcome, e.g., death or disability, of preterm infants.
- Hypoxic ventilatory depression and the proximity between the apneic and eupneic CO2 threshold are key to understanding its pathophysiology.
- Treatment should be incremental, starting with prone, head elevated positioning and caffeine administration, followed by nasal continuous positive airway pressure and synchronized nasal ventilation.

TABLE 23.1 Suggested Incremental Treatment Plan for Apnea of Prematurity

1st Step: Prone, 15-degree head-up tilt position

2nd Step: Caffeine*

3rd Step: Variable-flow CPAP or synchronized N-IPPV or N-HFOV

4th Step: Intubation and mechanical ventilation†

*Consider caffeine as first-line treatment in infants <29 weeks' GA/<1250 g.
†Doxapram may be considered by some neonatologists before intubation, but data are insufficient to give a clear recommendation.

References

1. Lemke RP, Idiong N, Al-Saedi S, Kwiatkowski K, Cates DB, Rigatto H. Evidence of a critical period of airway instability during central apneas in preterm infants. *Am J Respir Crit Care Med.* 1998;157:470–474.
2. Kianicka I, Diaz V, Dorion D, Praud JP. Coordination between glottic adductor muscle and diaphragm EMG activity in fetal lambs in utero. *J Appl Physiol.* 1998;84(5):1560–1565.
3. Abu-Osba YK, Mathew OP, Thach BT. An animal model for airway sensory deprivation producing obstructive apnea with postmortem findings of sudden infant death syndrome. *Pediatrics.* 1981;68:796–801.
4. Poets CF, Stebbens VA, Samuels MP, Southall DP. The relationship between bradycardia, apnea, and hypoxemia in preterm infants. *Pediatr Res.* 1993;34(2):144–147.
5. Daly M, Angell-James JE. Role of carotid-body chemoreceptors and their reflex interactions in bradycardia and cardiac arrest. *Lancet.* 1979;1(8919):764–767.
6. Finer NN, Barrington KJ, Hayes BJ, Hugh A. Obstructive, mixed, and central apnea in the neonate: physiologic correlates. *J Pediatr.* 1992;121:943–950.
7. Olinsky A, Bryan MH, Bryan AC. Influence of lung inflation on respiratory control in neonates. *J Appl Physiol.* 1974;36:426–429.
8. Kosch PC, Stark AR. Dynamic maintenance of end-expiratory lung volume in full-term infants. *J Appl Physiol: Respirat Environ Exercise Physiol.* 1984;57:1126–1133.
9. Gaertner VD, Waldmann AD, Davis PG, et al. Lung volume changes during apnoeas in preterm infants. *Arch Dis Child Fetal Neonatal Ed.* 2023;108(2):170–175.
10. Poets CF, Rau GA, Neuber K, Gappa M, Seidenberg J. Determinants of lung volume in spontaneously breathing preterm infants. *Am J Respir Crit Care Med.* 1997;155(2):649–653.
11. Tourneux P, Leke A, Kongolo G, et al. Relationship between functional residual capacity and oxygen desaturation during short central apneic events during sleep in "late preterm" infants. *Pediatr Res.* 2008;64(2):171–176.
12. Poets CF, Southall DP. Patterns of oxygenation during periodic breathing in preterm infants. *Early Human Dev.* 1991;26(1):1–12.
13. Sands SA, Edwards BA, Kelly VJ, Davidson MR, Wilkinson MH, Berger PJ. A model analysis of arterial oxygen saturation during apnea in preterm infants. *PLoS Comput Biol.* 2010;54:429–448.
14. Esquer C, Claure N, D'Ugard C, Wada Y, Bancalari E. Mechanisms of hypoxemia episodes in spontaneously breathing preterm infants after mechanical ventilation. *Neonatology.* 2008;94(2):100–104.
15. Hannam S, Ingram DM, Milner AD. A possible role for the Hering-Breuer deflation reflex in apnea of prematurity. *J Pediatr.* 1998;132:35–39.
16. Edwards BA, Sands SA, Feeney C, et al. Continuous positive airway pressure reduces loop gain and resolves periodic central apneas in the lamb. *Respir Physiol Neurobiol.* 2009;168(3):239–249.

17. Poets CF, Langner MU, Bohnhorst B. Effects of bottle feeding and two different methods of gavage feeding on oxygenation and breathing patterns in preterm infants. *Acta paediatrica.* 1997;86(4):419–423.

18. Peter CSSN, Bohnhorst B, Silny J, Poets CF. Gastroesophageal reflux and apnea of prematurity: no temporal relationship. *Pediatrics.* 2002;109:8–11.

19. Dorostkar PCAM, Baird TM, Rodriguez S, Martin RJ. Asystole and severe bradycardia in preterm infants. *Biol Neonate.* 2005;88:299–305.

20. Di Fiore JM, Arko M, Whitehouse M, Kimball A, Martin RJ. Apnea is not prolonged by acid gastroesophageal reflux in preterm infants. *Pediatrics.* 2005;116(5):1059–1063.

21. Montealegre-Pomar ADP, Charpak N. Randomized clinical trial of metoclopramide as prophylaxis of gastroesophageal reflux disease in preterm infants. *Paediatr Drugs.* 2021;23(6):591–599.

22. Heldt GP, McIlroy B. Distortion of chest wall and work of diaphragm in preterm infants. *J Appl Physiol.* 1987;62:164–169.

23. Heldt GP. Development of stability of the respiratory system in preterm infants. *J Appl Physiol.* 1988;65:441–444.

24. Numa AH, Newth CJL. Anatomic dead space in infants and children. *J Appl Physiol.* 1996;80:1485–1489.

25. Fairchild K, Mohr M, Paget-Brown A, et al. Clinical associations of immature breathing in preterm infants: part 1-central apnea. *Pediatr Res.* 2016;80(1):21–27.

26. Knill R, Bryan AC. An intercostal-phrenic inhibitory reflex in human newborn infants. *J Appl Physiol.* 1976;40:352–361.

27. Knill R, Andrews W, Bryan AC, Bryan MH. Respiratory load compensation in infants. *J Appl Physiol.* 1976;40(3):357–361.

28. Eastman NJ. Fetal blood studies. *Am J Obstetr Gynecol.* 1936:563–572.

29. Rigatto H, de la Torre Verduzco R, Cates DB. Effects of O_2 on the ventilatory response to CO_2 in preterm infants. *J Appl Physiol: Respir Environ Exercise Physiol.* 1975;39:896–899.

30. Martin RJ, Di Fiore JM, Davis RL, Miller MJ, Coles SK, Dick TE. Persistence of the biphasic ventilatory response to hypoxia in preterm infants. *J Pediatr.* 1998;132:960–964.

31. Rigatto H, Brady JP, de la Torre Verduzco R. Chemoreceptor reflexes in preterm infants: I. The effect of gestational and postnatal age on the ventilatory response to inhalation of 100% and 15% oxygen. *Pediatrics.* 1975;55:604–613.

32. Alvaro R, Alvarez J, Kwiatkowski K, Cates D, Rigatto H. Small preterm infants (<1500 g) have only a sustained decrease in ventilation in response to hypoxia. *Pediatr Res.* 1992;32:403–406.

33. Di Fiore JM, Walsh M, Wrage L, et al. Low oxygen saturation target range is associated with increased incidence of intermittent hypoxemia. *J Paediatr.* 2012;161(6):1047–1052.

34. Lagercrantz H, Ahlström H, Jonson B, Lindroth M, Svenningsen NA. *Critical Oxygen Level Below Which Irregular Breathing Occurs in Preterm Infants.* Pergamon Press; 1978:161–164.

35. Ramirez JM, Quellmalz UJA, Wilken B, Richter DW. The hypoxic response of neurones within the in vitro mammalian respiratory network. *J Physiol.* 1998;507:571–582.

36. Wilken B, Ramirez JM, Probst I, Richter DW, Hanefeld F. Anoxic ATP depletion in neonatal mice brainstem is prevented by creatine supplementation. *Arch Dis Child Fetal. Neonatal Ed.* 2000;82:F224–F227.

37. Wilken B, Ramirez JM, Richter DW, Hanefeld F. Supplemental creatine enhances hypoxic augmentation in vivo by preventing ATP depletion (abstract). *Eur J Pediatr.* 1998;157:178.

38. Bohnhorst B, Geuting T, Peter CS, Dördelmann M, Wilken B, Poets CF. Randomized, controlled trial of oral creatine supplementation (not effective) for apnea of prematurity. *Pediatrics.* 2004;113:e303–e307.

39. Khan A, Qurashi M, Kwiatkowski K, Cates D, Rigatto H. Measurement of the CO_2 apneic threshold in newborn infants: possible relevance for periodic breathing and apnea. *J Appl Physiol.* 2005;98(4):1171–1176.

40. Alvaro RE, Khalil M, Qurashi M, et al. CO(2) Inhalation as a Treatment for Apnea of Prematurity: A Randomized Double-Blind Controlled Trial. *J Pediatr.* 2012;160(2):252–257. e1.

41. Tappin DM, Ford RPK, Nelson KP, et al. Breathing, sleep state, and rectal temperature oscillations. *Arch Dis Child.* 1996;74:427–431.

42. Gozal D, Colin A, Daskalovic YI, Jaffe M. Environmental overheating as a cause of transient respiratory chemoreceptor dysfunction in an infant. *Pediatrics.* 1988;82:738–740.

43. Perlstein PH, Edwards NK, Sutherland JM. Apnea in premature infants and incubator-air-temperature changes. *N Engl J Med.* 1970;282:461–466.

44. Tourneux P, Cardot V, Museux N, et al. Influence of thermal drive on central sleep apnea in the preterm neonate. *Sleep.* 2008;31(4):549–556.

45. Thoppil CK, Belan MA, Cowen CP, Mathew OP. Behavioral arousal in newborn infants and its association with termination of apnea. *J Appl Physiol.* 1991;70:1479–1484.

46. Poets CF, Roberts RS, Schmidt B, et al. Association between intermittent hypoxemia or bradycardia and late death or disability in extremely preterm infants. *JAMA.* 2015;314(6):595–603.

47. Jensen EA, Whyte RK, Schmidt B, et al. Association between intermittent hypoxemia and severe bronchopulmonary dysplasia in preterm infants. *Am J Respir Crit Care Med.* 2021;204(10):1192–1199.

48. Di Fiore JM, Martin RJ, Li H, et al. Patterns of oxygenation, mortality, and growth status in the surfactant positive pressure and oxygen trial cohort. *J Pediatr.* 2017;186:49–56. e1.

49. Raffay TM, Dylag AM, Sattar A, et al. Neonatal intermittent hypoxemia events are associated with diagnosis of bronchopulmonary dysplasia at 36 weeks postmenstrual age. *Pediatr Res.* 2019;39(3):318–323.

50. Heimler R, Langlois J, Hodel DJ, Nelin LD, Sasidharan P. Effect of positioning on the breathing pattern of preterm infants. *Arch Dis Child.* 1992;67:312–314.

51. Martin RJ, Herrell N, Rubin D, Fanaroff A. Effect of supine and prone positions on arterial oxygen tension in the preterm infant. *Pediatrics.* 1979;63:528–531.

52. Bredemeyer SL, Foster JP. Body positioning for spontaneously breathing preterm infants with apnoea. *Cochrane Database Syst Rev.* 2012;6:CD004951.

53. Jenni OG, von Siebenthal K, Wolf M, Keel M, Duc G, Bucher HU. Effect of nursing in the head elevated tilt position (15) on the incidence of bradycardic and hypoxemic episodes in preterm infants. *Pediatrics.* 1997;100:622–625.

54. Bauschatz AS, Kaufmann CM, Haensse D, Pfister R, Bucher HU. A preliminary report of nursing in the three-stair-position to prevent apnoea of prematurity. *Acta Paediatr.* 2008;97(12):1743–1745.

55. Reher C, Kuny KD, Pantalitschka T, Urschitz MS, Poets CF. Randomised crossover trial of different postural interventions on bradycardia and intermittent hypoxia in preterm infants. *Arch Dis Child Fetal Neonatal Ed.* 2008;93(4):F289–291.

56. De Paoli AG, Davis PG, Faber B, Morley CJ. Devices and pressure sources for administration of nasal continuous positive airway pressure (NCPAP) in preterm neonates. *Cochrane Database Syst Rev.* 2008;(1):CD002977.

57. King BC, Gandhi BB, Jackson A, Katakam L, Pammi M, Suresh G. Mask versus prongs for nasal continuous positive airway pressure in preterm infants: A systematic review and meta-analysis. *Neonatology.* 2019;116:100–114.

58. Sreenan C, Lemke RP, Hudson-Mason A, Osiovich H. High-flow nasal cannulae in the management of apnea of prematurity: A comparison with conventional nasal continuous positive airway pressure. *Pediatrics.* 2001;107:1081–1083.

59. Manley BJ, Owen LS, Doyle LW, et al. High-flow nasal cannulae in very preterm infants after extubation. *N Engl J Med.* 2013;369(15):1425–1433.

60. Wilkinson D, Andersen C, O'Donnell CP, De Paoli AG, Manley BJ. High flow nasal cannula for respiratory support in preterm infants. *Cochrane Database Syst Rev.* 2016;2:CD006405.

61. Lemyre B, Davis PG, De Paoli AG, Kirpalani H. Nasal intermittent positive pressure ventilation (NIPPV) versus nasal continuous positive airway pressure (NCPAP) for preterm neonates after extubation. *Cochrane Database Syst Rev.* 2017;2:CD003212.

62. Pantalitschka T, Sievers J, Urschitz MS, Herberts T, Reher C, Poets CF. Randomised crossover trial of four nasal respiratory support systems for apnoea of prematurity in very low birthweight infants. *Arch Dis Child Fetal Neonatal Ed.* 2009;94(4):F245–248.

63. Gizzi C, Montecchia F, Panetta V, et al. Is synchronised NIPPV more effective than NIPPV and NCPAP in treating apnoea of prematurity (AOP)? A randomised cross-over trial. *Arch Dis Child Fetal Neonatal Ed.* 2015;100(1):F17–23.

64. Ruegger CM, Lorenz L, Kamlin COF, et al. The Effect of non-invasive high-frequency oscillatory ventilation on desaturations and bradycardia in very preterm infants: a randomized crossover trial. *J Pediatr.* 2018;201:269–273. e2.

65. Schmidt B, Roberts RS, Davis P, et al. Long-term effects of caffeine therapy for apnea of prematurity. *N Engl J Med.* 2007;357(19):1893–1902.

66. Schmidt B, Roberts RS, Davis P, et al. Caffeine therapy for apnea of prematurity. *N Engl J Med.* 2006;354(20):2112–2121.

67. Schmidt B, Anderson PJ, Doyle LW, et al. Survival without disability to age 5 years after neonatal caffeine therapy for apnea of prematurity. *JAMA.* 2012;307(3):275–282.

68. Schmidt B, Roberts RS, Anderson PJ, et al. Academic performance, motor function, and behavior 11 years after neonatal caffeine citrate therapy for apnea of prematurity: an 11-year follow-up of the CAP Randomized Clinical Trial. *JAMA Pediatr.* 2017;171(6):564–572.

69. Marcus CL, Meltzer LJ, Roberts RS, et al. Long-term effects of caffeine therapy for apnea of prematurity on sleep at school age. *Am J Respir Crit Care Med.* 2014;190(7):791–799.

70. Davis PG, Schmidt B, Roberts RS, et al. Caffeine for Apnea of Prematurity Trial: benefits may vary in subgroups. *J Pediatr.* 2010;156(3):382–387.

71. Rhein LM, Dobson NR, Darnall RA, et al. Effects of caffeine on intermittent hypoxia in infants born prematurely: a randomized clinical trial. *JAMA Pediatr.* 2014;168(3):250–257.

72. Oliphant EA, McKinlay CJ, McNamara D, Cavadino A, Alsweiler JM. Caffeine to prevent intermittent hypoxaemia in late preterm infants: randomised controlled dosage trial. *Arch Dis Child Fetal Neonatal Ed.* 2023;108(2):106–113.

73. Barrington K.J., Roberts R., Schmidt B., et al. The Caffeine for Apnea of Prematurity (CAP) Trial, analyses of dose effect. PAS 2010, Abstract-CD 2010.

74. Steer P, Flenady V, Shearman A, et al. High dose caffeine citrate for extubation of preterm infants: a randomised controlled trial. *Arch Dis Child Fetal Neonatal Ed.* 2004;89(6):F499–503.

75. McPherson C, Neil JJ, Tjoeng TH, Pineda R, Inder TE. A pilot randomized trial of high-dose caffeine therapy in preterm infants. *Pediatr Res.* 2015;78(2):198–204.

76. Kruszynski S, Stanaitis K, Brandes J, Poets CF, Koch H. Doxapram stimulates respiratory activity through distinct activation of neurons in the nucleus hypoglossus and the pre-Botzinger complex. *J Neurophysiol.* 2019;121(4):1102–1110.

77. Barrington KJ, Finer NN, Torok-Both G, Jamali F, Coutts RT. Dose-response relationship of doxapram in the therapy for refractory apnea of prematurity. *Pediatrics.* 1987;80:22–27.

78. Poets CF, Darraj S, Bohnhorst B. Effect of doxapram on episodes of apnoea, bradycardia and hypoxaemia in preterm infants. *Biol Neonate.* 1999;76(4):207–213.

79. Sreenan C, Etches PC, Demianczuk N, Robertson CMT. Isolated mental developmental delay in very low birth weight infants: association with prolonged doxapram therapy for apnea. *J Pediatr.* 2001;139:832–837.

80. Ten Hove CH, Vliegenthart RJ, Te Pas AB, et al. Long-term neurodevelopmental outcome after doxapram for apnea of prematurity. *Neonatology.* 2016;110(1):21–26.

81. Jordan GD, Themelis NJ, Messerly SO, Jarrett RV, Garcia J, Frank CG. Doxapram and potential benzyl alcohol toxicity: a moratorium on clinical investigation? *Pediatrics.* 1986;78(3):540–541.

24

Apnea of Infancy and Apparent Life-Threatening Events

Rosemary S.C. Horne

CHAPTER HIGHLIGHTS

- Apparent life-threatening events (ALTEs) are now termed brief resolved unexplained events (BRUEs) and are relatively common in infancy, particularly in infants <10 weeks of age and those born preterm.
- ALTEs (BRUEs) are common in infancy and it is often difficult to diagnose the cause, as most infants appear well by the time they present at the emergency department.
- A thorough history and details of the event together with a careful physical examination of the infant may provide clues to the underlying cause; however, frequently no cause can be determined.
- The most common causes of ALTEs (BRUEs) are gastroesophageal reflux, lower respiratory tract infection, and seizure and premature infants and those exposed to secondhand smoke are at increased risk.
- Most ALTEs (BRUEs) do not result in a serious diagnosis, and a single episode in a young infant usually does not require prolonged investigation or hospitalization.

Definitions of Apparent Life-Threatening Events and Brief Resolved Unexplained Events

In the 1970s, it was thought that apparent life-threatening events (ALTEs) were precursors to the sudden infant death syndrome (SIDS). These events, which were characterized by an acute and unexpected change in behavior with or without witnessed apnea, were referred to as near-miss for SIDS events.[1] In 1987, an expert panel sponsored by the National Institutes of Health developed the formerly widely accepted definition of an ALTE as "an episode that is frightening to the observer and that is characterized by some combination of apnea (central or occasionally obstructive), color change (usually cyanotic, but occasionally erythematous or plethoric), marked change in muscle tone (usually marked limpness), choking, or gagging."[2] The term ALTE was adopted to replace the term near-miss for SIDS as no substantial evidence could be found to link the two conditions.[2] During

the 1980s and 1990s, numerous studies were carried out investigating infants who presented with ALTE to try to identify causes and risk factors for SIDS; however, a link between the two has never been proven and there is substantial evidence that the two conditions are, in fact, not related.

In 2016, the American Academy of Pediatrics (AAP) issued a new practice guideline that recommended a third name change to brief resolved unexplained event (BRUE).[3] BRUE is used to describe an event occurring in an infant <1 year of age when the observer reports a sudden, brief, and now resolved episode of ≥1 of the following: (1) cyanosis or pallor; (2) absent, decreased or irregular breathing; (3) marked change in tone (hyper- or hypotonia); and (4) altered level of responsiveness. Moreover, it was recommended that BRUE should be diagnosed when there is no explanation for a qualifying event after conducting an appropriate history and physical examination.[3] The new guideline provides a decision tree to identify patients at lower risk based on history and physical examination and provides evidence-based guidelines for their evaluation and management. Higher risk patients, whose history and physical examination suggest a need for further examination, can be identified using this guideline, and a framework for their evaluation has recently been published.[4]

As the third name change to BRUE is recent, ALTE will be referred to when the literature reported is before 2016 and BRUE when recent literature is reported and this new term is used.

Relationship Between Apparent Life-Threatening Events and Sudden Infant Death Syndrome

There is substantial literature to show that there is no evidence that an ALTE is a precursor to SIDS.[2,5] This lack of association is evidenced by a number of findings including the temporal occurrence of the two events. SIDS invariably occurs during sleep and this finding has been included in the recent definition of the event.[6] An ALTE can occur during sleep, when awake, or during feeding,[7] and, in contrast to SIDS, most ALTEs have been reported to occur during the daytime[8–11] and while awake.[11] In most cases, observers of an infant experiencing an ALTE report that the event appeared life-threatening or that they thought that the infant had died, but that prompt intervention resulted in normalization of the child's appearance.[7]

This lack of association is further supported by the evidence that SIDS incidence has significantly decreased since the early 1990s in Western countries where campaigns to reduce the risks were introduced, whereas the incidence of ALTEs has remained unchanged.[12] In a study of 153 cases of ALTEs that were enrolled in the Collaborative Home Infant Monitoring Evaluation (CHIME) study between 1994 and 1998, it was reported that ALTE infants differed significantly from SIDS infants in four respects.[10] Fewer ALTE infants (9%) were small for gestational age at birth compared with 19% of SIDS infants;[13] fewer ALTE infants (19%) were born to teenage mothers, and this distribution was similar to the general population compared with 25% of SIDS mothers;[13] and ALTE infants were of a younger age, 74% under 2 months of age compared with 27%[14] and 24%.[15] SIDS and ALTE infants had similar rates of prematurity (≈20%) and exposure to maternal smoking (ALTE infants 36%[10] and SIDS infants 30–66%).[13–17] One estimate has suggested that 7% of SIDS cases were preceded by ALTE;[2] however, in the CHIME study only 1 of 153 ALTE infants subsequently died[10] and in a review of 8 studies and 643 infants 5 deaths (0.8%) were reported, with all infants having an underlying medical problem.[18]

Although ALTE is not a precursor to SIDS, one study found that the SIDS rate for infants with an ALTE was 10%, and in those infants who had experienced multiple ALTEs it rose to 28%.[19] The two entities do, however, share some common risk factors. In a study of 244 SIDS cases and 868 SIDS controls, the incidence of ALTE was 1.9% in SIDS controls compared with 7.4% in the infants who subsequently died of SIDS.[20] Furthermore, 33.3% of infants with ALTE who subsequently died from SIDS were exposed to both prenatal smoking and the prone sleeping position compared with 13% of ALTE survivors.[20] The study suggested that there may be a sub-population of ALTE infants who do not go on to die from SIDS because they were sleeping supine and not exposed to maternal smoking. In a study of 35 ALTE infants and 19 healthy control infants who underwent overnight polysomnography at 2–3 months, 5–6 months, and 8–9 months of age, arousal characteristics were examined.[21] All infants were born at term and were usual supine sleepers, and 18 of the ALTE infants had mothers who smoked. During non–rapid eye movement (NREM) sleep the ALTE infants had fewer total spontaneous arousals, cortical arousals, and subcortical activations at both 2–3 and 5–6 months of age compared to the control infants. ALTE infants with mothers who smoked had more obstructive apneas and more subcortical activations during rapid eye movement (REM) sleep. The same authors had previously reported that infants who subsequently died from SIDS had fewer cortical

arousals and more subcortical activations, especially during REM sleep;[22] thus they concluded that ALTE and SIDS victims had distinctly different arousal characteristics. In contrast, another polysomnographic study of 26 ALTE infants and 36 age-matched control infants studied at 3 months of age found that ALTE infants exhibited enhanced arousal mechanisms and increased NREM sleep discontinuity compared with controls.[23] Furthermore, normal infants showed a significant increase in cyclic alternating pattern (CAP) rate and a decrease in arousal index with age, whereas the ALTE infants showed no such correlation. The differences between the studies may have been due to the much lower incidence of maternal smoking (1/26) and the higher frequency of respiratory events (obstructive sleep apnea and periodic breathing) in the Miano and colleagues study.[23] Despite these differences, both studies identified that ALTE infants demonstrated an immaturity of sleep electroencephalogram (EEG) patterns that were most marked in NREM sleep, and both showed significant differences in arousal patterns from previous studies of SIDS infants.

Incidence of Apparent Life-Threatening Events

The incidence of ALTE has been estimated to be between 0.6 and 2.46 per 1,000 live births.[12,24–26] ALTEs account for 0.6–1.7% of all emergency department visits of patients <1 year of age[24–27] and 2.3% of pediatric hospitalizations in the United States.[28] The majority of ALTEs occur in infants <1 year of age, with a median age of 1–3 months,[18,26,29,30] and prematurely born infants are at increased risk.[26,31]

Causes of Apparent Life-Threatening Events (Brief Resolved Unexplained Events)

Over 80% of infants with ALTEs appear to have no acute distress when they are seen at the emergency department,[26,32] and no specific diagnosis can be found in up to 30% of those infants seen.[29] The common causes of ALTE (BRUE) are listed in Table 24.1.

In a systematic review of 23 publications with 20 different cohorts from 9 different countries and a total of 6,849 infants presenting with ALTE, 3.2% of infants were diagnosed with a serious bacterial infection, 5.0% with seizures, 0.4% as child abuse, and 0.3% with a metabolic disorder.[33] In another systematic review of eight nonrandomized descriptive studies,[24,25,34–38] the most common diagnoses were gastroesophageal reflux disease (GERD), which was reported in all studies and comprised 31% of total diagnoses; lower respiratory tract infection (LRTI) including "pertussis" and "respiratory syncytial virus infection" was reported in five studies and was 8% of all diagnoses; and seizure was reported in seven studies and 11% of diagnoses.[18] Other diagnoses were problems with ear, nose, and throat (3.6% of all diagnoses); cardiac problems (0.8%); urinary tract infection (1.1%); metabolic disease (1.5%); ingestion of drugs or toxins (1.5%); breath holding (2.3%); and factitious illness (0.3%). Only five ALTE episodes (0.7%) were

TABLE 24.1	Common Causes of Apparently Life-Threatening Events or Brief Resolved Unexplained Events

Most Common Causes

Gastroesophageal reflux
Infection (septicemia, urinary tract infection, gastroenteritis)
Volvulus
Intussusception
Dumping syndrome
Chemolaryngeal reflex
Aspiration and choking

Neurologic Problems

Convulsive disorders
Intracranial infection
Intracranial hypertension
Vasovagal reflexes
Congenital malformations of the brainstem
Muscular problems
Congenital central alveolar hypoventilation

Respiratory Problems

Apnea of infancy/breath-holding spells
Airway and pulmonary infection (respiratory syncytial virus, pertussis, pneumonia)
Congenital airway abnormalities
Airway obstruction
Obstructive sleep apnea

Cardiovascular Problems

Heart rhythm problems
Urea cycle defects
Galactosemia
Leigh or Reye syndrome
Nesidioblastosis
Menkes syndrome

Other Conditions

Excessive feeding volumes
Medications
Accidental smothering or asphyxia
Accidental carbon monoxide intoxication
Drug toxicity
Child abuse
Munchausen by proxy syndrome
Idiopathic apparent life-threatening event

Adapted from Kahn A. Recommended clinical evaluation of infants with an apparent life-threatening event. Consensus document of the European Society for the Study and Prevention of Infant Death, 2003. *Eur J Pediatr.* 2004;163(2):108–115; Fu LY, Moon RY. Apparent life-threatening events: an update. *Pediatr Rev.* 2012;33(8):361–368; quiz 368–369; Samuels MP. Apparent life-threatening events: Pathogenesis and management. In: Marcus CL, Carroll JM, Donnelly D, Loughlin GM, eds. *Sleep and Breathing in Children.* 2nd ed. Informa Healthcare; 2008:229–254; and Tieder JS, Bonkowsky JL, Etzel RA, Franklin WH, Gremse DA, Herman B, et al. Brief resolved unexplained events (formerly apparent life-threatening events) and evaluation of lower-risk infants. *Pediatrics.* 2016;137.

completely benign. Unknown diagnoses were reported in 7/8 studies and made up 23% of all diagnoses, and this varied widely from 9% to 83% between studies.[18]

When investigating the underlying causes of ALTE, child abuse should also be considered, as some studies have reported figures of up to 11%,[39] although other studies have reported the incidence to be around 2%.[40,41] In a study of infants diagnosed with abusive head trauma, over 30% of infants had been seen in the previous 3 weeks for other complaints including ALTE.[42]

Risk Factors for Apparent Life-Threatening Events (Brief Resolved Unexplained Event)

Studies have consistently identified a number of risk factors for ALTEs (BRUEs). ALTEs typically affect infants <1 year of age and usually <10 weeks of age, and there is a predisposition for more male infants to be affected.[43] Premature infants are at twice the risk, with a national survey in the Netherlands reporting that 29.5% of ALTE infants were born preterm compared with 13% being born preterm in the general population.[44] In a study of 625 infants admitted to Montreal Children's Hospital between 1996 and 2006 for ALTEs a similar proportion of 21% were born preterm.[27] Furthermore, the relative risk of having an extreme event (either a central apnea lasting >30 seconds or an extreme bradycardia heart rate [HR] <60 beats/min for 10 seconds) in infants <44 weeks post conceptional age (PCA) and HR <50 beats/min for 10 seconds in infants ≥44 weeks PCA while on a cardiorespiratory monitor was 6.3 (95% confidence interval [CI] 3.6–11.0) for preterm born infants. Other risk factors include exposure to secondhand cigarette smoke, pertussis, respiratory syncytial virus, or recent general anesthesia.[18,24,45]

Apparent Life-Threatening Events in the First 24 Hours After Birth

There have been reports of infants with ALTEs within the first day of life. A nationwide retrospective German study reported a rate of 2.6 per 100,000 live births of severe ALTEs requiring resuscitation and SIDS in the first 24 hours after birth.[46] Of the 17 infants who met the inclusion criteria, 7 infants died: 3 after unsuccessful resuscitation and 4 had initially been resuscitated but had treatment discontinued because of severe hypoxic brain damage. Of the 10 survivors, 6 were neurologically abnormal on discharge. Twelve infants were found lifeless, lying on their mother's breast/ abdomen or very close to and facing her, two were supine in their cots, two were being held by their fathers, and one was lying supine next to their mother. Among the 26 cases excluded from the analysis, 4 were preterm but otherwise met the inclusion criteria. A further three infants were resuscitated with vigorous stimulation only. A subsequent analysis of the data identified infants being in a potentially asphyxiating position and babies born to first-time mothers to be risk factors.[47] Another study published in the same year reported six cases of healthy term newborns (all with Apgar scores of 10 at both 5 and 10 minutes) who suffered an ALTE within 2 hours of delivery while in skin-to-skin contact with their mother; three of the six infants died.[48] A prospective French regional study reported a rate of ALTE and SIDS of 0.032 deaths per 1,000 live births within the first 2 hours after birth.[49] A similar study carried out in Stockholm found a much higher incidence of sudden unexpected post natal collapse of 38 per 100,000 live births within 24 hours of birth;[50] 16 of the 26 cases required resuscitation. Fifteen infants were found prone during skin-to-skin contact, 18 were primipara, 13 occurred during breastfeeding at <2 hours of age, and 3 occurred when the mother was using her mobile phone. Twenty-five of the 26 infants had a favorable neurologic outcome.[50] A recent study that monitored 100 term neonates for the first 2 hours after birth with pulse oximetry found desaturations (<85%) in 30% and prolonged desaturations in 25% of infants.[51] Significantly more desaturations were observed in infants who had been born by planned caesarian section and desaturations were also more frequent in infants diagnosed with neonatal infection and in infants born to a mother with gestational diabetes, although these did not reach statistical significance. These studies highlight that there are risks associated with early skin-to-skin contact or breastfeeding, especially when infants are not being closely observed by health care professionals.

Initial Assessment for Apparent Life-Threatening Events (Brief Resolved Unexplained Events)

In a consensus statement from the European Society for the Study and Prevention of Infant Death in 2004 it was concluded that "There was no standard minimal workup in the evaluation of ALTE."[7] The assessment of an infant who presents with an ALTE has been well reviewed in the literature.[7,11,33,52–55] A number of protocols for the initial examination have been published.[7,11,33,52–57]

The new clinical practice guideline published in May 2016 by the AAP[3] recommended the replacement of the term ALTE with BRUE, and provided an approach to evaluation that is based on the risk that an infant will have a repeat event or a serious underlying disorder and provides management recommendations for lower risk infants. By using the guideline, infants can be categorized as either lower risk on the basis of clinical history and physical examination or higher risk for whom further investigation and treatment is required. The new guideline is intended to foster a patient- and family-centered approach to care, reduce unnecessary and costly testing and interventions, and improve patient outcomes. Each key action statement is supported by a level of evidence, the benefit–harm relationship, and the strength of the recommendation.

The primary reason for the change in terminology and diagnosis was because of the imprecise nature of the original definition of ALTE, which was difficult to apply to clinical care.[3] The majority of infants are asymptomatic on presentation and these infants need to be distinguished from those exhibiting symptoms such as fever or respiratory distress. Furthermore, although the event was frightening to the

caregiver, most events are not life-threatening and are frequently a normal physiologic event such as periodic breathing, breath holding, or gastroesophageal reflux. Although events defined as ALTE rarely have serious underlying causes and do not recur, the name in itself cases anxiety for both clinicians and caregivers. It is anticipated that the replacement of the term "life-threatening" with "brief" and "resolved" will allay these concerns.

Clinicians should use the term BRUE to describe an event occurring in an infant <1 year of age when the observer describes a sudden, brief, and now resolved episode of ≥1 of the following:
- Cyanosis or pallor
- Absent, decreased, or irregular breathing
- Marked change in tone (hyper- or hypotonia)
- Altered level of responsiveness

In addition, also if there is no explanation for the event after conducting an appropriate history and medical examination. Factors that can be included in the diagnosis of a BRUE are listed in Table 24.2, and those that exclude a diagnosis of BRUE are listed in Table 24.3.[3]

Subsequently, the AAP released a framework for evaluation of the higher risk infant after a BRUE.[4] The criteria for a higher risk BRUE include the following:
- Age <60 days
- Prematurity: gestational age <32 weeks and PCA <45 weeks
- Recurrent event or occurring in clusters
- Duration of event ≥1 minute
- Cardiopulmonary resuscitation (CPR) required by trained medical provider
- Concerning historical features
- Concerning physical examination findings

Potential causes of high-risk BRUE are the same as for low-risk BRUE listed in Table 24.2 and potential evaluations are listed in Table 24.4. There is little evidence, however, to guide which high-risk BRUE infants will most likely benefit from hospitalization, and their management is challenging because of the diverse and extensive diagnostic possibilities and the potential presence of a serious underlying disorder.[4] It is particularly important that there is follow-up with these infants.

In summary, any evaluation should always start with a careful history of the event as reported by the observer, a review of the infant's past medical history, and a physical examination focusing on any evidence that might have caused or contributed to the event. Details of questions to be asked about the history of the infant and the event are listed in Table 24.4. If the event fits the definition of a BRUE, then the infant is deemed low risk and further investigation is deemed unnecessary.[3]

If, however, the description of the event and/or clinical history does not meet the criteria for BRUE then further investigations are required, as listed in Table 24.5. These include a full blood examination, blood glucose, serum electrolytes including calcium, and blood gases with serum bicarbonate and lactate should be done as soon as possible.

TABLE 24.2	Factors Included in the Definition of Brief Resolved Unexplained Event

Duration <1 minute; typically 20–30 seconds

Resolved

Patient returned to their baseline state of health after the event
Normal vital signs
Normal appearance

Unexplained

Not explained by an identifiable medical condition

Event Characterization

Cyanosis or pallor
Central cyanosis: blue or purple coloration of face, gums, and trunk
Central pallor: pale coloration of face or trunk
Absent, decreased, or irregular breathing
Central apnea
Obstructive apnea
Mixed obstructive apnea
Marked change in tone (hyper- or hypotonia)
Hypertonia
Hypotonia
Altered responsiveness
Loss of consciousness
Mental status change
Lethargy
Somnolence
Postictal phase

Adapted from Tieder JS, Bonkowsky JL, Etzel RA, Franklin WH, Gremse DA, Herman B, et al. Brief resolved unexplained events (formerly apparent life-threatening events) and evaluation of lower-risk infants. *Pediatrics*. 2016;137.

TABLE 24.3	Factors Excluded From the Definition of Brief Resolved Unexplained Event

Duration ≥1 minute

Resolved

At the time of medical evaluation:
Fever or recent fever
Tachypnea, bradypnea, apnea
Tachycardia or bradycardia
Hypotension, hypertension, or hemodynamic instability
Mental status changes, somnolence, lethargy
Hypotonia or hypertonia
Vomiting
Bruising, petechiae, or other signs of injury/trauma
Abnormal weight, growth, or head circumference
Noisy breathing (stridor, stertor, wheezing)
Repeat event(s)

Unexplained

Event consistent with gastroesophageal reflux, swallow dysfunction, nasal congestion, etc.
History or physical examination concerning for child abuse, congenital airway abnormality, etc.

Event Characterization

Cyanosis or pallor
Acrocyanosis or perioral cyanosis
Rubor
Absent, decreased, or irregular breathing
Periodic breathing of the newborn
Breath-holding spell
Marked change in tone (hyper- or hypotonia)
Hypertonia associated with crying, choking, or gagging due to gastroesophageal reflux or feeding problems
Tone changes associated with breath-holding spell
Tonic eye deviation or nystagmus
Tonic-clonic seizure activity
Infantile spasms
Altered responsiveness
Loss of consciousness associated with breath-holding spell

Adapted from Tieder JS, Bonkowsky JL, Etzel RA, Franklin WH, Gremse DA, Herman B, et al. Brief resolved unexplained events (formerly apparent life-threatening events) and evaluation of lower-risk infants. *Pediatrics*. 2016;137.

A urinary analysis and culture should also be performed. In most reviews a chest X-ray and tests to identify common respiratory viruses are also recommended. These tests are aimed at identifying a potential cause such as infection, hypocalcemia, hypomagnesemia, hypo- or hypernatremia leading to seizures, or hypo- or hyperkalemia leading to cardiac arrhythmias. Metabolic disorders account for 2–5% of all cases of ALTE and, if not identified and treated, can lead to long-term sequelae. As these serum biochemistry tests are routinely available and relatively inexpensive, they are recommended.[55] Urine toxicology screening is also important to identify both intentional and unintentional poisoning.[55] In a retrospective study of children <2 years of age presenting with ALTE, 8.4% had been given a medication that could have caused apnea, with 4.7% of children receiving over-the-counter cough and cold medication.[58] Importantly, none of the parents admitted to giving their children the medications, which were not recommended in children <2 years of age.

Around 30% of ALTE cases are attributed to GERD[18] and about 25% of children admitted for ALTE undergo an upper gastrointestinal fluoroscopy or swallowing test.[55] These tests are useful for diagnosing anatomical abnormalities that could contribute to ALTE but, as many normal infants suffer from reflux, they are not specific to ALTE. Esophageal pH monitoring with concurrent cardiorespiratory monitoring can identify periods of reflux associated with apnea and/or hypoxemia. As these tests are uncomfortable for the patient and not inexpensive, it has been suggested that these tests only be recommended if the ALTE infant history indicated frequent bouts of reflux, if the event was immediately following a feed, or if gastric contents were noted in the infant's mouth or nose by the caregiver during the event.[55]

In a review of 36 children's hospitals across the United States, there was large interhospital variability in all aspects of ALTE infant care; however, the most common tests requested after an ALTE were a full blood examination

TABLE 24.4   Details to Record of the History of the Potential BRUE

Personal and Family History

- Details of pregnancy, gestation at birth, delivery and neonatal health, usual sleeping and feeding habits, method of feeding
- Previous episodes of BRUE/ALTE
- Reflux? If yes obtain details including management
- Breathing problems? Noisy breathing or snoring?
- Normal development and growth?
- Any medical or surgical problems and previous evaluations
- Characteristics of other siblings with an ALTE; early death; SIDS; family history of genetic, metabolic, cardiac, or neurologic problems
- Parents' age, smoking and drinking habits. Usual medical treatments in the past 7 days. Details also of any other caregiver

Daily Routine

- Usual sleep conditions, including position put down and when found if event occurred during sleep. Bed/cot and bedding, sleep attire, room temperature, use of dummy/pacifier, or any sedative medications
- In breastfeeding mothers, did they take any prescription, over-the-counter, or herbal remedies within 24 hours of the event?

Events Immediately Preceding the Event

The events and minor symptoms that preceded the eventIncluding any episodes of fever, illness, medications, immunization, sleep restriction, or change in daily routine

Detailed Description of the Event

- Precise timing of the event, including approximate duration
- Relationship to feeding
- Exact place of the event (child's cot, parent's bed, car seat, parent's arms)
- The state of the infants when the event began – awake or asleep
- If asleep, infant's body position, type of bedding, whether face was covered or not. Specific details of the sleeping arrangements, own cot, parental bed, sofa, pram, etc. Was the infant in a co-sleeping situation?
- If awake, whether the infant was being fed, handled, crying, being bathed
- The reason the event was noticed – infant cry or other noise
- Was there anything unusual about the child before the event?
- Did the infant fall or experience any other trauma?
- Who discovered the infant or witnessed the event?
- The infant's appearance when found: were they conscious or not, muscle tone (rigid or floppy), vomiting, foreign body or milk in mouth or nose, sweating, skin temperature, lethargy, pupil size?
- Color (pallor, red, purple, blue), location of color changes – peripheral, whole body, around the mouth, tongue and palate, symmetric or asymmetric
- Respiratory effort – none, shallow, chocking, gasping, increased effort, nasal flaring, stridor, wheeze
- Movement and muscle tone – rigid, floppy, limp, jerking, convulsions
- How did the event stop – the event resolved spontaneously, required gentle stimulation, blowing air on face, vigorous stimulation, CPR
- Child's response to intervention
- Estimated time to recovery

Environmental History

- General housing, water damage or mold problems
- Exposure to tobacco smoke, toxic substances, drugs
- Family structure, individuals living in the home
- Support systems/access to needed resources
- Previous child protection services or law enforcement involvement

Considerations for Possible Child Abuse

- Multiple or changing versions of the history/circumstance
- History/circumstances inconsistent with child's developmental stage
- Incongruence between caregiver expectations and child's developmental stage, including assigning negative attributes to the child

Adapted from Kahn A. Recommended clinical evaluation of infants with an apparent life-threatening event. Consensus document of the European Society for the Study and Prevention of Infant Death, 2003. *Eur J Pediatr.* 2004;163(2):108–115; Scollan-Koliopoulos M, Koliopoulos JS. Evaluation and management of apparent life-threatening events in infants. *Pediatr Nurs.* 2010;36(2):77–83; quiz 84; Fu LY, Moon RY. Apparent life-threatening events: An update. *Pediatr Rev.* 2012;33(8):361–368; quiz 368–369; and Tieder JS, Bonkowsky JL, Etzel RA, Franklin WH, Gremse DA, Herman B, et al. Brief resolved unexplained events (formerly apparent life-threatening events) and evaluation of lower-risk infants. *Pediatrics.* 2016;137.

TABLE 24.5   Physical Examination Features to be Considered in the Evaluation of a Potential Brief Resolved Unexplained Event

General Appearance

- Craniofacial abnormalities
- Age-appropriate responsiveness to environment
- Appropriate growth, weight, and head circumference for age

Vital Signs

- Temperature, pulse, respiratory rate, blood pressure, oxygen saturation
- Skin color, evidence of injury, e.g., bruising or erythema
- Muscle tone, alertness, responsiveness

In the absence of identifiable risk factors and the description of the event meets the definition for BRUE, infants are at lower risk and laboratory studies, imaging studies, and other diagnostic procedures are unlikely to be useful or necessary. Recommend that the infant be discharged home after parent's fears have been addressed, notify the family primary care physician and advise follow-up, advise to re-consult if recurrence. Educate parents about BRUEs and offer resources for CPR training to caregiver.

If Event Does Not Fit the Definition of BRUE or Is Deemed High-Risk BRUE and the Physical Examination and Clinical History Were Not Normal

- Carry out investigation and manage as clinically indicated, usually with admission for at least 24 hours:
  - Cardiorespiratory monitoring and saturation recording
  - Complete blood count and differential
  - C-reactive protein levels
  - Sodium and potassium
  - Glucose and electrolytes
  - Magnesium and calcium
  - Blood glucose levels
  - Serum lactate
  - Urinalysis
  - Toxicology screen
  - Blood culture
  - Chest X-ray
  - ECG, CT, or MRI
  - Consider dilated fundoscopy or swallowing test or esophageal pH monitoring

If Event was Prolonged, Infant had Repetitive Events and Perceived Need for Strong Stimulation to Terminate Event

- As above
- If infant has fever or lethargy and does not appear normal on examination
- Also consider brain imaging
- Blood ammonia level
- Full metabolic work-up

Abbreviations: *CPR*, cardiorespiratory resuscitation; *BRUE*, brief resolved unexplained event; *ECG*, electrocardiogram; *CT*, computed tomography; *MRI*, magnetic resonance imaging.
Adapted from McGovern MC, Smith MB. Causes of apparent life threatening events in infants: A systematic review. *Arch Dis Child*. 2004;89(11):1043–1048; Al Khushi N, Cote A. Apparent life-threatening events: assessment, risks, reality. *Paediatr Respir Rev*. 2011;12(2):124–132; Merritt JL, 2nd, Quinonez RA, Bonkowsky JL, Franklin WH, Gremse DA, Herman BE, et al. A framework for evaluation of the higher-risk infant after a brief resolved unexplained event. *Pediatrics*. 2019;144.

(70%) and electrolytes (65%), chest X-ray (69%), electrocardiogram (36%), and upper gastrointestinal fluoroscopy or swallow testing (26%).[28]

Previously, McGovern and Smith[18] recommended inclusion of an EEG assessment in the initial investigation of ALTE based on the findings of their study that 11% of infants were diagnosed with seizures. However, in their review only two of seven revealed that the diagnosis of epilepsy was made from EEG. In a more recent study, only 3.6% of ALTE infants were diagnosed with epilepsy[39] and EEG only had a sensitivity for diagnosis of 15%. The majority of infants diagnosed had recurrent ALTE events within 1 month (71%) and 41% were diagnosed as having seizures within 1 week of the initial event. Recent recommendations suggest that, given the difficulty of obtaining an EEG in the emergency department setting and the low sensitivity for diagnosing epilepsy, EEG monitoring should be reserved for infants presenting with recurrent ALTE events.[55] In addition to EEG, neuroimaging can be used to help diagnose chronic epilepsy by identifying underlying brain anatomical abnormalities. Neuroimaging is also useful for identifying abusive head trauma. However, in a study by Bonkowsky and coworkers, when combined all neuroimaging techniques (cranial computed tomography [CT], magnetic resonance imaging [MRI], and ultrasound) only had a sensitivity of 6.7% for detecting chronic epilepsy.[39] Head CT is the most commonly ordered imaging study to investigate ALTE,[55] and one study found that ordering a head CT for all asymptomatic ALTE infants actually saved money from a medical payer perspective for identifying abusive head trauma.[59] However, as only 1–3% of all ALTE cases are due to abusive head trauma, many infants would be subjected to unnecessary irradiation if this practice was to be adopted, and it has been recommended that this assessment only be performed where abuse is suspected.[55] Two separate studies have identified that discrepancies in the reported history of the ALTE by different caregivers, or that the history changes over time or is confusing, was highly predictive of physical abuse.[60,61] In addition, delays in seeking medical attention, vomiting, and irritability were also predictive. It has been suggested that having multiple emergency department staff taking the history, looking for inconsistencies and for other symptoms of abuse such as retinal examinations and recent fractures, may help identify those infants who should be referred for CT scans.[55]

Should All Apparent Life-Threatening Events Infants be Admitted?

The question of whether an infant presenting at the emergency department with ALTE (BRUE) routinely requires hospital admission has been controversial; however, the new AAP guidelines have significantly clarified which infants are deemed low risk and should not be admitted. In the past, as it was thought that infants who had experienced an ALTE might subsequently go on to die from SIDS, infants were routinely admitted to hospital for diagnostic monitoring and frequently discharged home on an apnea/bradycardia monitor.[62] Some reviews of treatment for ALTE still strongly recommend admission.[24,56] It has been reported that in the United States the average length of hospital stay of an ALTE infant is 4.4 ± 5.6 (standard deviation [SD]) days with total charges of $15,567 ± $28,510 (SD).[28] In a retrospective study of 625 infants admitted following an ALTE, 13.6% had a subsequent extreme cardiorespiratory event and 85% of these occurred within the first 24 hours after admission and were attributed to respiratory tract infection.[27] In a prospective study of 66 infants, 14 of whom had perinatal risk factors and 16 of whom had had a previous ALTE, 12% had recurrent events within 24 hours of admission, 9% had events requiring moderate stimulation, and 3% required resuscitation.[63]

In the majority of cases presenting in the emergency department, the infants appear normal after a suspected ALTE (BRUE) at home, and there have been few studies to evaluate the benefit of hospital admission. In a recent multicenter observational cohort study of 832 infants, 84.4% of infants appeared well in the emergency department and 16.5% obviously required patient admission.[11] Criteria for

"obviously needed admission" were required supplemental oxygen for non–self-resolving hypoxia, intubation, ventilation, intravenous antibiotics for confirmed serious bacterial infection, antiepileptic drugs, or a positive test for respiratory syncytial virus or pertussis. Nearly 80% of infants were admitted, with more than 40% admitted to a monitored bed. Together with this criterion, two other factors, significant medical history and >1 ALTE in 24 hours, identified 89% of infants who ultimately had justifications for hospitalization. The use of the authors' published decision tree would have potentially reduced the number of admissions by 27% while missing 2% of patients who required hospital admission. In another large study of 300 infants, 76% were admitted but only 12% required significant intervention.[29] None of the infants died during their hospital stay or within 72 hours of discharge. Logistic regression identified prematurity, abnormal result on physical examination, color change to cyanosis, absence of symptoms of upper respiratory tract infection, and the absence of choking as predictors of significant intervention. When these predictors were used to form a clinical decision rule, 64% of infants could have been discharged home safely from the emergency department, reducing the hospitalization rate to 36%.[29] In an earlier smaller study of 59 patients, two "high-risk" factors that predicted the need for hospital admission were age <1 month and multiple ALTE in the past 24 hours.[64] They concluded that infants older than 1 month who had experienced a single ALTE could safely be discharged from the emergency department.

From the previously mentioned literature, it can be seen that there was still debate regarding whether or not all ALTE (BRUE) infants should be admitted. A 2012 review suggested that, in the light of findings that repeat events usually occurred within 24 hours, the majority of ALTE infants should be admitted for at least 23 hours with continuous cardiorespiratory monitoring, ideally with pulse oximetry and event recording.[55] However, if the event was the first ALTE experienced, when infants were not born preterm; had suffered a single event that was brief, not severe, and self-resolving; and if there was a probable cause such as GERD it was reasonable for the infant not to be admitted.[55]

As described at the beginning of this chapter, in 2016 the AAP published a new guideline to enable the identification of lower risk infants and to call these events BRUE. The guideline outlines the reasons for this reclassification and provides the background literature that supports the included decision tree for identifying these lower risk infants.[3] It is hoped that this new guideline will reduce unnecessary and costly medical interventions, improve patient outcomes, and foster a patient- and family-centered approach to care.

Long-Term Follow-Up: Home Monitoring

If it is decided that cardiorespiratory monitoring is required after discharge home, it should be aimed at assisting with diagnosis and management of ALTE (BRUE).[65] It is therefore important to use monitors that record respiration and

HR in conjunction with oxygen saturation so that central and obstructive respiratory events can we distinguished. In the CHIME study, the majority of significant events had a central component.[66]

There is still debate as to whether or not polysomnography should be routinely requested when investigating ALTE.[7,65] Disadvantages of polysomnography are that it is not readily available in all centers where ALTE infants might present, it frequently cannot be arranged immediately after admission, it is only for one night in duration, and it is costly to perform. It is, however, the gold standard for distinguishing central and obstructive respiratory events.

There is also still some debate as to whether or not ALTE infants should be sent home on cardiorespiratory monitors. In the 1980s, home cardiorespiratory monitoring became widely used to try to prevent SIDS; however, it is now no longer recommended.[5] Furthermore, the frequency of false alarms has the undesired effect of causing more anxiety for parents. For those infants who have suffered severe ALTE at home and who have underlying cardiorespiratory abnormalities that are not immediately treatable, home monitoring may be beneficial. Short periods of home monitoring with devices with which events can be subsequently downloaded can also assist with diagnosis. It has been documented that seizures, metabolic disorders, and Munchausen by proxy syndrome can be distinguished in infants who have had recurrent ALTEs.[67,68]

Impact of the New American Academy of Pediatrics Brief Resolved Unexplained Event Guidelines

Since the release of the AAP guidelines for the management of children with BRUE, there have been a number of studies that have evaluated the changes in management that have occurred. A study by Ramgopal and colleagues[69] used a multicenter administrative database to compare rates of admission, testing, revisits, and diagnoses of children diagnosed with BRUE or ALTE during 2015 with those in 2017. A total of 9,501 patients were included (5,608 in 2015 and 3,893 in 2017). The proportion of infants diagnosed with BRUE or ALTE decreased by ~25% in 2017 compared with 2015. The admission rate decreased by 5.7% (95% CI 3.8–7.5%) for infants aged 0–60 days and by 18% (95% CI 15.3–20.7%) for infants aged 61–365 days. In 2017, patients had lower rates of EEG, brain MRI, chest radiography, laboratory testing, and urine analysis compared with 2015.

In a retrospective analysis of the application of the new AAP BRUE criteria to infants younger than 1 year of age (n = 84) admitted for an ALTE between 2006 and 2016 to a single tertiary center in Italy, 42% were identified as not meeting the criteria for BRUE, 19% were low-risk BRUE and 39% were high-risk BRUE.[70] Only one low-risk BRUE infant had a subsequent BRUE during the follow-up period, but this infant was later diagnosed with a seizure disorder. There were no deaths or other significant

morbidities in any of the BRUE patients. Had the AAP BRUE guidelines been followed and low-risk BRUE infants not admitted there would have been an overall 20% saving in medical costs.[70]

In another retrospective review of patients (N = 406) who presented at an emergency department in the United States between 2014 and 2019 with a diagnosis of ALTE or BRUE, there was a significant reduction in admission to hospital, emergency department stay, and invasive tests between the pre- and post-AAP guideline cohorts.[71] Importantly, there were no increases in readmissions or repeat emergency department presentations.

In a study using data publicly available from the Pediatric Emergency Care Applied Research Network Core Data Project there were 9,009 cases identified by the International Classification of Diseases, Ninth Revision, Clinical Modification (ICD-9-CM) code for ALTE between 2009 and 2014.[72] After applying a modeling algorithm to develop a lower risk BRUE population sample, complete treatment and outcome variables were available for 3,116 subjects. The new AAP clinical guideline was followed in 1,974 (63.4%) cases and not followed in 1,142 (36.6%). The likelihood of hospital admission was significantly lower when the guideline was followed.[72]

There have been a number of subsequent studies that have all shown that since publication of the AAP BRUE guidelines there have been substantial reductions in testing, utilization of medications, admission rates, cost, and length of hospital stay, without a change in the revisit rates in the United States and other countries.[73–76]

Clinicians require evidence so that they can reassure parents with an infant diagnosed with BRUE that it is safe to return home from the emergency department with their baby. A recent meta-analysis of 12 studies published between 1999 and 2016 that included 3,005 infants, identified 12 deaths post event, of which 8 occurred within 4 months of the event.[77] This constitutes a post-event mortality rate of about 1 in 800 and provides evidence that the occurrence of a BRUE does not appear to increase a child's risk of death over the baseline risk of death in the first year of life, which is about 1 in 500. This meta-analysis provides an upper boundary of risk of death after a BRUE and supports the approach of not hospitalizing infants who present at the emergency department after a BRUE.[77]

CLINICAL PEARLS

- Apparent life-threatening events (ALTEs) are now termed brief resolved unexplained events (BRUEs) and are relatively common in infancy, particularly in infants <10 weeks of age and those born preterm.
- Diagnosis of the underlying cause is difficult.
- A thorough case history and detailed description of the event are essential.
- Most BRUEs do not result in a serious diagnosis and a single episode in a young infant usually does not require prolonged investigation.

Summary

ALTE (BRUE) is common in infancy and it is often difficult to diagnose the cause, as most infants appear well by the time they present at the emergency department. The definition of ALTE (BRUE) is also very subjective and depends on the firsthand report of the event by parents/caregivers and this adds to the difficulty of diagnosis. A thorough history and details of the event together with a careful physical examination of the infant may provide clues to the underlying cause. Most frequently, no cause can be determined and it is therefore difficult for clinicians to decide how intensively the infant should be investigated and for how long they should be monitored. The most common causes of ALTE (BRUE) are GER, LRTI, and seizure. Premature infants and those exposed to secondhand smoke are at increased risk. Most ALTEs (BRUEs) do not result in a serious diagnosis, and a single episode in a young infant usually does not require prolonged investigation or hospitalization. If the infant has had recurrent events and/or required vigorous stimulation, then admission and a battery of appropriate tests are required. It is no longer recommended that infants be monitored at home long term.

References

1. American Academy of Pediatrics American Academy of Pediatrics. Task Force on Prolonged Infantile Apnea. Prolonged infantile apnea: 1985. *Pediatrics.* 1985;76:129–131.

2. National Institutes of Health National Institutes of Health Consensus Development Conference on Infantile Apnea and Home Monitoring, Sept 29 to Oct 1, 1986. *Pediatrics.* 1987;79:292–299.

3. Tieder JS, Bonkowsky JL, Etzel RA, Franklin WH, Gremse DA, Herman B, et al. Brief resolved unexplained events (formerly apparent life-threatening events) and evaluation of lower-risk infants. *Pediatrics.* 2016:137.

4. Merritt 2nd JL, Quinonez RA, Bonkowsky JL, Franklin WH, Gremse DA, Herman BE, et al. A framework for evaluation of the higher-risk infant after a brief resolved unexplained event. *Pediatrics.* 2019:144.

5. American Academy of Pediatrics Apnea, sudden infant death syndrome, and home monitoring. *Pediatrics.* 2003;111:914–917.

6. Krous HF, Beckwith JB, Byard RW, Rognum TO, Bajanowski T, Corey T, et al. Sudden infant death syndrome and unclassified sudden infant deaths: A definitional and diagnostic approach. *Pediatrics.* 2004;114:234–238.

7. Kahn A. Recommended clinical evaluation of infants with an apparent life-threatening event. Consensus document of the European Society for the Study and Prevention of Infant Death, 2003. *Eur J Pediatr.* 2004;163:108–115.

8. Wennergren G, Milerad J, Lagercrantz H, Karlberg P, Svenningsen NW, Sedin G, et al. The epidemiology of sudden infant death syndrome and attacks of lifelessness in Sweden. *Acta Paediatr Scand.* 1987;76:898–906.

9. Kahn A, Blum D, Hennart P, Sellens C, Samson-Dollfus D, Tayot J, et al. A critical comparison of the history of sudden-death infants and infants hospitalised for near-miss for SIDS. *Eur J Pediatr.* 1984;143:103–107.

10. Esani N, Hodgman JE, Ehsani N, Hoppenbrouwers T. Apparent life-threatening events and sudden infant death syndrome: Comparison of risk factors. *J Pediatr.* 2008;152:365–370.

11. Kaji AH, Claudius I, Santillanes G, Mittal MK, Hayes K, Lee J, et al. Apparent life-threatening event: Multicenter prospective cohort study to develop a clinical decision rule for admission to the hospital. *Ann Emerg Med.* 2013;61:379–387.

12. Kiechl-Kohlendorfer U, Hof D, Peglow UP, Traweger-Ravanelli B, Kiechl S. Epidemiology of apparent life threatening events. *Arch Dis Child.* 2004;90:297–300.

13. Getahun D, Demissie K, Lu SE, Rhoads GG. Sudden infant death syndrome among twin births: United States, 1995–1998. *J Perinatol.* 2004;24:544–551.

14. Leach CE, Blair PS, Fleming PJ, Smith IJ, Platt MW, Berry PJ, et al. Epidemiology of SIDS and explained sudden infant deaths. CESDI SUDI Research Group. *Pediatrics.* 1999;104:e43.

15. Li DK, Petitti DB, Willinger M, McMahon R, Odouli R, Vu H, et al. Infant sleeping position and the risk of sudden infant death syndrome in California, 1997–2000. *Am J Epidemiol.* 2003;157:446–455.

16. Malloy MH. Size for gestational age at birth: Impact on risk for sudden infant death and other causes of death, USA 2002. *Arch Dis Child Fetal Neonatal Ed.* 2007;92:F473–F478.

17. Hauck FR, Herman SM, Donovan M, Iyasu S, Merrick Moore C, Donoghue E, et al. Sleep environment and the risk of sudden infant death syndrome in an urban population: The Chicago Infant Mortality Study. *Pediatrics.* 2003;111:1207–1214.

18. McGovern MC, Smith MB. Causes of apparent life threatening events in infants: A systematic review. *Arch Dis Child.* 2004;89:1043–1048.

19. Samuels MP, Poets CF, Noyes JP, Hartmann H, Hewertson J, Southall DP. Diagnosis and management after life threatening events in infants and young children who received cardiopulmonary resuscitation. *BMJ.* 1993;306:489–492.

20. Edner A, Wennborg M, Alm B, Lagercrantz H. Why do ALTE infants not die in SIDS? *Acta Paediatr.* 2007;96:191–194.

21. Franco P, Montemitro E, Scaillet S, Groswasser J, Kato I, Lin JS, et al. Fewer spontaneous arousals in infants with apparent life-threatening event. *Sleep.* 2011;34:733–743.

22. Kato I, Franco P, Groswasser J, Scaillet S, Kelmanson I, Togari H, et al. Incomplete arousal processes in infants who were victims of sudden death. *Am J Respir Crit Care Med.* 2003;168:1298–1303.

23. Miano S, Castaldo R, Ferri R, Peraita-Adrados R, Paolino MC, Montesano M, et al. Sleep cyclic alternating pattern analysis in infants with apparent life-threatening events: A daytime poly-somnographic study. *Clin Neurophysiol.* 2012;123:1346–1352.

24. Davies F, Gupta R. Apparent life threatening events in infants presenting to an emergency department. *Emerg Med J.* 2002;19:11–16.

25. Gray C, Davies F, Molyneux E. Apparent life-threatening events presenting to a pediatric emergency department. *Pediatr Emerg Care.* 1999;15:195–199.

26. Sahewalla R, Gupta D, Kamat D. Apparent Life-Threatening Events: An Overview. *Clin Pediatr (Phila).* 2016;55:5–9.

27. Al-Kindy HA, Gelinas JF, Hatzakis G, Cote A. Risk factors for extreme events in infants hospitalized for apparent life-threatening events. *J Pediatr.* 2009;154:332–337. 7.e1–e2.

28. Tieder JS, Cowan CA, Garrison MM, Christakis DA. Variation in inpatient resource utilization and management of apparent life-threatening events. *J Pediatr.* 2008;152:629–635. 35.e1–e2.

29. Mittal MK, Sun G, Baren JM. A clinical decision rule to identify infants with apparent life-threatening event who can be safely discharged from the emergency department. *Pediatr Emerg Care.* 2012;28:599–605.

30. DiMario Jr. FJ. Apparent life-threatening events: So what happens next? *Pediatrics.* 2008;122:190–191.

31. Myerberg DZ, Carpenter RG, Myerberg CF, Britton CM, Bailey CW, Fink BE. Reducing postneonatal mortality in West Virginia: A statewide intervention program targeting risk identified at and after birth. *Am J Public Health.* 1995;85:631–637.

32. Southall DP, Plunkett MC, Banks MW, Falkov AF, Samuels MP. Covert video recordings of life-threatening child abuse: Lessons for child protection. *Pediatrics.* 1997;100:735–760.

33. Al Khushi N, Cote A. Apparent life-threatening events: Assessment, risks, reality. *Paediatr Respir Rev.* 2011;12:124–132.

34. Laisne C, Rimet Y, Poujol A, Cornus P, Courcier D, Coze C, et al. [Apropos of 100 cases of malaise in infants]. *Ann Pediatr (Paris).* 1989;36:451–454.

35. Tal Y, Tirosh E, Even L, Jaffe M. A comparison of the yield of a 24 h versus 72 h hospital evaluation in infants with apparent life-threatening events. *Eur J Pediatr.* 1999;158:954.

36. Veereman-Wauters G, Bochner A, Van Caillie-Bertrand M. Gastroesophageal reflux in infants with a history of near-miss sudden infant death. *J Pediatr Gastroenterol Nutr.* 1991;12:319–323.

37. Tsukada K, Kosuge N, Hosokawa M, Umezu R, Murata M. Etiology of 19 infants with apparent life-threatening events: Relationship between apnea and esophageal dysfunction. *Acta Paediatr Jpn.* 1993;35:306–310.

38. Sheikh S, Stephen T, Frazer A, Eid N. Apparent life-threatening episodes in infants. *Clin Pulm Med.* 2000;7:81–84.

39. Bonkowsky JL, Guenther E, Filloux FM, Srivastava R. Death, child abuse, and adverse neurological outcome of infants after an apparent life-threatening event. *Pediatrics.* 2008;122:125–131.

40. Altman RL, Brand DA, Forman S, Kutscher ML, Lowenthal DB, Franke KA, et al. Abusive head injury as a cause of apparent life-threatening events in infancy. *Arch Pediatr Adolesc Med.* 2003;157:1011–1015.

41. Pitetti RD, Maffei F, Chang K, Hickey R, Berger R, Pierce MC. Prevalence of retinal hemorrhages and child abuse in children who present with an apparent life-threatening event. *Pediatrics.* 2002;110:557–562.

42. Jenny C, Hymel KP, Ritzen A, Reinert SE, Hay TC. Analysis of missed cases of abusive head trauma. *JAMA.* 1999;281:621–626.

43. Scollan-Koliopoulos M, Koliopoulos JS. Evaluation and management of apparent life-threatening events in infants. *Pediatr Nurs.* 2010;36:77–83. quiz 4.

44. Semmekrot BA, van Sleuwen BE, Engelberts AC, Joosten KF, Mulder JC, Liem KD, et al. Surveillance study of apparent life-threatening events (ALTE) in the Netherlands. *Eur J Pediatr.* 2010;169:229–236.

45. Carroll JL. Apparent life threatening event (ALTE) assessment. *Pediatr Pulmonol Suppl.* 2004;26:108–109.

46. Poets A, Steinfeldt R, Poets CF. Sudden deaths and severe apparent life-threatening events in term infants within 24 hours of birth. *Pediatrics.* 2011;127:e869–e873.

47. Poets A, Urschitz MS, Steinfeldt R, Poets CF. Risk factors for early sudden deaths and severe apparent life-threatening events. *Arch Dis Child Fetal Neonatal Ed.* 2012;97:F395–F397.

48. Andres V, Garcia P, Rimet Y, Nicaise C, Simeoni U. Apparent life-threatening events in presumably healthy newborns during early skin-to-skin contact. *Pediatrics.* 2011;127:e1073–e1076.

49. Dageville C, Pignol J, De Smet S. Very early neonatal apparent life-threatening events and sudden unexpected deaths: Incidence and risk factors. *Acta Paediatr.* 2008;97:866–869.

50. Pejovic NJ, Herlenius E. Unexpected collapse of healthy newborn infants: Risk factors, supervision and hypothermia treatment. *Acta Paediatr.* 2013;102680–628.

51. Burgmann DM, Foerster K, Klemme M, Delius M, Hubener C, Wisskott R, et al. Delivery room desaturations and bradycardia in the early postnatal period of healthy term neonates – A prospective observational study. *J Matern Fetal Neonatal Med.* 2020:1–5.

52. Hall KL, Zalman B. Evaluation and management of apparent life-threatening events in children. *Am Fam Physician.* 2005;71:2301–2308.

53. Brand DA, Altman RL, Purtill K, Edwards KS. Yield of diagnostic testing in infants who have had an apparent life-threatening event. *Pediatrics.* 2005;115:885–893.

54. Dewolfe CC. Apparent life-threatening event: A review. *Pediatr Clin North Am.* 2005;52:1127–1146. ix.

55. Fu LY, Moon RY. Apparent life-threatening events: An update. *Pediatr Rev.* 2012;33:361–368. quiz 8–9.

56. De Piero AD, Teach SJ, Chamberlain JM. ED evaluation of infants after an apparent life-threatening event. *Am J Emerg Med.* 2004;22:83–86.

57. Reix P, St-Hilaire M, Praud JP. Laryngeal sensitivity in the neonatal period: From bench to bedside. *Pediatr Pulmonol.* 2007;42:674–682.

58. Pitetti RD, Whitman E, Zaylor A. Accidental and nonaccidental poisonings as a cause of apparent life-threatening events in infants. *Pediatrics.* 2008;122:e359–e362.

59. Campbell KA, Berger RP, Ettaro L, Roberts MS. Cost-effectiveness of head computed tomography in infants with possible inflicted traumatic brain injury. *Pediatrics.* 2007;120:295–304.

60. Vellody K, Freeto JP, Gage SL, Collins N, Gershan WM. Clues that aid in the diagnosis of nonaccidental trauma presenting as an apparent life-threatening event. *Clin Pediatr (Phila).* 2008;47:912–918.

61. Guenther E, Powers A, Srivastava R, Bonkowsky JL. Abusive head trauma in children presenting with an apparent life-threatening event. *J Pediatr.* 2010;157:821–825.

62. Oren J, Kelly D, Shannon DC. Identification of a high-risk group for sudden infant death syndrome among infants who were resuscitated for sleep apnea. *Pediatrics.* 1986;77:495–499.

63. Santiago-Burruchaga M, Sanchez-Etxaniz J, Benito-Fernandez J, Vazquez-Cordero C, Mintegi-Raso S, Labayru-Echeverria M, et al. Assessment and management of infants with apparent life-threatening events in the paediatric emergency department. *Eur J Emerg Med.* 2008;15:203–208.

64. Claudius I, Keens T. Do all infants with apparent life-threatening events need to be admitted? *Pediatrics.* 2007;119:679–683.

65. Cote A. Home and hospital monitoring for ALTE. *Paediatr Respir Rev.* 2006;7(Suppl 1):S199–S201.

66. Ramanathan R, Corwin MJ, Hunt CE, Lister G, Tinsley LR, Baird T, et al. Cardiorespiratory events recorded on home monitors: Comparison of healthy infants with those at increased risk for SIDS. *JAMA.* 2001;285:2199–2207.

67. Cote A, Hum C, Brouillette RT, Themens M. Frequency and timing of recurrent events in infants using home cardiorespiratory monitors. *J Pediatr.* 1998;132:783–789.

68. Poets CF, Samuels MP, Noyes JP, Hewertson J, Hartmann H, Holder A, et al. Home event recordings of oxygenation, breathing movements, and heart rate and rhythm in infants with recurrent life-threatening events. *J Pediatr.* 1993;123:693–701.

69. Ramgopal S, Noorbakhsh KA, Callaway CW, Wilson PM, Pitetti RD. Changes in the management of children with brief resolved unexplained events (BRUEs). *Pediatrics.* 2019:144.

70. Colombo M, Katz ES, Bosco A, Melzi ML, Nosetti L. Brief resolved unexplained events: Retrospective validation of diagnostic criteria and risk stratification. *Pediatr Pulmonol.* 2019;54:61–65.

71. Sethi A, Baxi K, Cheng D, Laffey S, Hartman N, Heller K. Impact of guidelines regarding brief resolved unexplained events on care of patients in a pediatric emergency department. *Pediatr Emerg Care.* 2021;37:31468–e1472.

72. Oglesbee SJ, Roberts MH, Sapien RE. Implementing lower-risk brief resolved unexplained events guideline reduces admissions in a modelled population. *J Eval Clin Pract.* 2020;26:343–356.

73. Patra KP, Hall M, DeLaroche AM, Tieder JS. Impact of the AAP Guideline on Management of Brief Resolved Unexplained Events. *Hosp Pediatr.* 2022;12:780–791.

74. Ramgopal S, Colgan JY, Roland D, Pitetti RD, Katsogridakis Y. Brief resolved unexplained events: A new diagnosis, with implications for evaluation and management. *Eur J Pediatr.* 2022;181:463–470.

75. Gerber NL, Fawcett KJ, Weber EG, Patel R, Glick AF, Farkas JS, et al. Brief resolved unexplained event: Not just a new name for apparent life-threatening event. *Pediatr Emerg Care.* 2021;37:e1439–e1443.

76. Evers KS, Wellmann S, Donner BC, Ritz N. Apparent life-threatening events and brief resolved unexplained events: Management of children at a Swiss tertiary care center. *Swiss Med Wkly.* 2021;151:w30026.

77. Brand DA, Fazzari MJ. Risk of death in infants who have experienced a brief resolved unexplained event: A meta-analysis. *J Pediatr.* 2018;197:63–67.

25

Primary Snoring

Sonal Malhotra and Susanna A. McColley

CHAPTER HIGHLIGHTS

This chapter reviews primary snoring (PS), also called simple or habitual snoring. PS is diagnosed when snoring is not associated with apnea, hypopnea, respiratory effort-related arousals (RERAs), gas-exchange abnormalities, sleep disruptions, or daytime impairment. Thus, polysomnography (PSG) is required for diagnosis. Because there are no universal criteria for diagnosing, is it challenging to understand the true prevalence of the condition or its clinical impact in children. This chapter highlights considerations in diagnosis and management.

Primary Snoring

Snoring is noise produced during inspiration, and occasionally expiration, from the vibration of the soft tissues of the oropharyngeal walls that occurs because of changes in the configuration and muscle tone of the upper airway during sleep (Figs. 25.1 and 25.2). Snoring is the most common, and sometimes the only, presenting symptom of sleep-disordered breathing (SDB). A spectrum of SDB exists and is viewed on a continuum of severity based on the degree of upper airway narrowing and characterized on polysomnography (PSG) by apneas, hypopneas, respiratory effort-related arousals (RERAs), arousals, and gas exchange abnormalities. The spectrum ranges from primary snoring (PS) to upper airway resistance syndrome (UARS) to obstructive sleep apnea syndrome (OSAS).

PS, also referred to as simple or habitual snoring, is not associated with episodes of apnea, hypopnea, RERAs, hypoxemia, hypercapnia, sleep disruption or daytime impairment (daytime sleepiness/fatigue, inattentiveness or other related symptoms).[1] In children with habitual snoring, it is essential to discriminate PS from OSAS so that appropriate treatment and follow-up can be provided. It can be particularly difficult to assess neuropsychologic symptoms in young children who are rapidly developing. The diagnosis of PS is made by polysomnographic criteria with objective measurement of sleep and respiratory function, as clinical history alone cannot differentiate PS from OSAS.[2]

In a study of 83 snoring children referred to a tertiary pediatric sleep clinic, parents completed a standardized, nurse-administered questionnaire that asked questions regarding snoring frequency, observed apnea, struggling to breathe, and other daytime and nighttime symptoms. Children then underwent nocturnal PSG to assess for SDB. Although there were several differences in symptom frequencies between the children with PS and those with OSAS, both single and multiple questions showed poor sensitivity and specificity in differentiating PS and OSAS. Other studies demonstrate a similar inability of clinical history to differentiate PS from OSAS.[3–8]

Upper Airway Resistance Syndrome

The polysomnographic findings consistent with PS suggests that it is a benign condition because there are no aberrations in gas exchange abnormalities or sleep architecture. The definition also requires that the child has no adverse sleep-related or daytime sequelae. Because snoring affects approximately 10% of children, the presence of snoring without consequence is likely to occur. However, the original descriptions of PS occurred before the description of UARS, which was first reported by Guilleminault et al., in 1993.[9] To this day, the *International Classification of Sleep Disorders* still does not define UARS as its own distinct entity and reports UARS under the diagnosis of OSAS.[1] The lack of standardization in PSG measurement techniques and diagnostic criteria for UARS make it challenging to interpret the literature, and some children previously characterized as having PS may have actually had UARS.

UARS has been described as partial upper airway obstruction that is not associated with gas exchange abnormalities but is accompanied by repetitive RERAs (initially measured by changes in intrathoracic pressure via esophageal manometry) and responds positively to treatment in the same manner as OSAS.[10] Snoring occurs in most affected individuals, but physiologic findings of UARS have been noted in patients without snoring, particularly in those who have had palatal surgery for upper airway obstruction. UARS is associated with increased upper airway collapsibility during sleep.[11] Guilleminault and colleagues reported the clinical and polysomnographic (PSG) characteristics of UARS in 25 children who were referred for snoring, excessive daytime somnolence, and behavioral problems.[12] They demonstrated marked difference in the referred group compared with

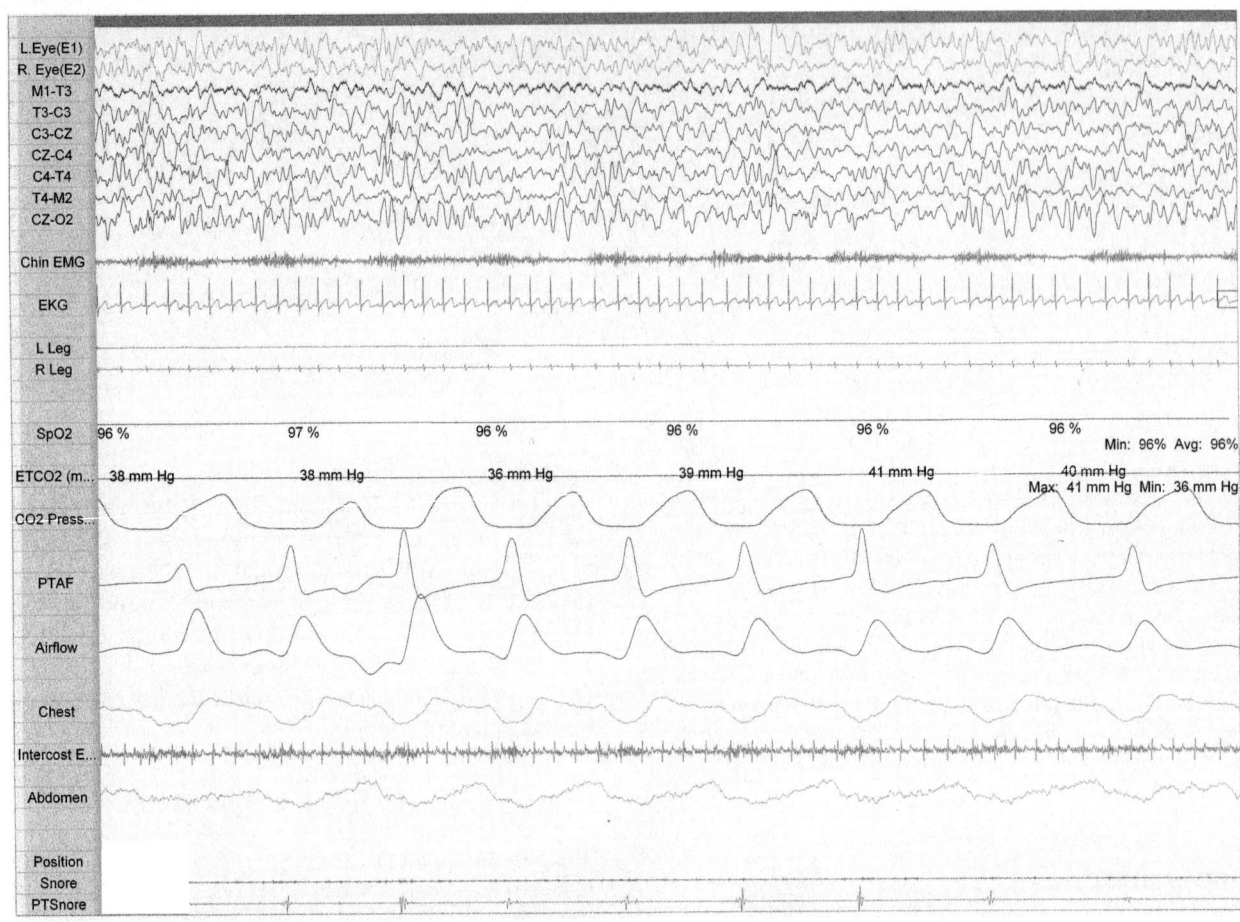

• **Fig. 25.1** Thirty-second epoch in N3 sleep from a 4-year-old girl referred for evaluation of snoring. Note the presence of snore artifact present in the chin electromyograph. This epoch demonstrates primary snoring without classic changes on electroencephalograph suggestive of an arousal.

25 healthy control children. Subsequently, numerous studies have demonstrated these PSG findings of UARS in adults with daytime somnolence. Daytime somnolence in adults with UARS is significantly improved with nasal continuous positive airway pressure therapy, as objectively measured by the multiple sleep latency test.[13]

In adults, excessive daytime somnolence has a number of significant sequelae, including an increased risk of motor vehicle and work-related accidents and impaired mood. Hypertension is also frequently seen in adults with UARS. Children identified as having UARS have a variety of daytime symptoms, including symptoms of attention-deficit/hyperactivity disorder (ADHD) and academic problems. Most studies of snoring have not defined or described UARS as a distinct clinical entity, and the true prevalence of UARS is unknown.[10] However, studies now suggest significant neurocognitive abnormalities in children with habitual snoring occur, including ADHD, academic problems, and behavior problems.[14–16] Children with polysomnographically confirmed PS may demonstrate reduced neurocognitive capabilities, particularly in the domains of attention, memory, and intelligence,[17] and decreased performance in several measures of language and visuospatial ability.[18]

Available data, however, do not allow clear separation between patients with UARS and those with OSAS.

Although sleep physiologists often view SDB as a spectrum with PS being the mildest and OSAS the most severe form, no studies demonstrate a clear relationship between the degree of SDB and symptoms or physiologic sequelae. The diagnosis of PS has traditionally been made on the basis of polysomnographic findings and requires the absence of daytime somnolence/fatigue. This definition does not account for those children with PS who may demonstrate daytime symptoms in the form of habitual mouth breathing or a dry mouth, symptoms that might reduce quality of life.[19,20] Additionally, no universal criteria for PS exists in the literature, making it impossible to understand the true impact of PS. This was shown in a review article by De Meyer et al., which reviewed past literature to investigate definitions used for PS in research practices. Although 29 out of the 30 selected papers actually defined PS in their manuscripts, definitions were inconsistent, with some including varying apnea-hypopnea index (AHI) thresholds (most often with an AHI >5), and others added inclusion criteria such as body mass index (BMI) and acoustical metrics.[21]

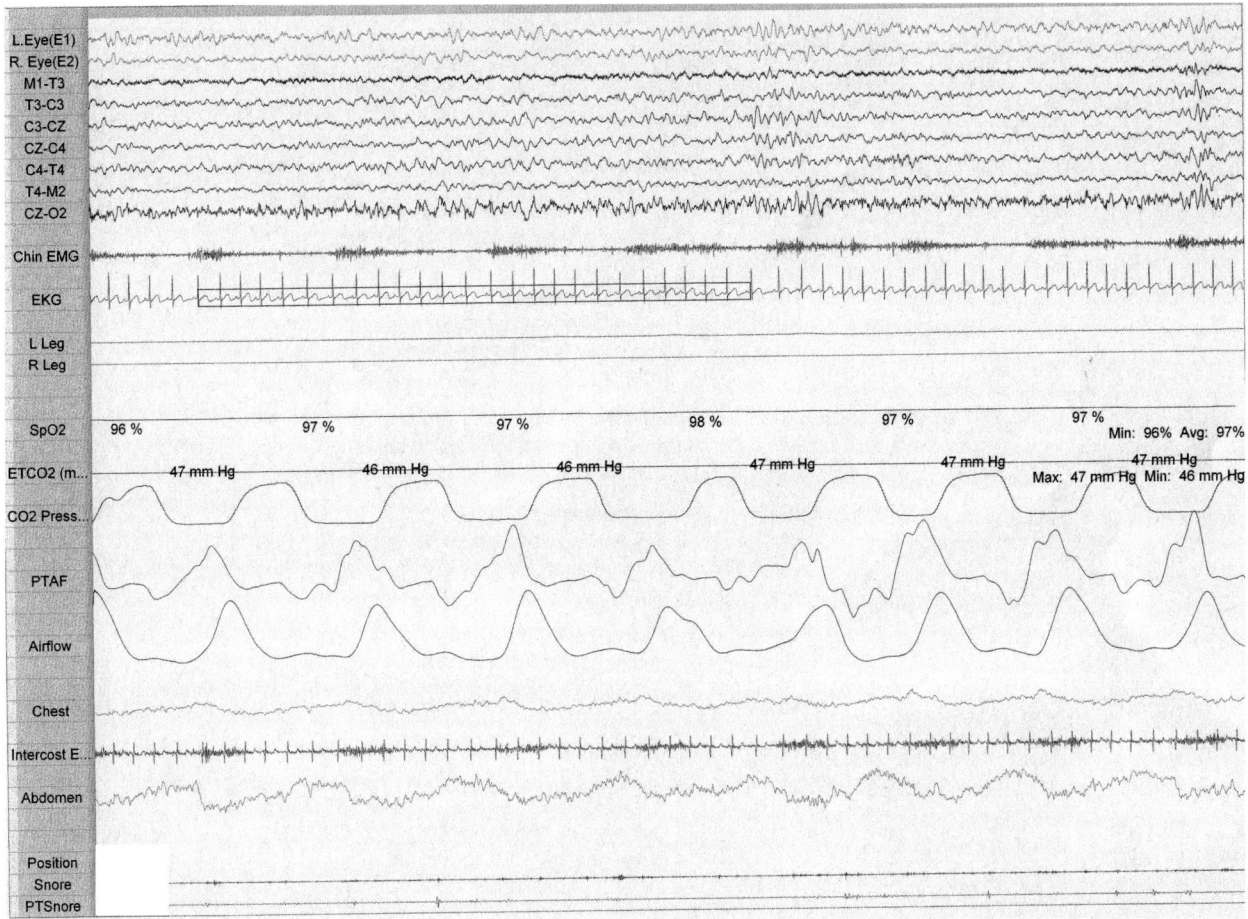

• **Fig. 25.2** Thirty-second epoch in N2 sleep from the same 4-year-old girl as in Fig. 25.1. Snore artifact is again noted in the chin electromyograph. However, theta bursts are associated with the snoring, suggestive of arousal and upper airway resistance.

Epidemiology

A number of epidemiologic studies from diverse populations and geographic locations have been published describing the prevalence of snoring in children. Most of these have used parental report by way of either questionnaire or interview format. Most have not included objective measurements of respiration during sleep, or they have included such measures on only a subset of children felt to be at high risk for OSAS. Additionally, there is no universally accepted, clear definition of snoring. Thus the prevalence of the condition may differ based on varying interpretations of the term "snoring" across cultures.[10]

A summary of representative epidemiologic studies of snoring in children is presented in Table 25.1. A recent meta-analysis by Lumeng and Chervin suggests the overall prevalence, as reported by parents, is 7.45%,[10] in contrast to the 40% frequency of regular snoring in adults. The same authors reported that the prevalence of habitual snoring ranges from a minimum of 2.4% in Turkey to a maximum of 34.5% in Italy. Within the same meta-analysis, the prevalence of OSAS is from 0.1% to 13%. The study presenting the prevalence of OSAS as 13% is a significant outlier,

with the diagnosis of OSAS based on oxygen desaturation index rather than standard measures. Excluding the 13%, the prevalence of OSAS ranges from 0.1% to 5.7%. None of these epidemiologic studies has attempted to distinguish UARS from PS. Rosen[22] studied 326 otherwise healthy children with snoring. Fifty-nine percent of the children had OSAS, 25% had PS, 6% had UARS, and 10% experienced no snoring. It is notable that 28% of the children in the study were obese. Racial and ethnic differences also contribute to varying prevalence of snoring in a given population.[7]

Natural History

Limited and inconsistent data are available regarding the natural history of PS in children. In 1998, Marcus and coworkers repeated PSG in 20 children 1–3 years after the initial diagnosis of PS.[36] All of these children had persistent snoring; in 20% snoring had increased, and in 70% there had been no change. Overall, there was no significant change in apnea index, oxyhemoglobin saturation, or peak end-tidal PCO_2. However, two children had mild OSAS on repeat testing. The authors concluded that most children

TABLE
25.1 **Epidemiology of Snoring in Children**

First Author (Year)	Number (Age Range)	Country	Methods*	Habitual Snoring† Prevalence	OSAS Prevalence
Corbo (1989)[23]	1,615 (6–13 yr)	Italy	Self-administered questionnaire	7.3%	Not examined
Teculescu (1992)[24]	190 (5–6.4 yr)	France	Interview questionnaire	10%	Not examined
Ali (1993)[25]	782 (4–5 yr)	England	Postal questionnaire; home overnight video and oximetry in a subset of "high risk" and control	12.1%	0.7%
Ali (1994)[26]	504 (7–10 yr)	England	Follow-up study of children in preceding study; repeat postal questionnaire only	11.4%	Not examined
Gislason (1995)[27]	454 (6 mo–6 yr)	Iceland	Postal questionnaire; overnight respiratory monitoring in children suspected of having sleep apnea	3.2%	2.9%
Hultcrantz (1995)[28]	500 (4 yr)	Sweden	Interview; PSG in children with habitual snoring	6.2%	Data incomplete
Smedje (1999)[29]	1,844 (5–7 yr)	Sweden	Self-administered questionnaire	7.7%	Not examined
Ferreira (2000)[30]	976 (6–11 yr)	Portugal	Self-administered questionnaire	8.6%	Not examined
Corbo (2001)[31]	2,209 (10–15 yr)	Italy	Self-administered questionnaire	5.6%	Not examined
Anuntaseree (2001)[32]	1,008 (6–13 yr)	Thailand	Self-administered questionnaire; PSG in patients snoring "most nights"	8.5%	0.7%
Zhang (2004)[33]	996 (4–12 yr)	Australia	Self-administered questionnaire	15.2%	Not examined
Tafur (2009)[34]	1,193 (6–12 yr)	Ecuador	Self-administered questionnaire	15.1%	Not examined
Li (2010)[35]	6,349 (5–14 yr)	China	Self-administered questionnaire	7.2%	Not examined
Goldstein (2011)[7]	346 (2–6 yr)	United States	Self-administered questionnaire	13.9%	Not examined

*All questionnaire and interview data were obtained from parents.
†Habitual snoring is defined as frequent or nightly snoring, or snoring ≥3 nights per week, in the absence of upper respiratory infection.
OSAS, Obstructive sleep apnea syndrome; *PSG*, polysomnography.

with PS do not progress to having OSAS, and those who do progress have only mild OSAS. Daytime symptoms in persistently snoring children were not reported.

Two additional studies had similar findings as Marcus and coworkers with cohorts of 31 and 9 children each, with a diagnosis of PS. Repeat PSG evaluations among these children with PS were obtained after 6 months and 3 years, respectively, and both studies concluded that PS in children does not evolve to OSAS over time.[37,38] Although Topol and Brooks found no overall changes in respiratory parameters in the nine children they studied with PS, the control group in this study had significantly better sleep efficiency and fewer brief arousals than the snoring group.[37] This suggests that some of the children diagnosed with PS may actually have had UARS. Urschitz and colleagues presented similar findings from a large-scale questionnaire-based study of 1,144 preschool children in Germany who were followed over a

1-year period.[20] At the 1-year follow-up, 48.8% of the former habitual snorers still reported snoring, with associated risk factors including decreased maternal education, the presence of a smoker in the household, loud snoring, and surgical intervention for snoring since the initial survey.[20]

In contrast to the above-mentioned studies, Albert et al., evaluated 70 children, aged 6–13 years, with an initial diagnosis of PS by PSG. Repeat PSG at their 4-year follow-up showed 26 children had progressed to OSA (obstructive apnea hypopnea index [OAHI] >1), out of which five children had moderate-to-severe disease (OAHI ≥5). Although 18 of the 70 total subjects had complete resolution of their snoring with normal PSG, 22 children remained at PS. In this study, PS had a high sensitivity (87.5%) and negative predictive value but showed poor specificity (45.2%) and positive predictive value when evaluating progression from PS to OSA. Even after adjusting for age, sex, persistently large tonsils, and persistent snoring, only the presence of persistent overweight/obesity was found to be associated with the progression of PS to OSA.[39] Therefore it should be noted that patients with PS may be at risk for developing OSAS over time.

Although some children with PS demonstrate resolution of their symptoms, Gozal and Pope demonstrated that a "learning debt" may develop in children who snore during early childhood.[16] In this large survey-based study, children in the bottom quartile of their seventh- or eighth-grade class were more likely to have snored during early childhood (odds ratio 2.79, confidence interval 1.88–4.15) and required a tonsillectomy for snoring as compared with the top-performing quartile members of their class. The authors suggested that children who experienced SDB during a period traditionally associated with major brain growth and substantial acquisition of cognitive and intellectual capabilities may in part undermine their capacity for future academic achievement.

These findings are consistent with the Urschitz et al. study where they evaluated 1,144 children who were habitual snorers and found evidence of impaired behavior. Pulse oximetry was used to access for intermittent hypoxia, parental questionnaire was used to evaluate for impaired behavior, and school performance was based on school report. There was a significant association between hyperactivity and inattentive behavior with daytime tiredness and sleepiness in children with habitual snoring, independent of intermittent hypoxemia. On follow-up, inattentive behavior and hyperactivity had significantly improved once PS had ceased.[40] Furthermore, recent studies suggest snoring status should be carefully analyzed regardless of AHI measures, as even occasional snoring is a predictor for adverse behavioral outcomes.[41]

Although there is increasing evidence that neurocognitive impairments are more frequent in children with PS when compared with children who have never snored, the underlying mechanism that explains the association remains not well understood. Intermittent hypoxia is an important contributing factor in children with OSA, but, by definition, this is absent in children with PS. Some postulate a combination of arousals, sleep fragmentation, and sleep disruption to play a vital role in PS.

Along with the potential long-term neurologic effects of PS, cardiovascular disturbances may be associated with PS. Studies of blood pressure (BP) abnormalities in children with PS give conflicting results. Kwok et al., demonstrated significantly increased systolic, diastolic and mean BP in 30 children with PS as compared with healthy controls matched by age, sex, and body size.[42] The TuCASA Study, a community-based sample of 239 non-Hispanic White and Hispanic preadolescent children, demonstrated an association between SDB, as diagnosed by unattended home PSG, and elevated BP.[43] Kaditis et al.[44] and Amin et al.[45] demonstrated no association between SDB and BP. Each of these studies had design limitations.

Li and colleagues[46] evaluated 190 children aged 6–13 years via overnight attended PSG and ambulatory BP monitoring. Systolic BP, diastolic BP, and mean arterial pressure were significantly increased in snoring subjects with PS as compared with healthy controls. As the severity of SDB increased, BP abnormalities worsened. Particularly notable was the increase in nocturnal diastolic BP in children with PS, which the authors attributed to an increase in sympathetic tone, similar to what is seen in OSAS. The authors conclude by stating that PS should no longer be considered entirely benign. Furthermore, there are now data to suggest that growth hormone secretion is impaired in children with PS,[47] illustrating a point made by Guilleminault and Lee: "chronic regular snoring always has had a health impact when we have investigated a child appropriately."[48]

Diagnosis

History and Physical Examination

A sleep history that includes questions regarding nocturnal snoring should be included in health maintenance and well-child care visits.[49] The hallmark of PS is nightly or near-nightly snoring without physiologic or neurologic consequences. Verifying the latter, however, may be difficult without objective neuropsychologic testing. Once a history of habitual snoring is elicited, additional history taking and physical examination serve to assess sleep-related or daytime symptoms that may be associated with significant upper airway obstruction during sleep. The sleep history should include questions about labored breathing during sleep, observed apnea, restless sleep, diaphoresis, enuresis, cyanosis, and behavioral or learning problems. A history of recurrent otitis media or tympanostomy tube placement may suggest habitual snoring.[50] A history of allergic rhinitis, wheezing, tonsillitis within the last 12 months, maternal education, atopy, and a parent with habitual snoring are risk factors for habitual snoring and should be identified.[20,23,51] An environmental history should be solicited for environmental tobacco smoke exposure and other particulate matter as air pollutants are associated with snoring.[50,51] Children who have numerous episodes of observed obstructive apnea, daytime somnolence, and problems with behavior, attention, or school performance require prompt referral for diagnostic testing and treatment for SDB.

The physical examination may be normal, or it may reveal signs of upper airway obstruction such as mouth breathing and tonsillar hypertrophy. Dolichocephaly and midface hypoplasia are associated with snoring and OSAS. Obesity is a predisposing factor to both snoring and OSAS, whereas growth failure may signify severe SDB.

Nocturnal Polysomnography

PS is currently defined by polysomnographic criteria. In scenarios where PS may be the only diagnosis on standard polysomnographic evaluation, it is important to note that habitual snorers are at increased risk for developing disease-related problems. A recent study compared sleep spindle activity, a marker of maturation of the thalamocortical regulatory pathways, in 20 children with PS and 20 age- and gender-matched PSG-confirmed nonsnoring controls. Children with PS exhibited significantly lower spindle activity when compared with their healthy counterparts.[52] This indicates there may be microstructural changes caused by disruption and fragmentation of sleep as a consequence of PS. The process underlying sleep spindles has been hypothesized to benefit cognitive function and has potential to be a neurobiologic indicator for level of cognitive development.[53] These findings reinforce that PS is not a benign diagnosis, and we must look beyond respiratory indices such as apneas, hypopneas, and RERAs when evaluating for SDB.

When differentiating PS from OSAS or UARS it is important to carefully evaluate sleep staging and the frequency of electroencephalographic (EEG) arousals. PS has shown impaired sleep architecture, including higher wake after sleep onset and N1 sleep in pubertal adolescents when compared with nonsnorers and lower percentage of rapid eye movement (REM) sleep in children who snore.[18,54] Although the gold standard for diagnosis of UARS is measurement of esophageal pressure, this technique is invasive. Other techniques have been evaluated but are not in widespread clinical use. There is evidence, however, suggesting the flattening of nasal pressure signal may be a useful tool in identifying upper airway resistance.

Additionally, no universal criteria for PS exists in the literature, making it impossible to understand the true impact of PS. This was shown in a review article by De Meyer et al., which reviewed past literature to investigate definitions used for PS in research practices. Although 29 out of the 30 selected papers actually defined PS in their manuscripts, definitions were inconsistent, with some including varying AHI thresholds (most often with an AHI >5), and others added inclusion criteria such as BMI and acoustical metrics.[21] The diagnosis of UARS is suggested by the presence of frequent arousals during the night.

A diagnosis of UARS should not be dependent only on the presence of visual EEG changes. Sophisticated assessments demonstrate sympathetic surges, EEG spectral power or cyclic alternating pattern score may change in the absence of typical EEG changes suggestive of an arousal.[55–57] Careful interpretation of the PSG is necessary to appreciate these changes and distinguish between PS and UARS. An otherwise asymptomatic snorer who has a normal PSG is diagnosed with PS. Normal cardiorespiratory function with frequent arousals is consistent with UARS. We propose that a child with normal PSG findings and abnormal daytime symptoms be given a working diagnosis of UARS, and treatment should be considered.

Treatment

Although PS is considered a benign condition, many studies have questioned this assumption and affected children should be reevaluated if symptoms, including learning or behavioral issues, increase over time. Historically, there have been no treatment recommended for children with PS, but one study looked at 248 children with PS defined by snoring and an AHI <3 events per hour of sleep with no evidence of increased work of breathing. Telephone interviews, age of interviewees at that time, and mean BMI Z-scores were recorded for later PSG. They compared data from children who did not undergo surgery ($N = 184$) with those who underwent surgery ($N = 64$) for SDB, finding that many of the untreated children had persistent SDB symptoms up to 5 years after the initial diagnosis. More importantly, 35% of those children with PS had symptoms of inattention/hyperactive behavior and sleepiness. Snoring duration was the most important factor linking them to long-term outcomes. In comparison, children who underwent surgery for PS had better outcomes including lower scores for sleepiness and inattention/behavioral subscales.[58] This study further supports the notion that pediatric SDB is a spectrum, and individual treatment such as weight management, household smoking cessation, and surgical options must be considered for patients based on their individual symptoms and physical findings, not on PSG findings alone.

Future Directions

Further studies of snoring in children are needed. The wide variability in published prevalence may be secondary to the influence of ethnicity and environment in different populations; further definition of prevalence differences would be useful in identifying patients at risk and in public health policy decisions. Better definition of the clinical consequences of snoring, and specific comparisons between patients with PS and those with UARS, are needed. Given the current, but limited, evidence of the long-term sequelae of snoring in children, more prospective studies are necessary to better identify and treat at-risk children.

CLINICAL PEARLS

- Snoring is the most common presenting symptom of SDB in children.
- A spectrum of snoring exists, ranging from PS to UARS to OSAS.
- History alone cannot distinguish PS from OSAS.
- Careful evaluation and treatment of snoring in children is necessary to avoid long-term sequelae.

References

1. American Academy of Sleep Medicine. *International Classification of Sleep Disorders*. 3rd ed. American Academy of Sleep Medicine; 2014.
2. Carroll JL, McColley SA, Marcus CL, et al. Inability of clinical history to distinguish primary snoring from obstructive sleep apnea syndrome in children. *Chest*. 1995;108:610–618.
3. Suen JS, Arnold JE, Brooks LJ. Adenotonsillectomy for treatment of obstructive sleep apnea in children. *Arch Otolaryngol Head Neck Surg*. 1995;121:525–530.

4. Nieminen P, Tolonen U, Lopponen H, et al. Snoring children: factors predicting sleep apnea. *Acta Otolaryngol Suppl.* 1997;529:190–194.

5. Leach J, Olson J, Hermann J, et al. Polysomnographic and clinical findings in children with obstructive sleep apnea. *Arch Otolaryngol Head Neck Surg.* 1992;118(7):741–744.

6. Wang RC, Elkins TP, Keech D, et al. Accuracy of clinical evaluation in pediatric obstructive sleep apnea. *Otolaryngol Head Neck Surg.* 1998;118:69–73.

7. Goldstein NA, Abramowitz T, Weedon J, et al. Racial/ethnic differences in the prevalence of snoring and sleep disordered breathing in young children. *J Clin Sleep Med.* 2011;7(2):163–171.

8. Spruyt K, Gozal D. Screening of pediatric sleep-disordered breathing: a proposed unbiased discriminative set of questions using clinical severity scales. *Chest.* 2012;142(6):1508.

9. Guilleminault C, Stoohs R, Clerk A, Cetel M, Maistros P. A cause of excessive daytime sleepiness. The upper airway resistance syndrome. *Chest.* 1993;104:781–787.

10. Lumeng JC, Chervin RD. Epidemiology of pediatric obstructive sleep apnea. *Proc Am Thorac Soc.* 2008;5:242–252.

11. Gold AR, Marcus CL, et al. Upper airway collapsibility during sleep in upper airway resistance syndrome. *Chest.* 2002;121:1531–1540.

12. Guilleminault C, Winkle R, Korobkin K, et al. Children and nocturnal snoring: evaluation of the effects of sleep related respiratory resistive load and daytime functioning. *Eur J Pediatr.* 1982;139:165–171.

13. Exar EN, Collop NA. The upper airway resistance syndrome. *Chest.* 1999;115:1127–1139.

14. Chervin R, Dillon J, Bassetti C, et al. Symptoms of sleep disorders, inattention, and hyperactivity in children. *Sleep.* 1997;20:1185–1192.

15. Gozal D. Sleep-disordered breathing and school performance in children. *Pediatrics.* 1998;102:616–620.

16. Gozal D, Pope Jr. DW. Snoring during early childhood and academic performance at ages 13–14 years. *Pediatrics.* 2001;107:1394–1399.

17. Blunden S, Lushington K, Kennedy D, et al. Behavior and neurocognitive performance in children aged 5–10 years who snore compared to controls. *J Clin Exp Neuropsychol.* 2000;22(5):554–568.

18. O'Brien LM, Mervis CB, Holbrook CR, et al. Neurobehavioral implications of habitual snoring in children. *Pediatrics.* 2004;114:44–49.

19. Ng DK, Chow PY, Kwok KL, et al. An update on childhood snoring. *Acta Paediatr.* 2006;95(9):1029–1035.

20. Urschitz MS, Guenther A, Eitner S, et al. Risk factors and natural history of habitual snoring. *Chest.* 2004;126:790–800.

21. De Meyer MMD, Jacquet W, Vanderveken OM, Marks LAM. Systematic review of the different aspects of primary snoring. *Sleep Med Rev.* 2019;45:88–94.

22. Rosen CL. Clinical features of obstructive sleep apnea in otherwise healthy children. *Pediatr Pulmonol.* 1999;27:403–409.

23. Corbo GM, Fuciarelli F, Foresi A, et al. Snoring in children: association with respiratory symptoms and passive smoking. *BMJ.* 1989;299:1491–1494.

24. Teculescu D, Caillier I, Perrin P, et al. Snoring in French preschool children. *Pediatr Pulmonol.* 1992;13:239–244.

25. Ali NJ, Pitson DJ, Stradling JR. Snoring, sleep disturbance, and behavior in 4–5-year-olds. *Arch Dis Child.* 1993;68:360–366.

26. Ali NJ, Pitson D, Stradling JR. Natural history of snoring and related behaviour problems between the ages of 4 and 7 years. *Arch Dis Child.* 1994;71:74–76.

27. Gislason T, Benediktsdottir B. Snoring apneic episodes and nocturnal hypoxemia among children 6 months to 6 years old. *Chest.* 1995;107:963–966.

28. Hultcrantz E, Lofstrand-Tidestrom B, Ahlquit-Rastad J. The epidemiology of sleep related breathing disorder in children. *Int J Pediatr Otorhinolaryngol.* 1995;32(Suppl):S63–S66.

29. Smedje H, Broman J-E, Hetta J. Parents' reports of disturbed sleep in 5–7 year old Swedish children. *Acta Paediatr.* 1999;88:858–865.

30. Ferreira AM, Clemente V, Gozal D, et al. Snoring in Portuguese primary school children. *Pediatrics.* 2000;106:E64.

31. Corbo GM, Forastiere F, Agabiti N, et al. Snoring in 9- to 15-year-old children: risk factors and clinical relevance. *Pediatrics.* 2001;108:1149–1154.

32. Anuntaseree W, Rookkapan K, Kuasirikul S, et al. Snoring and obstructive sleep apnea in Thai school-age children: prevalence and predisposing factors. *Pediatr Pulmonol.* 2001;32:222–227.

33. Zhang G, Spickett J, Rumchev K, et al. Snoring in primary school children and domestic environment: a Perth school based study. *Respir Res.* 2004;5:19.

34. Tafur A, Chérrez-Ojeda I, Patiño C, et al. Rhinitis symptoms and habitual snoring in Ecuadorian children. *Sleep Med.* 2009;10:1035–1039.

35. Li AM, Au CT, So HK, et al. Prevalence and risk factors of habitual snoring in primary school children. *Chest.* 2010;138:519–527.

36. Marcus CL, Hamer A, Loughlin GM. Natural history of primary snoring in children. *Pediatr Pulmonol.* 1998;26:6–11.

37. Topol HI, Brooks LJ. Follow-up of primary snoring in children. *J Pediatr.* 2001;138:291–293.

38. Nieminen P, Tolonen U, Löppönen H. Snoring and obstructive sleep apnea in children: a 6-month follow-up study. *Arch Otolaryngol Head Neck Surg.* 2000;126(4):481–486.

39. Li AM, Zhu Y, Chun TA, et al. Natural history of primary snoring in school-aged children a 4-year follow-up study. *Chest.* 2013;143(3):729–735.

40. Urschitz MS, Eitner S, Guenther A, et al. Habitual snoring, intermittent hypoxia, and impaired behavior in primary school children. *Pediatrics.* 2004;114(4):1041–1048.

41. Smith DL, Gozal D, Hunter SJ, Kheirandish-Gozal L. Frequency of snoring, rather than apnea-hypopnea index, predicts both cognitive and behavioral problems in young children. *Sleep Med.* 2017;34:170–178.

42. Kwok KL, Ng DK, Cheung YF. BP and arterial distensibility in children with primary snoring. *Chest.* 2003;123:1561–1566.

43. Enright PL, Goodwin JL, Sherrill DL, et al. Blood pressure elevation associated with sleep-related breathing disorder in a community sample of white and Hispanic children: the Tucson Children's Assessment of Sleep Apnea Study. *Arch Pediatr Adolesc Med.* 2003;157:901–904.

44. Kaditis AG, Alexopoulos EI, Kostadima E, et al. Comparison of blood pressure measurements in children with and without habitual snoring. *Pediatr Pulmonol.* 2005;39:408–414.

45. Amin RS, Carroll JL, Jeffries JL, et al. Twenty-four-hour ambulatory blood pressure in children with sleep-disordered breathing. *Am J Respir Crit Care Med.* 2004;169:950–956.

46. Li AM, Au CT, Ho C, et al. Blood pressure is elevated in children with primary snoring. *J Pediatr.* 2009;155:362–368.

47. Nieminen P, Löppönen T, Tolonen U, et al. Growth and biochemical markers of growth in children with snoring and obstructive sleep apnea. *Pediatrics.* 2002;109:e55.

48. Guilleminault C, Lee JH. Does benign "primary snoring" ever exist in children? *Chest.* 2004;126:1396–1398.

49. Subcommittee on Obstructive Sleep Apnea Syndrome. American Academy of Pediatrics. Clinical practice guideline: diagnosis and management of childhood obstructive sleep apnea syndrome. section on pediatric pulmonology. *Pediatrics.* 2002;109(4):704–712.

50. Gozal D, Kheirandish-Gozal L, Capdevila OS, et al. Prevalence of recurrent otitis media in habitually snoring school-aged children. *Sleep Med.* 2008;9:549–554.

51. Kalra M, LeMasters G, Bernstein D, et al. Atopy as a risk factor for habitual snoring at age 1 year. *Chest.* 2006;129:942–946.

52. Brockmann PE, Ferri R, Bruni O. Association of sleep spindle activity and sleepiness in children with sleep-disordered breathing. *J Clin Sleep Med.* 2020;16(4):583–589.

53. Gruber R, Wise MS. Sleep spindle characteristics in children with neurodevelopmental disorders and their relation to cognition. *Neural Plast.* 2016;2016:4724792.

54. Zhu Y, Au CT, Lam HS, et al. Sleep architecture in school-aged children with primary snoring. *Sleep Med.* 2014;15(3):303–308.

55. Bandla HP, Gozal D. Dynamic changes in EEG spectra during obstructive apnea in children. *Pediatr Pulmonol.* 2000;29(5):359–365.

56. Chervin RD, Shelgikar AV, Burns JW. Respiratory cycle-related EEG changes: response to CPAP. *Sleep.* 2012;35(2):203–209.

57. Tauman R, O'Brien LM, Mast BT, et al. Peripheral arterial tonometry events and electroencephalographic arousals in children. *Sleep.* 2004;27(3):502–506.

58. Borovich A, Sivan Y, Greenfeld M, Tauman R. The history of primary snoring in children: the effect of adenotonsillectomy. *Sleep Med.* 2016;17:13–17.

26

Obstructive Sleep Apnea Syndrome in Childhood: Pathophysiology and Clinical Characteristics

Asher Tal and Aviv Goldbart

CHAPTER HIGHLIGHTS

- Children with obstructive sleep apnea (OSA) suffer upper airway intermittent closures caused by both anatomic and physiologic factors.
- OSA consequences are increased work of breathing, intermittent hypoxemia, sleep fragmentation, and alveolar hypoventilation.
- OSA is associated with substantial morbidities, such as behavioral and cognitive impairment, growth retardation, and cardiovascular involvement.
- The significant improvement after treatment emphasizes the need for early diagnosis and treatment.
- Sleep-disordered breathing represents a spectrum of breathing disorders ranging from habitual snoring to OSA that disrupt nocturnal respiration and sleep architecture.

Definitions

The spectrum of obstructive sleep-disordered breathing (SDB) ranges from habitual snoring to upper airway resistance syndrome (UARS) and obstructive hypoventilation to intermittent occlusion of the upper airway, as seen in obstructive sleep apnea syndrome (OSAS). Habitual snoring ("always", "frequently," or ≥3 nights per week) may be associated with increased respiratory effort, without apnea, sleep disruption, or gas exchange alteration. UARS is characterized by increasingly negative intrathoracic pressures during inspiration that lead to arousals and sleep fragmentation, in the absence of readily perceived apneas, hypopneas, or oxygen desaturations. **Obstructive hypoventilation** is a pattern of persistent partial upper airway obstruction associated with hypercapnia and/or hypoxemia rather than cyclic discrete obstructive apneas.

OSAS is defined by the American Thoracic Society[1] as "a disorder of breathing during sleep characterized by prolonged partial upper airway obstruction and/or intermittent complete obstruction (obstructive apnea) that disrupts normal ventilation during sleep and normal sleep patterns."

Sleep apnea in children was well described as early as 1976 by Guilleminault et al.[2,3] SDB occurs in children of all ages, from neonates to adolescents, with a peak prevalence between 2 and 8 years of age. Habitual snoring occurs in 5–12% of children; the prevalence of SDB is estimated at 4–11%,[4] and the prevalence of obstructive sleep apnea (OSA) is estimated at 1–4%. SDB is more common among boys and among children who are obese.[4–7]

Pathophysiology

Transition to the sleep state normally results in elevation of upper airway resistance, mainly due to reduction in airway diameter, resulting from the reduced tone of the pharyngeal dilator and constrictor muscles. Normal sleep is characterized by relative hypoxemia and hypercapnia, particularly during REM sleep, when compared with wakefulness. This normal phenomenon is magnified in patients with underlying pulmonary (e.g., nocturnal asthma) or upper airway (e.g., OSA) disease. This is the result of the following physiologic factors:[8]

- Functional residual capacity is reduced during sleep, mainly during rapid eye movement (REM) sleep, leading to more rapid hypoxemia with apnea. This is due to decreased intercostal and upper airway muscle tone, particularly during REM sleep.
- Central ventilatory drive regulating upper airway tone and ventilatory response to hypoxia and hypercapnia decrease during normal sleep.
- Upper airway resistance increases during sleep as a result of the decrease in upper airway tone. Small increases in upper airway resistance can have a significant impact on breathing.

Children with OSA tend to have a narrow upper airway. The patency of the upper airway is determined by both anatomic and physiologic factors. The site of obstruction in children tends to be more distal than in adults, typically involving the oropharynx and hypopharynx. Magnetic resonance imaging (MRI) of upper airway structures confirmed that children with OSA have significantly larger adenoids and tonsils than those of controls. Arens et al.[9] described the region in which these two lymphoid tissues overlap to constitute the site with the smallest airway diameter as the "overlap region." The upper airway is rich in neural receptors, which play a part in controlling baseline muscle tone. Any loss in this tone, as occurs at sleep onset, contributes to increased pharyngeal resistance. During inspiration, many dilator upper airway muscles exhibit phasic respiratory activity. This phasic activation of the muscles of the nose, pharynx, and larynx occurs before diaphragm and intercostal muscle activity, suggesting preactivation of the upper airway muscles in preparation for the development of negative pressure.

The Starling Resistor Theory

Under conditions of negative interluminal pressure, collapse of the upper airway occurs variably during inspiration. The pattern of flow on the driving pressure occurs in "Starling resistors," which are a specific type of "collapsible tube" behavior (Fig. 26.1).[8] The model predicts that, under conditions of flow limitation, maximal inspiratory airflow is determined by the pressure changes upstream (nasal) from the collapsible site of the upper airway and is independent of the downstream (hypopharyngeal and tracheal) pressure generated by the diaphragm. The upper airway can be represented as a tube with a collapsible segment, the resistance of which is zero. The segments upstream and downstream from the collapsible segment each have a fixed diameter, resistance, and pressure. The upstream pressure can be approximated by the nasal pressure, and the downstream pressure can be approximated by the hypopharyngeal

pressure. In this model of the upper airway, inflow pressure at the airway opening (the nares) is atmospheric, and downstream pressure is equal to tracheal pressure. Collapse occurs when the pressure surrounding the collapsible segment of the upper airway (critical tissue pressure = P_{crit}) becomes greater than the pressure within the collapsible segment of the airway. In normal subjects with low upstream resistance or subatmospheric critical tissue pressure, hypopharyngeal pressure never drops to critical pressure; thus airflow is not limited and is largely determined by negative tracheal pressure. However, if hypopharyngeal pressure falls below critical pressure, maximal inspiratory flow reaches its maximum limitation and becomes independent of downstream pressure swings. Under these circumstances, nasal resistance and critical pressure determine maximal inspiratory flow as described by the equation:

$$VI_{max} = (P_N - P_{crit})/R_N$$

where VI_{max} is maximal inspiratory flow, P_N is nasal pressure, P_{crit} is critical tissue pressure, and R_N is nasal resistance. Airflow will become zero (i.e., the airway will occlude) when nasal pressure falls below critical pressure.

Normal infants and children have a narrower upper airway than adults. Nevertheless, they snore less and have fewer obstructive apneas. This could be due to either structural differences or differences in neuromotor regulation of the upper airway. It is difficult to determine critical pressure in normal children, as their upper airway is very resistant to collapse. Marcus et al. have shown that P_{crit} in children correlated with the severity of OSA.[10]

The upper airway in children with OSA is more collapsible compared with control subjects during wakefulness and sleep, and under general anesthesia. Several mechanisms may lead to more airway collapse in these subjects, including decreased motor tone, increased airway compliance, and excessive inspiratory driving pressures caused by proximal airway narrowing. This increased propensity of the airway to collapse should be reflected by increased motion of airway boundary during respiration as negative upper airway intraluminal pressure is increased. Using respiratory-gated MRI to quantify changes in shape and airway cross-section area during tidal breathing in children with OSA compared with control subjects, it has been shown that fluctuations in airway area during tidal breathing are significantly greater in subjects with OSA compared with control subjects.[11]

Resistive pressure loading is a probable explanation, although increased airway compliance may be a contributing factor. Studies using denervated upper airways have shown that when upper airway muscle function is decreased or absent, the airway is more prone to collapse.[12,13] Children have active upper airway dynamic responses to both negative pressure pulses and hypercapnia during sleep.[14] Normal children compensate for their smaller upper airway by increasing the ventilatory drive to their upper airway muscles. This compensatory mechanism may be absent or diminished in children with OSA.

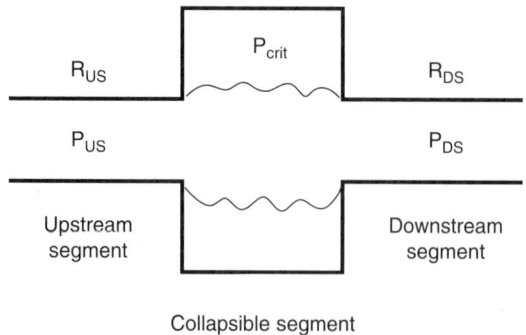

• **Fig. 26.1** Starling resistor model of the upper airway. The upper airway is represented as a tube with a collapsible segment. The upstream (nasal) and downstream (trachea) segments have fixed diameters and resistance (R_{US}, R_{DS}) and pressures (P_{US}, P_{DS}). Collapse occurs when the pressure surrounding the airway (P_{crit}) is greater than that within the airway. (Redrawn with permission from Marcus et al. Pathophysiology of OSAS in children. In: Loughlin GM, Carrol JL, Marcus CL, eds. *Sleep and Breathing in Children, a Developmental Approach.* Marcel Dekker; 2000:601-624.)

Physiological Consequences of OSA

Intermittent hypoxemia during sleep is common in children with OSA. Intermittent hypoxia may contribute to the increase in pulmonary pressure and the development of *cor pulmonale;* however, this effect will probably be more prominent with chronic hypoxemia. The more potentially serious consequences of intermittent hypoxemia are the behavioral and cognitive adverse effects on the brain. The relationship between the degree and duration of hypoxemia and neurologic and cardiopulmonary outcomes is not yet known.

Sleep fragmentation is a well-established consequence of OSA in adults but is much less determined in children. Although arousal from sleep is a protective reflex mechanism that restores breathing, an increase in the number of arousals per hour of sleep (arousal index) may cause sleep fragmentation and sympathetic activation.

Alveolar hypoventilation, or "obstructive hypoventilation," is the result of long periods of increased upper airway resistance and hypercapnia, with or without hypoxemia. Intermittent elevations in P_{CO_2} can exacerbate the effect of intermittent hypoxemia on neural tissue and can affect cerebral circulation and vasomotor activity.

Sleep Pattern in Children With OSA

The common phenotype of OSA in children is characterized by adenotonsillar hypertrophy in otherwise healthy children. It is well established that adult OSA is associated with altered sleep architecture, with an increase in stage N1 sleep, a decrease in deep sleep stages, and frequent arousals. Initial comparative polysomnography (PSG) data have revealed no consistent PSG differences before and after adenotonsillectomy.[1,4,6,7] Durdik et al., compared 94 children 3–8 years old with the common type of OSA to 55 healthy children controls, and found shorter stage N3 (slow-wave sleep) with a significantly longer stage N1 sleep.[15] In addition, children with untreated OSA exhibit decreased slow-wave activity level and slope during the night, indicating reduced sleep homeostasis. Adenotonsillectomy led to more physiologic sleep homeostasis in children with OSA.[16]

The etiology of OSA in children is multifactorial and is probably a combination of abnormal airway structure, decreased neuromuscular control, and genetic, hormonal, and metabolic factors (Fig. 26.2).

Airway structure is an important factor in pediatric OSA. Bony structure and soft tissue are two major contributing factors in determining upper airway patency.

Genetic syndromes that are associated with OSA include those producing micrognathia and those producing midfacial hypoplasia.

Pierre Robin sequence, consisting of micrognathia and posterior displacement of the tongue and soft palate, is frequently associated with SDB, presenting in early infancy, in the first few weeks of life.

Treacher Collins syndrome, caused by mutation in the region of 5q32-32.2 that codes for the treacle protein, is

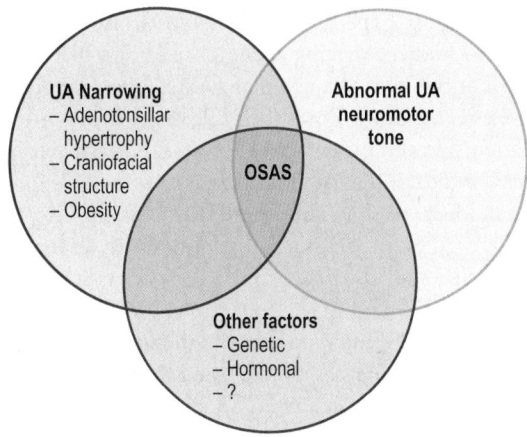

• **Fig. 26.2** Obstructive sleep apnea syndrome (*OSAS*) in children may result from a combination of factors. *UA*, Upper airway. (With permission from Smith PL, Schwartz AR, Gauda E, et al. The modulation of upper airway critical pressure during sleep. *Prog Clin Biolo Res.* 1990;345:253-258.)

characterized by mandibular hypoplasia, malar hypoplasia, antimongoloid slanting palpebral fissures, malformation of the auricles, and coloboma of the eyelid.

Midfacial hypoplasia syndromes include ***Crouzon syndrome, Apert syndrome,*** and ***Pfeiffer syndrome.***

Achondroplasia, an autosomal dominant skeletal dysplasia, is associated with OSA as the most common respiratory complication. About two-thirds of patients with achondroplasia present OSA.

Children with ***Down syndrome*** frequently present OSA because of their craniofacial structure: maxillary hypoplasia and small nose with low nasal bridge.[17] In addition, recurrent upper airway infections result in adenotonsillar hypertrophy.

Children with ***Arnold-Chiari malformation*** may be at risk for developing both central and OSA due to brainstem compression affecting respiratory drive and/or activation of the pharyngeal and laryngeal muscles that are enervated by cranial nerves IX and X.

Children with ***Prader-Willi syndrome,*** consisting of hypotonia, obesity, hypogonadism, and mental retardation, may also present OSA. In children with ***mucopolysaccharidoses,*** OSA is caused as a result of deposition of mucopolysaccharides in the airways, including the tongue, pharynx, trachea, and bronchi.

The high prevalence of habitual snoring in first-degree relatives of children with OSA, and documented familial aggregation of OSA, suggest a familial predisposition to this condition.[18,19] African Americans are at greater risk than Whites when controlling for age, sex, and body mass index, indicating *ethnicity* as another risk factor for OSA.[20]

Prematurity was also identified as a risk factor for OSA.[5,21] Former preterm infants are at increased risk to develop OSA in early infancy, possibly due to facial asymmetry, greater incidence of muscle hypotonia, or nasal obstruction after prolonged intubation.[22]

Adenotonsillar hypertrophy is the most common etiology of OSA in children, making adenotonsillectomy the first-line treatment at this age. The fact that most children significantly improve after surgery[23] proves their role in the etiology of OSA in children. However, the fact that cure is not achieved in all children[24] indicates that other factors are involved. The tonsils and adenoids increase in size from birth to about 12 years of age and are largest in relation to the underlying upper airway size between 3 and 6 years of age.[25] The correlation between adenotonsillar size and OSA is not strong. Whereas the severity of obstructive events was related to the size of the adenoids in one study,[26] other studies have failed to show a correlation between adenotonsillar size and OSA severity.[27]

OSA and Obesity

The presence of obesity in children significantly increases the risk of developing OSA.[28] The risk for residual OSA after adenotonsillectomy is markedly greater in obese children.[29] In addition, obesity-induced childhood OSA is different from OSA in otherwise healthy children with adenotonsillar hypertrophy. These observations resulted in a proposed differentiation between type I OSA (common type), associated with marked lymphadenoid hypertrophy without obesity, and type II OSA, associated with obesity with only mild lymphadenoid hypertrophy.[30]

OSA and Asthma

OSA has been identified as a risk factor for severe asthma in adults.[31,32] Asthma and OSA in children share multiple epidemiologic risk factors, and the prevalence of snoring is greater in asthmatic children. Asthma and OSA may coexist in children due to a shared relationship with atopy. SDB was recently reported as a modifiable risk factor for severe asthma in children.[33] The treatment of OSA appeared to be associated with substantial improvements in the severity of the underlying asthmatic condition.[34]

OSA and Inflammation

There is growing evidence indicating that adults and children with OSA present local (upper airway apparatus) inflammatory changes and systemic manifestations.[35] The measured inflammatory changes reflect activation of specific pathways such as the lipoxygenase pathway, which is involved in other inflammatory conditions that affect children, such as asthma and allergic rhinitis.

Goldbart et al.[36] suggested that an inflammatory process involving leukotriene (LT) expression and regulation occurs in children with OSA.[37,38] The main evidence of systemic inflammation associated with childhood OSA was the finding of elevated C-reactive protein (CRP) plasma levels. Tauman and others reported an increase in plasma CRP levels among American children with SDB, which correlated with apnea-hypopnea index (AHI), arterial oxygen saturation nadir, and arousal index measures.[39–41]

Several other inflammatory biomarkers were reported in children with OSA: interleukin (IL)-6, interferon-γ, IL-8 levels, tumor necrosis factor (TNF)-α, and fibrinogen.[42–44]

Activation of the transcription factor NF-κB, leading to elevation of its dependent genes (e.g., TNF-α), constitutes an important pathway linking OSA with systemic inflammation and end organ cardiovascular disease.[45]

Israel et al.[46] were able to show that NF-κB is locally and systemically activated in children with OSA, like in adults. The distinction between inflammatory mechanisms leading to OSA as opposed to the systemic/local inflammation resulting from the presence of OSA is difficult. The effect of adenotonsillectomy on CRP was assessed by investigators who found a significant decrease in its levels 3 months post-surgery. The authors reported a significant correlation between the change in hsCRP and a reduction in OSA severity after adenotonsillectomy.[41,47]

The importance of understanding the inflammatory mechanisms involved in the etiology of OSA is the potential role of anti-inflammatory drugs as an alternative, non-surgical treatment of OSA in children: intranasal corticosteroids[48] and LT modifiers. The results of the clinical studies performed so far support a therapeutic role for LT modifiers in pediatric non-severe OSA.[37,49,50]

OSA in Infants

More attention is directed recently to OSA in the very young. Chandrasekar et al. suggested that OSA in neonates is often multifactorial, caused by congenital malformation, airway abnormalities, neurologic disorders, and more.[51] Clinical presentation may be highly variable.

Stefanovski and colleagues have shown that central and obstructive AHI are significantly greater in healthy newborns than older children, with a spontaneous reduction in severity and type of events in the first 6 months of life.[52] At the age of 1 month, they found, in normal newborns, a total AHI (central plus obstructive) of 16.9 events per hour. Meta-analysis found a high AHI in healthy infants with significant heterogeneity. Rayasam described a group of 413 children under 3 years of age with OSA (based on PSG) and found that at this age they are most likely to be male and have gastroesophageal reflux disease, Down syndrome, and tonsillar hypertrophy.[53]

Diagnosis in young children should include overnight PSG and, in selected patients, also drug-induced sleep endoscopy.

Clinical Characteristics

OSA may present with nocturnal and/or diurnal symptoms (Box 26.1).

Nocturnal Symptoms

Snoring is the most characteristic presenting symptom of OSA in children.[54,55] Worsening is usually reported with

---

• BOX 26.1 **Symptoms of Obstructive Sleep Apnea Syndrome in Children**

Nocturnal

Snoring
Difficulty in breathing during sleep
Witnessed apnea
Restless sleep
Frequent awakenings
Night sweating
Nocturnal enuresis

Diurnal

Behavior problems
   Irritability
     Aggressiveness
Impaired cognitive function
    Poor school performance
Poor appetite
Daytime sleepiness

---

upper respiratory tract infections. In young children, compared with adults, snoring occurs in any position and is not necessarily worse in the supine position. Habitual snoring alone is not a specific symptom of OSA. Most children with habitual snoring do not progress to having OSA, and those who do so have only mild OSA. Several recent reports have indicated a significant impact of habitual snoring on behavioral and cognitive functions, even without polysomnographic evidence of OSA.

Difficulty in breathing during sleep is another frequent complaint of parents of children with OSAS. Parents usually describe paradoxical respiratory movements with "the abdomen going down when the thorax goes up."

Witnessed apnea is described by many parents, either spontaneously or after a direct question. The prevalence of parent report of apneic events during sleep is in the range of 0.2% to 4%.[4] Many parents describe the acoustic result of the sudden disappearance of snoring ending with a snort or gasp.

These first three symptoms are the most sensitive and specific for children with OSA. In the early 1980s, Brouillette[56] used these to create an "OSA Score" that practically showed that a child who snores every night, presents difficulties in breathing during sleep, and whose parent reported witnessing apneas, suffers from OSA. Unfortunately, whereas the positive predicted value of the OSA Score is high (50–75%), its negative predicted value is low (25–80%).

Restless sleep is the result of frequent arousals. Parents usually describe a child who disarranges sheets and blankets, moves a lot during sleep, and is found in strange postures during sleep, mainly with the neck hyperextended.

Frequent awakening is a very common parental complaint. Many parents accept it initially as a sign of being spoiled (many children move during sleep to their parents' bed), and they think the child is hungry or needs something to drink during sleep. As a result of the difficult breathing and numerous arousals and movements, *night sweating* is also common in children with OSA.

Nocturnal enuresis is reported in 8–47% of children with OSAS.[57] A recent study reported two-thirds of children with OSA with primary enuresis and one-third with secondary enuresis. The findings of a high prevalence of nocturnal enuresis in children with mild OSA indicate an increased risk of enuresis in children with sleep-disordered breathing, even without OSA. Retrospective data indicated a remarkable decrease in enuresis soon after adenotonsillectomy.[57–60]

Daytime Symptoms

In many children with OSA the presenting symptoms may be the result of disrupted sleep, namely *abnormal daytime functioning*. Whereas daytime sleepiness is a common symptom of OSA in adults, only the minority of pediatric OSA patients (<15%) present it. In fact, sleepiness and fatigue may present in young children as irritability, nervousness, and aggressiveness, as well as attention-deficit/hyperactivity disorder (ADHD) and poor school performance. This aspect of the impact of OSA in children is discussed in detail in Chapter 32.

Children with hypertrophied adenoids and tonsils may present with mouth breathing, recurrent upper respiratory infections, and hearing and speech problems. Morning headaches, a common complaint in adult patients with OSA, are much less common in children.

Clinical Consequences of OSA

The clinical consequences of OSA are probably the result of a combination of intermittent hypoxia, sleep fragmentation, and inflammation that are associated with sleep-disordered breathing. There is increasing evidence to support the association between OSA, SDB, and habitual snoring and ADHD in children.[61] Neurocognitive consequences associated with OSA are described in detail in Chapter 32.

Pulmonary hypertension is the most common cardiovascular complication in children with OSA. Initial case reports in the early 1960s indicated that in untreated cases of chronic nasopharyngeal obstruction, cardiomegaly, *cor pulmonale*, and pulmonary edema may develop.[62] Right ventricular dysfunction in children with OSA is reversible soon after adenotonsillectomy.[63] Cardiovascular consequences of OSA are described in Chapter 33.

Failure to thrive and *growth retardation* have been known as complications of OSA since the very first publications on this syndrome.[3] Three main factors contribute to the growth retardation: (1) low caloric intake; children with hypertrophied tonsils often present with poor appetite and dysphagia, resulting in poor caloric intake; (2) high energy expenditure due to increased work of breathing during sleep;[64] and (3) growth hormone (GH) secretion is impaired in children with OSA. Insulin-like growth factor (IGF)-1 was found to be low in children with OSA. Respiratory improvement after adenotonsillectomy results in weight gain and restores IGF-1 and GH secretion.[65,66]

Children with OSA are heavy users of health care services, indicating higher morbidity.[67] Children with OSA who were diagnosed at the age of 4 years have *greater respiratory morbidity and health care costs*, starting from the first year of life.[68] After adenotonsillectomy, health care cost significantly decreases because of reduced morbidity.[69] The reasons for higher costs before treatment are the result of an increase in the rates of hospitalization, emergency room referrals, and use of medications. Respiratory tract infections (upper and lower) are the most common causes of morbidity in children with OSA. A recent study reported that OSA represents a predisposing risk for community-acquired alveolar pneumonia in children under 5 years old.[70]

CLINICAL PEARLS

- Obstructive sleep apnea (OSA) is a disorder of breathing during sleep characterized by prolonged partial upper airway obstruction and/or intermittent complete obstruction that disrupts normal ventilation during sleep.
- Risk factors for OSA include adenotonsillar hypertrophy, craniofacial anomalies, familial predisposition, ethnicity, and prematurity.
- OSA has been associated with behavioral and cognitive impairment, growth retardation, and cardiovascular involvement.
- Treatment is essential and may include multiple options including nasal corticosteroids, leukotriene receptor antagonists, and/or adenotonsillectomy.

Summary

OSAS is a common disorder in children. Children with OSA tend to have a narrow and collapsible upper airway caused by both anatomic and physiologic factors. The consequences are increased work of breathing, intermittent hypoxemia, sleep fragmentation, and alveolar hypoventilation. In addition, OSA may be associated with local and systemic inflammation, obesity and asthma. Risk factors for OSA include adenotonsillar hypertrophy, craniofacial anomalies, familial predisposition, ethnicity, and prematurity. OSA is associated with substantial morbidities, such as behavioral and cognitive impairment, growth retardation, and cardiovascular involvement. The significant improvement after treatment emphasizes the need for early diagnosis and treatment. Understanding the pathophysiology, risk factors, daytime and nocturnal symptoms, and clinical implications of OSA in children is essential to early diagnosis and treatment of this common disorder.

References

1. American Thoracic Society Standards and indications for cardiopulmonary sleep studies in children. *Am J Respir Crit Care Med*. 1996;153:866–878.
2. Guilleminault C, Eldridge F, Simmons FB, et al. Sleep apnea in eight children. *Pediatrics*. 1976;58:28–31.
3. Guilleminault C, Korobkin R, Winkle R. A review of 50 children with obstructive sleep apnea syndrome. *Lung*. 1981;159:275–287.
4. Lumeng JC, Chervin RD. Epidemiology of pediatric obstructive sleep apnea. *Proc Am Thorac Soc*. 2008;5:242–252.
5. Rosen CL, Larkin EK, Kirchner HL, et al. Prevalence and risk factors for sleep-disordered breathing in 8- to 11 year-old children: association with race and prematurity. *J Pediatr*. 2003;142:383–389.
6. Corbo GM, Forastier F, Agabiti N, et al. Snoring in 9- to 15-year-old children: risk factors and clinical relevance. *Pediatrics*. 2001;108:1149–1154.
7. Tang JP, Rosen CL, Larkinn EK, et al. Identification of sleep-disordered breathing in children: variation with event definition. *Sleep*. 2002;25:72–79.
8. Marcus CL. Pathophysiology of OSAS in children. In: Loughlin GM, Carrol JL, Marcus CL, eds. *Sleep and Breathing in Children, A Developmental Approach*. Marcel Dekker; 2000:601–624.
9. Arens R, McDonough JM, Costarino AT, et al. Magnetic resonance imaging of the upper airway structure of children with obstructive sleep apnea syndrome. *Am J Respir Crit Care Med*. 2001;164:698–703.
10. Marcus CL, McColley SA, Carroll JL, Loughlin GM, Smith PL, Schwartz AR. Upper airway collapsibility in children with obstructive sleep apnea syndrome. *Appl Physiol*. 1994;77(2):918–924.
11. Arens R, Sin S, McDonough JM. Changes in upper airway size during tidal breathing in children with obstructive sleep apnea syndrome. *Am J Respir Crit Care Med*. 2005;171:1298–1304.
12. Smith PL, Schwartz AR, Gauda E, et al. The modulation of upper airway critical pressure during sleep. *Prog Clin Biol Res*. 1990;345:253–258.
13. Brouillette RT, Tach BT. A neuromuscular mechanism maintaining extrathoracic airway patency. *J Appl Physiol*. 1979;46:772–779.
14. Marcus CL, Fernandes Do Prado LB, Lutz J, et al. Dynamic responses to both negative pressure pulses and hypercapnia during sleep. *J Appl Physiol*. 2004;97:98–108.
15. Durdik P, Sujanska A, Suroviakova S, et al. Sleep architecture in children with common phenotype of obstructive sleep apnea. *J Clin Sleep Med*. 2018;14(1):9–14.
16. Ben Israel N, Zigel Y, Tal A, et al. Adenotonsillectomy improves slow wave activity in children with obstructive sleep apnea. *Eur Respir J*. 2011;37:1144–1150.
17. Marcus CL, Keens TG, Bautista DB, et al. Obstructive sleep apnea in children with Down syndrome. *Pediatrics*. 1991;88:132–139.
18. Pillar G, Lavie P. Assessment of the role of inheritance in sleep apnea syndrome. *Am J Respir Crit Car Med*. 1995;151:688–691.
19. Redline S, Tishler PV, Schuchter M, et al. Risk factors for sleep-disordered breathing in children: association with obesity, race, and respiratory problems. *Am J Respir Crit Care Med*. 1999;159:1527–1532.
20. Palmer LJ, Buxbaum SG, Larkin EK, et al. Whole genome scan for obstructive sleep apnea and obesity in African-American families. *Am J Respir Crit Care Med*. 2004;169:1314–1321.
21. Greenfeld M, Tauman R, DeRow A, Sivan Y. Obstructive sleep apnea syndrome to adenotonsillar hypertrophy in infants. *Int J Pediatr Otorhinolaryngol*. 2003;67:1055–1060.

22. Sharma PB, Baroody F, Gozal D, Lester LA. Obstructive sleep apnea in the formerly preterm infant: an overlooked diagnosis. *Front in Neurol.* 2011;2:75.

23. Tal A, Bar A, Leiberman A, Tarasiuk A. Sleep characteristics following adenotonsillectomy in children with obstructive sleep apnea syndrome. *Chest.* 2003;124:948–953.

24. Tauman R, Gulliver TE, Krishna J, et al. Persistence of obstructive sleep apnea syndrome in children after adenotonsillectomy. *J Pediatr.* 2006;149:803–808.

25. Jeans WD, Fernando DCJ, Maw AR, Leighton BC. A longitudinal study of the growth of the nasopharynx and its content in normal children. *Br J Radiol.* 1981;54:117–121.

26. Brooks LJ, Stephens B, Bacevic AM. Adenoid size is related to severity but not the number of obstructive apnea in children. *J Pediatr.* 1998;132:682–686.

27. Lam YY, Chan EY, Ng DK, et al. The correlation among obesity, apnea-hypopnea index, and tonsil size in children. *Chest.* 2006;130:1751–1756.

28. Verhulst SL, Schrauwen N, Haentiens D, et al. Sleep-disordered breathing in overweight and obese children and adolescents: prevalence, characteristics and the role of fat distribution. *Arch Dis Child.* 2007;92:205–208.

29. Bhattacharjee R, Kheirandish-Gozal L, Spruyt K, et al. Adenotonsillectomy outcomes in treatment of obstructive sleep apnea in children: a multicenter retrospective study. *Am J Respir Crit Care Med.* 2010;182:676–683.

30. Dayyat E, Kheirandish-Gozal L, Gozal D. Childhood obstructive sleep apnea: one or two distinct disease entity? *Sleep Med Clin.* 2007;2:433–444.

31. ten Brinke A, Sterk PJ, Masclee AA, et al. Risk factors of frequent exacerbations in difficult-to-treat asthma. *Eur Respir J.* 2005;26:812–818.

32. Julien JY, Martin JG, Ernest P, et al. Prevalence of obstructive sleep apnea-hypopnea in severe versus moderate asthma. *J Allergy Clin Immunol.* 2009;124:371–376.

33. Ross KR, Storfer-Isser A, Hart MA, et al. Sleep-disordered breathing is associated with asthma severity in children. *J Pediatr.* 2012;160(5):736–742.

34. Kheirandish-Gozal L, Dayyat EA, Eid NS, Morton RL, Gozal D. Obstructive sleep apnea in poorly controlled asthmatic children: effect of adenotonsillectomy. *Pediatr Pulmonol.* 2011;46:913–918.

35. Goldbart AD, Tal A. Inflammation and sleep-disordered breathing in children: a state-of the art review. *Pediatr Pulmonol.* 2008;43:1151–1160.

36. Goldbart AD, Goldman JL, Li RC, et al. Differential expression of cysteinyl leukotriene receptors 1 and 2 in tonsils of children with obstructive sleep apnea syndrome or recurrent infection. *Chest.* 2004;126:13–18.

37. Goldbart AD, Goldman JL, Veling MC, Gozal D. Leukotriene modifier therapy for mild sleep-disordered breathing in children. *Am J Respir Crit Care Med.* 2005;172:364–370.

38. Goldbart AD, Krishna J, Li RC, Serpero LD, Gozal D. Inflammatory mediators in exhaled breath condensate of children with obstructive sleep apnea syndrome. *Chest.* 2006;130:143–148.

39. Tauman R, Ivanenko A, O'Brien LM, Gozal D. Plasma C-reactive protein levels among children with sleep-disordered breathing. *Pediatrics.* 2004;113:e564–e569.

40. Kaditis AG, Alexopoulos EI, Kalampouka E, et al. Morning levels of C-reactive protein in children with obstructive sleep-disordered breathing. *Am J Respir Crit Care Med.* 2005;171:282–286.

41. Kheirandish-Gozal L, Capdevila OS, Tauman R, Gozal D. Plasma C-reactive protein in nonobese children with obstructive sleep apnea before and after adenotonsillectomy. *J Clin Sleep Med.* 2006;2:301–304.

42. Gozal D, Kheirandish-Gozal L, Sans Capdevila O, Kim J. TNF-alpha plasma levels are increased excessively in sleepy school-aged children with obstructive sleep apnea. *Sleep.* 2008;31:186.

43. Tam CS, Wong M, McBain R, Baily S, Waters KA. Inflammatory measures in children with obstructive sleep apnoea. *J Pediatr Child Health.* 2006;42:277–282.

44. Kaditis AG, Alexopoulos EI, Kalampouka E, et al. Morning levels of fibrinogen in children with sleep-disordered breathing. *Eur Respir J.* 2004;24:790–797.

45. Ryan S, Taylor CT, McNicholas WT. Selective activation of inflammatory pathways by intermittent hypoxia in obstructive sleep apnea syndrome. *Circulation.* 2005;112:2660–2667.

46. Israel LP, Benharoch D, Gopas J, Goldbart AD. A proinflammatory role for nuclear factor kappa b in childhood obstructive sleep apnea syndrome. *Sleep.* 2013;36(12):1947–1955.

47. Li AM, Chan MH, Yin J, et al. C-reactive protein in children with obstructive sleep apnea and the effects of treatment. *Pediatr Pulmonol.* 2008;43:34–40.

48. Brouillette RT, Manoukian JJ, Ducharme FM, et al. Efficacy of fluticasone nasal spray for pediatric obstructive sleep apnea. *J Pediatr.* 2001;138:838–844.

49. Goldbart AD, Greenberg-Dotan S, Tal A. Montelukast for children with obstructive sleep apnea: a double-blind, placebo-controlled study. *Pediatrics.* 2012;130(3):e575–e580.

50. Kheirandish-Gozal L, Bandla HP, Gozal D. Montelukast for children with obstructive sleep apnea: results of a double-blind, randomized, placebo-controlled trial. *Ann Am Thorac Soc.* 2016;13(10):1736–1741.

51. Chandrasekar I, Tabilzo MA, Witmans M, Cruz JM, Cummins Esterellado-Cruz. Obstructive sleep apnea in neonates. *Children (Basel).* 2022;9:419.

52. Stefanovski D, Tapia IE, Lioy J, Sengupta S, Mukhopadhay S, Cororan A, Conaglia MA, Cielo CM. Respiratory indices during sleep in healthy infants: a prospective longitudinal study and meta-analysis. *Sleep Med.* 2022;9:49–57.

53. Rayasam A, Johnson R, Lenahan D, Abjiay C, Mitchel R. Obstructive sleep apnea in children under 3 years of age. *Laryngoscope.* 2021;131:E2603–E2608.

54. Ali NJ, Piterson DJ, Stradling JR. Snoring, sleep disturbance, and behaviour in 4-5 year olds. *Arch Dis Child.* 1993;68:360–366.

55. Gisalson T, Benediktsdottir B. Snoring, apneic episodes, and nocturnal hypoxemia among children 6 months to 6 years old. *Chest.* 1995;107:963–966.

56. Brouillette R, Hanson D, David R, et al. A diagnostic approach to suspected obstructive sleep apnea in children. *J Pediatr.* 1984;105:10–14.

57. Brooks LJ, Topol HI. Enuresis in children with sleep apnea. *J Pediatr.* 2003;142:515–518.

58. Weider DJ, Sateia MJ, West RP. Nocturnal enuresis in children with upper airway obstruction. *Otolaryngol Head Neck Surg.* 1991;105:427–432.

59. Weissbach A, Leiberman A, Tarasiuk A, Tal A. Adenotonsillectomy improves enuresis in children with OSAS. *Int J Pediatr Otolaryngol.* 2006;80:1351–1356.

60. Jeyakumar A, Rahman SI, Armbrecht ES, Michell E. The association between sleep-disordered breathing and enuresis in children. *Laryngoscope.* 2012;122:1873–1877.

61. Chervin RD, Ruzicka DL, Giordani BJ, et al. Sleep-disordered breathing, behavior, and cognition in children before and after adenotonsillectomy. *Pediatrics.* 2006;117:e769–e778.

62. Sofer S, Weinhouse E, Tal A, et al. Cor pulmonale due to adenoid or tonsillar hypertrophy or both in children. *Chest.* 1988;93:119–122.

63. Tal A, Leiberman A, Margulis G, Sofer S. Ventricular dysfunction in children with obstructive sleep apnea: Radionuclide assessment. *Pediatr Pulmonol.* 1988;4:139–143.

64. Marcus CL, Carrol JL, Koerrner CB, et al. Determinants of growth in children with obstructive sleep apnea syndrome. *J Pediatr.* 1994;125:556–562.

65. Bar A, Tarasiuk A, Segev M, Philip A, Tal A. The effect of adenotonsillectomy on serum insulin-like growth factor-1 and growth in children with obstructive sleep apnea syndrome. *J Pediatr.* 1999;135:76–80.

66. Nieminen P, Lopponen T, Tolonen U, et al. Growth and biochemical markers of growth in children with snoring and obstructive sleep apnea. *Pediatrics.* 2002;109:e55.

67. Reuveni H, Simon T, Tal A, Elhayany A, Tarasiuk A. Health care services utilization in children with obstructive sleep apnea syndrome. *Pediatrics.* 2002;110:68–72.

68. Tarasiuk A, Greenberg-Dotan S, Simon-Tuval T, Freidman B, Goldbart A, Tal A, Reuveni H. Elevated morbidity and health care utilization in children with obstructive sleep apnea syndrome. *Am J Respir Crit Care Med.* 2007;175:55–61.

69. Tarasiuk A, Simon T, Tal A, Reuveni H. Adenotonsillectomy in children with obstructive sleep apnea syndrome reduces health care utilization. *Pediatrics.* 2004;113:351–356.

70. Goldbart AD, Tal A, Givon-Lavi N, Bar-Ziv J, Dagan R, Greenberg D. Sleep disordered breathing is a risk factor for community-acquired alveolar pneumonia in early childhood. *Chest.* 2012;141(5):1210–1215.

27

Diagnosis of Obstructive Sleep Apnea

ELIOT S. KATZ

CHAPTER HIGHLIGHTS

- Obstructive sleep apnea (OSA) is a continuous spectrum ranging from frank, intermittent occlusion (apnea), through partial obstruction (hypopnea), all the way to increased upper airway resistance (snoring) alone. OSA results in a combination of increased respiratory effort, intermittent hypoxemia, intermittent hypercapnia, and sleep fragmentation leading to cardiovascular, metabolic, and neurocognitive sequelae.

- Historically, pediatric obstructive sleep-disordered breathing was divided into four patterns based on polysomnographic findings, including OSA, upper airway resistance syndrome, obstructive hypoventilation (OH), and primary snoring (PS), though there is considerable overlap in clinical symptomatology and metabolic abnormalities.

- A personalized approach to the diagnosis of OSA includes consideration of the child's epidemiologic risk factors, genetics, clinical symptoms, physical examination, underlying medical conditions, validated questionnaires, imaging studies, laboratory testing, physiologic recordings, and the natural history of OSA in the child's particular context.

- There is a distinction to be made between polysomnographic OSA and clinically symptomatic OSA, recognizing that many snoring children are symptomatic from their increased upper airway resistance, but may not have polysomnographic evidence of frank, obstructive events that are scorable with present technology. Conversely, many children with mild polysomnographic OSA may not have discernible symptoms, which must be considered in selecting treatment options.

Introduction

Obstructive sleep apnea (OSA) is a common and serious cause of morbidity during childhood. OSA is recognized as a continuous spectrum ranging from frank, intermittent occlusion (apnea), through partial obstruction (hypopnea), all the way to increased upper airway resistance (snoring) alone. OSA results in a combination of increased respiratory effort, intermittent hypoxemia, intermittent hypercapnia, and sleep fragmentation leading to cardiovascular, metabolic, and neurocognitive sequelae. The pathophysiology of OSA includes anatomical abnormalities (craniofacial,

soft tissue, obesity), ventilatory control instability, arousal threshold, and neuromuscular control of the upper airway.

The new paradigm defines OSA by a combination of polysomnographic severity, biologic dysregulation, and clinical symptoms. A wide range of OSA patterns and severity have been associated with adverse effects in susceptible children; therefore a personalized medical approach requires consideration of the child's epidemiologic risk factors, genetics, clinical symptoms, physical examination, underlying medical conditions, validated questionnaires, imaging studies, laboratory testing, physiologic recordings, and the natural history of OSA in the child's particular context.

Nomenclature

The nomenclature for pediatric OSA is still evolving as the full range of the disorder is being elucidated. According to the latest 2014 *International Classification of Sleep Disorders, Third Edition* (ICSD-3)[1] pediatric OSA has two required criteria:

1. The presence of one or more of (1) snoring; (2) labored, paradoxical, or obstructed breathing during sleep; and (3) sleepiness, hyperactivity, behavioral problems, or learning problems.
2. Polysomnography demonstrates one or more of (1) ≥1 obstructive apnea, mixed apnea, or hypopnea per hour of sleep or (2) obstructive hypoventilation ([OH]; >25% of the total sleep time [TST] with an end-tidal carbon dioxide >50 torr) with one or more of snoring, flow limitation, or paradoxical thoracoabdominal motion.[1]

ICSD-3 also states that "the term upper airway resistance syndrome (UARS) is subsumed under this diagnosis because the pathophysiology does not significantly differ from that of OSA."[1] However, habitual snoring in the absence of other polysomnographic respiratory abnormalities in patients who have daytime symptoms is not specifically included in this diagnosis of OSA or in the ICSD-3 diagnosis of Snoring.

Snoring (habitual, primary, or simple):
1. Occurs without apnea, hypopnea, respiratory effort–related arousals, or hypoventilation.
2. Does not cause excessive daytime sleepiness or "other related symptoms."

3. Cannot report possible breathing pauses without objective measurement of breathing during sleep.[1]

As currently constituted, the ICSD-3 diagnostic criteria for Snoring requires that no daytime symptoms are present. Consequently, snoring children with daytime symptoms are presently excluded from a specific diagnosis despite the preponderance of clinical data supporting the association. In addition, a variety of abnormal breathing patterns have been associated with OSA in addition to apneas and hypopneas including tachypnea, increased respiratory effort, mouth breathing, and flow limitation that need to be incorporated into future nosology.[2,3]

This chapter will argue that there is a distinction to be made between polysomnographic OSA and clinically symptomatic OSA, recognizing that many snoring children are symptomatic from their increased upper airway resistance, but may not have polysomnographic evidence of frank, obstructive events that are scorable with present technology. Conversely, many children with mild polysomnographic OSA may not have discernible symptoms, which must be taken into account when considering treatment options. The determination as to whether snoring or OSA requires treatment is predicated on the clinical symptomatology, signs, laboratory markers, underlying medical conditions, likely natural history, and the polysomnographic severity.

Historically, pediatric obstructive sleep-disordered breathing was demarcated into four patterns based on the polysomnographic characteristics, though there is considerable overlap in clinical symptomatology and metabolic abnormalities, as follows:

- OSA is characterized by recurrent episodes of partial or complete airway narrowing with measurable decreases in airflow resulting in hypoxemia, hypercapnia, and/or respiratory arousal. The sleep fragmentation and gas exchange abnormalities observed with OSA may produce serious cardiovascular, metabolic, and neurobehavioral impairment.[4-6]

- UARS is characterized by brief, repetitive respiratory effort–related arousals (RERAs) during sleep in the absence of overt apnea, hypopnea, or gas exchange abnormalities[7] (Fig. 27.1). UARS may be associated with flow limitation, increased respiratory effort, mouth breathing, and changes in respiratory timing and muscle activity.[3] It has been linked to significant cognitive and behavioral sequelae in children including learning disabilities, attention-deficit/hyperactivity disorder, and aggressive behavior.[7,8]

- OH features prolonged increased upper airway resistance accompanied by hypercapnia, but not frank apnea or hypopnea.[9] Elevated carbon dioxide, in the absence of scorable obstructive events, was observed in 7% of a large cohort of snoring children with adenotonsillar hypertrophy.[10]

- Primary snoring (PS) is characterized by habitual snoring and increased respiratory effort in the absence of scorable

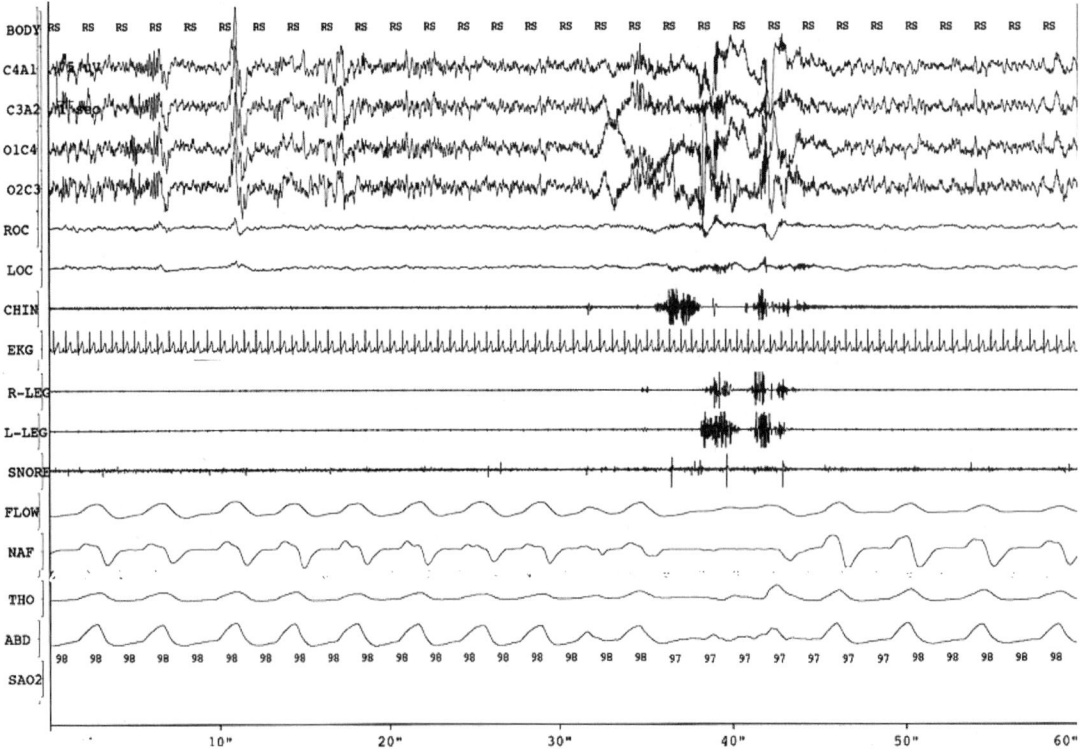

• **Fig. 27.1** A 60-second epoch from a 16-year-old with snoring and excessive daytime sleepiness. Note flow limitation in the nasal pressure tracing without a change in the thermistor leading to an electroencephalogram (EEG) arousal consistent with a respiratory effort–related arousal. Inspiration is upward. Abd, abdomen; Body, body position; Flow, thermistor; NAF, nasal pressure; RS, right side; SpO$_2$, pulse oximetry; Tho, thorax.

obstructive events, increased arousals, or gas exchange abnormalities. Though PS is sometimes defined as a benign condition, without polysomnographic abnormalities, recent evidence suggests that the increased respiratory effort in PS per se, independent of scorable obstructive events, may be associated with untoward neurobehavioral consequences.[11–13]

Some physicians have introduced the additional term "obstructive sleep-disordered breathing" as a clinical diagnosis that includes the entire spectrum from snoring to OSA, and reserve the term "obstructive sleep apnea" for patients with abnormal polysomnography.[14] Adopting this terminology permits a distinction to be made between snoring alone in the absence of other symptoms (primary or simple snoring), and snoring that is associated with discernible clinical or metabolic consequences.

Consideration of polysomnographic patterning may be useful in the personalized medical approach to OSA as certain intermediate phenotypes may be amenable to targeted therapy. For example, UARS may be associated with a low arousal threshold, OH with a high arousal threshold, and excessive obstructive cycling with ventilatory control instability.

The increased recognition of subtle neurocognitive impairments in children with OSA has forced clinicians to rethink the threshold level of disease requiring intervention. The diagnosis of pediatric OSA continues to evolve as more precise measures of sleep fragmentation, daytime consequences, and metabolic imbalances are introduced. The optimal methodology and criteria for the diagnosis of OSA requiring treatment in children has not been validated with outcomes data. It is clear that categorizing OSA severity by polysomnographic criteria alone (apnea-hypopnea index [AHI], gas exchange abnormalities, or sleep fragmentation) have proven unsatisfactory, because they fail to account for the individual trait susceptibility to the neurocognitive, cardiovascular, and metabolic sequelae of OSA. That is, the threshold level of OSA associated with adverse consequences varies widely among children; therefore considerable research effort has attempted to identify biomarkers to identify children at higher risk for OSA sequelae.

Clinical History

The high incidence of OSA in children mandates that screening inquiries about breathing disturbances during sleep ought to be a routine part of the primary care interview[15] (Table 27.1). Particular attention should be given to conditions known to exacerbate OSA such as craniofacial abnormalities, neuromuscular weakness, obesity, and genetic conditions. Epidemiologically, other important predictors of OSA in children are a history of prematurity (odds ratio 3), parental history of OSA, lower socioeconomic status, tobacco exposure,[16] and African American race (odds ratio 4). A parent typically provides the clinical history, with the patient oblivious to their condition, other than sometimes the complaint of excessive daytime

TABLE 27.1	Clinical History in Obstructive Sleep Apnea
Sleep	**Wakefulness**
Snoring	Poor school performance
Witnessed apnea	Behavior concerns
Gasping/choking noises	Hyperactivity
Work of breathing	Inattention
Paradoxical breathing	Excess daytime sleepiness
Enuresis	Age-inappropriate napping
Mouth breathing	Loud breathing
Restless sleep	Difficult to arouse from sleep
Diaphoresis	Mood disturbance
Hyperextended neck	Morning headache
Frequent awakenings	Failure to thrive
Dry mouth	Obesity
Sleep in seated position	Mouth breathing
Cyanosis	Craniofacial abnormalities
	Hypertension
	Adenotonsillar hypertrophy
	Adenoidal facies

sleepiness. Careful attention to the clinical presentation and polysomnographic patterning, in combination with supportive laboratory and questionnaire data, is required to accurately diagnose OSA severity to optimize surgical and medical management.[17] Risk factors for persistent OSA following adenotonsillectomy include obesity, male sex, severe baseline OSA, African American race, craniofacial anomalies, and neuromuscular weakness.

Nightly snoring is observed in most children with OSA. However, snoring may be absent in the setting of mouth breathing or craniofacial abnormalities, including Down syndrome, and especially in infants.[18] The incidence of habitual snoring (at least three times per week) has been reported in 12–15% of children,[19,20] but only 2–5% will have polysomnographic evidence of OSA. In one large study of children suspected to have OSA, snoring at least 5 days per week had a sensitivity of only 77% and a specificity of 48% for polysomnographic OSA.[21] A parental report of a snoring child is an accurate predictor of polysomnographic snoring, but not of OSA.[22] In addition, a population-based study using home-based polysomnography found that "loud snoring 1 to 2 times per week during the last month" was absent in at least 25% of children with documented OSA.[23] Snoring may be accompanied by labored breathing, hyperextension of the neck, and/or witnessed apneic pauses.

Excessive daytime sleepiness may be measured subjectively using the parent-completed and modified for children, Epworth Sleepiness Scale (ESS)[24] or the Pediatric

Sleep Questionnaire-Sleepiness Subscale (PSQ-SS[25]). Using the ESS, 28% of children with OSA had excessive daytime sleepiness.[24] Using the PSQ-SS, 43% of children with OSA were reportedly sleepy, but only a small correlation was found with objective testing.[25] Subjective reports of excessive daytime sleepiness are less common in young children with OSA, but are more often present in adolescents. Sleepiness had a sensitivity of 19% and a specificity of 88% for polysomnographic OSA.[21] Objective measurement of sleepiness with the multiple sleep latency test, reveals that only 13% of prepubertal children with OSA have a sleep latency <10 minutes.[26] However, the incidence of objective sleepiness is higher in obese children and those with more severe OSA.[26,27] Also, although not considered sleepy by adult standards, children with OSA may be relatively sleepier than normal children.[24]

Witnessed pauses during sleep in children had a sensitivity of only 42% and a specificity of 88% for polysomnographic OSA.[21] Additional nonspecific clinical findings are occasionally observed in children with OSA including failure to thrive, morning headaches, excessive nighttime sweating, and secondary enuresis. The neurocognitive consequences of OSA are nonspecific, such as cognitive deficits,[4] poor school performance,[28] behavioral disturbances, and hyperactivity.[29]

The primary underlying conditions predisposing toward OSA include obesity, micrognathia, midface hypoplasia, and neuromuscular weakness. Children with craniosynostosis, achondroplasia, and Down syndrome have midfacial hypoplasia and may have comorbid nasal anomalies contributing to the increased upper airway resistance. Children with micro- or retrognathia frequently experience glossoptosis including Treacher Collins, Stickler syndrome, and Nager syndrome. Weakness of the pharyngeal dilators is commonly observed in children with cerebral palsy and other generalized neuromuscular disorders.

Physical Examination

Physical examination in children with OSA may be normal, but frequently includes adenotonsillar hypertrophy, nasal passage narrowing, dysgnathia, or craniofacial abnormalities (Table 27.2). The majority of children with OSA are of normal height and weight, although both obesity and failure to thrive may occur. Though a longitudinal study documented that airway soft tissue peaks relative to airway size between 4 and 8 years of age,[30] the visualization of tonsillar size and airway configuration (Mallampati or Friedman classification) has an inconsistent correlation with AHI, symptoms, or response to adenotonsillectomy.[31–33] Tonsillar hypertrophy (defined as grade 3 or above; extending outside of the tonsillar pillars but not meeting at midline) had a sensitivity of only 77% and a specificity of 65% for polysomnographic OSA.[21]

Nasal resistance is an important determinant of OSA and may be amenable to specific surgical and medical therapies. Environmental allergies may be suspected on the basis

TABLE 27.2 Physical Examination in Obstructive Sleep Apnea

General
- Sleepiness
- Obesity
- Failure to thrive
- Neuromuscular weakness
- Genetic conditions

Head
- Swollen mucous membranes
- Deviated septum
- Adenoidal facies
- Infraorbital darkening
- Elongated midface
- Mouth breathing
- Tonsillar hypertrophy
- High arched palate
- Overjet
- Posterior buccal crossbite
- Crowded oropharynx
- Macroglossia
- Glossoptosis
- Midfacial hypoplasia
- Micrognathia/retrognathia
- Increased neck circumference

Cardiovascular
- Hypertension
- Loud P2
- Extremities
- Edema
- Clubbing (rare)

infraorbital darkening, a nasal crease, swollen nasal mucous membranes, nasal muscle atrophy, and elongated facial height ("adenoidal facies"). Additional common causes of nasal obstruction include a deviated septum or mucoid nasal discharge. Generally, chronic mouth breathing may give rise to a narrow, high-arched palate, and a crossbite. Malocclusion consisting of a posterior crossbite, reduced overbite, increased overbite, and increased overjet is also associated with OSA in children.[34,35] Evaluation of adenoid size using a mirror technique has an excellent correlation with direct visualization under sedation.[36]

Cardiovascular sequelae of OSA, such as cor pulmonale and congestive heart failure, are infrequently observed in current clinical practice, as heightened awareness has facilitated earlier diagnosis. Although blood pressure is statistically elevated in children with OSA, the wide range of normal makes this measurement a poor screening tool.[37,38] Hypertensive children with OSA have a decrease in blood pressure after adenotonsillectomy[39] and continuous positive airway pressure (CPAP).[40]

Questionnaires

The use of standardized screening questionnaires for OSA has been disappointing. Brouillette and colleagues presented a questionnaire aimed at distinguishing children with OSA from normal controls.[41] However, subsequent application of this and other questionnaires to a population of snoring children demonstrated a wide-ranging positive predictive value (48.3–76.9%) and negative predictive value (26.9–93%).[41–43] Although children with OSA are statistically more likely to have reported symptoms such as witnessed apnea, cyanosis, and/or labored breathing, no questionnaire has a sufficiently high positive predictive value and negative predictive value to be used as a primary diagnostic tool.[42] Thus the clinical history alone is insufficient to diagnose OSA among a population of snoring children.

Questionnaires have also been developed that incorporate questions relating to the consequences of OSA, including sleepiness, hyperactivity, and behavior. Compared with polysomnography, an affirmative response to at least one-third of questions on the 22 question PSQ had a sensitivity of 0.85 and a specificity of 0.87.[44,45] However, using the PSQ to screen for OSA in high-risk pediatric populations, including those with craniofacial and neuromuscular disorders, resulted in lower sensitivity.[46] Both generic[47] (Pediatric Quality of Life [PedsQL]) and disease-specific[48] (18-Item Obstructive Sleep Apnea tool [OSA-18]) quality-of-life questionnaires demonstrate impairments in quality of life in children with OSA, but are poor screening tools for OSA with a weak correlation with AHI.[49] Overall, questionnaires can provide essential information regarding cognitive and behavioral consequences of OSA that are omitted from polysomnography, but are poorly predictive of the AHI.[50]

Imaging Studies

Upper airway structural narrowing is an important determinant of OSA, and obstruction may be present at multiple levels, especially in children with craniofacial abnormalities. Polysomnography does not localize the level or levels of obstruction which limits its utility in predicting response to surgery. Imaging techniques may provide valuable anatomical information including dental cephalograms, lateral neck radiographs, and magnetic resonance imaging (MRI). Objective measurements of tonsil and adenoid size have a better correlation with AHI than visual inspection.[51] Complex postprocessing algorithms using computational fluid dynamics are being applied to predict obstruction and may in the future be helpful to guide therapy.[52]

Lateral neck radiographs or cephalometry encompass the nasopharynx to the upper trachea permitting evaluation of adenotonsillar size and the adjacent airway using low-dose radiation. The technique is limited by the upright acquisition and two-dimensional nature of the radiographs. The adenoid size determined by cephalometry was related to obstructive apnea duration and hypoxemia in one study,[53] and to apnea frequency in another.[54] Tonsillar size

determined from cephalometry, but not clinical examination, has been demonstrated to correlate well with AHI.[55] Cephalograms in children with OSA compared with controls demonstrated an increased anteroposterior jaw relationship, increased mandibular inclination in relation to the palatal line, increased facial height, a longer and thicker soft palate, smaller airway diameters, and lower hyoid bone position.[56,57]

Adenotonsillar enlargement is associated with chronic mouth breathing and therefore cephalometric changes that may predispose to future OSA, which argues for early intervention.[58] The measurement of the ratio of the width of the tonsil to the depth of the pharyngeal space by cephalometry was reported to have a good sensitivity and specificity for distinguishing mild from moderate/severe OSA in a small number of patients.[55] Adenoidal enlargement measured by cephalometry was present in over 80% of children with OSA but also in 42% with PS.[59] Though neck radiographs may be suggestive of adenoidal hypertrophy, direct visualization of the adenoids remains the diagnostic standard.[60] Lateral neck radiographs may also demonstrate enlargement of the lingual tonsil, which is commonly observed in Down syndrome.[61]

In children with OSA in whom the level of airway obstruction is uncertain, an MRI can provide valuable soft tissue and bony anatomical information. MRI of the upper airway in children with OSA compared with normal controls reveals a statistically smaller upper airway luminal volume and elongation of the soft palate, as well as enlarged tonsils and adenoids.[51,62] However, there is considerable overlap between the groups, rendering MRI a poor screening tool for OSA. In obese children, the presence of OSA was associated with increased upper airway lymphoid tissue, and the parapharyngeal fat pad, with the former correlating with the AHI.[63] Another MRI study demonstrated an excellent correlation between tonsillar size, pharyngeal airway volume, retropalatal cross-sectional area, and AHI.[64] In addition to these findings, a decrease in mandibular volume has been reported in children with OSA using MRI.[65] Overall, a poor relationship has been reported between the visual sizing of the tonsil[33] and the AHI, but MRI measurements of the tonsil demonstrate a more consistent relationship with the AHI.[51] Though useful in select cases, MRI testing is expensive and requires a long examination time that frequently requires sedation in young children. Moreover, the state of the airway muscle tone is different than that found during sleep and therefore airway function during wakefulness, or even sedation, may not be representative of that observed during natural sleep.

Dynamic imaging under sedation may demonstrate glossoptosis, particularly in children with macroglossia, micrognathia, or neuromuscular weakness.[66] Cine MRI has been demonstrated to localize the inspiratory narrowing level in children with OSA.[67,68] Anatomical localization of the site of obstruction with cine MRI may alter the therapeutic approach in some children with residual OSA following adenotonsillectomy or craniofacial facial anomalies. In a study of 15 children with Down syndrome and residual OSA following adenotonsillectomy, cine MRI demonstrated a variety of levels of obstruction including adenoidal regrowth, glossoptosis, soft palate collapse, hypopharyngeal collapse, macroglossia, and an enlarged lingual tonsil.[67,68] Another study of 36 children ranging from 3 to 18 years of age found the cine MRI identified a site of obstruction in 92% with residual OSA post-adenotonsillectomy, including lingual tonsillar hypertrophy and posterior displacement of the tongue.[69]

Airway Endoscopy

Adenotonsillar hypertrophy is the most common cause of OSA in children, but considerable obstruction is present at other sites, especially after adenotonsillectomy[70] and in children with craniofacial predispositions. A large meta-analysis demonstrated that following adenotonsillectomy only 60% of patients with have a normalization of their AHI (<1/hr), including only 39% of obese children[71]; otherwise normal children with residual OSA after adenotonsillectomy also have statistically smaller mandibles.[72] Other conditions at high risk for residual OSA post adenotonsillectomy include craniofacial abnormalities, obesity, and neuromuscular weakness. Direct visualization of the upper airway during wakefulness is commonly performed to determine the cause of OSA. A flexible fiberoptic endoscopic examination can be performed in the outpatient clinic setting to rapidly diagnose adenoidal enlargement, deviated septum, turbinate enlargement, choanal narrowing, pyriform aperture stenosis, vocal cord dysfunction, and laryngomalacia.

Drug-induced sedation endoscopy (DISE) has been widely adopted in children to identify the sites of airway narrowing and collapse allows for targeted surgical and non-surgical therapies. Under general anesthesia with spontaneous breathing, DISE utilizes a flexible endoscope inserted through the nose to evaluate the cross-sectional area at various levels including the nose, retropalatal area, oropharynx and hypopharynx. The sedation required to perform DISE alters the neuromuscular control of the upper airway; therefore this examination may not be fully representative of the sleeping airway. Though DISE is mostly reserved for children with persistent OSA, it has also been applied to surgically naïve children, especially those with underlying conditions predisposing to persistent OSA such as obesity, craniofacial abnormalities, and neurologic impairment. DISE in a population of 28 surgically naïve children <2 years of age demonstrated a preponderance of obstruction at the level of the adenoid and tonsil, but 50% of patients had obstruction at multiple levels.[73]

DISE has been shown to identify unsuspected sites of obstruction including deviated septum, turbinate hypertrophy, tongue-based collapse, or sleep-dependent laryngomalacia. In a large series of children with suspected OSA, DISE was reported to yield anatomical information in surgically naïve children that changed surgical management in 35% of patients.[74] In surgically naïve children with Down syndrome and OSA, DISE identified multilevel collapse in 85% of patients.[75] When DISE is used in children following adenotonsillectomy, most will have multilevel collapse,[76] and the most common sites of obstruction were the adenoids (55%), the supraglottis (49%), and the tongue base (46%).[77] The assessment of adenotonsillar dynamic collapse with DISE was a better predictor of response to adenotonsillectomy than awake tonsil size assessment.[78] Finally, DISE is required in children being considered for a hypoglossal nerve stimulator to rule out concentric pharyngeal collapse.

Metabolic Testing

Metabolic testing can be useful to identify those children at most risk for adverse consequences associated with OSA, in whom more aggressive therapy would be indicated. Urinary catecholamines are elevated in children with OSA, especially those with cognitive deficits.[79] Evidence for insulin resistance (glucose, insulin, hemoglobin A1c),[80] dyslipidemia (cholesterol, triglycerides, high-density lipoprotein [HDL], low-density lipoprotein [LDL]), endothelial dysfunction, and inflammation (C-reactive protein [CRP]) have been reported in children with OSA,[6,81–83] though obesity appears to be the most important risk factor.[84,85] Children with OSA have different baseline levels of proinflammatory cytokines and acute phase reactants (CRP, soluble CD-40 ligand) compared with normal controls.[86]

Molecular phenotyping targets that have been applied to children with OSA include urinary proteomics, inflammatory markers, and endothelial dysfunction. Both single nucleotide polymorphisms[87] and epigenetic changes[88] to the nitric oxide synthetase *(NOS)* gene have been reported in children with OSA. In a group of children with OSA, 31% had abnormal endothelial dysfunction measured by post-occlusive hyperemic responses, which was associated with higher methylation levels of the *eNOS* gene.[88] The *eNOS* gene is highly dependent on epigenetic modifications for expression that may be influenced by body habitus or environmental factors. The *FOXP3* gene regulates expression of T-regulatory lymphocytes, and its increased methylation has been reported in children with OSA.[89]

Children with OSA and endothelial dysfunction also had lower levels of serum adropin,[90] elevated angiopoietin-2,[91] elevated tyrosine kinase receptor TIE-2,[91] differentially expressed circulating microsomal microRNA,[92] and elevated lipoprotein-associated phospholipase A2 plasma activity levels.[5] Because endothelial dysfunction is believed to be a precursor of cardiovascular disease, its measurement may identify children at greatest risk for OSA-related morbidity. In addition, the APOE ε4 allele,[93] or certain nicotinamide adenine dinucleotide phosphate (NADPH) oxidase p22 subunit polymorphisms[94] are more likely in children with OSA that develop neurocognitive impairments. Children with OSA in combination with the tumor necrosis factor (TNF)-α-308G gene polymorphism are more likely to manifest excessive daytime sleepiness.[95]

Video/Audio Recordings

Diagnosing OSA using home audio recordings, in addition to a standard clinical history and physical examination, revealed a sensitivity of 71% and a specificity of 80%.[96] Though subtle forms of OSA are particularly difficult to evaluate using this technique, computer-aided processing of audio signals for regularity may improve predictive value.[97] Frequency domain analysis of the snoring signal has also shown promise in distinguishing OSA from PS.[98] Video recordings can also yield a noninvasive measure of movement and therefore arousal.[99–101] Video is also a useful adjunct to a comprehensive polysomnogram to evaluate body and head positioning, paradoxing, snoring, and mouth breathing. Studies correlating video scoring systems to standard polysomnography have been encouraging.[101] Future research will be necessary to validate the utility of a particular domiciliary video/audio study in a population with a well-characterized symptomatology.

Overnight Polysomnography

The clinical history and physical examination is poorly predictive of which snoring children have polysomnographic evidence for OSA.[102,103] Consequently, the American Academy of Pediatrics guideline encourages obtaining a polysomnogram in children that snore on a regular basis or referring to a sleep specialist or otolaryngologist for a more extensive evaluation.[15] Similarly, the American Academy of Sleep Medicine encourages routine polysomnograms before adenotonsillectomy to confirm the diagnosis and for assessment of perioperative risk.[104] By contrast, the American Academy of Otolaryngology guideline states that before performing tonsillectomy, the clinician should refer children with obstructive sleep-disordered breathing symptoms for polysomnography if the patients are <2 years of age or exhibit any of the following: obesity, Down syndrome, craniofacial abnormalities, neuromuscular disorders, sickle cell disease, or mucopolysaccharidoses.[105] Otherwise, children suspected of having OSA without these comorbidities should be referred for polysomnography if the need for tonsillectomy is uncertain or when there is discordance between the physical examination and the reported severity of the obstruction.[105]

Given that snoring in the absence of polysomnographic abnormalities may be associated with adverse outcomes, and that the treatment of these children is beneficial,[106] it is widespread practice to proceed with therapy without polysomnography. Nationally in the United States it has been estimated that 95% of children undergoing adenotonsillectomy for obstructive symptoms do so without confirmatory polysomnography. The decision as to whether to perform polysomnography depends on the extent of discernible clinical symptoms (inattentiveness, hyperactivity, mood disturbances, poor school performance, excessive daytime sleepiness), potential therapeutic options (airway soft tissue surgery, nasal allergy treatment, CPAP), comorbidities (obesity, craniofacial anomalies, neuromuscular weakness),

and patient preferences. Polysomnography may be useful to determine the need for surgery, adjust perioperative care, and to guide follow-up care. However, the majority of postoperative complications can be predicted by clinical factors including age, body mass index (BMI), and underlying medical conditions.[107] Children with moderate to severe OSA are unlikely to resolve without treatment. Polysomnography is also indicated for children with residual symptoms following adenotonsillectomy, severe OSA preoperatively, and underlying medical conditions. Drawbacks of relying on polysomnography include the considerable expense and lack of widespread availability. Also, polysomnography does not identify the site of obstruction, unequivocally determine which children ought to be treated, or determine the most appropriate therapy.

In the event that objective OSA testing is deemed necessary, polysomnography represents the gold standard for establishing the presence and severity of objective OSA in children.[15] Guidelines for performing laboratory-based polysomnography in children have been established.[108] Laboratory-based respiratory polygraphy (excluding electroencephalogram [EEG]) tends to underestimate the AHI enough to affect clinical decision making.[109] Home-based polygraphy has been reported to have an excellent concordance with lab-based studies,[110] but has also been reported to be missing key channels, especially nasal pressure, limiting the widespread application of this technology.[111]

The sleep laboratory should be a nonthreatening environment that comfortably accommodates a parent during the study. Personnel with pediatric training should record, score, and interpret the study. The use of sedatives and sleep deprivation[112] may worsen OSA, and are therefore not recommended. To the extent possible, sleep studies should conform to the child's usual sleep period. Young infants may reasonably be studied during the day, whereas adolescent studies should generally start later at night. The polysomnographic montage will vary with the patient's suspected disorder (Table 27.3).

TABLE 27.3	Example of Polysomnogram Montage
Electroencephalography (C_4-M_1, O_2-M_1, F_4-M_1)	
Electromyogram (chin, both legs)	
Electrooculogram (right/left)	
Electrocardiogram	
Respiratory inductance plethysmography	
Oximetry (2-second averaging), pulse waveform	
End-tidal PCO_2 (peak value, waveform)	
Flow: nasal pressure, oronasal thermistor	
Snore volume	
Body position sensor	
Video and audio taping	

Electroencephalogram

Consensus guidelines for analyzing sleep architecture have been established in infants, children, and adults.[108] Standard practice is to apply adult EEG criteria to children older than 2 months of age (48 weeks postconceptional age). Sleep staging establishes that an adequate amount of TST and sufficient rapid eye movement (REM) sleep were obtained on the night of the study, and demonstrates the presence or absence of sleep fragmentation. In addition to sleep staging, the EEG tracing is useful for scoring cortical arousals and detecting epileptiform discharges. Several reports indicated that children with snoring or even severe OSA may have normal sleep state distribution.[113,114] However, a large cohort (n = 559) comparing normal children to children with OSA revealed that OSA patients have increases in slow-wave sleep (23.5 vs. 28.8% TST), suggesting a greater pressure toward sleep, and decreases in REM sleep (22.3 vs. 17.3% TST).[115] Furthermore, these authors also observed a decline in the spontaneous arousal index in OSA patients versus controls (8.4 vs. 5.3/hr), indicating a homeostatic elevation in the arousal threshold.[115]

Arousal

Arousal from sleep is a protective reflex mechanism that restores airway patency through dilator muscle activation during a transient state of heightened vigilance. Both mechano- and chemoreceptors have a role in initiating the arousal response. Though arousals reverse the airway obstruction, they result in the untoward consequences of sleep fragmentation and sympathetic activation.[61] Polysomnographically, arousal is a graded phenomenon that may be associated with EEG changes,[108] increased airflow, elimination of airflow limitation, cessation of paradoxical breathing, tachycardia, movement, blood pressure elevation,[116] and autonomic activation.[117] By consensus, an electrocortical (EEG) arousal is defined as an abrupt shift in EEG frequency, including alpha, theta, and/or frequencies greater than 16 Hz that last at least 3 seconds, with at least 10 seconds of stable sleep preceding.[108] The interscorer agreement for standard EEG arousals in children is excellent with an intraclass correlation coefficient (ICC) of 0.90.[118] However, visible EEG arousals are present in only 18% and 51% of obstructive events in infants and children, respectively,[119] complicating the diagnosis of UARS in children. Adding Fz to the montage resulted in only an additional 3% of scorable EEG arousals.[120] Thus depending on the EEG arousal index alone for the diagnosis of UARS is unreliable. Frequency domain analysis may reveal evidence of EEG arousal not readily visible, and may be a clinically useful tool in the future.[121]

Obstructive events that terminate with autonomic activation, in the absence of visible EEG changes, are termed subcortical arousals. Autonomic measures that have been demonstrated to reliably identify subcortical arousals include heart rate variability, blood pressure elevations, pulse transit time, and peripheral arterial tonometry. The pulse transit time is a noninvasive measure that is inversely related to blood pressure and therefore subcortical arousals were reported to be a more sensitive measure of respiratory arousal compared with 3-second EEG arousals.[122] As a screening tool for OSA, the pulse transit time had a sensitivity of 81% and a specificity of 76%.[123] Subcortical arousals alone have been demonstrated to result in neurocognitive impairment in adults.[124]

Measures of Respiratory Movements

Thoracic and abdominal excursion is measured most commonly with respiratory inductive plethysmography (RIP). The classification of central and obstructive apneas is achieved by determining whether respiratory efforts are present during intervals of reduced flow. Uncalibrated RIP tracings may also be used to identify thoracoabdominal asynchrony, which is indicative of increased respiratory effort due to upper airway obstruction and OSA. Paradoxical breathing is normally seen in infants due to the high compliance of their chest wall, particularly during REM sleep, but is rare after 3 years of age.[125]

Esophageal manometry (P_{es}) represents the gold standard for quantifying respiratory effort and permits the detection of subtle, partially obstructive events that may produce sleep fragmentation.[126] However, P_{es} monitoring is uncomfortable and may itself alter the frequency of respiratory events.[127] The introduction of noninvasive, nasal pressure measurements has largely supplanted P_{es} in establishing the diagnosis of UARS (see Fig. 27.1). Nevertheless, esophageal manometry peak amplitude and percentage time spent lower than -10 cm H_2O has been reported to have a better correlation with behavioral outcomes than the traditional AHI with or without respiratory effort–related arousals.[128] Current practice is to reserve P_{es} monitoring for rare cases of children with diagnostic uncertainty even after standard overnight polysomnography.

Measures of Airflow

Airflow can be quantitatively measured using an oronasal mask and pneumotachograph. However, mask breathing is uncomfortable and has been shown to alter respiratory mechanics. Practically speaking, this methodology is restricted to research settings and to positive airway pressure titration studies. Thermistors provide qualitative measures of oronasal airflow by measuring the temperature of expired air. Though thermistors accurately indicate complete cessation of flow, they are not an accurate measure of tidal volume and therefore hypopnea.[129] Another drawback of the thermistor is its long-time constant that obscures the nuance of the flow profile making the evaluation of flow limitation impossible.[129]

Nasal cannula pressure recordings provide a minimally invasive, semiquantitative measure of airflow.[130,131] The resulting signal has been shown to be proportional to flow squared. Because nasal pressure measurements have a fast

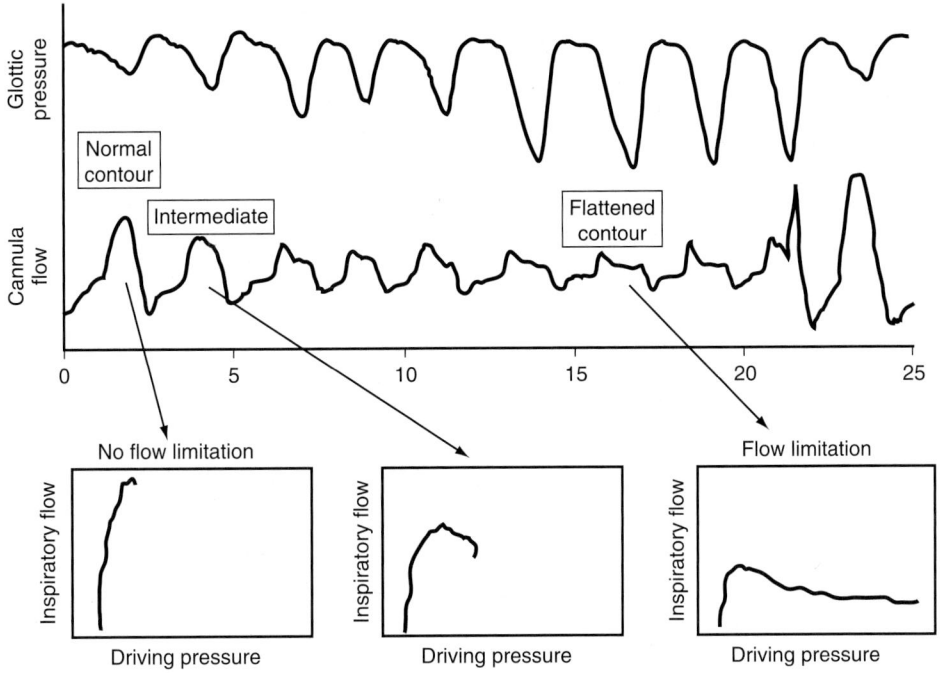

• **Fig. 27.2** Nasal cannula pressure tracing demonstrating that flow becomes independent of driving pressure during flow limited breaths. *(Reproduced with permission from Hosselet et al.[131])*

time constant, it is possible to detect flattening of the inspiratory nasal pressure signal (termed flow limitation) that occurs in a collapsible tube when flow becomes independent of driving pressure (Fig. 27.2). Limitations of the nasal cannula pressure recordings include obstruction of the tubing with secretions, mouth breathing (especially in children with adenoidal hypertrophy), and the possible increase in nasal resistance due to obstruction of the nares. In children, the reported signal quality has varied in laboratory-based studies. Trang and colleagues reported an overall uninterpretable nasal cannula signal during only 4% of TST.[132] However, 17% of subjects had uninterpretable signals for more than 20% of TST. In contrast, Serebrisky and colleagues reported adequate nasal cannula flow signals (>50% of TST) during sleep in only 71.8% of patients.[133] In a domiciliary study, the nasal cannula channel was not available overall for more than 50% of the night.[134] Verginis and colleagues compared the combination of the thermistor and nasal pressure measurement with either modality alone and found the combination significantly lowered the scoring of false-negative and false-positive obstructive events.[135]

Airflow may be approximated using RIP by considering that lung volume can be approximated by a two-compartment model (thoracic and abdomen excursion). RIP may be calibrated using an isovolume maneuver or a statistical technique and used to derive a "sum" channel proportional to tidal volume.[136] Thus the time derivative of the sum channel is proportional to flow. The RIP signal may therefore be analyzed for apnea, hypopnea, and flow limitation.[137] Our current practice is to combine RIP, nasal cannula pressure, capnometry, and an oronasal thermistor in

our laboratory-based studies to ensure that a flow signal is likely to be available throughout the night.

Gas Exchange

Pulse oximetry, which is based on the absorption spectra of hemoglobin, is the standard polysomnographic measure of hypoxemia. The relationship between the arterial oxygen tension and the SpO_2, the oxyhemoglobin curve, is sigmoidal. Patients with normal pulmonary function, whose baseline SpO_2 is on the flat portion of the curve, require large changes in PaO_2 to affect their SpO_2. By contrast, patients with parenchymal lung disease or obesity may be operating on the steep portion of the oxyhemoglobin curve, thereby experiencing a profound decline in SpO_2 with small decrements in PaO_2. In sickle cell disease, the oxyhemoglobin curve is variably shifted, thus limiting the utility of SpO_2 measurements in some patients.

The adequacy of ventilation can be assessed noninvasively during sleep by sampling CO_2 tension in expired air (capnography). Expired gas initially consists of dead space ventilation in the measuring apparatus as well as the physiologic dead space. In the setting of normal lungs, the terminal expired concentration of CO_2 reaches a plateau and reflects alveolar gas. The concentration of CO_2 in a given alveolus is predicated on the ventilation/perfusion relationship. In subjects with normal lung mechanics, end-tidal PCO_2 ($P_{ET}CO_2$) is approximately 2–5 mm Hg below the arterial $PaCO_2$ level.[138] However, in diseases with uneven ventilation/perfusion or altered alveolar time constants, such as cystic fibrosis, the $P_{ET}CO_2$ will not be an accurate measure of $PaCO_2$. Also, the rapid respiratory rates characteristic of infants may not permit the alveolar CO_2 to plateau; therefore it may underestimate the true CO_2 value.[139] The capnometry signal is prone to artifact due to nasal secretions obstructing the sampling cannula. Morielli and colleagues reported that 27% of polysomnographic epochs in their laboratory had a poor $P_{ET}CO_2$ waveform, stressing the importance of careful attention to technique.[139] Transcutaneous CO_2 ($TcCO_2$) monitors may be valuable in patients in whom $P_{ET}CO_2$ is not accurate, such as infants or patients with parenchymal lung disease.[139] Though absolute values of $TcCO_2$ are variable, the trend is proportional to the $PaCO_2$ with a lag of approximately 1 minute. Sleep is normally associated with a 4–6 mm Hg increase in $TcCO_2$.

Normative Polysomnographic Data

Normative data for the EEG and respiratory parameters of sleeping children are shown in Table 27.4.[113,140–143] In infants, longitudinal arterial oxygen saturation monitoring revealed a median SpO_2 baseline of 98%, but the SpO_2 was <90% during 0.51% of epochs.[144] Marcus and colleagues presented the respiratory data of 50 normal, nonobese children between 1 and 18 years of age (mean 9.7 ± 4.6), using a thermistor and $P_{ET}CO_2$ monitoring.[143] Nine subjects had at least one obstructive apneic event. One "normal" child had an apnea index of 3.1/hr, though he had a sibling with OSA. Including this outlier, an obstructive apnea index >1/hr was determined to be statistically abnormal. However, the threshold level at which the apnea index becomes clinically significant has not been established. Obstructive hypopneas are infrequently observed in normal children with the mean hypopnea index being 0.1–0.2/hr.[145,146] Acebo and colleagues also reported that hypopneas were rare in older children and adolescents.[142] Experience from our laboratory also indicates that hypopneas and respiratory

effort–related arousals occur infrequently in normal young children (<1.5/hr).

Normative data for esophageal manometry (ΔP_{es}) from 10 normal subjects in our laboratory, aged 2–11 years, showed that control subjects had a mean ΔP_{es} of −8 ± 2 cm H_2O (range −6 to −12), a peak ΔP_{es} of −12 ± 3 cm H_2O (range −9 to −9 cm H_2O), and had a $\Delta P_{es} \leq -10$ cm H_2O for 8 ± 12 % of breaths (range 3–61%).[122] Other investigators have considered ΔP_{es} swings of −8 to −14 cm H_2O as normal,[148] and suggested that normal children spend ≥10% of the night with inspiratory esophageal pressure swings ≤ -10 cm H_2O.[126] However, our data showed that two control patients spent 21% and 61% of the night with a $\Delta P_{es} \leq -10$ cm H_2O. Thus normative data from nonsnoring controls reveal considerable variability in respiratory effort. ΔP_{es} is lower in normal infants at 5–6 cm H_2O.[149]

Domiciliary Studies

Attended overnight polysomnography in a designated pediatric sleep laboratory represents the gold standard for the diagnosis of OSA in children.[150] However, such comprehensive testing is expensive, labor intensive, and not widely available. Recognizing that only 10–20% of children who snore will have OSA has prompted considerable interest in limited nap or unattended domiciliary studies. Polysomnography during a daytime nap may underestimate the degree of OSA.[151,152] REM sleep often does not occur during naps. Furthermore, obstructive respiratory events worsen as sleep progresses.[113] Thus, although the positive predictive value of an abnormal nap study is 100%, the negative predictive value is only 20%.[151,152] Home-based study devices may range in complexity from oximetry alone[153] to multichannel recordings.[154] Ambulatory studies may be used to evaluate oxygenation in infants with chronic lung disease, cystic fibrosis, restrictive lung diseases, and neuromuscular conditions. Goodwin and colleagues performed a

TABLE 27.4 Polysomnographic Data in Normal 3- to 8-Year-Old Children

Sleep		Respiratory	
EEG arousal index, n/hr	9.3 ± 4.8	Obstructive apnea index, n/hr TST	0.0 ± 0.1
Sleep efficiency, %	90 ± 7	Obstructive hypopnea index, n/hr TST	0.1 ± 0.1
Stage 1, %TST	5 ± 2	Central apneas with desaturation n/hr TST	0.6 ± 0.6
Stage 2, %TST	36 ± 6	$P_{ET}CO_2 \geq 50$ mm Hg, %TST	2.6 ± 11
Slow-wave sleep, %TST	25 ± 4	Peak $P_{ET}CO_2$, mm Hg	46 ± 3
REM sleep, %TST	21 ± 4	SpO_2 nadir, %	92 ± 4
REM cycles, n	4 ± 1	SpO_2 <90 (%TST)	0.04 ± 0.2
Awake, %TST	8 ± 7	SpO_2 <85 (%TST)	0.01 ± 0.05

Abbreviations: EEG, electroencephalogram; TST, total sleep time; SpO_2, oxygen saturation; $P_{ET}CO_2$, end-tidal carbon dioxide; mean ± SD; REM, rapid eye movement.
See references[122,140,142,143,147].

home-based study that was set up by a technician and then was completed unattended, with an excellent success rate of 91%.[155] Similarly, Rosen and colleagues performed 850 abbreviated home studies with 94% yielding technically satisfactory data.[23] A subset of 55 children also underwent laboratory-based polysomnography and the sensitivity and specificity of the home-based study to detect OSA as defined by an AHI >5/hr on the laboratory study, was 88% and 98%, respectively.[23] In a small group of children with Down syndrome (n = 19), home polygraphy was highly effective in diagnosing children with moderate to severe OSA compared with laboratory-based polysomnography.[156] Overall, the utility of ambulatory studies depends on the age group and channels acquired. As of 2017, the American Academy of Sleep Medicine position paper on home sleep studies concluded the following: "Use of a home sleep apnea test is not recommended for the diagnosis of OSA in children."[157]

Documenting oximeters should include an algorithm for artifact reduction using the plethysmograph waveform or heart rate detected by the oximeter. The oximetry channel alone has been compared with full polysomnography in a population of snoring children with adenotonsillar hypertrophy and demonstrated an excellent positive predictive value (97%), but a poor negative predictive ability (53%).[158] By contrast, Kirk and colleagues reported that overnight oximetry alone has a poor correlation with laboratory-based polysomnography.[159] Many children with OSA and clinically significant respiratory effort–related arousals will not demonstrate oxygen desaturation.[160] Oximetry is inadequate to diagnose a considerable percentage of pediatric OSA in which arousal or hypoventilation, rather than frank apnea or hypoxemia, predominate.[159] Changes in the pulse wave amplitude is thought to reflect changes in intrathoracic pressure that can aide in the diagnosis of obstructive events.[161] One report using smartphone-based oximetry incorporating photoplethysmogram dynamics reported a good sensitivity (80%, 85%, and 82%) and specificity (65%, 79%, and 91%) for detecting children with an AHI of ≥ 1, ≥ 5, and ≥ 10.[162] Using complex time- and frequency-domain techniques with oximeter recordings has demonstrated high correlations with the AHI determined with comprehensive polysomnography, and a high diagnostic accuracy for moderate and severe OSA.[163–165]

The peripheral arterial tonometer (PAT) is a noninvasive finger plethysmograph measuring pulsatile volume changes, and therefore sympathetic activity.[166] Sympathetic activation produces vasoconstriction of the cutaneous vasculature, attenuating the PAT signal. The specificity of the PAT as an arousal detection tool is enhanced by considering additional input variables, such as heart rate and oximetry.[167] The scoring of PAT arousals has been automated, and the technique validated using standard polysomnography.[168] The PAT arousal index was significantly correlated with the total EEG arousal index in children. PAT technology has been shown to be a robust ambulatory tool for diagnosing OSA, with a high correlation with laboratory-based studies.[168]

Night-to-Night Polysomnographic Variability

A single overnight polysomnogram is a well-recognized diagnostic tool used to determine the presence and severity of OSA in symptomatic children.[150] However, in adults an adaptation effect of the sleep laboratory environment, termed the "first night effect," has been reported to disrupt sleep architecture[169] and perhaps underestimate respiratory disturbance.[170] There are several pediatric studies that have documented consistency in the diagnosis of OSA using polysomnography from night to night.[169,171–173] In children, the clinical diagnosis of either OSA or PS remained the same in two polysomnogram studies 1–4 weeks apart.[171] Although the overall classification of subjects was unchanged, there were minimal changes in OSA severity between nights. This supports the view that a single polysomnographic night is sufficient for the diagnosis of OSA in otherwise normal, snoring children with adenotonsillar hypertrophy. No night-to-night systematic bias has been observed in any of the mean intersubject respiratory parameters.[169,171] The intrasubject respiratory parameters, however, demonstrated considerable variability, particularly in children with severe disease. The variability in respiratory parameters could not be accounted for by changes in body position or percent REM time. Among the sleep variables, a first night effect including increased wakefulness and a reduction of REM sleep was observed in one study as the result of adaptation to the sleep laboratory environment.[169] Circumstances in which a single study night may not be sufficient include studies with inadequate sleep duration, REM time, technical limitations in acquiring key channels, or if the parents report that the particular study night did not reflect a typical night's sleep.

Diagnostic and Event Classification

The optimal definition for respiratory events and clinical classification has not been established in children. There are few clinical studies evaluating the relative merit of specific event definitions in relation to clinical outcomes. The American Academy of Sleep Medicine scoring criteria for obstructive respiratory events are summarized in Table 27.5.[108] For children between 13 and 18 years, adult criteria may optionally be used if deemed appropriate. The polysomnographic OSA severity classification based on clinical experience is summarized in Table 27.6. However, well-designed outcomes studies are desperately needed to validate these criteria. Additional abnormal breathing patterns, including tachypnea and increased respiratory effort, have been described in children with OSA.[2] Normative data for respiratory effort–related arousals and flow limitation are scant in children, but these events appear to be uncommon. Nevertheless, the clinical classification of OSA severity in children cannot be exclusively based on AHI alone. Consideration of the AHI, flow limitation, SpO_2, $P_{ET}CO_2$, work of breathing,

TABLE 27.5	Respiratory Pattern Scoring
Obstructive apnea	Reduction of oronasal thermal airflow by ≥90% lasting ≥2 missed breaths with persistent respiratory effort (alternative flow signal includes nasal pressure, capnogram, respiratory inductance plethysmography)
Obstructive hypopnea	Reduction in the nasal pressure amplitude ≥30% for at greater than or equal a two-breath duration with a desaturation ≥3%, or arousal and one or more of snoring, inspiratory flattening of nasal pressure, or thoracoabdominal paradox not seen during the pre-event baseline
Respiratory effort–related arousal	Sequence not meeting the criteria for apnea or hypopnea lasting ≥2 breaths leading to an arousal with one or more of increasing respiratory effort, flattening of the inspiratory nasal pressure, or elevation of end-tidal CO_2 above pre-event baseline
Hypoventilation	End-tidal or transcutaneous CO_2 >50 mm Hg for >25% total sleep time
Central apnea	Absence of oronasal airflow without respiratory effort and either ≥20 seconds' duration or ≥2 missed breaths duration and is associated with either arousal, decrease in heart rate (50/min for 5 seconds or <60/min for 15 seconds in infants), or ≥3% desaturation

and arousal indices, in conjunction with the clinical picture, also contribute to the diagnosis of OSA severity.

Phenotyping/Endotyping Classification

OSA may be categorized by the relative contribution of the physiologic traits including anatomy, arousal threshold, ventilatory control, and neuromuscular compensation. All patients experiencing OSA must have some level of airway collapsibility. However, airway dimensions alone in children has little relation to the severity of OSA as estimated by the AHI.[51] Thus the development of OSA depends on additional nonanatomical factors including overly sensitive ventilatory control, low pharyngeal dilator muscle activity/responsiveness, and/or a lower respiratory arousal threshold. The importance of nonanatomical mechanisms varies considerably between OSA patients, potentially allowing individualized targeted therapy.

Standard polysomnographic metrics may also be suggestive of a particular endotype. If obstructive apneas account for >90% of the total AHI, the patient is very likely to have a severe anatomical deficit with an airway critical closing pressure of >2 cm H_2O.[174] OSA patients with a combination of central, mixed, and obstructive events[175]

or significant non-REM (NREM) obstructive apnea[176] are likely to have a prominent component of ventilatory control instability. A low arousal threshold has been reported in patients with AHI <30, oxygen desaturation nadir >82.5%, and a hypopnea:apnea ratio >58.3%.[177] Routine polysomnography has also been used to estimate the intermediate phenotypes of muscle responsiveness,[178,179] airway collapsibility,[178,179] arousal threshold,[179,180] and ventilatory control instability.[176,179] Nontraditional polysomnographic patterns that have also been associated with OSA-related morbidity include the hypoxic burden,[181,182] REM-related OSA,[183,184] positional OSA,[185] neural network–based automated analysis of oximetry,[163] sleep fragmentation,[185] periodic leg movements,[186] and TST with arterial oxygen saturation <90%.[187]

Airway anatomy has been quantitated in children using the critical closing pressure, MRI,[188] cephalograms, photographs,[189] and physical examination. Anatomy could be further divided into craniofacial structure (mostly nose, mandible, and maxilla), soft tissue size (adenoids and tonsils), and airway inflammation. Anything that increases upper airway resistance predisposes toward OSA, and provides a potential target for therapy. The patients' therapeutic level of CPAP is strongly predictive of their critical closing pressure; therefore it may be useful to identify patients with mild airway collapsibility in whom non-CPAP therapies are more likely to be effective.[190]

Children with OSA may also be clinically triaged based on their anatomy, adenotonsillectomy for soft tissue enlargement, rapid maxillary expansion for a constricted maxilla, mandibular distraction osteometry for micrognathia, and turbinate reduction for swollen nasal mucous membranes. Other factors that may contribute to the anatomy endotype include obesity, fat distribution, lung volumes, and fluid shifts in the supine position. It has also been proposed that pediatric OSA be broadly divided into two types: type 1 is associated with adenotonsillar hypertrophy and a lean body habitus, and type 2 associated with obesity and milder adenotonsillar enlargement. Clinically, the type 1 patients are more likely to have hyperactivity, and the type 2 patients express more excessive daytime sleepiness, mood disorders, cardiovascular, and metabolic morbidities.[191]

OSA patients may also be divided polysomnographically into those with positional apnea (AHI supine at least double nonsupine) and nonpositional OSA. In adults, positional OSA is observed in 30–56% of patients, who are mostly younger and leaner.[192] In children, positional OSA is observed in only approximately 18% of children with OSA, and the incidence is higher in obese and older children.[185]

An elevated loop gain or increased ventilatory instability results in an overshoot decreasing carbon dioxide, therefore decreasing pharyngeal muscle activity. Identifying OSA patients with a prominent high loop gain component may identify patients likely to respond to loop gain–reducing therapies including supplemental oxygen,[192]

TABLE 27.6   Diagnostic Classification and Severity of Obstructive Sleep Apnea in Children >1 Year of Age

	oAHI (Events/hr)	SpO_2 Nadir (%)	$P_{ET}CO_2$ Peak (torr)	$P_{ET}CO_2$ >50 torr (%TST)	Arousals (Events/hr)
Primary snoring	≤1	>92	≤53	<25%	EEG <12
Upper airway resistance syndrome	≤1	>92	≤53	<25%	RERA >1 EEG >12
Mild OSA	1–4	86–91	>53	10–24%	EEG > 12
Moderate OSA	5–10	76–85	>60	25–49%	EEG > 12
Severe OSA	>10	≤75	>65	≥50%	EEG > 12

Abbreviations: SpO_2, arterial oxygen saturation; $P_{ET}CO_2$, end-tidal PCO_2; EEG, electrocortical; RERA, respiratory effort–related arousal; TST, total sleep time; oAHI, obstructive apnea-hypopnea index; OSA, obstructive sleep apnea.

carbon dioxide,[194] and acetazolamide.[195] Methodologies to estimate loop gain from standard polysomnographic recordings have been reported.[176] A component of loop gain is the "plant gain," which can be easily estimated from a standard polysomnography recording, and represents the change in blood gases for a given change in ventilation.[196] The plant gain was reported to be increased in pediatric patients with OSA compared with asthmatics without OSA.[196] A cluster analysis revealed a distinct phenotype of asthmatic children with more severe OSA, worse pulmonary function, increased plant gain, and decreased controller gain.[196]

A lower arousal threshold predisposes toward OSA by more rapidly increasing ventilatory drive in response to airway loading resulting in ventilatory overshoot that contributes to cyclic obstructions. Adult OSA patients with a low arousal threshold can be identified polysomnographically by an oxygen saturation nadir >82.5% and a proportion of obstructive events that are hypopneas of >58.3%.[177] The arousal threshold may be increased using trazadone[197] or eszopiclone,[198] resulting in a lower AHI. Combination therapy with supplemental oxygen and eszopiclone may be effective in a subset of OSA patients.[199]

Ancillary Testing

The diagnosis of OSA is firmly established using polysomnography, and ancillary testing is rarely indicated. Further screening may be useful to facilitate the perioperative care, guide therapy, and to exclude underlying conditions (Table 27.7). For example, concern regarding right ventricular dysfunction may necessitate an electrocardiogram (ECG) or echocardiogram. Occasionally, chronic intermittent hypoxemia may induce polycythemia, whereas persistent hypercarbia can elevate serum bicarbonate. Routine pulmonary function testing is not indicated in children suspected of having OSA unless restrictive or obstructive lung disease is suspected. Other promising but understudied tools for identifying OSA in children include nasal rhinometry[200] and acoustic pharyngometry.[201]

TABLE 27.7   Ancillary Diagnostic Studies in Obstructive Sleep Apnea

Serum Markers

- CRP
- HOMA
- Hematocrit
- Serum bicarbonate

Imaging

- Brain MRI
- Anteroposterior and lateral neck radiograph
- Upper airway CT/MRI (craniofacial)
- Cine MRI
- Dynamic fluoroscopy

Sleep Monitoring

- MSLT

Miscellaneous

- Echocardiogram
- Neurocognitive testing
- Electrocardiogram
- Pulmonary function testing

Abbreviations: CRP, C-reactive protein; HOMA, homeostatic model assessment; MRI, magnetic resonance imaging; CT, computed tomography; MSLT, multiple sleep latency test.

Special Considerations in Infants

The pathophysiology of OSA in infants frequently differs from that observed in older children with infants having a higher likelihood of congenital anomalies of the upper airway including laryngomalacia, choanal atresia, laryngeal webs, and pyriform aperture stenosis, in addition to gastroesophageal reflux, hypotonia, and other issues.[202] Therefore direct endoscopic visualization of the upper airway is a helpful part of the diagnostic workup to establish nasal size, adenoidal volume, laryngeal stability/anatomy, mucosal swelling, and vocal cord function. Infants with OSA may not snore[18] and many snoring infants do not have OSA.[203] Therefore polysomnography should be performed to confirm the diagnosis and establish the severity. Polysomnographically, normative data are different in infants with respect to REM sleep percentage, respiratory rate, oximetry, and the arousal index compared with older children.[147,202] Occasional scored obstructive apneas and hypopneas (nap obstructive AHI 4.9/hr,[204] overnight obstructive apnea index 2.3/hr[205]) may be observed in otherwise normal infants, indicating the need to modify the obstructive AHI criteria in this age group.

Conclusions

A personalized approach to the diagnosis of pediatric OSA requires consideration of clinical symptoms, physical examination, comorbid conditions, laboratory markers, and objective physiologic sleep testing. The traditional paradigm of defining OSA by polysomnographic criteria alone fails to account for the idiosyncratic trait susceptibility that includes lifestyle choices (diet, exercise, sleep hygiene), genetics, symptoms, and pathophysiologic endotypes that contribute to the adverse sequelae. Pediatric OSA patterns are highly variable, including intermittent obstruction, increased respiratory effort, flow limitation, tachypnea, snoring alone, and/or gas exchange abnormalities. These patterns have been associated with variable degrees of autonomic and cortical disruptions of sleep homeostasis. Many snoring children will become symptomatic and require treatment despite the absence of scorable obstructive apneas and hypopneas. It is also important to recognize the breadth of symptoms beyond excessive daytime sleepiness, including hyperactivity, cognitive impairment, poor school performance, and mood disorders. Conversely, some children with mild polysomnographic OSA may be completely asymptomatic and reasonably managed with watchful waiting. By consensus, children with moderate to severe polysomnographic OSA and those with symptoms or comorbidities should be treated more aggressively. Additional evaluation using imaging, awake fiberoptic endoscopy, and DISE are also indicated in select patients. Careful phenotyping of children suspected of having OSA to localize the level of obstruction, arousal threshold, or ventilatory control instability may be helpful in determining the natural history of the condition and to guide therapy.

CLINICAL PEARLS

- The diagnosis of obstructive sleep apnea requires consideration of the apnea hypopnea index, respiratory effort, gas exchange, and sleep architecture.
- Normative data for infants indicates that occasional obstructive events are present and therefore the diagnostic criteria for obstructive sleep apnea must be modified.
- Laboratory-based polysomnography remains the gold-standard for the diagnosis for obstructive sleep apnea in children.

References

1. American Academy of Sleep Medicine. *International Classification of Sleep Disorders*. 3rd ed. American Academy of Sleep Medicine; 2014.
2. Guilleminault C, Li K, Khramtsov A, Palombini L, Pelayo R. Breathing patterns in prepubertal children with sleep-related breathing disorders. *Arch Pediatr Adol Med*. 2004;158(2):153–161.
3. Guilleminault C, Huang Y, Chin W-C, Okorie C. The nocturnal-polysomnogram and "non-hypoxic sleep-disordered-breathing" in children. *Sleep Med*. 2018;60:31–44.
4. Hunter SJ, Gozal D, Smith DL, Philby MF, Kaylegian J, Kheirandish-Gozal L. Effect of sleep-disordered breathing severity on cognitive performance measures in a large community cohort of young school-aged children. *Am J Resp Crit Care Med*. 2016;194(6):739–747.
5. Kheirandish-Gozal L, Philby MF, Qiao Z, Khalyfa A, Gozal D. Endothelial dysfunction in children with obstructive sleep apnea is associated with elevated lipoprotein-associated phospholipase A2 plasma activity levels. *JAMA*. 2017;6(2):e004923.
6. Patinkin ZW, Feinn R, Santos M. Metabolic consequences of obstructive sleep apnea in adolescents with obesity: A systematic literature review and meta-analysis. *Child Obes*. 2017;13(2):102–110.
7. Guilleminault C, Stoohs R, Clerk A, Cetel M, Maistros P. A cause of excessive daytime sleepiness. The upper airway resistance syndrome. *Chest*. 1993;104(3):781–787.
8. Guilleminault C, Kirisoglu C, Poyares D, et al. Upper airway resistance syndrome: A long-term outcome study. *J Psych Res*. 2006;40(3):273–279.
9. Rosen CL, D'Andrea L, Haddad GG. Adult criteria for obstructive sleep apnea do not identify children with serious obstruction. *Am Rev Resp Dis*. 1992;146(5 Pt 1):1231–1234.
10. Paruthi S, Rosen CL, Wang R, et al. End-tidal carbon dioxide measurement during pediatric polysomnography: Signal quality, association with apnea severity, and prediction of neurobehavioral outcomes. *Sleep*. 2015;38(11):1719–1726.
11. Smith DL, Gozal D, Hunter SJ, Kheirandish-Gozal L. Frequency of snoring, rather than apnea–hypopnea index, predicts both cognitive and behavioral problems in young children. *Sleep Med*. 2017;34:170–178.
12. Bourke R, Anderson V, Yang JSC, et al. Cognitive and academic functions are impaired in children with all severities of sleep-disordered breathing. *Sleep Med*. 2011;12(5):489–496.
13. Brockmann PE, Urschitz MS, Schlaud M, Poets CF. Primary snoring in school children: Prevalence and neurocognitive impairments. *Sleep Breath*. 2011;16(1):23–29.
14. Benedek P, Balakrishnan K, Cunningham MJ, et al. International Pediatric Otolaryngology group (IPOG) consensus on the diagnosis and management of pediatric obstructive sleep apnea (OSA). *Int J Pediatr Otorhinolaryngol*. 2020;138:110276.
15. Marcus CL, Brooks LJ, Draper KA, et al. Diagnosis and management of childhood obstructive sleep apnea syndrome. *Pediatrics*. 2012;130(3):576–584.
16. Weinstock TG, Rosen CL, Marcus CL, et al. Predictors of obstructive sleep apnea severity in adenotonsillectomy candidates. *Sleep*. 2014:1–9.
17. Wilson K, Lakheeram I, Morielli A, Brouillette R, Brown K. Can assessment for obstructive sleep apnea help predict post-adenotonsillectomy respiratory complications? *Anesthesiology*. 2002;96(2):313–322.

18. Anderson ICW, Sedaghat AR, McGinley BM, Redett RJ, Boss EF, Ishman SL. Prevalence and severity of obstructive sleep apnea and snoring in infants with Pierre Robin sequence. *Cleft Palate Craniofac J*. 2011;48(5):614–618.

19. Ali NJ, Pitson DJ, Stradling JR. Snoring, sleep disturbance, and behaviour in 4–5 year olds. *Arch Dis Child*. 1993;68(3):360.

20. Tang JPL, Rosen CL, Larkin EK, et al. Identification of sleep-disordered breathing in children: Variation with event definition. *Sleep*. 2002;25(1):72–79.

21. Kang K-T, Weng W-C, Lee C-H, et al. Detection of pediatric obstructive sleep apnea syndrome: History or anatomical findings? *Sleep Med*. 2015;16(5):617–624.

22. Preutthipan A, Chantarojanasiri T, Suwanjutha S, Udomsubpayakul U. Can parents predict the severity of childhood obstructive sleep apnoea? *Acta Paediatr*. 2000;89(6):708–712.

23. Rosen CL, Larkin EK, Kirchner HL, et al. Prevalence and risk factors for sleep-disordered breathing in 8- to 11-year-old children: Association with race and prematurity. *J Pediatr*. 2003;142(4):383–389.

24. Melendres CS, Lutz JM, Rubin ED, Marcus CL. Daytime sleepiness and hyperactivity in children with suspected sleep-disordered breathing. *Pediatrics*. 2004;114(3):768–775.

25. Chervin RD, Weatherly RA, Ruzicka DL, et al. Subjective sleepiness and polysomnographic correlates in children scheduled for adenotonsillectomy vs other surgical care. *Sleep*. 2006;29(4):495–503.

26. Gozal D, Wang M, Pope DW. Objective sleepiness measures in pediatric obstructive sleep apnea. *Pediatrics*. 2001;108(3):693–697.

27. Gozal D, Kheirandish-Gozal L. Obesity and excessive daytime sleepiness in prepubertal children with obstructive sleep apnea. *Pediatrics*. 2009;123(1):13–18.

28. Gozal D. Sleep-disordered breathing and school performance in children. *Pediatrics*. 1998;102(3):616–620.

29. Guilleminault C, Winkle R, Korobkin R, Simmons B. Children and nocturnal snoring: Evaluation of the effects of sleep related respiratory resistive load and daytime functioning. *Eur J Pediatr*. 2012;139(3):165–171.

30. Jeans WD, Fernando DCJ, Maw AR, Leighton BC. A longitudinal study of the growth of the nasopharynx and its contents in normal children. *Br J Radiol*. 1981;54:117–121.

31. Lam Y, Chan EYT, Ng DK, et al. The correlation among obesity, apnea-hypopnea index, and tonsil size in children. *Chest*. 2006;130(6):1751–1756.

32. Mitchell RB, Garetz S, Moore RH, et al. The use of clinical parameters to predict obstructive sleep apnea syndrome severity in children. *JAMA Otolaryngol Head Neck Surg*. 2015;141(2):130–137.

33. Nolan J, Brietzke SE. Systematic review of pediatric tonsil size and polysomnogram-measured obstructive sleep apnea severity. *Otolaryngol Head Neck Surg*. 2011;144(6):844–850.

34. Galeotti A, Festa P, Viarani V, et al. Prevalence of malocclusion in children with obstructive sleep apnoea. *Orthod Craniofac Res*. 2018;21(4):242–247.

35. Pirila-Parkkinen K, Pirttiniemi P, Nieminen P, Tolonen U, Pelttari U, Lopponen H. Dental arch morphology in children with sleep-disordered breathing. *Eur J Orthod*. 2009;31(2):160–167.

36. Zalzal HG, Carr M, Kohler W, Coutras SW. Adenoid size by drug induced sleep endoscopy compared to nasopharyngeal mirror exam. *Int J Pediatr Otorhinolaryngol*. 2018;112:75–79.

37. Marcus CL, Greene MG, Carroll JL. Blood pressure in children with obstructive sleep apnea. *Am J Resp Crit Care*. 2012;157(4):1098–1103.

38. Kang K-T, Chiu S-N, Weng W-C, Lee P-L, Hsu W-C. Comparisons of office and 24-hour ambulatory blood pressure monitoring in children with obstructive sleep apnea. *J Pediatr*. 2017;182(177–183):e2.

39. Kang K-T, Chiu S-N, Lin C-Y, Weng W-C, Lee P-L, Hsu W-C. Trajectory of ambulatory blood pressure after adenotonsillectomy in children with obstructive sleep apnea: Comparison at 3- and 6-month follow-up. *Sleep Med*. 2019;65: 127–133.

40. DelRosso LM, King J, Ferri R. Systolic blood pressure elevation in children with obstructive sleep apnea is improved with positive airway pressure use. *J Pediatr*. 2018;195:102–107. e1.

41. Brouillette R, Hanson D, David R, et al. A diagnostic approach to suspected sleep apnea in children. *J Pediatr*. 1984;105:10–14.

42. Spruyt K, Gozal D. Screening of pediatric sleep-disordered breathing a proposed unbiased discriminative set of questions using clinical severity scales. *Chest*. 2012;142(6):1508–1515.

43. Carroll JL, McColley SA, Marcus CL, Curtis S, Loughlin GM. Inability of clinical history to distinguish primary snoring from obstructive sleep apnea syndrome in children. *Chest*. 1995;108(3):610–618.

44. Chervin RD, Weatherly RA, Garetz SL, et al. Pediatric Sleep Questionnaire: Prediction of sleep apnea and outcomes. *Arch Otolaryngol Head Neck Surg*. 2007;133(3):216–222.

45. Chervin RD, Hedger K, Dillon JE, Pituch KJ. Pediatric Sleep Questionnaire (PSQ): Validity and reliability of scales for sleep-disordered breathing, snoring, sleepiness, and behavioral problems. *Sleep Med*. 2000;1(1):21–32.

46. Pabary R, Goubau C, Russo K, Laverty A, Abel F, Samuels M. Screening for sleep-disordered breathing with Pediatric Sleep Questionnaire in children with underlying conditions. *J Sleep Res*. 2019;28(5):e12826.

47. Crabtree VM, Varni JW, Gozal D. Health-related quality of life and depressive symptoms in children with suspected sleep-disordered breathing. *Sleep*. 2004;27(6):1131–1138.

48. Garetz SL, Mitchell RB, Parker PD, et al. Quality of life and obstructive sleep apnea symptoms after pediatric adenotonsillectomy. *Pediatrics*. 2015;135(2):e477–e486.

49. Øverland B, Berdal H, Akre H. Correlations between disease-specific quality of life and polysomnographic findings in children with obstructive sleep apnea. *Int J Pediatr Otorhinolaryngol*. 2020;134:1–4.

50. Patel AP, Meghji S, Phillips JS. Accuracy of clinical scoring tools for the diagnosis of pediatric obstructive sleep apnea. *Laryngoscope*. 2019;5(5 pt 1):242–210.

51. Arens R, McDonough JM, Costarino AT, et al. Magnetic resonance imaging of the upper airway structure of children with obstructive sleep apnea syndrome. *Am J Resp and Crit Care Med*. 2001;164(4):698–703.

52. Wootton DM, Luo H, Persak SC, et al. Computational fluid dynamics endpoints to characterize obstructive sleep apnea syndrome in children. *J App Physiol*. 2014;116(1):104–112.

53. Brooks LJ, Stephens BM, Bacevice AM. Adenoid size is related to severity but not the number of episodes of obstructive apnea in children. *J Pediatr*. 1998;132(4):682–686.

54. Jain A, Sahni JK. Polysomnographic studies in children undergoing adenoidectomy and/or tonsillectomy. *J Laryngol Otol*. 2002;116(9):711–715.

55. Li AM, Wong E, Kew J, Hui S, Fok TF. Use of tonsil size in the evaluation of obstructive sleep apnoea. *Arch Dis Child.* 2002;87(2):156–159.

56. Pirila-Parkkinen K, Lopponen H, Nieminen P, Tolonen U, Pirttiniemi P. Cephalometric evaluation of children with nocturnal sleep-disordered breathing. *Eur J Orthod.* 2010;32(6):662–671.

57. Yap B, Kontos A, Pamula Y, et al. Differences in dentofacial morphology in children with sleep disordered breathing are detected with routine orthodontic records. *Sleep Med.* 2019;55:109–114.

58. Özdemir H, Altin R, Söğüt A, et al. Craniofacial differences according to AHI scores of children with obstructive sleep apnoea syndrome: Cephalometric study in 39 patients. *Pediatr Radiol.* 2004;34(5):393–399.

59. Xu J, Hu H, Sun H, et al. Clinical evaluation in predicting childhood obstructive sleep apnea. *Chest.* 2006;130(6):1765–1771.

60. Mlynarek A, Tewfik MA, Hagr A, et al. Lateral neck radiography versus direct video rhinoscopy in assessing adenoid size. *J Otolaryngol.* 2005;33(6):360.

61. Sedaghat AR, Flax-Goldenberg RB, Gayler BW, Capone GT, Ishman SL. A case-control comparison of lingual tonsillar size in children with and without down syndrome. *Laryngoscope.* 2012;122(5):1165–1169.

62. Schwab RJ, Kim C, Bagchi S, et al. Understanding the anatomic basis for obstructive sleep apnea syndrome in adolescents. *Am J Resp Crit Care Med.* 2015;191(11):1295–1309.

63. Arens R, Sin S, Nandalike K, et al. Upper airway structure and body fat composition in obese children with obstructive sleep apnea syndrome. *Am J Crit Care Med.* 2011;183(6):782–787.

64. Fregosi RF, Quan SF, Kaemingk KL, et al. Sleep-disordered breathing, pharyngeal size and soft tissue anatomy in children. *J App Physiol.* 2003;95(5):2030–2038.

65. Cappabianca S, Iaselli F, Negro A, et al. Magnetic resonance imaging in the evaluation of anatomical risk factors for pediatric obstructive sleep apnoea–hypopnoea: A pilot study. *Int J Pediatr Otorhinolaryngol.* 2013;77(1):69–75.

66. Donnelly LF, Strife JL, Myer CM. Glossoptosis (posterior displacement of the tongue) during sleep: A frequent cause of sleep apnea in pediatric patients referred for dynamic sleep fluoroscopy. *Am J Roentgenol.* 2000;175(6):1557–1560.

67. Donnelly LF, Shott SR, LaRose CR, Chini BA, Amin RS. Causes of persistent obstructive sleep apnea despite previous tonsillectomy and adenoidectomy in children with Down syndrome as depicted on static and dynamic cine MRI. *Am J Roentgenol.* 2004;183(1):175–181.

68. Shott SR, Donnelly LF. Cine magnetic resonance imaging: Evaluation of persistent airway obstruction after tonsil and adenoidectomy in children with Down syndrome: Cine magnetic resonance imaging: Evaluation of persistent airway obstruction after tonsil and adenoidectomy in children with Down syndrome. *Laryngoscope.* 2010;114(10):1724–1729.

69. Isaiah A, Kiss E, Olomu P, Koral K, Mitchell RB. Characterization of upper airway obstruction using cine MRI in children with residual obstructive sleep apnea after adenotonsillectomy. *Sleep Med.* 2018;50:79–86.

70. Bhattacharjee R, Kheirandish-Gozal L, Spruyt K, et al. Adenotonsillectomy outcomes in treatment of obstructive sleep apnea in children. *Am J Resp Crit Care Med.* 2010;182(5):676–683.

71. Friedman M, Wilson M, Lin H-C, Chang H-W. Updated systematic review of tonsillectomy and adenoidectomy for treatment of pediatric obstructive sleep apnea/hypopnea syndrome. *Otolaryngol Head Neck Surg.* 2009;140(6):800–808.

72. Maeda K, Tsuiki S, Nakata S, Suzuki K, Itoh E, Inoue Y. Craniofacial contribution to residual obstructive sleep apnea after adenotonsillectomy in children: A preliminary study. *J Clin Sleep Med.* 2014:1–5.

73. Boudewyns A, Heyning PV, de, Verhulst S. Drug-induced sedation endoscopy in children <2 years with obstructive sleep apnea syndrome: Upper airway findings and treatment outcomes. *Eur Arch Otorhinolaryngol.* 2017;274(5):2319–2325.

74. Gazzaz MJ, Isaac A, Anderson S, Alsufyani N, Alrajhi Y, El-Hakim H. Does drug-induced sleep endoscopy change the surgical decision in surgically naïve non-syndromic children with snoring/sleep disordered breathing from the standard adenotonsillectomy? A retrospective cohort study. *J Otolaryngol Head Neck Surg.* 2017;46(1):12.

75. Maris M, Verhulst S, Saldien V, Heyning PV, de, Wojciechowski M, Boudewyns A. Drug-induced sedation endoscopy in surgically naive children with Down syndrome and obstructive sleep apnea. *Sleep Med.* 2016;24:63–70.

76. Wootten CT, Chinnadurai S, Goudy SL. Beyond adenotonsillectomy: Outcomes of sleep endoscopy-directed treatments in pediatric obstructive sleep apnea. *Int J Pediatr Otorhinolaryngol.* 2014;78(7):1158–1162.

77. Raposo D, Menezes M, Rito J, et al. Drug-induced sleep endoscopy in pediatric obstructive sleep apnea. *Otolaryngol Head Neck Surg.* 2021;164(2):414–421.

78. Lam DJ, Krane NA, Mitchell RB. Relationship between drug-induced sleep endoscopy findings, tonsil size, and polysomnographic outcomes of adenotonsillectomy in children. *Otolaryngol Head Neck Surg.* 2019;161(3):507–513.

79. Kheirandish-Gozal L, McManus CJT, Kellermann GH, Samiei A, Gozal D. Urinary neurotransmitters are selectively altered in children with obstructive sleep apnea and predict cognitive morbidity. *Chest.* 2013;143(6):1576–1583.

80. Peña-Zarza JA, Peña MD, la, Yañez A, et al. Glycated hemoglobin and sleep apnea syndrome in children: Beyond the apnea–hypopnea index. *Sleep Breath.* 2018;22(1):205–210.

81. Alonso-Álvarez ML, Terán-Santos J, Martinez MG, et al. Metabolic biomarkers in community obese children: Effect of obstructive sleep apnea and its treatment. *Sleep Med.* 2017;37:1–9.

82. Kheirandish-Gozal L, Capdevila OS, Tauman R, Gozal D. Plasma C-reactive protein in nonobese children with obstructive sleep apnea before and after adenotonsillectomy. *J Clin Sleep Med.* 2006;15:301–304.

83. Zhang F, Wu Y, Feng G, Ni X, Xu Z, Gozal D. Polysomnographic correlates of endothelial function in children with obstructive sleep apnea. *Sleep Med.* 2018;52:45–50.

84. Tauman R, O'Brien LM, Ivanenko A, Gozal D. Obesity rather than severity of sleep-disordered breathing as the major determinant of insulin resistance and altered lipidemia in snoring children. *Pediatrics.* 2005;116(1):e66–e73.

85. Eyck AV, Hoorenbeeck KV, Winter BYD, Gaal LV, Backer WD, Verhulst SL. Sleep-disordered breathing, systemic adipokine secretion, and metabolic dysregulation in overweight and obese children and adolescents. *Sleep Med.* 2017;30:52–56.

86. Smith DF, Hossain MM, Hura A, et al. Inflammatory milieu and cardiovascular homeostasis in children with obstructive sleep apnea. *Sleep.* 2017;40(4):1264–1268.

87. Chatsuriyawong S, Gozal D, Kheirandish-Gozal L, et al. Polymorphisms in nitric oxide synthase and endothelin genes

among children with obstructive sleep apnea. *BMC Med Genomics*. 2013;6:29.

88. Kheirandish-Gozal L, Khalyfa A, et al. Endothelial dysfunction in children with obstructive sleep apnea is associated with epigenetic changes in the eNOS gene. *Chest*. 2013;143(4):971–977.

89. Kim J, Bhattacharjee R, Khalyfa A, et al. DNA methylation in inflammatory genes among children with obstructive sleep apnea. *Am J Resp Crit Care Med*. 2012;185(3):330–338.

90. Gozal D, Kheirandish-Gozal L, Bhattacharjee R, et al. Circulating adropin concentrations in pediatric obstructive sleep apnea: Potential relevance to endothelial function. *J Pediatr*. 2013;163(4):1122–1126.

91. Gozal D, Khalyfa A, Qiao Z, et al. Angiopoietin-2 and soluble tie-2 receptor plasma levels in children with obstructive sleep apnea and obesity. *Obesity*. 2017;25(6):1083–1090.

92. Khalyfa A, Kheirandish-Gozal L, Khalyfa AA, et al. Circulating plasma extracellular microvesicle microRNA cargo and endothelial dysfunction in children with obstructive sleep apnea. *Am J Resp Crit Care Med*. 2016;194(9):1116–1126.

93. Gozal D, Capdevila OS, Kheirandish-Gozal L, Crabtree VM. APOE epsilon 4 allele, cognitive dysfunction, and obstructive sleep apnea in children. *Neurology*. 2007;69(3):243–249.

94. Gozal D, Khalyfa A, Capdevila OS, Kheirandish-Gozal L, Khalyfa AA, Kim J. Cognitive function in prepubertal children with obstructive sleep apnea: A modifying role for NADPH oxidase p22 subunit gene polymorphisms? *Antiox Red Signal*. 2012;16(2):171–177.

95. Khalyfa A, Serpero L, Kheirandish-Gozal L, Capdevila O, Gozal D. TNF-α gene polymorphisms and excessive daytime sleepiness in pediatric obstructive sleep apnea. *J Pediatr*. 2011;158(1):77–82.

96. Lamm C, Mandeli J, Kattan M. Evaluation of home audiotapes as an abbreviated test for obstructive sleep apnea syndrome (OSAS) in children. *Pediatr Pulmonol*. 1999;27(4):267–272.

97. Potsic WiP Comparison of polysomnography and sonography for assessing regularity of respiration during sleep in adenotonsillar hypertrophy. *Laryngoscope*. 1987;97:1430–1437.

98. Mccombe AW, Kwok V, Hawke WM. An acoustic screening test for obstructive sleep apnoea. *Clin Otolaryngology Allied Sci*. 1995;20(4):348–351.

99. Mograss MA, Ducharme FM, Brouillette RT. Movement/arousals. Description, classification, and relationship to sleep apnea in children. *Am J Resp Crit Care Med*. 1994;150(6 Pt 1):1690–1696.

100. Morielli A, Ladan S, Ducharme FM, Brouillette RT. Can sleep and wakefulness be distinguished in children by cardiorespiratory and videotape recordings? *Chest*. 1996;109(3):680–687.

101. Sivan Y, Kornecki A, Schonfeld T. Screening obstructive sleep apnoea syndrome by home videotape recording in children. *Eur Resp J*. 1996;9(10):2127–2131.

102. Brietzke SE, Katz ES, Roberson DW. Can history and physical examination reliably diagnose pediatric obstructive sleep apnea/hypopnea syndrome? A systematic review of the literature. *Otolaryngol Head Neck Surg*. 2016;131(6):827–832.

103. Certal V, Catumbela E, Winck JC, Azevedo I, Teixeira-Pinto A, Costa-Pereira A. Clinical assessment of pediatric obstructive sleep apnea: A systematic review and meta-analysis. *Laryngoscope*. 2012;122(9):2105–2114.

104. Wise MS, Nichols CD, Grigg-Damberger MM, et al. Executive summary of respiratory indications for polysomnography in children: An evidence-based review. *Sleep*. 2011;34(3):389–398.

105. Mitchell RB, Archer SM, Ishman SL, et al. Clinical Practice Guideline: Tonsillectomy in Children (Update)—Executive Summary. *Otolaryngol Head Neck Surg*. 2018;160(2):187–205.

106. Giordani B, Hodges EK, Guire KE, et al. Changes in neuropsychological and behavioral functioning in children with and without obstructive sleep apnea following tonsillectomy. *J Int Neuropsychol Soc*. 2012;18(02):212–222.

107. Saur JS, Brietzke SE. Polysomnography results versus clinical factors to predict post-operative respiratory complications following pediatric adenotonsillectomy. *Int J Pediatr Otorhinolaryngol*. 2017;98:136–142.

108. Berry RB, Quan SF, Abreu AR, et al. *The AASM Manual for the Scoring of Sleep and Associated Events: Rules, Terminology, and Technical Specifications*. American Academy of Sleep Medicine; 2020.

109. Tan H-L, Gozal D, Ramirez HM, Bandla HPR, Kheirandish-Gozal L. Overnight polysomnography versus respiratory polygraphy in the diagnosis of pediatric obstructive sleep apnea. *Sleep*. 2014;37(2):255–260.

110. Alonso-Álvarez ML, Terán-Santos J, Carbajo EO, et al. Reliability of home respiratory polygraphy for the diagnosis of sleep apnea in children. *Chest*. 2015;147(4):1020–1028.

111. Gudnadottir G, Hafsten L, Redfors S, Ellegård E, Hellgren J. Respiratory polygraphy in children with sleep-disordered breathing. *J Sleep Res*. 2019;28(6):e12856.

112. Canet E, Gaultier C, D'Allest AM, Dehan M. Effects of sleep deprivation on respiratory events during sleep in healthy infants. *J Appl Physiol*. 2002;66(3):1158–1163.

113. Goh DY, Galster P, Marcus CL. Sleep architecture and respiratory disturbances in children with obstructive sleep apnea. *Am J Resp Crit Care Med*. 2000;162(2 Pt 1):682–686.

114. Fuentes-Pradera MA, Botebol G, Sánchez-Armengol Á, et al. Effect of snoring and obstructive respiratory events on sleep architecture in adolescents. *Arch Pediatr Adol Med*. 2003;157(7):649–654.

115. Tauman R, O'Brien LM, Holbrook CR, Gozal D. Sleep pressure score: A new index of sleep disruption in snoring children. *Sleep*. 2004;27(2):274–278.

116. Davies RJ, Vardi-Visy K, Clarke M, Stradling JR. Identification of sleep disruption and sleep disordered breathing from the systolic blood pressure profile. *Thorax*. 1993;48(12):1242–1247.

117. Somers VK, Dyken ME, Clary MP, Abboud FM. Sympathetic neural mechanisms in obstructive sleep apnea. *J Clin Invest*. 1995;96(4):1897–1904.

118. Wong TK, Galster P, Lau TS, Lutz JM, Marcus CL. Reliability of scoring arousals in normal children and children with obstructive sleep apnea syndrome. *Sleep*. 2004;27(6):1139–1145.

119. McNamara F, Issa FG, Sullivan CE. Arousal pattern following central and obstructive breathing abnormalities in infants and children. *J Appl Physiol*. 1996;81(6):2651–2657.

120. Kaleyias J, Grant M, Darbari F, Ajagbe O, Cepelowicz-Rajter J, Kothare SV. Detection of cortical arousals in children using frontal EEG leads in addition to conventional central leads. *J Clin Sleep Med*. 2006;2(3):305–308.

121. Bandla HP, Gozal D. Dynamic changes in EEG spectra during obstructive apnea in children. *Pediatr Pulmonol*. 2000;29(5):359–365.

122. Katz ES, Lutz J, Black C, Marcus CL. Pulse transit time as a measure of arousal and respiratory effort in children with sleep-disordered breathing. *Pediatr Res*. 2003;53(4):580–588.

123. Brietzke SE, Katz ES, Roberson DW. Pulse transit time as a screening test for pediatric sleep-related breathing disorders. *Arch Otolaryngol Head Neck Surg.* 2007;133(10):980–984.

124. Martin SE, Wraith PK, Deary IJ, Douglas NJ. The effect of nonvisible sleep fragmentation on daytime function. *Am J Resp Crit Care Med.* 1997;155(5):1596–1601.

125. Gaultier C, Praud JP, Canet E, Delaperche MF, D'Allest AM. Paradoxical inward rib cage motion during rapid eye movement sleep in infants and young children. *J Dev Physiol.* 1987;9(5):391–397.

126. Guilleminault C, Pelayo R, Leger D, Clerk A, Bocian RC. Recognition of sleep-disordered breathing in children. *Pediatrics.* 1996;98(5):871–882.

127. Groswasser Scaillon Rebuffat Naso-oesophageal probes decrease the frequency of sleep apnoeas in infants. *J Sleep Res.* 2000;9(2):193–196.

128. Chervin RD, Ruzicka DL, Hoban TF, et al. Esophageal pressures, polysomnography, and neurobehavioral outcomes of adenotonsillectomy in children. *Chest.* 2012;142(1):101–110.

129. Farré R, Montserrat JM, Rotger M, Ballester E, Navajas D. Accuracy of thermistors and thermocouples as flow-measuring devices for detecting hypopnoeas. *Eur Resp J.* 1998;11(1):179–182.

130. Norman RG, Ahmed MM, Walsleben JA, Rapoport DM. Detection of respiratory events during NPSG: Nasal cannula/pressure sensor versus thermistor. *Sleep.* 1997;20(12):1175–1184.

131. Hosselet JJ, Norman RG, Ayappa I, Rapoport DM. Detection of flow limitation with a nasal cannula/pressure transducer system. *Am J Resp Crit Care Med.* 1998;157(5):1461–1467.

132. Trang H, Leske V, Gaultier C. Use of nasal cannula for detecting sleep apneas and hypopneas in infants and children. *Am J Resp Crit Care Med.* 2002;166(4):464–468.

133. Serebrisky D, Cordero R, Mandeli J, Kattan M, Lamm C. Assessment of inspiratory flow limitation in children with sleep-disordered breathing by a nasal cannula pressure transducer system. *Pediatr Pulmonol.* 2002;33(5):380–387.

134. Poels PJP, Schilder AGM, Berg S, van den, Hoes AW, Joosten KFM. Evaluation of a new device for home cardiorespiratory recording in children. *Arch Otolaryngol Head Neck Surg.* 2003;129(12):1281–1284.

135. Verginis N, Davey MJ, Horne RSC. Scoring respiratory events in paediatric patients: Evaluation of nasal pressure and thermistor recordings separately and in combination. *Sleep Med.* 2010;11(4):400–405.

136. Sackner MA, Watson H, Belsito AS, et al. Calibration of respiratory inductive plethysmograph during natural breathing. *J Appl Physiol.* 1989;66(1):410–420.

137. Griffiths A, Maul J, Wilson A, Stick S. Improved detection of obstructive events in childhood sleep apnoea with the use of the nasal cannula and the differentiated sum signal. *J Sleep Res.* 2005;14(4):431–436.

138. Bhavani-Shankar K, Moseley H, Kumar AY, Delph Y. Capnometry and anaesthesia. *Can J Anaesth.* 2008;39(6):617–632.

139. Morielli A, Desjardins D, Brouillette RT. Transcutaneous and end-tidal carbon dioxide pressures should be measured during pediatric polysomnography. *Am Rev Resp Dis.* 1993;148(6 Pt 1):1599–1604.

140. Montgomery-Downs HE, O'Brien LM, Gulliver TE, Gozal D. Polysomnographic characteristics in normal preschool and early school-aged children. *Pediatrics.* 2006;117(3):741–753.

141. Uliel S, Tauman R, Greenfeld M, Sivan Y. Normal polysomnographic respiratory values in children and adolescents. *Chest.* 2004;125(3):872–878.

142. Acebo C, Millman RP, Rosenberg C, Cavallo A, Carskadon MA. Sleep, breathing, and cephalometrics in older children and young adults. *Chest.* 1996;109(3):664–672.

143. Marcus CL, Omlin KJ, Basinski DJ, et al. Normal polysomnographic values for children and adolescents. *Am Rev Resp Dis.* 1992;146:1235–1239.

144. Hunt CE, Corwin MJ, Lister G, et al. Longitudinal assessment of hemoglobin oxygen saturation in healthy infants during the first 6 months of age. *J Pediatr.* 2010;135(5):580–586.

145. Witmans MB, Keens TG, Ward SLD, Marcus CL. Obstructive hypopneas in children and adolescents normal values. *Am J Resp Crit Care Med.* 2003;168:1540.

146. Wang G, Xu Z, Tai J, et al. Normative values of polysomnographic parameters in Chinese children and adolescents: A cross-sectional study. *Sleep Med.* 2016:27–28. 49–53.

147. Traeger N, Schultz B, Pollock AN, Mason T, Marcus CL, Arens R. Polysomnographic values in children 2–9 years old: Additional data and review of the literature. *Pediatr Pulmonol.* 2005;40(1):22–30.

148. Miyazaki S, Itasaka Y, Yamakawa K, Okawa M, Togawa K. Respiratory disturbance during sleep due to adenoid-tonsillar hypertrophy. *Am J Otolaryngol.* 2003;10(2):143–149.

149. Skatvedt O, Grøgaard J. Infant sleeping position and inspiratory pressures in the upper airways and oesophagus. *Arch Dis Child.* 1994;71(2):138.

150. Aurora RN, Zak RS, Karippot A, et al. Practice parameters for the respiratory indications for polysomnography in children. *Sleep.* 2011;34(3):379–388.

151. Saeed MM, Keens TG, Stabile MW, Bolokowicz J, Ward SLD. Should children with suspected obstructive sleep apnea syndrome and normal nap sleep studies have overnight sleep studies? *Chest.* 2000;118(2):360–365.

152. Marcus CL, Keens TG, Ward SLD. Comparison of nap and overnight polysomnography in children. *Pediatr Pulmonol.* 1992;13(1):16–21.

153. Cooper BG, Veale D, Griffiths CJ, Gibson GJ. Value of nocturnal oxygen saturation as a screening test for sleep apnoea. *Thorax.* 1991;46(8):586.

154. Redline S, Tosteson T, Boucher MA, Millman RP. Measurement of sleep-related breathing disturbances in epidemiologic studies. *Chest.* 1991;100(5):1281–1286.

155. Goodwin JL, Enright PL, Kaemingk KL, et al. Feasibility of using unattended polysomnography in children for research–report of the Tucson Children's Assessment of Sleep Apnea study (TuCASA). *Sleep.* 2001;24(8):937–944.

156. Ikizoglu NB, Kiyan E, Polat B, Ay P, Karadag B, Ersu R. Are home sleep studies useful in diagnosing obstructive sleep apnea in children with down syndrome? *Pediatr Pulmonol.* 2019;54(10):1–6.

157. Kirk V, Baughn J, et al. American Academy of Sleep Medicine Position Paper for the Use of a Home Sleep Apnea Test for the Diagnosis of OSA in Children. *J Clin Sleep Med.* 2017;13(10):1199–1203.

158. Brouillette RT, Morielli A, Leimanis A, Waters KA, Luciano R, Ducharme FM. Nocturnal pulse oximetry as an abbreviated testing modality for pediatric obstructive sleep apnea. *Pediatrics.* 2000;105(2):405–412.

159. Kirk VG, Bohn SG, Flemons WW, Remmers JE. Comparison of home oximetry monitoring with laboratory polysomnography in children. *Chest*. 2003;124(5):1702–1708.

160. Guilleminault C, Pelayo R, Léger D, Clerk A, Bocian RCZ. Recognition of sleep-disordered breathing in children. *Pediatrics*. 1996;98(5):871–882.

161. Sommermeyer D, Zou D, Grote L, Hedner J. Detection of sleep disordered breathing and its central/obstructive character using nasal cannula and finger pulse oximeter. *J Clin Sleep Med*. 2012;08(05):527–533.

162. Garde A, Hoppenbrouwer X, Dehkordi P, et al. Pediatric pulse oximetry-based OSA screening at different thresholds of the apnea-hypopnea index with an expression of uncertainty for inconclusive classifications. *Sleep Med*. 2018;60:45–52.

163. Hornero R, Kheirandish-Gozal L, Gutiérrez-Tobal GC, et al. Nocturnal oximetry–based Evaluation of habitually snoring children. *Am J Resp Crit Care Med*. 2017;196(12):1591–1598.

164. Vaquerizo-Villar F, Álvarez D, Kheirandish-Gozal L, et al. Wavelet analysis of oximetry recordings to assist in the automated detection of moderate-to-severe pediatric sleep apnea-hypopnea syndrome. *PLoS One*. 2018;13(12):e0208502.

165. Crespo A, Álvarez D, Kheirandish-Gozal L, et al. Assessment of oximetry-based statistical classifiers as simplified screening tools in the management of childhood obstructive sleep apnea. *Sleep Breath*. 2018;22(4):1063–1073.

166. Pillar G, Bar A, Shlitner A, Schnall R, Shefy J, Lavie P. Autonomic arousal index: An automated detection based on peripheral arterial tonometry. *Sleep*. 2002;25(5):543–549.

167. O'Donnell CP, Allan L, Atkinson P, Schwartz AR. The effect of upper airway obstruction and arousal on peripheral arterial tonometry in obstructive sleep apnea. *Am J Resp Crit Care Med*. 2002;166(7):965–971.

168. Bar A, Pillar G, Dvir I, Sheffy J, Schnall RP, Lavie P. Evaluation of a portable device based on peripheral arterial tone for unattended home sleep studies. *Chest*. 2003;123(3):695–703.

169. Scholle S, Scholle HC, Kemper A, et al. First night effect in children and adolescents undergoing polysomnography for sleep-disordered breathing. *Clin Neurophysiol*. 2003;114(11):2138–2145.

170. Bon OL, Hoffmann G, Tecco J, et al. Mild to moderate sleep respiratory events. *Chest*. 2000;118(2):353–359.

171. Katz ES, Greene MG, Carson KA, et al. Night-to-night variability of polysomnography in children with suspected obstructive sleep apnea. *J Pediatr*. 2002;140(5):589–594.

172. Li AM, Wing YK, Cheung A, et al. Is a 2-night polysomnographic study necessary in childhood sleep-related disordered breathing? *Chest*. 2004;126(5):1467–1472.

173. Verhulst SL, Schrauwen N, Backer WAD, Desager KN. First night effect for polysomnographic data in children and adolescents with suspected sleep disordered breathing. *Arch Dis Child*. 2006;91(3):233–237.

174. Gleadhill IC, Schwartz AR, Schubert N, Wise RA, Permutt S, Smith PL. Upper airway collapsibility in snorers and in patients with obstructive hypopnea and apnea. *Am J Respir Dis*. 1991;143:1300–1303.

175. Xie A, Bedekar A, Skatrud JB, Teodorescu M, Gong Y, Dempsey JA. The heterogeneity of obstructive sleep apnea (predominant obstructive vs pure obstructive apnea). *Sleep*. 2011;34(6):745–750.

176. Terrill PI, Edwards BA, Nemati S, et al. Quantifying the ventilatory control contribution to sleep apnoea using polysomnography. *Eur Resp J*. 2015;45(2):1–11.

177. Edwards BA, Eckert DJ, McSharry DG, et al. Clinical predictors of the respiratory arousal threshold in patients with obstructive sleep apnea. *Am J Resp Crit Care Med*. 2014;190(11):1293–1300.

178. Sands SA, Edwards BA, Terrill PI, et al. Phenotyping pharyngeal pathophysiology using polysomnography in patients with obstructive sleep apnea. *Am J Resp Crit Care Med*. 2018;197(9):1187–1197.

179. Eckert DJ, White DP, Jordan AS, Malhotra A, Wellman A. Defining phenotypic causes of obstructive sleep apnea. *Identification of novel therapeutic targets. Am J Resp Crit Care Med*. 2013;188(8):996–1004.

180. Sands SA, Terrill PI, Edwards BA, et al. Quantifying the arousal threshold using polysomnography in obstructive sleep apnea. *Sleep*. 2017;41(1):996–999.

181. Azarbarzin A, Sands SA, White DP, Redline S, Wellman A. The hypoxic burden: A novel sleep apnoea severity metric and a predictor of cardiovascular mortality—Reply to "The hypoxic burden: Also known as the desaturation severity parameter. *Eur Heart J*. 2019;40:1149–1152.

182. Azarbarzin A, Sands SA, Stone KL, et al. The hypoxic burden of sleep apnoea predicts cardiovascular disease-related mortality: The Osteoporotic Fractures in Men study and the Sleep Heart Health Study. *Eur Heart J*. 2018;40(14):1149–1157.

183. Varga AW, Mokhlesi B. REM obstructive sleep apnea: Risk for adverse health outcomes and novel treatments. *Sleep Breath*. 2019;23(2):1–11.

184. Mokhlesi B, Hagen EW, Finn LA, Hla KM, Carter JR, Peppard PE. Obstructive sleep apnoea during REM sleep and incident non-dipping of nocturnal blood pressure: A longitudinal analysis of the Wisconsin Sleep Cohort. *Thorax*. 2015;70(11):1062–1069.

185. Verhulst E, Clinck I, Deboutte I, Vanderveken O, Verhulst S, Boudewyns A. Positional obstructive sleep apnea in children: Prevalence and risk factors. *Sleep Breath*. 2019;130(3):1–8.

186. Lutsey PL, McClelland RL, Duprez D, et al. Objectively measured sleep characteristics and prevalence of coronary artery calcification: The Multi-Ethnic Study of Atherosclerosis Sleep study. *Thorax*. 2015;70(9):880–887.

187. Labarca G, Campos J, Thibaut K, Dreyse J, Jorquera J. Do T90 and SaO₂ nadir identify a different phenotype in obstructive sleep apnea? *Sleep Breath*. 2019;23(3):1007–1010.

188. Sutherland K, Schwab RJ, Maislin G, et al. Facial phenotyping by quantitative photography reflects craniofacial morphology measured on magnetic resonance imaging in Icelandic sleep apnea patients. *Sleep*. 2014;37(5):959–968.

189. Sutherland K, Lee RWW, Chan TO, Ng S, Hui DS, Cistulli PA. Craniofacial phenotyping in Chinese and Caucasian patients with sleep apnea: Influence of ethnicity and sex. *J Clin Sleep Med*. 2018;14(07):1143–1151.

190. Landry SA, Joosten SA, Eckert DJ, et al. Therapeutic CPAP level predicts upper airway collapsibility in patients with obstructive sleep apnea. *Sleep*. 2017;40(6):1300–1308.

191. Dayyat E, Kheirandish-Gozal L, Gozal D. Childhood obstructive sleep apnea: One or two distinct disease entities? *Sleep Med Clin*. 2007;2(3):433–444.

192. Oksenberg A, Gadoth N, Töyräs J, Leppänen T. Prevalence and characteristics of positional obstructive sleep apnea (POSA) in patients with severe OSA. *Sleep Breath.* 2019;112(43):1–9.

193. Wellman A, Malhotra A, Jordan AS, Stevenson KE, Gautam S, White DP. Effect of oxygen in obstructive sleep apnea: Role of loop gain. *Resp Phys Neurobiol.* 2008;162(2):144–151.

194. Xie A, Teodorescu M, Pegelow DF, et al. Effects of stabilizing or increasing respiratory motor outputs on obstructive sleep apnea. *J Appl Phys.* 2013;115(1):22–33.

195. Edwards BA, Sands SA, Eckert DJ, et al. Acetazolamide improves loop gain but not the other physiological traits causing obstructive sleep apnoea. *J Physiol.* 2012;590(5):1199–1211.

196. He Z, Armoni-Domany K, Nava-Guerra L, et al. Phenotype of ventilatory control in children with moderate to severe persistent asthma and obstructive sleep apnea. *Sleep.* 2019;42(9):731–710.

197. Smales ET, Edwards BA, Deyoung PN, et al. Trazodone effects on obstructive sleep apnea and non-REM arousal threshold. *Ann Am Thor Soc.* 2015;12(5):758–764.

198. Eckert DJ, Owens RL, Kehlmann GB, et al. Eszopiclone increases the respiratory arousal threshold and lowers the apnoea/hypopnoea index in obstructive sleep apnoea patients with a low arousal threshold. *Clin Sci (London).* 2011;120(12):505–514.

199. Landry SA, Joosten SA, Sands SA, et al. Response to a combination of oxygen and a hypnotic as treatment for obstructive sleep apnoea is predicted by a patient's therapeutic CPAP requirement. *Respirology.* 2017;22(6):1219–1224.

200. Rizzi M, Onorato J, Andreoli A, et al. Nasal resistances are useful in identifying children with severe obstructive sleep apnea before polysomnography. *Int J Pediatr Otorhinolaryngol.* 2002;65(1):7–13.

201. Monahan KJ, Larkin EK, Rosen CL, Graham G, Redline S. Utility of noninvasive pharyngometry in epidemiologic studies of childhood sleep-disordered breathing. *Am J Resp Crit Care Med.* 2002;165(11):1499–1503.

202. Katz ES, Mitchell RB, D'Ambrosio CM. Obstructive sleep apnea in infants. *Am J Resp Crit Care Med.* 2012;185(8):805–816.

203. Kahn A, Groswasser J, Sottiaux M, et al. Clinical symptoms associated with brief obstructive sleep apnea in normal infants. *Sleep.* 1993;16(5):409–413.

204. Kanack MD, Nakra N, Ahmad I, Vyas RM. Normal neonatal sleep defined. Refining patient selection and interpreting sleep outcomes for mandibular distraction. *Plast Reconstr Surg Glob Open.* 2022;10:e4031.

205. Daftary AS, Jalou HE, Shively L, Slaven JE, Davis SD. Polysomnography reference values in healthy newborns. *J Clin Sleep Med.* 2019;15:437–443.

28

Ambulatory Monitoring in Pediatric Obstructive Sleep Apnea

Deborah Michelle Brooks and Lee J. Brooks

CHAPTER HIGHLIGHTS

- Obstructive respiratory disorders range from primary snoring to obstructive sleep apnea.
- The gold-standard for diagnosing Obstructive sleep apnea in children is an in-lab polysomnography.
- An inconclusive (or even negative home test) necessitates and in-lab PSG to verify the results.

Introduction

Obstructive sleep apnea (OSA) is common in children and first-line treatment typically consists of surgical intervention (adenotonsillectomy). To get an idea of which children would most benefit from surgery, their sleep apnea must be quantified and categorized (by the number and type of respiratory events, degree of hypoxemia, hypercapnia, and sleep fragmentation, etc.). While in adults there are many options for sleep apnea monitoring, including some that can be done in the comfort of the patient's home, the same does not apply to children. An in-lab polysomnogram (PSG) is the safest and best way to monitor a child's sleep apnea. In some situations where resources are scarce, the physician can perform a risk/benefit analysis and use a home-monitoring option on a child, but in the case of an inconclusive or even a negative home test, a PSG performed in a sleep laboratory is recommended.

Obstructive Sleep Apnea in Children

As covered in detail in other chapters, sleep apnea is a disorder in which breathing starts and stops repeatedly during sleep. Apneas can be classified as either obstructive or central, depending on where the breathing dysregulation originates. This chapter will briefly mention central sleep apneas but will focus primarily on OSA in children.

Obstructive respiratory sleep disorders in children represent a continuum, ranging from habitual snoring to OSA.[1] Primary snoring, which needs to be distinguished from OSA, is defined as snoring without obstructive apneas, frequent arousals from sleep, or gas exchange abnormalities. OSA, in contrast, is characterized by recurrent episodes of partial or complete airway obstruction associated with arousals, awakenings, and/or oxyhemoglobin desaturations during sleep.[2–5]

OSA affects 1–4% of children with the main risk factors being adenotonsillar hypertrophy, obesity, craniofacial abnormalities, and neuromuscular diseases.[6–8] It is usually worse during rapid eye movement (REM) sleep.[9,10] While OSA occurs in youth of all ages, it is thought to be most common in preschool-age children because the tonsils and adenoids are the largest compared with the size of their airway. Primary snoring is more common still and occurs in 3–12% of preschool-age children.[5] Children are typically brought to their pediatrician for complaints of noisy breathing, snoring, cessation of breathing, increased body movements during sleep, and increased nocturnal awakenings.[3] Daytime sleepiness and neurobehavioral problems are sometimes also noted.[5,6,11]

OSA in children is associated with significant morbidity, including periodic hypoxia, hypercarbia, increased respiratory effort, intrathoracic pressure changes, neurocognitive impairment, behavioral problems, failure to thrive, and cor pulmonale, so it is important to recognize and diagnose the condition in a timely fashion.[1,4,5,11,12] It is also very important, especially in small children, to know whether or not central sleep apnea is present, as this can change management.[7]

According to the American Academy of Pediatrics Subcommittee on Obstructive Sleep Apnea, the goals of diagnosis are to identify children at risk for adverse outcomes, avoid unnecessary intervention in patients not at risk for adverse outcomes, and evaluate which patients are at risk for perioperative complications so that appropriate precautions can be taken. Because OSA in children is usually caused by hypertrophy of the tonsils and adenoids, treatment with adenotonsillectomy is typically effective.[11,13] Severe OSA is associated with higher risk for perioperative complications, and even residual OSA after surgery, so accurate preoperative assessment of the presence and severity of OSA is essential.[2,14] For those children who are not surgical candidates or who did not respond to surgery, continuous positive airway

311

pressure (CPAP) is an option.[5] Treatment of OSA can result in improvements in behavior and cognitive abilities.[15]

Gold Standard for Diagnosis: In-Lab Polysomnogram (PSG)

PSG performed overnight in a sleep lab is the gold standard for diagnosing OSA in children.[1,2,4–7,10] PSG includes simultaneous recording of electroencephalogram (EEG), electrooculogram, electrocardiogram (ECG), submental and leg electromyogram, oronasal thermistor, nasal pressure, thoracic and abdominal wall movement sensors, end-tidal and/or transcutaneous CO_2, and pulse oximetry, all under the continuous observation of a trained technologist.[9] These channels are used to measure, among other things, the presence of obstructive, mixed, and central apneas, which is especially important in the pediatric population (particularly with patients with neuromuscular disorders) where hypoventilation is possible.[4,10,16] The sensors can also determine partial airway obstruction, oxyhemoglobin desaturations, and sleep architecture.[10]

The clinical practice guidelines on the diagnosis and management of childhood OSA by the American Academy of Pediatrics noted that if an in-lab PSG is not available, clinicians may order alternative diagnostic tests (discussed later); however, prescribers need to be aware of the sensitivity and specificity of the test used and consider proceeding to a full PSG if the results are inconclusive.[4]

Full in-lab PSGs are preferred because they provide an objective measure of disturbances in respiratory parameters and sleep architecture and can differentiate primary snoring from sleep apneas while determining the severity of the apneas.[4] They can also differentiate OSA from other sleep disorders, including movement disorders and parasomnias.

Despite the gold standard designation, in-lab PSGs do have their pitfalls. Full PSGs are expensive, time-consuming, inconvenient, and may be limited in their availability, which may lead to long wait times.[1,2,4,6,12,17] Thus, other options have been suggested.

A nap PSG is typically a 4-hour or shorter PSG, often during the daytime. This is most commonly used in infants. It has been shown to generally underestimate sleep-disordered breathing in children.[3] While a nap PSG may be useful if the results are strongly positive, an overnight study is still required if a nap PSG is negative. The difference in predictive value between the nap and overnight studies can be attributed to the decreased amount of time in REM sleep during naps as well as the decrease in total sleep time.[9]

Factors in Diagnosis

A commonly used index of the severity of respiratory events is the apnea-hypopnea index (AHI; number of respiratory events per hour of sleep). The *International Classification of Sleep Disorders, Third Edition* (ICSD-3) defines pediatric OSA as an AHI ≥1 or a pattern of obstructive hypoventilation defined as at least 25% of total sleep time with hypercapnia (PaCO₂

>50 mm Hg) in association with snoring, flattening of the nasal pressure waveform, or paradoxical respiratory efforts.[2] However, these criteria are controversial. Early studies did not include hypopneas and/or central events. An AHI >1.5 has been shown to be statistically abnormal in some studies, while it seems that physiologic abnormalities such as hypertension may not be seen until the AHI >5[18] (Table 28.1).

Can Ambulatory Monitoring Provide the Essential Elements to Diagnose Obstructive Sleep Apnea in Children?

While the 2017 American Academy of Sleep Medicine (AASM) guidelines do not support the use of home sleep apnea testing for the diagnosis of OSA in children, they have approved the use of portable monitors as an alternative to PSG in certain situations based on the doctor's clinical judgment (taking into account access to available diagnostic tools, individual patient circumstances, and available treatment options).[2,16,19]

To replace laboratory-based PSG, home-based studies need to be reliable and well tolerated by the children.[13] In general, abbreviated diagnostic techniques tend to be helpful if the results are positive but they have a poor predictive value if the results are negative; thus, children with a negative portable study are still recommended to undergo a more comprehensive evaluation including full in-laboratory PSG. Portable studies are also of limited use in evaluating the severity of the OSA, which limits their ability to predict perioperative morbidity.[5,15] The European Respiratory Society is somewhat more liberal and allows video PSG, nap PSG, respiratory polygraphy (RP), and nocturnal pulse oximetry as tools to diagnose OSA, although they still list in-lab PSG as the gold standard for diagnosis.[1]

Despite their low sensitivity and specificity, portable monitoring devices have some advantages.[15] They are generally feasible and reproducible, if not as accurate as full PSGs.

Home studies are initially less expensive, more convenient, and more accessible, with theoretically less "first night effect."[4] However, these benefits may be mitigated by the need to repeat a full PSG either because of questionable results or a technically inadequate study.

Portable Monitoring Classifications

In 1994, the AASM Portable Monitoring Task Force classified diagnostic monitoring into four categories, of which types 2–4 are applicable to home testing.[4]

Type 1

Type 1 monitoring is a fully attended PSG with seven or more channels, completed in a laboratory setting.[4] This is considered the gold-standard for diagnosing OSA because it provides an objective, quantitative evaluation

TABLE 28.1   Traditional Polysomnogram Components and Their Importance

PSG components	Measurements	Why It Is Important
EEG	Sleep vs. wakefulness, sleep architecture	Can identify seizure activity Determine total sleep time which is the denominator for apnea-hypopnea index Determine if events happen during wake or sleep (e.g., baby crying may mimic apnea)
EOG	Eye movements	Differentiates REM, non-REM, and wakefulness
Submental EMG	Pharyngeal muscles (genioglossus)	Demonstrates atony, which differentiates REM sleep from wakefulness
Leg EMG	Leg movements	Measures periodic limb movements during sleep
Oronasal thermistor	Exhaled air temperature	Temperature during exhalation is higher than inhalation, shows the presence of airflow
Thoracic and abdominal movement sensor	Chest and abdominal movement	Differentiates obstructive vs. central event
Pulse oximeter	Oxyhemoglobin saturation	Extent and duration of hypoxemia, identifies hypopneas
ECG	Heart rate and rhythm	Helps identify bradycardias and more severe arrhythmias
Video	Body movements, extraneous events causing an arousal	Helps identify wakefulness vs. sleep, especially in infants Helps identify body movements, whether tonic-clonic suggesting seizures, periodic limb movements, or other movements
Nasal capnograph or transcutaneous CO_2 monitor	CO_2	Identifies hypoventilation
Laryngeal microphone	Snoring sounds	Presence of snoring

Abbreviations: ECG, electrocardiogram; EEG, electroencephalogram; EMG, electromyogram; EOG, electrooculogram; PSG, polysomnogram; REM, rapid eye movement.

of disturbances of respiratory and sleep patterns.[15] Type 1 PSGs also allows patients to be stratified according to their severity, helping to determine which children are at risk for perioperative complications. *Recommendation: PSG is the gold standard for diagnosis and assessment of severity in OSA and other sleep disorders.*

Type 2

Type 2 monitoring consists of an unattended PSG with seven or more channels.[4] This is essentially a "PSG in the home" and generally includes EEG as well as respiratory monitoring. These ambulatory PSGs are appropriate and reliable in some adults, but they should not be used for the exclusive evaluation of severe OSA in children, especially preschool children, because they rarely include capnography.[12,15] Portable PSGs are feasible in older children and had no significant difference in respiratory parameters compared with in-lab PSG, but the type 2 monitors have a high error rate in children <5 years old.[4,9,15] Under research conditions, with a trained staff to go to the child's home and apply the sensors, there is a high degree of technically acceptable recordings.[4,16]

Type 2 studies are still quite labor intensive and expensive as a technologist must travel to the home to set up and take down the equipment. The scoring is no different from in-lab PSGs.[4] Video recordings are not always included with home PSG, nor is CO_2 monitoring, which is particularly important in children in whom there is concern about hypoventilation, such as those with neuromuscular disease, underlying lung disease, or obesity hypoventilation. Other limitations for these home PSGs include possible interference from siblings, lack of electrical outlets near the child's bed, signal artifacts caused by home technology, and insufficient battery life if the unit was unplugged (say for a bathroom trip) and not replugged.[4] In many cases, even if caregivers noted that sensors came off overnight, few attempted to replace them. Nasal cannula–based flow signals are often suboptimal with no sleep technologist continuously monitoring the patient.[4,8] Any cost advantage of type 2 monitoring may be mitigated by the need for a technologist to set up the devices in the home, and the not infrequent need to perform full PSG anyway because of an inconclusive home study.

At this time, only one device has been approved by the U.S. Food and Drug Administration (FDA) as a type 2 home-monitoring device but it is only approved in adults. This device is designed to be applied by a layperson after receiving instruction from a trained professional. It consists of a nasal pressure cannula and thermistor, chest and abdominal belts, digital probe for oximetry, and an ECG lead. It shows mixed results in pediatric studies when compared with laboratory PSG with good sensitivity when worn in the sleep lab, but only 70% sensitivity in the home.[11] The AHI was not comparable to PSG in children, and this device is not approved by the FDA for use in children.[11]

Recommendation: Type 2 studies may be useful in older children and adults when there is a high clinical suspicion for straightforward, uncomplicated OSA, but if negative the child may still need an in-lab PSG. Type 2 monitors work best when a trained professional goes to the child's house to place the sensors and instruct the family.

Type 3

Type 3 portable monitoring devices are more limited than types 1 and 2. These studies typically include only 4–7 channels, usually without EEG monitoring of sleep stages.[4,15] The AASM recommends that at a minimum, a type 3 monitor, also known as RP, should record the presence of airflow, respiratory efforts, and oxyhemoglobin saturation.[7,19] Home RP is accepted and used effectively in adults. Although more research in children is needed, type 3 portable monitoring may offer a viable alternative in the diagnosis of otherwise healthy children with moderate to severe OSA, particularly in settings where access to PSG is scarce or unavailable.[4] These studies can identify an AHI that highly correlates to a level 1 PSG, especially in older children aged 12–17.[8] The type 3 device also demonstrated relatively high sensitivity and specificity to diagnose OSA with AHI >10, but was inferior to PSG in mild and moderate cases of OSA. These research studies, however, were enhanced by having a sleep technologist present at the child's home.[8] These devices must be used judiciously because hypoventilation cannot be assessed without a CO_2 monitor, hypopneas cannot be accurately assessed without EEG monitoring for arousals, and sleep time and time in REM sleep cannot be assessed without EEG monitoring. Similar to type 2 monitors, the percentage of successful recordings is higher if set up by trained staff.[4]

Type 3 monitors have been studied in special populations including children with Down syndrome, Prader-Willi syndrome, and neuromuscular disorders; notably, hypoventilation could not be detected using these monitors. Half of the muscular dystrophy patients had incomplete or falsely low CO_2 values because of missing data, mouth breathing, or signal loss.[9,16] Additionally, many children, especially younger children, could not tolerate the sensors and, even with detailed oral and written instructions, the caregivers were unable to place the sensors adequately.[13] Because of the high specificity but low sensitivity, a negative test necessitates an

in-lab PSG.[7] If the child is sleeping poorly, a type 3 monitor, which cannot stage sleep, may miss obstructive events as those events tend to cluster during REM sleep.[4] Additional limitations include that total recording time, rather than total sleep time, is used for the denominator for AHI.[12] When an RP is performed in-laboratory, it tends to use the same equipment as the PSG (minus certain signals). In comparison, home RPs are designed to be portable and, while similar, they are not the same as the in-laboratory equipment; thus they may yield poorer results than even these studies suggest.[4] Any cost advantage of type 3 monitoring may be mitigated by the need for a technologist to set up the devices in the home, and the not infrequent need to perform full PSG anyway because of an inconclusive home study.

Recommendation: Type 3 portable monitoring devices may be useful in older children with a strong history and physical examination that are suggestive of severe OSA. It should not be used in children <3 years of age and only sparingly in children <12 years of age because of its high failure rate in these populations. It should not be used in patients in whom hypoventilation is likely or suspected, including Down syndrome and neuromuscular, craniofacial, or skeletal syndromes. If inconclusive, a conventional PSG should be performed. Results are improved if a trained professional sets up the sensors at the beginning of the night.

Type 4

Type 4 portable monitoring consists of only one to two signal channels, traditionally, but not exclusively, with pulse oximetry as one of the measurements.[4] The second channel may be ECG/heart rate, peripheral arterial tonometry (PAT), or chest wall movement. As with other portable monitoring systems, type 4 monitors have a good positive predictive value in patients with a high pretest probability for OSA but a poor negative predictive value, indicating that oximetry is useful when results are positive, but if the test is negative the patient still requires a full PSG.[5,11] Overall, single-channel recording has not been shown to correlate well with in-lab PSG for the diagnosis of OSA.[11,17] Oximetry alone is generally insufficient because of the higher rate of inconclusive test results, especially considering that children with OSA can experience arousals and sleep fragmentation and not develop desaturations. Children also tend to move around in their sleep, which can result in motion artifacts.[15] Pulse oximetry alone also cannot differentiate between obstructive and central respiratory events.[11] Type 4 monitoring can be useful to help in the prioritization of treatment and can play a more central role in resourcing poor areas where PSGs are not available.[4] It is most useful in children being treated with home oxygen to determine the feasibility of stopping oxygen therapy. *Recommendation: Type 4 portable monitoring cannot replace laboratory PSG because of its poor sensitivity, and it is not sufficient for the identification of OSA in otherwise healthy children. If the result is negative or inconclusive, it necessitates a full PSG* (Tables 28.2 and 28.3).

TABLE 28.2   Comparison of Obstructive Sleep Apnea Monitoring Devices

Components	Type 1 (in-lab PSG)	Type 2 (Unattended PSG)	Type 3 (RP)	Type 4 (1–2 channels)
EEG	✓	✓		
EOG	✓	✓		
Submental EMG	✓	✓		
Leg EMG	✓	✓		
Oronasal thermistor	✓	✓	✓	
Thoracic and abdominal movement sensor	✓	✓	✓	
Pulse oximetry	✓	✓	✓	✓
ECG	✓	✓		
Video	✓	✓ (Usually not included)	✓ (Usually not included)	
Nasal CO_2 capnograph or transcutaneous CO_2 monitor	✓	✓ (Usually not included)	✓ (Usually not included)	
Laryngeal microphone for snoring sounds	✓	✓		

Abbreviations: ECG, electrocardiogram; EEG, electroencephalogram; EMG, electromyogram; EOG, electrooculogram; PSG, polysomnogram; RP, respiratory polygraphy.

TABLE 28.3	Advantages and Limitations of Portable Monitoring Devices			
	Type 1 PSG	**Type 2 Portable Monitoring Device**	**Type 3 Portable Monitoring Device**	**Type 4 Portable Monitoring Device**
Advantages	"Gold standard"; Can identify hypopneas, hypoventilation, movement disorders	More convenient for families Theoretically less first night effect because child is sleeping at home	More convenient for families Theoretically less first night effect because child is sleeping at home	Inexpensive, small, convenient
Limitations	Expensive Labor intensive	Expensive Labor intensive Less useful in young children Signals can be lost overnight	Less sensitive and specific Does not typically measure CO_2 so cannot determine hypoventilation	Poor sensitivity overall, poor negative predictive value Cannot differentiate obstructive from central apneas

Abbreviation: PSG, polysomnogram.

Other Monitoring Options

In addition to the more standard portable monitoring devices, there are other methods in use to determine the presence and severity of OSA in children. While these methods will be described briefly, it is important to note that none can fully replace a full in-lab PSG for diagnosis of OSA in children.

The first step in evaluating OSA in children, in addition to laboratory or ambulatory monitoring, is a thorough sleep history, and physical examination. A thorough sleep history should include any report of nightly snoring, labored breathing, observed apneas, restless sleep, diaphoresis, enuresis, cyanosis, excessive daytime sleepiness, and behavioral or learning problems. The history is best obtained from the person who observes the child sleeping on a regular basis, which may be a sibling who shares a bedroom with the patient. Physical examination should pay special attention to the anatomy of the pharynx, including size of the tonsils and a thorough cardiovascular exam. Be aware that the findings on physical examination during wakefulness are often normal, or nonspecific related to adenotonsillar hypertrophy. And while adenotonsillar hypertrophy is a major risk factor for OSA in children, numerous studies have shown that there is no relation between the size of the tonsils and adenoids on inspection and the presence of OSA; it is a combination of the size and the neuromuscular tone of the upper airway that leads to OSA.[20] In addition to the standard history and physical, several questionnaires have been developed to screen for OSA, although they too generally exhibit low sensitivity and specificity.[7] Sleep Clinical Score is a composite score derived from the physical examination, subjective symptoms, and clinical history, and this combination has been shown to correlate relatively well with AHI on PSG.[4] The overall performance on questionnaires supports their use more as a screening tool than as a diagnostic agent, such that a negative score would be unlikely to mislabel a child

with OSA as being healthy, but a positive score would be unlikely to accurately diagnose a particular child with certainty.[15] While this is all important information, history and physical alone have a poor sensitivity and specificity in diagnosing sleep apnea.[5,14,15] Radiographic studies are usually not helpful to make a diagnosis, but a lateral neck film may suggest a treatment approach.

Other types of portable monitoring include the following. Certain *radiologic studies* have been used to help diagnose OSA. For example, the presence of airway narrowing on a lateral neck radiograph increases the probability of predicting OSA on PSG.[15] *Acoustic pharyngometry* uses reflected sound waves administered through the mouth to assess the size of the pharynx, but its accuracy has been questioned.[21] When sound waves are applied through the nose *(acoustic rhinometry)*, nasal resistance may be assessed; a high nasal resistance suggests an increased risk for OSA.[22] *Objective snoring evaluations* independent from a history and physical examination generally do not correlate well with the degree of OSA, as the loudness of the snoring does not necessarily correlate with the degree of obstructive apnea.[15] Snoring may disappear following surgery such as adenotonsillectomy, yet OSA may persist if the baseline OSA was severe.

Studies have found changes in *cardiovascular parameters* (heart rate, heart rate variability, pulse transit time, and PAT) in children with OSA, but the sensitivities and specificities are variable and they cannot be recommended for clinical use at this point by themselves.[15] PAT assesses changes in peripheral arterial volume as a surrogate measure of transient elevations of sympathetic tone associated with arousals. This, combined with a pulse oximeter and actigraphy, provides a relatively high degree of correlation sleep variables when compared with PSG in adults, and in children with severe OSA.[4,23]

Using *pulmonary function tests (PFTs)*, a "sawtoothed" pattern of the maximal expiratory flow-volume loop has been suggested to screen for OSA in adults, but young children may have difficulty performing the maneuver.[15]

Some studies have tried to use *urinary/serum proteomic analysis* for screening and in a highly selected population, urinary proteins did have a high sensitivity and specificity, although more studies are needed.[15,24]

Currently Experimental Noncontact Methods for Assessing Sleep-Disordered Breathing in the Home

Audio and videotaping, facilitated by the near-universal presence of cell phones with videotaping capabilities, shows a number of discrepancies in screening for and diagnosing OSA in children.[5] Home video may be a useful first step in the clinical evaluation of children with suspected OSA,[3] with a generally high sensitivity and medium specificity. The most useful information gleaned from the recording is differentiating snoring from other respiratory noises. Limitations of video recording include that neither sleep state, nor other parameters, are monitored.[3] *Audio* recording alone is inferior to video because it only monitors one variable, the presence of noisy breathing.[3]

Investigators have also attempted to use video game modalities to assess sleep in the home, namely the *Microsoft Kinect* video game system. (Of note, this game system is not being manufactured for video game purposes anymore but it continues to be used for monitoring of various medical issues.) The system has three optical sensors to provide body tracking, three-dimensional (3D) body reconstruction, skeletal tracking, and joint tracking to detect respiratory activity, particularly visualizing paradoxical movements of the thorax and abdomen, and monitoring limb movements. It cannot alone detect oxygen saturation levels, arousals, or changes in heart rate. One study showed that this system can accurately measure respiratory movements under minimal light conditions and therefore detect apneas in even young children, although more studies are necessary.[25]

Radar has also been examined as a noncontact monitoring device for OSA making use of the Doppler effect. However, this requires that the system be within 1 m of the patient. If radio frequency identification technology (RFID) is used sensors are still required on the patient's body, which may be uncomfortable and are prone to distortion by the patient's movement and signal interference.[25]

Thermal video cameras have also been used to detect carbon dioxide emissions or to determine skin temperature differences between inhalation and exhalation. However, these measurements are affected by head position, movement artifact, and anything that might cover the face such as a blanket.[25]

Image sequence analysis uses optical flow of the chest surface captured by a video camera, but lighting conditions are a major drawback and the data had to be interpreted after

the video was analyzed, so abnormal events cannot be captured in real time.[25]

3D surface information of the patient's chest and abdomen captured by time-of-flight cameras for detecting respiratory motion is also affected by noise and motion artifact and is quite expensive.[25]

Capacitor-based systems detect static charge contained within bedding material and can discern breathing movements, but studies so far have had limited success with children.[4]

Sheets and mats with pressure, vibration, and sound sensors also exist although the *pressure-sensing sheets* can detect central, but not obstructive apneas. *Vibration-sensing mats* underestimate the AHI in adults.[4] A newer device, the Sonomat, a mattress pad with both sound and movement sensors, is showing some promise in identifying both obstructive and central apneas in children.[26] Last, *noncontact biomotion sensors* can use radio waves to measure movement and respiration from the bedside table and were found useful in adults with an AHI >15.[4]

Children Are Not Small Adults

Many of the previously mentioned ambulatory monitoring devices work well in adults but not in children, and generally, home sleep testing has been shown to be noninferior to in-lab PSG for adults. Why is it different in children?[11] Children are fundamentally different from the adults they will become and they experience a different kind of OSA. Partial airway obstruction is more common, and oxygen desaturation is less common, in children with OSA compared with adults.[17] These episodes may be missed completely by oximetry-based monitoring.[17] Additionally, the cutoffs for clinically significant OSA are higher in adults, thus eliminating the need for discrimination between low and very low AHI values.[9] Scoring is also different between children and adults, where the pediatric scoring allows the opportunity to score a hypopnea if the event is associated with an arousal, rather than just oxyhemoglobin desaturation, thus EEG monitoring is essential.[2] The lack of EEG or CO_2 monitoring on home testing may therefore result in significant underestimation of the presence and severity of OSA in children.[2] Children also sleep differently and are notably more restless during sleep and children with OSA have more movement arousals than age-matched controls, increasing artifact signal.[17] Additionally, monitors with leads can increase the risk of strangulation and entrapment for young children.[25] Children are also generally less tolerant of the machine and their body sizes and cognitive and emotional maturity can vary widely, so it is more difficult to predict who will be able to tolerate the numerous sensors.[2] In addition, the first-line treatment for adults is CPAP, which is generally noninvasive, whereas the treatment in children is usually surgery. The baseline AHI predicts the response to surgery[14] and perioperative complications so it is important to know the severity, not just the presence, of OSA in children.[27–30] Home sleep apnea testing has made a significant impact in adult sleep medicine but, unfortunately, these results cannot be extrapolated to children, especially because children may have a greater susceptibility to develop comorbid consequences with OSA.[4]

Conclusion

While portable home monitoring of OSA is accepted and validated in adults, it is not recommended at this time for the diagnosis of OSA in children. However, the ultimate judgment regarding this, and any specific care, must be made by the physician, considering the individual circumstances of the patient, the available diagnostic tools, and the accessible treatment options.[2] This is not to say that home monitoring will never be appropriate in children, but given the few validated studies and conflicting results in children, in-lab PSG remains the gold standard for diagnosing and evaluating OSA in children.

CLINICAL PEARLS

- The primary treatment for children with OSA is surgery (usually adenotonsillectomy), as opposed to CPAP in adults.
- The more severe the OSA is in any particular child, the more likely surgical complications are to occur, which is why it is very important to accurately label the severity of the OSA.
- Primary snoring differs from OSA in the primary snoring does not cause arousals, apneas, or blood-gas abnormalitiess.

References

1. Michelet M, Blanchon S, Guinand S, Ruchonnet-Metrailler I, Mornand A, Van HC, Corbelli R. Successful home respiratory polygraphy to investigate sleep-disordered breathing in children. *Sleep Med.* 2020;68:146–152.
2. Kirk V, Baughn J, D'Andrea L, Friedman N, Galion A, Garetz S, Malhotra R. American Academy of Sleep Medicine Position Paper for the Use of a Home Sleep Apnea Test for the Diagnosis of OSA in Children. *J Clin Sleep Med.* 2017;13(10):1199–1203.
3. Sivan Y, Kornecki A, Scholfeld T. Screening obstructive sleep apnoea syndrome by home videotape recording in children. *Eur Respir J.* 1996;9:2127–2131.
4. Tan HL, Kheirandish-Gozal L, Gozal D. Pediatric home sleep apnea testing slowly getting there. *Chest.* 2015, December;148(6):1382–1395.
5. American Academy of Pediatrics Section on Pediatric Pulmonology, Subcommittee on Obstructive Sleep Apnea. Clinical Practice Guideline: Diagnosis and Management of Childhood Obstructive Sleep Apnea Syndrome. *Pediatrics.* 2002;109:704–712.
6. Pavone M, Verrillo E, Cutrera R, Salerno T, Soldini S, Brouillette R. Night-to-night consistency of at-home nocturnal pulse oximetry testing for obstructive sleep apnea in children. *Pediatr Pulmonol.* 2013;48:754–760.
7. Alonso-Alvarez ML, Teran-Santos J, Carbajo EO, Cordero-Guevara JA, Navazo-Eguia AI, Kheirandish-Gozal L, Gozal D. Reliability of home respiratory polygraphy for the diagnosis of sleep apnea in children. *Chest.* 2015;147(4):1020–1028.
8. Bhattacharjee R. Ready for primetime? Home sleep apnea tests for children. *J Clin Sleep Med.* 2019;155:685–686.
9. Katidis A, Alonso Alvarez ML, Boudewyns A, Abel F, Alexopoulos E, Ersu R, Verhulst S. ERS statement on obstructive sleep disordered breathing in 1- to 23-month-old children. *Eur Respir J.* 2017;50(6):1700985.
10. Morielle A, Ladan S, Ducharme F, Brouillette R. Can sleep and wakefulness be distinguished in children by cardiorespiratory and videotape recordings? *Chest.* 1996, March;109(3):680–687.
11. Scalzitti N, Hansen S, Maturo S, Lospinoso J, O'Connor P. Comparison of home sleep apnea testing versus laboratory polysomnography for the diagnosis of obsturctive sleep apnea in children. *Int J Pediatr Otorhinolaryngol.* 2017;100:44–51.
12. Suzuki M, Furukawa T, Sugimoto A, Kotani R, Hosogaya R. Comparison of diagnostic reliability of out-of-center sleep tests for obstructive sleep apnea between adults and children. *Int J Pediatr Otorhinolaryngol.* 2017;94:54–58.
13. Poels P, Schilder A, van den Berg S, Hoes A, Joosten K. Evaluation of a new device for home cardiorespiratory recording in children. *Arch Otolaryngol Head Neck Surg.* 2003, Dec;129:1281–1284.
14. Suen JS, Arnold JE, Brooks LJ. Adenotonsillectomy for treatment of obstructive sleep apnea in children. *Arch Otolaryngol Head Neck Surg.* 1995;121:525–530.
15. Marcus C, Brooks L, Davidson Ward S, Draper K, Gozal D, Halbower A, Spruyt K. Diagnosis and management of childhood obstructive sleep apnea syndrome. *Am Acad Pediatr.* 2012, September;130(3):e714–e755.
16. Hassan F, D'Andrea L. Best and safest care versus care closer to home. *J Clin Sleep Med.* 2018;14(12):1973–1974.
17. Kirk V, Bohn S, Flemons W, Remmers J. Comparison of home oximetry with laboratory polysomnogrpahy in children. *Chest.* 2003, November;124(5):1702–1708.
18. Brooks DM, Brooks LJ. Reevaluating norms for childhood obstructive sleep apnea. *J Clin Sleep Med.* 2019;15(11):1557–1558.
19. Masoud A, Patwari P, Adavadkar P, Arantes H, Park C, Carley D. Validation of the MediByte portable monitor for the diagnosis of sleep apnea in pediatric patients. *J Clin Sleep Med.* 2019, May;15(5):733–742.
20. Brooks LJ, Stephens BM, Bacevice M. Adenoid size is related to severity but not the number of episodes of obstructive apnea in children. *J Pediatr.* 1994;132(4):682–686.
21. Brooks L. Acoustic reflectance. In: Marcus C, Carroll JL, Donnelly D, Loughlin GM, eds. *Sleep and Breathing in Children.* CRC Press; 2008.
22. Okun MN, Hadjiangelis N, Green D, Hedli LC, Lee KC, Krieger AC. Acoustic rhonometry in pediatric sleep apnea. *Sleep Breath.* 2010;14:43–49.
23. Tanphaichitr A, Thianboonsong A, Banhiran W, Vathanophas V, Ungkanont K. Watch peripheral arterial tonometry in the diagnosis of pediatric obstructive sleep apnea. *Otolaryngol Head Neck Surg.* 2018;159(1):166–172.

24. Feliciano A, Millic Torres V, Vaz F, Carvalho AS, Matthiesen R, Pinto P, Penque D. Overview of proteonomics studies in obstructive sleep apnea. *Sleep Med*. 2015, April;16(4):437–445.

25. Al-Naji A, Gibson K, Lee SH, Chahl J. Real time monitoring of children using the microsoft kinect sensor: A pilot study. *Sensors*. 2017;17(2):286.

26. Norman MB, Pithers SM, Teng AY, Waters KA, Sullivan CC. Validation of the Sonomat against PSG and quantitative measurement of partial upper airway obstruction in children with sleep-disordered breathing. *Sleep*. 2017, March;40(3). https://doi.org/10.1093/sleep/zsx017.

27. Kasle D, Virbalas J, Bent JP, Cheng J. Tonsillectomies and respiratory complications in children: A look at pre-op polysomnography risk factors and post-op admissions. *Int J Pediatr Otorhinolaryngol*. 2016, September;88:224–227.

28. Hamada M, Iida M. Home monitoring using portable polysomnography for perioperative assessment of pediatric obstructive sleep apnea syndrome. *J Exp Clin Med*. 2012;37(3):66–70.

29. Isaiah A, Pereira K, Das G. Polysomnography and treatment-related outcomes of childhood sleep apnea. *Pediatrics*. 2019, October;144(4):e20191097.

30. Quan S, Goodwin J, Babar S, Kaemingk K, Enright P, Rosen G, Morgan W. Sleep architecture on normal Caucasian and Hispanic children aged 6–11 years recorded during unattended home polysomnography: Experience from the Tucson Children's Assessment of Sleep Apnea Study (TuCASA). *Sleep Med*. 2013;4:13–19.

29

Cognitive and Behavioral Consequences of Obstructive Sleep Apnea

LOUISE M. O'BRIEN

CHAPTER HIGHLIGHTS

- Sleep-disordered breathing in children is common and associated with impaired behavior and cognition.
- Behavioral manifestations are the most robust sequelae.
- Children with behavioral difficulties should be evaluated for underlying sleep disturbance prior to a diagnosis of ADHD.
- Adenotonsillectomy improves behavior but there is no clear evidence that cognition improves post-surgery.

OBJECTIVES

- Habitual snoring and obstructive sleep apnea are common in children and associated with neurobehavioral morbidity.
- Insults may manifest years later, suggestive of a window of vulnerability in developing children.
- However, there is no consistent phenotype and no dose–response relationships; indeed, mild sleep-disordered breathing is often associated with poor outcomes.
- Polysomnographic findings alone may not be sufficient for identifying children in need of treatment; symptoms and behavioral disturbances should also be considered.
- Treatment interventions such as adenotonsillectomy appear to improve behavioral morbidities but not cognitive abilities.

Introduction

Sleep-disordered breathing (SDB) describes a range of breathing problems during sleep from habitual snoring to obstructive sleep apnea (OSA). It is a frequent condition characterized by repeated events of partial or complete upper airway obstruction during sleep, resulting in disruption of normal ventilation, hypoxemia, and sleep. The estimated population prevalence for SDB by varying constellations of parent-reported symptoms on questionnaire has been reported to be 4–11%, whereas OSA diagnosed by varying criteria on diagnostic studies is approximately 1–4%.[1] However, OSA is believed to be more common in preschoolers between 3 and 5 years, when lymphoid tissue growth is

at a peak.[2] Although OSA was first described by McKenzie over a century ago,[3] it was not until the mid-1970s that it was recognized in children.[4] Using polysomnography (PSG) in eight children aged 5–14 years, Guilleminault and colleagues published the first detailed report of children with adenotonsillar hypertrophy and OSA and suggested that surgery may eliminate their clinical symptoms.[4] Since this initial report there has been considerable research in this area and it is now clear that OSA in children is a distinct disorder from the OSA that occurs in adults, in particular with respect to gender distribution, clinical manifestations, polysomnographic findings, and treatment.[5–7] OSA is frequently diagnosed in association with adenotonsillar hypertrophy, and is also common in obese children and those with craniofacial abnormalities and neurologic disorders affecting upper airway patency.[8,9] During sleep, the patency of the upper airway is controlled by complex interactions between upper airway resistance, the tone of pharyngeal dilator muscles, pharyngeal collapsibility, and negative intraluminal pressure generated by inspiratory muscles;[10] disruption in this interplay can result in airway collapse.

The primary symptom of OSA is frequent snoring and while snoring is not normal, as it indicates the presence of heightened upper airway resistance, many snoring children may have primary snoring (i.e., habitual snoring without alterations in sleep architecture, alveolar ventilation, and oxygenation). Nonetheless, definitive criteria that allow for reliable distinction between primary snoring and OSA and the threshold at which morbidity occurs remain elusive. PSG remains the gold standard for the definitive diagnosis of OSA, because clinical history and physical examination are insufficient to confirm its presence or severity.[11,12]

The implications of SDB in children are multifaceted and potentially complex. If left untreated or, alternatively, if treated late, pediatric SDB may lead to substantial morbidity that affects multiple target organs and systems, which may not be completely reversed with appropriate treatment. There is now a wealth of literature showing strong and significant associations between parental report and/or objective measures of SDB with a range of neurobehavioral, cognitive, and psychiatric problems. The potential consequences of SDB in children include behavioral disturbances and learning deficits,[13–22] psychiatric symptoms,[23–27] autonomic dysfunction,[28–33] and cardiovascular dysfunction.[34–39] This chapter will focus on the behavioral and cognitive consequences of SDB.

Behavior

Behavioral dysregulation is the most commonly encountered comorbidity of SDB. As described later, the vast majority of studies consistently report, mostly robust, associations between SDB symptoms, or objective measures of SDB, and hyperactivity, impulsivity, and attention-deficit/hyperactivity disorder (ADHD)-like symptoms.

Hyperactivity

Hyperactivity is commonly reported in both children with habitual snoring,[15–17,40–45] and those in whom SDB was formally diagnosed by PSG.[15,42,46–50] Despite differences in the definition of snoring or PSG-confirmed SDB, many studies support the relationship between snoring/SDB and hyperactive behaviors even when hyperactivity is measured with a range of parent-report tools, including the Conners' Parent Rating Scales,[16,17,42,44,45,47] the Child Behavior Checklist,[42,44–47] or the Behavioral Assessment Scale for Children.[22,41]

Notably, while it has been previously reported that a trend toward a dose response may exist between reported snoring frequency and hyperactive behavior,[16] more recent evidence suggests that the impact of SDB on behavior is greatest in those with the mildest degree of severity.[50] Smith and colleagues[50] conducted PSG and behavioral assessments in over 1,000 5- to 7-year-old children and subdivided participants into four groups based on the apnea-hypopnea index (AHI; respiratory events per hour of total sleep time) as follows: group 1, nonsnoring and AHI <1; group 2, habitual snoring and AHI <1; group 3, habitual snoring and AHI 1–5; and group 4, habitual snoring and AHI >5. Compared with controls (group 1), habitual snorers with AHI <1 (group 2) were the most behaviorally impaired. Moreover, differences between the habitual snoring group and those with more severe sleep pathology were rarely significant. These findings thus suggest that children who snore may be at increased risk for development of behavioral concerns independent of the severity of SDB. Additional analyses by the same authors examined snoring and AHI separately (rather than defining groups by snoring and AHI measures together) and found that snoring status was a significant predictor of impaired behavior even when adjustment was made for AHI severity.[45] Of interest, more frequent snoring was associated with poorer behavioral outcomes regardless of AHI severity, but higher AHI was associated with fewer problems in hyperactive behaviors. The authors postulated that snoring should not be assumed to represent a lower severity of SDB; instead it should be examined as a potential predictor of relevant outcomes.[45] These findings further emphasize the importance of including snoring status and not just PSG-derived metrics in assessments of behavioral outcomes in pediatric SDB.

Inattention

Attention, which is a prerequisite to optimal learning, is a critical behavior arising from brain mechanisms and can be categorized as sustained, selective, and divided attention, thus representing a cluster of variables, each of which contributes to learning and memory. Inattentive behaviors identified by parental report have been observed in children with habitual snoring[16,17,45,50] and PSG-defined SDB,[46,49,51] although this finding is not as robust as the associations with hyperactivity. Different categories of attention, for example, selective and sustained attention, can also be measured using objective assessments such as auditory or visual continuous performance tests (CPTs) and therefore may provide more robust assessment than parental report. Such studies have shown that even children with mild SDB exhibit some deficits in attention compared with controls.[44,45,50,52]

A small study of Australian children found that both selective and sustained attention measured objectively using the auditory CPT were found to be impaired in children with habitual snoring compared with controls.[53] Similarly, in New Zealand, Galland and colleagues[54] found that compared with a normal population, children with objectively confirmed SDB, compared with those without, had significantly higher scores on a visual CPT for inattention and impulsivity albeit within the average range of a normal nonclinical score. Inattention scores have also been reported to be higher in a U.S.-based cohort of primary snoring children, even after accounting for AHI severity, similar to the hyperactivity findings described earlier from the same group.[45,50] Importantly, more severe disease does not appear to be correlated with worse attention scores. Moreover, in a recent study of primary school-aged children in Finland, snoring time on PSG was quantified and children were defined as primary snorers if their parents reported frequent snoring at least three nights per week and their PSG demonstrated an obstructive AHI index <1 with snoring time >1.5% of sleep time. These children had significantly more attention problems than controls.[44] Collectively, these findings point to snoring as a key factor associated with development of inattentive behaviors and that increased severity of SDB is not associated with increased severity of inattention dysregulation.

In addition to standard inattention evaluations, event-related potential (ERP) recordings using a high-density array during an oddball attention task have also shown objective evidence of impaired attention in children with SDB.[51] Because ERP patterns strongly correlate with learning, reading, and school performance, the authors postulated that their findings suggested that brain changes associated with pediatric SDB have the potential to be used to determine which children might require earlier diagnosis or treatment. Nonetheless, some studies fail to observe differences in visual attention.[41,55] Emancipator and colleagues[56] proposed that the CPT might either not be sufficiently sensitive in children who are not obviously sleepy or possibly, with the increase in time children now spend playing video games, such CPT tools might be less discriminating. Indeed, while the CPT typically has excellent face validity (measuring the ability to sustain attention for an extended period of time), the psychometric validity is often low to moderate with wide heterogenicity in sensitivity and specificity between different tests.[57,58]

Aggressive Behaviors

In addition to hyperactivity and inattention, aggressive and bullying behaviors have also been associated with SDB. According to the Centers for Disease Control and Prevention (CDC), "… nearly 30% of American adolescents reported at least moderate bullying experiences as the bully, victim, or both."[59] Aggressive behaviors present a major challenge not only for schools, which often have local, state, and national programs to address this issue, but also for society, as aggressive children are at high risk for future psychiatric symptoms, such as depression, and delinquency, violence, substance abuse, criminality, and intimate partner violence.[60,61] Clearly, the causes of aggressive behaviors are complex and include social, biologic, and cultural factors; however, there is now emerging evidence that sleep problems might play a role.

In a large population-based study of over 3,000 5-year-old children, those with symptoms of SDB were twice as likely to have parentally reported aggressive behaviors,[40] which is similar to a study that also adjusted for comorbid hyperactivity and stimulant use.[62] A report specifically designed to query parents of aggressive elementary school children as well as nonaggressive controls about symptoms of SDB, found that aggressive children were twice as likely to have SDB symptoms compared with nonaggressive children.[27] Notably, daytime sleepiness rather than snoring appeared to drive the relationship with aggressive behavior, which suggests that other causes of daytime sleepiness, such as poor sleep hygiene, are also important. In children with objectively confirmed SDB, aggressive behaviors are more frequent than in children without SDB,[49] even when SDB is mild.[63] Individuals with aggressive behaviors also have electroencephalogram (EEG) slowing during wakefulness,[64,65] which might reflect deficient levels of arousal or excessive daytime sleepiness, likely mediated via the prefrontal cortex.[66]

Of note, short sleep duration, which perhaps might partially explain sleepiness, and sleep difficulties have been found to be associated with aggressive behaviors in young children[67,68] and adolescents.[69] In the latter study of seventh through ninth graders in Japan, nocturnal sleep duration was associated with bullying status, including being a victim and being bully-victim, particularly in junior high school students, as was irregular bedtimes.[69] Poor sleep is also a risk factor for suicidal ideation and suicide attempts in adolescents.[70,71]

Parent Versus Teacher Report of Behavior

There are conflicting findings on the association between SDB and behavior depending on whether behavioral reports are provided by parents or teachers. The literature regarding teacher reports is small compared with parental reports. Some studies report elevated hyperactive behaviors on both parent and teacher scales,[41,72] whereas others found only elevated hyperactive behaviors on parent scales.[22,27,44] Kohler and colleagues[73] have performed a direct comparison of parent and teacher reports in children with SDB. They found that both parents and teachers report more problematic behavior, which is predominantly internalizing such as anxious and withdrawn behavior, somatic complaints, and social and affective problems. In addition, parents reported a greater severity and range of behaviors. Overall, the concordance for individual children was poor. The limited number of studies that have collected teacher reports, the different tools used, and the sample sizes involved make it difficult to reach conclusions regarding classroom behavior. However, despite the inconsistencies, the teacher-report studies published to date appear to support a role for SDB in at least some areas of behavioral regulation.

Sleep-Disordered Breathing and Attention-Deficit/Hyperactivity Disorder

ADHD is the most commonly diagnosed pediatric mental health disorder in North America, and sleep problems are one of the most frequently reported comorbidities in these children. The major features of ADHD (e.g., inattention, hyperactivity, and impulsivity) are also frequent manifestations of childhood SDB and, conversely, comorbid sleep problems are highly prevalent in ADHD. Therefore it is unsurprising that the relationship between SDB and ADHD is of great interest. Children with habitual snoring are significantly more likely to have higher scores on ADHD scales compared with nonsnoring controls,[44,45,50,74] yet the severity of SDB as measured by PSG is inconsistent in its relationship with ADHD symptoms.[45,47,50,75] A meta-analysis, including children diagnosed with SDB who were examined for ADHD as well as children diagnosed with ADHD who were evaluated for SDB, found that there was an overall relationship between SDB and ADHD symptoms that improve with adenotonsillectomy.[76] Moreover, children with ADHD may exhibit symptoms of other sleep disorders, such as periodic limb movements, restless legs syndrome, delayed sleep phase syndrome, and initiation and maintenance insomnia as well as poor sleep hygiene and daytime sleepiness.[77–80]

Multiple studies have shown that children with ADHD demonstrate a number of parentally reported sleep problems,[79–82] with a frequency up to five times greater than that of otherwise healthy children.[83] Children with ADHD have been reported to snore more than their peers,[84–86] snoring possibly being more common in children with the hyperactive/impulsive subtype of ADHD.[87] However, polysomnographic data are less clear in terms of an association between PSG-defined SDB and ADHD.[88–90] One study in China reported that approximately 30% of children with OSA had ADHD; OSA symptom scores were higher in children with comorbid ADHD compared with OSA alone and a higher frequency of respiratory events, and more severe hypoxia was found in children with concomitant ADHD than in those with OSA alone.[91] However, other studies have found no relationship between ADHD and OSA.[88,90]

Methodologic issues may be at least in part related to such inconsistencies, particularly because the majority of studies did not use criteria from the *Diagnostic and Statistical Manual of Mental Disorders* (DSM) for ADHD; instead, they relied on parental report of hyperactivity symptoms. In one study of school-aged children that did use formal criteria, diagnoses of ADHD were found in almost a third of children.[92] However, a meta-analysis,[75] which included studies utilizing rigorous criteria for ADHD, suggested that the AHI in the three objective studies retained in the meta-analysis[93–95] were not very elevated (1.0, 5.8, and 3.57, respectively). Nonetheless, using a pediatric AHI threshold of 1,[96] these values suggest that SDB may indeed be more frequent in children with ADHD compared with controls. Interestingly, children with ADHD and an AHI between 1 and 5 have been reported to improve more following adenotonsillectomy than after stimulant treatment.[23,97,98] This raises questions about appropriate screening and intervention in these children and suggests that children presenting with behavioral difficulties should be evaluated for sleep problems and snoring prior to a diagnosis of ADHD[50,78] as both sleep regulation and ADHD likely share common neural correlates.[99]

Cognition

Studies of the associations between SDB and behavioral deficits are vast and demonstrate robust associations as described previously, but the cognitive impact of SDB is less well understood. Cognition is a mental act or process by which knowledge is acquired, including awareness, perception, intuition, and reasoning. It is often used interchangeably with intelligence; however, cognitive processes can be influenced by intelligence and generally show an age-dependent performance increase, whereas intelligence typically refers to developmental differences between individuals.[100] Lower-order cognitive processes, which include perceptual motor learning, visual short-term memory, and selective attention, can be measured by tasks such as reaction times or problem-solving. Intelligence, on the other hand, is indirectly inferred typically via psychometric testing. A detailed discussion of the associations between sleep, cognition, and intelligence has been published.[101]

One of the fundamental roles of sleep is believed to involve learning, memory consolidation, and brain plasticity;[102] thus sleep disruption has the potential to impair cognition while awake. Indeed, many studies, but not all, find some differences in cognition of children with and without SDB. Of note, however, the vast majority of studies in this area are from a limited age range, often elementary school age, thus limiting the conclusions that can be drawn. Moreover, in adolescents, Frye and colleagues have recently reported that central obesity, as measured by dual-energy X-ray absorptiometry, is more strongly associated with

neurocognitive and behavioral problems in adolescents than is SDB alone.[103] This finding is not completely captured with less precise measures of obesity and supports that SDB and its associated neurobehavioral morbidity are related to underlying metabolic dysfunction as early as adolescence.[103]

Intelligence

The intelligence quotient (IQ) is often reported in studies of SDB, although findings are not consistent. Lower IQ scores have been reported in children with SDB compared with controls, although in most studies (but not all),[104] these scores are typically still within the normal range.[17,40,53,63,104–108] One study of Australian children awaiting adenotonsillectomy found that compared with healthy nonsnoring children, the snoring children had a 10-point reduction in IQ.[109] Of course, the clinical significance of this remains to be shown for a high-functioning child, but a 10-point IQ difference could be rather significant in children performing at a lower level. Several studies fail to support findings of differences in full-scale IQ,[110–112] although some have found lower scores for verbal IQ (language skills) in children with SDB.[111,112] A systematic review of 13 studies found that although OSA may lower overall cognitive performance in children, in most cases it remains well within normal limits.[113]

Lack of robust findings between SDB and IQ is perhaps not surprising given that measurement of IQ is complex and, in essence, measures performance across several tasks rather than a focus on a particular area of cognition. Standardized vocabulary tests, as a proxy measure of IQ and an excellent predictor of cognition and academic success,[114] have demonstrated that the difference in scores between children with and without SDB may be equivalent to the impact of lead exposure.[115] These findings have the potential for great clinical significance. Nonetheless, there are many other factors that clearly impact a child's IQ that require consideration in studies of SDB, including genetics, parental education level, and biologic and environmental factors.[116]

Memory

Significantly lower performance on measures of memory have been reported in 5-year-old children with symptoms of SDB compared with asymptomatic children,[55] and assessment of working memory in children aged 8–12 years with OSA revealed that those with OSA had poorer performance on both tasks of basic storage and central executive components in the verbal domain of working memory compared with matched controls.[117] Data from PSG in the latter study also suggested that the AHI and oxygen saturation nadir were associated with verbal working memory performance. A study of memory recall in children with and without SDB[118] found that memory recall to a picture was impaired in children at an immediate memory assessment and as a follow-up assessment the following day. Notably, the children with SDB also demonstrated declines in recall performance, which suggests that children with SDB require more time and additional learning opportunities to reach immediate and longer-term recall performance and that these children may have slower information processing and/or secondary memory problems perhaps due to inefficient encoding.[119] Indeed, changes in basic perceptual processes that underlie higher-order functions have been shown to be impaired in pediatric SDB, even when performance is not altered on standard measures of memory.[120]

Nonetheless, there is little consistency between the severity of OSA and measures of memory in children. Although some studies do support a relationship with SDB and memory impairment,[53,106,121,122] multiple studies have failed to find evidence for memory impairment in children with SDB.[17,105,123] Inconsistencies in memory findings are likely related to the type of memory measured (such as verbal memory or working memory). Indeed, working memory has been found to correlate with intellectual function better than short-term memory, which is a component of working memory.[124] In addition, many reports provide only a cumulative memory score rather than address specific processes involved in memory acquisition. Of note, an Australian study of children aged 7–12 years with SDB reported that parents of children with less severe SDB tended to overestimate their child's deficits, possibly as a reflection of behavior, suggesting that observation of deficits in working memory may be largely dependent on the method of assessment, and that children with SDB may not be as impaired as previously believed.[125] A recent review suggested that there is currently "insufficient evidence of deficits in visual and verbal long-term memory, short-term or working memory storage, and working memory capacity in children with OSA."[113]

Academic Performance

Good academic performance is often essential for future career success and many studies have reported on deficits in academic performance in children with SDB. The term "academic performance" encompasses a range of achievements/abilities and it can be assessed by various means including mathematical abilities, spelling, reading, writing, and overall school grade. In a landmark study of first-grade children, Gozal[19] found a six- to ninefold increase in gas-exchange abnormalities in the lowest performing tenth percentile.

Several studies have reported lower grades in mathematics, spelling, reading, and science[22,126–130] in children and adolescents with SDB compared with controls, even when intermittent hypoxemia is absent,[129] which suggests that primary snoring may impact academic achievement. It is also possible that the presence of hypoxemia may affect the threshold of respiratory events associated with performance deficits, as the threshold for respiratory disturbances associated with learning problems may be lower in the presence of hypoxemia.[131] For example, in the absence of hypoxemia, a respiratory disturbance index >5 has been associated with parent reporting of learning problems in young children; however, when the presence of hypoxemia was used to define

the respiratory event, a respiratory disturbance index >1 was associated with learning problems.[131] A study of obese adolescents in New Zealand found that those with OSA performed significantly worse on math scores, but this association became nonsignificant when controlling for IQ, age, gender, and body mass index (BMI) Z-score.[130] Notably, IQ was the strongest predictor in this association, a covariate that most other studies do not account for. Children with SDB have also been found to perform lower than controls on a phonologic processing test,[105,132] which measures phonologic awareness, a skill that is critical for learning to read. In addition, processes that may underlie memory encoding and storage will also impact academic performance.[119,120]

We should also be reminded that the vast majority of current literature focuses on young school-aged children. A minority of studies include adolescents, a unique developmental stage where challenges differ considerably from young children and where any SDB-associated behavioral difficulties may result in significant impairment in school performance at a critical time for future success.[130,133] In addition to verbal problems, poor academic achievement may also be affected by inattention difficulties due to the complex brain associations involved. School problems may underscore more extensive behavioral disturbances, such as restlessness, aggressive behavior, excessive daytime sleepiness, and poor test performances.[124]

Measurement of school performance is inherently difficult, and the role of SDB difficult to tease out, as it really represents a number of factors, which include age, socioeconomic status (SES), home environment, genetics, behavior, and cognition.[22] Unsurprisingly, when some of the latter variables are accounted for, a number of studies fail to find evidence of an association between SDB and academic performance.[56,106,130,134,135]

Executive Functions

Executive function encompasses cognitive processes, including memory, planning, problem-solving, verbal reasoning, inhibition, mental flexibility, and multitasking, which are crucial for normal psychologic and social development. Executive function is complex and it is difficult to isolate certain executive functions from other cognitive abilities; despite this, executive dysfunction is often reported in children with SDB compared with controls.[13,41,104,112] A large community-based study of 5- to 7-year-old children that utilized PSGs classified children as nonsnoring controls (AHI <1), habitual snoring with AHI <1, habitual snoring with AHI 1–5, and habitual snoring with AHI >5. Results showed that executive skills differed across the groups, with a dose–response effect whereby those with AHI >5 were more impaired than the other groups, but only with the arrow subtest of executive measures.[108] In an age-matched group of 31 children aged 6–16 years, worse performance was observed in category fluency, but not letter fluency, problem-solving, planning, or inhibitory control in children with OSA compared with controls.[104] However, a study in snoring preschool children found substantially lower performance on executive function dimensions such as inhibition, working memory, and planning compared with controls.[136] Nonetheless, although many studies find some components of executive functions are worse in children with OSA versus those without, specific executive domains that appear to be particularly affected are not well defined.[113]

Causality

The vast majority of studies provide cross-sectional data on associations between SDB and learning and behavior. Although a proportion of children will have resolution of OSA during the transition to adolescence and young adulthood, and approximately one-third of primary snorers will develop OSA,[137] obesity is a significant risk factor for persistent OSA.[137,138] Indeed, obesity treatment in a group of adolescents with OSA demonstrated that a reduction in BMI was significantly associated with a decrease in AHI after 6 months.[139] Several longitudinal studies as well as treatment intervention trials now exist for children with SDB and these are described in the following paragraphs.

Longitudinal Evidence

The vast majority of published studies report cross-sectional findings, which while important, provide no information on the direction of the proposed relationships. Data from a case-control study of seventh- and eighth-grade children with poor school performance have demonstrated that these children were more likely than others in their grades to have snored frequently and loudly during their early childhood.[140] In a prospective 4-year follow-up study,[141] snoring and symptoms of SDB were strong risk factors for the future development or exacerbation of hyperactive behaviors, with habitual snoring at baseline increasing the risk for hyperactivity at follow-up by more than fourfold, especially in boys. Results were independent of hyperactivity at baseline and stimulant use as well as SDB symptoms at follow-up. A Canadian study of infants assessed quarterly from the age of 3 months until 2 years of age found that parent-reported symptoms of SDB were related to behavioral morbidity and that persistent SDB predicted the greatest magnitude of behavioral problems.[142] Moreover, although the trajectories of SDB phenotypes were important for internalizing but not for externalizing behaviors, there were no significant associations between home-PSG and parent-reported behavior problems.[142]

In support of these findings, a study from the Avon Longitudinal Study of Parents and Children[143] examined the effects of snoring, apnea, and mouth-breathing patterns on behavior, from infancy through 7 years in more than 11,000 children. By 4 years, symptomatic children were 20–60% more likely to exhibit behavioral difficulties consistent with a clinical diagnosis; by 7 years, they were 40–100% more likely, even after controlling for 15 major confounders.[14] Furthermore, SDB effects at 4 years were as predictive of behavioral difficulties at 7 years, and the worst symptoms were associated with the worst behavioral outcomes, with hyperactivity being most affected. Together, these findings suggest that damage done years earlier may be visible as a behavioral phenotype only years later and alludes to the belief that there may be a "window of vulnerability" in developing humans.

Treatment Interventions

In the past decade, there have been a number of treatment intervention studies. Adenotonsillectomy is typically the first-line therapy in children and residual OSA is believed to occur in up to 13–29% of low-risk children and up to 75% in higher-risk groups, for example, in obese individuals.[144] In one of the first intervention studies, first-grade children in the lowest tenth percentile were screened for SDB and parents were advised to seek treatment if their child had gas-exchange abnormalities.[19] Children's school grades were obtained in first grade and also during follow-up in second grade; children who had evidence of SDB and had received treatment had significantly improved school grades, whereas those who had declined treatment did not have significant improvement. The same group[140] showed that middle-school children with academic performance in the lowest 25% of their class were more likely to have snored during their preschool years and to have required adenotonsillectomy for snoring compared with schoolmates in the top 25% of class.

In a prospective 1-year follow-up of neurobehavioral outcomes in 5- to 12-year-old children with OSA, Chervin and colleagues[92] found that those who had adenotonsillectomy were more hyperactive and more likely to have ADHD, as diagnosed by a child psychiatrist, at baseline compared with controls. By 1 year postintervention there were no differences between groups and children who underwent adenotonsillectomy had substantial improvement in all measures (control children did not improve in any measure). Notably, 28% of children scheduled for adenotonsillectomy had ADHD at baseline, compared with 7% of controls, and at the 1-year follow-up, 50% no longer met the criteria for an ADHD diagnosis. No improvement was seen with the control children. Moreover, PSG variables did not predict neurobehavioral improvement, only sleepiness.[92]

In subsequent studies of children with adenotonsillar hypertrophy and ADHD identified by parental questionnaire, adenotonsillectomy has considerably reduced ADHD symptoms (hyperactive, inattentive, and impulsive behaviors) with more significant reductions occurring 3–6 months postsurgery.[145–149] Collectively, these findings suggest that children with ADHD who also have enlarged tonsils and adenoids may gain significant clinical improvement in ADHD symptoms from adenotonsillectomy and that greater improvement may occur in children with mild SDB compared with children prescribed methylphenidate.[97] Indeed, Huang and colleagues[97] postulated that recognition and surgical treatment of underlying mild SDB in children with ADHD may prevent unnecessary long-term methyl-phenidate use and the associated potential side effects. The first randomized controlled trial that was designed to evaluate the efficacy of early adenotonsillectomy (versus watchful waiting with supportive care) on neurobehavioral measures in 5- to 9-year-old children with OSA was published in 2013 (the Childhood Adenotonsillectomy Trial [CHAT]).[150] Although adenotonsillectomy did not significantly improve attention or executive function, it did reduce symptoms and improve behavior. A secondary analysis of this cohort revealed that selective attention improved in the intervention group[151] and the post randomization changes in most behavioral outcome measures between baseline and follow-up assessments were partially mediated by the changes in the parentally reported symptom scores, without contribution from any of the polysomnographic variables.[152]

Cognitive function appears to improve at follow-up, approximately 6–12 months later for executive function,[153,154] multiple subtests including general conceptual ability, verbal and nonverbal ability, phonologic processing and naming,[153–155] IQ,[154,156] attention, as measured by continuous performance assessment,[72,92] visual attention and processing speed,[157] matrix analogies, sequential and simultaneous processing scales, and mental processing scales,[158] with medium to large effect sizes.[158] However, not all studies report significant improvement in cognitive measures following treatment.[54,159] An Australian study showed a wide range of cognitive deficits in 3- to 12-year-old children at baseline, including IQ, language, and executive function, which did not improve to control levels following adenotonsillectomy.[109] The magnitude of the deficits persisted at the 6-month follow-up with a mean full-scale IQ difference of 10 points between children with SDB and controls. Of particular note, the fluid reasoning, knowledge, quantitative reasoning, visuospatial and working memory composite scores, and corresponding verbal and nonverbal subtest scores were all significantly reduced in children with SDB compared with controls at both baseline and follow-up. In addition, composite scores for attention/executive function (specifically planning, inhibition, auditory and visual attention), language (phonologic processing), and sensorimotor function and memory (especially narrative memory) were significantly reduced in children with SDB at both baseline and follow-up. The finding that measures of executive function remain significantly lower in children with SDB following adenotonsillectomy is supported by another study,[157] although mean postoperative scores in the latter study were lower than preoperative scores.

Many prior studies were limited by small sample sizes, nonrandomized design, or lack of controls. Nonetheless, the large randomized controlled CHAT trial[150] observed no significant difference between either the early adenotonsillectomy or watchful waiting groups in the change from baseline to follow-up in attention or executive function. However, in almost half of the children in the watchful waiting group the PSG parameters normalized by 7 months, which suggests that many children may improve without therapy.[160]

These findings were supported by a subsequent study of children aged 3–13 years with OSA where cognitive and behavioral disturbances were partially resolved 1 year following adenotonsillectomy.[161] However, improvements in the cognitive and behavioral variables did not significantly differ from normal development, and were independent of the resolution of respiratory disorders.[161] Most studies have focused on school-aged children. The Preschool Obstructive Sleep Apnea Tonsillectomy and Adenoidectomy (POSTA) study[162] was undertaken in Australian preschool children (3–5 years old) with the goal of evaluating whether adenotonsillectomy improved intellectual function after (early) adenotonsillectomy.[163] In this randomized controlled trial of 141 young children, evaluations at 12 months post adenotonsillectomy demonstrated that although global IQ scores improved over time for both groups, no change in global IQ was attributable to the intervention (adenotonsillectomy). Similar to the CHAT trial,[150] however, the POSTA trial[163] did show improvement in sleep variables as well as behavioral measures. Nonetheless, in another recent study from Australia of 3-to 12-year-olds undergoing adenotonsillectomy, compared with controls the surgical group did not demonstrate any improvements in behavior at either 6 months or 48 months postsurgery, despite showing improvements in sleep parameters and quality of life by 6 months, which were maintained at 48 months.[164]

Lack of improvement post adenotonsillectomy may be somewhat unexpected. However, it should be noted that children undergoing adenotonsillectomy for non-SDB and SDB reasons perform worse on specific cognitive measures such as short-term attention, visuospatial ability, memory, and arithmetic academic achievement compared with control children.[165] Interestingly, children without SDB may have more consistent and larger deficits compared with those with SDB.[166] At 12-month follow-up in the study by Giordani and colleagues,[166] measures of verbal abstraction ability, arithmetic calculations, visual and verbal learning, verbal delayed recall, sustained attention, and another measure of visual delayed recall demonstrated declines in ability, and measures of executive function and academic performance improved, whereas other measures did not improve over time.[166] The authors suggested that their findings question the expectation that adenotonsillectomy resolves the majority of deficits in children with SDB, which has the potential to translate into a significant lifetime impact later in life.

Despite some of the persuasive arguments noted previously, it should be noted that there are some arguments against a causal relationship between SDB and neurobehavior. Importantly, there is no consistent phenotype, there is a lack of expected relationships as well as dose–response across studies, and the response to treatment is not entirely clear. In addition, there is added complexity that arises from the developmental context in which these studies are conducted, as compensatory mechanisms to an insult may occur in these children. Nonetheless, there may be an argument for treatment initiation for children with mild

SDB particularly because core aspects of executive development appear vulnerable, which may contribute to progressive delays in achievement and educational morbidity.[108] Moreover, a recent study in Australian preschool children has shown that regardless of whether children had primary snoring or OSA diagnosed by PSG, the symptoms, behavior, and cognition are the same in these groups.[20] These authors concluded that symptoms and behavioral disturbances should be considered in addition to PSG findings when determining the need for treatment.

Studies of positive airway pressure (PAP) therapy are limited in children with regards to neurobehavioral outcomes and have inconsistent findings. Some PAP studies have demonstrated improvements in attention and behavior,[167] as well as memory and motor speed,[168] but not in other measures of neurobehavior. In a study of obese adolescents nonadherent participants showed worsening neurobehavioral functioning over time, whereas PAP users showed stable or improved functioning, similar to controls.[169] Obesity is present in a large proportion of children with OSA and these individuals often have persistent OSA after treatment.[170] Alternative approaches have been suggested including drug-induced sleep endoscopy (DISE), which allows direct visualization of the upper airway obstruction and can provide diagnostic information about an individual's unique disease phenotype.[171] Indeed, DISE has been reported to identify alternate site of collapse and to change management in 24–35% of children[172,173] with a high (91%) success rate of OSA resolution.[172] This therapy could ultimately be used to personalize therapy and improve outcomes of pediatric OSA.[174]

Potential Mechanisms

The most plausible mechanisms of behavioral and cognitive deficits in children with SDB include intermittent hypoxia and sleep fragmentation, the two main components of SDB that likely impact the prefrontal cortex. The importance of executive dysfunction and the involvement of the prefrontal cortex in SDB have been reviewed[175] and a model linking sleep disruption, hypoxemia, and disruption of the prefrontal cortex was proposed. The prefrontal cortex is believed to play a critical role in the regulation of arousal, sleep, affect, and attention in children.[176] Indeed, disturbances of prefrontal inhibitory functions have been implicated in deficits observed in children with ADHD,[177] and neuroimaging studies in ADHD have supported specific impairments in prefrontal cortical functioning.[178,179]

Hypoxemia even in the absence of SDB is known to impact cognition.[180] Animal models demonstrate that intermittent hypoxia during sleep induces neuronal cell loss and impairs spatial memory[181–183] and that early development might be a particularly vulnerable time.[184] Interestingly,

data from a brain imaging study have shown that neuronal metabolites are altered in children with SDB in the hippocampal and right frontal cortical regions,[104] the very areas that are implicated in executive function and cognition.

Similarly, sleep fragmentation or deprivation does not only affect those with SDB; such disruption in the absence of SDB has also been shown to impact behavior and cognition.[185–191] Indeed, children with daytime sleepiness have been shown to have significantly more hyperactivity, inattention, and conduct problems as well as worse measures of processing speed and working memory.[192] In addition, aggressive elementary school children have been reported to be more likely to have daytime sleepiness than their peers.[27]

Chronic intermittent hypoxia and sleep fragmentation as observed in SDB result in large amounts of reactive oxygen species production, which induce excessive activation of oxidative stress responses, including lipid peroxidation, protein oxidation, and DNA oxidation, which may then result in dysfunction of the mitochondria, endoplasmic reticulum, and endothelial cells, along with massive inflammatory responses[193–197] with resultant chronic damage of neuronal cells. The cerebral cortex and hippocampus are particularly vulnerable to such insults and neurobehavioral dysfunction is likely the end result.[194] Neuroimaging techniques have shown that children with moderate to severe OSA have extensive cortical gray matter volume reductions in areas that control cognition[198] and reduced neuronal metabolites in the hippocampi.[104] Changes in cortical thickness are also present in children with OSA and likely indicate disrupted neural developmental processes.[199] Regions with thicker cortices may reflect inflammation or astrocyte activation and both the thinning and thickening may contribute to the cognitive and behavioral dysfunction frequently observed in pediatric OSA.[199]

CLINICAL PEARLS

- Habitual snoring and obstructive sleep apnea are common in children and associated with neurobehavioral morbidity.
- Insults may manifest years later, suggestive of a window of vulnerability in developing children.
- However, there is no consistent phenotype and no dose–response relationships; indeed, mild sleep-disordered breathing is often associated with poor outcomes.
- Polysomnographic findings alone may not be sufficient for identifying children in need of treatment; symptoms and behavioral disturbances should also be considered.
- Treatment interventions such as adenotonsillectomy appear to improve behavioral morbidities but not cognitive abilities.

Summary

There is now a wealth of robust data that support a role for SDB in behavioral deficits, particularly mild SDB, in children, as well as less consistent evidence to support its role in cognitive deficits. Current data are mixed with regards to the reversibility of such dysfunction with treatment, perhaps due to brain plasticity or genetic/environmental interactions. In the randomized controlled trials of adenotonsillectomy, while treatment normalized polysomnographic measures in most children, a proportion of children in the control groups also demonstrated normalization of sleep measures. Nonetheless, behavior scores appear to improve following intervention although there is currently no clear evidence that cognition improves with adenotonsillectomy. Obese children are at particularly high risk of residual OSA posttreatment, which raises the question of alternative, personalized approaches that have now begun to be investigated.

References

1. Lumeng JC, Chervin RD. Epidemiology of pediatric obstructive sleep apnea. *Proc Am Thorac Soc.* 2008;5(2):242–252.
2. Alsubie HS, BaHammam AS Obstructive sleep apnoea: Children are not little adults. *Paediatr Respir Rev.* 2017;21:72–79.
3. McKenzie M. *A Manual of Diseases of the Throat and Nose, Including the Pharynx, Larynx, Trachea Oesophagus. Nasal Cavities, and Neck.* Churchill; 1880.
4. Guilleminault C, Eldridge FL, Simmons FB, Dement WC. Sleep apnea in eight children. *Pediatrics.* 1976;58(1):23–30.
5. Rosen CL, D'Andrea L, Haddad GG. Adult criteria for obstructive sleep apnea do not identify children with serious obstruction. *Am Rev Respir Dis.* 1992;146(5 Pt 1):1231–1234.
6. Lo Bue A, Salvaggio A, Insalaco G. Obstructive sleep apnea in developmental age. A narrative review. *Eur J Pediatr.* 2020;179(3):357–365.
7. Carroll JL, Loughlin GM. Diagnostic criteria for obstructive sleep apnea syndrome in children. *Pediatr Pulmonol.* 1992;14(2):71–74.
8. Kaditis A, Kheirandish-Gozal L, Gozal D. Algorithm for the diagnosis and treatment of pediatric OSA: A proposal of two pediatric sleep centers. *Sleep Med.* 2012;13(3):217–227.
9. ElMallah M, Bailey E, Trivedi M, Kremer T, Rhein LM. Pediatric obstructive sleep apnea in high-risk populations: Clinical implications. *Pediatr Ann.* 2017;46(9):e336–e339.
10. Remmers JE, deGroot WJ, Sauerland EK, Anch AM. Pathogenesis of upper airway occlusion during sleep. *J Appl Physiol Respir Environ Exerc Physiol.* 1978;44(6):931–938.
11. Carroll JL, McColley SA, Marcus CL, Curtis S, Loughlin GM. Inability of clinical history to distinguish primary snoring from obstructive sleep apnea syndrome in children. *Chest.* 1995;108(3):610–618.
12. Brietzke SE, Katz ES, Roberson DW. Can history and physical examination reliably diagnose pediatric obstructive sleep apnea/ hypopnea syndrome? A systematic review of the literature. *Otolaryngol Head Neck Surg.* 2004;131(6):827–832.
13. Archbold KH, Giordani B, Ruzicka DL, Chervin RD. Cognitive executive dysfunction in children with mild sleep-disordered breathing. *Biol Res Nurs.* 2004;5(3):168–176.
14. Bonuck K, Freeman K, Chervin RD, Xu L. Sleep-disordered breathing in a population-based cohort: Behavioral outcomes at 4 and 7 years. *Pediatrics.* 2012;129(4):e857–e865.
15. Chervin RD, Archbold KH. Hyperactivity and polysomnographic findings in children evaluated for sleep-disordered breathing. *Sleep.* 2001;24(3):313–320.
16. Chervin RD, Archbold KH, Dillon JE, et al. Inattention, hyperactivity, and symptoms of sleep-disordered breathing. *Pediatrics.* 2002;109(3):449–456.
17. O'Brien LM, Mervis CB, Holbrook CR, et al. Neurobehavioral implications of habitual snoring in children. *Pediatrics.* 2004;114(1):44–49.
18. Spruyt K, O'Brien LM, Macmillan Coxon AP, Cluydts R, Verleye G, Ferri R. Multidimensional scaling of pediatric sleep breathing problems and bio-behavioral correlates. *Sleep Med.* 2006;7(3):269–280.
19. Gozal D. Sleep-disordered breathing and school performance in children. *Pediatrics.* 1998;102(3 Pt 1):616–620.
20. Chawla J, Harris MA, Black R, et al. Cognitive parameters in children with mild obstructive sleep disordered breathing. *Sleep Breath.* 2021;25(3):1625–1634.
21. Owens JA. Neurocognitive and behavioral impact of sleep disordered breathing in children. *Pediatr Pulmonol.* 2009;44(5):417–422.
22. Beebe DW, Ris MD, Kramer ME, Long E, Amin R. The association between sleep disordered breathing, academic grades, and cognitive and behavioral functioning among overweight subjects during middle to late childhood. *Sleep.* 2010;33(11):1447–1456.
23. Dillon JE, Blunden S, Ruzicka DL, et al. DSM-IV diagnoses and obstructive sleep apnea in children before and 1 year after adenotonsillectomy. *J Am Acad Child Adolesc Psychiatry.* 2007;46(11):1425–1436.
24. Park KM, Kim SY, Sung D, et al. The relationship between risk of obstructive sleep apnea and other sleep problems, depression, and anxiety in adolescents from a community sample. *Psychiatry Res.* 2019;280:112504.
25. Tseng WC, Liang YC, Su MH, Chen YL, Yang HJ, Kuo PH. Sleep apnea may be associated with suicidal ideation in adolescents. *Eur Child Adolesc Psychiatry.* 2019;28(5):635–643.
26. Yilmaz E, Sedky K, Bennett DS. The relationship between depressive symptoms and obstructive sleep apnea in pediatric populations: A meta-analysis. *J Clin Sleep Med.* 2013;9(11):1213–1220.
27. O'Brien LM, Lucas NH, Felt BT, et al. Aggressive behavior, bullying, snoring, and sleepiness in schoolchildren. *Sleep Med.* 2011;12(7):652–658.
28. O'Brien LM, Gozal D. Autonomic dysfunction in children with sleep-disordered breathing. *Sleep.* 2005;28(6):747–752.
29. Nisbet LC, Yiallourou SR, Nixon GM, et al. Nocturnal autonomic function in preschool children with sleep-disordered breathing. *Sleep Med.* 2013;14(12):1310–1316.

30. Nisbet LC, Yiallourou SR, Walter LM, Horne RS. Blood pressure regulation, autonomic control and sleep disordered breathing in children. *Sleep Med Rev.* 2014;18(2):179–189.

31. Chaidas K, Tsaoussoglou M, Theodorou E, Lianou L, Chrousos G, Kaditis AG. Poincaré plot width, morning urine norepinephrine levels, and autonomic imbalance in children with obstructive sleep apnea. *Pediatr Neurol.* 2014;51(2):246–251.

32. Hakim F, Gozal D, Kheirandish-Gozal L. Sympathetic and catecholaminergic alterations in sleep apnea with particular emphasis on children. *Front Neurol.* 2012;3:7.

33. Zhang F, Wu Y, Feng G, Ni X, Xu Z, Gozal D. Polysomnographic correlates of endothelial function in children with obstructive sleep apnea. *Sleep Med.* 2018;52:45–50.

34. Horne RS, Yang JS, Walter LM, et al. Elevated blood pressure during sleep and wake in children with sleep-disordered breathing. *Pediatrics.* 2011;128(1):e85–e92.

35. Bixler EO, Vgontzas AN, Lin HM, et al. Blood pressure associated with sleep-disordered breathing in a population sample of children. *Hypertension.* 2008;52(5):841–846.

36. Hinkle J, Connolly HV, Adams HR, Lande MB. Severe obstructive sleep apnea in children with elevated blood pressure. *J Am Soc Hypertens.* 2018;12(3):204–210.

37. Brooks DM, Kelly A, Sorkin JD, et al. The relationship between sleep-disordered breathing, blood pressure, and urinary cortisol and catecholamines in children. *J Clin Sleep Med.* 2020;16(6):907–916.

38. Gallucci M, Gessaroli M, Bronzetti G, et al. Cardiovascular issues in obstructive sleep apnoea in children: A brief review. *Paediatr Respir Rev.* 2020

39. Hui W, Slorach C, Guerra V, et al. Effect of Obstructive sleep apnea on cardiovascular function in obese youth. *Am J Cardiol.* 2019;123(2):341–347.

40. Gottlieb DJ, Vezina RM, Chase C, et al. Symptoms of sleep-disordered breathing in 5-year-old children are associated with sleepiness and problem behaviors. *Pediatrics.* 2003;112(4):870–877.

41. Beebe DW, Wells CT, Jeffries J, Chini B, Kalra M, Amin R. Neuropsychological effects of pediatric obstructive sleep apnea. *J Int Neuropsychol Soc.* 2004;10(7):962–975.

42. Rosen CL, Storfer-Isser A, Taylor HG, Kirchner HL, Emancipator JL, Redline S. Increased behavioral morbidity in school-aged children with sleep-disordered breathing. *Pediatrics.* 2004;114(6):1640–1648.

43. Urschitz MS, Eitner S, Guenther A, et al. Habitual snoring, intermittent hypoxia, and impaired behavior in primary school children. *Pediatrics.* 2004;114(4):1041–1048.

44. Hagstrom K, Saarenpaa-Heikkila O, Himanen SL, Lampinlampi AM, Rantanen K. Neurobehavioral Outcomes in School-Aged Children with Primary Snoring. *Arch Clin Neuropsychol.* 2020;35(4):401–412.

45. Smith DL, Gozal D, Hunter SJ, Kheirandish-Gozal L. Frequency of snoring, rather than apnea-hypopnea index, predicts both cognitive and behavioral problems in young children. *Sleep Med.* 2017;34:170–178.

46. Bourke RS, Anderson V, Yang JS, et al. Neurobehavioral function is impaired in children with all severities of sleep disordered breathing. *Sleep Med.* 2011;12(3):222–229.

47. Zhao Q, Sherrill DL, Goodwin JL, Quan SF. Association Between Sleep Disordered Breathing and Behavior in School-Aged Children: The Tucson Children's Assessment of Sleep Apnea Study. *Open Epidemiol J.* 2008;1:1–9.

48. Jackman AR, Biggs SN, Walter LM, et al. Sleep-disordered breathing in preschool children is associated with behavioral, but not cognitive, impairments. *Sleep Med.* 2012;13(6):621–631.

49. Mulvaney SA, Goodwin JL, Morgan WJ, Rosen GR, Quan SF, Kaemingk KL. Behavior problems associated with sleep disordered breathing in school-aged children–the Tucson children's assessment of sleep apnea study. *J Pediatr Psychol.* 2006;31(3):322–330.

50. Smith DL, Gozal D, Hunter SJ, Philby MF, Kaylegian J, Kheirandish-Gozal L. Impact of sleep disordered breathing on behaviour among elementary school-aged children: A cross-sectional analysis of a large community-based sample. *Eur Respir J.* 2016;48(6):1631–1639.

51. Barnes ME, Gozal D, Molfese DL. Attention in children with obstructive sleep apnoea: An event-related potentials study. *Sleep Med.* 2012;13(4):368–377.

52. Blunden S, Lushington K, Kennedy D, Martin J, Dawson D. Behavior and neurocognitive performance in children aged 5–10 years who snore compared to controls. *J Clin Exp Neuropsychol.* 2000;22(5):554–568.

53. Kennedy JD, Blunden S, Hirte C, et al. Reduced neurocognition in children who snore. *Pediatr Pulmonol.* 2004;37(4):330–337.

54. Galland BC, Dawes PJ, Tripp EG, Taylor BJ. Changes in behavior and attentional capacity after adenotonsillectomy. *Pediatr Res.* 2006;59(5):711–716.

55. Gottlieb DJ, Chase C, Vezina RM, et al. Sleep-disordered breathing symptoms are associated with poorer cognitive function in 5-year-old children. *J Pediatr.* 2004;145(4):458–464.

56. Emancipator JL, Storfer-Isser A, Taylor HG, et al. Variation of cognition and achievement with sleep-disordered breathing in full-term and preterm children. *Arch Pediatr Adolesc Med.* 2006;160(2):203–210.

57. Berger I, Slobodin O, Cassuto H. Usefulness and Validity of continuous performance tests in the diagnosis of attention-deficit hyperactivity disorder children. *Arch Clin Neuropsychol.* 2017;32(1):81–93.

58. Pan XX, Ma HW, Dai XM. [Value of integrated visual and auditory continuous performance test in the diagnosis of childhood attention deficit hyperactivity disorder]. *Zhongguo Dang Dai Er Ke Za Zhi.* 2007;9(3):210–212.

59. Hamburger M.E., Basile K.C., Vivolo A.M. Measuring Bullying, Victimization, Perpetration, and Bystander Experiences: A Compendium of Assessment Tools. Centers for Disease Control and Prevention;2011.

60. Kumpulainen K, Rasanen E. Children involved in bullying at elementary school age: Their psychiatric symptoms and deviance in adolescence. An epidemiological sample. *Child Abuse Negl.* 2000;24(12):1567–1577.

61. Ttofi MM, Farrington DP. Risk and protective factors, longitudinal research, and bullying prevention. *New Dir Youth Dev.* 2012;2012(133):85–98.

62. Chervin RD, Dillon JE, Archbold KH, Ruzicka DL. Conduct problems and symptoms of sleep disorders in children. *J Am Acad Child Adolesc Psychiatry.* 2003;42(2):201–208.

63. Bourke R, Anderson V, Yang JS, et al. Cognitive and academic functions are impaired in children with all severities of sleep-disordered breathing. *Sleep Med.* 2011;12(5):489–496.

64. Forssman H, Frey TS. Electroencephalograms of boys with behavior disorders. *Acta Psychiatr Neurol Scand.* 1953;28(1):61–73.

65. Konicar L, Radev S, Silvoni S, et al. Balancing the brain of offenders with psychopathy? Resting state EEG and

electrodermal activity after a pilot study of brain self-regulation training. *PLoS One.* 2021;16(1):e0242830.

66. Thomas M, Sing H, Belenky G, et al. Neural basis of alertness and cognitive performance impairments during sleepiness. I. Effects of 24 h of sleep deprivation on waking human regional brain activity. *J Sleep Res.* 2000;9(4):335–352.

67. Komada Y, Abe T, Okajima I, et al. Short sleep duration and irregular bedtime are associated with increased behavioral problems among Japanese preschool-age children. *Tohoku J Exp Med.* 2011;224(2):127–136.

68. Ivanenko A, Crabtree VM, Obrien LM, Gozal D. Sleep complaints and psychiatric symptoms in children evaluated at a pediatric mental health clinic. *J Clin Sleep Med.* 2006;2(1):42–48.

69. Tochigi M, Nishida A, Shimodera S, et al. Irregular bedtime and nocturnal cellular phone usage as risk factors for being involved in bullying: A cross-sectional survey of Japanese adolescents. *PLoS One.* 2012;7(9):e45736.

70. Bernert RA, Hom MA, Iwata NG, Joiner TE. Objectively assessed sleep variability as an acute warning sign of suicidal ideation in a longitudinal evaluation of young adults at high suicide risk. *J Clin Psychiatry.* 2017;78(6):e678–e687.

71. Mars B, Heron J, Klonsky ED, et al. Predictors of future suicide attempt among adolescents with suicidal thoughts or non-suicidal self-harm: A population-based birth cohort study. *Lancet Psychiatry.* 2019;6(4):327–337.

72. Landau YE, Bar-Yishay O, Greenberg-Dotan S, Goldbart AD, Tarasiuk A, Tal A. Impaired behavioral and neurocognitive function in preschool children with obstructive sleep apnea. *Pediatr Pulmonol.* 2012;47(2):180–188.

73. Kohler MJ, Kennedy JD, Martin AJ, Lushington K. Parent versus teacher report of daytime behavior in snoring children. *Sleep Breath.* 2013;17(2):637–645.

74. Kim KM, Kim JH, Kim D, et al. Associations among high risk for sleep-disordered breathing, related risk factors, and attention deficit/hyperactivity symptoms in elementary school children. *Clin Psychopharmacol Neurosci.* 2020;18(4):553–561.

75. Cortese S, Faraone SV, Konofal E, Lecendreux M. Sleep in children with attention-deficit/hyperactivity disorder: Meta-analysis of subjective and objective studies. *J Am Acad Child Adolesc Psychiatry.* 2009;48(9):894–908.

76. Sedky K, Bennett DS, Carvalho KS. Attention deficit hyperactivity disorder and sleep disordered breathing in pediatric populations: A meta-analysis. *Sleep Med Rev.* 2014;18(4):349–356.

77. Gruber R, Xi T, Frenette S, Robert M, Vannasinh P, Carrier J. Sleep disturbances in prepubertal children with attention deficit hyperactivity disorder: A home polysomnography study. *Sleep.* 2009;32(3):343–350.

78. Wajszilber D, Santiseban JA, Gruber R. Sleep disorders in patients with ADHD: Impact and management challenges. *Nat Sci Sleep.* 2018;10:453–480.

79. Miano S, Amato N, Foderaro G, et al. Sleep phenotypes in attention deficit hyperactivity disorder. *Sleep Med.* 2019;60:123–131.

80. Martins R, Scalco JC, Ferrari Junior GJ, Gerente J, Costa MDL, Beltrame TS. Sleep disturbance in children with attention-deficit hyperactivity disorder: A systematic review. *Sleep Sci.* 2019;12(4):295–301.

81. Frye SS, Fernandez-Mendoza J, Calhoun SL, Vgontzas AN, Liao D, Bixler EO. Neurocognitive and behavioral significance of periodic limb movements during sleep in adolescents with attention-deficit/hyperactivity disorder. *Sleep.* 2018;41(10):zsy129.

82. Becker SP, Langberg JM, Eadeh HM, Isaacson PA, Bourchtein E. Sleep and daytime sleepiness in adolescents with and without ADHD: Differences across ratings, daily diary, and actigraphy. *J Child Psychol Psychiatry.* 2019;60(9):1021–1031.

83. Owens JA, Maxim R, Nobile C, McGuinn M, Msall M. Parental and self-report of sleep in children with attention-deficit/hyperactivity disorder. *Arch Pediatr Adolesc Med.* 2000;154(6):549–555.

84. Chin WC, Huang YS, Chou YH, et al. Subjective and objective assessments of sleep problems in children with attention deficit/hyperactivity disorder and the effects of methylphenidate treatment. *Biomed J.* 2018;41(6):356–363.

85. O'Brien LM, Holbrook CR, Mervis CB, et al. Sleep and neurobehavioral characteristics of 5- to 7-year-old children with parentally reported symptoms of attention-deficit/hyperactivity disorder. *Pediatrics.* 2003;111(3):554–563.

86. Liu X, Liu ZZ, Liu BP, Sun SH, Jia CX. Associations between sleep problems and ADHD symptoms among adolescents: Findings from the Shandong Adolescent Behavior and Health Cohort (SABHC). *Sleep.* 2020;43(6):zsz294.

87. LeBourgeois MK, Avis K, Mixon M, Olmi J, Harsh J. Snoring, sleep quality, and sleepiness across attention-deficit/hyperactivity disorder subtypes. *Sleep.* 2004;27(3):520–525.

88. Choi J, Yoon IY, Kim HW, Chung S, Yoo HJ. Differences between objective and subjective sleep measures in children with attention deficit hyperactivity disorder. *J Clin Sleep Med.* 2010;6(6):589–595.

89. Sadeh A, Pergamin L, Bar-Haim Y. Sleep in children with attention-deficit hyperactivity disorder: A meta-analysis of polysomnographic studies. *Sleep Med Rev.* 2006;10(6):381–398.

90. Accardo JA, Marcus CL, Leonard MB, Shults J, Meltzer LJ, Elia J. Associations between psychiatric comorbidities and sleep disturbances in children with attention-deficit/hyperactivity disorder. *J Dev Behav Pediatr.* 2012;33(2):97–105.

91. Wu J, Gu M, Chen S, et al. Factors related to pediatric obstructive sleep apnea-hypopnea syndrome in children with attention deficit hyperactivity disorder in different age groups. *Medicine (Baltimore).* 2017;96(42):e8281.

92. Chervin RD, Ruzicka DL, Giordani BJ, et al. Sleep-disordered breathing, behavior, and cognition in children before and after adenotonsillectomy. *Pediatrics.* 2006;117(4):e769–e778.

93. Huang YS, Chen NH, Li HY, Wu YY, Chao CC, Guilleminault C. Sleep disorders in Taiwanese children with attention deficit/hyperactivity disorder. *J Sleep Res.* 2004;13(3):269–277.

94. Cooper J, Tyler L, Wallace I, Burgess KR. No evidence of sleep apnea in children with attention deficit hyperactivity disorder. *Clin Pediatr (Phila).* 2004;43(7):609–614.

95. Golan N, Pillar G. [The relationship between attention deficit hyperactivity disorder and sleep-alertness problems]. *Harefuah.* 2004;143(9):676–680. 693.

96. Chervin RD. How many children with ADHD have sleep apnea or periodic leg movements on polysomnography? *Sleep.* 2005;28(9):1041–1042.

97. Huang YS, Guilleminault C, Li HY, Yang CM, Wu YY, Chen NH. Attention-deficit/hyperactivity disorder with obstructive sleep apnea: A treatment outcome study. *Sleep Med.* 2007;8(1):18–30.

98. Fallah R, Arabi Mianroodi A, Eslami M, Khanjani N. Does Adenotonsillectomy alter symptoms of attention deficit hyperactivity disorder in children? *Iran J Otorhinolaryngol.* 2020;32(113):359–364.

99. Shen C, Luo Q, Chamberlain SR, et al. What is the link between attention-deficit/hyperactivity disorder and sleep

disturbance? A multimodal examination of longitudinal relationships and brain structure using large-scale population-based cohorts. *Biol Psychiatry*. 2020;88(6):459–469.

100. Anderson M. *Marrying Intelligence and Cognition – A Developmental View*. Cambridge University Press; 2005.

101. Geiger A, Achermann P, Jenni OG. Sleep, intelligence and cognition in a developmental context: Differentiation between traits and state-dependent aspects. *Prog Brain Res*. 2010;185:167–179.

102. Walker MP. The role of sleep in cognition and emotion. *Ann NY Acad Sci*. 2009;1156:168–197.

103. Frye SS, Fernandez-Mendoza J, Calhoun SL, et al. Neurocognitive and behavioral functioning in adolescents with sleep-disordered breathing: A population-based, dual-energy X-ray absorptiometry study. *Int J Obes (Lond)*. 2018;42(1):95–101.

104. Halbower AC, Degaonkar M, Barker PB, et al. Childhood obstructive sleep apnea associates with neuropsychological deficits and neuronal brain injury. *PLoS Med*. 2006;3(8):e301.

105. O'Brien LM, Mervis CB, Holbrook CR, et al. Neurobehavioral correlates of sleep-disordered breathing in children. *J Sleep Res*. 2004;13(2):165–172.

106. Kaemingk KL, Pasvogel AE, Goodwin JL, et al. Learning in children and sleep disordered breathing: Findings of the Tucson Children's Assessment of Sleep Apnea (tuCASA) prospective cohort study. *J Int Neuropsychol Soc*. 2003;9(7):1016–1026.

107. Miano S, Paolino MC, Urbano A, et al. Neurocognitive assessment and sleep analysis in children with sleep-disordered breathing. *Clin Neurophysiol*. 2011;122(2):311–319.

108. Hunter SJ, Gozal D, Smith DL, Philby MF, Kaylegian J, Kheirandish-Gozal L. Effect of sleep-disordered breathing severity on cognitive performance measures in a large community cohort of young school-aged children. *Am J Respir Crit Care Med*. 2016;194(6):739–747.

109. Kohler MJ, Lushington K, van den Heuvel CJ, Martin J, Pamula Y, Kennedy D. Adenotonsillectomy and neurocognitive deficits in children with sleep disordered breathing. *PLoS One*. 2009;4(10):e7343.

110. Calhoun SL, Mayes SD, Vgontzas AN, Tsaoussoglou M, Shifflett LJ, Bixler EO. No relationship between neurocognitive functioning and mild sleep disordered breathing in a community sample of children. *J Clin Sleep Med*. 2009;5(3):228–234.

111. Aronen ET, Liukkonen K, Simola P, et al. Mood is associated with snoring in preschool-aged children. *J Dev Behav Pediatr*. 2009;30(2):107–114.

112. Lewin DS, Rosen RC, England SJ, Dahl RE. Preliminary evidence of behavioral and cognitive sequelae of obstructive sleep apnea in children. *Sleep Med*. 2002;3(1):5–13.

113. da Silva Gusmao Cardoso T, Pompeia S, Miranda MC. Cognitive and behavioral effects of obstructive sleep apnea syndrome in children: A systematic literature review. *Sleep Med*. 2018;46:46–55.

114. Lezak MD, Howieson DB, Loring DW. *Neuropsychological Assessment*. 4th ed. Oxford University Press; 2004.

115. Suratt PM, Barth JT, Diamond R, et al. Reduced time in bed and obstructive sleep-disordered breathing in children are associated with cognitive impairment. *Pediatrics*. 2007;119(2):320–329.

116. Plomin R, Deary IJ. Genetics and intelligence differences: Five special findings. *Mol Psychiatry*. 2015;20(1):98–108.

117. Lau EY, Choi EW, Lai ES, et al. Working memory impairment and its associated sleep-related respiratory parameters in children with obstructive sleep apnea. *Sleep Med*. 2015;16(9):1109–1115.

118. Kheirandish-Gozal L, De Jong MR, Spruyt K, Chamuleau SA, Gozal D. Obstructive sleep apnoea is associated with impaired pictorial memory task acquisition and retention in children. *Eur Respir J*. 2010;36(1):164–169.

119. Spruyt K, Capdevila OS, Kheirandish-Gozal L, Gozal D. Inefficient or insufficient encoding as potential primary deficit in neurodevelopmental performance among children with OSA. *Dev Neuropsychol*. 2009;34(5):601–614.

120. Key AP, Molfese DL, O'Brien L, Gozal D. Sleep-disordered breathing affects auditory processing in 5-7-year-old children: Evidence from brain recordings. *Dev Neuropsychol*. 2009;34(5):615–628.

121. Rhodes SK, Shimoda KC, Waid LR, et al. Neurocognitive deficits in morbidly obese children with obstructive sleep apnea. *J Pediatr*. 1995;127(5):741–744.

122. Maski K, Steinhart E, Holbrook H, Katz ES, Kapur K, Stickgold R. Impaired memory consolidation in children with obstructive sleep disordered breathing. *PLoS One*. 2017;12(11):e0186915.

123. Blunden S, Lushington K, Lorenzen B, Martin J, Kennedy D. Neuropsychological and psychosocial function in children with a history of snoring or behavioral sleep problems. *J Pediatr*. 2005;146(6):780–786.

124. Trosman I, Trosman SJ. Cognitive and Behavioral Consequences of Sleep Disordered Breathing in Children. *Med Sci (Basel)*. 2017;5(4):30.

125. Biggs SN, Bourke R, Anderson V, et al. Working memory in children with sleep-disordered breathing: Objective versus subjective measures. *Sleep Med*. 2011;12(9):887–891.

126. Kim JK, Lee JH, Lee SH, Hong SC, Cho JH. School performance and behavior of Korean elementary school students with sleep-disordered breathing. *Ann Otol Rhinol Laryngol*. 2011;120(4):268–272.

127. Ravid S, Afek I, Suraiya S, Shahar E, Pillar G. Sleep disturbances are associated with reduced school achievements in first-grade pupils. *Dev Neuropsychol*. 2009;34(5):574–587.

128. Goyal A, Pakhare AP, Bhatt GC, Choudhary B, Patil R. Association of pediatric obstructive sleep apnea with poor academic performance: A school-based study from India. *Lung India*. 2018;35(2):132–136.

129. Urschitz MS, Guenther A, Eggebrecht E, et al. Snoring, intermittent hypoxia and academic performance in primary school children. *Am J Respir Crit Care Med*. 2003;168(4):464–468.

130. Tan E, Healey D, Schaughency E, Dawes P, Galland B. Neurobehavioural correlates in older children and adolescents with obesity and obstructive sleep apnoea. *J Paediatr Child Health*. 2014;50(1):16–23.

131. Goodwin JL, Kaemingk KL, Fregosi RF, et al. Clinical outcomes associated with sleep-disordered breathing in Caucasian and Hispanic children–the Tucson Children's Assessment of Sleep Apnea study (TuCASA). *Sleep*. 2003;26(5):587–591.

132. Lundeborg I, McAllister A, Samuelsson C, Ericsson E, Hultcrantz E. Phonological development in children with obstructive sleep-disordered breathing. *Clin Linguist Phon*. 2009;23(10):751–761.

133. Beebe DW, Miller N, Kirk S, Daniels SR, Amin R. The association between obstructive sleep apnea and dietary choices among obese individuals during middle to late childhood. *Sleep Med*. 2011;12(8):797–799.

134. Chervin RD, Clarke DF, Huffman JL, et al. School performance, race, and other correlates of sleep-disordered breathing in children. *Sleep Med*. 2003;4(1):21–27.

135. Mayes SD, Calhoun SL, Bixler EO, Vgontzas AN. Nonsignificance of sleep relative to IQ and neuropsychological scores in predicting academic achievement. *J Dev Behav Pediatr.* 2008;29(3):206–212.

136. Karpinski AC, Scullin MH, Montgomery-Downs HE. Risk for sleep-disordered breathing and executive function in preschoolers. *Sleep Med.* 2008;9(4):418–424.

137. Li AM, Zhu Y, Au CT, Lee DLY, Ho C, Wing YK. Natural history of primary snoring in school-aged children: A 4-year follow-up study. *Chest.* 2013;143(3):729–735.

138. Chan KC, Au CT, Hui LL, Ng SK, Wing YK, Li AM. How OSA evolves from childhood to young adulthood: Natural history from a 10-year follow-up study. *Chest.* 2019;156(1):120–130.

139. Andersen IG, Holm JC, Homoe P. Impact of weight-loss management on children and adolescents with obesity and obstructive sleep apnea. *Int J Pediatr Otorhinolaryngol.* 2019;123:57–62.

140. Gozal D, Pope Jr. DW. Snoring during early childhood and academic performance at ages thirteen to fourteen years. *Pediatrics.* 2001;107(6):1394–1399.

141. Chervin RD, Ruzicka DL, Archbold KH, Dillon JE. Snoring predicts hyperactivity four years later. *Sleep.* 2005;28(7):885–890.

142. Tamana SK, Smithson L, Lau A, et al. Parent-reported symptoms of sleep-disordered breathing are associated with increased behavioral problems at 2 years of age: The Canadian Healthy Infant Longitudinal Development Birth Cohort Study. *Sleep.* 2018;41(1):zsx177.

143. Golding J, Pembrey M, Jones R, Team AS. ALSPAC–the Avon Longitudinal Study of Parents and Children. I. Study methodology. *Paediatr Perinat Epidemiol.* 2001;15(1):74–87.

144. Gozal D, Tan HL, Kheirandish-Gozal L. Treatment of obstructive sleep apnea in children: Handling the unknown with precision. *J Clin Med.* 2020;9(3):888.

145. Ahmadi MS, Poorolajal J, Masoomi FS, Haghighi M. Effect of adenotonsillectomy on attention deficit-hyperactivity disorder in children with adenotonsillar hypertrophy: A prospective cohort study. *Int J Pediatr Otorhinolaryngol.* 2016;86:193–195.

146. Ayral M, Baylan MY, Kinis V, et al. Evaluation of hyperactivity, attention deficit, and impulsivity before and after adenoidectomy/adenotonsillectomy surgery. *J Craniofac Surg.* 2013;24(3):731–734.

147. Dadgarnia MH, Baradaranfar MH, Fallah R, Atighechi S, Ahsani AH, Baradaranfar A. Effect of adenotonsillectomy on ADHD symptoms of children with adenotonsillar hypertrophy. *Acta Med Iran.* 2012;50(8):547–551.

148. Amiri S, AbdollahiFakhim S, Lotfi A, Bayazian G, Sohrabpour M, Hemmatjoo T. Effect of adenotonsillectomy on ADHD symptoms of children with adenotonsillar hypertrophy and sleep disordered breathing. *Int J Pediatr Otorhinolaryngol.* 2015;79(8):1213–1217.

149. Aksu H, Gunel C, Ozgur BG, Toka A, Basak S. Effects of adenoidectomy/adenotonsillectomy on ADHD symptoms and behavioral problems in children. *Int J Pediatr Otorhinolaryngol.* 2015;79(7):1030–1033.

150. Marcus CL, Moore RH, Rosen CL, et al. A randomized trial of adenotonsillectomy for childhood sleep apnea. *N Engl J Med.* 2013;368(25):2366–2376.

151. Taylor HG, Bowen SR, Beebe DW, et al. Cognitive Effects of adenotonsillectomy for obstructive sleep apnea. *Pediatrics.* 2016;138(2):e20154458.

152. Isaiah A, Spanier AJ, Grattan LM, Wang Y, Pereira KD. Predictors of behavioral changes after adenotonsillectomy in pediatric obstructive sleep apnea: A secondary analysis of a randomized clinical trial. *JAMA Otolaryngol Head Neck Surg.* 2020;146(10):900–908.

153. Yu Y, Chen YX, Liu L, Yu ZY, Luo X. Neuropsychological functioning after adenotonsillectomy in children with obstructive sleep apnea: A meta-analysis. *J Huazhong Univ Sci Technolog Med Sci.* 2017;37(3):453–461.

154. Song SA, Tolisano AM, Cable BB, Camacho M. Neurocognitive outcomes after pediatric adenotonsillectomy for obstructive sleep apnea: A systematic review and meta-analysis. *Int J Pediatr Otorhinolaryngol.* 2016;83:205–210.

155. Montgomery-Downs HE, Crabtree VM, Gozal D. Cognition, sleep and respiration in at-risk children treated for obstructive sleep apnoea. *Eur Respir J.* 2005;25(2):336–342.

156. Ezzat WF, Fawaz S, Abdelrazek Y. To what degree does adenotonsillectomy affect neurocognitive performance in children with obstructive sleep apnea hypopnea syndrome due to adenotonsillar enlargement? *ORL J Otorhinolaryngol Relat Spec.* 2010;72(4):215–219.

157. Hogan AM, Hill CM, Harrison D, Kirkham FJ. Cerebral blood flow velocity and cognition in children before and after adenotonsillectomy. *Pediatrics.* 2008;122(1):75–82.

158. Friedman BC, Hendeles-Amitai A, Kozminsky E, et al. Adenotonsillectomy improves neurocognitive function in children with obstructive sleep apnea syndrome. *Sleep.* 2003;26(8):999–1005.

159. Li HY, Huang YS, Chen NH, Fang TJ, Lee LA. Impact of adenotonsillectomy on behavior in children with sleep-disordered breathing. *Laryngoscope.* 2006;116(7):1142–1147.

160. Burton MJ, Goldstein NA, Rosenfeld RM. Cochrane Corner: Extracts from The Cochrane Library: Tonsillectomy or Adenotonsillectomy versus Non-Surgical Management for Obstructive Sleep-Disordered Breathing in Children. *Otolaryngol Head Neck Surg.* 2016;154(4):581–585.

161. Esteller E, Barcelo M, Segarra F, Estivill E, Girabent-Farres M. [Neurocognitive and behavioral disturbances after adenotonsillectomy in obstructive sleep apnea syndrome]. *An Pediatr (Barc).* 2014;80(4):214–220.

162. Waters KA, Chawla J, Harris MA, et al. Rationale for and design of the "POSTA" study: Evaluation of neurocognitive outcomes after immediate adenotonsillectomy compared to watchful waiting in preschool children. *BMC Pediatr.* 2017;17(1):47.

163. Waters KA, Chawla J, Harris MA, et al. Cognition after early tonsillectomy for mild OSA. *Pediatrics.* 2020;145:2.

164. Lushington K, Kennedy D, Martin J, Kohler M. Quality-of-life but not behavior improves 48-months post-adenotonsillectomy in children with SDB. *Sleep Med.* 2021;81:418–429.

165. Giordani B, Hodges EK, Guire KE, et al. Neuropsychological and behavioral functioning in children with and without obstructive sleep apnea referred for tonsillectomy. *J Int Neuropsychol Soc.* 2008;14(4):571–581.

166. Giordani B, Hodges EK, Guire KE, et al. Changes in neuropsychological and behavioral functioning in children with and without obstructive sleep apnea following Tonsillectomy. *J Int Neuropsychol Soc.* 2012;18(2):212–222.

167. Marcus CL, Radcliffe J, Konstantinopoulou S, et al. Effects of positive airway pressure therapy on neurobehavioral outcomes in children with obstructive sleep apnea. *Am J Respir Crit Care Med.* 2012;185(9):998–1003.

168. Yuan HC, Sohn EY, Abouezzeddine T, et al. Neurocognitive functioning in children with obstructive sleep apnea syndrome: A pilot study of positive airway pressure therapy. *J Pediatr Nurs.* 2012;27(6):607–613.

169. Beebe DW, Byars KC. Adolescents with obstructive sleep apnea adhere poorly to positive airway pressure (PAP), but PAP users show improved attention and school performance. *PLoS One.* 2011;6(3):e16924.

170. Alonso-Alvarez ML, Teran-Santos J, Navazo-Eguia AI, et al. Treatment outcomes of obstructive sleep apnoea in obese community-dwelling children: The NANOS study. *Eur Respir J.* 2015;46(3):717–727.

171. Wilcox LJ, Bergeron M, Reghunathan S, Ishman SL. An updated review of pediatric drug-induced sleep endoscopy. *Laryngoscope Investig Otolaryngol.* 2017;2(6):423–431.

172. Boudewyns A, Verhulst S, Maris M, Saldien V, Van de Heyning P. Drug-induced sedation endoscopy in pediatric obstructive sleep apnea syndrome. *Sleep Med.* 2014;15(12):1526–1531.

173. Gazzaz MJ, Isaac A, Anderson S, Alsufyani N, Alrajhi Y, El-Hakim H. Does drug-induced sleep endoscopy change the surgical decision in surgically naive non-syndromic children with snoring/sleep disordered breathing from the standard adenotonsillectomy? A retrospective cohort study. *J Otolaryngol Head Neck Surg.* 2017;46(1):12.

174. Keefe KR, Patel PN, Levi JR. The shifting relationship between weight and pediatric obstructive sleep apnea: A historical review. *Laryngoscope.* 2019;129(10):2414–2419.

175. Beebe DW, Gozal D. Obstructive sleep apnea and the prefrontal cortex: Towards a comprehensive model linking nocturnal upper airway obstruction to daytime cognitive and behavioral deficits. *J Sleep Res.* 2002;11(1):1–16.

176. Dahl RE. The impact of inadequate sleep on children's daytime cognitive function. *Semin Pediatr Neurol.* 1996;3(1):44–50.

177. Chelune GJ, Ferguson W, Koon R, Dickey TO. Frontal lobe disinhibition in attention deficit disorder. *Child Psychiatry Hum Dev.* 1986;16(4):221–234.

178. Arnsten AF, Rubia K. Neurobiological circuits regulating attention, cognitive control, motivation, and emotion: Disruptions in neurodevelopmental psychiatric disorders. *J Am Acad Child Adolesc Psychiatry.* 2012;51(4):356–367.

179. Cortese S, Castellanos FX. Neuroimaging of attention-deficit/hyperactivity disorder: Current neuroscience-informed perspectives for clinicians. *Curr Psychiatry Rep.* 2012;14(5):568–578.

180. Bass JL, Corwin M, Gozal D, et al. The effect of chronic or intermittent hypoxia on cognition in childhood: A review of the evidence. *Pediatrics.* 2004;114(3):805–816.

181. Gozal D, Daniel JM, Dohanich GP. Behavioral and anatomical correlates of chronic episodic hypoxia during sleep in the rat. *J Neurosci.* 2001;21(7):2442–2450.

182. Row BW, Kheirandish L, Cheng Y, Rowell PP, Gozal D. Impaired spatial working memory and altered choline acetyltransferase (CHAT) immunoreactivity and nicotinic receptor binding in rats exposed to intermittent hypoxia during sleep. *Behav Brain Res.* 2007;177(2):308–314.

183. Nair D, Dayyat EA, Zhang SX, Wang Y, Gozal D. Intermittent hypoxia-induced cognitive deficits are mediated by NADPH oxidase activity in a murine model of sleep apnea. *PLoS One.* 2011;6(5):e19847.

184. Row BW, Kheirandish L, Neville JJ, Gozal D. Impaired spatial learning and hyperactivity in developing rats exposed to intermittent hypoxia. *Pediatr Res.* 2002;52(3):449–453.

185. van der Heijden KB, Vermeulen MCM, Donjacour C, et al. Chronic sleep reduction is associated with academic achievement and study concentration in higher education students. *J Sleep Res.* 2018;27(2):165–174.

186. Agostini A, Carskadon MA, Dorrian J, Coussens S, Short MA. An experimental study of adolescent sleep restriction during a simulated school week: Changes in phase, sleep staging, performance and sleepiness. *J Sleep Res.* 2017;26(2):227–235.

187. Sun W, Ling J, Zhu X, Lee TM, Li SX. Associations of weekday-to-weekend sleep differences with academic performance and health-related outcomes in school-age children and youths. *Sleep Med Rev.* 2019;46:27–53.

188. Phillips AJK, Clerx WM, O'Brien CS, et al. Irregular sleep/wake patterns are associated with poorer academic performance and delayed circadian and sleep/wake timing. *Sci Rep.* 2017;7(1):3216.

189. Thomas JH, Burgers DE. Sleep is an eye-opener: Behavioral causes and consequences of hypersomnolence in children. *Paediatr Respir Rev.* 2018;25:3–8.

190. Sadeh A, Gruber R, Raviv A. Sleep, neurobehavioral functioning, and behavior problems in school-age children. *Child Dev.* 2002;73(2):405–417.

191. Astill RG, Van der Heijden KB, Van Ijzendoorn MH, Van Someren EJ. Sleep, cognition, and behavioral problems in school-age children: A century of research meta-analyzed. *Psychol Bull.* 2012;138(6):1109–1138.

192. Calhoun SL, Fernandez-Mendoza J, Vgontzas AN, et al. Learning, attention/hyperactivity, and conduct problems as sequelae of excessive daytime sleepiness in a general population study of young children. *Sleep.* 2012;35(5):627–632.

193. Lavie L. Oxidative stress in obstructive sleep apnea and intermittent hypoxia–revisited–the bad ugly and good: Implications to the heart and brain. *Sleep Med Rev.* 2015;20:27–45.

194. Zhou L, Chen P, Peng Y, Ouyang R. Role of oxidative stress in the neurocognitive dysfunction of obstructive sleep apnea syndrome. *Oxid Med Cell Longev.* 2016;2016:9626831.

195. Clinton JM, Davis CJ, Zielinski MR, Jewett KA, Krueger JM. Biochemical regulation of sleep and sleep biomarkers. *J Clin Sleep Med.* 2011;7(5 Suppl):S38–S42.

196. Silva RH, Abilio VC, Takatsu AL, et al. Role of hippocampal oxidative stress in memory deficits induced by sleep deprivation in mice. *Neuropharmacology.* 2004;46(6):895–903.

197. Nair D, Zhang SX, Ramesh V, et al. Sleep fragmentation induces cognitive deficits via nicotinamide adenine dinucleotide phosphate oxidase-dependent pathways in mouse. *Am J Respir Crit Care Med.* 2011;184(11):1305–1312.

198. Philby MF, Macey PM, Ma RA, Kumar R, Gozal D, Kheirandish-Gozal L. Reduced regional grey matter volumes in pediatric obstructive sleep apnea. *Sci Rep.* 2017;7:44566.

199. Macey PM, Kheirandish-Gozal L, Prasad JP, et al. Altered regional brain cortical thickness in pediatric obstructive sleep apnea. *Front Neurol.* 2018;9:4.

30

Cardiovascular Consequences of Obstructive Sleep Apnea

Raouf Samy Amin

CHAPTER HIGHLIGHTS

- Abnormal neural, inflammatory, and hormonal factors have been implicated in the initiation and progression of cardiovascular disease in children with sleep-disordered breathing.
- Children with SDB who are at risk for cardiovascular consequences may exhibit chemo/baroreflex dysfunction, abnormal renin-angiotensin-aldosterone system-mediated feedback control, increased highly reactive free oxygen radicals, and insulin resistance.
- These abnormalities manifest as elevated blood pressure readings, cardiac remodeling, including ventricular hypertrophy, and endothelial dysfunction including arterial dilation.
- As a consequence, early intervention to prevent cardiovascular comorbidities by treating pediatric sleep-disordered breathing proactively may have significant long-term benefits.

Introduction

Our knowledge about the link between sleep-disordered breathing (SDB) and cardiovascular dysfunction in children has grown significantly in the last 3 decades.[1-4] Cardiovascular research in children with SDB has focused primarily on disease mechanisms and has not yet provided unequivocal evidence of cardiovascular morbidity. Nevertheless, small differences in cardiovascular functions between children with SDB and healthy controls have been described recently. The clinical significance of these early childhood observations in terms of cardiovascular morbidity either during childhood or in adult life has yet to be explained. It is also worth noting that the changes in structure and functions of the cardiovascular system are not universally observed across population including races, ethnic background, socioeconomic status, and body habitus. Therefore, future research that focuses on better understanding of the contributions of environmental, genetic, and socioeconomic conditions depends on the observations made to date. This chapter will describe the most recent evidence-based understanding of

cardiovascular dysfunction in children with SDB. Proposed hypothetical mechanisms of cardiovascular disease in SDB and evidence of end organ damage in childhood SDB that have been investigated to date will be discussed (Fig. 30.1).

Normal Sleep and Cardiovascular System

Normal sleep is associated with sleep stages related cardiovascular and autonomic changes.[5,6] Progressive reduction of heart rate (HR), blood pressure (BP), and stroke volume during non–rapid eye movement (NREM) sleep is synchronized with reduced sympathetic nervous system activity (SNA).[7] During REM sleep, sympathetic drive increases markedly with consequent increase in vascular resistance, which results in increased BP and HR.[7] Fig. 30.2 shows BP and SNA changes recorded directly from peripheral nerves in humans during normal sleep (Fig. 30.2).[7] Although exact significance of cyclical and rhythmic alteration in cardiovascular functions during NREM and REM sleep cycle is not well understood, it is believed to be critical for normal cardiovascular health.

SDB and Cardiovascular System

Repetitive apneas during sleep disrupt the physiologic changes in the cardiovascular and autonomic nervous systems.[8-10] Increased SNA during episodes of apnea is associated with increased systemic BP, pulmonary arterial pressure, and left ventricular (LV) afterload (Fig. 30.3).[9,11] Hypoxemia and hypercapnia during SDB events are major contributors to chemoreflex-mediated increase in SNA and cardiovascular changes.[9] Negative intrathoracic pressures during upper airway obstruction in SDB events affect intrathoracic hemodynamics including LV transmural pressure and LV afterload.[12] LV relaxation and LV filling may also be affected by the negative intrathoracic pressure.[13,14] In addition, negative intrathoracic pressure alters aortic pressure, inducing stretch of the aortic wall, activating aortic baroreceptors and thus buffering sympathetic activation during obstructive sleep apnea (OSA).[15,16] On resumption of

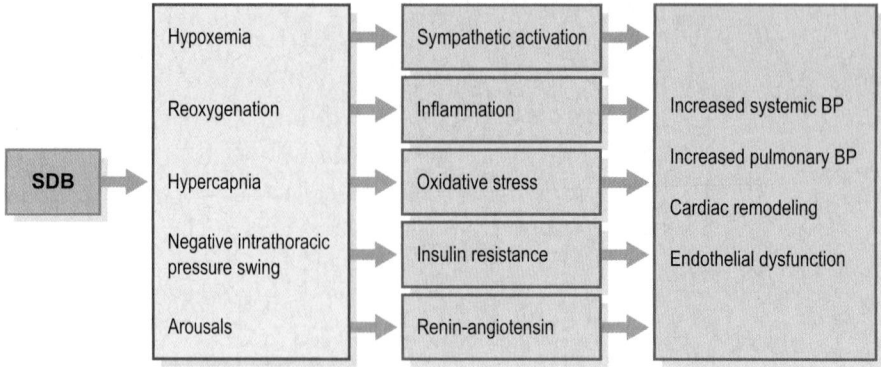

• **Fig. 30.1** Mechanisms of cardiovascular disease in sleep-disordered breathing *(SDB)*. The schematic shows hypothetical mechanisms of cardiovascular diseases in SDB and cardiovascular dysfunction in children with SDB. BP, blood pressure.

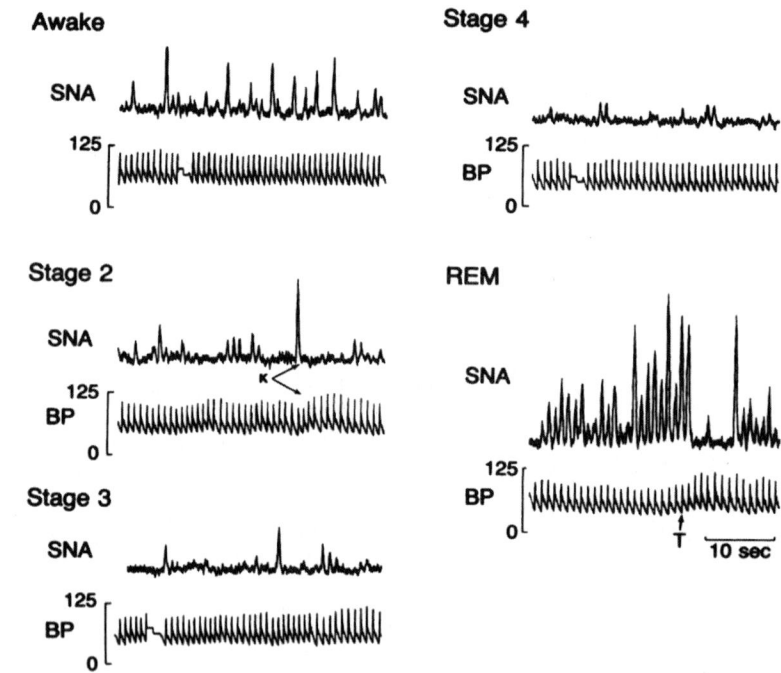

• **Fig. 30.2** Blood pressure *(BP)* and sympathetic nerve activity *(SNA)* during non–rapid eye movement (NREM) and REM sleep in a healthy human. SNA and BP progressive reduced during the deeper stage of non-REM sleep. REM sleep is associated with a striking increase in SNA.[7]

breathing, increased venous return distends the right ventricle, reducing LV compliance due to leftward shift of interventricular septum and thus LV diastolic filling.[12] Increased stroke volume on resumption of breathing at the time when systemic vascular resistance is highest elicits further increase in BP. SDB events are commonly associated with arousals from sleep. Arousal may also contribute to the acute increases in BP at termination of SDB events.[17] Repetitive nocturnal arousals cause sleep fragmentation that may also be associated with daytime cardiovascular dysfunction.

Mechanisms of Cardiovascular Diseases in SDB

A number of neural, inflammatory, and hormonal abnormalities are evident in children with SDB. These are implicated in the initiation and progression of cardiac and vascular disease conditions.

Neural Mechanisms

Neural control of the circulation represents the integrated response to diverse reflexes including baroreflex, chemoreflex, and low-pressure cardiopulmonary reflexes. The interaction between cardiovascular and respiratory variables constitutes an important influence on neurally mediated changes in cardiac and vascular control (Fig. 30.4). Interactions between these reflexes in conditions of hypoxemia and hypercapnia during episodes of OSA are implicated as the primary mechanisms of cardiovascular dysfunction in children with SDB.

Chemoreflex and Cardiovascular System

Chemoreflexes exert profound influences on respiratory, autonomic, and cardiovascular functions during apnea events.[18] The central chemoreceptors are located on the

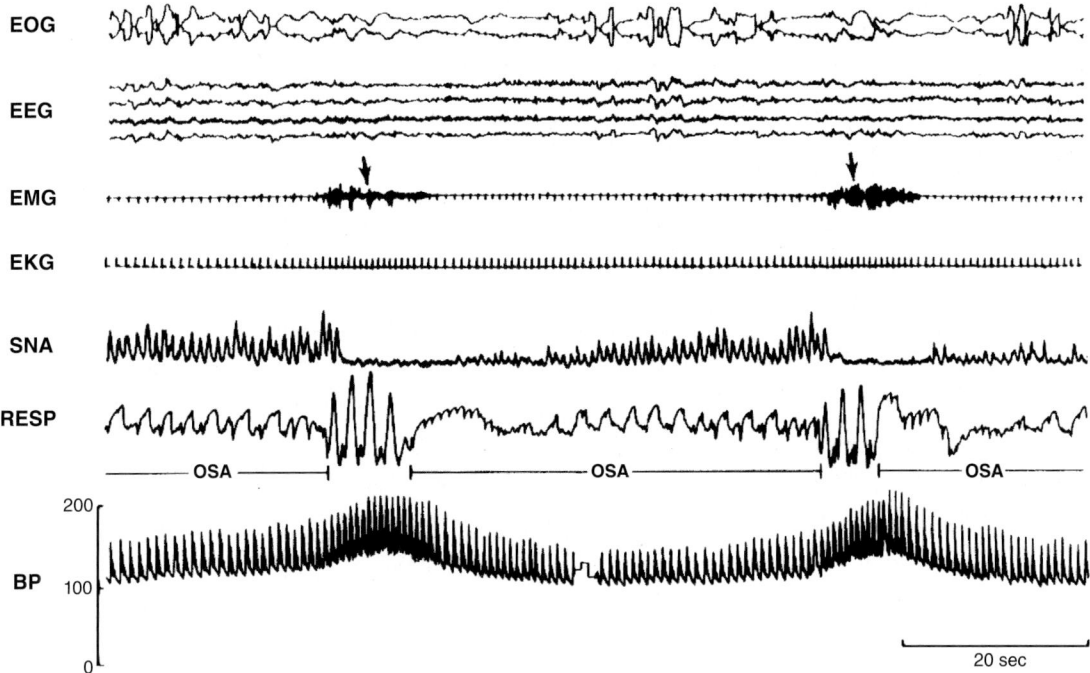

EOG

EEG

EMG

EKG

SNA

RESP

OSA OSA OSA

BP 200 100 0

20 sec

• **Fig. 30.3** Acute effects of apnea during sleep on sympathetic nerve activity and blood pressure. Apnea is associated with progressive arterial deoxygenation and sympathetic activation. Resumption of breathing and arousal at the end of apnea increases stroke volume and heart rate and a consequent increase in arterial pressure.[9]

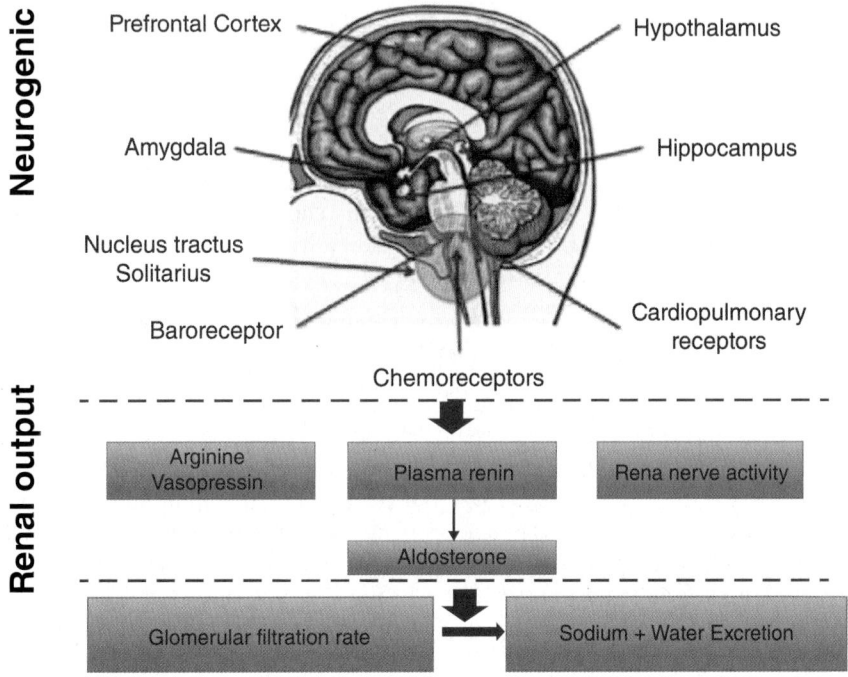

Neurogenic

Prefrontal Cortex
Hypothalamus
Amygdala
Hippocampus
Nucleus tractus Solitarius
Baroreceptor
Cardiopulmonary receptors

Chemoreceptors

Renal output

Arginine Vasopressin | Plasma renin | Rena nerve activity
Aldosterone
Glomerular filtration rate | Sodium + Water Excretion

• **Fig. 30.4** Interaction of baroreflex and chemoreflex for central nervous system control of the cardiovascular and renal systems.

ventral surface of the medulla and are vital for cardiorespiratory control.[19,20] The peripheral chemoreceptors are located in the carotid bodies that respond primarily to hypoxemia to produce hyperventilation, tachycardia, and increased sympathetic vasoconstrictor activity.[21,22] Peripheral chemoreceptor activation as a result of cessation of breathing during OSA elicits simultaneous activation of vascular sympathetic and cardiac vagal drives with consequent cardiac slowing and increased BP. Hypercapnia primarily acts through the central chemoreceptors in the brainstem,

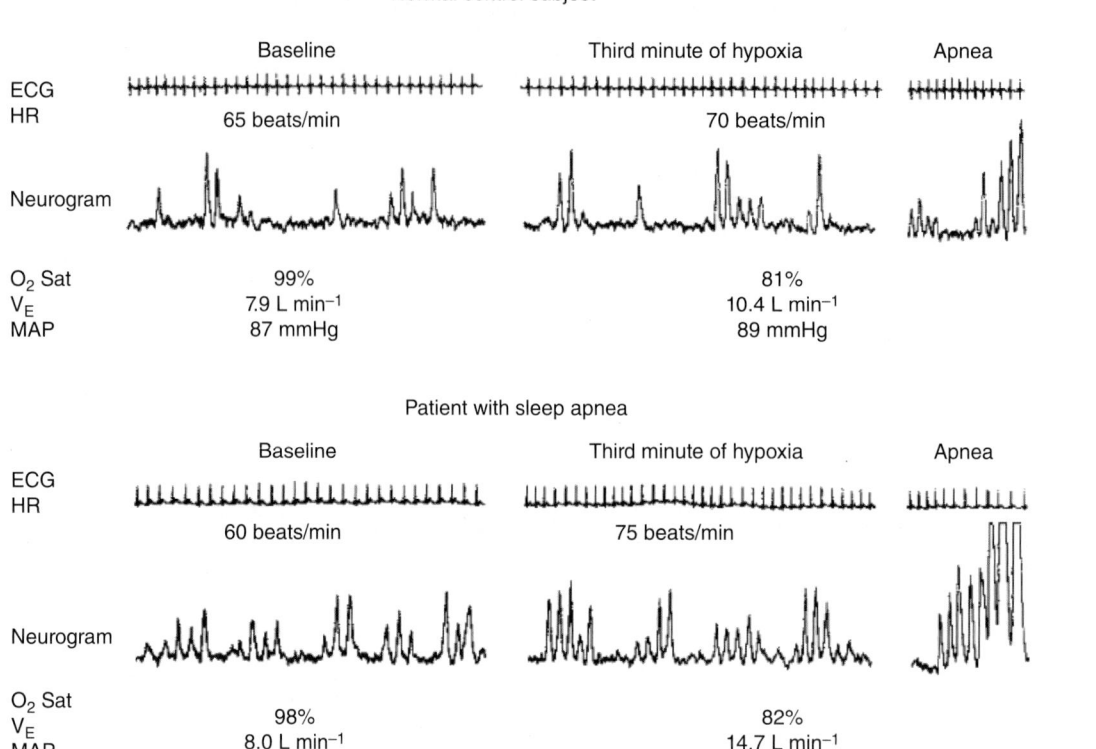

Normal control subject

	Baseline	Third minute of hypoxia	Apnea

ECG
HR   65 beats/min   70 beats/min

Neurogram

O₂ Sat   99%   81%
Vᴇ   7.9 L min⁻¹   10.4 L min⁻¹
MAP   87 mmHg   89 mmHg

Patient with sleep apnea

	Baseline	Third minute of hypoxia	Apnea

ECG
HR   60 beats/min   75 beats/min

Neurogram

O₂ Sat   98%   82%
Vᴇ   8.0 L min⁻¹   14.7 L min⁻¹
MAP   81 mmHg   89 mmHg

10 s

• **Fig. 30.5** Ventilation, heart rate, blood pressure, and sympathetic nerve activity during rest and responses to apnea during hypoxia. Note exaggerated sympathetic responses to apnea during hypoxia in a patient with obstructive sleep apnea.

but also in part through the peripheral chemoreceptors, to produce hyperventilation and increased sympathetic traffic to peripheral blood vessels.[23] Interestingly, hypercapnia does not induce vagally mediated bradycardia as seen during hypoxia. Hypoxemia and hypercapnia administered simultaneously causes synergistic increase in minute ventilation.[24] Sympathetic activation is also greater than that induced by either of the individual stimuli alone. During OSA, combined hypoxemic-hypercapnic stimuli potentiate the chemoreflex-mediated neural and circulatory responses (Fig. 30.5). There is now strong evidence that after exposure to hypoxia there is a time-dependent increase in the sensitivity of the carotid chemoreceptors, and muscle sympathetic nerve activity and eventually hypertension. Intermittent hypoxia has an even more sensitizing effect on the carotid chemoreceptors as a result of a more dominant effect of pro-oxidant HIF1α relative to the antioxidant effect of HIF2α.[25] The resulting sustained increase in oxidative stress, as well as local inflammation around the chemoreceptors, systemically lead to increased chemosensitivity, systemic vasocontraction, and endothelial dysfunction. Animal studies suggest that increased frequency of arousals and sleep fragmentation may also play an essential role in hyperactivity of the peripheral chemoreceptors.[26]

Hyperactivity of the peripheral chemoreceptors contributes significantly to the pathogenesis of hypertension in adult patients with OSA.[27] However, the role of

chemoreceptors in cardiovascular morbidity in children is yet to be clearly understood, particularly, that maturation of the chemoreceptors influences its sensitivity with aging leading to gradual attenuation of the hypoxic response.[28]

Baroreflex and Cardiovascular System

Baroreflexes provide critical negative feedback control of arterial pressure.[18] Arterial baroreceptors are nerve endings innervating large arteries. Changes in arterial pressure in the aorta and carotid arteries alter vascular stretch and thus frequency of baroreceptor inhibitory impulse to the brainstem. Increased baroreceptor activity during a rise in BP triggers reflex inhibition of sympathetic activity, parasympathetic activation, and subsequent decrease in vascular resistance and HR. Conversely, a decrease in arterial pressure reduces baroreceptor afferent discharge and triggers a reflex increase in sympathetic activity, parasympathetic inhibition, and vascular resistance and HR. Thus reduced baroreflex function may be associated with abnormal control of autonomic and circulatory functions. Asphyxia alone increases BP and alters the baroreflex control of HR.[29] Indeed, impairment of baroreflex modulation of vascular control is associated with the presence of OSA in adults.[30] In children, baroreflex gain decreases with increase severity of OSA.[31] Furthermore, the normal monotonic increase in baroreflex gain during the sleep period is not observed in children with an OSA and apnea-hypopnea

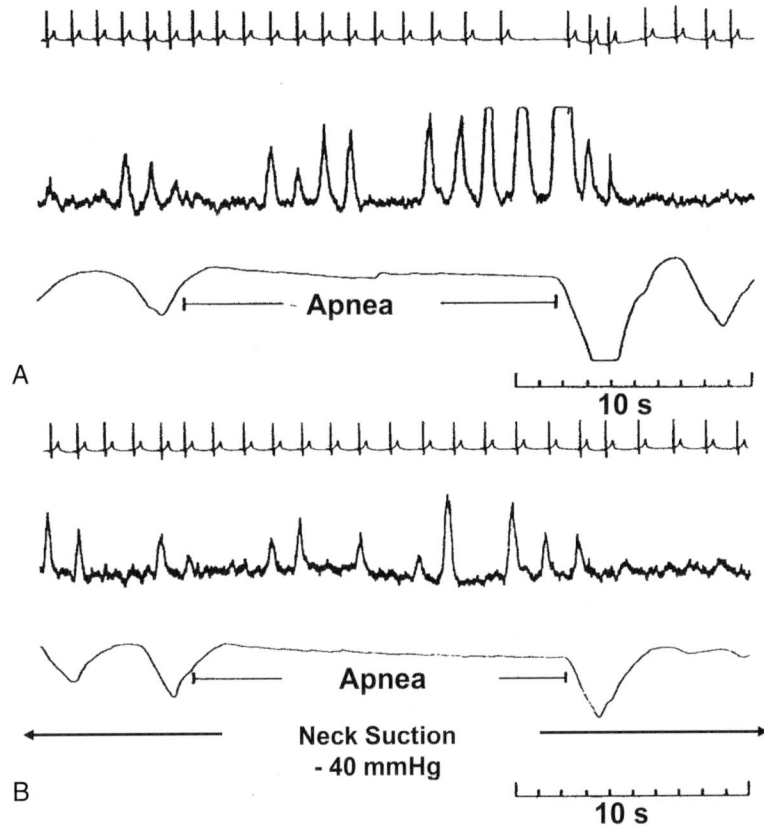

• **Fig. 30.6** Role of carotid arterial baroreflex on chemoreflex-mediated bradycardic and sympathetic responses. Activation of the carotid baroreceptor reflex by neck suction attenuates sympathetic responses to apnea. Note that arterial baroreflex not only regulates the cardiac and vascular functions, but it also has critical inhibitory effects on chemoreflex-mediated sympathetic responses.[36]

index (AHI) greater than 5/hr[31] (Fig. 30.10). Treatment of OSA with adenotonsillectomy leads to improved baroreflex gain, restored monotonic increase in baroreflex during sleep, and decrease in BP and BP variability.[32]

Baroreflex and Chemoreflex Interactions

The baroreflex has a significant role on the chemoreflex-mediated responses to hypoxemia. Baroreflex activation inhibits both ventilatory and vasoconstrictor responses to peripheral chemoreflex stimulation.[33] In the presence of hypoxia, the vasoconstrictor response to chemoreceptor activation may be exaggerated as a result of diminished baroreflex gain.[34] Alternatively, activation of chemoreceptors in the face of hypoxia may lead to resetting of baroreflex control of both HR and sympathetic activity to higher pressures without changes in baroreflex sensitivity.[35]

Increased BP activates arterial baroreceptors and causes bradycardia.[36] Chemoreflex activation in the setting of apnea also elicits bradycardia. The bradycardia response is attenuated when chemoreflex activation and apnea occur in a setting of increased baroreflex activation. Thus the arterial baroreflex inhibits not only the chemoreflex-mediated sympathetic vasoconstrictor response, but also the vagal bradycardic response (Fig. 30.6).[36] The normal buffering influence of the baroreflex

may be diminished in patients with SDB,[36] resulting in excessive potentiation of chemoreflex sensitivity with consequent exaggerated sympathetic activation and/or bradyarrhythmias during hypoxemia and apnea. Interaction of chemoreceptor and baroreceptor reflexes by hypoxia and hypercapnia during repeated episodes of OSA could be a mechanism for increased BP and promoting hypertension in OSA.[37]

Cortical Modulation of Baroreflex and Chemoreflex

Central command continuously modulates the baroreflex and chemoreflex-mediated cardiovascular and autonomic functions.[38,39] This modulation is important for BP variability during sleep and daytime activities. Although it is well-known that sympathetic vasomotor tone originates from structures within the medulla oblongata, the intramedullary network(s) of neurons that mediate cardiovascular reflexes and generation of sympathetic vasomotor tone may also be modulated by the activity of neurons within various hypothalamic structures, within the dorsal and ventral pons including the parabrachial/Kölliker-Fuse nuclei complex and A5 cell group, the midbrain periaqueductal gray area, and adjacent cuneiform nucleus, the central nucleus of the amygdala. Specific regions of the cerebral cortex such as the medial prefrontal cortex and the insular cortex modulate the autonomic drive to the heart and blood vessels to control HR and BP (Fig. 30.4). The interaction of the cortical, subcortical brain areas and the brainstem autonomic centers is important for the control of circulatory functions. There are structural changes of these regions that occur during brain development that may also influence the modulation of cardiovascular reflexes.[40] It is yet to be determined whether intermittent hypoxemia in OSA may alter the maturation trajectories of the cortical and subcortical regions and their abilities to modulate the sympathetic vasomotor tone.

Renin-Angiotensin-Aldosterone System Activation

The renin-angiotensin-aldosterone system (RAS) is important for the regulation of extracellular fluid volume and thus BP (Fig. 30.4).[41] Angiotensin II (ANG-II) is a potent vasoconstrictor that acts directly on vascular smooth muscle cells, causing vasoconstriction. ANG-II also regulates blood volume by increasing aldosterone production. Combined effects of ANG-II on vascular resistance and extracellular fluid volume play an important role on BP regulation. Renin released from the kidney is regulated by renal sympathetic nerves. Hypoxia is associated with increased level of sympathetic nerve and ANG-II.[42,43] OSA patients have higher ANG-II concentrations compared with healthy subjects.[44] Recent studies suggest that resistant hypertension in adults with OSA is associated with activation of the RAS.[45,46] A recent meta-analysis of the effects of OSA in adults on RAS suggested that ANG-II levels were significantly higher in OSA than in controls, whereas aldosterone levels were significantly higher in OSA with hypertension than normotensive subjects with OSA.[47] In a study of the renin-BP relationship in children with OSA, the normal negative association between renin level and BP was present only in control subjects of normal weight. There was absence of the negative association between renin level and BP in children with OSA and in overweight children, suggesting that both obesity and OSA significantly affect the RAS-mediated control of BP. Dysfunction of the RAS-mediated feedback control of BP may be a potential mechanism for elevated BP and thus development of hypertension and resistant hypertension in children with OSA, particularly in overweight and obese individuals.[48] The RAS also affects 24-hour ambulatory BP in children.[41] The role of RAS for BP regulation in children with OSA is still not well understood.

Systemic and Local Inflammation in SDB

The evidence of increased systemic inflammatory markers in children with SDB is emerging.[49] Chronic low-grade inflammation has been linked to pathophysiology of cardiovascular diseases in SDB.[50,51] Patients with OSA have increased levels of interleukin-6, tumor necrosis factor α, and C-reactive protein (CRP).[52] The combination of

Geometric Mean Values of CRP, mg/L*			
	Unadjusted	Partially Adjusted[†]	Fully Adjusted[‡]
AHI <1	0.42 (0.33–0.54)	0.43 (0.33–0.56)	0.50 (0.40–0.63)
AHI 1–4.9	0.56 (0.36–0.88)	0.54 (0.34–0.86)	0.43 (0.29–0.66)
AHI 5–14.9	1.48 (0.62–3.53)	1.37 (0.56–3.34)	0.97 (0.43–2.16)
AHI ⬚15	3.11 (1.38–7.03)	2.73 (1.17–6.37)	1.66 (0.76–3.60)

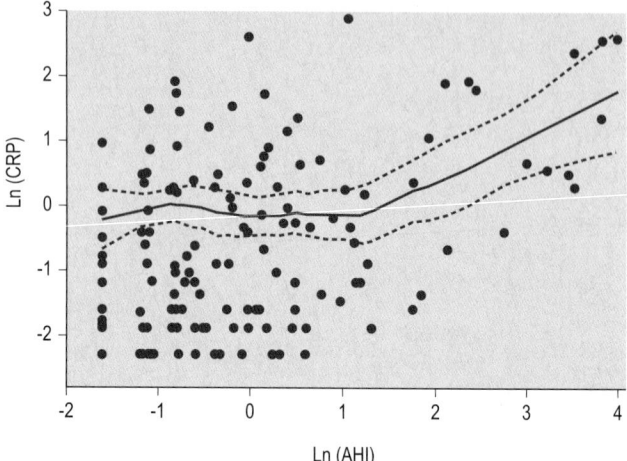

• **Fig. 30.7** Plasma C-reactive protein *(CRP)* levels in adolescents with obstructive sleep apnea (OSA) and normal controls. Adolescents with OSA, particularly with severe OSA (apnea-hypopnea index *[AHI]* > 5 events/hr) have significantly higher CRP levels. Elevated CRP levels in these patients are directly proportional to the severity of OSA as measured by AHI. *Values are geometric means (95% confidence interval) of CRP (mg/L) values in unadjusted and adjusted models. †Adjusted for age, sex, race. ‡Adjusted for age, sex, race, body mass index [BMI] percentile (BMI percentile).[56]

hypoxemia and sleep deprivation in patients with SDB may lead to increased levels of inflammatory markers. CRP may itself contribute to vascular disease by inhibiting nitric oxide synthase and increasing cell adhesion molecule expression.[53,54] The clinical significance of low-grade inflammation in children with OSA was demonstrated by two studies showing a significant association between markers of inflammation, vessel stiffness, and carotid artery structure and function.[55] A recent study in 143 adolescents reported an elevated level of CRP in SDB, and the levels were directly related to the severity of nocturnal hypoxemia independent of body mass index (Fig. 30.7).[56] Several studies did not find any significant association between CRP and SDB.[57,58] The conflicting results were in part attributed to the difference in the degree of adiposity between the study populations.

Local inflammation of upper airway has an important role in modulating airway patency.[59] Sputum in children with SDB showed increased neutrophils compared with controls and the level of neutrophils correlated significantly and positively with the severity of SDB.[60] Infiltration of inflammatory cells in the muscular layer of the pharynx has also been described in patients with SDB.[61] Active processes of nerve degeneration and regeneration and muscular damage in patents with SDB suggest that inflammation might negatively impact the function of upper airway tissues. However, its role in modulating upper airway collapsibility in patients with SDB is not fully investigated. Local inflammatory response in the upper airway may be associated with mechanical trauma induced by large intraluminal pharyngeal pressure swings, tissue vibration, and eccentric muscle contraction. Recent studies on the relationship between local inflammation and airway collapsibility suggests an important role of surface tension of upper airway lining fluid for generation of a force that hinders airway opening.[62,63] However, the exact mechanisms underlying the upregulation of inflammatory processes within the upper airway are not clear.

Oxidative Stress and Coagulation in SDB

Hypoxemia and reperfusion during repetitive nocturnal apneas may generate highly reactive free oxygen radicals.[64] Ischemia-reperfusion injury to the vascular wall may result in increased risk for atherosclerosis.[65] Low oxygen tension is a trigger for activation of polymorphonuclear neutrophils and release of free oxygen radicals. In SDB, repeated cycles of arterial oxygen desaturation and reoxygenation occur in response to apneas followed by hyperventilation. Treatment of OSA reduces production of free radicals.[66] Increased platelet and platelet aggregability increases in patients with OSA and reduces after treatment of SDB.[67,68] Increased hematocrit, nocturnal and daytime fibrinogen levels, and blood viscosity in SDB may also contribute to any predisposition to clot formation and cardiovascular morbidity.[69] Treatment of SDB reduces factor VII clotting activity and suggests that SDB may indeed be causally related to increased coagulability.[70] Oxidative stress and inflammatory markers in the exhaled breath condensate is increased in children with SDB.[71] Oxidant and antioxidant defense mechanisms are altered in children with obstructive adenotonsillar hypertrophy, and this alteration improves after tonsillectomy.[72]

Metabolic Syndrome and Insulin Resistance in SDB

Childhood SDB has been linked to metabolic syndrome.[73] Increased sympathetic activation in OSA may be associated with insulin resistance.[74,75] OSA patients have higher fasting blood glucose, insulin, and hemoglobin A1C levels, independent of body weight.[76] The severity of OSA appears to be correlated with the degree of insulin resistance.[77] Severe OSA is accompanied by a fivefold increase in the risk of overt diabetes mellitus.[78] Impaired glucose tolerance in OSA, independent of the effects of obesity per se, may be linked to sleep deprivation and sympathetic activation. Recent studies suggests increased risk for insulin resistance in children with OSA that correlate with the level of inflammatory biomarkers.[77,79]

SDB-Related Cardiac and Vascular Dysfunction

Unlike adults, children with SDB have minimal cardiovascular dysfunction that primarily includes abnormality in BP regulation and minimal changes in cardiac structure and function.

Elevated Systemic Arterial Pressure and Hypertension in SDB

Children with SDB have elevated BP compared with healthy children during nighttime sleep and even during daytime resting conditions (Fig. 30.8).[80-84] Simple snoring in children without SDB is also associated with increased daytime resting BP. Levels of increased systolic and diastolic BP in these patients are directly associated with the respiratory disturbance index.[83] Increased 24-hour BP variability during wakefulness and sleep are also associated with the presence of SDB in children.[81] In addition, SDB severity measured by desaturation during sleep and AHI are also associated with increased daytime and nocturnal BP variability.[81] It is very important to note that the level of BP in children with SDB reported in several cross-sectional studies did not reach a level that is considered clinically significant (Fig. 30.9).[85] Unlike adult patients with SDB, hypertension in children and adolescents is not independently associated with SDB. However, advanced stage of SDB may be associated with hypertension. BP load is a measure of hypertension and measured by percentage of BP measurements exceeding the 95th percentile during 24-hour BP monitoring.[81] A recent study in 140 children with AHI > 5 events/hr, nightly snoring, and tonsillar hypertrophy reported an increase in BP load and morning BP surge.[81] Significant reduction of 24-hour ambulatory BP is observed after treatment of SDB with adenotonsillectomy.[86] Although exact mechanisms of increased BP in children with SDB are not clear, reduced baroreflex during nighttime and daytime might be a potential candidate (Fig. 30.10).[31] It is unlikely that minimal increase in BP and variability in BP in children with SDB will lead to significant cardiac dysfunction. Whether early childhood SDB may predispose to BP deregulation in children and adolescents has yet to be demonstrated.

Elevated Pulmonary Arterial Pressure and Pulmonary Hypertension in SDB

Evidence of the presence of pulmonary hypertension in children with SDB are limited. Several case reports and studies with small sample size suggested statistically significant increase in pulmonary arterial pressure in SDB.[87,88] These studies are limited by either the procedures for diagnosis of SDB or by technique for measurements of pulmonary arterial pressure. Increased prevalence of echocardiographic diagnosis of cor pulmonale has been reported in children with adenotonsillar hypertrophy and snoring.[88] Both the absence[89] and presence[90] of pulmonary hypertension children with adenotonsillar hypertrophy and OSA are reported. However, significant improvement of pulmonary hypertension after treatment of SDB has been reported[87,91] (Fig. 30.11). A recent retrospective study demonstrated a prevalence of pulmonary hypertension by echocardiography in 8.2% of children with severe OSA.[92] Complete resolution or significant improving of cor pulmonale after treatment of SDB was described in several studies.[93]

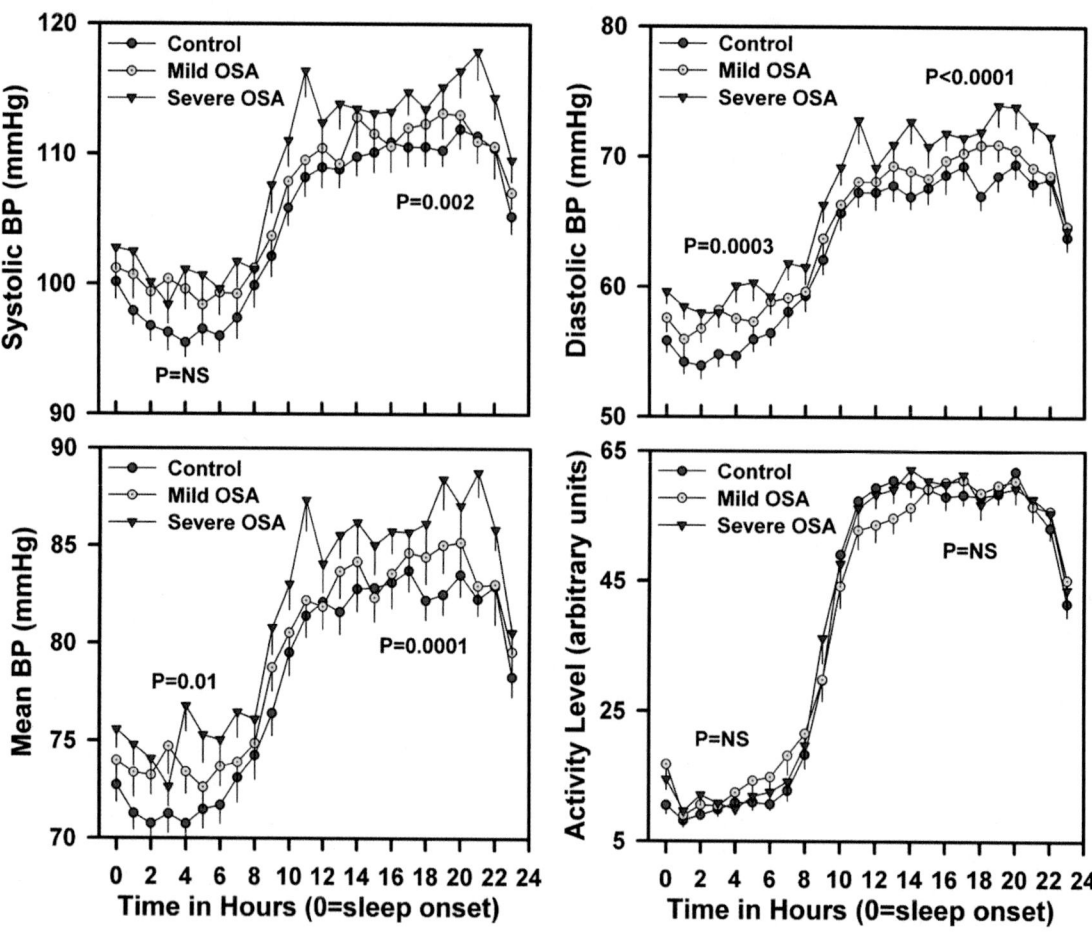

• **Fig. 30.8** Elevated blood pressure (BP) during 24-hour activated adjusted ambulatory BP monitoring in children with mild and severe sleep-disordered breathing. Children with severe obstructive sleep apnea have significantly higher BP compared with control during nighttime sleep and daytime activity.[81]

Cardiac Remodeling: Structural and Functional Changes of the Heart in SDB

Presence of LV hypertrophy has been described in children with SDB.[94] LV mass and relative wall thickness are significantly greater in normotensive children with OSA compared with children with primary snoring (Fig. 30.12).[94] An AHI of 10 is associated with a sixfold increased risk for hypertrophy. LV posterior wall thickness also correlated with the severity of SDB measured by respiratory disturbance index. Severity of SDB is directly related to the level of decrease in LV diastolic function.[95] Recently, impaired right ventricular function was also reported in children with adenotonsillar hypertrophy.[96] Brain natriuretic peptide, a hormone released by ventricular myocytes in response to pressure and volume overload, was increased in children with snoring and correlated with severity of SDB.[97,98] In otherwise healthy children, those with more severe SDB (AHI > 5 events/hr) had echocardiographic evidence of increased LV wall thickness. Thus severity of SDB may determine the presence of cardiac functional and structural changes. LV end-diastolic dimension and thickness of interventricular septum are significantly greater in children with SDB compared with control children. Adenotonsillectomy was associated with

a reduction in LV dimension and posterior wall and septal thicknesses. However, pre- and postadenotonsillectomy differences for LV dimension and ventricular septal thickness were not statistically significant.[99] Improvement of LV ejection fraction after treatment of OSA was also described recently.[95] The mechanism of LV hypertrophy in children with OSA is not well understood. Hypoxia-induced activation of the RAS may be linked to cardiac remodeling in patients with SDB.[100] Similarly, the degree of reversibility of abnormal LV geometry after treatment has not been comprehensively examined. In a recent study that included 373 children with and without OSA, diastolic function of the left ventricle was diminished in children with OSA compared with controls.[92] Adenotonsillectomy led to improvement of diastolic function 6 months postoperatively.[92]

Endothelial Dysfunction in SDB

Endothelial dysfunction is associated with cardiovascular morbidity in SDB.[101] Flow-mediated dilatation of the brachial artery is an indirect measure of endothelial dysfunction, which is elevated in SDB and normalized after treatment with continuous positive airway pressure. Endothelin, a marker of endothelial injury, is elevated in

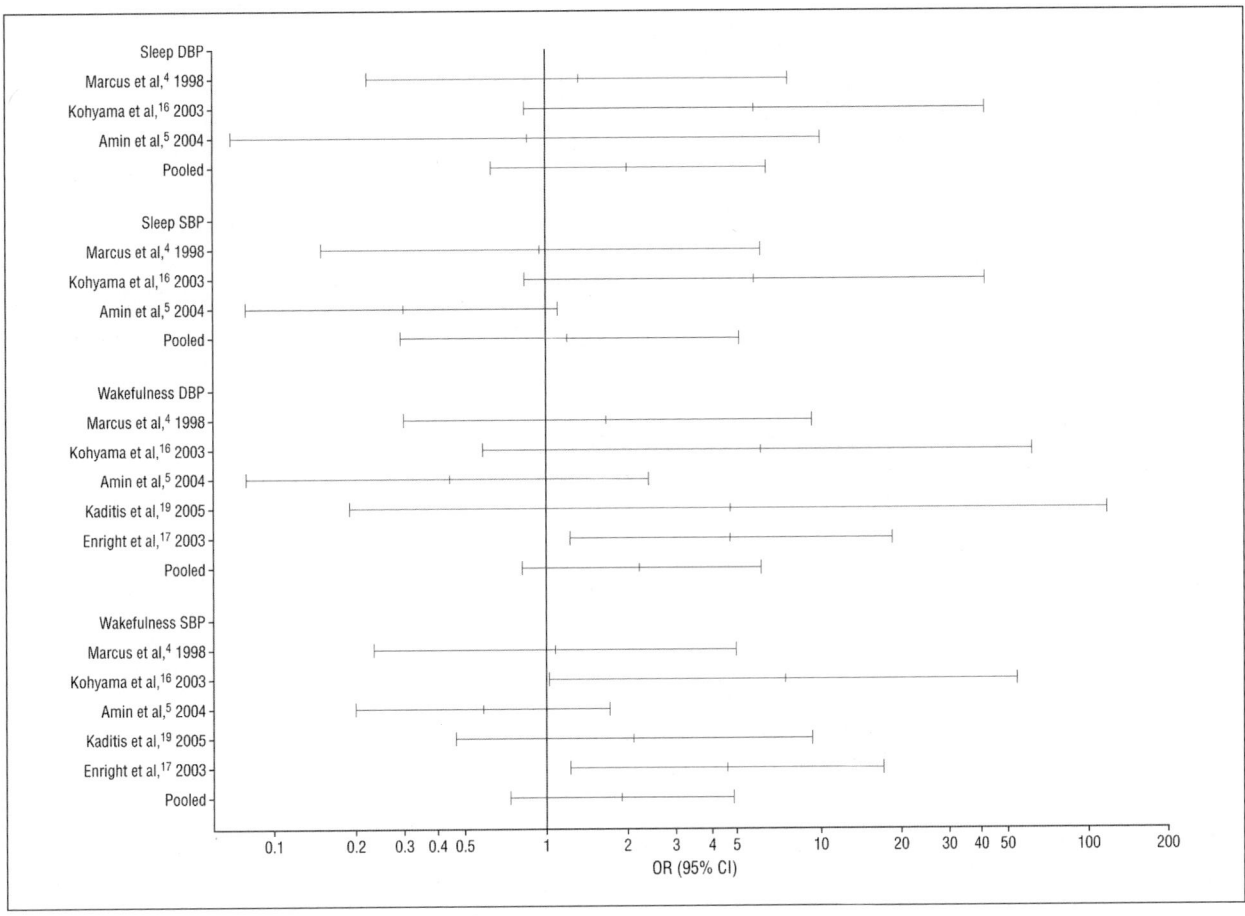

• **Fig. 30.9** Meta-analysis on blood pressure (BP) in children with sleep-disordered breathing (SDB) showing the relationship between severity of SDB and risk of elevated BP. An odds ratio (OR) estimate is given for each study, with the corresponding 95% confidence interval indicated by the error bars. The random-effects pooled ORs are shown. The horizontal axis is plotted on a log scale. Note that there is no evidence showing that moderate to severe SDB in childhood increases the risk of elevated BP.[85] DBP, Diastolic blood pressure; SBP, systolic blood pressure.

SDB.[102,103] The hypoxia, hypercapnia, and pressor surges accompanying obstructive apneic events may serve as potent stimuli for the release of vasoactive substances and an impairment of endothelial function. Elevated levels of endothelin in response to the hypoxemia of SDB may contribute to sustained vasoconstriction and other cardiovascular changes and endothelial dysfunction.[104] Recent study in children with SDB reported that both obesity and OSA can independently increase the risk for endothelial dysfunction, and the concurrence of both markedly increases the risk (Fig. 30.13).[105,106] Mechanisms of endothelial dysfunction in children are not clear. Inflammatory mediators are known to play an important role in vascular injury.[107] Thus elevated inflammatory mediators in children with SDB might be associated with endothelial dysfunction.

Conclusion

Existence of significant cardiovascular dysfunction in pediatric SDB population has been recognized recently. Cardiovascular research in these parents primarily focuses on the comparison of cardiovascular risk factors between children with SDB and controls. Collective evidence in children with SDB, particularly severe forms of SDB, suggests an increase in several established risk factors for cardiovascular disease (CVD). Nevertheless, there are controversies on the level of biomarkers and effectiveness of treatment to reverse the cardiovascular risk. Primary reasons for these controversies are the presence of conditions that also affect cardiovascular risk, such as age, race, body habitus, and socioeconomic conditions. In addition, it is not clear whether differences in those biomarkers will cause any long-term cardiovascular morbidity in children with SDB. There are limited longitudinal studies on the effects of SDB on cardiovascular outcomes in children. A clear understanding of disease mechanisms in SDB known to elicit cardiac and vascular damage may provide a rationale for early intervention to prevent cardiovascular morbidity in childhood and adult life. In the absence of definitive evidence of cardiovascular risk in children with SDB, cautions should be taken for generalized therapeutic intervention to improve cardiovascular outcomes. Thus the benefit of treating SDB in children should be considered on an individualized basis.

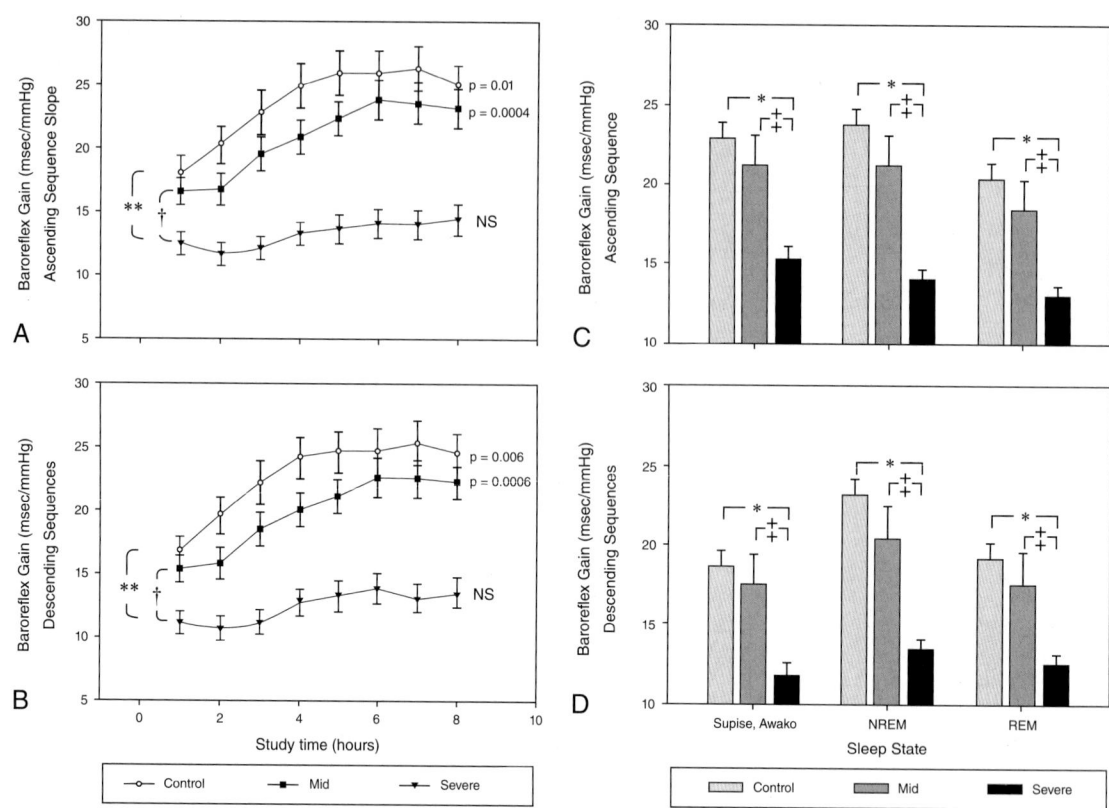

• **Fig. 30.10** Decreased baroreflex sensitivity during awake and sleep in children with sleep-disordered breathing (SDB), particularly evident in children with severe SDB.[31]

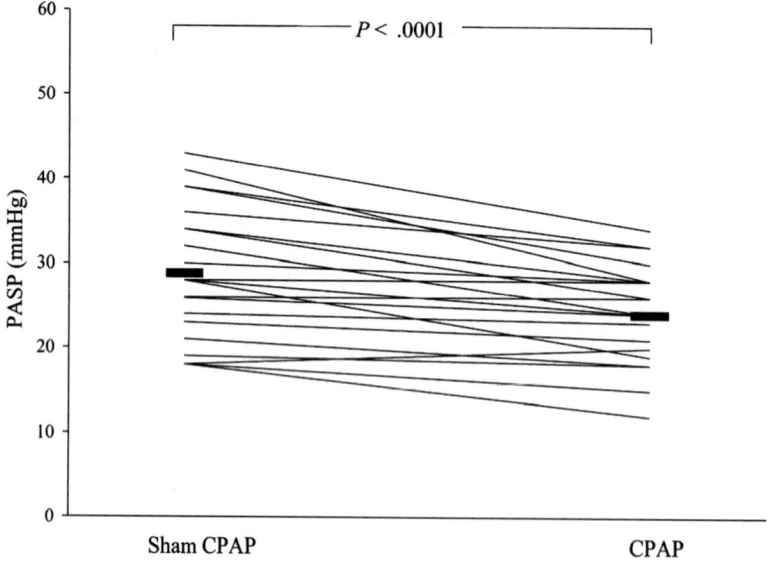

• **Fig. 30.11** Pulmonary artery systolic pressure *(PASP)* measured by Doppler echocardiography before and after 3-month sham treatment or 3-month effective continuous positive airway pressure *(CPAP)* treatment in 21 patients with obstructive sleep apnea. Significant reduction in pulmonary arterial pressure is observed after only 3 months of effective treatment.[91]

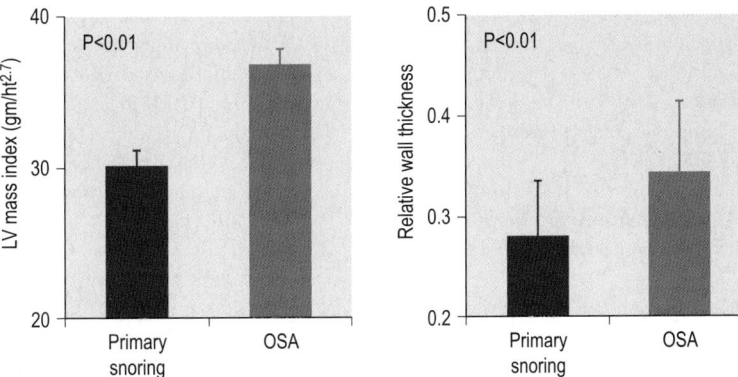

• **Fig. 30.12** Cardiac modeling in children with sleep-disordered breathing. Children with obstructive sleep apnea *(OSA)* have significantly elevated left ventricular *(LV)* mass and relative wall thickness compared with matched children with primary snoring.[94]

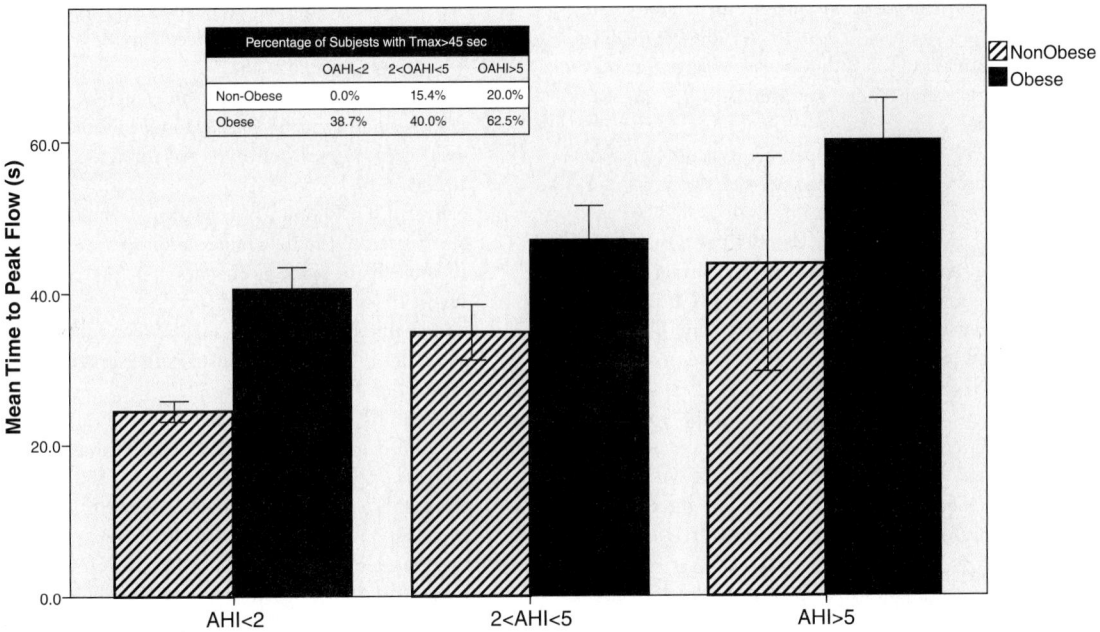

• **Fig. 30.13** Endothelial function in obese and non-obese children with and without obstructive sleep apnea (OSA). Obesity alone, OSA alone, and combination of both obesity and OSA in children are associated with significant endothelial dysfunction.[106]

CLINICAL PEARLS

- Children with severe forms of sleep-disordered breathing (SDB) tend to experience an increase in several established risk factors for cardiovascular disease.
- Increased systemic blood pressure (BP), increased pulmonary BP, cardiac remodeling, and endothelial dysfunction are some of the hypothetical long-term cardiovascular concerns associated with SDB.
- SDB is also associated with altered central nervous system processes (such as the sympathetic nervous system, baroreflexes, and chemoreflexes), which adversely affect both cardiovascular and renal system function.
- Further research is necessary to characterize definitive evidence of the association between cardiovascular risk and SDB in children.

References

1. O'Driscoll DM, Horne RS, Davey MJ, et al. Increased sympathetic activity in children with obstructive sleep apnea: cardiovascular implications. *Sleep Med.* 2011;12(5):483–488.
2. Bhattacharjee R, Kheirandish-Gozal L, Pillar G, Gozal D. Cardiovascular complications of obstructive sleep apnea syndrome: evidence from children. *Prog Cardiovasc Dis.* 2009;51(5):416–433.
3. Kwok KL, Ng DK, Chan CH. Cardiovascular changes in children with snoring and obstructive sleep apnoea. *Ann Acad Med Singapore.* 2008;37(8):715–721.
4. Baharav A, Kotagal S, Rubin BK, Pratt J, Akselrod S. Autonomic cardiovascular control in children with obstructive sleep apnea. *Clin Auton Res.* 1999;9(6):345–351.
5. A Monti, C Medigue, H Nedelcoux, P Escourrou. Autonomic control of the cardiovascular system during sleep in normal subjects. *Eur J Appl Physiol.* 2002;87(2):174–181.

6. Penzel T, Wessel N, Riedl M, et al. Cardiovascular and respiratory dynamics during normal and pathological sleep. *Chaos*. 2007;17(1):015116.

7. Somers VK, Dyken ME, Mark AL, Abboud FM. Sympathetic-nerve activity during sleep in normal subjects [see comments]. *N Engl J Med*. 1993;328(5):303–307.

8. Tilkian AG, Guilleminault C, Schroeder JS, Lehrman KL, Simmons FB, Dement WC. Hemodynamics in sleep-induced apnea. Studies during wakefulness and sleep. *Ann Intern Med*. 1976;85(6):714–719.

9. Somers VK, Dyken ME, Clary MP, Abboud FM. Sympathetic neural mechanisms in obstructive sleep apnea. *J Clin Invest*. 1995;96(4):1897–1904.

10. Morgan BJ. Acute and chronic cardiovascular responses to sleep disordered breathing. *Sleep*. 1996;19(10 Suppl):S206–S209.

11. Sajkov D, Cowie RJ, Thornton AT, Espinoza HA, McEvoy RD. Pulmonary hypertension and hypoxemia in obstructive sleep apnea syndrome. *Am J Respir Crit Care Med*. 1994;149(2 Pt 1):416–422.

12. Shiomi T, Guilleminault C, Stoohs R, Schnittger I. Leftward shift of the interventricular septum and pulsus paradoxus in obstructive sleep apnea syndrome. *Chest*. 1991;100(4):894–902.

13. Stoohs R, Guilleminault C. Cardiovascular changes associated with obstructive sleep apnea syndrome. *J Appl Physiol*. 1992;72(2):583–589.

14. Virolainen J, Ventila M, Turto H, Kupari M. Effect of negative intrathoracic pressure on left ventricular pressure dynamics and relaxation. *J Appl Physiol*. 1995;79(2):455–460.

15. Morgan BJ, Denahan T, Ebert TJ. Neurocirculatory consequences of negative intrathoracic pressure vs. asphyxia during voluntary apnea. *J Appl Physiol*. 1993;74(6):2969–2975.

16. Somers VK, Dyken ME, Skinner JL. Autonomic and hemodynamic responses and interactions during the Mueller maneuver in humans. *J Auton Nerv Syst*. 1993;44(2-3):253–259.

17. Morgan BJ, Crabtree DC, Puleo DS, Badr MS, Toiber F, Skatrud JB. Neurocirculatory consequences of abrupt change in sleep state in humans. *J Appl Physiol*. 1996;80(5):1627–1636.

18. Shamsuzzaman AS, Somers VK. Cardiorespiratory interactions in neural circulatory control in humans. *Ann N Y Acad Sci*. 2001;940:488–499.

19. Guyenet PG. Neural structures that mediate sympathoexcitation during hypoxia. *Respir Physiol*. 2000;121(2-3):147–162.

20. Taylor EW, Jordan D, Coote JH. Central control of the cardiovascular and respiratory systems and their interactions in vertebrates. *Physiol Rev*. 1999;79(3):855–916.

21. Wade JG, Larson CP, Jr, Hickey RF, Ehrenfeld WK, Severinghaus JW. Effect of carotid endarterectomy on carotid chemoreceptor and baroreceptor function in man. *N Engl J Med*. 1970;282(15):823–829.

22. Somers VK, Mark AL, Zavala DC, Abboud FM. Influence of ventilation and hypocapnia on sympathetic nerve responses to hypoxia in normal humans. *J Appl Physiol*. 1989;67(5):2095–2100.

23. Gelfand R, Lambertsen CJ. Dynamic respiratory response to abrupt change of inspired CO2 at normal and high PO2. *J Appl Physiol*. 1973;35(6):903–913.

24. Somers VK, Mark AL, Zavala DC, Abboud FM. Contrasting effects of hypoxia and hypercapnia on ventilation and sympathetic activity in humans. *J Appl Physiol*. 1989;67(5):2101–2106.

25. Semenza GL, Prabhakar NR. The role of hypoxia-inducible factors in carotid body (patho) physiology. *J Physiol*. 2018;596(15):2977–2983.

26. Ferreira CB, Schoorlemmer GH, Rocha AA, Cravo SL. Increased sympathetic responses induced by chronic obstructive sleep apnea are caused by sleep fragmentation. *J Appl Physiol (1985)*. 2020;129(1):163–172.

27. Loredo JS, Clausen JL, Nelesen RA, Ancoli-Israel S, Ziegler MG, Dimsdale JE. Obstructive sleep apnea and hypertension: are peripheral chemoreceptors involved? *Med Hypotheses*. 2001;56(1):17–19.

28. Gauda EB, McLemore GL. Premature birth, homeostatic plasticity and respiratory consequences of inflammation. *Respir Physiol Neurobiol*. 2020;274:103337.

29. Cooper VL, Bowker CM, Pearson SB, Elliott MW, Hainsworth R. Effects of simulated obstructive sleep apnoea on the human carotid baroreceptor-vascular resistance reflex. *J Physiol*. 2004;557(Pt 3):1055–1065.

30. Narkiewicz K, Pesek CA, Kato M, Phillips BG, Davison DE, Somers VK. Baroreflex control of sympathetic nerve activity and heart rate in obstructive sleep apnea. *Hypertension*. 1998;32(6):1039–1043.

31. McConnell K, Somers VK, Kimball T, et al. Baroreflex gain in children with obstructive sleep apnea. *Am J Respir Crit Care Med*. 2009;180(1):42–48.

32. Crisalli JA, McConnell K, Vandyke RD, et al. Baroreflex sensitivity after adenotonsillectomy in children with obstructive sleep apnea during wakefulness and sleep. *Sleep*. 2012;35(10):1335–1343.

33. Heistad DD, Abboud FM, Mark AL, Schmid PG. Interaction of baroreceptor and chemoreceptor reflexes. Modulation of the chemoreceptor reflex by changes in baroreceptor activity. *J Clin Invest*. 1974;53(5):1226–1236.

34. Kronsbein H, Gerlach DA, Heusser K, et al. Testing individual baroreflex responses to hypoxia-induced peripheral chemoreflex stimulation. *Clin Auton Res*. 2020.

35. Halliwill JR, Morgan BJ, Charkoudian N. Peripheral chemoreflex and baroreflex interactions in cardiovascular regulation in humans. *J Physiol*. 2003;552(Pt 1):295–302.

36. Somers VK, Dyken ME, Mark AL, Abboud FM. Parasympathetic hyperresponsiveness and bradyarrhythmias during apnoea in hypertension. *Clin Auton Res*. 1992;2(3):171–176.

37. Cooper VL, Pearson SB, Bowker CM, Elliott MW, Hainsworth R. Interaction of chemoreceptor and baroreceptor reflexes by hypoxia and hypercapnia—a mechanism for promoting hypertension in obstructive sleep apnoea. *J Physiol*. 2005;568 (Pt 2):677–687.

38. Gianaros PJ, Onyewuenyi IC, Sheu LK, Christie IC, Critchley HD. Brain systems for baroreflex suppression during stress in humans. *Hum Brain Mapp*. 2012;33(7):1700–1716.

39. Netzer F, Bernard JF, Verberne AJ, et al. Brain circuits mediating baroreflex bradycardia inhibition in rats: an anatomical and functional link between the cuneiform nucleus and the periaqueductal grey. *J Physiol*. 2011;589(Pt 8):2079–2091.

40. DiFrancesco MW, Shamsuzzaman A, McConnell KB, et al. Age-related changes in baroreflex sensitivity and cardiac autonomic tone in children mirrored by regional brain gray matter volume trajectories. *Pediatr Res*. 2018;83(2):498–505.

41. Harshfield GA, Pulliam DA, Alpert BS, Stapleton FB, Willey ES, Somes GW. Ambulatory blood pressure patterns in children and adolescents: influence of renin-sodium profiles. *Pediatrics*. 1991;87(1):94–100.

42. Foster GE, Hanly PJ, Ahmed SB, Beaudin AE, Pialoux V, Poulin MJ. Intermittent hypoxia increases arterial blood pressure in

humans through a renin-angiotensin system–dependent mechanism. *Hypertension*. 2010;56(3):369–377.

43. Ip SP, Chan YW, Leung PS. Effects of chronic hypoxia on the circulating and pancreatic renin-angiotensin system. *Pancreas*. 2002;25(3):296–300.

44. Barcelo A, Elorza MA, Barbe F, Santos C, Mayoralas LR, Agusti AG. Angiotensin converting enzyme in patients with sleep apnoea syndrome: plasma activity and gene polymorphisms. *Eur Respir J*. 2001;17(4):728–732.

45. Dudenbostel T, Calhoun DA. Resistant hypertension, obstructive sleep apnoea and aldosterone. *J Hum Hypertens*. 2012;26(5):281–287.

46. Di Murro A, Petramala L, Cotesta D, et al. Renin-angiotensin-aldosterone system in patients with sleep apnoea: prevalence of primary aldosteronism. *J Renin Angiotensin Aldosterone Syst*. 2010;11(3):165–172.

47. Jin ZN, Wei YX. Meta-analysis of effects of obstructive sleep apnea on the renin-angiotensin-aldosterone system. *J Geriatr Cardiol*. 2016;13(4):333–343.

48. Shamsuzzaman A, Szczesniak RD, Fenchel MC, Amin RS. Plasma renin levels and renin-blood pressure relationship in normal-weight and overweight children with obstructive sleep apnea and matched controls. *Sleep Med*. 2015;16(1):101–106.

49. Gozal D, Kheirandish-Gozal L. Cardiovascular morbidity in obstructive sleep apnea: oxidative stress, inflammation, and much more. *Am J Respir Crit Care Med*. 2008;177(4):369–375.

50. Danesh J, Whincup P, Walker M, et al. Low grade inflammation and coronary heart disease: prospective study and updated meta-analyses. *BMJ*. 2000;321(7255):199–204.

51. Smith SCJr, Anderson JL, Cannon 3rd RO, et al. CDC/AHA Workshop on markers of inflammation and cardiovascular disease: application to clinical and public health practice: report from the clinical practice discussion group. *Circulation*. 2004;110(25):e550–e553.

52. Dyugovskaya L, Lavie P, Hirsh M, Lavie L. Activated CD8+ T-lymphocytes in obstructive sleep apnoea. *Eur Respir J*. 2005;25(5):820–828.

53. Venugopal SK, Devaraj S, Yuhanna I, Shaul P, Jialal I. Demonstration that C-reactive protein decreases eNOS expression and bioactivity in human aortic endothelial cells. *Circulation*. 2002;106(12):1439–1441.

54. Woollard KJ, Phillips DC, Griffiths HR. Direct modulatory effect of C-reactive protein on primary human monocyte adhesion to human endothelial cells. *Clin Exp Immunol*. 2002;130(2):256–262.

55. Smith DF, Hossain MM, Hura A, et al. Inflammatory milieu and cardiovascular homeostasis in children with obstructive sleep apnea. *Sleep*. 2017;40(4).

56. Larkin EK, Rosen CL, Kirchner HL, et al. Variation of C-reactive protein levels in adolescents: association with sleep-disordered breathing and sleep duration. *Circulation*. 2005;111(15):1978–1984.

57. Guilleminault C, Li KK, Khramtsov A, Pelayo R, Martinez S. Sleep disordered breathing: surgical outcomes in prepubertal children. *Laryngoscope*. 2004;114(1):132–137.

58. Kaditis AG, Alexopoulos EI, Kalampouka E, et al. Morning levels of C-reactive protein in children with obstructive sleep-disordered breathing. *Am J Respir Crit Care Med*. 2005;171(3):282–286.

59. Dusser DJ, Djokic TD, Borson DB, Nadel JA. Cigarette smoke induces bronchoconstrictor hyperresponsiveness to substance P and inactivates airway neutral endopeptidase in the guinea pig. Possible role of free radicals. *J Clin Invest*. 1989;84(3):900–906.

60. Li AM, Hung E, Tsang T, et al. Induced sputum inflammatory measures correlate with disease severity in children with obstructive sleep apnoea. *Thorax*. 2007;62(1):75–79.

61. Boyd JH, Petrof BJ, Hamid Q, Fraser R, Kimoff RJ. Upper airway muscle inflammation and denervation changes in obstructive sleep apnea. *Am J Respir Crit Care Med*. 2004;170(5):541-6.

62. Kirkness JP, Madronio M, Stavrinou R, Wheatley JR, Amis TC. Surface tension of upper airway mucosal lining liquid in obstructive sleep apnea/hypopnea syndrome. *Sleep*. 2005;28(4):457–463.

63. Kirkness JP, Madronio M, Stavrinou R, Wheatley JR, Amis TC. Relationship between surface tension of upper airway lining liquid and upper airway collapsibility during sleep in obstructive sleep apnea hypopnea syndrome. *J Appl Physiol*. 2003;95(5):1761–1766.

64. Dean RT, Wilcox I. Possible atherogenic effects of hypoxia during obstructive sleep apnea. *Sleep*. 1993;16(8 Suppl):S15–S21. discussion S-2.

65. Halliwell B. The role of oxygen radicals in human disease, with particular reference to the vascular system. *Haemostasis*. 1993;23(Suppl 1):118–126.

66. Schulz R, Mahmoudi S, Hattar K, et al. Enhanced release of superoxide from polymorphonuclear neutrophils in obstructive sleep apnea. Impact of continuous positive airway pressure therapy. *Am J Respir Crit Care Med*. 2000;162(2 Pt 1):566–570.

67. Kim J, Bhattacharjee R, Kheirandish-Gozal L, Spruyt K, Gozal D. Circulating microparticles in children with sleep disordered breathing. *Chest*. 2011;140(2):408–417.

68. Sanner BM, Konermann M, Tepel M, Groetz J, Mummenhoff C, Zidek W. Platelet function in patients with obstructive sleep apnoea syndrome. *Eur Respir J*. 2000;16(4):648–652.

69. Kaditis AG, Alexopoulos EI, Kalampouka E, et al. Morning levels of fibrinogen in children with sleep-disordered breathing. *Eur Respir J*. 2004;24(5):790–797.

70. Chin K, Ohi M, Kita H, et al. Effects of NCPAP therapy on fibrinogen levels in obstructive sleep apnea syndrome. *Am J Respir Crit Care Med*. 1996;153(6 Pt 1):1972–1976.

71. Malakasioti G, Alexopoulos E, Befani C, et al. Oxidative stress and inflammatory markers in the exhaled breath condensate of children with OSA. *Sleep Breath*. 2012;16(3):703–708.

72. Dogruer ZN, Unal M, Eskandari G, et al. Malondialdehyde and antioxidant enzymes in children with obstructive adenotonsillar hypertrophy. *Clin Biochem*. 2004;37(8):718–721.

73. Redline S, Storfer-Isser A, Rosen CL, et al. Association between metabolic syndrome and sleep-disordered breathing in adolescents. *Am J Respir Crit Care Med*. 2007;176(4):401–408.

74. Hannon TS, Lee S, Chakravorty S, Lin Y, Arslanian SA. Sleep-disordered breathing in obese adolescents is associated with visceral adiposity and markers of insulin resistance. *Int J Pediatr Obes*. 2011;6(2):157–160.

75. Li AM, Chan MH, Chan DF, et al. Insulin and obstructive sleep apnea in obese Chinese children. *Pediatr Pulmonol*. 2006;41(12):1175–1181.

76. Vgontzas AN, Papanicolaou DA, Bixler EO, et al. Sleep apnea and daytime sleepiness and fatigue: relation to visceral obesity, insulin resistance, and hypercytokinemia. *J Clin Endocrinol Metab*. 2000;85(3):1151–1158.

77. Deboer MD, Mendoza JP, Liu L, Ford G, Yu PL, Gaston BM. Increased systemic inflammation overnight correlates with

insulin resistance among children evaluated for obstructive sleep apnea. *Sleep Breath.* 2012;16(2):349–354.

78. Elmasry A, Lindberg E, Berne C, et al. Sleep-disordered breathing and glucose metabolism in hypertensive men: a population-based study. *J Intern Med.* 2001;249(2):153–161.

79. Siriwat R, Wang L, Shah V, Mehra R, Ibrahim S. Obstructive sleep apnea and insulin resistance in children with obesity. *J Clin Sleep Med.* 2020;16(7):1081–1090.

80. Weber SA, Santos VJ, Semenzati Gde O, Martin LC. Ambulatory blood pressure monitoring in children with obstructive sleep apnea and primary snoring. *Int J Pediatr Otorhinolaryngol.* 2012;76(6):787–790.

81. Amin R, Somers VK, McConnell K, et al. Activity-adjusted 24-hour ambulatory blood pressure and cardiac remodeling in children with sleep disordered breathing. *Hypertension.* 2008;51(1):84–91.

82. Xu Z, Li B, Shen K. Ambulatory blood pressure monitoring in chinese children with obstructive sleep apnea/hypopnea syndrome. *Pediatr Pulmonol.* 2012

83. Leung LC, Ng DK, Lau MW, et al. Twenty-four-hour ambulatory BP in snoring children with obstructive sleep apnea syndrome. *Chest.* 2006;130(4):1009–1017.

84. Ng DK, Leung LC, Chan CH. Blood pressure in children with sleep-disordered breathing. *Am J Respir Crit Care Med.* 2004;170(4):467. author reply -8.

85. Zintzaras E, Kaditis AG. Sleep-disordered breathing and blood pressure in children: a meta-analysis. *Arch Pediatr Adolesc Med.* 2007;161(2):172–178.

86. Ng DK, Wong JC, Chan CH, Leung LC, Leung SY. Ambulatory blood pressure before and after adenotonsillectomy in children with obstructive sleep apnea. *Sleep Med.* 2010;11(7):721–725.

87. Brown OE, Manning SC, Ridenour B. Cor pulmonale secondary to tonsillar and adenoidal hypertrophy: management considerations. *Int J Pediatr Otorhinolaryngol.* 1988;16(2):131–139.

88. Wilkinson AR, McCormick MS, Freeland AP, Pickering D. Electrocardiographic signs of pulmonary hypertension in children who snore. *Br Med J (Clin Res Ed).* 1981;282(6276):1579–1581.

89. Li AM, Hui S, Wong E, Cheung A, Fok TF. Obstructive sleep apnoea in children with adenotonsillar hypertrophy: prospective study. *Hong Kong Med J.* 2001;7(3):236–240.

90. Miman MC, Kirazli T, Ozyurek R. Doppler echocardiography in adenotonsillar hypertrophy. *Int J Pediatr Otorhinolaryngol.* 2000;54(1):21–26.

91. Arias MA, Garcia-Rio F, Alonso-Fernandez A, Martinez I, Villamor J. Pulmonary hypertension in obstructive sleep apnoea: effects of continuous positive airway pressure: a randomized, controlled cross-over study. *Eur Heart J.* 2006;27(9):1106–1113.

92. Maloney MA, Ward SLD, Su JA, et al. Prevalence of pulmonary hypertension on echocardiogram in children with severe obstructive sleep apnea. *J Clin Sleep Med.* 2022;18(6):1629–1637.

93. Hunt CE, Brouillette RT. Abnormalities of breathing control and airway maintenance in infants and children as a cause of cor pulmonale. *Pediatr Cardiol.* 1982;3(3):249–256.

94. Amin RS, Kimball TR, Bean JA, et al. Left ventricular hypertrophy and abnormal ventricular geometry in children and adolescents with obstructive sleep apnea. *Am J Respir Crit Care Med.* 2002;165(10):1395–1399.

95. Amin RS, Kimball TR, Kalra M, et al. Left ventricular function in children with sleep-disordered breathing. *Am J Cardiol.* 2005;95(6):801–804.

96. Duman D, Naiboglu B, Esen HS, Toros SZ, Demirtunc R. Impaired right ventricular function in adenotonsillar hypertrophy. *Int J Cardiovas Imaging.* 2008;24(3):261–267.

97. Kaditis AG, Alexopoulos EI, Hatzi F, et al. Overnight change in brain natriuretic peptide levels in children with sleep-disordered breathing. *Chest.* 2006;130(5):1377–1384.

98. Sans Capdevila O, Crabtree VM, Kheirandish-Gozal L, Gozal D. Increased morning brain natriuretic peptide levels in children with nocturnal enuresis and sleep-disordered breathing: a community-based study. *Pediatrics.* 2008;121(5):e1208–e1214.

99. Gorur K, Doven O, Unal M, Akkus N, Ozcan C. Preoperative and postoperative cardiac and clinical findings of patients with adenotonsillar hypertrophy. *Int J Pediatr Otorhinolaryngol.* 2001;59(1):41–46.

100. Miwa Y, Sasaguri T. Hypoxia-induced cardiac remodeling in sleep apnea syndrome: involvement of the renin-angiotensin-aldosterone system. *Hypertens Res.* 2007;30(12):1147–1149.

101. Lavie L. Sleep apnea syndrome, endothelial dysfunction, and cardiovascular morbidity. *Sleep.* 2004;27(6):1053–1055.

102. Phillips BG, Narkiewicz K, Pesek CA, Haynes WG, Dyken ME, Somers VK. Effects of obstructive sleep apnea on endothelin-1 and blood pressure. *J Hypertens.* 1999;17(1):61–66.

103. Grimpen F, Kanne P, Schulz E, Hagenah G, Hasenfuss G, Andreas S. Endothelin-1 plasma levels are not elevated in patients with obstructive sleep apnoea. *Eur Respir J.* 2000;15(2):320–325.

104. Allen SW, Chatfield BA, Koppenhafer SA, Schaffer MS, Wolfe RR, Abman SH. Circulating immunoreactive endothelin-1 in children with pulmonary hypertension. Association with acute hypoxic pulmonary vasoreactivity. *Am Rev Respir Dis.* 1993;148(2):519–522.

105. Bhattacharjee R, Alotaibi WH, Kheirandish-Gozal L, Capdevila OS, Gozal D. Endothelial dysfunction in obese non-hypertensive children without evidence of sleep disordered breathing. *BMC Pediatr.* 2010;108

106. Bhattacharjee R, Kim J, Alotaibi WH, Kheirandish-Gozal L, Capdevila OS, Gozal D. Endothelial dysfunction in children without hypertension: potential contributions of obesity and obstructive sleep apnea. *Chest.* 2012;141(3):682–691.

107. Gozal D, Kheirandish-Gozal L, Serpero LD, Sans Capdevila O, Dayyat E. Obstructive sleep apnea and endothelial function in school-aged nonobese children: effect of adenotonsillectomy. *Circulation.* 2007;116(20):2307–2314.

31

Metabolic Consequences of Sleep-Disordered Breathing

David Gozal

CHAPTER HIGHLIGHTS

- The prevalence of childhood obesity is increasing worldwide at an alarming rate – ranging from 12-22% depending on age range.
- Sleep duration and regularity are compromised in the setting of childhood obesity with short sleep and obstructive sleep apnea as some of the common sleep-related comorbidities.
- There is a bi-directional relationship between obstructive sleep apnea and obesity as obesity is a risk factor for obstructive sleep apnea and obstructive sleep apnea may promote obesity and associated metabolic consequences including dyslipidemia, abnormal insulin sensitivity, increased systemic blood pressure elevations, liver dysfunction, and metabolic syndrome.

Introduction

Epidemiologic studies over the last several decades have conclusively demonstrated that both the prevalence and severity of being overweight and obese in children and adolescents have clearly been increasing worldwide, even if some deceleration in such trends has emerged more recently, possibly as the result of public health campaigns aiming to curb the alarming rates of obesity in childhood.[1–4] Indeed, reported obesity prevalence was 12.7% among 2- to 5-year-olds, 20.7% among 6- to 11-year-olds, and 22.2% among 12- to 19-year-olds.[5–8] Childhood obesity is also more common among certain populations, particularly underserved communities.

Indeed obesity prevalence was reported by the Centers for Disease Control and Prevention (CDC) as 26.2% among Hispanic children, 24.8% among non-Hispanic Black children, 16.6% among non-Hispanic White children, and 9.0% among non-Hispanic Asian children (https://www.cdc.gov/obesity/data/childhood.html; accessed last on May 19th, 2022). A major consequence of this obesity epidemic has been the concomitant increase in the prevalence of obesity-associated morbidities, and previously infrequent conditions such as metabolic syndrome, cardiovascular disease, non-alcoholic liver steatosis, depression, and decreased quality of life, which have all begun to emerge, even among the youngest of the children.[9–12]

Sleep Curtailment, Irregular Sleep, and Obesity

The increasingly demanding life pace of technology-driven societies has radically changed the way we sleep, as well as the way our children sleep. Over a period of 100 years or so, the overall duration of sleep in children has steadily declined.[13–15] Although the reasons underlying these trends in sleep curtailment are multifactorial,[16–18] reductions in sleep duration have also been accompanied by increased irregularity in sleep schedules. There is now compelling evidence linking the progressive decrements in sleep duration and sleep regularity to the reciprocal increases observed in the prevalence of childhood obesity.[19–28] However, the associations between obesity and sleep have not been consistently reported by all studies,[29] raising the possibility that the current definitions of short sleep and insufficient sleep are quite arbitrary, and therefore operate as a confounder rather than a true causal pathway.[30–32] Furthermore, additional confounding factors that play a role in the propensity for obesity may begin in early life,[33] such that extrication of the role of sleep may not be trivial. In a cross-sectional and longitudinal study, Chaput and collaborators reported that only those subjects who exhibited the combination of short sleep duration, highly disinhibited eating behaviors, and low dietary calcium intake had significantly higher body mass index (BMI).[34] Based on the previously mentioned considerations, it is clear that intervention trials aiming to establish whether restoration of sleep quality and quantity will ameliorate metabolic and ponderal indices in children are needed.[35–43] It is also noteworthy that sleep-associated changes in BMI appear to be primarily affecting those children whose BMI is already elevated.[44]

Some of the putative biologic pathways linking sleep duration and regularity to obesity clearly involve alterations in some of the neuropeptides that regulate appetite both peripherally and centrally. In addition, the contribution of perturbations in circadian timing cannot be overlooked.[45] For example, increased levels of ghrelin, reduced levels of leptin, and reduced central biologic activity of orexin have all been identified in experimental sleep restriction paradigms, and will lead to increased food intake, and reduced satiety.[46,47] Furthermore, disruptions of the circadian clock have been implicated in perturbations within a complex network of metabolic pathways that not only affect regulatory central nervous system (CNS) regions such as in the hypothalamus, but also alter metabolic processes in peripheral tissues.[48,49]

Unfortunately, in-depth exploration of these pathways in the context of childhood is almost completely lacking; furthermore, we should keep in mind that both sleep duration and body weight trajectory are determined by a multitude of factors, such as sociodemographic, socioeconomic, familial, or genetic (e.g., family structure, overweight parent) and individual (e.g., health behavior, physical activity, health status, stress levels) factors (Fig. 31.1).[50–52] Regardless, we need to be cognizant that obese children are 1.5- to 2-fold (odds ratios

ranging from 1.15–11) more likely of being short sleepers,[53,54] and that any interventions seeking to modify sleep patterns in children are less likely to succeed if implemented later in childhood, because both sleep regularity and sleep duration are consistently preserved across long periods of time, even in children.[55] Thus, sleep interventions need to be implemented early in life; therefore identification of which children are at risk during infancy and early childhood is essential before any prospective interventions to prolong and regularize sleep are implemented. Such interventional studies are clearly required to delineate the potentially causal role of sleep in the context of BMI regulation and metabolic homeostasis.

Obesity as a Risk Factor of Obstructive Sleep Apnea

Since the early descriptions of obstructive sleep apnea (OSA) in the pediatric age range, a clear change has occurred, with a majority of the patients being evaluated in most pediatric sleep centers fulfilling the criteria for being either overweight

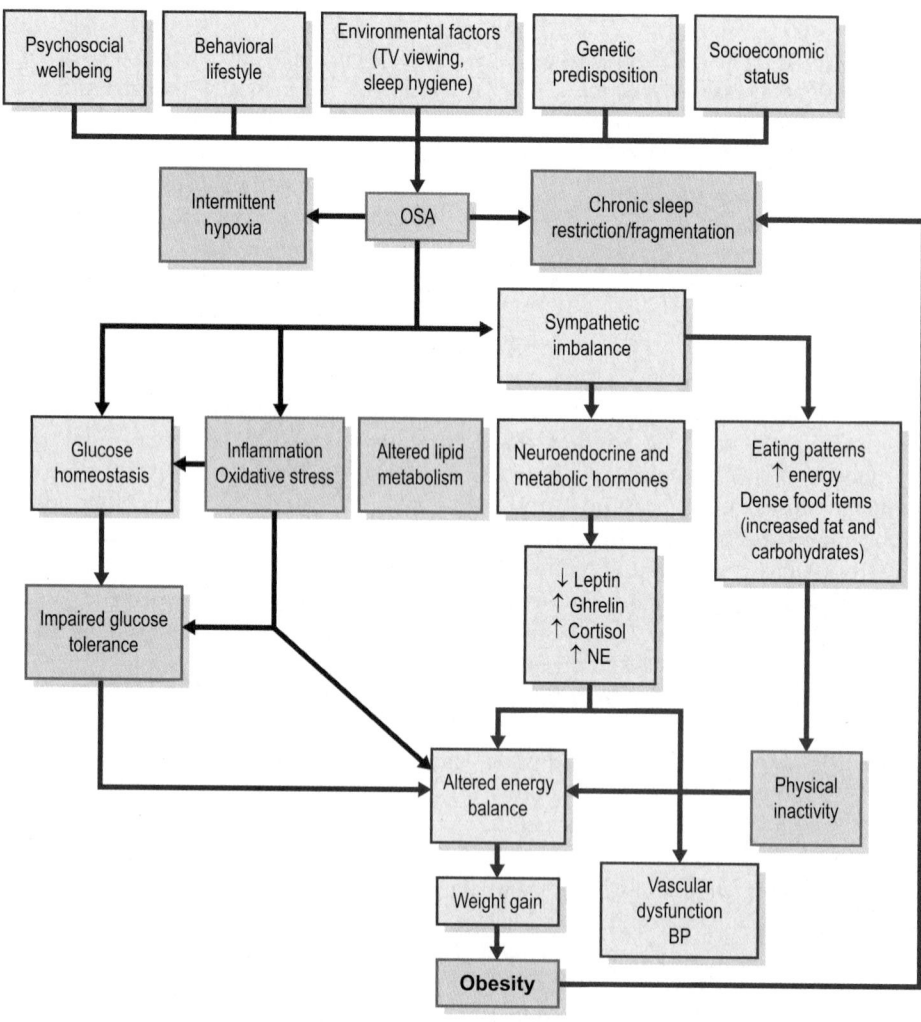

• **Fig. 31.1** Schematic diagram illustrating the potential interactions between sleep, obstructive sleep apnea, obesity, and metabolic dysfunction in children. BP, Blood pressure; NE, norepinephrine; OSA, obstructive sleep apnea.

or obese.[56] This is not surprising, considering that the risk of OSA in obese children is markedly increased.[57] In a case-control study design, Redline and colleagues examined risk factors for sleep-disordered breathing in children aged 2–18 years, and found that the risk among obese children was increased 4- to 5-fold.[58] In fact, for every increment in BMI by 1 kg/m[2] beyond the mean BMI for age and gender, the risk of OSA syndrome (OSAS) increased by 12%. Similar trends demonstrating increased risk of OSA among obese and overweight children have been consistently reported in many countries.[59–68] A community-based study exploring the risk of OSA in a non-referral cohort of obese children in Spain revealed a prevalence of OSA in the 30–40% range contingent upon the criteria used.[69]

The frequent presence of upper airway narrowing in obese children could result from fatty infiltration of upper airway structures and tongue, whereas subcutaneous fat deposits in the anterior neck region and other cervical structures will undoubtedly contribute and exert collapsing forces promoting increased pharyngeal collapsibility.[70,71] Interestingly, Arens and collaborators have shown that obese children exhibit enlarged lymphadenoid tissues in the upper airway, the latter potentially reflecting the result of systemic low-grade inflammatory processes that accompany the obese state.[72,73] Obesity may also affect lung volumes through mass loading of the respiratory system,[74] and increased adipose tissue deposition in the abdominal and thoracic walls and around the viscera will increase the overall respiratory load, and reduce intrathoracic volumes and diaphragmatic excursion, particularly when in the supine position. Thus, obesity will lead to decreased lung volumes and oxygen reserve and will augment the work of breathing during sleep.

Obesity is also associated with peripheral and central leptin tissue resistance, resulting in reduced biologic effectiveness despite elevation of circulating leptin levels.[75–77] The unique properties of leptin as a potent respiratory stimulant with both central and peripheral chemoreceptor modulatory properties are therefore markedly dampened by the emergence of leptin resistance, and may precipitate the gradual onset of attenuated respiratory reflexes, particularly during sleep.[78,79] Obesity can be accompanied by fragmented sleep that will progressively increase the arousal threshold, thereby potentially aggravating the duration of upper airway obstruction events.[80]

Obstructive Sleep Apnea May Promote Obesity and Its Consequences

Although there is currently only incipient evidence, it is plausible to assume that the presence of OSA could promote or aggravate obesity or its consequences (see Fig. 31.1). This concept has developed in recent years whereby the presence of OSA would promote weight gain and obesity, via sleep fragmentation and associated daytime sleepiness.[81–84] The presence of sleepiness is likely to reduce overall daily physical activity,[85] particularly in those children at risk for obesity.

In addition, the degree of daytime sleepiness resulting from OSA is amplified in obese children.[86]

Similar to obesity, OSA should now be viewed as a low-grade systemic inflammatory disease, and the coexistence of obesity and OSA further exacerbates the magnitude of the inflammatory responses.[87–92] Thus, OSA is viewed as a major risk factor for development of metabolic syndrome in children (see also Chapter 18).

Obstructive Sleep Apnea Potentiates Alterations in Serum Lipids in Children

In a large series of studies in adult patients, OSA has been identified as a risk factor for dyslipidemia and insulin resistance.[93–95] However, because most adult OSA patients are obese, it is nearly impossible to determine the exact contribution of OSA on lipid metabolism.

The evidence in children linking OSA to lipid alterations is relatively scarce. In a study of 135 children (many of them obese), no associations emerged between polysomnographic indices of OSA severity and fasting serum lipids, even though strong association was apparent between BMI and lipid levels.[96] Verhulst and coworkers[97] showed significant correlations between the degree of oxyhemoglobin desaturation (but not the respiratory disturbance index) and serum lipid and cholesterol levels among 104 relatively older obese children (42% post-pubertal), even when controlling for gender, puberty, and body mass index. In a retrospective study of Greek children evaluated for suspected OSA, Alexopoulos and colleagues[98] reported that the risk of low high-density lipoprotein (HDL) cholesterol was 3-fold higher in non-obese children with moderate to severe OSA compared with those children with mild OSA or primary snoring. In a prospective cohort study of adolescents recruited from the general community, Redline and colleagues[99] reported a 6-fold increase in the risk for developing metabolic syndrome in those individuals with OSA. Furthermore, OSA in these adolescent subjects was closely associated with serum low-density lipoprotein (LDL) concentrations. In a more recent study, Zong and collaborators further confirmed the existence of putative inverse associations between HDL cholesterol and apnea-hypopnea index (AHI) in a small cohort of 44 children in China.[100]

In a prospective study of 62 consecutive prepubertal obese and non-obese children with OSA, surgical adenotonsillectomy resulted in improvements of OSA in all children, but normalization of the respiratory disturbances during sleep occurred only in a fraction. In non-obese children, surgical removal of adenoids and tonsils led to significant improvements in LDL, HDL, and LDL/HDH levels, and overall similar findings occurred in obese children with OSA after treatment, in the absence of any significant changes in BMI. These findings suggest that the improvements in serum lipids can be ascribed to OSA rather than obesity. Apolipoprotein B serum levels were improved in both non-obese and obese groups following surgery, and all lipids were correlated with measures of OSA severity.[101] In more recent studies focused on non-obese children with OSA, significant associations emerged with a large number of recognized cardiometabolic risk factors. Indeed, in a study on 128 school-age children (mean age 9.7 ± 3.4 years) diagnosed with OSA and 213 controls (mean age 9.5 ± 3.4 years) significant associations between inflammation markers and OSA severity indicators were found along with increased transaminase, glucose, uric acid, and insulin levels when compared with healthy children.[102] Similarly, in a study from South Korea that included 273 participants of all ages (ages 0–18 years), obesity was strongly associated with OSA severity, and HDL cholesterol levels were significantly lower in the OSA group irrespective of the presence of obesity, even after adjusting for body mass index.[103] Together, these findings strongly support that disrupted sleep and episodic hypoxia in the context of OSAS impose substantial changes in lipid regulatory mechanisms in children.

Because not every child with OSA will manifest alterations in serum lipids, it is possible that genetic factors may contribute. To examine this issue, Bhushan and colleagues[104] assessed gene variants in the fatty acid-binding protein 4 (FABP4) gene, which plays a major role in inflammation and metabolism, particularly in the regulation of the intracellular processing of lipids in critical tissues such as adipose tissues and macrophages. Children with OSA had elevated concentrations of FABP4 in plasma, and the presence of the rs1054135 polymorphism in the FABP4 gene was associated with elevated levels of FABP4 and serum lipids, even after adjustment of BMI, suggesting that genetic predisposition may contribute to impaired lipid homeostasis in children with OSA.

Obstructive Sleep Apnea Adversely Affects Insulin Sensitivity

In 110 non-obese children, Kaditis and colleagues[105] found no correlations between the severity of OSAS and fasting insulin or homeostatic model assessment (HOMA) levels, with serum lipids not being reported. However, most other studies have found that OSA imposes independent alterations on insulin sensitivity, particularly if obesity is present.[101] In a small cohort of obese Latino males, the presence of OSA with corresponding sleep fragmentation and intermittent hypoxemia was associated with metabolic impairments manifesting as increased insulin resistance.[106] Similar results were reported by Canapari and coworkers who also pointed out the importance of visceral fat mass in the associations between OSA and insulin resistance.[107]

Obstructive Sleep Apnea Imposes Increased Risk for Systemic Blood Pressure Elevations

See Chapter 30.

Obstructive Sleep Apnea and Non-Alcoholic Hepatic Steatosis

The potential adverse effects of OSA on liver function, particularly when underlying obesity is present, have

been critically explored by Mirrakhimov and Polotsky in a murine model.[108] In a study from our laboratory, we showed that the prevalence of elevated liver enzymes in serum of obese patients was significantly higher if OSA was concurrently present, and that effective treatment of OSA ameliorated liver function tests, indicating that sleep-disordered breathing may serve as a catalyst of non-alcoholic hepatic steatosis via its oxidant stress and inflammatory effects.[109] Similar findings were subsequently reported in another study.[110]

Obstructive Sleep Apnea and Metabolic Syndrome

From the individually analyzed effects of OSA described earlier, it becomes apparent that when obesity is present, the risk for developing metabolic syndrome is markedly exacerbated by the concurrent presence of OSA. [101,111–119] However, although the bidirectional interactions between OSAS and obesity appear to be irrefutable, well-controlled interventional trials aiming to assess the implications of treating one of the disorders to ameliorate the other have yet to be conducted. There is now little doubt that the usual treatment of OSA, i.e., surgical adenotonsillectomy, is associated with a much higher failure rate in obese children,[120,121] and initial encouraging studies would suggest that weight loss promotes beneficial effects on OSA severity as well as on metabolic function.[122,123] Indeed, in a study in Brazil, 76 adolescents with obesity were recruited and underwent a 9- to 12-month diet and exercise intervention.[123] OSA was associated with increased insulin resistance and higher blood pressure without any detectable effects on lipid profiles. Implementation of the dietary and exercise lifestyle intervention was effective in decreasing metabolic risk whether or not the respiratory disturbance was corrected. In another study in our group, Koren and collaborators[124] evaluated 69 young children (mean age 6 years and 70% non-obese) with OSA. The children underwent baseline overnight polysomnography, anthropometric and metabolic measurements, adenotonsillectomy, and follow-up testing after an average of 8 months after surgery. Surgical adenotonsillectomy improved insulin resistance and led to increases in HDL cholesterol levels. If residual OSA was present, it was predicted by BMI Z-score and fasting insulin levels. If insulin levels after surgery remained elevated, they were associated with obesity measures rather than with measures of sleep-disordered breathing. It is important, however, to emphasize that clinical diagnosis of metabolic syndrome in children and adolescents should be viewed preferentially as a conceptual framework for detection of risk factors centered around obesity and insulin resistance rather than considered as a syndrome that is defined by absolute "all-or-none" specific criteria.[125]

Together, the deleterious interplay between obesity and OSA on metabolic function needs to be viewed as an extremely concerning consequence of these two conditions, particularly in the context of the potentially long-term effects that can ensue.[126,127]

CLINICAL PEARLS

- Alterations in sleep patterns and duration may contribute to the increased prevalence and severity of obesity in children and adolescents.
- OSA and obesity interact to increase the severity and morbid consequences of each other, possibly via their shared effects on the recruitment and potentiation of inflammatory pathways.
- Not every child with OSA will manifest metabolic dysfunction, suggesting that genetic and environmental factors may also play a role.
- Randomized, controlled intervention trials are urgently needed to more conclusively delineate the causative roles played by sleep and OSA in metabolic function in children and adolescents.

References

1. Magarey AM, Daniels LA, Boulton TJ. Prevalence of overweight and obesity in Australian children and adolescents: Reassessment of 1985 and 1995 data against new standard international definitions. *Med J Aust.* 2001;174:561–564.
2. Lobstein T, Baur L, Uauy R. IASO International Obesity Task Force. Obesity in children and young people: A crisis in public health. *Obes Rev.* 2004;Suppl. 1:1–4.
3. Oza-Frank R, Hade EM, Norton A, et al. Trends in body mass index among Ohio's third-grade children: 2004–2005 to 2009–2010. *J Acad Nutr Diet.* 2013;113(3):440–446.
4. Smith SM, Craig LC, Raja AE, et al. Growing up before growing out: Secular trends in height, weight and obesity in 5–6-year-old children born between 1970 and 2006. *Arch Dis Child.* 2013;98(4):269–273.
5. Ogden CL, Flegal KM, Carroll MD, et al. Prevalence and trends in overweight among US children and adolescents, 1999–2000. *JAMA.* 2002;288:1728–1732.
6. Edwards KL, Clarke GP, Ransley JK, et al. Serial cross-sectional analysis of prevalence of overweight and obese children between 1998 and 2003 in Leeds, UK, using routinely measured data. *Public Health Nutr.* 2010;25:1–6.
7. Broyles S, Katzmarzyk PT, Srinivasan SR, et al. The pediatric obesity epidemic continues unabated in Bogalusa, Louisiana. *Pediatrics.* 2010;125(5):900–905.
8. Claire Wang Y, Gortmaker SL, Taveras EM. Trends and racial/ethnic disparities in severe obesity among US children and adolescents, 1976–2006. *Int J Pediatr Obes.* 2011 Feb;6(1):12–20.
9. Luepker RV, Jacobs DR, Prineas RJ, et al. Secular trends of blood pressure and body size in a multi-ethnic adolescent population: 1986 to 1996. *J Pediatr.* 1999;134:668–674.
10. Daniels SR, Arnett DK, Eckel RH, et al. Overweight in children and adolescents: Pathophysiology, consequences, prevention, and treatment. *Circulation.* 2005;111:1999–2012.
11. Barlow SE, Dietz WH. Obesity Evaluation and Treatment: Expert Committee Recommendations. The Maternal and Child Health Bureau, Health Resources and Services Administration and the Department of Health and Human Services. *Pediatrics.* 1998;102:e29.
12. Biro FM, Wien M. Childhood obesity and adult morbidities. *Am J Clin Nutr.* 2010;91(5):1499S–1505S.
13. Matricciani LA, Olds TS, Blunden S, et al. Never enough sleep: A brief history of sleep recommendations for children. *Pediatrics.* 2012;129(3):548–556.
14. Krueger PM, Friedman EM. Sleep duration in the United States: A cross-sectional population-based study. *Am J Epidemiol.* 2009;169(9):1052–1063.
15. National Sleep Foundation. Sleep in America Poll – Sleep in Children Survey. https://www.sleepfoundation.org/how-sleep-works/sleep-facts-statistics.
16. Jones CH, Ball HL. Napping in English preschool children and the association with parents' attitudes. *Sleep Med.* 2013;14(4):352–358.
17. Foley LS, Maddison R, Jiang Y, et al. Presleep activities and time of sleep onset in children. *Pediatrics.* 2013;131(2):276–282.
18. Koulouglioti C, Cole R, Moskow M, et al. The longitudinal association of young children's everyday routines to sleep duration. *J Pediatr Health Care.* 2014 Jan–Feb;28(1):80–87.
19. Wang Y, Beydoun MA. The obesity epidemic in the United States – gender, age, socioeconomic, racial/ethnic, and geographic characteristics: A systematic review and meta-regression analysis. *Epidemiol Rev.* 2007;29:6–28.
20. Chen X, Beydoun MA, Wang Y. Is sleep duration associated with childhood obesity? A systematic review and meta-analysis. *Obesity (Silver Spring).* 2008;16(2):265–274.
21. Marshall NS, Glozier N, Grunstein RR. Is sleep duration related to obesity? A critical review of the epidemiological evidence. *Sleep Med Rev.* 2008;12(4):289–298.
22. Taheri S, Thomas GN. Is sleep duration associated with obesity – Where do U stand? *Sleep Med Rev.* 2008;12(4):299–302.
23. Spruyt K, Gozal D. The underlying interactome of childhood obesity: The potential role of sleep. *Child Obes.* 2012;8(1):38–42.
24. Spruyt K, Molfese DL, Gozal D. Sleep duration, sleep regularity, body weight, and metabolic homeostasis in school-aged children. *Pediatrics.* 2011;127(2):e345–e352.
25. Golley RK, Maher CA, Matricciani L, et al. Sleep duration or bedtime? Exploring the association between sleep timing behaviour, diet and BMI in children and adolescents. *Int J Obes (Lond).* 2013;37(4):546–551.
26. Jarrin DC, McGrath JJ, Drake CL. Beyond sleep duration: Distinct sleep dimensions are associated with obesity in children and adolescents. *Int J Obes (Lond).* 2013;37(4):552–558.
27. Chahal H, Fung C, Kuhle S, et al. Availability and night-time use of electronic entertainment and communication devices are associated with short sleep duration and obesity among Canadian children. *Pediatr Obes.* 2013;8(1):42–51.
28. O'Dea JA, Dibley MJ, Rankin NM. Low sleep and low socioeconomic status predict high body mass index: A 4-year longitudinal study of Australian schoolchildren. *Pediatr Obes.* 2012;7(4):295–303.
29. Nielsen LS, Danielsen KV, Sørensen TI. Short sleep duration as a possible cause of obesity: Critical analysis of the epidemiological evidence. *Obes Rev.* 2011;12(2):78–92.
30. Calamaro CJ, Park S, Mason TB, et al. Shortened sleep duration does not predict obesity in adolescents. *J Sleep Res.* 2010;19(4):559–566.
31. Sun Y, Sekine M, Kagamimori S. Lifestyle and overweight among Japanese adolescents: The Toyama Birth Cohort Study. *J Epidemiol.* 2009;19(6):303–310.
32. Grandner MA, Patel NP, Gehrman PR, et al. Problems associated with short sleep: Bridging the gap between laboratory and epidemiological studies. *Sleep Med Rev.* 2010;14(4):239–247.

33. Monasta L, Batty GD, Cattaneo A, et al. Early-life determinants of overweight and obesity: A review of systematic reviews. *Obes Rev.* 2010;11(10):695–708.

34. Chaput JP, Leblanc C, Pérusse L, et al. Risk factors for adult overweight and obesity in the Quebec Family Study: Have we been barking up the wrong tree? *Obesity (Silver Spring).* 2009;17(10):1964–1970.

35. Cizza G, Marincola P, Mattingly M, et al. Treatment of obesity with extension of sleep duration: A randomized, prospective, controlled trial. *Clin Trials.* 2010;7(3):274–285.

36. Olsen NJ, Larsen SC, Rohde JF, Stougaard M, Händel MN, Specht IO, Heitmann BL. Effects of the healthy start randomized intervention on psychological stress and sleep habits among obesity-susceptible healthy weight children and their parents. *PLoS One.* 2022 Mar 10;17(3):e0264514.

37. Saidi O, Rochette E, Del Sordo G, Doré É, Merlin É, Walrand S, Duché P. Eucaloric balanced diet improved objective sleep in adolescents with obesity. *Nutrients.* 2021 Oct 10;13(10):3550.

38. Hudson JL, Zhou J, Campbell WW. Adults Who Are Overweight or Obese and Consuming an Energy-Restricted Healthy US-Style Eating Pattern at Either the Recommended or a Higher Protein Quantity Perceive a Shift from "Poor" to "Good" Sleep: A Randomized Controlled Trial. *J Nutr.* 2020 Dec 10;150(12):3216–3223.

39. Campos M, Pomeroy J, Mays MH, Lopez A, Palacios C. Intervention to promote physical activation and improve sleep and response feeding in infants for preventing obesity early in life, the baby-act trial: Rationale and design. *Contemp Clin Trials.* 2020 Dec;99:106185.

40. Perkin MR, Bahnson HT, Logan K, Marrs T, Radulovic S, Craven J, Flohr C, Lack G. Association of Early Introduction of Solids With Infant Sleep: A Secondary Analysis of a Randomized Clinical Trial. *JAMA Pediatr.* 2018 Aug 6; 172(8):e180739.

41. Yackobovitch-Gavan M, Machtei A, Lazar L, Shamir R, Phillip M, Lebenthal Y. Randomised study found that improved nutritional intake was associated with better sleep patterns in pre-pubertal children who were both short and lean. *Acta Paediatr.* 2018 Apr;107(4):666–671.

42. Rangan A, Zheng M, Olsen NJ, Rohde JF, Heitmann BL. Shorter sleep duration is associated with higher energy intake and an increase in BMI z-score in young children predisposed to overweight. *Int J Obes (Lond).* 2018 Jan;42(1):59–64.

43. Taylor BJ, Gray AR, Galland BC, Heath AM, Lawrence J, Sayers RM, Cameron S, Hanna M, Dale K, Coppell KJ, Taylor RW. Targeting sleep, food, and activity in infants for obesity prevention: An RCT. *Pediatrics.* 2017 Mar;139(3): e20162037.

44. Bayer O, Rosario AS, Wabitsch M, et al. Sleep duration and obesity in children: Is the association dependent on age and choice of the outcome parameter? *Sleep.* 2009;32(9):1183–1189.

45. Bass J, Takahashi JS. Circadian integration of metabolism and energetics. *Science.* 2010;330(6009):1349–1354.

46. Zheng H, Berthoud H-R. Neural systems controlling the drive to eat: Mind versus metabolism. *Physiology.* 2008;23(2): 75–83.

47. Mavanji V, Teske JA, Billington CJ, et al. Elevated sleep quality and orexin receptor mRNA in obesity-resistant rats. *Int J Obes (Lond).* 2010;34(11):1576–1588.

48. Maury E, Ramsey KM, Bass J. Circadian rhythms and metabolic syndrome: From experimental genetics to human disease. *Circ Res.* 2010;106(3):447–462.

49. Eckel-Mahan KL, Patel VR, Mohney RP, et al. Coordination of the transcriptome and metabolome by the circadian clock. *Proc Natl Acad Sci U S A.* 2012;109(14):5541–5546.

50. Reilly JJ, Armstrong J, Dorosty AR, et al. Early life risk factors for obesity in childhood: Cohort study. *BMJ.* 2005;330(7504):1357.

51. Flynn MA, McNeil DA, Maloff B, et al. Reducing obesity and related chronic disease risk in children and youth: A synthesis of evidence with "best practice" recommendations. *Obes Rev.* 2006;7(Suppl. 1):7–66.

52. Sekine M, Yamagami T, Handa K, et al. A dose–response relationship between short sleeping hours and childhood obesity: Results of the Toyama birth cohort study. *Child Care Health Dev.* 2002;28(2):163–170.

53. Padez C, Mourao I, Moreira P, et al. Long sleep duration and childhood overweight/obesity and body fat. *Am J Hum Biol.* 2009;21(3):371–376.

54. Taveras EM, Rifas-Shiman SL, Oken E, et al. Short sleep duration in infancy and risk of childhood overweight. *Arch Pediatr Adol Med.* 2008;162(4):305–311.

55. Touchette Â, Petit D, Tremblay RE, et al. Associations between sleep duration patterns and overweight/obesity at age 6. *Sleep.* 2008;31(11):1507–1514.

56. Dayyat E, Kheirandish-Gozal L, Gozal D. Childhood obstructive sleep apnea: One or two distinct disease entities? *Sleep Med Clin.* 2007;2(3):433–444.

57. Arens R, Muzumdar H. Childhood obesity and obstructive sleep apnea syndrome. *J Appl Physiol.* 2010;108 (2):436–444.

58. Redline S, Tishler PV, Schluchter M, et al. Risk factors for sleep-disordered breathing in children. Associations with obesity, race, and respiratory problems. *Am J Respir Crit Care Med.* 1999;159(5 Pt 1):1527–1532.

59. Wing YK, Hui SH, Pak WM, et al. A controlled study of sleep related disordered breathing in obese children. *Arch Dis Child.* 2003;88:1043–1047.

60. Kalra M, Inge T, Garcia V, et al. Obstructive sleep apnea in extremely overweight adolescents undergoing bariatric surgery. *Obes Res.* 2005;13:1175–1179.

61. Kahn A, Mozin MJ, Rebuffat E, et al. Sleep pattern alterations and brief airway obstructions in overweight infants. *Sleep.* 1989;12:430–438.

62. Shine NP, Coates HL, Lannigan FJ. Obstructive sleep apnea, morbid obesity, and adenotonsillar surgery: A review of the literature. *Int J Ped Otolaryngol.* 2005;69:1475–1482.

63. Bixler EO, Vgontzas AN, Lin HM, et al. Sleep disordered breathing in children in a general population sample: Prevalence and risk factors. *Sleep.* 2009;32(6):731–736.

64. Verhulst SL, Franckx H, Van Gaal L, et al. The effect of weight loss on sleep-disordered breathing in obese teenagers. *Obesity (Silver Spring).* 2009;17(6):1178–1183.

65. Dayyat E, Kheirandish-Gozal L, Sans Capdevila O, et al. Obstructive sleep apnea in children: Relative contributions of body mass index and adenotonsillar hypertrophy. *Chest.* 2009;136(1):137–144.

66. Brunetti L, Tesse R, Miniello VL, et al. Sleep-disordered breathing in obese children: The southern Italy experience. *Chest.* 2010;137(5):1085–1090.

67. Kohler MJ, Thormaehlen S, Kennedy JD, et al. Differences in the association between obesity and obstructive sleep apnea among children and adolescents. *J Clin Sleep Med.* 2009;5(6):506–511.

68. Mitchell RB, Boss EF. Pediatric obstructive sleep apnea in obese and normal-weight children: Impact of adenotonsillectomy on quality-of-life and behavior. *Dev Neuropsychol.* 2009;34(5):650–661.

69. Alonso-Álvarez M, Cordero-Guevara JA, Terán-Santos J, Gonzalez Martinez M, Jurado-Luque MJ, Corral-Peñafiel J, Duran-Cantolla J, Kheirandish-Gozal L, Gozal D. and the Spanish Sleep Network. Obstructive sleep apnea in obese community dwelling children: The NANOS study. *Sleep.* 2014;37(5):943–949.

70. White DP, Lombard RM, Cadieux RJ, et al. Pharyngeal resistance in normal humans: Influence of gender, age, and obesity. *J Appl Physiol.* 1985;58:365–371.

71. Horner RL, Mohiaddin RH, Lowell DG, et al. Sites and sizes of fat deposits around the pharynx in obese patients with obstructive sleep apnoea and weight matched controls. *Eur Respir J.* 1989;2:613–622.

72. Arens R, Sin S, Nandalike K, et al. Upper airway structure and body fat composition in obese children with obstructive sleep apnea syndrome. *Am J Respir Crit Care Med.* 2011;183(6):782–787.

73. Kheirandish-Gozal L. Fat and lymphadenoid tissues: A mutually obstructive combination. *Am J Respir Crit Care Med.* 2011;183(6):694–695.

74. Naimark A, Cherniack RM. Compliance of the respiratory system and its components in health and obesity. *J Appl Physiol.* 1960;15:377–382.

75. Aygun AD, Gungor S, Ustundag B, et al. Proinflammatory cytokines and leptin are increased in serum of prepubertal obese children. *Mediators Inflamm.* 2005;2005(3):180–183.

76. Reinehr T, Kratzsch J, Kiess W, et al. Circulating soluble leptin receptor, leptin, and insulin resistance before and after weight loss in obese children. *Int J Obes (Lond).* 2005;29:1230–1235.

77. Celi F, Bini V, Papi F, et al. Leptin serum levels are involved in the relapse after weight excess reduction in obese children and adolescents. *Diabetes Nutr Metab.* 2003;16:306–311.

78. Polotsky VY, Smaldone MC, Scharf MT, et al. Impact of interrupted leptin pathways on ventilatory control. *J Appl Physiol.* 2004;96:991–998.

79. Arens R, Marcus CL. Pathophysiology of upper airway obstruction: A developmental perspective. *Sleep.* 2004;27(5):997–1019.

80. Beebe DW, Lewin D, Zeller M, et al. Sleep in overweight adolescents: Shorter sleep, poorer sleep quality, sleepiness, and sleep-disordered breathing. *J Pediatr Psychol.* 2007;32(1):69–79.

81. Gozal D, Wang M, Pope Jr. DW. Objective sleepiness measures in pediatric obstructive sleep apnea. *Pediatrics.* 2001;108(3):693–697.

82. Tauman R, O'Brien LM, Holbrook CR, et al. Sleep pressure score: A new index of sleep disruption in snoring children. *Sleep.* 2004;27(2):274–278.

83. Melendres MC, Lutz JM, Rubin ED, et al. Daytime sleepiness and hyperactivity in children with suspected sleep-disordered breathing. *Pediatrics.* 2004;114(3):768–775.

84. Chervin RD, Weatherly RA, Ruzicka DL, et al. Subjective sleepiness and polysomnographic correlates in children scheduled for adenotonsillectomy vs other surgical care. *Sleep.* 2006;29(4):495–503.

85. Spruyt K, Sans Capdevila O, Serpero LD, et al. Dietary and physical activity patterns in children with obstructive sleep apnea. *J Pediatr.* 2010;156(5):724–730. 730.e1–730.e3.

86. Gozal D, Kheirandish-Gozal L. Obesity and excessive daytime sleepiness in prepubertal children with obstructive sleep apnea. *Pediatrics.* 2009;123(1):13–18.

87. Gozal D, Serpero LD, Sans Capdevila O, et al. Systemic inflammation in non-obese children with obstructive sleep apnea. *Sleep Med.* 2008;9(3):254–259.

88. Tauman R, Ivanenko A, O'Brien LM, et al. Plasma C-reactive protein levels among children with sleep-disordered breathing. *Pediatrics.* 2004;113(6):e564–e569.

89. Gozal D. Sleep, sleep disorders and inflammation in children. *Sleep Med.* 2009;10(Suppl. 1):S12–S16.

90. Khalyfa A, Capdevila OS, Buazza MO, et al. Genome-wide gene expression profiling in children with non-obese obstructive sleep apnea. *Sleep Med.* 2009;10(1):75–86.

91. Kim J, Bhattacharjee R, Snow AB, et al. Myeloid-related protein 8/14 levels in children with obstructive sleep apnoea. *Eur Respir J.* 2010;35(4):843–850.

92. Gozal D, Serpero LD, Kheirandish-Gozal L, et al. R. Sleep measures and morning plasma TNF-alpha levels in children with sleep-disordered breathing. *Sleep.* 2010;33(3):319–325.

93. Davies RJ, Turner R, Crosby J, et al. Plasma insulin and lipid levels in untreated obstructive sleep apnoea and snoring; their comparison with matched controls and response to treatment. *J Sleep Res.* 1994;3(3):180–185.

94. Punjabi NM, Sorkin JD, Katzel LI, et al. Sleep-disordered breathing and insulin resistance in middle-aged and overweight men. *Am J Respir Crit Care Med.* 2002;165(5):677–682.

95. Ip MS, Lam B, Ng MM, Lam WK, Tsang KW, Lam KS. Obstructive sleep apnea is independently associated with insulin resistance. *Am J Respir Crit Care Med.* 2002;165(5):670–676.

96. Tauman R, O'Brien LM, Ivanenko A, et al. Obesity rather than severity of sleep-disordered breathing as the major determinant of insulin resistance and altered lipidemia in snoring children. *Pediatrics.* 2005;116(1):e66–e73.

97. Verhulst SL, Schrauwen N, Haentjens D, et al. Sleep-disordered breathing and the metabolic syndrome in overweight and obese children and adolescents. *J Pediatr.* 2007;150(6):608–612.

98. Alexopoulos EI, Gletsou E, Kostadima E, et al. Effects of obstructive sleep apnea severity on serum lipid levels in Greek children with snoring. *Sleep Breath.* 2011;15(4):625–631.

99. Redline S, Storfer-Isser A, Rosen CL, et al. Association between metabolic syndrome and sleep-disordered breathing in adolescents. *Am J Respir Crit Care Med.* 2007;176(4):401–408.

100. Zong J, Liu Y, Huang Y, et al. Serum lipids alterations in adenoid hypertrophy or adenotonsillar hypertrophy children with sleep disordered breathing. *Int J Pediatr Otorhinolaryngol.* 2013;77(5):717–720.

101. Gozal D, Capdevila OS, Kheirandish-Gozal L. Metabolic alterations and systemic inflammation in obstructive sleep apnea among nonobese and obese prepubertal children. *Am J Respir Crit Care Med.* 2008;177(10):1142–1149.

102. Di Sessa A, Messina G, Bitetti I, Falanga C, Farello G, Verrotti A, Carotenuto M. Cardiometabolic risk profile in non-obese children with obstructive sleep apnea syndrome. *Eur J Pediatr.* 2022;181(4):1689–1697.

103. Kang EK, Jang MJ, Kim KD, Ahn YM. The association of obstructive sleep apnea with dyslipidemia in Korean children and adolescents: A single-center, cross- sectional study. *J Clin Sleep Med.* 2021 Aug 1;17(8):1599–1605.

104. Bhushan B, Khalyfa A, Spruyt K, et al. Fatty-acid binding protein 4 gene polymorphisms and plasma levels in children with obstructive sleep apnea. *Sleep Med*. 2011;12(7):666–671.

105. Kaditis AG, Alexopoulos EI, Damani E, et al. Obstructive sleep-disordered breathing and fasting insulin levels in non-obese children. *Pediatr Pulmonol*. 2005;40(6):515–523.

106. Lesser DJ, Bhatia R, Tran WH, et al. Sleep fragmentation and intermittent hypoxemia are associated with decreased insulin sensitivity in obese adolescent Latino males. *Pediatr Res*. 2012;72(3):293–298.

107. Canapari CA, Hoppin AG, Kinane TB, et al. Relationship between sleep apnea, fat distribution, and insulin resistance in obese children. *J Clin Sleep Med*. 2011;7(3):268–273.

108. Mirrakhimov AE, Polotsky VY. Obstructive sleep apnea and non-alcoholic fatty liver disease: Is the liver another target? *Front Neurol*. 2012;3:149.

109. Kheirandish-Gozal L, Sans Capdevila O, Kheirandish E, et al. Elevated serum aminotransferase levels in children at risk for obstructive sleep apnea. *Chest*. 2008;133(1):92–99.

110. Verhulst SL, Jacobs S, Aerts L, et al. Sleep-disordered breathing: A new risk factor of suspected fatty liver disease in overweight children and adolescents? *Sleep Breath*. 2009;13(2):207–210.

111. Verhulst SL, Rooman R, Van Gaal L, et al. Is sleep-disordered breathing an additional risk factor for the metabolic syndrome in obese children and adolescents? *Int J Obes (Lond)*. 2009;33(1):8–13.

112. Koren D, Gozal D, Philby MF, Bhattacharjee R, Kheirandish-Gozal L. Impact of obstructive sleep apnoea on insulin resistance in nonobese and obese children. *Eur Respir J*. 2016 Apr;47(4):1152–1161.

113. Siriwat R, Wang L, Shah V, Mehra R, Ibrahim S. Obstructive sleep apnea and insulin resistance in children with obesity. *J Clin Sleep Med*. 2020 Jul15;16(7):1081–1090.

114. Bhatt SP, Guleria R, Kabra SK. Metabolic alterations and systemic inflammation in overweight/obese children with obstructive sleep apnea. *PLoS One*. 2021 Jun 4;16(6):e0252353.

115. Alonso-Álvarez ML, Terán-Santos J, Gonzalez Martinez M, Cordero-Guevara JA, Jurado-Luque MJ, Corral-Peñafiel J, Duran-Cantolla J, Ordax Carbajo E, MasaJimenez F, Kheirandish-Gozal L, Gozal D. Spanish Sleep Network. Metabolic biomarkers in community obese children: Effect of obstructive sleep apnea and its treatment. *Sleep Med*. 2017 Sep;37:1–9.

116. Katz SL, MacLean JE, Hoey L, Horwood L, Barrowman N, Foster B, Hadjiyannakis S, Legault L, Bendiak GN, Kirk VG, Constantin E. Insulin Resistance and Hypertension in Obese Youth With Sleep-Disordered Breathing Treated With Positive Airway Pressure: A Prospective Multicenter Study. *J Clin Sleep Med*. 2017 Sep 15;13(9):1039–1047.

117. Gozal D, Khalyfa A, Qiao Z, Smith DL, Philby MF, Koren D, Kheirandish-Gozal L. Angiopoietin-2 and soluble Tie-2 receptor plasma levels in children with obstructive sleep apnea and obesity. *Obesity (Silver Spring)*. 2017 Jun;25(6):1083–1090.

118. Van Eyck A, Van Hoorenbeeck K, De Winter BY, Van Gaal L. De Backer W, Verhulst SL. Sleep-disordered breathing, systemic adipokine secretion, and metabolic dysregulation in overweight and obese children and adolescents. *Sleep Med*. 2017 Feb;30:52–56.

119. Tsaoussoglou M, Bixler EO, Calhoun S, et al. Sleep-disordered breathing in obese children is associated with prevalent excessive daytime sleepiness, inflammation, and metabolic abnormalities. *J Clin Endocrinol Metab*. 2010;95(1):143–150.

120. Tauman R, Gulliver TE, Krishna J, et al. Persistence of obstructive sleep apnea syndrome in children after adenotonsillectomy. *J Pediatr*. 2006;149(6):803–808.

121. Bhattacharjee R, Kheirandish-Gozal L, Spruyt K, et al. Adenotonsillectomy outcomes in treatment of OSA in children: A multicenter retrospective study. *Am J Respir Crit Care Med*. 2010;182(5):676–683.

122. Verhulst SL, Franckx H, Van Gaal L, et al. The effect of weight loss on sleep-disordered breathing in obese teenagers. *Obesity (Silver Spring)*. 2009;17(6):1178–1183.

123. Roche J, Corgosinho FC, Isacco L, Scheuermaier K, Pereira B, Gillet V, Moreira GA, Pradella-Hallinan M, Tufik S, de Mello MT, Mougin F, Dâmaso AR, Thivel D. A multidisciplinary weight loss intervention in obese adolescents with and without sleep-disordered breathing improves cardiometabolic health, whether SDB was normalized or not. *Sleep Med*. 2020 Nov;75:225–235.

124. Koren D, Gozal D, Bhattacharjee R, Philby MF, Kheirandish-Gozal L. Impact of adenotonsillectomy on insulin resistance and lipoprotein profile in nonobese and obese children. *Chest*. 2016 Apr;149(4):999–1010.

125. Serbis A, Giapros V, Galli-Tsinopoulou A, Siomou E. Metabolic syndrome in children and adolescents: Is there a universally accepted definition? Does it matter? *Metab Syndr Relat Disord*. 2020 Dec;18(10):462–470.

126. Hanevold C, Hooper SR, Ingelfinger JR, Lande MB, Martin LJ, Meyers K, Mitsnefes M, Rosner B, Samuels J, Flynn JT. Cardiovascular risk factors and target organ damage in adolescents: The SHIP AHOY Study. *Pediatrics*. 2022 May 3 e2021054201.

127. Jacobs Jr DR, Woo JG, Sinaiko AR, Daniels SR, Ikonen J, Juonala M, Kartiosuo N, Lehtimäki T, Magnussen CG, Viikari JSA, Zhang N, Bazzano LA, Burns TL, Prineas RJ, Steinberger J, Urbina EM, Venn AJ, Raitakari OT, Dwyer T. Childhood cardiovascular risk factors and adult cardiovascular events. *N Engl J Med*. 2022;386(20):1877–1888.

32

Sleep-Disordered Breathing in Cystic Fibrosis and Asthma

Theresa Annette Laguna and Avani Shah

CHAPTER HIGHLIGHTS

- Sleep-disordered breathing is common in children with chronic lung disease and it can significantly impact quality of life and cognitive development.
- Cystic fibrosis can impact sleep through symptoms directly related to the disease or indirectly through the burden of treatment.
- There is a strong association between sleep-disordered breathing and asthma, with treatment of either disorder influencing the outcome of the other.
- Understanding and addressing the factors that affect poor sleep quality in children with asthma can improve asthma morbidity, quality of life, and school performance.
- Primary care providers should ask patients with chronic lung disease directly about sleep and have a low threshold for a screening polysomnogram or referral to a specialist.

Sleep-Disordered Breathing in Cystic Fibrosis and Asthma

It is well studied that sleep disruption and sleep-disordered breathing (SDB) negatively impact quality of life, school performance, and cognitive function in children in the absence of chronic disease.[1] In the setting of a multisystem, progressive genetic disease like cystic fibrosis (CF) or a chronic inflammatory disease like asthma, the contribution of sleep abnormalities to the clinical course and overall prognosis should not be overlooked.[2] Providers and multidisciplinary care team members should be familiar with the signs and symptoms of sleep abnormalities and should have a strategy with which to approach, diagnose, and treat SDB in children affected by these disorders characterized by obstructive lung disease and chronic airway inflammation.

Introduction to Cystic Fibrosis

CF is an autosomal recessive disease that causes abnormal chloride transport across the apical surface of epithelial cells throughout the body.[3] Inadequate or absent chloride transport results in thick, tenacious secretions that clog ducts and glands in multiple organs including the lungs, sinuses, pancreas, liver, and reproductive organs.[3] The lungs are frequently impacted, where mucus stasis contributes to a cycle of infection, inflammation, and destruction that results in significant morbidity and early mortality. Children with CF typically have progressive obstructive lung disease and pancreatic insufficiency in addition to the likelihood of developing such complications as malnutrition, sinus disease, nasal polyps, liver failure, and CF-related diabetes (CFRD).[3] Significant advances in clinical care and the development of medications targeting the underlying genetic defect in CF have resulted in increased life expectancy; however, CF care remains burdensome and time-consuming.[4] People with CF often devote hours per day to respiratory treatments and require frequent medical care to improve their prognosis in the setting of this life-shortening disease.

Factors Affecting Sleep in Cystic Fibrosis

Given the multisystem nature of the disease, sleep may be adversely impacted in CF through a multitude of factors. CF-related sinus disease including inflammation of the nasal mucosa and nasal polyps may contribute to mouth breathing, snoring, and airway obstruction.[5] Chronic, obstructive lung disease may cause mucus production, recurrent infections and frequent, daytime and nighttime cough.[6,7] Symptoms of gastrointestinal distress such as constipation, abdominal pain, gastroesophageal reflux (GERD), flatulence, or frequent stooling may be intermittent or constant and flare up during sleep.[7] Malnutrition may necessitate nighttime drip feedings through a gastrostomy tube, resulting in increased fluid intake overnight and excessive need for urination.[8] Glucose dysregulation, including CFRD, can result in nocturnal polyuria as well.[8,9] Side effects from medications frequently used in the treatment of CF (i.e., prednisone and albuterol) can disrupt sleep and cause insomnia.[10] Finally, headaches or abdominal pain frequently impact sleep and quality of life in children with chronic disease.[11] When asked directly about sleep habits and challenges through qualitative interviews, children with CF and their parents identified common themes, the majority of which were related to CF directly or required therapeutic care.[12] Children with CF have additional risk factors for having SDB even when they are well, and it is imperative that care providers develop the awareness and the tool kit necessary to address these concerns.[13]

Polysomnography Findings in Cystic Fibrosis

Screening for SDB in children with CF is not commonplace. Although assessing for symptoms of snoring and obstructive sleep apnea (OSA) is recommended by the American Academy of Pediatrics (AAP) for all children, there are no additional recommendations for children with CF. Both acute (i.e., CF pulmonary exacerbations) and chronic (i.e., polyps, progressive lung disease) risk factors exist that raise the level of concern for sleep abnormalities that should drive a low threshold for screening.

Poor Sleep Quality

Children with CF have poor sleep quality with difficulties initiating sleep, frequent awakenings, lower total sleep time, snoring, trouble breathing, and daytime sleepiness and fatigue that has been documented both subjectively and objectively.[8,14–16] Reasons for this are likely multifactorial; however, these findings appear to be present even during times of clinical stability. Strikingly, 80% of children with CF without symptoms of illness coughed during two nights of monitoring, which is substantially higher than 5% of "normal" children.[17] In children with CF, frequent awakenings and less total sleep time were associated with a lower forced expiratory volume in one second (FEV_1), a lower baseline oxygen saturation, CFRD, nocturnal gastrostomy tube feedings, and behavioral concerns (Fig. 32.1).[7,8,18] Children with a lower FEV_1% predicted had lower sleep efficiency that correlated with the degree of lung disease (Fig. 32.2).[15] Importantly, poor sleep quality is associated with reduced quality of life and lower mood in children with CF, and insomnia is associated with anxiety and depression in adults with CF,[19] highlighting the importance of interventions to address it.[2]

Tachypnea

Compared with healthy controls, children with CF have been noted to have a higher respiratory rate in non–rapid eye movement (NREM) sleep.[14] Interestingly, a higher respiratory rate during sleep was negatively correlated with FEV_1.[20] In children with CF where nutrition is key to prolonged survival, increased respiratory work can divert valuable calories to support breathing instead of promoting growth and nutrition. The clinical significance of this should not be minimized.

Nocturnal Hypoxemia

Disorders of oxygenation (hypoxemia) have been well documented in children with CF from infants to adolescents.[6,14,21–23] Physiologic hypotheses for nocturnal hypoxemia include reduced lung volumes (i.e., reduced functional residual capacity [FRC]) secondary to hypoventilation during REM sleep, ventilation and perfusion mismatch, and upper airway obstructive pathology.[22] Although nocturnal hypoxemia is common in CF children with evidence of pulmonary inflammation and/or an infective pulmonary exacerbation, lower oxygen saturations can also be found in asymptomatic CF children compared with healthy controls.[5,7,18,24] As the obstructive lung disease in CF progresses, lung function as measured by FEV_1 declines. Although it is widely known that adults with CF and severe lung disease have nocturnal hypoxemia, even children with mild to moderate lung disease can have clinically relevant nocturnal symptoms.[5,18,22,25,26] An FEV_1% predicted <64% has been demonstrated to be predictive of nocturnal hypoxemia, prompting health care providers to consider overnight pulse oximetry or polysomnogram (PSG) to evaluate for gas exchange abnormalities during sleep.[18,21] A resting, awake oxygen saturation of <94% also may be beneficial in predicting those people with CF who may desaturate during sleep (Fig. 32.3).[27] Given such devastating clinical complications as pulmonary hypertension and cor pulmonale, it is important for health care providers to assess for predictors of nocturnal hypoxemia and be vigilant about monitoring oxygen saturations in children with CF, even those who are asymptomatic or with mild lung disease.[28]

Nocturnal Hypercapnia

While noted to be more common in adults with CF, children and adolescents with CF can also experience impaired ventilation and hypercapnia during sleep.[16,20] Hypercapnia has been associated with more severe lung disease (i.e., lower FEV_1), poor subjective sleep quality, and hypoxemia[20] in early adolescence. Although hypercapnia can be detected on overnight PSGs in children with CF, the long-term implications of this has yet to be determined and requires further investigation.[20] While there are some data that noninvasive ventilation (NIV) may be a useful adjunct to other airway clearance techniques in adults with CF, there is a need for additional research to understand its long-term role and/or benefit in children.[29,30]

Obstructive Sleep Apnea. SDB defined by the loss or decrease of airflow during sleep due to obstruction in the upper airway despite adequate continued respiratory effort is more common in young children with CF compared with healthy controls.[5] In a study of infants and children with CF in a healthy state, 70% were found to have mild to moderate OSA defined by an apnea-hypopnea index (AHI) >2 and 46% of this cohort had an AHI ≥5.[5] Given the risk factors for OSA present in children with CF (i.e., nasal obstruction, inflammation of nasal mucosa/sinuses or polyps, mouth breathing, and tonsillar hypertrophy), health care providers should have a low threshold for PSG and/or referral for

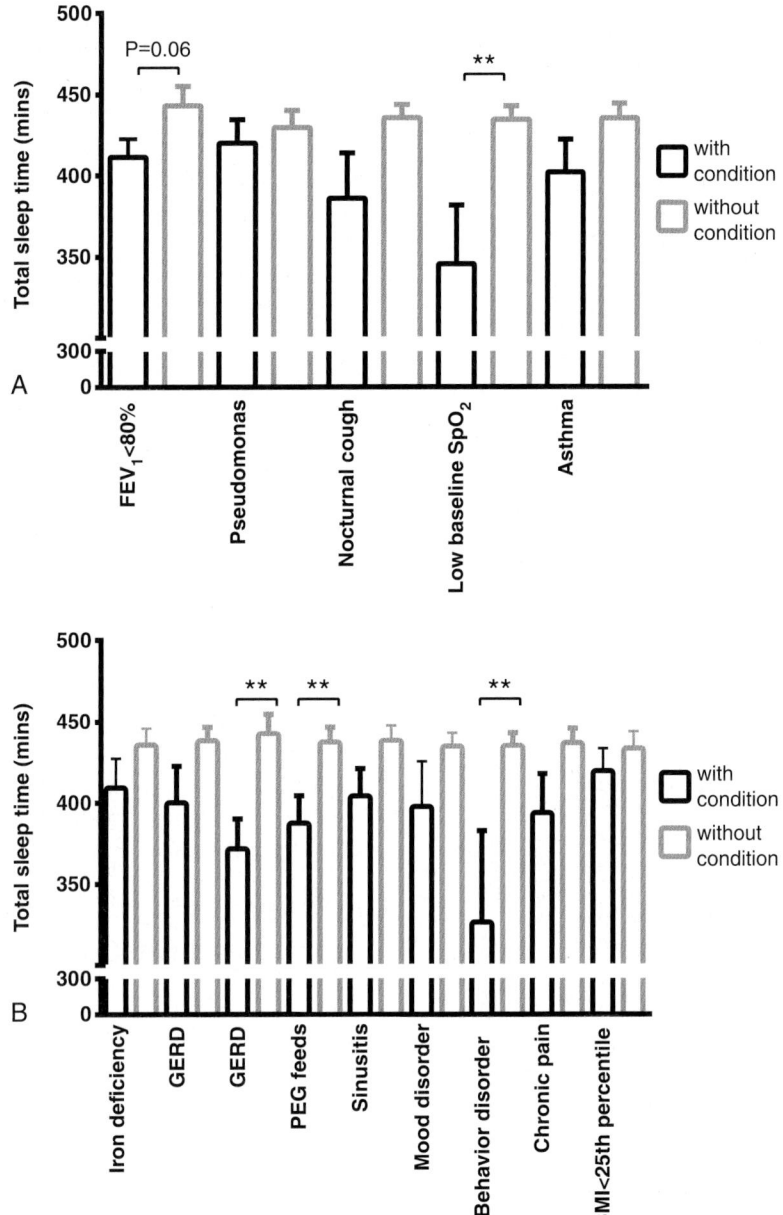

• **Fig. 32.1** Total sleep time of children with cystic fibrosis (CF), with and without (A) respiratory comorbidities, or (B) non-respiratory comorbidities. Data presented as mean ± SEM. *$p \leq 0.05$, **$p \leq 0.01$. FEV$_1$, forced expiratory volume in 1 second; GERD, gastroesophageal reflux; PEG, percutaneous endoscopic gastrostomy; BMI, body mass index.[8]

adenotonsillectomy (AT) for signs and symptoms of OSA given the potential for sleep disruption.[5]

Conclusions

Children with CF frequently have disrupted sleep and poor sleep quality that directly impacts their quality of life, even in the setting of minimal or mild lung disease.[2,8,15] While guidelines are not yet in place to identify the age at which to start screening children with CF for SDB, sleep disruption is both significant and consequential. Health care providers should be vigilant about asking children and families questions about sleep hygiene and referring early to sleep

medicine for evaluation and/or PSG. While the advent of new therapies that treat the underlying defect in CF may improve sleep as well, the full impact of these drugs remains to be seen.[31] Given sleep disturbances in CF begin early in the course of CF, health care providers should learn to identify risk factors in this vulnerable population.

Introduction to Asthma

Asthma is one of the most prevalent diseases in childhood affecting approximately 6 million children in the United States. Uncontrolled asthma accounts for 80,000 hospitalizations and over 500,000 emergency room visits per year.[32] Asthma is a chronic respiratory disease characterized by recurrent episodes of wheezing, shortness of breath, cough, and chest tightness often associated with an identified trigger. Pathophysiologic features include

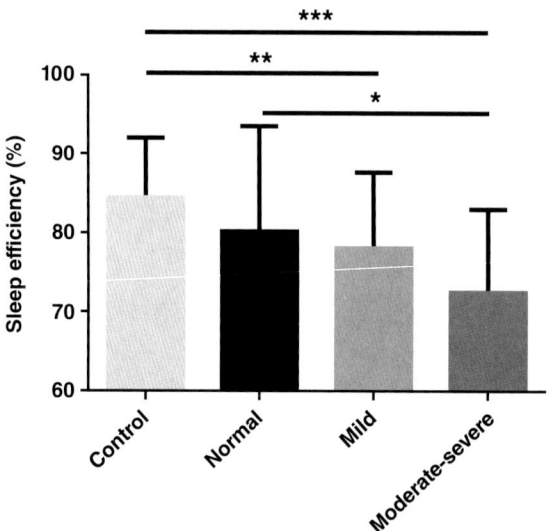

Lung function severity group

• **Fig. 32.2** Sleep efficiency of control children and children with cystic fibrosis (CF) across three different groups of forced expiratory volume in 1 second (FEV$_1$ [normal ≥90%, mild 70–89%, moderate-severe <70%]). A significant difference was found in the children with CF across the three groups ($p = 0.03$) after controlling for sex, age, and socioeconomic status (SES; univariate analysis). A significant difference was measured between CF patients with normal lung function versus CF patients with moderate-severe lung function (*p <0.05). A significant difference also was measured between control children and CF patients with mild (**p <0.01) and moderate-severe (***p <0.001) lung function but not with those with normal lung function ($p = 0.08$).[15]

airway hyperreactivity with bronchoconstriction, airway inflammation, and the formation of mucus plugs.[33] If left untreated, these features eventually lead to fixed airway obstruction and airway remodeling that results in a significant decline in lung function and increased risk for morbidity and mortality from asthma.[34] Poorly controlled asthma can have significant effects on sleep in children as a result of nocturnal symptoms as well as physiologic changes that occur with circadian variations. Symptoms of asthma often include nocturnal cough and nocturnal awakenings leading to sleep disruption and poor sleep quality. In addition, the relationship between SDB and asthma, and their influence on each other in children, is well established. This section will review what is known about SDB and asthma and will discuss the impact of asthma on sleep quality.

Asthma and Sleep-Disordered Breathing

Asthma and SDB have both increased in prevalence worldwide over the last few decades.[35,36] This concurrent increase in prevalence and the overlap in pathophysiology of these disorders has led to further investigation of an association and possible causal relationship between asthma and SDB. For the purposes of this chapter, SDB will refer to snoring, upper airway resistance syndrome, and OSA. OSA will refer to the diagnosis made by PSG criteria established at the time of the referenced study.

Pathophysiologic Overlap Between Asthma and Sleep-Disordered Breathing

Asthma and SDB are both disorders of airway inflammation, the former of the lower airway and the latter of the upper airway. Airway oxidative stress and the release of inflammatory mediators have been implicated in the

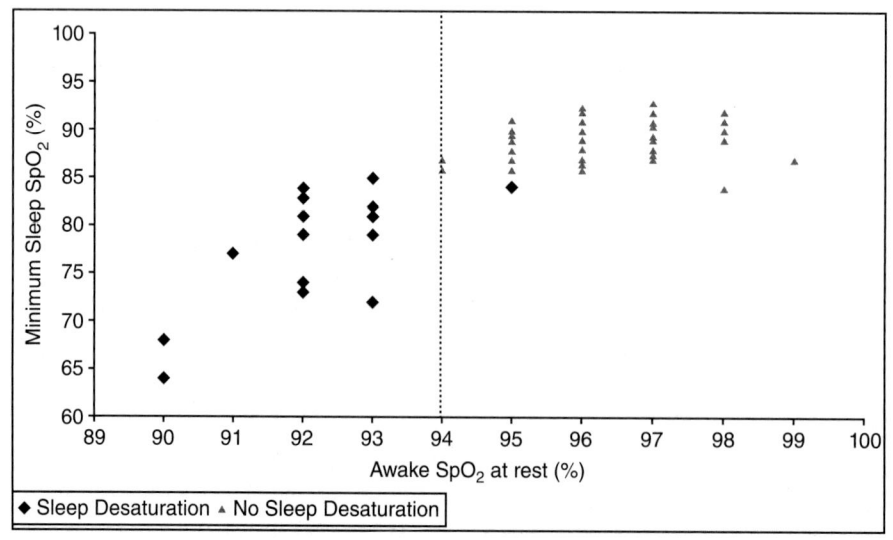

• **Fig. 32.3** Relationship between the minimum sleep SpO$_2$ and awake SpO$_2$ at rest in sitting position in people with cystic fibrosis (CF). The *vertical dotted line* represents the threshold (awake SpO$_2$ = 94%) that best separates patients who did desaturate (*filled diamond*) and who did not desaturate (*filled triangle*).[27]

pathogenesis of both disorders. Elevated concentrations of leukotriene B4, cysteinyl leukotrienes, and 8-isoprostane, an oxidative stress marker, have been detected in exhaled breath condensate in children with asthma and SDB.[37,38] In addition, cysteinyl leukotrienes may play a role in the development of adenotonsillar hyperplasia, one of the leading factors that contributes to SDB in children. Treatment for both asthma and SDB involves leukotriene antagonists and topical steroids, further strengthening the evidence of their similar pathophysiology.[39] Furthermore, OSA, a more severe form of SDB, may exacerbate asthma by altering oropharyngeal reflexes, increasing intrathoracic pressure, and increasing cholinergic tone, thereby promoting bronchoconstriction.[40]

The Association of Asthma and Sleep-Disordered Breathing

Given the overlap in the pathophysiology of asthma and SDB, there has been significant interest in understanding the association of these two disorders and exploring a possible causal relationship. A systematic review by Brockmann and colleagues evaluated studies in children less than 18 years old with a diagnosis of asthma and SDB. The diagnosis of these disorders was based on questionnaires except for in two studies in which PSGs were used. SDB included children with snoring, upper airway resistance syndrome, and OSA. This review studied over 45,000 children and found that SDB was two times more likely in children with asthma than in children without asthma (Fig. 32.4).[41] Goldstein and coworkers determined the prevalence of SDB in children with and without asthma and associated behavioral problems.[42] SDB was determined by the Pediatric Sleep Questionnaire

(PSQ), behavior was assessed by the Child Behavior Checklist (CBCL), and asthma severity was determined by the National Heart, Lung, and Blood Institute (NHLBI) asthma guidelines.[43] The prevalence of snoring was more than double in patients with asthma than those without asthma; however, asthma did not predict behavioral problems unlike SDB, which was an independent predictor of a positive CBCL. Furthermore, an association with severity of asthma and likelihood of developing SDB has been established. In this same study, children with more severe asthma had an increased odds ratio for snoring and a positive PSQ suggesting a dose-dependent relationship.[42] In addition, a large study of inner-city adolescents showed that the odds of reporting SDB symptoms increased with asthma severity (determined by NHLBI guidelines)[43] and, interestingly, results comparing daytime severity and nighttime severity were similar suggesting that even without nocturnal symptoms, patients with asthma are at risk of developing SDB.[44] It is important to note that in most of these studies SDB was diagnosed by patient questionnaire and not by PSG. Given this, it is possible that nocturnal symptoms of SDB may be mistaken for asthma symptoms, related to other diagnoses, or inaccurately reported and vice versa.

Polysomnography and Asthma

Studies that have used PSGs and other objective measures to diagnose SDB have also found associations between asthma and SDB. One such study found the prevalence of SDB to be higher in patients with asthma than in the general population. This study evaluated for OSA in poorly controlled asthmatics by PSG and found a prevalence of 63% for OSA compared with 4% in the general

Study or Subgroup	Asthmatics Events	Total	Control Events	Total	Weight	Odds Ratio M-H, Random, 95% CI
Bidad 2006	24	201	205	2699	5.8%	1.6496 [1.0524, 2.5858]
Chng 2004	135	1427	451	8380	12.5%	1.8370 [1.5024, 2.2461]
Corbo 2001	13	94	110	1343	3.6%	1.7990 [0.9705, 3.3349]
Desager 2005	38	83	224	860	5.6%	2.3976 [1.5168, 3.7899]
Ersu 2004	18	179	161	1968	4.8%	1.2548 [0.7512, 2.0961]
Fadzil 2012	14	48	68	502	3.1%	2.6280 [1.3410, 5.1504]
Hoskyns 1994	8	21	2	12	0.5%	3.0769 [0.5319, 17.7979]
Kaditis 2010	74	210	52	232	6.3%	1.8835 [1.2391, 2.8631]
Li 2010	138	636	2280	19516	12.8%	2.0948 [1.7262, 2.5422]
Lu 2003	43	273	59	701	6.3%	2.0343 [1.3355, 3.0989]
Marshall 2007	25	61	31	152	3.4%	2.7106 [1.4221, 5.1663]
Pescatore 2013	267	345	613	881	9.5%	1.4965 [1.1195, 2.0005]
Ramagopal 2008	30	74	67	162	4.2%	0.9668 [0.5525, 1.6918]
Sulit 2005	33	121	92	600	5.6%	2.0707 [1.3103, 3.2721]
Urschitz 2004	4	52	110	1017	1.5%	0.6871 [0.2431, 1.9421]
Vallery 2004	71	337	142	1316	8.8%	2.2068 [1.6114, 3.0221]
Verhulst 2007	51	89	161	563	5.6%	3.3511 [2.1196, 5.2982]
Total (95% CI)		4251		40904	100.0%	1.9071 [1.6721, 2.1751]
Total events	986		4828			

Heterogeneity: Tau² = 0.03; Chi² = 26.23, df = 16 (P = 0.05); I² = 39%
Test for overall effect: Z = 9.62 (P < 0.00001)

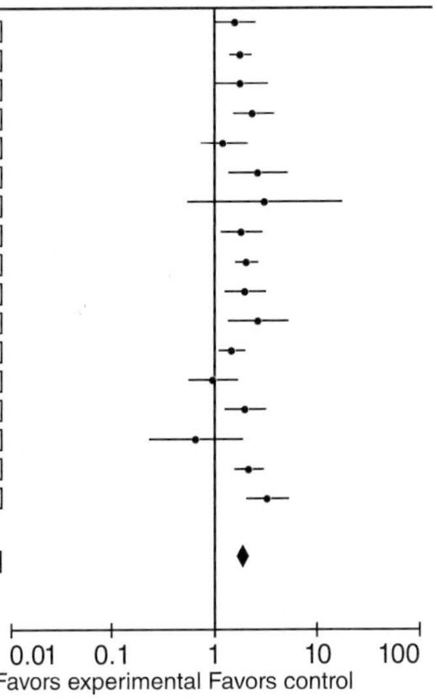

• **Fig. 32.4** Forest plot of the association of asthma and sleep-disordered breathing (SDB).[41] CI, confidence interval.

pediatric population.[45] Additionally, in a study of 50 African-American children, poorly controlled asthma was associated with an increase in the AHI by 8.8.[46] In another study of 108 children with asthma, where SDB was determined by snoring and overnight pulse oximetry, children with SDB showed 3.6 times higher odds of having severe asthma. In this study, severity of asthma was determined by level of therapy, symptom burden, and health care utilization.[47] Finally, it is possible that patients with asthma and OSA may have a different OSA phenotype. A study by Gutierrez and colleagues found that in PSGs of patients with OSA and asthma, the asthma patients had worse maximal oxygen desaturation during REM sleep, a higher REM-obstructive AHI, and a higher prevalence of REM-related OSA than the patients with OSA but without asthma.[48]

Sleep-Disordered Breathing as a Risk Factor for Asthma and Asthma Severity

It is possible that there is more than just an association between SDB and asthma, as SDB has been shown to be a risk factor for the development of asthma. Sulit and colleagues found that children with SDB had almost twice the odds of developing wheeze than those without SDB.[49] Furthermore, an epidemiologic study of more than 20,000 children showed that habitual snoring and OSA were significant predictors of asthma.[50] Additionally, the presence of SDB or OSA may affect asthma control and severity of asthma exacerbations. Ginis and coworkers studied over 400 children with asthma and found that SDB was an independent risk factor for poor asthma control.[51] In a study of over 25,000 children hospitalized with asthma, patients with OSA had a significantly longer length of stay suggesting that they had a higher level of nocturnal hypoxia and hypoventilation during their asthma episodes.[52] Similar to this finding, another study found that in patients with asthma that were not in an acute exacerbation, nocturnal ventilatory control was reduced in children who also had OSA when compared with children who only had asthma.[53]

Asthma, Sleep-Disordered Breathing, and Causality

Though there is a clear association with asthma and SDB, no studies have been able to definitively conclude a causal relationship between SDB and asthma. Castro-Rodriguez and colleagues used the Bradford Hill criteria (the most common epidemiology criteria for causality) to test if the relationship between asthma and SDB is causal. This method tests nine criteria including strength, consistency, specificity, temporality, biologic gradient, plausibility, coherence, experiment, and analogy to determine causality. The authors concluded that though eight of nine criteria were fulfilled, no study showed temporality or directionality between asthma and SDB, so establishing a causal relationship was not possible based on known evidence.[54]

Sleep-Disordered Breathing Treatment and Asthma

Though a causal relationship between SDB and asthma has not been proven, studies evaluating asthma outcomes following treatment of SDB suggest that these disorders do influence each other. In the study previously mentioned that used PSG to diagnose OSA, AT was performed in asthmatic children with OSA. On 1-year follow-up, annual number of exacerbations, weekly use of bronchodilators, and asthma symptom scores decreased significantly in these children. However, it should be noted that in this study, the control group used were children with asthma and not OSA so there was no comparison between children with asthma and OSA who did not receive treatment.[45] A systematic review by Brockmann and coworkers also evaluated the impact of treatment and management of SDB and asthma. Among 32 studies with over 140,000 patients, the authors found several studies that investigated the effect of AT on asthma control. In all of these studies, AT was associated with reduction in acute asthma exacerbations, asthma-related emergency room visits, and asthma-related hospitalizations (Fig. 32.5A and B).[55] There was also an association with reduction in

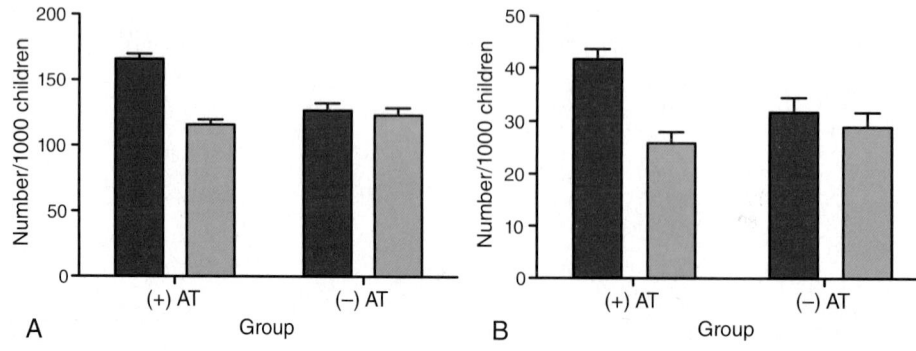

• **Fig. 32.5** Annual incidence of acute asthma exacerbation (A) and acute status asthmaticus (B). *Red bars* represent 1 year prior to adenotonsillectomy (AT) in AT+ children or first year of follow-up in AT− children; *green bars* represent 1 year after AT or second year of follow-up.[55]

asthma prescription refills of bronchodilators, systemic steroids, and leukotriene receptor antagonists.[40]

Asthma and Sleep Quality

Children with asthma, even those who do not have SDB, are at high risk for poor sleep quality and missed sleep.[56] Forty-one percent of children with asthma have intermittent nocturnal symptoms and an even higher percentage have persistent nocturnal symptoms. Nocturnal symptoms are an obvious reason for sleep disruption in these patients.[57] Other reasons that may account for poor sleep in patients with asthma include circadian variations of lung function, supine posture, air temperature, allergens in the bedroom, hormonal variations, and diurnal variations of lung inflammation.[56,58,59] In addition, environmental factors and comorbid conditions can contribute to poor sleep in asthmatic children. Many asthma patients reside in urban environments where sleep may also be disrupted by poor sleep hygiene, noise disturbance, external stressors, and frequent relocation. Triggers for allergic rhinitis, a frequent contributor to poor asthma control, are also prevalent in the urban environment and can impact sleep. In addition, external stressors can lead to symptoms of anxiety, which also affect sleep quality.[60–62]

Abnormal sleep in patients with asthma who do not have SDB has also been shown by PSG. Studies have shown abnormal findings on PSG, problems with sleep quality, and consequent daytime dysfunction in asthma patients without a diagnosis of SDB. In one study, patients with controlled and uncontrolled asthma who underwent PSGs had more nocturnal awakenings, a higher mean wakefulness after sleep onset, and less REM sleep than normative values.[57] In addition, in a study comparing PSG findings in asthma patients with and without OSA, patients with asthma but not OSA had significantly longer sleep latency and less slow-wave sleep compared with non-asthmatics.[63]

Furthermore, poor sleep quality and missed sleep can affect asthma outcomes. Studies have shown that missed sleep is an indicator of asthma morbidity and poorly controlled asthma. Daniel and colleagues reported an association of missed sleep with frequent school absences, more activity limitations, and lower quality of life scores in urban children with asthma. In addition, they found that of those asthma patients with anxiety, there was an even stronger association of missed sleep and asthma morbidity. Given that poor sleep can result in increased asthma morbidity, fatigue, and daytime sleepiness, the high frequency of sleep disruption in patients with asthma underscores the importance of determining sleep quality when evaluating these patients.[56]

Conclusions

Based on numerous investigations, asthma and SDB are clearly associated. SDB can be a risk factor for developing asthma, and treatment of SDB can influence asthma outcomes. Additionally, sleep disturbances in patients with asthma without SDB can lead to daytime dysfunction even when asthma is well controlled. This strong association coupled with the known effects of poor sleep quality on asthma outcomes highlights the importance of a comprehensive assessment of sleep in patients with asthma. Similarly, the prevalence of asthma among patients with SDB necessitates the implementation of screening for asthma in patients with symptoms of SDB. Therapy for one disorder may influence the outcome of the other, requiring a multifaceted approach to the care for patients with symptoms of SDB and for patients with asthma. The impact of improved sleep on quality of life, academic performance, and cognitive function makes screening for these disorders critical for clinicians seeing patients with sleep and respiratory problems.

CLINICAL PEARLS

- Children with cystic fibrosis frequently have disrupted sleep and poor sleep quality that directly impacts their quality of life even in the setting of mild or minimal lung disease.
- Health care providers should have a low threshold for screening overnight oximetry studies and/or polysomnograms in children with cystic fibrosis.
- There is an overlap in inflammatory pathophysiology between asthma and sleep-disordered breathing.
- The known effects of sleep-disordered breathing and poor sleep quality on asthma outcomes highlights the importance of a comprehensive assessment of sleep in children with asthma.

References

1. Spruyt K. A review of developmental consequences of poor sleep in childhood. *Sleep Med.* 2019;60:3–12.
2. Vandeleur M, Walter LM, Armstrong DS, Robinson P, Nixon GM, Horne RSC. Quality of life and mood in children with cystic fibrosis: Associations with sleep quality. *J Cyst Fibros.* 2018;17(6):811–820.
3. Goetz D, Ren CL. Review of cystic fibrosis. *Pediatr Ann.* 2019;48(4):e154–e161.
4. Egan ME. Cystic fibrosis transmembrane conductance receptor modulator therapy in cystic fibrosis, an update. *Curr Opin Pediatr.* 2020;32(3):384–388.
5. Spicuzza L, Sciuto C, Leonardi S, La Rosa M. Early occurrence of obstructive sleep apnea in infants and children with cystic fibrosis. *Arch Pediatr Adolesc Med.* 2012;166(12):1165–1169.
6. van der Giessen L, Loeve M, de Jongste J, Hop W, Tiddens H. Nocturnal cough in children with stable cystic fibrosis. *Pediatr Pulmonol.* 2009;44(9):859–865.
7. Amin R, Bean J, Burklow K, Jeffries J. The relationship between sleep disturbance and pulmonary function in stable pediatric cystic fibrosis patients. *Chest.* 2005;128(3):1357–1363.
8. Vandeleur M, Walter LM, Armstrong DS, Robinson P, Nixon GM, Horne RSC. What keeps children with cystic fibrosis awake at night? *J Cyst Fibros.* 2017;16(6):719–726.
9. Suratwala D, Chan JS, Kelly A, Meltzer LJ, Gallagher PR, Traylor J, et al. Nocturnal saturation and glucose tolerance in children with cystic fibrosis. *Thorax.* 2011;66(7):574–578.

10. Daniel LC, Li Y, Kloss JD, Reilly AF, Barakat LP. The impact of dexamethasone and prednisone on sleep in children with acute lymphoblastic leukemia. *Support Care Cancer.* 2016;24(9):3897–3906.

11. Allen JM, Graef DM, Ehrentraut JH, Tynes BL, Crabtree VM. Sleep and Pain in pediatric illness: A conceptual review. *CNS Neurosci Ther.* 2016;22(11):880–893.

12. Canter KS, Strang A, Franklin M, Wilks S, Geiser D, Okonak K, et al. A Qualitative exploration of sleep habits and intervention needs among youth with cystic fibrosis. *J Clin Psychol Med Settings.* 2022;29(1):44–53.

13. Jagpal SK, Jobanputra AM, Ahmed OH, Santiago TV, Ramagopal M. Sleep-disordered breathing in cystic fibrosis. *Pediatr Pulmonol.* 2021;56(Suppl 1):S23–S31.

14. Paranjape SM, McGinley BM, Braun AT, Schneider H. Polysomnographic markers in children with cystic fibrosis lung disease. *Pediatrics.* 2015;136(5):920–926.

15. Vandeleur M, Walter LM, Armstrong DS, Robinson P, Nixon GM, Horne RSC. How well do children with cystic fibrosis sleep? An actigraphic and questionnaire-based study. *J Pediatr.* 2017;182:170–176.

16. Fauroux B, Pepin JL, Boelle PY, Cracowski C, Murris-Espin M, Nove-Josserand R, et al. Sleep quality and nocturnal hypoxaemia and hypercapnia in children and young adults with cystic fibrosis. *Arch Dis Child.* 2012;97(11):960–966.

17. Munyard P, Bush A. How much coughing is normal? *Arch Dis Child.* 1996;74(6):531–534.

18. de Castro-Silva C, de Bruin VM, Cavalcante AG, Bittencourt LR, de Bruin PF. Nocturnal hypoxia and sleep disturbances in cystic fibrosis. *Pediatr Pulmonol.* 2009;44(11):1143–1150.

19. Mulette P, Ravoninjatovo B, Guguen C, Barbe C, Ancel J, Dury S, et al. Insomnia in adults with cystic fibrosis: strong association with anxiety/depression and impaired quality of life. *BMC Pulm Med.* 2021;21(1).108

20. Waters KA, Lowe A, Cooper P, Vella S, Selvadurai H. A cross-sectional analysis of daytime versus nocturnal polysomnographic respiratory parameters in cystic fibrosis during early adolescence. *J Cyst Fibros.* 2017;16(2):250–257.

21. Isaiah A, Daher A, Sharma PB, Naqvi K, Mitchell RB. Predictors of sleep hypoxemia in children with cystic fibrosis. *Pediatr Pulmonol.* 2019;54(3):273–279.

22. Tepper RS, Skatrud JB, Dempsey JA. Ventilation and oxygenation changes during sleep in cystic fibrosis. *Chest.* 1983;84(4):388–393.

23. Villa MP, Pagani J, Lucidi V, Palamides S, Ronchetti R. Nocturnal oximetry in infants with cystic fibrosis. *Arch Dis Child.* 2001;84(1):50–54.

24. van der Giessen L, Bakker M, Joosten K, Hop W, Tiddens H. Nocturnal oxygen saturation in children with stable cystic fibrosis. *Pediatr Pulmonol.* 2012;47(11):1123–1130.

25. Ramos RT, Salles C, Daltro CH, Santana MA, Gregorio PB, Acosta AX. Sleep architecture and polysomnographic respiratory profile of children and adolescents with cystic fibrosis. *J Pediatr (Rio J).* 2011;87(1):63–69.

26. Dobbin CJ, Bartlett D, Melehan K, Grunstein RR, Bye PT. The effect of infective exacerbations on sleep and neurobehavioral function in cystic fibrosis. *Am J Respir Crit Care Med.* 2005;172(1):99–104.

27. Perin C, Fagondes SC, Casarotto FC, Pinotti AF, Menna Barreto SS, Dalcin Pde T. Sleep findings and predictors of sleep desaturation in adult cystic fibrosis patients. *Sleep Breath.* 2012;16(4):1041–1048.

28. Ziegler B, Perin C, Casarotto FC, Fagondes SC, Menna-Barreto SS, Dalcin PTR. Pulmonary hypertension as estimated by Doppler echocardiography in adolescent and adult patients with cystic fibrosis and their relationship with clinical, lung function and sleep findings. *Clin Respir J.* 2018;12(2):754–761.

29. Moran F, Bradley JM, Piper AJ. Non-invasive ventilation for cystic fibrosis. *Cochrane Database Syst Rev.* 2017;2(2):Cd002769.

30. Milross MA, Piper AJ, Dwyer TJ, Wong K, Bell SC, Bye PTP. Non-invasive ventilation versus oxygen therapy in cystic fibrosis: A 12-month randomized trial. *Respirology.* 2019;24(12):1191–1197.

31. McCormick J, Cho DY, Lampkin B, Richman J, Hathorne H, Rowe SM, et al. Ivacaftor improves rhinologic, psychologic, and sleep-related quality of life in G551D cystic fibrosis patients. *Int Forum Allergy Rhinol.* 2019;9(3):292–297.

32. Centers for Disease Control and Prevention. Most Recent National Asthma Data. Published [2018]. Updated March 24, [2020]. https://www.cdc.gov/asthma/most_recent_national_asthma_data.htm

33. Banasiak NC. Understanding the relationship between asthma and sleep in the pediatric population. *J Pediatr Health Care.* 2016;30(6):546–550.

34. King GG, James A, Harkness L, Wark PAB. Pathophysiology of severe asthma: We've only just started. *Respirology.* 2018;23(3):262–271.

35. Pearce N, Aït-Khaled N, Beasley B, Mallol J, Keil U, Mitchell E, Robertson C, the ISAAC Phase Three Study Group Worldwide trends in the prevalence of asthma symptoms: Phase III of the International Study of Asthm and Allergies in Childhood (ISAAC). *Thorax.* 2007;62(9):758–766.

36. Lumeng JC, Chervin RD. Epidemiology of pediatric obstructive sleep apnea. *Proc Am Thoracic Soc.* 2008;5(2):242–252.

37. Caballero Balanzá S, Martorell Aragonés A, Cerdá Mir JC, Belda Ramírez J, Navarro Iváñez R, Navarro Soriano A, et al. Leukotriene B4 and 8-isoprostane in exhaled breath condensate of children with episodic and persistent asthma. *J Investig Allergol Clin Immunol.* 2010;20(3):237–243.

38. Goldbart AD, Krishna J, Li RC, Serpero LD, Gozal D. Inflammatory mediators in exhaled breath condensate of children with obstructive sleep apnea syndrome. *Chest.* 2006;130(1):143–148.

39. Malakasioti G, Gourgoulianis K, Chrousos G, Kaditis A. Interactions of obstructive sleep-disordered breathing with recurrent wheezing or asthma and their effects on sleep quality. *Pediatr Pulmonol.* 2011;46(11):1047–1054.

40. Brockmann P, Sanchez T, Castro-Rodriguez JA. Sleep-disordered breathing in children with asthma: A systematic review on the impact of treatment. *J Asthma Allergy.* 2016;9:83–91.

41. Brockmann PE, Bertrand P, Castro-Rodriguez JA. Influence of asthma on sleep disordered breathing in children: A systematic review. *Sleep Med Rev.* 2014;18(5):393–397.

42. Expert Panel Report 3 (EPR-3) Guidelines for the Diagnosis and Management of Asthma–Summary Report 2007. *J Allergy Clin Immunol.* 2007;120(5):S94–S138.

43. Goldstein NA, Aronin C, Kantrowitz B, Hershcopf R, Fishkin S, Lee H, et al. The prevalence of sleep-disordered breathing in children with asthma and its behavioral effects. *Pediatr Pulmonol.* 2015;50(11):1128–1136.

44. Zandieh SO, Cespedes A, Ciarleglio A, Bourgeois W, Rapoport DM, Bruzzese J-M. Asthma and subjective sleep disordered breathing in a large cohort of urban adolescents. *J Asthma.* 2017;54(1):62–68.

45. Kheirandish-Gozal L, Dayyat EA, Eid NS, Morton RL, Gozal D. Obstructive sleep apnea in poorly controlled asthmatic children: Effect of adenotonsillectomy. *Pediatr Pulmonol.* 2011;46(9):913–918.

46. Ramagopal M, Mehta A, Roberts DW, Wolf JS, Taylor RJ, Mudd KE, et al. Asthma as a predictor of obstructive sleep apnea in urban African-American children. *J Asthma.* 2009;46(9):895–899.

47. Ross KR, Storfer-Isser A, Hart MA, Kibler AMV, Rueschman M, Rosen CL, et al. Sleep-disordered breathing is associated with asthma severity in children. *J Pediatr.* 2012;160(5):736–742.

48. Gutierrez MJ, Zhu J, Rodriguez-Martinez CE, Nino CL, Nino G. Nocturnal phenotypical features of obstructive sleep apnea (OSA) in asthmatic children. *Pediatr Pulmonol.* 2013;48(6):592–600.

49. Sulit LG, Storfer-Isser A, Rosen CL, Kirchner HL, Redline S. Associations of obesity, sleep-disordered breathing, and wheezing in children. *Am J Respir Crit Care Med.* 2005;171(6):659–664.

50. Li L, Xu Z, Jin X, Yan C, Jiang F, Tong S, et al. Sleep-disordered breathing and asthma: Evidence from a large multicentric epidemiological study in China. *Respir Res.* 2015;16(1):56.

51. Ginis T, Akcan FA, Capanoglu M, Toyran M, Ersu R, Kocabas CN, et al. The frequency of sleep-disordered breathing in children with asthma and its effects on asthma control. *J Asthma.* 2017;54(4):403–410.

52. Shanley LA, Lin H, Flores G. Factors associated with length of stay for pediatric asthma hospitalizations. *J Asthma.* 2015;52(5):471–477.

53. He Z, Armoni Domany K, Nava-Guerra L, Khoo MCK, Difrancesco M, Xu Y, et al. Phenotype of ventilatory control in children with moderate to severe persistent asthma and obstructive sleep apnea. *Sleep.* 2019;42(9):zsz130.

54. Castro-Rodriguez JA, Brockmann PE, Marcus CL. Relation between asthma and sleep disordered breathing in children: Is the association causal? *Paediatr Respir Rev.* 2017;22:72–75.

55. Bhattacharjee R, Choi BH, Gozal D, Mokhlesi B. Association of adenotonsillectomy with asthma outcomes in children: A longitudinal database analysis. *PLoS Med.* 2014;11(11):e1001753.

56. Daniel LC, Boergers J, Kopel SJ, Koinis-Mitchell D. Missed sleep and asthma morbidity in urban children. *Ann Allergy, Asthma Immunol.* 2012;109(1):41–46.

57. Fagnano M, Bayer AL, Isensee CA, Hernandez T, Halterman JS. Nocturnal asthma symptoms and poor sleep quality among urban school children with asthma. *Acad Pediatr.* 2011;11(6):493–499.

58. Kavanagh J, Jackson DJ, Kent BD. Sleep and asthma. *Curr Opin Pulm Med.* 2018;24(6):569–573.

59. Litinski M, Scheer FAJL, Shea SA. Influence of the circadian system on disease severity. *Sleep Med Clin.* 2009;4(2):143–163.

60. Martin SR, Boergers J, Kopel SJ, McQuaid EL, Seifer R, LeBourgeois M, et al. Sleep hygiene and sleep outcomes in a sample of urban children with and without asthma. *J Pediatr Psychol.* 2017;42(8):825–836.

61. Koinis-Mitchell D, Kopel SJ, Boergers J, Ramos K, LeBourgeois M, McQuaid EL, et al. Asthma, allergic rhinitis, and sleep problems in urban children. *J Clin Sleep Med.* 2015;11(02):101–110.

62. Daphne K-M, Julie B, Sheryl JK, Elizabeth LM, Michael LF, Monique L. Racial and ethnic disparities in sleep outcomes among urban children with and without asthma. *Sleep Health.* 2019;5(6):532–538.

63. Teng Y-K, Chiang L-C, Lue K-H, Chang S-W, Wang L, Lee S-P, et al. Poor sleep quality measured by polysomnography in non-obese asthmatic children with or without moderate to severe obstructive sleep apnea. *Sleep Med.* 2014;15(9):1062–1067.

33

Sleep-Disordered Breathing and Allergic Disorders

JOONG KI CHO and ANNA FISHBEIN

CHAPTER HIGHLIGHTS

- Allergic diseases have increased in prevalence and incidence over the past few decades.
- There is a bidirectional relationship between sleep and allergy-related factors.
- Medications associated with treatment of allergic diseases, including asthma, allergic rhinitis, and atopic dermatitis, can have a significant impact on sleep.
- For children with sleep disordered breathing (SDB) and allergic disease, sleep providers should work in close consultation with their allergist colleagues to ensure the treatment of both SDB and allergic disease are optimized.

This chapter provides a primer on allergic disease for the pediatric sleep medicine practitioner. The overlap of allergies and sleep is presented with research on epidemiology, clinical and mechanistic features of allergic disease, sleep-disordered breathing (SDB), and other sleep-disturbing conditions. Given most allergic disease has nocturnal flares, circadian mechanisms and sleep disturbance are common. Allergic Th2 inflammation might also be triggered by sleep disturbance and SDB, contributing to the viscous bidirectional relationship with allergic disease flare.

This chapter is organized by the most common allergic diseases, such as asthma, allergic rhinitis (AR), and atopic dermatitis (AD), and other allergic conditions (such as chronic rhinosinusitis [CRS] and urticaria). For each disease, we present an evidence-based approach to assessment by describing the clinical presentation, the impact on sleep. and the treatment approach. We outline treatment algorithms for each allergic disease.

Highlights from the chapter include the following:

- Sleep-disordered breathing (SDB) is common in children with allergic diseases (up to 88.5%) in asthma/AR patients. It might even predispose to the development of asthma.
- There is a bidirectional relationship between the inflammatory upregulation and disease flares in allergic disease and SDB.
- Sleep medicine providers should consider therapy personalized to comorbid allergic conditions. Therapies for allergic

disease are outlined in Table 33.1, including key side effects and efficacy for sleep. Referral to an allergist should be considered to help with diagnosis and management.

Introduction to Allergic Disease

Allergic diseases like asthma, AR, and AD are prevalent in the United States and have been increasing in incidence for the past few decades.[1-5] The prevalence of asthma in American children is 8.4%,[6] AR is up to 40%,[7,8] and AD is 10–20%.[9,10] AD is usually the first manifestation of atopy,[10] with 60% of children diagnosed in the first year of life.[11] Food allergy also commonly presents at <1 year of age. The allergic or "atopic march" can then progress to asthma (usually by 3–4 years of age) and finally AR (often by 7–8 years of age).[12,13] Allergic diseases, most notably asthma, disproportionately afflict urban minority children, particularly African Americans and persons of Puerto Rican descent.[6,14] Given the high prevalence of allergic disease in children, particularly in urban minority youth, it is important for pediatric sleep medicine providers to have basic knowledge of allergic disease and how it impacts sleep. In this chapter we will provide a background of SDB and allergy, and review the three most common allergic conditions that impact sleep. For asthma, AR, and AD we will (1) define the condition, (2) discuss the mechanism and clinical overlap with sleep/SDB, and (3) will briefly discuss treatment. Finally, we conclude the chapter with a discussion of other allergic conditions and their relationship with sleep and SDB.

Sleep-Disordered Breathing and Allergy

SDB is frequently encountered in pediatric allergy patients, most commonly co-occurring in asthma and AR; 88.5% of children at risk of sleep-related breathing disorders (based on Pediatric Sleep Questionnaire [PSQ] screening) were diagnosed with both AR and asthma.[15] SDB encompasses disorders that have abnormal respiratory patterns or insufficient ventilation during sleep, such as mouth breathing due to nasal obstruction, upper airways resistance syndrome, snoring, and obstructive sleep apnea (OSA).[16] SDB prevalence in the general pediatric population (apnea-hypopnea index [AHI] >10 and 5) is 1.6 and 10.3%, respectively.[17] Given the pathophysiology of uncontrolled AR causing upper airway resistance and/or obstruction and asthma causing ventilation defects and abnormal respiratory patterns, treatment of SDB should also include identification and treatment of the patient's underlying allergic conditions.

Furthermore, asthma guidelines recommend screening for SDB in poorly controlled asthma.[18] Assessment of AR severity is defined in part by the presence of sleep-related impairment on the most broadly used tool (Allergic Rhinitis and its Impact on Asthma [ARIA] guidelines).[19] One

systematic review in asthmatics noted average odds of 2–3 for SDB across 11 studies.[20] As pointed out by this paper, SDB can be variably defined as an outcome measure (presence of snoring, AHI >1.5, etc.).

Screening for SDB is possible via the PSQ, a 22-item questionnaire validated in children 2–18 years of age.[21] Questions capture domains of breathing (such as observed apneas), sleepiness, behavior (such as fidgeting), and other associated symptoms/risk factors (such as obesity). In 54 subjects with polysomnography (PSG)-confirmed sleep-related breathing disorder, a score of 0.33 on this PSQ SDB subscale was 85% sensitive and 87% specific for SDB.[22] Given SDB is distinct from asthma yet can have a great deal of overlap in symptomatology, it might not be surprising that the PSQ is

TABLE 33.1　Common Therapeutics for Allergic Disease and Impact on Sleep

Allergic disease	Treatment	Key side effect considerations	Comments on indication/benefits in sleep
Asthma	Inhaled corticosteroids (ICS), e.g., fluticasone, budesonide	• Thrush in mouth • Potential decreased linear growth	• First-line therapy • Decreases nocturnal awakenings
	Combination inhaler with ICS + long-acting β-agonist (LABA), e.g., fluticasone/salmeterol, budesonide/formoterol	• Same as ICS • Possible mild tachycardia with LABA	• Good option for step-up therapy or in moderate/severe disease
	Montelukast (leukotriene receptor antagonist)	• Black box warning for suicidal ideations	• Not generally used as monotherapy, best in combination with ICS • Good choice for children with concomitant OSA
	Omalizumab (first FDA-approved systemic therapy for pediatric asthma)	• Injection-related side effects • Required 30-minute observation period due to anaphylaxis risk	• Case reports suggest also improves OSA • Generally believed to decrease nocturnal awakenings
	Adenotonsillectomy	• Surgical risks	• In comorbid OSA/SDB, improves nocturnal asthma symptoms and SDB
Allergic rhinitis	First-generation antihistamines, e.g., Benadryl, hydroxyzine	• Drying (anticholinergic) effect on skin/mucous membranes • Sedating	• Not generally recommended for allergic rhinitis, short half-life • Potential for hypersomnolence, appears to decrease sleep-onset latency • Potential tolerance
	Second-generation antihistamines, e.g., fexofenadine, cetirizine, loratadine	• ~20% risk of sedating effect (cetirizine)	• First-line therapy • Improve patient-/parent-reported sleep disturbance, sleep interference and quality of life • Can be taken PRN
	Intranasal corticosteroid, e.g., fluticasone propionate and mometasone	• Epistaxis, more common with incorrect use • Very theoretical effect on linear growth	• Most effective of first-line treatments • Decreases upper airways resistance to improve sleep quality
	Intranasal antihistamine/combination with intranasal steroid	• Can be sedating like oral antihistamine	• Nice adjunctive therapy, best used as combination therapy with intranasal steroid • Provides only temporary relief • Not clear impact on sleep
	Montelukast	• See above	• Not first line • Potentially Improves daytime somnolence and fatigue
	Allergen immunotherapy (subcutaneous or sublingual)	• Local reactions or anaphylaxis • Time-consuming	• Improvement in sleep quality by patient report

TABLE 33.1 Common Therapeutics for Allergic Disease and Impact on Sleep—Cont'd

Allergic disease	Treatment	Key side effect considerations	Comments on indication/benefits in sleep
Atopic dermatitis	Topical corticosteroid, e.g., hydrocortisone 2.5% ointment, triamcinolone 0.1% ointment	• Reversible side effects: skin thinning, telangiectasia, abnormal hair growth • Non-reversible, with long-term higher potency use: striae	• First-line treatment • Understudied in sleep, but likely improves sleep quality by improving disease severity
	Topical calcineurin inhibitor, e.g., tacrolimus 0.1% ointment, pimecrolimus 1% cream	• Black box warning for malignancy risk (from animal studies, but not clearly true in humans)	• Second-line treatment • Improvement in patient-report of sleep
	Topical PDE-4 inhibitor, i.e., crisaborole ointment 2%	• Burning/stinging with application	• Improvement based on one parent-reported question on sleep disturbance
	Melatonin	• Might flare asthma and ↑ allergic inflammation • Can be sedating	• Reduction in sleep-onset latency • Improved sleep quality
	First-generation antihistamines	• Same as above	• Classically hydroxyzine is used, also with antipruritic effects • Only recommended for short-term use • Not good data to support efficacy in sleep, might decrease sleep-onset latency, but does not appear to improve other aspects of sleep quality
	Dupilumab (newest FDA-approved systemic therapy in children ≥6-year-olds)	• Conjunctivitis • Injection site reactions	• Likely improves sleep quality • Very effective to reduce eczema severity, indicated only for moderate/severe disease

OSA, obstructive sleep apnea; *FDA*, U.S. Food and Drug Administration; *SDB*, sleep-disordered breathing; *PRN*, as needed.

sensitive (0.82) but not specific (0.13) for SDB in children with asthma.[22] This affirms that PSQ is an effective screening tool, but PSG is still necessary to differentiate asthma-induced wheezing with SDB-associated snoring and apnea.[23]

Bidirectional Relationship between Sleep and Allergy

Allergic inflammatory mediators, interleukin (IL)-4, IL-5, and IL-13, are released and perpetuated by "allergic" Th2 cells.[24,25] These cytokines can increase arousals, produce aberrations in rapid eye movement (REM) sleep, increase REM latency, and decrease REM duration.[26] Sleep disturbance itself can also result in pro-Th2 inflammatory release, thereby contributing to the vicious cycle between sleep disturbance and exacerbation of allergic disease. In fact, adenotonsillar regrowth after surgery is more common in children with asthma,[27] and this might be in part due to the allergic inflammatory cascade.

Seventy-two percent of allergists inquire about sleep quality[16] because when allergy patients report poor sleep or daytime fatigue, these are signs of poor disease control.[28] Maladapted sleep habits can develop in allergic patients, and allergic disease has a common pattern of nocturnal flare, making poor sleep efficiency common.[29,30] Indeed, fragmented sleep impairs cognition, attention, school performance, and might be one mechanism for the increased

risk of obesity.[31] Circadian rhythms and circadian immunology play a large mechanistic role in the interaction between allergic disease and sleep; we refer the reader to another book chapter for a more detail on that topic.[32]

From the perspective of a practicing sleep medicine physician who is evaluating a child with excessive daytime sleepiness, one study found in their modeling that asthma history is actually a bigger risk factor for excessive daytime sleepiness than PSG-measured sleep derangements.[33] In a study of urban children with asthma, children with more comorbid conditions (such as obesity and AR) were at a greater risk for shorter sleep duration and more school absences.[34] With regards to sleep disturbance causing allergic disease, one study found that short sleep duration (<6.8 hours) is associated with increased risk of developing food allergy (odds ratio [OR] 1.9, 1.3 – 2.7).[35] Another longitudinal study found that being overtired in childhood due to sleep disturbance resulted in increased odds of rhinitis (2.59; 95% confidence interval [CI] 1.31–5.11) at adolescence.[36]

Asthma

Clinical Presentation of Asthma

Asthma is a chronic inflammatory disease of the lower respiratory tract characterized by bronchial hyperreactivity and episodic partially reversible lower airway obstruction.[18] Most children present with a history of persistent cough, wheezing, chest tightness, or shortness of breath. Family history of atopy is common. Classic triggers include viral illness, exercise, allergens, and irritants. Although bronchial provocation can be performed to prove airway hyperreactivity, this test is rarely ordered in clinical practice due to risk and expense. Per guidelines, for the diagnosis a clinician should establish a history consistent with episodic airways obstruction/hyperresponsiveness that is reversible. Reversibility is usually defined by $\geq 12\%$ improvement in forced expiratory volume in 1 second (FEV_1) after administration of short-acting β_2-agonist (SABA). Alternative diagnoses should be ruled out.[18] If there is no access to spirometry to measure lung function objectively, clinical history of bronchodilator responsiveness is sufficient to make the diagnosis.

Asthma affects boys more than girls in early childhood with prevalence rates shifting during adolescence.[37] Given many children are transient wheezers in early childhood, the diagnosis of asthma is usually not made before 3 years of age.[38] Asthma severity is defined depending on guidelines reviewed,[39,40] but in general it is considered persistent once daily inhaled corticosteroid (ICS) is required to maintain control. We generally discuss the "rule of 2s" to assess control. If children are coughing more than two times per week or need SABA more than two times per week (except pre-exercise), then this indicates inadequate control.[18,41]

Nocturnal Asthma Fragments Sleep and Is Exacerbated by Sleep-Disordered Breathing

Asthma classically flares at night with a prevalence rate of 34–40%.[42,43] Nocturnal asthma flare occurs when lung function has a physiologic nadir, ~4 a.m.[44] In fact, several studies have demonstrated that day/night differences in lung function are ~10% in healthy controls, and 25–50% in asthmatics.[45,46] These nocturnal flares can result in significant sleep disturbance. It is important to note many parents will not think much of their child's nocturnal cough if they "sleep through it," so the clinician must specifically query about these episodes. Asthma can cause significant sleep fragmentation and increased time spent awake,[47] and, in fact, even with good asthma control there might still be poor sleep.[48] This can lead to an increased risk of school truancy and worse school performance.[43] Sleep-related impairment is also a big concern in children with asthma, with a strong association between lung function and sleep quality,[49] and one small study (n = 21 asthmatics) found worse performance on memory and concentration tasks compared with controls (N = 18).[49,50] Unfortunately the vicious cycle of poor sleep can also exacerbate asthma as demonstrated in one pilot study of adolescents,[51] and poor sleep quality might even worsen asthma symptoms the following day.[52] Interventions to improve sleep hygiene, such as encouraging a patient to sleep in their own bed[53] and decreasing screen time, might increase sleep duration and decrease insomnia.[54]

As discussed previously, SDB is a common comorbidity in asthma, and children with SDB have 3.62-fold increased odds of developing severe asthma.[55] OSA is also a common comorbidity in asthma, and more severe asthmatics tend to have more severe OSA.[56] Importantly, treatment of pediatric OSA can actually improve asthma control.[57]

Treatment Considerations in Asthma

The goals of asthma treatment include improving quality of life by decreasing morbidity (decreasing symptoms of day/night cough, improving daytime function, improving exercise tolerance) and reducing risk of exacerbation.[18,58] According to the National Heart, Lung, and Blood Institute (NHLBI) guidelines for control in children, nighttime symptoms are acceptable no more than one time per month.[59]

Personalized treatment and action plans should be evidence based and in-clinic teaching for children and parents should emphasize triggers (cigarette smoke, allergens, exercise, viral illness, strong scents, etc.) as well as adherence and adequate technique when using ICS. As part of guidelines-based care, recognition and treatment of comorbidities, such as AR, OSA, etc., is crucial to asthma control.[40] Asthma control is primarily assessed by patient-reported measures, such as the Asthma Control Test.[60] Objective lung function assessment of control (such as with spirometry) can also be crucial in children who are "poor perceivers."[59] NHLBI guidelines recommend a "step-up" or "step-down" approach with disease control assessed every 3 months.[39] Consideration of other factors is prudent in determining when to adjust therapy, i.e., step-down therapy is not usually recommended during the fall/winter.

Classically patients are initiated on ICS to gain control of their disease. In patients with milder or seasonally flared asthma, ICS can be used as a "yellow zone" plan only. ICS is crucial for asthma control and should be used if needed, but it is important to counsel patients that long-term studies have found long-term use (particularly in prepubescent children) might be associated with decreased height by about 1 cm and does not have any long-term benefit of preserving lung function.[61–63] In terms of step-up therapy from those on low/mid-potency ICS, generally long-acting β_2-agonists (LABAs) are the most effective strategy,[64] and in African American children, higher dose ICS or ICS + LABA is effective.[65] Leukotriene receptor antagonists (LRTAs), specifically montelukast, is another option for "add-on" therapy that appears to be of particular benefit in those with comorbid OSA. This might be because cysteinyl leukotriene receptor-1 is overexpressed in adenotonsillar cells in children with OSA,[66] and montelukast appears to decrease adenoid size,[67,68] resulting in decreased AHI in children with mild OSA.[69] Given the new black box warning on montelukast for side effects of aggression, depression, suicidal thinking, and behavioral issues,[70] it is important to counsel parents prior to prescription. As a side point, evening administration of LTRA is recommended due to its relative short half-life and possibly better efficacy in combatting the nocturnal upregulation of leukotrienes.[71]

Another consideration in asthma with comorbid OSA, is the potential benefit of adenotonsillectomy (AT). One small study found that 60% of asthmatic children were able to eliminate all of their asthma therapies and 28% able to eliminate some of their therapies after AT.[72] AT was also found to reduce the frequency of asthma exacerbations and bronchodilator usage in children with poorly controlled asthma and OSA, a finding not seen in children without OSA.[73] The Childhood Adenotonsillectomy Trial (CHAT) study has demonstrated the benefit of AT for sleep-related outcomes in OSA,[74] and a new study, Pediatric Adenotonsillectomy Trial for Snoring (PATS), is addressing the benefit of AT for mild OSA and SDB.[75]

Allergic Rhinitis

Clinical Presentation of Allergic Rhinitis

AR, also called allergic rhinoconjunctivitis when the eyes are involved, is triggered by specific IgE (sIgE) to aeroallergens in the environment.[76] Often rhinitis is "mixed" meaning it is also exacerbated by irritants, such as extremely cold weather, and not just allergens. Allergens that commonly trigger AR in younger children are indoor, such as pet dander and dust mite, as they have not yet had time to become allergic to outdoor seasonal allergens. Whereas older children are often allergic to indoor and outdoor allergens (mold, weed, pollens). Symptomatic AR usually begins by 7 years of age.[77] The natural history of AR is that it tends to become more persistent and worsen throughout childhood.[78]

Allergic Rhinitis Impairs Sleep Quality and Increased Nasal Airway Resistance Contributes to Sleep-Disordered Breathing

Sleep problems are common in children with AR, with up to 88% of children with AR having some degree of sleep impairment.[79] Parent-report of sleep disturbance in a study of 67 children with AR was significantly associated with sleepiness, poor perceived cognitive function, anxiety, fatigue, depression, and worse peer relationships.[80] A classic paper on this topic showed that allergic sensitization (positive allergy skin test) is common in children who snore (35%), and OSA was more common in the sensitization population.[81] This is likely due to the "one airway" in which inflammatory mediators as a result of rhinitis induce edema and resistance throughout the airway.

The mechanism of the nocturnal flare in AR peaking in early morning hours (classically ~6 a.m.) is due to dependent edema while laying down throughout the night, increased pollen counts in the early morning, and upregulated inflammation in peripheral blood/tissues as a response to cortisol nadir.[82,83] In fact, pollen counts on the day of PSG can influence the study in children with AR.[84]

Nasal congestion in AR leads to increased airway resistance and sometimes frank nasal obstruction, resulting in obligate mouth breathing. Mouth breathing can result in adenoid facies, characterized by retrognathia and a high arched palate, exacerbating sleep apnea.[85] In a meta-analysis on the prevalence of AR in SDB, children with SDB or OSA had concomitant AR 40.8% and 45% of the time, respectively, giving 2.12 times higher odds of AR in children with versus without SDB.[86] AR may be a contributor to adenotonsillar hypertrophy,[87] and in children with sleep apnea post-AT, the presence of AR can lead to persistently poor quality of life.[88]

Treatment of Allergic Rhinitis

Treatment of AR should initially focus on identification and avoidance of aeroallergen triggers. For example, in patients with dust mite allergy, dust mite covers and dust mite avoidance measures can be implemented.

As far as pharmacotherapy, intranasal corticosteroids are generally considered as first-line treatment for moderate to severe AR in children ≥3 years old due to their efficacy at inducing apoptosis of eosinophils and significantly shrinking nasal tissue swelling.[89] Several systematic reviews summarize the clinical benefits of nasal steroids in children with AR that combat the most common symptoms, including sneezing, itching, rhinorrhea, and congestion, and shrink adenotonsillar tissue.[90,91] They are superior to antihistamines in their efficacy and also improve sleep-related symptoms including daytime fatigue and somnolence.[82,90]

Second-generation (non-sedating) antihistamines are generally the first initiated treatment for mild AR in children due to ease of use, easy on and off, and lack of side effects. Although they do not shrink tissue swelling, they do relieve symptoms of pruritus and can improve comfort.[89] Second-generation antihistamines have been shown to improve sleep and quality of life.[92] As mentioned with asthma, LTRAs like montelukast can be effective in improving daytime somnolence and daytime fatigue over placebo,[93] but they are not recommended as monotherapy AR because nasal steroids are more effective.[94]

Subcutaneous allergen immunotherapy ("allergy shots") is an effective therapy for those inadequately controlled on pharmacotherapy. Sublingual immunotherapy (SLIT) is a newer easy approach, but is only effective for mild disease.[89]

Atopic Dermatitis

Clinic Presentation of Atopic Dermatitis

AD, also commonly called eczema, is the most common inflammatory skin condition of childhood. Some refer to it as the "itch that rashes." Due to the hallmark symptom of itch and the nocturnal flare of disease, sleep disturbance is rampant and can be referred to as "nocturnal eczema."[95] Although AD is more common in young children, and the disease tends to get better over time, newer data suggest 20–50% of cases persist into adulthood.[96,97]

Atopic Dermatitis Is a Sleep-Disturbing Condition

Several studies affirm that AD causes sleep disturbance in ~60% of children and much higher in times of disease flare, with consistently reported sleep fragmentation and sometimes prolonged sleep-onset latency.[95] Furthermore, AD can wax and wane and can be exacerbated by many triggers, including viral illness. Although allergies can exacerbate AD, such as foods, or dust mite/pets in the home environment, they are rarely the only cause. Families should be counseled that it is chronic disease requiring chronic treatment, and attempts to isolate "the cause" are unlikely to be successful. Importantly in AD or AR, inpatient sleep studies might not always capture the degree of sleep disturbance the condition can inflict due to the relatively sterile environment.

The burden of sleep disturbance in AD correlates strongly with disease severity and those with moderate to severe disease experience ~50 minutes more wake after sleep onset on actigraphy than healthy controls.[98] Scratching appears to peak ~3 hours after sleep onset,[99] and it appears to be highest during transitional sleep (N1 and N2) compared with N3.[100,101] When differentiating from periodic limb movement disorder (PLMD) on PSG, it can be helpful to look for scratching movements during wake. Additionally, PLMD versus AD appears to have increased limb movements and arousals during N2 sleep.[101] It is important, even in AD that is quiescent, to query about a history, because sleep disturbance can still be present.[102]

Although AD has been associated with SDB in terms of snoring, it is not clear how much that is due to underlying atopy and other allergic conditions.[103] OSA is also comorbid with AD, and the IL-6 upregulation in OSA can trigger Th2 cytokine upregulation to induce AD flare.[104]

Treatment of Atopic Dermatitis

Treatment of AD itself can certainly improve sleep, and therapy should be approached based on disease severity and existing guidelines.[105] For all levels of severity, therapy should start with good basic skin care, frequent moisturization, and adjuvant therapies such as nighttime wet wraps and bleach baths.[106] Although first-generation antihistamines, such as hydroxyzine, are frequently used to induce sedation and might decrease sleep-onset latency, there is no data showing they improve sleep maintenance and decrease nocturnal scratching/sleep fragmentation.[99] Prescription topical corticosteroids are the first-line therapy after basic skin care, and are safe to use even in infants. Feared side effects, such as skin thinning, telangiectasias, and abnormal hair growth are rare and reversible.[107] Topical non-steroidal agents, such as calcineurin inhibitors like pimecrolimus might improve sleep (as shown on a one-question visual analog scale)[108] as does the PDE-4 inhibitor crisaborole.[109] Newer systemic

therapies, such as dupilumab have been shown to improve sleep quality based on one-question surveys.[110] Objective sleep data to demonstrate the expected aspects of improvement on these therapies are still needed.

Although melatonin has been shown to be proinflammatory in asthma,[111] one group found a significant reduction in AD disease severity scores and improved sleep-onset latency by ~20 minutes.[112,113]

Other Allergic Conditions to Consider

Chronic Rhinosinusitis

CRS is defined by at least 12 weeks of sinusitis symptoms and abnormal finding on endoscopy or on sinus computed tomography (CT).[114] Because sinuses are still developing and pneumatizing throughout childhood, CRS is less common in children compared with adults. However, CRS in children still accounts for 5.6 million outpatient visits.[115,116] CRS is burdensome on quality of life,[117] and although little data exist in children about sleep in CRS, it is presumed to have a significant impact as extrapolated from the adult literature. In adults, 60–75% of people with CRS report poor sleep with specific symptoms of excessive daytime sleepiness, difficulty initiating sleep, difficulty maintaining sleep, snoring, and early morning awakenings.[118–121] CRS can occur with or without nasal polyps, and in children the presence of nasal polyps necessitates an evaluation for cystic fibrosis.

In CRS practice parameters, sleep apnea is considered a common factor associated with CRS.[114] This is because 11–15% of the U.S. population of CRS patients also have physician-diagnosed OSA,[118,121,122] suggesting a shared common inflammatory link (upregulated IL-6).[123] It is not surprising that the presence of nasal polys compared with those without polyps is associated with a twofold higher risk of sleep disturbance, due to their presence increasing upper airways resistance.[124]

Initial treatment of CRS should take a conservative approach, such as elevating the head of the bed and intranasal corticosteroid and sinus rinses.[125] Antibiotics are minimally effective in acute sinusitis, and for CRS can be considered with major disease flares.[126] After conservative measures fail, patients can be evaluated for surgical management, and in older children this might mean functional endoscopic sinus surgery (FESS). In a study of 344 adult CRS patients who underwent FESS, they found improvements in all sleep-related measures including difficulty falling asleep, waking up tired, waking up at night, lack of a good night's sleep, and fatigue over the average 14.5-month follow-up period.[127]

Urticaria

Urticaria, also known as hives, is common with a cumulative prevalence of 15% by age 10 years.[126] It can be sleep disturbing especially when it lasts for more than 6 weeks, which is known as chronic idiopathic urticaria (CIU).[128]

Among adolescents with CIU, 78% reported waking at least once in the night.[129] To our knowledge there are no pediatric studies evaluating the concurrence of SDB in CIU, but one study in adults with CIU found a concurrence in 25% of patients.[130] First-line treatment of CIU is non-sedating antihistamines, and for more severe cases systemic therapy is warranted. Specifically, omalizumab (approved by the U.S. Food and Drug Administration for ≥12-year-olds for CIU, and ≥6-year-olds for asthma) is highly effective for CIU, but it does require monthly intravenous (IV) infusion with 30 minutes of observation due to risk of anaphylaxis (<1%).[114]

Conclusion

In summary, allergic disease is a common occurrence and has significant comorbidity with SDB and other sleep-related conditions, such as parasomnias.[131–134] Poor parental sleep is also commonly seen and should be something the clinician queries. Sleep medicine providers should consider the impact of allergic disease on sleep and personalize treatment to address allergic disease in conjunction with other sleep pathologies. Consultation with an allergist should be considered in difficult to treat cases.

> **CLINICAL PEARLS**
>
> - Allergy disorders, such as asthma, allergic rhinitis, and atopic dermatitis, are commonly observed in children with sleep-disordered breathing (SDB).
> - Inflammatory cytokines are increased in allergy disorders, which in turn can increase arousals at night and adversely affect REM sleep (increased REM sleep latency and decreased REM sleep duration).
> - In addition, exacerbations in asthma, allergic rhinitis and atopic dermatitis can significantly disrupt sleep duration and quality.
> - Treatment of the allergy disorder along with SBD treatment is critical as SBD treatment is inadequate with adenotonsillar regrowth after surgery often being observed in children with untreated allergy disorders.

References

1. Burr ML, Butland BK, King S, Vaughan-Williams E. Changes in asthma prevalence: Two surveys 15 years apart. *Arch Dis Child.* 1989;64(10):1452–1456.
2. Aberg N. Asthma and allergic rhinitis in Swedish conscripts. *Clin Exp Allergy.* 1989;19(1):59–63.
3. Robertson CF, Heycock E, Bishop J, Nolan T, Olinsky A, Phelan PD. Prevalence of asthma in Melbourne schoolchildren: Changes over 26 years. *BMJ.* 1991;302(6785):1116–1118.
4. Silverberg JI. Public health burden and epidemiology of atopic dermatitis. *Dermatol Clin.* 2017;35(3):283–289.
5. Backman H, Räisänen P, Hedman L, et al. Increased prevalence of allergic asthma from 1996 to 2006 and further to 2016-results from three population surveys. *Clin Exp Allergy.* 2017;47(11):1426–1435.
6. Akinbami LJ, Moorman JE, Bailey C, et al. Trends in asthma prevalence, health care use, and mortality in the United States, 2001–2010. *NCHS Data Brief.* 2012;94:1–8.
7. Derebery J, Meltzer E, Nathan RA, et al. Rhinitis symptoms and comorbidities in the United States: Burden of rhinitis in America survey. *Otolaryngol Head Neck Surg.* 2008;139(2):198–205.
8. Settipane RA. Demographics and epidemiology of allergic and nonallergic rhinitis. *Allergy Asthma Proc.* 2001;22(4):185–189.
9. Silverberg JI, Garg NK, Paller AS, Fishbein AB, Zee PC. Sleep disturbances in adults with eczema are associated with impaired overall health: A US population-based study. *J Invest Dermatol.* 2015;135(1):56–66.
10. Shaw TE, Currie GP, Koudelka CW, Simpson EL. Eczema prevalence in the United States: Data from the 2003 National Survey of Children's Health. *J Invest Dermatol.* 2011;131(1):67–73.
11. Kay J, Gawkrodger DJ, Mortimer MJ, Jaron AG. The prevalence of childhood atopic eczema in a general population. *J Am Acad Dermatol.* 1994;30(1):35–39.
12. Davidson WF, Leung DYM, Beck LA, et al. Report from the National Institute of Allergy and Infectious Diseases workshop on "Atopic dermatitis and the atopic march: Mechanisms and interventions. *J Allergy Clin Immunol.* 2019;143(3):894–913.
13. Czarnowicki T, Krueger JG, Guttman-Yassky E. Novel concepts of prevention and treatment of atopic dermatitis through barrier and immune manipulations with implications for the atopic march. *J Allergy Clin Immunol.* 2017;139(6):1723–1734.
14. Fishbein AB, Lee TA, Cai M, et al. Sensitization to mouse and cockroach allergens and asthma morbidity in urban minority youth: Genes-environments and Admixture in Latino American (GALA-II) and Study of African-Americans, Asthma, Genes, and Environments (SAGE-II). *Ann Allergy Asthma Immunol.* 2016;117(1):43–49. e41.
15. Perikleous E, Steiropoulos P, Nena E, et al. Association of Asthma and Allergic Rhinitis With Sleep-Disordered Breathing in Childhood. *Front Pediatr.* 2018;6:250.
16. Shusterman D, Baroody FM, Craig T, Friedlander S, Nsouli T, Silverman B. Role of the allergist-immunologist and upper airway allergy in sleep-disordered breathing. *J Allergy Clin Immunol Pract.* 2017;5(3):628–639.
17. Redline S, Tishler PV, Schluchter M, Aylor J, Clark K, Graham G. Risk factors for sleep-disordered breathing in children. Associations with obesity, race, and respiratory problems. *Am J Respir Crit Care Med.* 1999;159(5 Pt 1):1527–1532.
18. Expert Panel Report 3 (EPR-3) Guidelines for the Diagnosis and Management of Asthma-Summary Report 2007. *J Allergy Clin Immunol.* 2007;120(5 Suppl):S94–S138..
19. Demoly P, Calderon MA, Casale T, et al. Assessment of disease control in allergic rhinitis. *Clin Transl Allergy.* 2013;3(1):7.
20. Sánchez T, Castro-Rodríguez JA, Brockmann PE. Sleep-disordered breathing in children with asthma: A systematic review on the impact of treatment. *J Asthma allergy.* 2016;9:83–91.
21. Chervin RD, Hedger K, Dillon JE, Pituch KJ. Pediatric sleep questionnaire (PSQ): Validity and reliability of scales for sleep-disordered breathing, snoring, sleepiness, and behavioral problems. *Sleep Med.* 2000;1(1):21–32.
22. Ehsan Z, Kercsmar CM, Collins J, Simakajornboon N. Validation of the pediatric sleep questionnaire in children with asthma. *Pediatr Pulmonol.* 2017;52(3):382–389.

23. Marcus CL, Brooks LJ, Draper KA, et al. Diagnosis and management of childhood obstructive sleep apnea syndrome. *Pediatrics*. 2012;130(3):576–584.

24. Akdis CAS SH. Allergy and the immunologic basis of atopic disease. In: Kliegman RM, St, Geme JW, Schor NF, Behrman RE, eds. *Nelson Textbook of Pediatrics*. 20th ed. Elsevier; 2016:1074–1978.

25. Mukundan TH. Screening for allergic disease in child with sleep disorder and screening for sleep disturbance in allergic disease. In: Fishbein A, Sheldon SH, eds. *Allergy and Sleep: Basic Principles and Clinical Practice*. Springer; 2019.

26. Thompson A, Sardana N, Craig TJ. Sleep impairment and daytime sleepiness in patients with allergic rhinitis: The role of congestion and inflammation. *Ann Allergy Asthma Immunol*. 2013;111(6):446–451.

27. Huo Z, Shi J, Shu Y, Xiang M, Lu J, Wu H. The relationship between allergic status and adenotonsillar regrowth: A retrospective research on children after adenotonsillectomy. *Sci Rep*. 2017;7:46615.

28. Craig TJ, Teets S, Lehman EB, Chinchilli VM, Zwillich C. Nasal congestion secondary to allergic rhinitis as a cause of sleep disturbance and daytime fatigue and the response to topical nasal corticosteroids. *J Al. lergy Clin Immunol*. 1998;101(5):633–637.

29. Camfferman D, Kennedy JD, Gold M, Martin AJ, Winwood P, Lushington K. Eczema, sleep, and behavior in children. *J Clin Sleep Med*. 2010;6(6):581–588.

30. Liu J, Zhang X, Zhao Y, Wang Y. The association between allergic rhinitis and sleep: A systematic review and meta-analysis of observational studies. *PLoS One*. 2020;15(2):e0228533.

31. Combs D, Goodwin JL, Quan SF, Morgan WJ, Parthasarathy S. Longitudinal differences in sleep duration in Hispanic and Caucasian children. *Sleep Med*. 2016;18:61–66.

32. Nurcicek Padem AF. Overview and understanding of human circadian immunology. In: Fishbein A, Sheldon SH, eds. *Allergy and Sleep*. Springer; 2019:43–58.

33. Calhoun SL, Vgontzas AN, Fernandez-Mendoza J, et al. Prevalence and risk factors of excessive daytime sleepiness in a community sample of young children: The role of obesity, asthma, anxiety/depression, and sleep. *Sleep*. 2011;34(4):503–507.

34. Reynolds KC, Boergers J, Kopel SJ, Koinis-Mitchell D. Featured article: Multiple comorbid conditions, sleep quality and duration, and academic performance in urban children with asthma. *J Pediatr Psychol*. 2018;43(9):943–954.

35. Wang X, Gao X, Yang Q, et al. Sleep disorders and allergic diseases in Chinese toddlers. *Sleep Med*. 2017;37:174–179.

36. Jernelöv S, Lekander M, Almqvist C, Axelsson J, Larsson H. Development of atopic disease and disturbed sleep in childhood and adolescence–a longitudinal population-based study. *Clin Exp Allergy*. 2013;43(5):552–559.

37. Keller T, Hohmann C, Standl M, et al. The sex-shift in single disease and multimorbid asthma and rhinitis during puberty – a study by MeDALL. *Allergy*. 2018;73(3):602–614.

38. Stein RT, Holberg CJ, Morgan WJ, et al. Peak flow variability, methacholine responsiveness and atopy as markers for detecting different wheezing phenotypes in childhood. *Thorax*. 1997;52(11):946–952.

39. National Asthma Education and Prevention Program TEPotDaMoA. Expert Panel Report 3: Guidelines for the Diagnosis and Management of Asthma. 2007.

40. Global Strategy for Asthma Management and Prevention. 2017 GINA Report, Global Strategy for Asthma Management and Prevention. 2017.

41. Bergeron C, Al-Ramli W, Hamid Q. Remodeling in asthma. *Proc Am Thorac Soc*. 2009;6(3):301–305.

42. Strunk RC, Sternberg AL, Bacharier LB, Szefler SJ. Nocturnal awakening caused by asthma in children with mild-to-moderate asthma in the childhood asthma management program. *J Allergy Clin Immunol*. 2002;110(3):395–403.

43. Diette GB, Markson L, Skinner EA, Nguyen TT, Algatt-Bergstrom P, Wu AW. Nocturnal asthma in children affects school attendance, school performance, and parents' work attendance. *Arch Pediatr Adolesc Med*. 2000;154(9):923–928.

44. Sutherland ER. Nocturnal asthma. *J Allergy Clin Immunol*. 2005;116(6):1179–1186. quiz 1187.

45. Barnes P, FitzGerald G, Brown M, Dollery C. Nocturnal asthma and changes in circulating epinephrine, histamine, and cortisol. *N Engl J Med*. 1980;303(5):263–267.

46. Meltzer AA, Smolensky MH, D'Alonzo GE, Harrist RB, Scott PH. An assessment of peak expiratory flow as a surrogate measurement of FEV1 in stable asthmatic children. *Chest*. 1989;96(2):329–333.

47. Fagnano M, Bayer AL, Isensee CA, Hernandez T, Halterman JS. Nocturnal asthma symptoms and poor sleep quality among urban school children with asthma. *Acad Pediatr*. 2011;11(6):493–499.

48. Khassawneh B, Tsai SC, Meltzer LJ. Polysomnographic characteristics of adolescents with asthma and low risk for sleep-disordered breathing. *Sleep Breath*. 2019;23(3):943–951.

49. Sadeh A, Horowitz I, Wolach-Benodis L, Wolach B. Sleep and pulmonary function in children with well-controlled, stable asthma. *Sleep*. 1998;21(4):379–384.

50. Stores G, Ellis AJ, Wiggs L, Crawford C, Thomson A. Sleep and psychological disturbance in nocturnal asthma. *Arch Dis Child*. 1998;78(5):413–419.

51. Meltzer LJ, Faino A, Szefler SJ, Strand M, Gelfand EW, Beebe DW. Experimentally manipulated sleep duration in adolescents with asthma: Feasibility and preliminary findings. *Pediatr Pulmonol*. 2015;50(12):1360–1367.

52. Hanson MD, Chen E. The temporal relationships between sleep, cortisol, and lung functioning in youth with asthma. *J Pediatr Psychol*. 2008;33(3):312–316.

53. Meltzer LJ, Ullrich M, Szefler SJ. Sleep duration, sleep hygiene, and insomnia in adolescents with asthma. *J Allergy Clin Immunol Pract*. 2014;2(5):562–569.

54. Dewald-Kaufmann JF, Oort FJ, Meijer AM. The effects of sleep extension and sleep hygiene advice on sleep and depressive symptoms in adolescents: A randomized controlled trial. *J Child Psychol Psychiatry*. 2014;55(3):273–283.

55. Ross KR, Storfer-Isser A, Hart MA, et al. Sleep-disordered breathing is associated with asthma severity in children. *J Pediatr*. 2012;160(5):736–742.

56. Nguyen-Hoang Y, Nguyen-Thi-Dieu T, Duong-Quy S. Study of the clinical and functional characteristics of asthmatic children with obstructive sleep apnea. *J Asthma Allergy*. 2017;10:285–292.

57. Prasad B, Nyenhuis SM, Weaver TE. Obstructive sleep apnea and asthma: Associations and treatment implications. *Sleep Med Rev*. 2014;18(2):165–171.

58. Papi A, Brightling C, Pedersen SE, Reddel HK. Asthma. *Lancet*. 2018;391(10122):783–800.

59. Witmans M. Asthma treatment outcome measures. In: Fishbein A, Sheldon SH, eds. *Allergy and Sleep: Basic Principles and Clinical Practice*. Springer; 2019:185–193.

60. Sangvai S, Hersey SJ, Snyder DA, et al. Implementation of the asthma control test in a large primary care network. *Pediatr Qual Saf.* 2017;2(5):e038.

61. Pruteanu AI, Chauhan BF, Zhang L, Prietsch SO, Ducharme FM. Inhaled corticosteroids in children with persistent asthma: Dose-response effects on growth. *Cochrane Database Syst Rev.* 2014(7):Cd009878.

62. Zhang L, Prietsch SO, Ducharme FM. Inhaled corticosteroids in children with persistent asthma: Effects on growth. *Evid Based Child Health.* 2014;9(4):829–930.

63. Kelly HW, Sternberg AL, Lescher R, et al. Effect of inhaled glucocorticoids in childhood on adult height. *N Engl J Med.* 2012;367(10):904–912.

64. Lemanske RF, Jr., Mauger DT, Sorkness CA, et al. Step-up therapy for children with uncontrolled asthma receiving inhaled corticosteroids. *N Engl J Med.* 2010;362(11):975–985.

65. Wechsler ME, Szefler SJ, Ortega VE, et al. Step-up therapy in Black children and adults with poorly controlled asthma. *N Engl J Med.* 2019;381(13):1227–1239.

66. Goldbart AD, Goldman JL, Li RC, Brittian KR, Tauman R, Gozal D. Differential expression of cysteinyl leukotriene receptors 1 and 2 in tonsils of children with obstructive sleep apnea syndrome or recurrent infection. *Chest.* 2004;126(1):13–18.

67. Goldbart AD, Greenberg-Dotan S, Tal A. Montelukast for children with obstructive sleep apnea: A double-blind, placebo-controlled study. *Pediatrics.* 2012;130(3):e575–e580..

68. Kheirandish-Gozal L, Bandla HP, Gozal D. Montelukast for children with obstructive sleep apnea: Results of a double-blind, randomized, placebo-controlled trial. *Ann Am Thorac Soc.* 2016;13(10):1736–1741.

69. Kheirandish L, Goldbart AD, Gozal D. Intranasal steroids and oral leukotriene modifier therapy in residual sleep-disordered breathing after tonsillectomy and adenoidectomy in children. *Pediatrics.* 2006;117(1):e61–e66..

70. Dykewicz MS, Wallace DV, Baroody F, et al. Treatment of seasonal allergic rhinitis: An evidence-based focused 2017 guideline update. *Ann Allergy Asthma Immunol.* 2017;119(6):489–511. e441.

71. Singulair Product Monograph. Canada; Merck-Frosst Canada; 2004.

72. Saito H, Asakura K, Hata M, Kataura A, Morimoto K. Does adenotonsillectomy affect the course of bronchial asthma and nasal allergy? *Acta Otolaryngol Suppl.* 1996;523:212–215.

73. Kheirandish-Gozal L, Dayyat EA, Eid NS, Morton RL, Gozal D. Obstructive sleep apnea in poorly controlled asthmatic children: Effect of adenotonsillectomy. *Pediatr Pulmonol.* 2011;46(9):913–918.

74. Marcus CL, Moore RH, Rosen CL, et al. A randomized trial of adenotonsillectomy for childhood sleep apnea. *N Engl J Med.* 2013;368(25):2366–2376.

75. Wang R, Bakker JP, Chervin RD, et al. Pediatric Adenotonsillectomy Trial for Snoring (PATS): Protocol for a randomised controlled trial to evaluate the effect of adenotonsillectomy in treating mild obstructive sleep-disordered breathing. *BMJ Open.* 2020;10(3):e033889.

76. Adkinson NF. *Middleton's Allergy Principles and Practice.* Mosby Elsevier; 2009.

77. Meltzer EO. Allergic rhinitis: Burden of illness, quality of life, comorbidities, and control. *Immunol Allergy Clin North Am.* 2016;36(2):235–248.

78. Westman M, Stjärne P, Asarnoj A, et al. Natural course and comorbidities of allergic and nonallergic rhinitis in children. *J Allergy Clin Immunol.* 2012;129(2):403–408.

79. Koinis-Mitchell D, Craig T, Esteban CA, Klein RB. Sleep and allergic disease: A summary of the literature and future directions for research. *J Allergy Clin Immunol.* 2012;130(6):1275–1281.

80. Dass K, Petrusan AJ, Beaumont J, Zee P, Lai JS, Fishbein A. Assessment of sleep disturbance in children with allergic rhinitis. *Ann Allergy Asthma Immunol.* 2017;118(4):505–506.

81. McColley SA, Carroll JL, Curtis S, Loughlin GM, Sampson HA. High prevalence of allergic sensitization in children with habitual snoring and obstructive sleep apnea. *Chest.* 1997;111(1):170–173.

82. Lunn M, Craig T. Rhinitis and sleep. *Sleep Med Rev.* 2011;15(5):293–299.

83. Craig TJ, McCann JL, Gurevich F, Davies MJ. The correlation between allergic rhinitis and sleep disturbance. *J Allergy Clin Immunol.* 2004;114(5 Suppl):S139–S145..

84. Walter LM, Tamanyan K, Nisbet L, et al. Pollen levels on the day of polysomnography influence sleep disordered breathing severity in children with allergic rhinitis. *Sleep Breath.* 2019;23(2):651–657.

85. Rappai M, Collop N, Kemp S, deShazo R. The nose and sleep-disordered breathing: What we know and what we do not know. *Chest.* 2003;124(6):2309–2323.

86. Cao Y, Wu S, Zhang L, Yang Y, Cao S, Li Q. Association of allergic rhinitis with obstructive sleep apnea: A meta-analysis. *Medicine (Baltimore).* 2018;97(51):e13783.

87. Sadeghi-Shabestari M, Jabbari Moghaddam Y, Ghaharri H. Is there any correlation between allergy and adenotonsillar tissue hypertrophy? *Int J Pediatr Otorhinolaryngol.* 2011;75(4):589–591.

88. Kim DK, Han DH. Impact of allergic rhinitis on quality of life after adenotonsillectomy for pediatric sleep-disordered breathing. *Int Forum Allergy Rhinol.* 2015;5(8):741–746.

89. Dykewicz MS, Wallace DV, Amrol DJ, et al. Rhinitis 2020: A Practice Parameter Update. *J Allergy Clin Immunol.* 2020

90. Weiner JM, Abramson MJ, Puy RM. Intranasal corticosteroids versus oral H1 receptor antagonists in allergic rhinitis: Systematic review of randomised controlled trials. *BMJ.* 1998;317(7173):1624–1629.

91. Bitar MA, Nassar J, Dana R. Is the effect of topical intranasal steroids on obstructive adenoids transient or long-lasting? Case series and systematic review of literature. *J Laryngol Otol.* 2016;130(4):357–362.

92. Murray JJ, Nathan RA, Bronsky EA, Olufade AO, Chapman D, Kramer B. Comprehensive evaluation of cetirizine in the management of seasonal allergic rhinitis: Impact on symptoms, quality of life, productivity, and activity impairment. *Allergy Asthma Proc.* 2002;23(6):391–398.

93. Santos CB, Hanks C, McCann J, Lehman EB, Pratt E, Craig TJ. The role of montelukast on perennial allergic rhinitis and associated sleep disturbances and daytime somnolence. *Allergy Asthma Proc.* 2008;29(2):140–145.

94. Seidman MD, Gurgel RK, Lin SY, et al. Clinical practice guideline: Allergic rhinitis. *Otolaryngol Head Neck Surg.* 2015;152(1 Suppl):S1–S43.

95. Fishbein AB, Vitaterna O, Haugh IM, et al. Nocturnal eczema: Review of sleep and circadian rhythms in children with atopic dermatitis and future research directions. *J Allergy Clin Immunol.* 2015;136(5):1170–1177.

96. Kim JP, Chao LX, Simpson EL, Silverberg JI. Persistence of atopic dermatitis (AD): A systematic review and meta-analysis. *J Am Acad Dermatol.* 2016;75(4):681–687. e611.

97. Margolis JS, Abuabara K, Bilker W, Hoffstad O, Margolis DJ. Persistence of mild to moderate atopic dermatitis. *JAMA Dermatol.* 2014;150(6):593–600.

98. Fishbein AB, Mueller K, Kruse L, et al. Sleep disturbance in children with moderate/severe atopic dermatitis: A case-control study. *J Am Acad Dermatol.* 2018;78(2):336–341.

99. Fishbein AB, Lin B, Beaumont J, Paller AS, Zee P. Nocturnal movements in children with atopic dermatitis have a timing pattern: A case control study. *J Am Acad Dermatol.* 2018

100. Savin JA, Paterson WD, Oswald I. Scratching during sleep. *Lancet.* 1973;2(7824):296–297.

101. Treister AD, Stefek H, Grimaldi D, et al. Sleep and limb movement characteristics of children with atopic dermatitis coincidentally undergoing clinical polysomnography. *J Clin Sleep Med.* 2019;15(8):1107–1113.

102. Reuveni H, Chapnick G, Tal A, Tarasiuk A. Sleep fragmentation in children with atopic dermatitis. *Arch Pediatr Adolesc Med.* 1999;153(3):249–253.

103. Chng SY, Goh DY, Wang XS, Tan TN, Ong NB. Snoring and atopic disease: A strong association. *Pediatr Pulmonol.* 2004;38(3):210–216.

104. Vinaya Soundararajan JL, Anna B, Fishbein. Sleep apnea and skin. *Curr Sleep Med Rep.* 2020

105. Fishbein AB, Silverberg JI, Wilson EJ, Ong PY. Update on atopic dermatitis: Diagnosis, severity assessment, and treatment selection. *J Allergy Clin Immunol Pract.* 2020;8(1):91–101.

106. Boguniewicz M, Fonacier L, Guttman-Yassky E, Ong PY, Silverberg J, Farrar JR. Atopic dermatitis yardstick: Practical recommendations for an evolving therapeutic landscape. *Ann Allergy Asthma Immunol.* 2018;120(1):10–22. e12.

107. Fishbein AB, Mueller K, Lor J, Smith P, Paller AS, Kaat A. Systematic review and meta-analysis comparing topical corticosteroids with vehicle/moisturizer in childhood atopic dermatitis. *J Pediatr Nurs.* 2019;47:36–43.

108. Bieber T, Vick K, Fölster-Holst R, et al. Efficacy and safety of methylprednisolone aceponate ointment 0.1% compared to tacrolimus 0.03% in children and adolescents with an acute flare of severe atopic dermatitis. *Allergy.* 2007;62(2):184–189.

109. Simpson EL, Paller AS, Boguniewicz M, et al. Crisaborole Ointment improves quality of life of patients with mild to moderate atopic dermatitis and their families. *Dermatol Ther (Heidelb).* 2018;8(4):605–619.

110. Paller AS, Bansal A, Simpson EL, et al. Clinically meaningful responses to dupilumab in adolescents with uncontrolled moderate-to-severe atopic dermatitis: Post-hoc analyses from a randomized clinical trial. *Am J Clin Dermatol.* 2020;21(1):119–131.

111. Sutherland ER, Martin RJ, Ellison MC, Kraft M. Immunomodulatory effects of melatonin in asthma. *Am J Respir Crit Care Med.* 2002;166(8):1055–1061.

112. Chang YS, Lin MH, Lee JH, et al. Melatonin supplementation for children with atopic dermatitis and sleep disturbance: A randomized clinical trial. *JAMA Pediatr.* 2016;170(1):35–42.

113. Chang YS, Chou YT, Lee JH, et al. Atopic dermatitis, melatonin, and sleep disturbance. *Pediatrics.* 2014;134(2):e397–e405..

114. Bernstein JA, Lang DM, Khan DA, et al. The diagnosis and management of acute and chronic urticaria: 2014 update. *J Allergy Clin Immunol.* 2014;133(5):1270–1277.

115. Hamilos DL. Drivers of chronic rhinosinusitis: Inflammation versus infection. *J Allergy Clin Immunol.* 2015;136(6):1454–1459.

116. Gilani S, Shin JJ. The burden and visit prevalence of pediatric chronic rhinosinusitis. *Otolaryngol Head Neck Surg.* 2017;157(6):1048–1052.

117. Cheng BT, Smith SS, Fishbein AB. Functional burden and limitations in children with chronic sinusitis. *Pediatr Allergy Immunol.* 2020;31(1):103–105.

118. Alt JA, Smith TL, Mace JC, Soler ZM. Sleep quality and disease severity in patients with chronic rhinosinusitis. *Laryngoscope.* 2013;123(10):2364–2370.

119. Alt JA, Smith TL, Schlosser RJ, Mace JC, Soler ZM. Sleep and quality of life improvements after endoscopic sinus surgery in patients with chronic rhinosinusitis. *Int Forum Allergy Rhinol.* 2014;4(9):693–701.

120. Bengtsson C, Lindberg E, Jonsson L, et al. Chronic rhinosinusitis impairs sleep quality: Results of the GA2LEN Study. *Sleep.* 2017;40(1).

121. Jiang RS, Liang KL, Hsin CH, Su MC. The impact of chronic rhinosinusitis on sleep-disordered breathing. *Rhinology.* 2016;54(1):75–79.

122. Hui JW, Ong J, Herdegen JJ, et al. Risk of obstructive sleep apnea in African American patients with chronic rhinosinusitis. *Ann Allergy Asthma Immunol.* 2017;118(6):685–688. e681.

123. Salahi N, Mirkarimi S, Fares S, et al. A biomarker for obstructive sleep apnea in chronic rhinosinusitis. *J Allergy Clin Immunol.* 2019;143(2):AB86.

124. Serrano E, Neukirch F, Pribil C, et al. Nasal polyposis in France: Impact on sleep and quality of life. *J Laryngol Otol.* 2005;119(7):543–549.

125. Shahid SK. Rhinosinusitis in children. *ISRN Otolaryngol.* 2012;2012851–831.

126. Peters AT, Spector S, Hsu J, et al. Diagnosis and management of rhinosinusitis: A practice parameter update. *Ann Allergy Asthma Immunol.* 2014;113(4):347–385.

127. El Rassi E, Mace JC, Steele TO, Alt JA, Smith TL. Improvements in sleep-related symptoms after endoscopic sinus surgery in patients with chronic rhinosinusitis. *Int Forum Allergy Rhinol.* 2016;6(4):414–422.

128. Tanaka T, Hiragun M, Hide M, Hiragun T. Analysis of primary treatment and prognosis of spontaneous urticaria. *Allergol Int.* 2017;66(3):458–462.

129. Mathias SD, Tschosik EA, Zazzali JL. Adaptation and validation of the Urticaria Patient Daily Diary for adolescents. *Allergy Asthma Proc.* 2012;33(2):186–190.

130. Perkowska J, Kruszewski J, Gutkowski P, Chciałowski A, Kłos K. Occurrence of sleep-related breathing disorders in patients with chronic urticaria at its asymptomatic or oligosymptomatic stages. *Postepy Dermatol Alergol.* 2016;33(1):63–67.

131. Loekmanwidjaja J, Carneiro ACF, Nishinaka MLT, et al. Sleep disorders in children with moderate to severe persistent allergic rhinitis. *Braz J Otorhinolaryngol.* 2018;84(2):178–184.

132. Gupta MA, Gupta AK. Sleep-wake disorders and dermatology. *Clin Dermatol.* 2013;31(1):118–126.

133. Shani-Adir A, Rozenman D, Kessel A, Engel-Yeger B. The relationship between sensory hypersensitivity and sleep quality of children with atopic dermatitis. *Pediatr Dermatol.* 2009;26(2):143–149.

134. Cicek D, Halisdemir N, Dertioglu SB, Berilgen MS, Ozel S, Colak C. Increased frequency of restless legs syndrome in atopic dermatitis. *Clin Exp Dermatol.* 2012;37(5):469–476.

34

Treatment of Children with Obstructive Sleep Apnea Syndrome

Iris A. Perez and Sally Davidson Ward

CHAPTER HIGHLIGHTS

- Adenotonsillectomy is the mainstay of treatment of obstructive sleep apnea (OSA) in children and it is curative in most; follow-up directed at persistent symptoms or complications of OSA is indicated.
- Typically developing children with mild OSA due to adenotonsillar hypertrophy maybe observed (watchful waiting) or placed on pharmacologic therapy.
- Careful attention to risk factors for perioperative complications of adenotonsillectomy with plans for hospital observation of high-risk patients is key to minimizing adverse outcomes.
- Parental and patient education regarding positive airway pressure (PAP) therapy and mask acclimatization well in advance of the initial titration sleep study are important in subsequent adherence.
- Select patients who are intolerant of continuous PAP (CPAP) may be successfully treated with high-flow nasal cannula and other surgical approaches, in addition to adenotonsillectomy.

Introduction

Obstructive sleep apnea (OSA) is a common childhood sleep-related disorder resulting from an anatomically or functionally narrowed upper airway. The most common etiologies include adenotonsillar hypertrophy, obesity, and craniofacial malformations.[1–4] When left untreated, childhood OSA can lead to significant morbidity and may lay the foundation for adult cardiovascular and metabolic disease, thus effective treatment may confer a lifelong benefit. In this chapter we review the different treatment options for OSA, their indications, efficacy, and limitations in the pediatric population.

Treatment Options

Adenotonsillectomy

Most children with OSA will be treated with adenotonsillectomy (AT) as first-line therapy. AT results in improvement not only in symptoms,[5–7] but also in sleep quality and homeostasis,[5] daytime behavior,[7] neurocognitive functioning,[6,8] and overall quality of life.[5,7] Modest neurocognitive improvements have been found in the areas of non-verbal reasoning, selective attention, and fine motor skills in school-aged children.[8] These improvements can persist up to 1 year after AT in preschool children with OSA.[9] AT can lead to weight gain with associated increase in growth markers (insulin-like growth factor 1 [IGF-1] and insulin-like growth factor binding protein 3 [IGFBP-3]).[10–13] It is associated with improved right ventricular function,[14,15] resolution of tachycardia and decreased pulse rate variability,[16] and significant improvement in ambulatory blood pressure,[17–19] particularly for those who are hypertensive.[18]

Unfortunately, up to 29% of children will have persistence of OSA following AT.[20,21] Factors that contribute to persistent or residual OSA after AT are listed in Table 34.1.[20–22] In this group of patients, postoperative polysomnography (PSG) will help identify the response to AT and the additional treatments needed for residual OSA.[21]

Patients with mild OSA and without comorbidities generally do well post operatively from a respiratory standpoint. Complications following AT include postoperative bleeding, infection, upper airway obstruction secondary to airway edema, pulmonary edema, hypoxemia or respiratory failure requiring admission to the intensive care unit, need for oral or nasal airway, and reintubation or noninvasive ventilation.[23–25] Pulmonary complication rate ranges between 5% and 38%.[25–30] Risk factors for pulmonary complications following AT are listed in Table 34.2.[25–33] These are the children who will benefit from overnight hospitalization for observation following AT. In one study SpO_2 <90% on preoperative PSG predicted postoperative oxygen requirement.[32] Cardiac disease, airway anomalies, and young age have been reported as strong predictors for sentinel respiratory events following AT in medically complex children.[26] One study reported an intensive care admission rate of 2.4% in a group of children with known risk factors for respiratory complications. Of these patients, about 1% required unanticipated transfer to the pediatric intensive

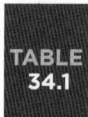

TABLE 34.1	Risk Factors for Residual or Persistent Obstructive Sleep Apnea After Adenotonsillectomy

- Obesity
- Asthma
- Down syndrome
- Cerebral palsy
- Neuromuscular weakness
- Gastroesophageal reflux disease
- High preoperative apnea-hypopnea index ≥20/hr
- Age (>7 years)
- Craniofacial abnormalities

TABLE 34.2	Risk Factors for Pulmonary Complications Following Adenotonsillectomy

- Age
- <3 years
- Black race
- Severe obstructive sleep apnea syndrome (profound hypoxemia (SpO$_2$ <80%, apnea-hypopnea index >10, significant hypoventilation)
- Oxygen desaturation index, total sleep time <90%, SpO$_2$ nadir
- Morbid obesity
- Neuromuscular disease
- Pulmonary hypertension
- Congenital heart disease
- Down syndrome
- Craniofacial anomalies
- Airway anomalies
- Asthma
- Sickle cell disease
- Failure to thrive
- History of respiratory compromise or anesthesia complications

care unit (PICU).[23] Dexamethasone administration and a reduction in opioid administration following AT have been found to reduce the incidence of recurrent hypoxemia and major respiratory medical intervention.[34]

Polysomnography Prior to Adenotonsillectomy

Preoperative PSG is important in identifying the presence and severity of OSA because symptoms, physical examination, and laboratory tests do not predict PSG findings in children. PSG findings will also help determine the type of therapy for the patient. PSG evidence of minimal respiratory disturbance is associated with low risk for perioperative complications supporting the decision to perform AT in an ambulatory center. Because increased preoperative obstructive apnea-hypopnea index (AHI) and low SpO$_2$ nadir are highly predictive of pulmonary complications post-surgery, performing AT without the PSG can put children at risk for unexpected postoperative complications. Further, because elevated preoperative AHI is predictive of residual OSA, PSG prior to AT will help identify patients who will need close follow-up and further evaluation.[20,21]

Inpatient versus Outpatient

The decision to perform surgery in the ambulatory setting is not straightforward and different professional societies with a vested interest in the safety of children undergoing AT recommend inpatient monitoring for patients at risk for respiratory complications (see Table 34.2), such as children younger than age 3 or those with severe OSA (AHI ≥10 or oxygen saturation nadir <80%, or both).[21,35] The American Society of Anesthesiologists implements a scoring system to estimate a patient's increased perioperative risk from OSA and offers guidance in determining which patients can be safely managed in an outpatient versus inpatient setting.[36] Important components of the risk assessment include sleep apnea status, nature of surgery (airway surgery under general anesthesia receives a score of 3), requirement for postoperative opioids, use of noninvasive positive pressure ventilation (NPPV) pre- and postoperatively, and resting PaCO$_2$ >50 mm Hg. A score of 4 may indicate increased perioperative risk, whereas ≥5 suggests significant risk. Patient's age, coexisting disease, adequacy of post-discharge observation, and capabilities of the outpatient facility are also important factors in the determination of the location of the surgery.[36] De and colleagues found significant residual OSA and sleep architecture abnormalities on the night following AT in obese children with severe OSA.[37] Additionally, the severity of the OSA and SpO$_2$ nadir were similar to the preoperative indices,[37] thus highlighting the importance of overnight hospital stay for observation the night following AT in patients with obesity. In summary, patients who are at higher risk for postoperative complications will require a higher level of care and should be admitted for overnight observation and may even require the intensive cardiorespiratory monitoring afforded by a PICU. In one study, about 45% of the patients with planned ICU stays required respiratory support and about 30% of the patients experienced complications.[38]

At present, elective admission to the PICU is generally under the discretion of the clinical team.[39] Some report that only a select group of children will require admission to PICU after AT.[40,41] In one series, 39% of children admitted to the PICU who had an uneventful post-anesthetic care unit period did not require any high-level care.[41] Lavin and colleagues used oxygen requirements more than 2 LPM between 2 and 24 hours postoperatively, more than two desaturation events in a 2-hour period, or more than hourly nursing interventions, as the definition of needing ICU resources.[40] Associated clinical features such as young age, gastrointestinal comorbidities/gastrostomy tube status, technologic dependence (positive airway pressure [PAP]), viral infections, a history of reflux, an oxygen saturation nadir of <80% on preoperative PSG, and neuromuscular disorders can predict need for PICU care post-AT.[38,40,42] In one study, preoperative PSG oxygen desaturation index (ODI), SpO$_2$ nadir, and total sleep time (TST) with SpO$_2$ <90% predicted PICU in children with severe OSA.[25]

Uvulopalatopharyngoplasty

Some children with associated neuromuscular disability, i.e., cerebral palsy or Down syndrome, may benefit from more extensive surgical procedures such as uvulopalatopharyngoplasty (UPPP).[43–46] In one study, 77% of children with neurologic impairment and moderate to severe OSA who were treated with UPPP with AT did not require further intervention.[44] These patients require monitoring as they are at risk for residual OSA.

Skeletal Advancement Procedures in Children with Craniofacial Abnormalities

Infants and children with craniofacial abnormalities and severe OSA can benefit with skeletal advancement procedures to avoid tracheostomy or facilitate decannulation. Two procedures performed in children include mandibular distraction osteogenesis (MDO) or mandibular advancement surgeries (MAS) and rapid maxillary expansion (RME).

Mandibular Distraction Osteogenesis/Mandibular Advancement Surgeries

Patients with micrognathia or retrognathia have upper airway obstruction from retropositioning of the base of the tongue, compromising the hypopharyngeal space. MDO has been shown to be successful in patients with micro- and retrognathia with severe OSA. This procedure improves the position of the tongue in the posterior pharynx by lengthening the mandible and bringing its muscular insertions forward thus increasing the anteroposterior dimension of the airway. This has allowed relief of symptoms and avoidance of a tracheostomy in infants or children with OSA[47–50] and allowed decannulation in those who are already tracheostomy dependent.[51,52] In one systematic review, MAS or MDO for mandibular insufficiency resulted in dramatic improvement from very severe to mild OSA with reduction in the AHI from 41 to 4.5 events per hour and increase in mean oxygen saturation nadir from 77–91%.[53] In one study, 84% of infants with Robin sequence and severe OSA who had external MDO during the neonatal period had 50% reduction in obstructive AHI, but all had residual OSA with 48% having persistent severe OSA following surgery,[54] emphasizing the need for pre- and postoperative PSG. Complications associated with MDO include neurosensory disturbances, minor infection, device failure, anterior open bite, permanent dental damage, and skeletal relapse.[55]

Rapid Maxillary Expansion

Some patients with OSA and maxillofacial malformation and dental malocclusion may benefit from RME, which is an orthodontic procedure that widens the palate by gradual distraction osteogenesis. Bone distraction at the midpalatal suture widens the maxilla and increases the volume of the nasal cavity, thus decreasing nasal resistance. Following this procedure, patients have shown improvement in symptoms, AHI, arousal index, and with almost normalized sleep architecture up to 24 months following completion of the treatment.[56–59] Short-term (<3 years) follow-up of children who have undergone RME have shown improvement in AHI and oxygen saturation with greater improvement seen in those who have small tonsils or are status post-AT than those with coexisting tonsillar hypertrophy.[60] However, in one study, although there was improvement in oxygenation at the 12-month follow-up, there was residual/persistent OSA in 6/11 patients (55%).[61] Thus, close monitoring with periodic PSG for documentation of resolution of OSA is essential.

Other surgical procedures include maxillomandibular advancement for midface hypoplasia, as well as tongue reduction, genioglossal advancement, or hyoid myotomy and suspension, which are aimed at relieving retroglossal obstruction. These are infrequently performed in children and are generally only indicated in those with craniofacial malformations or syndromes. Ultimately, in children with severe OSA who have failed standard therapies, positive pressure therapy or tracheostomy may be required.

Hypoglossal Nerve Stimulation

Hypoglossal nerve stimulation is a treatment option that is of increasing use in adults who are intolerant of PAP therapy. There are three surgically unilaterally implanted components involved in hypoglossal nerve stimulation: (1) a sensing lead implanted in the region of the fourth intercostal region between the internal and external intercostal muscles, (2) a neurostimulator implanted 2–4 cm below the clavicle, and (3) a stimulation lead placed in the medial XII nerve branch. The hypoglossal nerve stimulator delivers an electrical impulse to the anterior branches of the hypoglossal nerve through the stimulation lead in response to respiration detected by the sensing lead resulting in tongue base protrusion and thus alleviating obstruction.[62] The device is only activated by the patient at the onset of sleep. On follow-up of patients treated with hypoglossal nerve stimulation, adult patients showed clinically significant improvements in OSA severity, daytime sleepiness, and sleep-related quality of life. Older age, higher preoperative AHI, and lower body mass index (BMI) were associated with greater improvements.[63] Currently, the utility of hypoglossal nerve stimulation in the pediatric population has not been demonstrated other than in adolescents with Down syndrome and OSA.[64,65]

Positive Pressure Therapy

PAP therapy, i.e., continuous positive airway pressure (CPAP) or bilevel positive airway pressure (BPAP), is a highly effective means of treatment in children with OSA. PAP is the treatment of choice for patients who do not improve sufficiently following AT or when surgery is not possible or indicated. It offers temporary treatment for those awaiting surgery. It is often used for patients with OSA related to obesity, Down syndrome, craniofacial disorders, and neuromuscular disorders such as cerebral palsy.[21]

AT remains the first line of treatment for OSA in most situations; however, residual symptoms may persist in up to one-third of children[66] with some studies reporting an even higher failure rate.[67] When a PSG reveals an AHI of more than five events per hour following AT, then PAP should be considered.[68] A titration study should be performed in the sleep laboratory with a technician in attendance. Although not yet approved by the U.S. Food and Drug Administration, there are studies documenting the efficacy of off-label autotitrating CPAP use in children.[69-71]

Practice guidelines for detailed, step-by-step, titration strategies for positive pressure therapy in adults and children have been proposed in the Clinical Guidelines for the Manual Titration of Positive Airway Pressure in Patients with OSA sponsored by the American Academy of Sleep Medicine.[72] Four separate algorithms for CPAP and BPAP titrations for patients less than and greater than 12 years of age, respectively, are presented. These can be adapted for use in the sleep laboratory to guide technicians in decision making throughout the night. The goal for an optimal titration is to reduce the AHI to <5 events per hour with supine rapid eye movement (REM) sleep recorded at the selected pressure. Evidence-based guidelines for the selection of continuous versus BPAP therapy are lacking for OSA. Studies have not found an advantage in adherence or outcome in either adults or children.[73] The practice of the authors is to use bilevel therapy when high pressures (>14 cm H_2O) are needed to relieve airway obstruction or the patient complains of intolerably high pressure during the study. Bilevel therapy is also utilized for OSA in the face of hypoventilation with coexisting respiratory muscle weakness, or with extreme obesity, or in those with prolonged central apneas in which a backup rate is needed. Supplemental oxygen may be required with coexisting pulmonary disease when hypoxemia persists despite control of obstructive events and hypoventilation.

The most important consideration in selecting the PAP interface is patient comfort. Generally nasal masks are preferred over nasal-oral (full-face) masks in the pediatric population as there is less chance for gaseous distension of the stomach or aspiration if emesis occurs. However, some patients have marked nasal occlusion and/or significant mouth breathing and a nasal-oral mask is the only route available. Some patients will prefer nasal prongs or "pillows," especially if they have a strong preference to sleep on their side. The head gear should be snug but not tight. Some redness of the skin in the morning related to the interface that fades during the day is acceptable, but persistent tenderness or erythema over the nasal bridge is not, as it can lead to painful skin breakdown and thus must be addressed quickly. Covering the site with a hydrocolloid gel dressing is helpful as an interim solution. Masks should fit such that air leak, or the mask itself, does not irritate the eyes.

At each follow-up, potential problems with the interface and other complications associated with the therapy that may interfere with usage are discussed. It is helpful if the PAP device is brought to each clinic visit for troubleshooting or adjustment of settings. Complications such as nasal dryness or congestion, epistaxis, eye irritation, skin compromise, gastric distension, emesis in those patients using a full-face mask, and mouth breathing with excessive leak in those using nasal mask or prongs are addressed. Nasal steroids and/or warm humidification can help relieve nasal obstruction and improve adherence. Skin complications can be avoided by regular follow-up to assess mask fit and by changing the interface from time to time. Monitoring of facial growth for the development of midface hypoplasia related to nightly pressure from the mask interface has been suggested. In one study, children with a mean age of 10 years who were adherent to CPAP therapy for 2.5 years were found to develop midface retrusion and dental abnormalities.[74] There is now an increasing array of interfaces available for infants and children, allowing for periodic switches to prevent skin complications and pressure from the mask interfaces. At this time, in the United States, FDA-approved interfaces are only available for children age 2 years and older. Some countries have interfaces available for even younger children and infants; however, in the United States these devices are used "off-label" at the discretion of the prescribing physician, and this information should be shared with parents.

When the decision has been made to institute PAP, one of the most important considerations is preparing the child and family for the use of the therapy on a nightly basis. This approach varies with the age and developmental level of the child. The patient and family should be educated about the titration study, the PAP equipment, and the interface with verbal and written material in advance.[73] The medical care team must convey a high level of confidence and trust in the parents' abilities to master the techniques, and more importantly in their ability to work with their child to use the therapy each night. A parental approach that is consistent, committed, and calm should be emphasized. Patients ideally should be fitted with and given an appropriate interface to wear at home at bedtime for practice and desensitization prior to the titration study. The interface is worn without being attached to the tubing or positive pressure device so there is no flow or pressure. Parents are encouraged to build this into the child's usual bedtime routine. An age-appropriate reward system (behavior modification) for wearing the interface is often helpful. Child developmental psychologists with expertise in sleep medicine can guide desensitization in difficult cases. In this way when the patient arrives for the titration study, the focus can be on identifying the correct settings to achieve adequate gas exchange, normal respiratory pattern, and optimal sleep quality. Similar to adults, split studies are possible with typically developing adolescents; the educational session need not be as extensive and can be accomplished with a prestudy explanation or video.[75,76]

Pressure titration is affected by the age of the child. Younger children generally do not tolerate pressures at the higher range (>15 cm H_2O), and in general OSA can be managed with pressures lower than this. Children are also

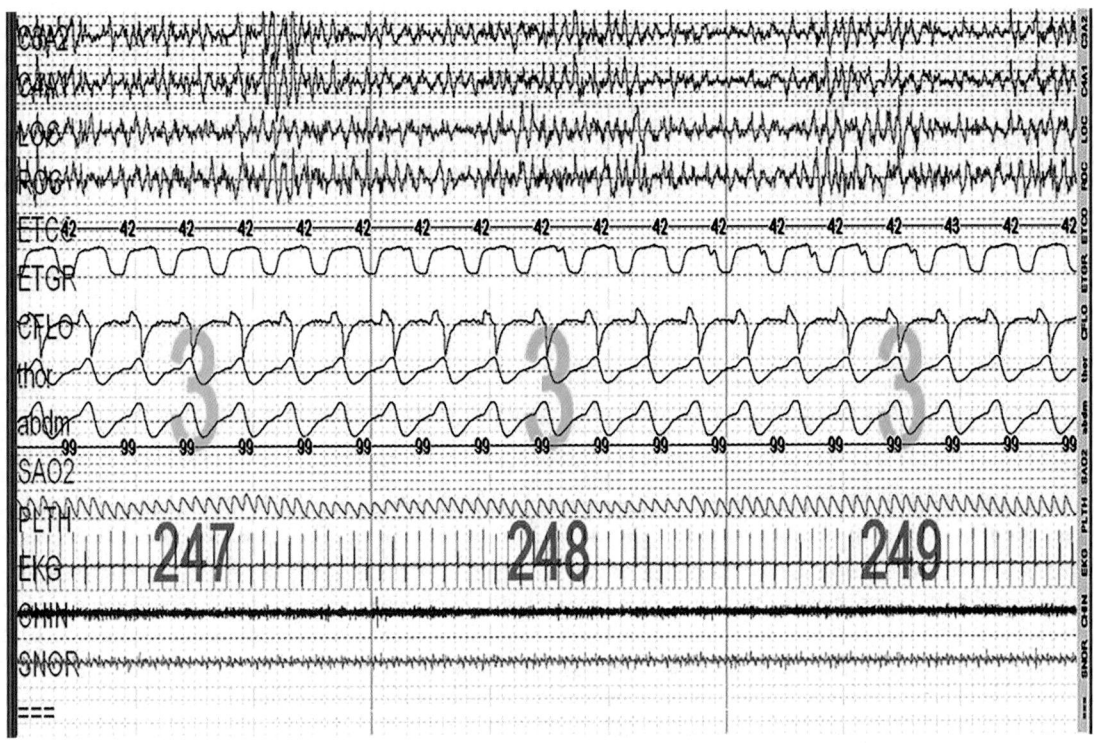

• **Fig. 34.1** $P_{ET}CO_2$ monitoring during continuous positive airway pressure (CPAP) titration polysomnography.

poorly tolerant of painful procedures; thus gas exchange should be monitored noninvasively. The use of end-tidal CO_2 monitoring during the titration study can provide an accurate measure of ventilation. A small end-tidal CO_2 catheter is placed at one of the nares under the mask interface. Readings are deemed accurate when a plateau is present in the waveform (Fig. 34.1). If the plateau is lost the catheter can be repositioned at the first wakefulness opportunity. Because the catheter is small, the interface seal is not disrupted. However, subjects who use nasal prongs or pillows as their preferred interface cannot be monitored in this way and gas exchange must be inferred from SpO_2 measurements or transcutaneous CO_2 measurements.

Some children with OSA who are very young or have developmental disabilities cannot communicate with the polysomnographic technician or respiratory therapist to express discomfort with the interface or the pressures. Technicians and therapists who are skilled in working with children of all ages and abilities are required for a successful PAP titration in the pediatric sleep lab. Understanding that a patient's discomfort can have different origins and working carefully with the child and parent to minimize fear and maximize comfort require patience and skills that develop over years of experience. Reducing pressures, selecting a different interface, and changing the patient's position should all be tried. However, there are occasions, despite advance preparation, when the child's inability to cooperate prevents completion of an adequate titration. If OSA is not severe, a further period of time acclimating in the home setting can be tried. The PAP interface and device can be

used for a short time each night in the home on the best-tolerated pressure levels identified during the study with a gradual increase in the time used each night. When use has increased to more than 4–6 hours per night the laboratory titration can be repeated to identify optimal pressures. If the clinical situation dictates a more rapid initiation of therapy, then hospitalization would be indicated.

Expert opinion recommends periodic retitration studies for children treated with PAP. This is logically based on the notion that children are growing and developing and that these changes may interact with upper airway anatomy and neuromuscular function such that positive pressure needs may increase or decrease. Thus, younger patients would need more frequent reevaluations than older children. Repeat titration should be performed after surgeries of the upper airway, significant change in weight, and certainly if new symptoms indicating poor control of OSA or tolerance of PAP arise. Very limited data are available to guide the frequency of routine repeat titration studies in children.

Perioperative Use

OSA increases the risk of poor outcomes with surgery requiring general anesthesia.[77] PAP has been proposed as a strategy for stabilization of patients with severe OSA in the perioperative period prior to AT and prior to other elective surgical procedures.[78] Data are lacking regarding the cost-effectiveness and efficacy of this approach, but there is some evidence in the adult literature documenting decreased surgical risk in patients with OSA treated with preoperative PAP in preparation for elective surgery.[36,79] Use of PAP for

4–6 weeks prior to surgery has been recommended.[77,80] As is typical for any indication for PAP, strategies and technologies to improve adherence remain critical needs.

Adherence

Adherence to PAP is a major problem in patients with OSA both in children and adults. Ideally, adherence should be determined objectively via machine download information. Information regarding patient use rather than the time the unit is simply turned on is needed. In one study, treatment with PAP was associated with high drop-out rate (one-third of children) before 6 months and with mean nightly use of only 5.3 hours in those who were deemed adherent. This is brief considering the long sleep hours in children.[73] Behavioral therapy, in conjunction with ongoing support and close follow-up, increased adherence to PAP in children.[81,82] Uong and coworkers identified 70% PAP adherence in a retrospective study of 27 cognitively intact children with residual OSA post-AT (adherence defined as more than 4 hours nightly use at least 5 nights per week determined objectively by machine counter clock/meter). They found that adherence in terms of days of use was better in patients with more severe OSA and in those with the greatest decrease in AHI with PAP. Age, gender, race, BMI, and PAP mode did not affect adherence. Parental report of adherence correlated with the meter readings.[83] The initial use of PAP during the first week of use was a predictor of subsequent use in a prospective study of 30 children, including those with developmental disability. This emphasizes the importance of starting out on the "right foot" as outlined previously. The authors commented that using PAP at low, perhaps subtherapeutic pressures, during sleep prior to formal titration, may interfere with subsequent adherence.[84] Demographic factors impacting adherence were found by DiFeo and coworkers with maternal education being the greatest predictor of higher use, whereas African American race and older patient age predicted poorer adherence. The children studied had a number of underlying conditions and 23% had developmental disabilities. In general, adherence was rated suboptimal for the group as a whole with an average use of 3 hours per night and 22 days per month.[85] Designing effective strategies to enhance PAP adherence would be facilitated by an understanding of perceived barriers on the part of parents and patients. Simon and colleagues devised a questionnaire evaluating barriers to PAP use and identified a number of psychosocial issues including embarrassment, forgetfulness, and denial as frequently playing a role.[86] A reasonable hypothesis has been that patients would find BPAP to be more comfortable than CPAP with greater ease of exhalation and synchrony with natural breathing patterns; furthermore that increased comfort would improve adherence. Marcus and coworkers examined this relationship in two studies, the first comparing BPAP and CPAP and the second comparing CPAP with a bilevel technology that includes pressure relief. Neither study identified better adherence in the bilevel group and adherence was suboptimal in both groups despite efficacy.[73,87] As clinical experience with autoPAP

devices accumulates in the pediatric population, it will be important to understand the characteristics of this approach in terms of adherence and efficacy.

Clearly a major challenge for the pediatric sleep medicine community is to refine methods of increasing adherence to PAP therapy. The therapy itself is safe and effective, and the potential to reduce both childhood comorbidities and the early development of adult cardiovascular disease is of extraordinary value to the individual child and society.

Supplemental Oxygen

Supplemental oxygen can relieve hypoxemia in patients with OSA while awaiting definitive therapy or in patients in whom no other treatment option is available.[88] In those with long-term hypercapnia, oxygen must be used with caution and preferably started during the PSG when gas exchange is carefully monitored or during hospitalization with blood gas monitoring. Infants treated with supplemental oxygen had significant improvement in oxygen saturation nadir associated with obstructive events without adverse effect on alveolar hypoventilation.[89]

High-Flow Nasal Cannula

High-flow nasal cannula (HFNC) offers an alternative treatment option for patients with OSA who are intolerant to PAP therapy. With HFNC, high-flow heated and humidified air is delivered through the nose, with oxygen added to achieve the desired FiO_2 thus continuously flushing the dead space of the upper airways with gas flow. Because the flow rate is greater than the normal inspiratory flow rate, it decreases upper airway collapse and creates PAP in the airways. It has been found to lessen respiratory events, improve oxygenation, and provide clinical benefits for children with moderate to severe OSA who cannot tolerate CPAP.[90–92] Amaddeo and coworkers report a protocol of initiating HFNC at home. In their study, the nasal cannula was sized where nasal cannula to nares ratio was 80%. The device was initially set at 1 L/kg/min with a maximum flow of 20 L/min, temperature 34°C and FiO_2 21%. A titration study was performed when the patient was tolerating 4 hours of sleep per night for 1 week at home. During the titration study pressure signal was obtained via the outlet of a t-tube.[90] In another study, a thermal oronasal sensor was used for scoring hypopneas as the nasal pressure transducer is unreliable. In this study, <50% of the cross-sectional area of the nares was occluded by the nasal prongs to allow for intentional leak. Initial flow was 5 L/min or 15 L/min for pediatric- or adult-sized cannula and titrated in 5–15 L/min increments, respectively, based on symptoms of snoring, labored respirations, oxygen desaturations, etc., until disordered breathing was normalized or recommended maximum flow was reached (20 L/min for pediatric-sized and 50 L/min for adult-sized cannula). Supplemental oxygen was added if hypoxemia or desaturations persisted at maximum flow of room air.[92]

Development of pneumothorax or pneumomediastinum has been described as a complication of HFNC in some patients with significant hyperinflation. In HFNC, air pressure is not regulated and the high flow tends to increase end-expiratory volume. Although the risk of pneumothorax is considered low for OSA, HFNC should be used with caution in those with coexisting obstructive lung disease.[91,93,94]

Anti-Inflammatory Therapies

Anti-inflammatory therapies, i.e. nasal steroids[95–97] and montelukast,[98,99] alone or in combination[100,101] can be an option in the management of mild OSA resulting in improvement in symptoms and reduction in adenoid size.[97] Combined montelukast and intranasal budesonide may help children with residual mild OSA following AT.[102] In children treated with nasal steroids, clinical improvement may persist up to 9 months after the completion of therapy[96] and reduction in adenoid size may persist 8 weeks after discontinuation of therapy.[97] In a prospective study of subjects scheduled for surgery, intranasal fluticasone resulted in significant improvement such that 76% of the patients were no longer considered surgical candidates.[103] Goldbart and colleagues demonstrated the abundant expression of glucocorticoid receptors[104] and cysteinyl leukotriene receptors[105,106] in adenotonsillar tissue from children with OSA. There is reduction in proliferative responses, increased cellular apoptosis, and decreased release of proinflammatory cytokines in tonsils or adenoids from children with OSA treated with intranasal steroids[107,108] and leukotriene receptor antagonists.[109]

Oral Appliances

Oral appliances enlarge the upper airway by positioning the mandible and tongue forward including the mandibular repositioning and tongue retaining devices. Two small trials in children with OSA showed improvement in symptoms and polysomnographic AHI.[110,111] Side effects associated with oral appliance therapies include excessive salivation,[110] dry mouth, and tooth and/or jaw discomfort.[112] Although frequently used in the adult population with snoring or mild to moderate OSA syndrome and a recommended treatment to those who prefer alternate therapy or intolerant to CPAP,[113] there is insufficient data at present to state that it is effective in children.[114] Furthermore, there are no long-term data to support the use of oral appliances before full maturation of the jaw and teeth.

Weight Loss/Role of Bariatric Surgery

Weight loss and lifestyle intervention can be an effective treatment for mild OSA associated with being overweight or obesity,[115,116] although, there is a significant rate of relapse even in the most aggressive weight loss therapies

including use of pharmacotherapy. For this reason, bariatric surgery may play a role. A few studies of bariatric surgery in adolescents show promising short-term outcome with early weight loss, improvement of OSA and of the associated medical comorbidities (i.e., hypertension and metabolic syndrome), improvement in quality of life, and near complete resolution of OSA.[117–119] One study of obese children and adolescents with a median BMI of 47.4 kg/m^2 who underwent laparoscopic sleeve gastrectomy showed short-term weight loss in more than 90% of the patients. Twenty of 22 patients with OSA had resolution of symptoms.[120] With these results, it can be assumed that if bariatric surgery can provide a long-term effective reduction of body weight, it can also lead to successful improvement of OSA. However, adult studies showed that despite remarkable weight loss, many patients had residual OSA following bariatric surgery.[121,122]

Criteria for metabolic and bariatric surgery in adolescents include (1) BMI ≥35 kg/m^2 or 120% of the 95th percentile with clinically significant comorbid conditions such as OSA (AHI >5), type 2 diabetes, hypertension, non-alcoholic steatohepatosis, or BMI ≥40 kg/m^2 or 140% of the 95th percentile (whichever is lower) and (2) multidisciplinary team assessment that the patient and family have the ability and motivation to adhere to recommended treatments pre- and postoperatively, including consistent use of micronutrient supplements.[123] Contraindications to bariatric surgery for the adolescent include (1) a medically correctable cause of obesity; (2) an ongoing substance abuse problem (within the preceding year); (3) a medical, psychiatric, psychosocial, or cognitive condition that prevents adherence to postoperative dietary and medication regimens; and (4) current or planned pregnancy within 12–18 months of the procedure.[123]

Watchful Waiting

Children with mild OSA due to adenotonsillar hypertrophy and without comorbidities may do well with close observation and monitoring (watchful waiting). In the Childhood Adenotonsillectomy Trial (CHAT), children 5–9 years of age with mild to moderate OSA, with 42% of those considered to be surgical candidates, showed PSG-documented resolution of OSA after 7 months of observation. In this study, baseline predictors of spontaneous resolution were lower AHI, small waist and neck circumference, low symptom burden, and little snoring.[124] Improvement in attention or executive function did not differ between watchful waiting group and the children who had AT,[7] but there was less improvement in behavior, quality of life, or polysomnographic outcomes in the watchful waiting group.[7] In a randomized trial of otherwise healthy children aged 2–4 years of age, the differences in improvement in obstructive AHI between those who had AT and watchful waiting was small,[125] suggesting that even younger children with mild OSA may benefit from watchful waiting.

Specific Populations

Obesity

The prevalence of OSA is estimated at 13–59% in obese children. OSA can be severe with frequent obstructive events, profound hypoxemia, and significant hypoventilation. AT is the first line of treatment. These patients are at risk for hypoventilation; thus oxygen and narcotics should be used judiciously postoperatively. Obese children are at risk for residual OSA following AT or other surgical upper airway interventions[12,126] and frequently require treatment with PAP therapy even after AT. Thus, setting realistic goals and emphasizing preoperative weight management should be a part of the treatment plan.[126]

Down Syndrome

OSA is highly prevalent in Down syndrome, affecting 50–76% of patients.[127,128] About half of these children have moderate to severe OSA.[128,129] Risk factors for OSA in Down syndrome include midface and mandibular hypoplasia, large tongue, pharyngomalacia, laryngomalacia, subglottic stenosis, tracheal stenosis, obesity, and hypothyroidism.[129,130] The primary treatment is AT, but risk of persistent or residual OSA is significant.[131–133] In one study, AT alone resulted in only 51% reduction in the preoperative AHI.[134] In Down syndrome patients, lingual tonsillar hypertrophy, large tongue base, laryngomalacia, and epiglottic collapse also contribute to OSA;[135–137] thus other sleep surgeries such as lingual tonsillectomy, tongue base reduction, and supraglottoplasty maybe indicated.[131] Drug-induced sleep endoscopy is requisite to identify areas of obstruction and direct surgical therapies. PAP can provide effective therapy in those with residual OSA or with persistent hypoventilation.[138,139] Those who are intolerant to CPAP may benefit with HFNC.[92] Hypoglossal nerve stimulation may afford a potential therapeutic option for those with refractory OSA after AT who are unable to tolerate PAP therapy.[64,65] Thyroid disease is common and present in 4–18% of Down syndrome patients;[127] thus periodic evaluation of thyroid function in addition to the annual monitoring is indicated when OSA exists.[140] Medication therapy alone (i.e., intranasal steroid or montelukast or in combination) has not been demonstrated to be effective in Down syndrome patients, including those with mild OSA.[141]

Prader-Willi Syndrome

OSA is highly prevalent in patients with Prader-Willi syndrome with a rate of 80%.[142] Risk factors for OSA include obesity, hypotonia, micrognathia, altered ventilatory control, and hypothyroidism. AT generally results in OSA improvement but residual OSA is common.[143,144] A recent systematic review found improvement in quality of life as well as polysomnographic resolution of OSA to AHI <1.5 in 20% and improvement from moderate to severe OSA to mild or resolved (AHI <5) in 67% post-AT.[144] However, it is also associated with considerable risk of postoperative complications of which velopharyngeal insufficiency is the most

common.[144,145] Central apneas may manifest in some children post operatively, thus it is essential to repeat PSG.[143] Growth hormone (GH) therapy plays a critical role in the management of Prader-Willi syndrome patients. GH is associated with growth of lymphoid tissues and may worsen OSA; however, theoretically, the promotion of lean body mass and improved hypotonia could also be beneficial for reduction in OSA risk or severity. PSG is required before starting GH and 8–10 weeks after initiating treatment.[146]

Infancy

Infants can have OSA from nasal obstruction, craniofacial abnormalities, laryngomalacia, subglottic stenosis, or gastroesophageal reflux disease.[3,147,148] Therapy is directed to the underlying cause.[148] Those who are not stable or are not candidates for surgery can be placed on supplemental oxygen, if hypoxemia is present. Supplemental oxygen has been found to improve the hypoxemia without associated alveolar hypoventilation.[89] PAP therapy is limited in this age group as it is not well tolerated and there is not an array of appropriate nasal interfaces. Adenoidectomy has been found to relieve OSA and failure to thrive.[149] Tongue lip adhesion,[150–153] MDO,[47–49] or nasopharyngeal tube[154] may relieve OSA in infants with micrognathia and Robin sequence. Infants with laryngomalacia and mild symptoms may be observed as this usually improves with maturation. However, those with moderate to severe OSA and/or associated feeding difficulties and poor growth will require supraglottoplasty.[155,156] Although supraglottoplasty can significantly improve PSG outcomes in laryngomalacia, residual mild to moderate OSA exists in most children postoperatively[157–159] emphasizing the need for periodic evaluation post-surgery. HFNC can also be considered in infants with OSA.

Gastroesophageal reflux disease (GERD) is common in infants and worsens OSA via increased inflammation of the upper airway.[3,160] It is strongly associated with laryngomalacia.[161] Most often, medical management with acid suppression is sufficient.

CLINICAL PEARLS

- Careful attention to risk factors for perioperative complications of adenotonsillectomy with plans for hospital observation of high-risk patients is key to minimizing adverse outcomes.
- Parental and patient education regarding PAP therapy well in advance of the initial titration study is very important in subsequent adherence.
- Not all patients will be cured following adenotonsillectomy, and follow-up directed at persistent symptoms or complications of OSA is indicated.
- A very high index of suspicion for OSA is needed for overweight and obese children; OSA may represent a modifiable risk factor in this population for the reduction of for serious cardiovascular and metabolic disease in later life.

Summary

AT is the mainstay of treatment of OSA in children and it is curative in most. About one-third of patients will have residual or persistent OSA and will require additional therapies. Most children with OSA can be treated with AT in the ambulatory surgery center. Knowledge of risk factors for respiratory complications and risk assessment strategies has allowed clinicians to determine safety of surgery in the outpatient setting. Children at high risk for postoperative complications require inpatient postoperative monitoring and treatment. In addition to AT, OSA can be successfully treated with other surgical approaches and by the use of PAP including HFNC. Typically developing children with mild OSA due to adenotonsillar hypertrophy maybe observed (watchful waiting) or placed on pharmacologic therapy. Because OSA has significant concurrent comorbidities and may be a precursor to serious adult disease, effective treatment is imperative. Reliance on PAP as the mainstay of long-term therapy requires additional efforts on behalf of the sleep medicine community to help patients achieve optimal adherence. The importance of preventing childhood obesity cannot be overemphasized.

References

1. Lumeng JC, Chervin RD. Epidemiology of pediatric obstructive sleep apnea. *Proc Am Thorac Soc.* 2008;5(2):242–252. https://doi.org/10.1513/pats.200708-135MG.

2. Selvadurai S, Voutsas G, Propst EJ, Wolter NE, Narang I. Obstructive sleep apnea in children aged 3 years and younger: Rate and risk factors. *Paediatr Child Health.* 2020;25(7):432–438. https://doi.org/10.1093/pch/pxz097.

3. Katz ES, Mitchell RB, D'Ambrosio CM. Obstructive sleep apnea in infants. *Am J Respir Crit Care Med.* 2012;185(8):805–816. https://doi.org/10.1164/rccm.201108-1455CI.

4. Spilsbury JC, Storfer-Isser A, Rosen CL, Redline S. Remission and incidence of obstructive sleep apnea from middle childhood to late adolescence. *Sleep.* 2015;38(1):23–29. https://doi.org/10.5665/sleep.4318.

5. Constantin E, Kermack A, Nixon GM, Tidmarsh L, Ducharme FM, Brouillette RT. Adenotonsillectomy improves sleep, breathing, and quality of life but not behavior. *J Pediatr.* 2007;150(5):540–546. https://doi.org/10.1016/j.jpeds.2007.01.026.

6. Friedman BC, Hendeles-Amitai A, Kozminsky E, et al. Adenotonsillectomy improves neurocognitive function in children with obstructive sleep apnea syndrome. *Sleep.* 2003;26(8):999–1005. https://doi.org/10.1093/sleep/26.8.999.

7. Marcus CL, Moore RH, Rosen CL, et al. A Randomized trial of adenotonsillectomy for childhood sleep apnea. *N Engl J Med.* 2013;368(25):2366–2376. https://doi.org/10.1056/nejmoa1215881.

8. Taylor H.G., Bowen S.R., Beebe D.W., et al. Cognitive effects of adenotonsillectomy for obstructive sleep apnea. 2016;138(2):e20154458.

9. Landau YE, Bar-Yishay O, Greenberg-Dotan S, Goldbart AD, Tarasiuk A, Tal A. Impaired behavioral and neurocognitive function in preschool children with obstructive sleep apnea. *Pediatr Pulmonol.* 2012;47(2):180–188. https://doi.org/10.1002/ppul.21534.

10. Bonuck KA, Freeman K, Henderson J. Growth and growth biomarker changes after adenotonsillectomy: Systematic review and metaanalysis. *Arch Dis Child.* 2009;94(2):83–91. https://doi.org/10.1136/adc.2008.141192.

11. Kiris M, Muderris T, Celebi S, Cankaya H, Bercin S. Changes in serum IGF-1 and IGFBP-3 levels and growth in children following adenoidectomy, tonsillectomy or adenotonsillectomy. *Int J Pediatr Otorhinolaryngol.* 2010;74(5):528–531. https://doi.org/10.1016/j.ijporl.2010.02.014.

12. Beauchamp MT, Regier B, Nzuki A, et al. Weight change before and after adenotonsillectomy in children: An analysis based upon pre-surgery body mass category. *Clin Otolaryngol.* 2020;45(5):739–745. https://doi.org/10.1111/coa.13568.

13. Katz ES, Moore RH, Rosen CL, et al. Growth after adenotonsillectomy for obstructive sleep apnea: An RCT. *Pediatrics.* 2014;134(2):282–289. https://doi.org/10.1542/peds.2014-0591.

14. Koc S, Aytekin M, Kalay N, et al. The effect of adenotonsillectomy on right ventricle function and pulmonary artery pressure in children with adenotonsillar hypertrophy. *Int J Pediatr Otorhinolaryngol.* 2012;76(1):45–48. https://doi.org/10.1016/j.ijporl.2011.09.028.

15. Ingram DG. Singh AV, Ehsan Z, Birnbaum BF. Obstructive sleep apnea and pulmonary hypertension in children. Paediatr Respir Rev. 2017;23:33–39. https://doi.org/10.1016/j.prrv.2017.01.001.

16. Constantin E, McGregor CD, Cote V, Brouillette RT. Pulse rate and pulse rate variability decrease after adenotonsillectomy for obstructive sleep apnea. *Pediatr Pulmonol.* 2008;43(5):498–504. https://doi.org/10.1002/ppul.20811.

17. Ng DK, Wong JC, hong Chan C, Leung LCK, yu. Leung S. Ambulatory blood pressure before and after adenotonsillectomy in children with obstructive sleep apnea. *Sleep Med.* 2010;11(7):721–725. https://doi.org/10.1016/j.sleep.2009.10.007.

18. Hsu WC, Kang KT, Chiu SN, Weng WC, Lee PL, Lin CY. 24-Hour ambulatory blood pressure after adenotonsillectomy in childhood sleep apnea. *J Pediatr.* 2018;199:112–117. https://doi.org/10.1016/j.jpeds.2018.03.072.

19. Kuo YL, Kang KT, Chiu SN, Weng WC, Lee PL, Hsu WC. Blood pressure after surgery among obese and nonobese children with obstructive sleep apnea. *Otolaryngol Head Neck Surg.* 2015;152(5):931–940. https://doi.org/10.1177/0194599815573927.

20. Bhattacharjee R, Kheirandish-Gozal L, Spruyt K, et al. Adenotonsillectomy outcomes in treatment of obstructive sleep apnea in children: A multicenter retrospective study. *Am J Respir Crit Care Med.* 2010;182(5):676–683. https://doi.org/10.1164/rccm.200912-1930OC.

21. Marcus CL, Brooks LJ, Draper KA, et al. Diagnosis and management of childhood obstructive sleep apnea syndrome. *Pediatrics.* 2012;130(3):576–584. https://doi.org/10.1542/peds.2012-1671.

22. O'Brien LM, Sitha S, Baur LA, Waters KA. Obesity increases the risk for persisting obstructive sleep apnea after treatment in children. *Int J Pediatr Otorhinolaryngol.* 2006;70(9):1555–1560. https://doi.org/10.1016/j.ijporl.2006.04.003.

23. Tweedie DJ, Bajaj Y, Ifeacho SN, et al. Peri-operative complications after adenotonsillectomy in a UK pediatric tertiary referral centre. *Int J Pediatr Otorhinolaryngol.* 2012;76(6):809–815. https://doi.org/10.1016/j.ijporl.2012.02.048.

24. Sanders JC, King MA, Mitchell RB, Kelly JP. Perioperative complications of adenotonsillectomy in children with obstructive sleep apnea syndrome. *Anesth Analg.* 2006;103(5):1115–1121. https://doi.org/10.1213/01.ane.0000244318.77377.67.

25. Molero-Ramirez H, Kakazu MT, Baroody F, Bhattacharjee R. Polysomnography parameters assessing gas exchange best predict postoperative respiratory complications following adenotonsillectomy in children with severe OSA. *J Clin Sleep Med.* 2019;15(09):1251–1259. https://doi.org/10.5664/jcsm.7914.

26. Katz SL, Monsour A, Barrowman N, et al. Predictors of postoperative respiratory complications in children undergoing adenotonsillectomy. *J Clin Sleep Med.* 2020;16(1):41–48. https://doi.org/10.5664/JCSM.8118.

27. Ye J, Liu H, Zhang G, Huang Z, Huang P, Li Y. Postoperative respiratory complications of adenotonsillectomy for obstructive sleep apnea syndrome in older children: Prevalence, risk factors, and impact on clinical outcome. *J Otolaryngol Head Neck Surg.* 2009;38(1):49–58.

28. Spencer DJ, Jones JE. Complications of adenotonsillectomy in patients younger than 3 years. *Arch Otolaryngol Head Neck Surg.* 2012;138(4):335–339. https://doi.org/10.1001/archoto.2012.1.

29. Hill CA, Litvak A, Canapari C, et al. A pilot study to identify pre- and peri-operative risk factors for airway complications following adenotonsillectomy for treatment of severe pediatric OSA. *Int J Pediatr Otorhinolaryngol.* 2011;75(11):1385–1390. https://doi.org/10.1016/j.ijporl.2011.07.034.

30. McColley SA, April MM, Carroll JL, Naclerio RM, Loughlin GM. Respiratory compromise after adenotonsillectomy in children with obstructive sleep apnea. *Arch Otolaryngol Neck Surg.* 1992;118(9):940–943. https://doi.org/10.1001/archotol.1992.01880090056017.

31. Thongyam A, Marcus CL, Lockman JL, et al. Predictors of perioperative complications in higher risk children after adenotonsillectomy for obstructive sleep apnea: A prospective study. *Otolaryngol Head Neck Surg (United States).* 2014;151(6):1046–1054. https://doi.org/10.1177/0194599814552059.

32. Keamy DG, Chhabra KR, Hartnick CJ. Predictors of complications following adenotonsillectomy in children with severe obstructive sleep apnea. *Int J Pediatr Otorhinolaryngol.* 2015;79(11):1838–1841. https://doi.org/10.1016/j.ijporl.2015.08.021.

33. Kalra M, Buncher R, Amin RS. Asthma as a risk factor for respiratory complications after adenotonsillectomy in children with obstructive breathing during sleep. *Ann Allergy, Asthma Immunol.* 2005;94(5):549–552. https://doi.org/10.1016/S1081-1206(10)61132-5.

34. Raghavendran S, Bagry H, Detheux G, Zhang X, Brouillette RT, Brown KA. An anesthetic management protocol to decrease respiratory complications after adenotonsillectomy in children with severe sleep apnea. *Anesth Analg.* 2010;110(4):1093–1101. https://doi.org/10.1213/ANE.0b013e3181cfc435.

35. Mitchell RB, Archer SM, Ishman SL, et al. Clinical Practice Guideline: Tonsillectomy in Children (Update)—Executive Summary. *Otolaryngol Head Neck Surg (United States).* 2019;160(2):187–205. https://doi.org/10.1177/0194599818807917.

36. American Society of Anesthesiologists Task Force on Perioperative Management of Patients with Obstructive Sleep Apnea. Practice guidelines for the perioperative management of patients with obstructive sleep apnea. *Anesthesiology.* 2014;120(2):268–286. doi:10.1097/ALN.0000000000000053

37. De A, Waltuch T, Gonik NJ, et al. Sleep and breathing the first night after adenotonsillectomy in obese children with obstructive sleep apnea. *J Clin Sleep Med.* 2017;13(06):805–811. https://doi.org/10.5664/jcsm.6620.

38. Allen DZ, Worobetz N, Lukens J, et al. Outcomes intensive care unit placement following pediatric adenotonsillectomy. *Int J Pediatr Otorhinolaryngol.* 2020;129:109736. https://doi.org/10.1016/j.ijporl.2019.109736.

39. Cheong RCT, Bowles P, Moore A, Watts S. Peri-operative management of high-risk paediatric adenotonsillectomy patients: A survey of 35 UK tertiary referral centres. *Int J Pediatr Otorhinolaryngol.* 2017;96:28–34. https://doi.org/10.1016/j.ijporl.2017.03.001.

40. Lavin JM, Smith C, Harris ZL, Thompson DM. Critical care resources utilized in high-risk adenotonsillectomy patients. *Laryngoscope.* 2019;129(5):1229–1234. https://doi.org/10.1002/lary.27623.

41. Levi E, Alvo A, Anderson BJ, Mahadevan M. Postoperative admission to paediatric intensive care after tonsillectomy. *SAGE Open Med.* 2020;8 https://doi.org/10.1177/2050312120922027. 2050312120922027.

42. Vandjelovic ND, Briddell JW, Crippen MM, Schmidt RJ. Evaluating pediatric intensive care unit utilization after tonsillectomy. *Int J Pediatr Otorhinolaryngol.* 2020;128:109693. https://doi.org/10.1016/j.ijporl.2019.109693.

43. Wiet GJ, Bower C, Seibert R, Griebel M. Surgical correction of obstructive sleep apnea in the complicated pediatric patient documented by polysomnography. *Int J Pediatr Otorhinolaryngol.* 1997;41(2):133–143. https://doi.org/10.1016/S0165-5876(97)00065-7.

44. Kerschner JE, Lynch JB, Kleiner H, Flanary VA, Rice TB. Uvulopalatopharyngoplasty with tonsillectomy and adenoidectomy as a treatment for obstructive sleep apnea in neurologically impaired children. *Int J Pediatr Otorhinolaryngol.* 2002;62(3):229–235. https://doi.org/10.1016/S0165-5876(01)00623-1.

45. Jacobs JN, Gray RF, Todd NW. Upper airway obstruction in children with down syndrome. *Arch Otolaryngol Head Neck Surg.* 1996;122(9):945–950. https://doi.org/10.1001/archotol.1996.01890210025007.

46. Kosko JR, Derkay CS. Uvulopalatopharyngoplasty: Treatment of obstructive sleep apnea in neurologically impaired pediatric patients. *Int J Pediatr Otorhinolaryngol.* 1995;32(3):241–246. https://doi.org/10.1016/0165-5876(95)01178-E.

47. Lin SY, Halbower AC, Tunkel DE, Vanderkolk C. Relief of upper airway obstruction with mandibular distraction surgery: Long-term quantitative results in young children. *Arch Otolaryngol Head Neck Surg.* 2006;132(4):437–441. https://doi.org/10.1001/archotol.132.4.437.

48. Wittenborn W, Panchal J, Marsh JL, Sekar KC, Gurley J. Neonatal distraction surgery for micrognathia reduces obstructive apnea and the need for tracheotomy. *J Craniofac Surg.* 2004;15(4):623–630. https://doi.org/10.1097/00001665-200407000-00018.

49. Scott AR, Tibesar RJ, Lander TA, Sampson DE, Sidman JD. Mandibular distraction osteogenesis in infants younger than 3

months. *Arch Facial Plast Surg*. 2011;13(3):173–179. https://doi.org/10.1001/archfacial.2010.114.

50. Hammoudeh J, Bindingnavele VK, Davis B, et al. Neonatal and infant mandibular distraction as an alternative to tracheostomy in severe obstructive sleep apnea. *Cleft Palate Craniofac J*. 2012;49(1):32–38. https://doi.org/10.1597/10-069.

51. Rachmiel A, Srouji S, Emodi O, Aizenbud D. Distraction osteogenesis for tracheostomy dependent children with severe micrognathia. *J Craniofac Surg*. 2012;23(2):459–463. https://doi.org/10.1097/SCS.0b013e3182413db8.

52. Williams JK, Maull D, Grayson BH, Longaker MT, McCarthy JG. Early decannulation with bilateral mandibular distraction for tracheostomy-dependent patients. *Plast Reconstr Surg*. 1999;103(1):48–57. https://doi.org/10.1097/00006534-19990 1000-00009.

53. Noller MW, Guilleminault C, Gouveia CJ, et al. Mandibular advancement for pediatric obstructive sleep apnea: A systematic review and meta-analysis. *J Cranio-Maxillofacial Surg*. 2018;46(8):1296–1302. https://doi.org/10.1016/j.jcms.2018.04.027.

54. Ehsan Z, Weaver KN, Pan BS, Huang G, Hossain MM, Simakajornboon N. Sleep outcomes in neonates with pierre robin sequence undergoing external mandibular distraction: A longitudinal analysis. *Plast Reconstr Surg*. 2020;146(5):1103–1115. https://doi.org/10.1097/PRS.0000000000007289.

55. Verlinden CRA, Van De Vijfeijken SECM, Tuinzing DB, Jansma EP, Becking AG, Swennen GRJ. Complications of mandibular distraction osteogenesis for developmental deformities: A systematic review of the literature. *Int J Oral Maxillofac Surg*. 2015;44(1):44–49. https://doi.org/10.1016/j.ijom.2014.09.007.

56. Villa MP, Rizzoli A, Miano S, Malagola C. Efficacy of rapid maxillary expansion in children with obstructive sleep apnea syndrome: 36 months of follow-up. *Sleep Breath*. 2011;15(2):179–184. https://doi.org/10.1007/s11325-011-0505-1.

57. Monini S, Malagola C, Villa MP, et al. Rapid maxillary expansion for the treatment of nasal obstruction in children younger than 12 years. *Arch Otolaryngol Head Neck Surg*. 2009;135(1):22–27. https://doi.org/10.1001/archoto.2008.521.

58. Villa MP, Malagola C, Pagani J, et al. Rapid maxillary expansion in children with obstructive sleep apnea syndrome: 12-month follow-up. *Sleep Med*. 2007;8(2):128–134. https://doi.org/10.1016/j.sleep.2006.06.009.

59. Villa MP, Rizzoli A, Rabasco J, et al. Rapid maxillary expansion outcomes in treatment of obstructive sleep apnea in children. *Sleep Med*. 2015;16(6):709–716. https://doi.org/10.1016/j.sleep.2014.11.019.

60. Camacho M, Chang ET, Song SA, et al. Rapid maxillary expansion for pediatric obstructive sleep apnea: A systematic review and meta-analysis. *Laryngoscope*. 2017;127(7):1712–1719. https://doi.org/10.1002/lary.26352.

61. Buccheri A, Chinè F, Fratto G, Manzon L. Rapid maxillary expansion in obstructive sleep apnea in young patients: Cardio-respiratory monitoring. *J Clin Pediatr Dent*. 2017;41(4):312–316. https://doi.org/10.17796/1053-4628-41.4.312.

62. Strollo PJ, Soose RJ, Maurer JT, et al. Upper-airway stimulation for obstructive sleep apnea. *N Engl J Med*. 2014;370(2):139–149. https://doi.org/10.1056/nejmoa1308659.

63. Kent DT, Carden KA, Wang L, Lindsell CJ, Ishman SL. Evaluation of hypoglossal nerve stimulation treatment in obstructive sleep apnea. *JAMA Otolaryngol Head Neck Surg*. 2019;145(11):1044–1052. https://doi.org/10.1001/jamaoto.2019.2723.

64. Diercks GR, Keamy D, Kinane TB, et al. Hypoglossal nerve stimulator implantation in an adolescent with down syndrome and sleep apnea. *Pediatrics*. 2016;137(5): https://doi.org/10.1542/peds.2015-3663. e20153663–e20153663.

65. Caloway CL, Diercks GR, Keamy D, et al. Update on hypoglossal nerve stimulation in children with down syndrome and obstructive sleep apnea. *Laryngoscope*. 2020;130(4): E263–E267. https://doi.org/10.1002/lary.28138.

66. Mitchell RB. Adenotonsillectomy for obstructive sleep apnea in children: Outcome evaluated by pre- and postoperative polysomnography. *Laryngoscope*. 2007;117(10):1844–1854. https://doi.org/10.1097/MLG.0b013e318123ee56.

67. Tauman R, Gulliver TE, Krishna J, et al. Persistence of obstructive sleep apnea syndrome in children after adenotonsillectomy. *J Pediatr*. 2006;149(6):803–808. https://doi.org/10.1016/j.jpeds.2006.08.067.

68. Capdevila OS, Kheirandish-Gozal L, Dayyat E, Gozal D. Pediatric obstructive sleep apnea: Complications, management, and long-term outcomes. *Proc Am Thorac Soc*. 2008;5(2):274–282. https://doi.org/10.1513/pats.200708-138MG.

69. Khaytin I, Tapia IE, Xanthopoulos MS, et al. Auto-titrating CPAP for the treatment of obstructive sleep apnea in children. *J Clin Sleep Med*. 2020;16(6):871–878. https://doi.org/10.5664/jcsm.8348.

70. Marshall MJ, Bucks RS, Hogan AM, et al. Auto-adjusting positive airway pressure in children with sickle cell anemia: Results of a phase I randomized controlled trial. *Haematologica*. 2009;94(7):1006–1010. https://doi.org/10.3324/haematol.2008.005215.

71. Palombini L, Pelayo R, Guilleminault C. Efficacy of automated continuous positive airway pressure in children with sleep-related breathing disorders in an attended setting. *Pediatrics*. 2004;113(5):e412–e417. https://doi.org/10.1542/peds.113.5.e412.

72. Kushida CA, Chediak A, Berry RB, et al. Clinical guidelines for the manual titration of positive airway pressure in patients with obstructive sleep apnea. *J Clin Sleep Med*. 2008;4(2):157–171. https://doi.org/10.5664/jcsm.27133.

73. Marcus CL, Rosen G, Ward SLD, et al. Adherence to and effectiveness of positive airway pressure therapy in children with obstructive sleep apnea. *Pediatrics*. 2006;117(3):e442–e451. https://doi.org/10.1542/peds.2005-1634.

74. Roberts SD, Kapadia H, Greenlee G, Chen ML. Midfacial and dental changes associated with nasal positive airway pressure in children with obstructive sleep apnea and craniofacial conditions. *J Clin Sleep Med*. 2016;12(4):469–475. https://doi.org/10.5664/jcsm.5668.

75. Waters K. Interventions in the paediatric sleep laboratory: The use and titration of respiratory support therapies. *Paediatr Respir Rev*. 2008;9(3):181–191. https://doi.org/10.1016/j.prrv.2008.01.003.

76. Evans C, Hensley R, Waters K. *Interventions in the pediatric sleep laboratory. Fundamentals of Sleep Technology*. 2nd ed. Wolters Kluwer; 2012.

77. Jain SS, Dhand R. Perioperative treatment of patients with obstructive sleep apnea. *Curr Opin Pulm Med*. 2004;10(6):482–488. https://doi.org/10.1097/01.mcp.0000143968.41702.f0.

78. Rosen GM, Muckle RP, Mahowald MW, Goding GS, Ullevig C. Postoperative respiratory compromise in children with obstructive sleep apnea syndrome: Can it be

anticipated? *Pediatrics.* 1994;93(5):784–788. https://doi.org/10.1097/00132586-199502000-00061.

79. Mutter TC, Chateau D, Moffatt M, Ramsey C, Roos LL, Kryger M. A matched cohort study of postoperative outcomes in obstructive sleep apnea: Could preoperative diagnosis and treatment prevent complications? *Anesthesiology.* 2014;121(4):707–718. https://doi.org/10.1097/ALN.0000000000000407.

80. Mehta Y, Manikappa S, Juneja R, Trehan N. Obstructive sleep apnea syndrome: Anesthetic implications in the cardiac surgical patient. *J Cardiothorac Vasc Anesth.* 2000;14(4):449–453. https://doi.org/10.1053/jcan.2000.7948.

81. O'Donnell AR, Bjornson CL, Bohn SG, Kirk VG. Compliance rates in children using noninvasive continuous positive airway pressure. *Sleep.* 2006;29(5):651–658. https://doi.org/10.1093/sleep/29.5.651.

82. Koontz KL, Slifer KJ, Cataldo MD, Marcus CL. Improving pediatric compliance with positive airway pressure therapy: The impact of behavioral intervention. *Sleep.* 2003;26(8):1010–1015. https://doi.org/10.1093/sleep/26.8.1010.

83. Uong EC, Epperson M, Bathon SA, Jeffe DB. Adherence to nasal positive airway pressure therapy among school-aged children and adolescents with obstructive sleep apnea syndrome. *Pediatrics.* 2007;120(5):e1203–e1211. https://doi.org/10.1542/peds.2006-2731.

84. Nixon GM, Mihai R, Verginis N, Davey MJ. Patterns of continuous positive airway pressure adherence during the first 3 months of treatment in children. *J Pediatr.* 2011;159(5):802–807. https://doi.org/10.1016/j.jpeds.2011.04.013.

85. DiFeo N, Meltzer LJ, Beck SE, et al. Predictors of positive airway pressure therapy adherence in children: A prospective study. *J Clin Sleep Med.* 2012;8(3):279–286. https://doi.org/10.5664/jcsm.1914.

86. Simon SL, Duncan CL, Janicke DM, Wagner MH. Barriers to treatment of paediatric obstructive sleep apnoea: Development of the adherence barriers to continuous positive airway pressure (CPAP) questionnaire. *Sleep Med.* 2012;13(2):172–177. https://doi.org/10.1016/j.sleep.2011.10.026.

87. Marcus CL, Beck SE, Traylor J, et al. Randomized, double-blind clinical trial of two different modes of positive airway pressure therapy on adherence and efficacy in children. *J Clin Sleep Med.* 2012;8(1):37–42. https://doi.org/10.5664/jcsm.1656.

88. Aljadeff G, Gozal D, Bailey-Wahl SL, Burrell B, Keens TG, Ward SLD. Effects of overnight supplemental oxygen in obstructive sleep apnea in children. *Am J Respir Crit Care Med.* 1996;153(1):51–55. https://doi.org/10.1164/ajrccm.153.1.8542162.

89. Brockbank J, Leon-Astudillo C, Che D, et al. Supplemental oxygen for treatment of infants with obstructive sleep apnea. *J Clin Sleep Med.* 2019;15(8):1115–1123. https://doi.org/10.5664/jcsm.7802.

90. Amaddeo A, Khirani S, Frapin A, Teng T, Griffon L, Fauroux B. High-flow nasal cannula for children not compliant with continuous positive airway pressure. *Sleep Med.* 2019;63:24–28. https://doi.org/10.1016/j.sleep.2019.05.012.

91. Joseph L, Goldberg S, Shitrit M, Picard E. High-flow nasal cannula therapy for obstructive sleep apnea in children. *J Clin Sleep Med.* 2015;11(9):1007–1010. https://doi.org/10.5664/jcsm.5014.

92. Hawkins S, Huston S, Campbell K, Halbower A. High-Flow, Heated, Humidified Air Via Nasal Cannula Treats CPAP-Intolerant Children With Obstructive Sleep Apnea. *J Clin Sleep Med.* 2017 Aug 15;13(8):981–989. http://doi: 10.5664/jcsm.6700. PMID: 28728621; PMCID: PMC5529135.

93. Hegde S, Prodhan P. Serious air leak syndrome complicating high-flow nasal cannula therapy: A report of 3 cases. *Pediatrics.* 2013;131(3):e939–e944. https://doi.org/10.1542/peds.2011-3767.

94. Hough JL, Pham TMT, Schibler A. Physiologic effect of high-flow nasal cannula in infants with bronchiolitis. *Pediatr Crit Care Med.* 2014;15(5):e214–e219. https://doi.org/10.1097/PCC.0000000000000112.

95. Brouillette RT, Manoukian JJ, Ducharme FM, et al. Efficacy of fluticasone nasal spray for pediatric obstructive sleep apnea. *J Pediatr.* 2001;138(6):838–844. https://doi.org/10.1067/mpd.2001.114474.

96. Alexopoulos EI, Kaditis AG, Kalampouka E, et al. Nasal corticosteroids for children with snoring. *Pediatr Pulmonol.* 2004;38(2):161–167. https://doi.org/10.1002/ppul.20079.

97. Kheirandish-Gozal L, Gozal D. Intranasal budesonide treatment for children with mild obstructive sleep apnea syndrome. *Pediatrics.* 2008;122(1):e149–e155. https://doi.org/10.1542/peds.2007-3398.

98. Goldbart AD, Greenberg-Dotan S, Tal A. Montelukast for children with obstructive sleep apnea: A double-blind, placebo-controlled study. *Pediatrics.* 2012;130(3):e575–e580. https://doi.org/10.1542/peds.2012-0310.

99. Kheirandish-Gozal L, Bandla HPR, Gozal D. Montelukast for children with obstructive sleep apnea: Results of a double-blind, randomized, placebo-controlled trial. *Ann Am Thorac Soc.* 2016;13(10):1736–1741. https://doi.org/10.1513/AnnalsATS.201606-432OC.

100. Kheirandish-Gozal L, Bhattacharjee R, Bandla HPR, Gozal D. Antiinflammatory therapy outcomes for mild OSA in children. *Chest.* 2014;146(1):88–95. https://doi.org/10.1378/chest.13-2288.

101. Liming BJ, Ryan M, Mack D, Ahmad I, Camacho M. Montelukast and nasal corticosteroids to treat pediatric obstructive sleep apnea: A systematic review and meta-analysis. *Otolaryngol Head Neck Surg (United States).* 2019;160(4):594–602. https://doi.org/10.1177/0194599818815683.

102. Kheirandish L, Goldbart AD, Gozal D. Intranasal steroids and oral leukotriene modifier therapy in residual sleep-disordered breathing after tonsillectomy and adenoidectomy in children. *Pediatrics.* 2006;117(1):e61–e66. https://doi.org/10.1542/peds.2005-0795.

103. Demirhan H, Aksoy F, Özturan O, Yildirim YS, Veyseller B. Medical treatment of adenoid hypertrophy with "fluticasone propionate nasal drops." *Int J Pediatr Otorhinolaryngol.* 2010;74(7):773–776. https://doi.org/10.1016/j.ijporl.2010.03.051.

104. Goldbart AD, Veling MC, Goldman JL, Li RC, Brittian KR, Gozal D. Glucocorticoid receptor subunit expression in adenotonsillar tissue of children with obstructive sleep apnea. *Pediatr Res.* 2005;57(2):232–236. https://doi.org/10.1203/01.PDR.0000150722.34561.E6.

105. Goldbart AD, Goldman JL, Li RC, Brittian KR, Tauman R, Gozal D. Differential expression of cysteinyl leukotriene receptors 1 and 2 in tonsils of children with obstructive sleep apnea syndrome or recurrent infection. *Chest.* 2004;126(1):13–18. https://doi.org/10.1378/chest.126.1.13.

106. Kaditis AG, Ioannou MG, Chaidas K, et al. Cysteinyl leukotriene receptors are expressed by tonsillar T cells of children with obstructive sleep apnea. *Chest.* 2008;134(2):324–331. https://doi.org/10.1378/chest.07-2746.

107. Kheirandish-Gozal L, Serpero LD, Dayyat E, et al. Corticosteroids suppress in vitro tonsillar proliferation in children with obstructive sleep apnoea. *Eur Respir J.* 2009;33(5):1077–1084. https://doi.org/10.1183/09031936.00130608.

108. Esteitie R, Emani J, Sharma S, Suskind DL, Baroody FM. Effect of fluticasone furoate on interleukin 6 secretion from adenoid tissues in children with obstructive sleep apnea. *Arch Otolaryngol Head Neck Surg.* 2011;137(6):576–582. https://doi.org/10.1001/archoto.2011.86.

109. Dayyat E, Serpero LD, Kheirandish-Gozal L, et al. Leukotriene pathways and in vitro adenotonsillar cell proliferation in children with obstructive sleep apnea. *Chest.* 2009;135(5):1142–1149. https://doi.org/10.1378/chest.08-2102.

110. Villa MP, Bernkopf E, Pagani J, Broia V, Montesano M, Ronchetti R. Randomized controlled study of an oral jaw-positioning appliance for the treatment of obstructive sleep apnea in children with malocclusion. *Am J Respir Crit Care Med.* 2002;165(1):123–127. https://doi.org/10.1164/ajrccm.165.1.2011031.

111. Modesti-Vedolin G, Chies C, Chaves-Fagondes S, Piza-Pelizzer E, Lima-Grossi M. Efficacy of a mandibular advancement intraoral appliance (MOA) for the treatment of obstructive sleep apnea syndrome (OSAS) in pediatric patients: A pilot-study. *Med Oral Patol Oral y Cir Bucal.* 2018;23(6):e656–e663. https://doi.org/10.4317/medoral.22580.

112. de Almeida FR, Lowe AA, Tsuiki S, et al. Long-term compliance and side effects of oral appliances used for the treatment of snoring and obstructive sleep apnea syndrome. *J Clin Sleep Med.* 2005;1(2):143–152. https://doi.org/10.5664/jcsm.8978.

113. Ramar K, Dort LC, Katz SG, et al. Clinical practice guideline for the treatment of obstructive sleep apnea and snoring with oral appliance therapy: An update for 2015. *J Clin Sleep Med.* 2015;11(7):773–828. https://doi.org/10.5664/jcsm.4858.

114. Carvalho FR, Lentini-Oliveira DA, Prado LBF, Prado GF, Carvalho LBC. Oral appliances and functional orthopaedic appliances for obstructive sleep apnoea in children. *Cochrane Database Syst Rev.* 2016;2016(10). https://doi.org/10.1002/14651858.CD005520.pub3.

115. Verhulst SL, Franckx H, Van Gaal L, De Backer W, Desager K. The effect of weight loss on sleep-disordered breathing in obese teenagers. *Obesity.* 2009;17(6):1178–1183. https://doi.org/10.1038/oby.2008.673.

116. Tuomilehto HPI, Seppä JM, Partinen MM, et al. Lifestyle intervention with weight reduction: First-line treatment in mild obstructive sleep apnea. *Am J Respir Crit Care Med.* 2009;179(4):320–327. https://doi.org/10.1164/rccm.200805-669OC.

117. Kalra M, Inge T, Garcia V, et al. Obstructive sleep apnea in extremely overweight adolescents undergoing bariatric surgery. *Obes Res.* 2005;13(7):1175–1179. https://doi.org/10.1038/oby.2005.139.

118. Amin R, Simakajornboon N, Szczesniak R, Inge T. Early improvement in obstructive sleep apnea and increase in orexin levels after bariatric surgery in adolescents and young adults. *Surg Obes Relat Dis.* 2017;13(1):95–100. https://doi.org/10.1016/j.soard.2016.05.023.

119. Holterman AX, Browne A, Dillard BE, et al. Short-term outcome in the first 10 morbidly obese adolescent patients in the FDA-approved trial for laparoscopic adjustable gastric banding. *J Pediatr Gastroenterol Nutr.* 2007;45(4):465–473. https://doi.org/10.1097/MPG.0b013e318063eef6.

120. Alqahtani AR, Antonisamy B, Alamri H, Elahmedi M, Zimmerman VA. Laparoscopic sleeve gastrectomy in 108 obese children and adolescents aged 5 to 21 years. *Ann Surg.* 2012;256(2):266–273. https://doi.org/10.1097/SLA.0b013e318251e92b.

121. Greenburg DL, Lettieri CJ, Eliasson AH. Effects of surgical weight loss on measures of obstructive sleep apnea: A meta-analysis. *Am J Med.* 2009;122(6):535–542. https://doi.org/10.1016/j.amjmed.2008.10.037.

122. Lettieri CJ, Eliasson AH, Greenburg DL. Persistence of obstructive sleep apnea after surgical weight loss. *J Clin Sleep Med.* 2008;4(4):333–338. https://doi.org/10.5664/jcsm.27233.

123. Pratt JSA, Browne A, Browne NT, et al. ASMBS pediatric metabolic and bariatric surgery guidelines, 2018. *Surg Obes Relat Dis.* 2018;14(7):882–901. https://doi.org/10.1016/j.soard.2018.03.019.

124. Chervin RD, Ellenberg SS, Hou X, et al. Prognosis for spontaneous resolution of OSA in children. *Chest.* 2015;148(5):1204–1213. https://doi.org/10.1378/chest.14-2873.

125. Fehrm J, Nerfeldt P, Browaldh N, Friberg D. Effectiveness of adenotonsillectomy vs watchful waiting in young children with mild to moderate obstructive sleep apnea: A randomized clinical trial. *JAMA Otolaryngol Head Neck Surg.* 2020;146(7):647–654. https://doi.org/10.1001/jamaoto.2020.0869.

126. Scheffler P, Wolter NE, Narang I, et al. Surgery for obstructive sleep apnea in obese children: Literature review and meta-analysis. *Otolaryngol Head Neck Surg (United States).* 2019;160(6):985–992. https://doi.org/10.1177/0194599819829415.

127. Bull MJ, Committee on Genetics. Health supervision for children with Down syndrome. *Pediatrics.* 2011;128(2):393–406. https://doi.org/10.1542/peds.2011-1605.

128. Lee C-F, Lee C-H, Hsueh W-Y, Lin M-T, Kang K-T. Prevalence of obstructive sleep apnea in children with Down syndrome: A meta-analysis. *J Clin Sleep Med.* 2018;14(5):867–875. https://doi.org/10.5664/jcsm.7126.

129. Chamseddin BH, Johnson RF, Mitchell RB. Obstructive sleep apnea in children with Down Syndrome: Demographic, clinical, and polysomnographic features. *Otolaryngol Neck Surg.* 2019;160(1):150–157. https://doi.org/10.1177/0194599818797308.

130. Lal C, White DR, Joseph JE, van Bakergem K, LaRosa A. sleep-disordered breathing in Down syndrome. *Chest J.* 2015;147(2):570. https://doi.org/10.1378/chest.14-0266.

131. Ong AA, Atwood CM, Nguyen SA, et al. Down syndrome and pediatric obstructive sleep apnea surgery: A national cohort. *Laryngoscope.* 2018;128(8):1963–1969. https://doi.org/10.1002/lary.27063.

132. Farhood Z, Isley JW, Ong AA, et al. Adenotonsillectomy outcomes in patients with Down syndrome and obstructive sleep apnea. *Laryngoscope.* 2017;127(6):1465–1470. https://doi.org/10.1002/lary.26398.

133. Best J, Mutchnick S, Ida J, Billings KR. Trends in management of obstructive sleep apnea in pediatric patients with Down syndrome. *Int J Pediatr Otorhinolaryngol.* 2018;110:1–5. https://doi.org/10.1016/j.ijporl.2018.04.008.

134. Nation J, Brigger M. The efficacy of adenotonsillectomy for obstructive sleep apnea in children with Down syndrome: A systematic review. *Otolaryngol Head Neck Surg.* 2017;157(3):401–408. https://doi.org/10.1177/0194599817703921.

135. Sedaghat AR, Flax-Goldenberg RB, Gayler BW, Capone GT, Ishman SL. A case-control comparison of lingual tonsillar size in children with and without down syndrome. *Laryngoscope.* 2012;122(5):1165–1169. https://doi.org/10.1002/lary.22346.

136. Guimaraes CVA, Donnelly LF, Shott SR, Amin RS, Kalra M. Relative rather than absolute macroglossia in patients with Down syndrome: Implications for treatment of obstructive sleep apnea. *Pediatr Radiol.* 2008;38(10):1062–1067. https://doi.org/10.1007/s00247-008-0941-7.

137. Maris M, Verhulst S, Saldien V, Van de Heyning P, Wojciechowski M, Boudewyns A. Drug-induced sedation endoscopy in surgically naive children with Down syndrome and obstructive sleep apnea. *Sleep Med.* 2016;24:63–70. https://doi.org/10.1016/j.sleep.2016.06.018.

138. Nehme Bsc J, Laberge R, Pothos M, et al. Treatment and persistence/recurrence of sleep-disordered breathing in children with Down syndrome. *Pediatr Pulmonol.* 2019;54:1291–1296. https://doi.org/10.1002/ppul.24380.

139. Dudoignon B, Amaddeo A, Frapin A, et al. Obstructive sleep apnea in Down syndrome: Benefits of surgery and noninvasive respiratory support. *Am J Med Genet A.* 2017;173(8):2074–2080. https://doi.org/10.1002/ajmg.a.38283.

140. Rosen D. Severe hypothyroidism presenting as obstructive sleep apnea. *Clin Pediatr (Phila).* 2010;49(4):381–383. https://doi.org/10.1177/0009922809351093.

141. Yu W, Sarber KM, Howard JJM, et al. Children with down syndrome and mild OSA: Treatment with medication versus observation. *J Clin Sleep Med.* 2020;16(6):899–906. https://doi.org/10.5664/jcsm.8358.

142. Sedky K, Bennett DS, Pumariega A. Prader Willi syndrome and obstructive sleep apnea: Co-occurrence in the pediatric population. *J Clin Sleep Med.* 2014;10(4):403–409. https://doi.org/10.5664/jcsm.3616.

143. Meyer SL, Splaingard M, Repaske DR, Zipf W, Atkins J, Jatana K. Outcomes of adenotonsillectomy in patients with Prader-Willi syndrome. *Arch Otolaryngol Head Neck Surg.* 2012;138(11):1047–1051. https://doi.org/10.1001/2013.jamaoto.64.

144. Clements AC, Dai X, Walsh JM, et al. Outcomes of adenotonsillectomy for obstructive sleep apnea in Prader-Willi Syndrome: Systematic review and meta-analysis. *Laryngoscope.* 2021;131(4):898–906. https://doi.org/10.1002/lary.28922.

145. Crockett DJ, Ahmed SR, Sowder DR, Wootten CT, Chinnadurai S, Goudy SL. Velopharyngeal dysfunction in children with Prader-Willi syndrome after adenotonsillectomy. *Int J Pediatr Otorhinolaryngol.* 2014;78(10):1731–1734. https://doi.org/10.1016/j.ijporl.2014.07.034.

146. Duis J, van Wattum PJ, Scheimann A, et al. A multidisciplinary approach to the clinical management of Prader-Willi syndrome. *Mol Genet Genomic Med.* 2019;7(3):e514. https://doi.org/10.1002/mgg3.514.

147. Ramgopal S, Kothare SV, Rana M, Singh K, Khatwa U. Obstructive sleep apnea in infancy: A 7-year experience at a pediatric sleep center. *Pediatr Pulmonol.* 2014;49(6):554–560. https://doi.org/10.1002/ppul.22867.

148. Leonardis RL, Robison JG, Otteson TD. Evaluating the management of obstructive sleep apnea in neonates and infants. *JAMA Otolaryngol Head Neck Surg.* 2013;139(2):139–146. https://doi.org/10.1001/jamaoto.2013.1331.

149. Shatz A. Indications and outcomes of adenoidectomy in infancy. *Ann Otol Rhinol Laryngol.* 2004;113(10):835–838. https://doi.org/10.1177/000348940411301011.

150. Papoff P, Guelfi G, Cicchetti R, et al. Outcomes after tongue-lip adhesion or mandibular distraction osteogenesis in infants with Pierre Robin sequence and severe airway obstruction. *Int J Oral Maxillofac Surg.* 2013;42(11):1418–1423. https://doi.org/10.1016/j.ijom.2013.07.747.

151. Sedaghat AR, Anderson ICW, McGinley BM, Rossberg MI, Redett RJ, Ishman SL. Characterization of obstructive sleep apnea before and after tongue-lip adhesion in children with micrognathia. *Cleft Palate-Craniofacial J.* 2012;49(1):21–26. https://doi.org/10.1597/10-240.

152. Resnick CM, Dentino K, Katz E, Mulliken JB, Padwa BL. Effectiveness of tongue-lip adhesion for obstructive sleep apnea in infants with robin sequence measured by polysomnography. *Cleft Palate-Craniofacial J.* 2016;53(5):584–588. https://doi.org/10.1597/15-058.

153. Viezel-Mathieu A, Safran T, Gilardino MS. A systematic review of the effectiveness of tongue lip adhesion in improving airway obstruction in children with pierre robin sequence. *J Craniofac Surg.* 2016;27(6):143–1456. https://doi.org/10.1097/SCS.0000000000002721.

154. Whitaker IS, Koron S, Oliver DW, Jani P. Effective management of the airway in the Pierre Robin syndrome using a modified nasopharyngeal tube and pulse oximetry. *Br J Oral Maxillofac Surg.* 2003;41(4):272–274. https://doi.org/10.1016/S0266-4356(03)00100-1.

155. Cockerill CC, Frisch CD, Rein SE, Orvidas LJ. Supraglottoplasty outcomes in children with Down syndrome. *Int J Pediatr Otorhinolaryngol.* 2016;87:87–90. https://doi.org/10.1016/j.ijporl.2016.05.022.

156. Landry AM, Thompson DM. Laryngomalacia: Disease presentation, spectrum, and management. *Int J Pediatr.* 2012;2012:753526. https://doi.org/10.1155/2012/753526.

157. B. B, S.R. H, D.M. T, J.W. S. Improvement in polysomnography outcomes after isolated supraglottoplasty in children with Occult Laryngomalacia. *Sleep.* 2016.

158. Bhushan B, Schroeder JW, Billings KR, Giancola N, Thompson DM. Polysomnography outcomes after supraglottoplasty in children with obstructive sleep apnea. *Otolaryngol Head Neck Surg (United States).* 2019;161(4):694–698. https://doi.org/10.1177/0194599819844512.

159. Farhood Z, Ong AA, Nguyen SA, Gillespie MB, Discolo CM, White DR. Objective outcomes of supraglottoplasty for children with laryngomalacia and obstructive sleep apnea ameta-analysis. *JAMA Otolaryngol Head Neck Surg.* 2016;142(7):665–671. https://doi.org/10.1001/jamaoto.2016.0830.

160. Shepherd KL, James AL, Musk AW, Hunter ML, Hillman DR, Eastwood PR. Gastro-oesophageal reflux symptoms are related to the presence and severity of obstructive sleep apnoea. *J Sleep Res.* 2011;20(1 Pt 2):241–249. https://doi.org/10.1111/j.1365-2869.2010.00843.x.

161. Giannoni C, Sulek M, Friedman EM, Duncan III NO. Gastroesophageal reflux association with laryngomalacia: A prospective study. *Int J Pediatr Otorhinolaryngol.* 1998;43(1):11–20. https://doi.org/10.1016/s0165-5876(97)00151-1.

35

The Otolaryngologist Approach to Obstructive Sleep Apnea

Laura Petrauskas and Fuad M. Baroody

CHAPTER HIGHLIGHTS

- Sleep disordered breathing and obstructive sleep apnea are common occurrences in the pediatric age group and can lead to significant physiologic and behavioral/cognitive sequalae.
- Sleep questionnaires are useful in identifying patients with sleep disordered breathing.
- Polysomnography is the gold standard in the diagnosis of obstructive sleep apnea.
- Although adenotonsillectomy leads to improvement in sleep disordered breathing, many children will have residual disease after surgery.

Introduction

Sleep-disordered breathing (SDB) is a relatively common problem in childhood and is a spectrum of severity ranging from primary snoring to hypoventilation and obstructive sleep apnea (OSA). The prevalence of primary snoring in children is around 10%, and the prevalence of OSA ranges from 1% to 4%.[1] Adenotonsillar hypertrophy is a common underlying problem and adenotonsillectomy is considered the first step in the surgical management of children with OSA. Thus, the otolaryngologist plays a significant role in the diagnosis and management of children with SDB. This chapter will attempt to discuss the approach used by most otolaryngologists in treating this problem.

History

Nighttime Symptoms

Snoring is an almost universal symptom in children with OSA. Observers will describe mouth breathing, and pauses or interruptions in breathing regularity followed by a deep catch-up breath. Choking and awakenings are common and so is enuresis. Children sleep in unusual positions such as half sitting with pillows to support them as well as with neck hyperextension, which improves airway patency. The sleep is restless with frequent repositioning. Some children

will experience retractions and paradoxical inward rib cage motion but cyanosis is not seen. Many of these symptoms will worsen during upper respiratory tract infections as these are usually associated with adenotonsillar enlargement.

Many children with OSA manifest with enuresis. In a systematic review of articles between 1980 and 2010, Jeyakumar and colleagues studied the incidence of enuresis and resolution after treatment of OSA.[2] In 12 studies involving 3,550 children with SDB, 33% had enuresis. Furthermore, it seems that the chance of having any or frequent enuresis increases significantly with increasing obstructive events as documented by polysomnogram (PSG).[3]

Daytime Symptoms and Sequalae

Daytime symptoms of OSA extend beyond the obstructive realm and are likely related to the negative impact on sleep in affected children. Symptoms related to obstruction include mouth breathing, nasal obstruction, rhinorrhea, and hyponasality. Less commonly, children may have dysphagia. OSA has a negative impact on quality of life (QoL) in children. In a meta-analysis looking at the impact of OSA on QoL using standardized questionnaires, Baldassari and colleagues showed significantly lower (worse QoL) scores in children with OSA compared with healthy children.[4] The impact extended to multiple domains including physical functioning, role limitations-emotional, bodily pain, behavior, general health perceptions, parental impact-emotional, parental impact-time, and family activities. The same analysis showed that children with OSA had similar QoL scores compared with children with juvenile rheumatoid arthritis with the exception of the subscales of parental impact-emotional and parental impact-time, which were worse in children with OSA. There was a significant improvement in QoL when evaluated in the short term (1.6–5.5 months) and the long term (6–16 months) following adenotonsillectomy.

Another manifestation of OSA in children is cognitive dysfunction and behavioral problems. In a review of available studies, behavioral problems described in children with SDB were reduced attention, hyperactivity, increased aggression, irritability, emotional and peer problems, and somatic complaints.[5] Neurocognitive dysfunction manifestations include a generalized reduction in the speed of information processing and diminished capacity in basic neurocognitive skills including memory, immediate recall, visuospatial functions, attention and vigilance, mental flexibility, and intelligence.[5] Several studies suggested an elevated incidence of SDB, ranging from 25–57%, among children and adolescents diagnosed with attention-deficit/hyperactivity disorder (ADHD) symptoms.[6] Sedky and colleagues used meta-analysis to study the relation between ADHD and SDB in children and adolescents.[6] The results suggested that a medium relationship exists between SDB and ADHD symptoms and that a medium improvement is found in ADHD symptoms following adenotonsillectomy. The negative impact of SDB on school performance was demonstrated by a study performed in academically low performing children.[7] A single night recording of pulse oximetry and transcutaneous partial pressure of carbon dioxide and a detailed sleep questionnaire were used to identify children with sleep-associated gas exchange abnormalities. The parents of these children were advised on treatment and almost half of them pursued adenotonsillectomy for those children. School grades were then compared before and after intervention. The only group that had a significant improvement in school grades was the group of children with OSA who underwent adenotonsillectomy. The children with OSA who did not undergo any therapy, and the other two groups of children with primary snoring and no sleep problems also did not achieve any improvement in school grades during the same observation period.

Whereas growth retardation was recognized in children with OSA earlier on,[8,9] it is now unusual to see significant growth retardation in these children, likely due to better and faster diagnosis of OSA. However, this is still observed in correlation with OSA as evidenced by a study of Mediterranean children.[10] When compared with a control cohort, many criteria of growth failure were statistically significantly higher in the children with OSA, and these improved after adenotonsillectomy. Multiple small studies have reported an increase in blood pressure in children with OSA and SDB with a variable relationship to obesity.[11–13] A meta-analysis of five articles focused on the impact of OSA on blood pressure and found that moderate to severe SDB was associated with an 87% higher risk of elevated systolic blood pressure and a 121% higher risk of elevated diastolic blood pressure compared with mild or no SDB.[14] However, the association was not statistically significant and there was a great deal of heterogeneity among the studies. There is consensus among the field that more and larger studies are needed to better elucidate this relationship.

Recurrent hypoxic and hypercapnic episodes in OSA elevate pulmonary vascular resistance and can lead to pulmonary hypertension with subsequent right ventricular remodeling and cor pulmonale. Indeed, around 37% of children with OSA have been shown to have evidence of right ventricular dysfunction.[15,16] There is also some

evidence of left ventricular dysfunction in children with OSA.[17] Furthermore, elevated carbon dioxide from airway obstruction can result in blood flow redistribution in the central nervous system with negative sequalae.

Physical Exam

The physical exam is an important part of the evaluation of children with SDB. Height, weight, and body mass index (BMI) are critical to identify children with obesity, which is an important comorbidity of OSA in many children. Pulse oximetry measurement is not routinely performed in the otolaryngologist's office as most patients are not expected to have desaturations during wakefulness. Although blood pressure measurement is not routinely obtained in an otolaryngology office, it is important to record this parameter in patients with OSA. This is particularly relevant in obese patients. Careful observation of general appearance with specific evaluation of craniofacial structure is essential. Special attention should be paid to midface hypoplasia, retrognathia, micrognathia, and adenoid facies. It is also common to detect high arched palate and excessive vertical growth of the maxilla, a narrow maxillary transverse arch width, and high palatal vault anatomy in children with chronic airway obstruction and mouth breathing. It is also important to help identify syndromic facies (Down syndrome, Treacher Collins, Crouzon, etc.), which might be associated with an increased incidence of OSA. Noisy breathing with open mouth posture and stertor is also important to note and usually warrants a more careful assessment for symptoms of SDB.

The upper airway evaluation is the most relevant in the office. Clearly assessment of tonsillar size is important and is usually classified as 1+ (tonsils barely visible within the tonsillar pillars), 2+ (tonsils seen outside the pillars but not touching the uvula), 3+ (tonsils outside the pillars and touching the uvula), and 4+ (tonsils touching each other in the midline). Relationship of the position of the tongue to the palatal structures, the uvula, and the tonsils has been graded in adults by two classifications. The Mallampati classification was originally described as a guide to facility of intubation and is based on the structures that are able to be viewed in the oropharynx with the patient at rest with the tongue protruded.[18] The classification involves four classes: class I (full visibility of tonsils, uvula, and soft and hard palate), class II (upper part of the tonsils, uvula, and soft and hard palate are visible), class III (base of the uvula and soft and hard palate are visible), class IV (hard palate is only visible structure) (Fig. 35.1). The higher the class, the more the obstruction. Friedman modified the classification and coined the Friedman tongue position classification (FTP), which is performed in natural position with the mouth open and the tongue kept inside the mouth.[19] The FTP also has four classes: FTP I (tonsils, uvula, and soft and hard palate are visible), FTP IIa (upper part of tonsils, uvula, and soft and hard palate visible), FTP IIb (base of uvula and soft and hard palate visible), FTP III (proximal soft palate and hard palate visible but distal soft palate not seen), FTP IV (only hard palate is visible) (Fig. 35.2). A meta-analysis has subsequently shown that both classifications are significantly

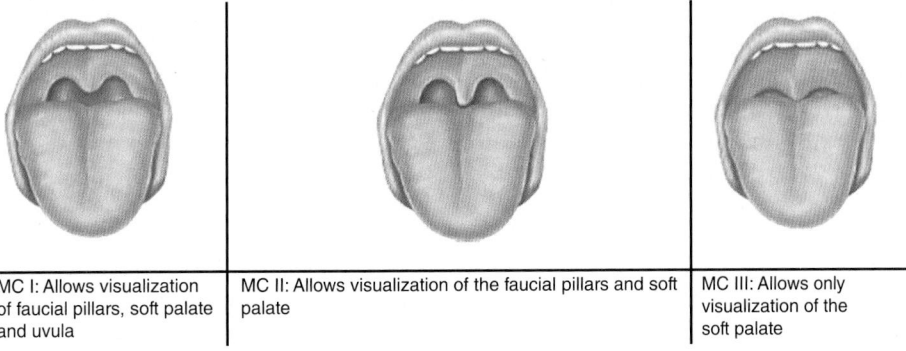

MC I: Allows visualization of faucial pillars, soft palate and uvula

MC II: Allows visualization of the faucial pillars and soft palate

MC III: Allows only visualization of the soft palate

• **Fig. 35.1** Mallampati classification.[20]

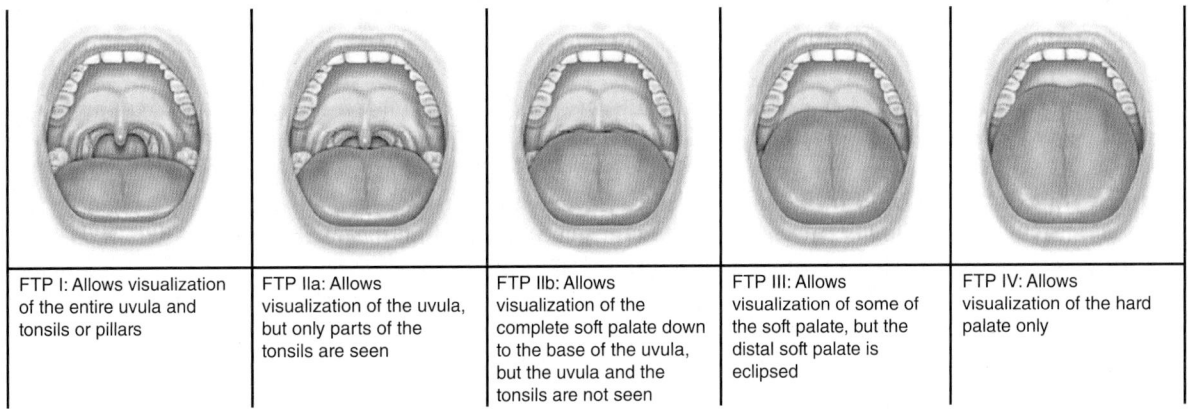

FTP I: Allows visualization of the entire uvula and tonsils or pillars

FTP IIa: Allows visualization of the uvula, but only parts of the tonsils are seen

FTP IIb: Allows visualization of the complete soft palate down to the base of the uvula, but the uvula and the tonsils are not seen

FTP III: Allows visualization of some of the soft palate, but the distal soft palate is eclipsed

FTP IV: Allows visualization of the hard palate only

• **Fig. 35.2** Friedman tongue position classification.[20]

correlated with predicting OSA severity as determined by the apnea-hypopnea index (AHI) with the FTP system yielding a slightly higher correlation with AHI.[20] Although these classifications are studied in adults, they might be useful for older children, especially adolescents. In fact, in a retrospective review of a group of older children, the Mallampati score was shown to be a good predictor of OSA on PSG with the odds ratio of having OSA increasing by more than 6-fold for every point increase in the score.[21]

Assessment of adenoid size is not always necessary as evidence of OSA and large tonsils is often enough reason to move forward with adenotonsillectomy irrespective of adenoid size. It becomes important to assess the adenoids when the main complaints are those of nasal obstruction or if evidence of OSA is present but the tonsils are small. This can be achieved by nasal endoscopy in the office or lateral neck film in the radiology suite. If laryngeal abnormalities are suspected, a full laryngoscopy is performed.

Chest exam is useful and might identify the presence of pectus excavatum, which might suggest chronic airway obstruction. Clearly, general physical exam is important especially in cases of poor motor tone, cerebral palsy, or other neurologic or craniofacial abnormalities that are often associated with OSA.

Sleep Questionnaires

As many children snore but a smaller portion have true OSA that warrants intervention, many questionnaires have

been developed in an attempt to distinguish primary snoring from OSA. The Pediatric Sleep Questionnaire (PSQ) has been shown to be a reliable instrument for identification of OSA in children from 2–18 years. It has a sensitivity of 81–85% and a specificity of 87%.[22] Another questionnaire commonly used by otolaryngologists is the OSA-18, which is a disease-specific QoL questionnaire.[23] This tool was validated against a 90-minute daytime nap sleep study with an overall correlation of the OSA-18 score with respiratory disturbance index (RDI; R = 0.43) found to be statistically and clinically significant.[23] When the predictive value of the OSA-18 was investigated in relation to PSGs in children, it showed poor validity in detecting and predicting pediatric OSA.[24] The analysis suggested that the majority of children with severe OSA would not be correctly diagnosed if the OSA-18 were used as a dominant diagnostic tool. It is, however, a useful tool to evaluate QoL in children with OSA as it includes assessments of emotional symptoms, daytime function, and caregiver concerns.[23] Another tool is the Clinical Assessment Score-15 (CAS-15), which contains 10 history and 5 physical exam items and can be completed in an office visit in 10 minutes.[25] In an attempt to evaluate the generalizability of this tool, a multi-institutional study was performed assessing the reliability of the CAS-15 in predicting PSG-documented OSA.[26] A score ≥32 on the CAS-15 had a sensitivity of 69.0%, a specificity of 63.4%, a positive predictive value of 88.7%, and a negative predictive value of 32.9% in predicting positive PSG.[26] In a recent meta-analysis of the diagnostic accuracy of screening questionnaires for OSA in children, Parenti and colleagues evaluated 13 studies and concluded that PSQ had higher sensitivity (0.76) than OSA-18 (0.56), whereas OSA-18 exhibited higher specificity (0.73) than PSQ (0.43).[27] It is clear from the above that more refinement of these tools is required to help better predict results of PSGs.

Polysomnography

PSG is the gold standard for the detection of OSA and is best performed in a pediatric sleep laboratory with technical staff trained to work with children. It involves monitoring several variables that allow quantitation of airway obstruction and accompanying hypoxemia. Details pertaining to the actual test are found elsewhere in this book. In a survey of practice patterns among otolaryngologists, 90% of children in the United States are treated for SDB based on clinical assessment without a PSG.[28] We also know that clinical history, physical exam, and questionnaires do not necessarily always predict a positive PSG. Based on these facts and considering the ease of performance of PSG across the country, there are slightly different recommendations related to the performance of a PSG in a child with SDB. The 2012 American Academy of Pediatrics Clinical Practice Guidelines recommend that PSG be obtained prior to adenotonsillectomy to differentiate OSA from primary snoring.[29] The clinical practice guideline from the American Academy of Otolaryngology-Head and Neck Surgery differs.[30] It recommends a PSG prior to adenotonsillectomy in the child suspected of having SDB if they are <2 years of age, or if they exhibit any of the following: obesity, Down syndrome, craniofacial abnormalities, neuromuscular disorders, sickle cell disease, or mucopolysaccharidoses.[30] Furthermore, a PSG is recommended in children without any of the previously listed comorbidities whenever the need for tonsillectomy is uncertain or when there is discordance between the physical exam and the reported severity of obstructive SDB.[30] Even with the less restrictive American Academy of Otolaryngology-Head and Neck Surgery Guidelines, adherence is pretty low (20%) and the most consistent predictor of obtaining a PSG prior to adenotonsillectomy is being young (1–3 years).[31] Most experts agree on the following determination of severity of OSA based on the AHI, which represents the number of obstructive events per hour of sleep as follows: AHI <1 is considered a normal PSG with no evidence of OSA, AHI between 1 and 5 events an hour is mild OSA, between 5 and 10 events per hour is moderate, and AHI >10 events per hour is severe OSA.

Medical Therapy for Obstructive Sleep Apnea in Children

The most commonly used therapies that have evidence-based support in the literature for the treatment of OSA in children are leukotriene modifiers (montelukast is the most commonly studied) and intranasal steroids. The

earliest data are from a randomized placebo-controlled parallel study using intranasal fluticasone propionate for 6 weeks in a small number of children with OSA.[32] They showed a significant reduction in the AHI from 10.7 to 5.8 in the fluticasone group compared with a change from 10.9 to 13.1 in the placebo group. Another small placebo-controlled parallel study with mometasone furoate used for 4 months in children with OSA showed a significant reduction of obstructive AHI (2.7–1.7) in the active group compared with placebo, which showed an increase in obstructive AHI (2.5–2.9).[33] Kheirandish-Gozal and Gozal completed a double-blind, randomized, placebo-controlled, crossover trial in children with OSA.[34] They treated the children with intranasal budesonide or placebo for 6 weeks, then allowed a 2-week washout followed by crossover therapy with the other spray for another 6 weeks. There was a significant decrease in obstructive AHI (3.7–1.3) in the children who received budesonide for 6 weeks compared with the placebo-treated children who had an increase in their obstructive AHI (2.9–4.0). More importantly, in the children initially treated with budesonide, sleep apnea remained controlled as evidenced by the PSG obtained 8 weeks after cessation of active therapy.

A systematic review and meta-analysis evaluating the benefit of either montelukast or the combination of montelukast and intranasal steroids identified six articles that met inclusion criteria.[35] Of these, five studies involving 166 children evaluated montelukast alone and found a 55% improvement in the AHI from 6.2 to 2.8 events per hour. One of the five studies did not show a significant reduction of AHI with montelukast.[36] Of note, the duration of montelukast therapy in these studies was between 12 and 16 weeks. Two studies with 502 children evaluated the effects of montelukast with intranasal corticosteroids on pediatric OSA and found a 70% improvement in AHI from 4.7 to 1.4 events per hour. One of these studies with the largest number of children involved a retrospective design.[37]

Based on the previously mentioned data, it is reasonable to offer medical therapy as an option for patients with mild OSA without significant sequalae; however, several considerations come to mind. It is important to note that none of these medications are approved by the U.S. Food and Drug Administration (FDA) for OSA. Furthermore, a few years back, the FDA issued a black box warning for montelukast in relation to neuropsychiatric events that range from agitation, sleep disturbances, anxiousness, and depression to suicidal events.[38] It is therefore very important to discuss these potential side effects with the parents before initiating therapy. The other concern that parents often bring up is duration of therapy. It is reasonable, based on the data available, to treat children for 12 weeks with either montelukast or intranasal steroids or the combination. If there is no benefit perceived, an adenotonsillectomy should be pursued. If the parents perceive benefit, continuing these agents seems reasonable. It is hard to determine length of therapy as a natural course related to resolution of OSA is not well investigated. Parents who are not interested in prolonged medical therapy might opt instead for a more definitive resolution of OSA with adenotonsillectomy. This is a shared decision-making process that should involve the parents.

Adenotonsillectomy for Obstructive Sleep Apnea in Children

Removal of tonsils and adenoids (adenotonsillectomy) is the traditional treatment for OSA in children and leads to improvement in symptoms in most cases. In addition to improving PSG findings, tonsillectomy and adenoidectomy (T&A) also improves symptoms, QoL, and sequalae. In a meta-analysis of studies looking at the effect of TA on QoL, Todd and colleagues included 37 articles for qualitative analysis and 3 for quantitative synthesis.[39] There was a robust improvement in QoL after adenotonsillectomy in the short term (<6 months). The persistence of QoL improvement after the 6-month time point was unclear, with studies showing mixed results. As mentioned earlier, many children with OSA have enuresis. In their systematic review, Jeyakumar and colleagues included seven studies that evaluated the incidence of enuresis before and after adenotonsillectomy in children with SDB.[2] The prevalence of enuresis went from 31% before surgery to 16% after adenotonsillectomy, a significant reduction. Asthma frequently coexists with OSA, and a database analysis showed a reduction in acute asthma exacerbations and acute status asthmaticus in a group of children with asthma and adenotonsillectomy compared with a similar group of children with asthma who did not undergo an adenotonsillectomy.[40] Kohli and colleagues performed a systematic review of asthma outcomes after adenotonsillectomy in children with SDB and identified four articles that were included in the qualitative synthesis.[41] All included studies found clinically significant reductions in markers for asthma severity (respiratory medication use, emergency room visits for asthma-related symptoms, overall asthma symptoms, and asthma-related exacerbations) after adenotonsillectomy.

An important prospective trial evaluated the benefit of adenotonsillectomy versus watchful waiting in children with sleep apnea.[42] The Childhood Adenotonsillectomy Trial (CHAT) involved children 5–9 years of age who, overall, had mild OSA with median AHI <5 for the group and no child was included in the study if they had desaturations <90% for 2% or longer of total sleep time. Children underwent PSGs and cognitive and behavioral testing at baseline and 7 months after randomization. Early adenotonsillectomy resulted in a significant reduction of symptoms, behavioral outcomes, QoL, and PSG findings compared with the watchful waiting group, but did not lead to any significant improvement of attention or executive function. Also important in this study is that normalization of sleep study (AHI <2) occurred in a significantly higher percentage (79%) of the children randomized to the adenotonsillectomy arm, but 46% of the children in the watchful waiting group also achieved normalization of their PSGs. Similar results were obtained from a meta-analysis of 11 studies that compared adenotonsillectomy with watchful waiting.[43] In a more recent study, improvement in PSG indices was more favorable in the adenotonsillectomy group compared with the watchful waiting group and the changes between the groups were accentuated in children with moderate OSA.[44]

Post operative Management

Adenotonsillectomy is a painful procedure, and the pain can often last >1 week.[45] Post operative pain can lead to additional issues including poor intake by mouth (PO), dehydration, emergency department visits, and phone calls to the physician's office. One study showed that 6.3% of children had visits to the emergency room following adenotonsillectomy with the most common reasons being pain, dehydration, fever, nausea/vomiting, and bleeding.[46,47] The financial costs of these unplanned visits are not insignificant with an average cost of $1,420.[48] In addition these visits are emotionally stressful to parents, caregivers, and patients.

Although adenotonsillectomy is one of the most commonly performed pediatric surgeries, post operative pain management remains incredibly varied among surgeons. The clinical practice guidelines strongly recommend clinicians advise parents to give acetaminophen and ibuprofen for pain control,[30] and studies show that this regimen provides adequate pain control.[49,50]

Acetaminophen (Tylenol)

Acetaminophen is one of the most commonly prescribed medications for pain control after adenotonsillectomy.[51] A double-blind, randomized control trial comparing acetaminophen versus acetaminophen and codeine showed that there was no difference in pain control among the two groups. However, the acetaminophen-only group had statistically significant higher PO intake than the combination treatment group on the sixth post operative day.[52] Another study also demonstrated that parental assessment of pain was not rated as poorly controlled when comparing opioid versus non-opioid pain regimens.[53]

Non-Steroidal Antiinflammatory Drugs

Ibuprofen is effective for control of post-tonsillectomy pain and is recommended as part of the clinical practice guidelines.[51] However, concerns among clinicians remain regarding the association of ibuprofen with post-tonsillectomy hemorrhage, a potentially fatal complication. A recent non-inferiority randomized control trial could not exclude a higher rate of bleeding associated with ibuprofen when comparing it with acetaminophen,[54] and other studies have suggested similar results.[55,56] Of note, a large retrospective cohort from the children's hospital of Philadelphia compared the rate of bleeding post-adenotonsillectomy in children before and after the implementation of ibuprofen for post-tonsillectomy management.[57] Although they showed that there was no significant increase in the incidence of bleeding after ibuprofen use, there was a significant increase in the severity of bleeding as demonstrated by a 3-fold increase in the transfusion rate in these patients.

Alternatively, other studies, including a meta-analysis, suggested that there is no association between ibuprofen and increased rates of post-tonsillectomy hemorrhage.[58,59] In summary, the use of ibuprofen alternating with acetaminophen is recommended by the otolaryngology clinical practice guidelines,[30] and is one of the most popular pain regimens following pediatric tonsillectomy. Impact on post-tonsillectomy hemorrhage is still being debated.

Opioids

In the past, codeine had been prescribed frequently to children following adenotonsillectomy.[51] In 2009, the FDA reviewed the use of the drug following a reported death.[60] They identified 10 deaths and 3 overdoses in children treated with codeine between 1969 and 2012.[61] Eight of 13 events occurred in children who received codeine after adenotonsillectomy. Subsequently, FDA placed a black box warning on the use of codeine and tramadol in pediatric patients undergoing adenotonsillectomy.[62,63] This is likely related to the respiratory depressive effect of opioids, which is exaggerated in children with OSA, especially those who have significant hypoxemia on preoperative sleep studies.[64] A randomized control trial comparing morphine and the combination of acetaminophen and ibuprofen found a significantly increased number of respiratory events following adenotonsillectomy in the morphine group and no differences in pain control or bleeding reinforcing the respiratory depressive of opioids in children with OSA.[65]

Codeine and tramadol are metabolized to morphine by the enzyme cytochrome P450 (CYP450) 2D6. Genotypic variations lead to different phenotypes causing some patients to be ultrarapid metabolizers resulting in respiratory depression after codeine ingestion.[51] The clinical practice guidelines strongly recommend against prescription of codeine or medications containing codeine to children undergoing adenotonsillectomy under the age of 12.[30] One study looking at 110 patients undergoing tonsillectomy showed no differences in pain levels, readmissions, or bleeding rates when comparing ibuprofen and codeine, and in fact showed less nausea with ibuprofen.[66] Oxycodone and morphine are also options for post operative pain relief as they are metabolized by a different pathway.[51] However, all opioids also come with a concern for respiratory depression.

Steroids

The benefit of a single intraoperative dose of dexamethasone in children undergoing tonsillectomy is well documented and has been shown to reduce post operative nausea and vomiting. Other benefits include the reduction of throat pain and increased likelihood to advance to a soft diet early after surgery.[67,68] Numerous studies have shown benefits of steroids following adenotonsillectomy; however, they are limited by varying constraints including retrospective nature, lack of placebo comparison, inclusion of adults, or varying types of steroids and doses.[69,70] A recent randomized control trial found that one dose of post operative dexamethasone on post operative day 3 for children undergoing adenotonsillectomy demonstrated significant reduction in pain, as well as post operative phone calls and emergency department visits.[71] Ongoing studies are continuing to investigate the use of post operative steroids for additional pain control.

Persistent Obstructive Sleep Apnea After Adenotonsillectomy

Recent data suggest that while OSA is improved in most children after adenotonsillectomy, many do not achieve complete resolution as defined by AHI <1. Friedman and colleagues performed a systematic review of the literature until 2008 and identified 23 studies where adenotonsillectomy was used as the only modality of treatment for OSA in patients <20 years of age and where pre- and post-operative PSGs were obtained.[72] The meta-analysis included 1,079 subjects with a mean age of 6.5 years. When cure was assessed by each individual study as an AHI ≤5, the treatment success of adenotonsillectomy was 66.3%. However, when cure was defined as AHI <1, treatment success with adenotonsillectomy was only 59.8%. In these studies, mean AHI preoperatively ranged from 6.9 to 69.3 and mean AHI post operatively ranged from 0.3 to 14.2. Furthermore, all the studies showed a reduction in post operative AHI compared with the preoperative value. A later retrospective study evaluated otherwise healthy children undergoing adenotonsillectomy for OSA who had pre- and post operative PSGs at six pediatric sleep centers in the United States and two in Europe.[73] Multivariate linear modeling was used to assess the contributions of specific demographic factors on persistent OSA post-adenotonsillectomy. A total of 578 children were evaluated and they had a significant reduction in AHI from 18.2 to 4.1 events per hour after surgery. Treatment success gauged by AHI <1/hr was 27% and success gauged as AHI <5/hr was 78.4%. Age (particularly over 7 years) and BMI Z-score were the most significant contributors to post-operative AHI. Asthma, and preoperative AHI (i.e., severity of OSA preoperatively), were more modest but significant contributors. In another retrospective study in 70 children under age 3, adenotonsillectomy led to a significant reduction of AHI from 34 to 5.7 events per hour with 79% of children having AHI ≤5 post operatively and 41% having a post operative AHI ≤1.[74] In this series, the only predictor of OSA post operatively was severity of OSA preoperatively as obesity was not prevalent in this young cohort. Similar conclusions were reached by Mitchell and colleagues who demonstrated that none of a group of children with preoperative AHI <10 had persistent sleep apnea post operatively.[75] In contrast 36% of the children with a preoperative AHI >20 had persistent sleep apnea post operatively.

Obesity has been found to be associated with persistent sleep apnea after adenotonsillectomy and is supported by numerous studies that show persistent OSA in up to 51–66% of patients.[76–78] Using drug-induced sleep endoscopy (DISE) in these children, Coutras and colleagues found that obese children with persistent sleep apnea after adenotonsillectomy were more likely to have obstruction due to adenoid regrowth and lingual tonsil hypertrophy (LTH).[79]

There have been many studies that show that children with Down syndrome are more likely to have sleep apnea and have persistent sleep apnea after adenotonsillectomy. The rate of persistent disease in these reports ranges from 47% to 58%.[80,81] Children with craniofacial abnormalities are also more likely to have sleep apnea and show persistent symptoms after adenotonsillectomy.[82–84]

The clinical practice guidelines recommend that physicians counsel parents about the possibility of persistence or recurrence of OSA.[30] On reassessment it is important to perform a detailed history assessing for signs and symptoms of OSA and to perform a head and neck exam to evaluate for anatomical sites of obstruction. Examples of potential obstruction seen on exam include turbinate hypertrophy, retrognathia, large tongue base, and redundant palatal tissue.[85] In addition, the practitioner can consider sleep questionnaires, flexible laryngoscopy, DISE, cine magnetic resonance imaging (MRI), and repeat PSG in assisting with reevaluation.[86]

Sleep Endoscopy

DISE was introduced in 1991 as a way to evaluate sites of airway obstruction and collapse using flexible nasopharyngoscopy.[87] It is currently used in adults to help determine site-specific areas of collapse and inform surgery to improve sleep apnea. The velum, oropharynx, tongue base, and epiglottis (VOTE) classification system is commonly used in adults to rate DISE findings.[88] A systematic review comparing DISE with awake exam showed that the surgical treatment plan changed 50% of the time after DISE; however, studies looking at surgical outcomes after DISE are limited.[89] There are many available DISE scoring systems used in adults and children. In a systematic review of such systems, 44 studies were evaluated that included 5,784 patients.[90] Most of the studies focused on adult airway evaluation (80%) with 14% focusing on children and the rest including a combination of adults and children. There were 21 scoring systems reported in the included studies with the two most common being the VOTE classification and the Pringle and Croft system. The most common upper airway sites evaluated among the 21 scoring systems were the tongue base, lateral pharynx/oropharynx, palate, epiglottis/supraglottis, and hypopharynx. Less commonly included sites were the larynx, velum, nose, tongue, adenoids, and nasopharynx. Only pediatric studies included evaluation of the adenoids and obstruction at the nasopharynx, which were frequently reported for children. Unfortunately, the most common grading systems (the VOTE and Pringle and Croft scales) do not include evaluation of the nose or

nasopharynx. Thus, there is currently no single grading system for DISE in children, and most agree that evaluation of the nose and nasopharynx should be included in any such system.

Sleep endoscopy is performed under sedation with the goal of mimicking the natural state of sleep. Ideal conditions for this exam would maintain spontaneous ventilation, be repeatable, minimize excessive secretions, and be short duration.[91] The medications used to achieve these outcomes vary substantially and a recent review found that dexmedetomidine and ketamine may be the most ideal options for pediatric patients.[92] Further studies will need to be performed, particularly in children, to find the optimal regimen and standardize the procedure.

Recently, an expert consensus statement was assembled by the American Academy of Otolaryngology-Head and Neck surgery whereby authors reviewed available and relevant literature and reached consensus related to DISE in children.[93] Consensus was achieved on obtaining a PSG prior to DISE to confirm the diagnosis of OSA. They also agreed that DISE is indicated in children with OSA and small tonsils, and useful for children with persistent OSA after adenotonsillectomy to help plan additional surgery. They advocated performing DISE in children with persistent OSA before they are considered for additional pharyngeal or other surgery. They also agreed that there was limited utility in performing DISE in children with AHI <2, and that the role of DISE at the time of adenotonsillectomy is limited in children with OSA and adenotonsillar hypertrophy without risk factors for persistent OSA post operatively. However, if children had high risk for persistent OSA post operatively, DISE at the time of adenotonsillectomy does identify additional obstruction beyond the tonsils and adenoids. Finally, children with OSA and small tonsils who have some degree of obstruction at the tonsillar level observed during DISE would benefit from a tonsillectomy. As to protocols in pediatric DISE, there was consensus that photo and video documentation was useful and would facilitate future research and that jaw thrusting and other maneuvers used to facilitate visualization could be used during the procedure. Topical nasal decongestion was discouraged as it could alter the findings, and evaluation of the airway beyond the glottis was justified and indicated in children with signs and symptoms suggesting tracheal or bronchial pathology. As for sedation protocols for pediatric DISE, the panel members agreed that either propofol or dexmedetomidine were optimal forms of sedation for use in pediatric DISE and that the level of sedation during pediatric DISE should be titrated to audible snoring, an obstructive breathing pattern, or both. While inhalational agents may be used for induction purposes, it was recommended that they be discontinued for the diagnostic portion of the study. DISE in pediatrics should evaluate and grade obstruction at the following sites: nasal airway (including nasal cavities, nasopharynx), palate/velum, pharyngeal airway (including lateral oropharyngeal wall and tongue base), and supraglottic larynx.

The most common indication for DISE in children remains facilitating the identification of airway obstruction in children with persistent OSA after adenotonsillectomy. Sites of obstruction include the inferior turbinates, adenoid regrowth, velum, lateral oropharynx, and tongue base with one review of 162 children showing that 100% had at least one site of obstruction identified in this context.[94] Evolving indications include performing DISE for children with OSA and small tonsils as well as in children with high risk of persistent disease after adenotonsillectomy. Evidence for these indications is still scarce. Chen and He evaluated the impact of DISE-directed tonsillectomy in children with OSA and small tonsils.[95] The active group had planned adenoidectomy and additional tonsillectomy based on DISE findings of significant lateral wall collapse, and the control group had adenoidectomy only with no DISE performed. Forty-five percent of the children in the active group had significant lateral wall collapse when evaluated with DISE and underwent tonsillectomy in addition to the initially planned adenoidectomy. Results showed a significant improvement in the RDI at 6 months and 1 year following DISE-directed tonsillectomy for children with small tonsils compared with the control group. As for utilizing DISE in children at high risk of persistent OSA after adenotonsillectomy, Ulualp evaluated children with severe OSA with DISE at the time of adenotonsillectomy and performed additional expansion pharyngoplasty when indicated by DISE findings.[96] They showed larger improvements in the AHI in children who had additional palatal surgery performed when compared with patients who were treated with adenotonsillectomy alone (control). Further randomized control, prospective studies with larger sample sizes are still needed to validate these evolving indications and better position DISE in the surgical management of OSA in children.

Additional Surgical Alternatives

Palate Surgery

Lateral pharyngeal wall collapse has been shown to be a common contributor to airway obstruction in children with OSA.[97] Surgery to address the palate in adults has been shown to have good outcomes for treatment of OSA and many types of palatal surgeries that have been described including lateral pharyngoplasty, expansion sphincter pharyngoplasty (ESP), uvulopalatopharyngoplasty (UPPP), and combinations of those procedures.[98–101] Small studies looking at palatal surgeries in children have shown potential benefit. Ulualp and colleagues compared the outcome of modified ESPs added to adenotonsillectomy with adenotonsillectomy alone in a group of children with severe OSA.[96] The decision to pursue ESP was guided by DISE that showed lateral pharyngeal wall collapse. Results showed

that whereas both groups lowered their AHI postoperatively, the postoperative AHI of the modified ESP group was significantly lower than that of the adenotonsillectomy group. Furthermore, cure rate (AHI <1) was higher in the ESP group. Another study found adenotonsillectomy with UPPP to be successful for neurologically impaired children.[102] However, a randomized study comparing standard adenotonsillectomy with adenotonsillectomy with suturing of tonsillar pillars found no significant difference in the outcomes of obstructive AHI between the groups.[103]

Lingual Tonsillectomy and Base of Tongue Surgeries

Based on studies using DISE, it is evident that LTH and tongue base obstruction are significant contributors to persistent sleep apnea after adenotonsillectomy.[79,104] The most common surgical option to address LTH or tongue base obstruction is lingual tonsillectomy. The goal of the procedure is to reduce the lingual tonsil tissue to create more space within the airway. A variety of methods including sharp dissection, microdebrider, CO_2 laser, cryotherapy, coblation, and suction cautery have been described.[105] Rivero and Durr conducted a systematic review and meta-analysis of five studies evaluating the impact of lingual tonsillectomy for persistent OSA after initial adenotonsillectomy in 132 pediatric patients.[106] They showed that lingual tonsillectomy was associated with a significant decrease in AHI and increase in minimal oxygen saturation. The overall success rate defined as AHI <5 was 52% suggesting that complete resolution was rare. Complications are comparable to those of adenotonsillectomy and include airway obstruction due to tongue base edema, hemorrhage, and poor oral intake.[107,108]

A few studies of combined lingual tonsillectomy with open midline glossectomy showed improvement in AHI in both syndromic and non-syndromic children.[109,110] In one study, obesity, either pre- or postoperatively, was associated with worse outcomes.[110] Another option for tongue base surgery is transoral robotic surgery (TORS) tongue base reduction, which has been shown to be an effective treatment option of OSA in adults.[111] Few studies have used transoral robotic tongue base resection in pediatrics and have found success.[112,113] A systematic review and meta-analysis looking at nine papers reporting tongue base surgeries in pediatrics found that AHI improved by 48.5% in all patients but more so in non-syndromic compared with syndromic children (59.2% vs. 40% improvement).[114] They concluded that non-syndromic children, and those with BMI <25, had the best outcomes. In addition they found that >90% of the patients had previously undergone adenotonsillectomy, indicating that tongue base reduction is not a first-line treatment option for OSA.

In conclusion, we know that LTH is a significant contributor to residual OSA after adenotonsillectomy, and options for these patients can include lingual tonsillectomy or tongue base reduction surgeries; however, outcomes are not perfect, and further studies are indicated.

Supraglottoplasty

Laryngomalacia or collapse of supraglottic structures into the airway can be associated with OSA.[115] Supraglottoplasty is a surgical procedure that removes redundant tissue in the supraglottis. When laryngomalacia is present, studies show that supraglottoplasty can be performed and is associated with statistically significant reduction in AHI.[116,117] However, most studies have small sample sizes and, as with other treatments, patients with other comorbidities were found to have worse outcomes.[117] Camacho and colleagues performed a systematic review and meta-analysis evaluating the effect of isolated supraglottoplasty on indices of OSA in children.[118] They identified 13 studies with 138 patients: 64 with sleep exclusive laryngomalacia (older children) and 74 with congenital laryngomalacia (younger children). In both groups AHI was reduced and low sats were improved significantly after supraglottoplasty. However, cure rate (AHI <1/hr) was 10.5% in the patients with sleep-exclusive laryngomalacia and 26.5% in the congenital laryngomalacia group suggesting, as with most of additional procedures, that supraglottoplasty is helpful but not perfect in achieving complete resolution of OSA. Comparable results with 88% of patients having residual disease were obtained from another review of four studies looking at supraglottoplasty for OSA.[119]

Hypoglossal Nerve Stimulator

The hypoglossal nerve stimulator has been shown to be a safe and effective surgical option for adults who meet criteria as an alternative to continuous positive airway pressure (CPAP). Median AHI scores were decreased by 68% in the Stimulation Therapy for Apnea Reduction (STAR) trial.[120] The procedure consists of implanting a nerve stimulator on the hypoglossal nerve that is linked to a receiver with a sensing lead in the chest wall to stimulate tongue protrusion with expiration. In the pediatric world, studies of hypoglossal nerve stimulators have been done in patients with Down syndrome. Results show that it is well tolerated and effective with reduction in AHI by 56–85%.[121,122] In addition, preliminary studies show that improvement is maintained for up to 44–58 months post operatively.[123] The device has recently been approved by the FDA to treat patients with Down syndrome who are at least 13 years and older and cannot be effectively treated with CPAP.

Mandibular Distraction

Patients with craniofacial abnormalities such as retrognathia or micrognathia can present with variable degrees of airway obstruction. They are also at high risk for persistent and severe OSA. Some of the more common conditions include Pierre Robin sequence, Treacher Collins, Nager syndrome, velocardiofacial syndrome, and Pfeiffer syndrome.[124] Initially introduced in 1992, mandibular distraction osteogenesis (MDO) involves mandibular osteotomies, insertion of an internal or external distractor device, and gradual lengthening of the mandible with the ultimate goal to relieve tongue base obstruction.[125] A meta-analysis of 37 pediatric studies found significant improvement following distraction with AHI decreases from 41 to 4.5 events per hour.[126] However, the meta-analysis notes significant heterogeneity within the studies and comments on the need for research on long-term outcomes. This option is currently not used routinely for children with OSA and is reserved for conditions where a small or retruded jaw is contributing to airway obstruction.

Tracheotomy

Although tracheostomy is the definitive treatment for OSA in adults,[127] it is not frequently used due to the many associated morbidities and mortalities. In pediatrics, it is an uncommon indication for primary treatment of OSA, and is reserved for severe, refractory cases. The majority of patients have some other comorbidity. In one retrospective study describing the characteristics of pediatric patients undergoing tracheostomy for OSA (AHI >10) in four tertiary care academic children's hospitals, 29 children aged <18 years were examined.[128] Seventy-nine percent of the patients either had a craniofacial deformity, hypotonia resulting from a neurologic disorder, or laryngomalacia and the majority were tracheostomy dependent for >24 months. A systematic review of pediatric tracheostomy outcomes for OSA found few studies with quantitative data but were able to conclude that tracheostomy does lead to significant improvement in OSA, and that the majority of these patients were syndromic.[129]

Conclusions

In summary, OSA in children is a common disorder with behavioral and hemodynamic sequalae that have a significant negative impact on QoL. The gold standard for diagnosis is a PSG, but clinical history and physical exam are a very important part of the evaluation. Adenotonsillectomy remains the initial treatment of choice in these patients with medical therapy available in instances of mild disease with minimal sequalae. Although adenotonsillectomy is highly effective in most children, not all achieve complete resolution of disease after the procedure. Children with residual OSA post-adenotonsillectomy can be treated medically or evaluated with DISE to identify other sites of obstruction that might be amenable to further surgical options. Although these improve OSA in children, they are often not completely curative. Orthodontic procedures such as rapid maxillary expansion as well as CPAP are also options but are beyond the scope of this chapter and are not discussed.

CLINICAL PEARLS

- Although sleep questionnaires are useful in identifying the negative impact of sleep disordered breathing on quality of life, they are not a substitute for polysomnography in the accurate diagnosis of obstructive sleep apnea.
- Mild obstructive sleep apnea can be treated with montelukast, intranasal steroids or a combination of these 2 agents.
- Drug induced sleep endoscopy is useful in delineating potential causes of persistent obstructive sleep apnea after adenotonsillectomy.

References

1. Lumeng JC, Chervin RD. Epidemiology of pediatric obstructive sleep apnea. *Proc Am Thorac Soc.* 2008;5(2):242–252.
2. Jeyakumar A, Rahman SI, Armbrecht ES, Mitchell R. The association between sleep-disordered breathing and enuresis in children. *Laryngoscope.* 2012;122:1873–1877.
3. Brooks LJ, Topol HI. Enuresis in children with sleep apnea. *J Pediatr.* 2003;142(5):515–518.
4. Baldassari CM, Mitchell RB, Schubert C, Rudnick EF. Pediatric obstructive sleep apnea and quality of life: A meta-analysis. *Otolaryngol Head Neck Surg.* 2008;138:265–273.
5. Mitchell RB, Kelly J. Behavior, neurocognition and quality of life in children with sleep-disordered breathing. *Int J Pediatr Otorhinolaryngol.* 2006;70:395–406.
6. Sedky K, Bennett DS, Carvalho KS. Attention deficit hyperactivity disorder and sleep disordered breathing in pediatric populations: A meta-analysis. *Sleep Med Rev.* 2014;18:349–356.
7. Gozal D. Sleep-disordered breathing and school performance in children. *Pediatrics.* 1998;102(3 Pt 1):616–620.
8. Lind MG, Lundell BP. Tonsillar hyperplasia in children. A cause of obstructive sleep apneas, CO_2 retention and retarded growth. *Arch Otolaryngol.* 1982;108(10):650–654.
9. Marcus CL, Carroll JL, Koerrner CB, Hamer A, Lutz J, Loughlin GM. Determinants of growth in children with obstructive sleep apnea syndrome. *J Pediatr.* 1994;125(4):556–562.
10. Estellera E, Villatoroa JC, Agüeroa A, Lopeza R, Matiñóa E, Argemic J, Girabent-Farrés M. Obstructive sleep apnea syndrome and growth failure. *Int J Pediatr Otorhinolaryngol.* 2018;108:214–218.
11. Marcus CL, Greene MG, Carroll JL. Blood pressure in children with obstructive sleep apnea. *Am J Respir Crit Care Med.* 1998;157:1098–1103.
12. Kohyama J, Ohinata JS, Hasegawa T. Blood pressure in sleep disordered breathing. *Arch Dis Child.* 2003;88(2):139–142.
13. Amin RS, Carroll JS, Jeffries JL, Grone C, Bean JA, Chini B, et al. Twenty four hour ambulatory blood pressure in children with sleep disordered breathing. *Am J Respir Crit Care Med.* 2004;169(8):950–956.
14. Zintzaras E, Kaditis A. Sleep-disordered breathing and blood pressure in children. A meta-analysis. *Arch Pediatr Adolesc Med.* 2007;161:172–178.
15. Sofer S, Weinhouse E, Tal A, Wanderman KL, Margulis G, Leiberman A, et al. Cor pulmonal due to adenoidal or tonsillar hypertrophy or both in children. Noninvasive diagnosis and follow up. *Chest.* 1988;93(1):119–122.
16. Tal A, Leiberman A, Margulis G, Sofer S. Ventricular dysfunction in children with obstructive sleep apnea: radionuclide assessment. *Pediatr Pulmonol.* 1988;4(3):139–143.
17. Amin RS, Kimball TR, Kalra M, Jeffries JL, Carroll JL, Bean JA, et al. Left ventricular function in children with sleep-disordered breathing. *Am J Cardiol.* 2005;95(6):801–804.
18. Mallampati SR, Gatt SP, Gugino LD, et al. A clinical sign to predict difficult tracheal intubation: A prospective study. *Can Anaesth Soc J.* 1985;32:429–434.
19. Friedman M, Tanyeri H, La Rosa M, et al. Clinical predictors of obstructive sleep apnea. *Laryngoscope.* 1999;109(12):1901–1907.
20. Friedman M, Hamilton C, Samuelson CG, Lundgren ME, Pott T. Diagnostic value of the Friedman tongue position and Mallampati classification for obstructive sleep apnea: A meta-analysis. *Otolaryngol Head Neck Surg.* 2013;148(4):540–547.
21. Kumar HVM, Schroeder JW, Gang Z, Sheldon SH. Mallampati score and pediatric obstructive sleep apnea. *J Clin Sleep Med.* 2014;10(9):985–990.
22. Chervin RD, Hedger K, Dillon JE, Pituch KJ. Pediatric sleep questionnaire (PSQ): Validity and reliability of scales for sleep-disordered breathing, snoring, sleepiness, and behavioral problems. *Sleep Med.* 2000;1:21–32.
23. Franco RA, Rosenfeld RM, Rao M. Quality-of-life for children with obstructive sleep apnea. *Otolaryngol Head Neck Surg.* 2000;123:9–16.
24. Borgstrom A, Nerfeldt P, Friberg D. Questionnaire OSA-18 has poor validity compared to polysomnography in pediatric obstructive sleep apnea. *Int J Pediatr Otorhinolaryngol.* 2013;77:1864–1868.
25. Goldstein NA, Stefanov DG, Graw-Panzer KD, et al. Validation of a clinical assessment score for pediatric sleep-disordered breathing. *Laryngoscope.* 2012;122:2096–2104.
26. Goldstein NA, Friedman NR, Nardone HC, Aljasser A, Tobey ABJ, Don D, Baroody FM, Lam DJ, Goudy S, Ishman SL, Arganbright JA, Baldassari C, Schreinemakers JBS, Wine TM, Ruszkay NJ, Alammar A, Shaffer AD, Koempel JA, Weedon J. The generalizability of the clinical assessment Score-15 for pediatric sleep-disordered breathing. *Laryngoscope.* 2020;130:2256–2262.
27. Parenti SI, Fiordelli A, Bartolucci ML, Martina S, D'Anto V, Alessandri-Bonetti G. Diagnostic accuracy of screening questionnaires for obstructive sleep apnea in children: A systematic review and meta-analysis. *Sleep Med Rev.* 2021;57:101464.
28. Mitchell RB, Pereira KD, Friedman NR. Sleep-disordered breathing in children: Survey of current practice. *Laryngoscope.* 2006;116:956–958.
29. Marcus CL, Brooks LJ, Draper KA, Gozal D, Halbower AC, Jones J, Schechter MS, Sheldon SH, Spruyt K, Davidson Ward S, Lehmann C, Shiffman RN. Diagnosis and management of childhood obstructive sleep apnea syndrome. *Pediatrics.* 2012;130(3):576–584.
30. Mitchell RB, Archer SM, Ishman SL, Rosenfeld RM, Coles S, Finestone SA, Friedman NR, Giordano T, Hildrew DM, Kim TW, Lloyd RM, Parikh SR, Shulman ST, Walner DL, Walsh SA, Nnacheta LC. Clinical Practice Guideline: Tonsillectomy in children (update). *Otolaryngol Head Neck Surg.* 2019;160(1S):S1–S42.
31. Lam DJ, Shea SA, Weaver EM, Mitchell RB. Predictors of obtaining polysomnography among otolaryngologists prior to

adenotonsillectomy for childhood sleep-disordered breathing. *J Clin Sleep Med.* 2018;14(8):1361–1367.

32. Brouillette RT, Manoukian JJ, Ducharme FM, Oudjhane K, Earle LG, Ladan S, Morielli A. Efficacy of fluticasone nasal spray for pediatric obstructive sleep apnea. *J Pediatr.* 2001;138(6):838–844.

33. Chan CCK, Au CT, Lam HS, Lee DLY, Wing YK, Li AM. Intranasal corticosteroids for mild childhood obstructive sleep apnea- a randomized, placebo-controlled study. *Sleep Med.* 2015;16(3):358–363.

34. Kheirandish-Gozal L, Gozal D. Intranasal budesonide treatment for children with mild obstructive sleep apnea syndrome. *Pediatrics.* 2008;122:e149–e155.

35. Liming BJ, Ryan M, Mack D, Ahmad I, Camacho M. Montelukast and nasal corticosteroids to treat pediatric obstructive sleep apnea: A systematic review and meta-analysis. *Otolaryngol Head Neck Surg.* 2019;160(4):594–602.

36. Sunkonkit K, Sritippayawan S, Veeravikrom M, et al. Urinary cysteinyl leukotriene E4 level and therapeutic response to montelukast in children with mild obstructive sleep apnea. *Asian Pac J Allergy Immunol.* 2017;35:233–238.

37. Kheirandish-Gozal L, Bhattacharjee R, Bandla HPR, et al. Antiinflammatory therapy outcomes for mild OSA in children. *Chest.* 2014;146:88–95.

38. Clarridge K, Chin S, Eworuke E, Seymour S. A boxed warning for Montelukast: The FDA perspective. *J Allergy Clin Immunol Pract.* 2021 Jul;9(7):2638–2641.

39. Todd CA, Bareiss AK, McCoul ED, Rodriguez KH. Adenotonsillectomy for obstructive sleep apnea and quality of life: Systematic review and meta-analysis. *Otolaryngol Head Neck Surg.* 2017;157(5):767–773.

40. Bhattacharjee R, Choi BH, Gozal D, Mokhlesi B. Association of adenotonsillectomy with asthma outcomes in children: A longitudinal database analysis. *PLoS Med.* 2014;11(11):e1001753.

41. Kohli N, DeCarlo D, Goldstein NA, Silverman J. Asthma outcomes after adenotonsillectomy: A systematic review. *Int J Pediatr Otorhinolaryngol.* 2016;90:107–112.

42. Marcus CL, Moore RH, Rosen CL, Giordani B, Garetz SL, Taylor HG, Mitchell RB, Amin R, Katz ES, Arens R, Paruthi S, Muzumdar H, Gozal D, Hattiangadi Thomas N, Ware J, Beebe D, Snyder K, Elden L, Sprecher RC, Willging P, Jones D, Bent JP, Hoban T, Chervin RD, Ellenberg SS, Redline S, Childhood Adenotonsillectomy Trial (CHAT). A randomized trial of adenotonsillectomy for childhood sleep apnea. *N Engl J Med.* 2013;368(25):2366–2376.

43. Chinnadurai S, Jordan AK, Sathe NA, Fonnesbeck C, McPheeters ML, Francis DO. Tonsillectomy for obstructive sleep-disordered breathing: A meta-analysis. *Pediatrics.* 2017;139(2).e20163491

44. Fehrm J, Nerfeldt P, Browaldh N, Friberg D. Effectiveness of adenotonsillectomy vs watchful waiting in young children with mild to moderate obstructive sleep apnea. A randomized clinical trial. *JAMA Otolaryngol Head Neck Surg.* 2020;146(7):647–654.

45. Warnock FF, Lander J. Pain progression, intensity and outcomes following tonsillectomy. *Pain.* 1998;75(1):37–45.

46. Curtis JL, Harvey DB, Willie S, Narasimhan E, Andrews S, Henrichsen J, Van Buren NC, Srivastava R, Meier JD. Causes and costs for ED visits after pediatric adenotonsillectomy. *Otolaryngol Head Neck Surg.* 2015;152(4):691–696.

47. Shay S, Shapiro NL, Bhattacharyya N. Revisit rates and diagnoses following pediatric tonsillectomy in a large multistate population. *Laryngoscope.* 2015;125(2):457–461.

48. Duval M, Wilkes J, Korgenski K, Srivastava R, Meier J. Causes, costs, and risk factors for unplanned return visits after adenotonsillectomy in children. *Int J Pediatr Otorhinolaryngol.* 2015;79(10):1640–1646.

49. Liu C, Ulualp SO. Outcomes of an alternating ibuprofen and acetaminophen regimen for pain relief after tonsillectomy in children. *Ann Otol Rhinol Laryngol.* 2015;124(10):777–781.

50. Bedwell JR, Pierce M, Levy M, Shah RK. Ibuprofen with acetaminophen for postoperative pain control following tonsillectomy does not increase emergency department utilization. *Otolaryngol Head Neck Surg.* 2014;151(6):963–966.

51. Tan GX, Tunkel DE. Control of pain after tonsillectomy in children. *JAMA Otolaryngol Head Neck Surg.* 2017;143(9):937–942.

52. Moir MS, Bair E, Shinnick P, Messner A. Acetaminophen versus acetaminophen with codeine after pediatric tonsillectomy. *Laryngoscope.* 2000;110(11):1824–1827.

53. Adler AC, Mehta DK, Messner AH, Salemi JL, Chandrakantan A. Parental assessment of pain control following pediatric adenotonsillectomy: Do opioids make a difference? *Int J Pediatr Otorhinolaryngol.* 2020;134:110045.

54. Diercks GR, Comins J, Bennett K, Gallagher TQ, Brigger M, Boseley M, Gaudreau P, Rogers D, Setlur J, Keamy D, Cohen MS, Hartnick C. Comparison of ibuprofen vs acetaminophen and severe bleeding risk after pediatric tonsillectomy. *JAMA Otolaryngol Head Neck Surg.* 2019;145(6):494–500.

55. D'Souza JN, Schmidt RJ, Xie Li, Adelman JP, Nardone HC. Postoperative nonsteroidal anti-inflammatory drugs and risk of bleeding in pediatric intracapsular tonsillectomy. *Int J Pediatr Otorhinolaryngol.* 2015;79(9):1472–1476.

56. Swanson RT, Schubart JR, Carr MM. Association of ibuprofen use with post-tonsillectomy bleeding in older children. *Am J Otolaryngol.* 2018;39(5):618–622.

57. Mudd PA, Thottathil P, Giordano T, Wetmore RF, Elden L, Jawad AF, Ahumada L, Galvez JA. Association between ibuprofen use and severity of surgically managed posttonsillectomy hemorrhage. *JAMA Otolaryngol Head Neck Surg.* 2017;143(7):712–717.

58. Pfaff JA, Hsu K, Chennupati SK. The use of ibuprofen in posttonsillectomy analgesia and its effect on posttonsillectomy hemorrhage rate. *Otolaryngol Head Neck Surg.* 2016;155(3):508–513.

59. Losorelli SD, Scheffler P, Qian ZJ, Lin HFC, Truong MT. Posttonsillectomy ibuprofen: Is there a dose-dependent bleeding risk? *Laryngoscope.* 2021;132(7):1473–1481.

60. Ciszkowski C, Madadi P, Phillips MS, Lauwers AE, Koren G. Codeine, ultrarapid-metabolism genotype, and postoperative death. *New Engl J Med.* 2009;361(8):827–828.

61. Kuehn BM. FDA: No codeine after tonsillectomy for children. *JAMA.* 2013;309(11):1100.

62. US Food and Drug Administration. FDA Drug Safety Communication: FDA evaluating the risks of using the pain medicine tramadol in children aged 17 and younger. http://www.fda.gov. 2015. Accessed 21.09.15.

63. US Food and Drug Administration. FDA Drug Safety Communication: FDA restricts use of prescription codeine pain and cough medicines and tramadol pain medicines in children;

recommends against use in breastfeeding women. http://www.fda.gov. 2017. Accessed 20.04.17.

64. Brown KA, Laferriere A, Lakheeram I, Moss IR. Recurrent Hypoxemia In Children Is Associated With Increased Analgesic Sensitivity To Opiates. *Anesthesiology.* 2006;105(4):665–669.

65. Kelly LE, Sommer DD, Ramakrishna J, Hoffbauer S, Arbab-Tafti S, Reid D, Maclean J, Koren G. Morphine or ibuprofen for post-tonsillectomy analgesia: A randomized trial. *Pediatrics.* 2015;135(2):307–313.

66. St Charles CS, Matt BH, Hamilton MM, Katz BP. A comparison of ibuprofen versus acetaminophen with codeine in the young tonsillectomy patient. *Otolaryngol Head Neck Surg.* 1997;117(1):76–82.

67. Steward DL, Grisel J, Meinzen-Derr J. Steroids for improving recovery following tonsillectomy in children. *Cochrane Database Syst Rev.* 2011;8:CD003997.

68. Gao W, Zhang QR, Jiang L, Geng JY. Comparison of local and intravenous dexamethasone for postoperative pain and recovery after tonsillectomy. *Otolaryngol Head Neck Surg.* 2015;152:530–535.

69. Park SK, Kim J, Kim JM, Yeon JY, Shim WS, Lee DW. Effects of Oral Prednisolone on Recovery after Tonsillectomy. *Laryngoscope.* 2014;125(1):111–117.

70. Redmann AJ, Maksimoski M, Brumbaugh C, Ishman SL. The Effect of postoperative steroids on post-tonsillectomy pain and need for postoperative physician contact. *Laryngoscope.* 2018;128(9):2187–2192.

71. Greenwell AG, Isaiah A, Pereira KD. Recovery after Adenotonsillectomy-do steroids help? Outcomes from a randomized controlled trial. *Otolaryngol Head Neck Surg.* 2021;165(1):83–88.

72. Friedman M, Wilson M, Lin HC, Chang HW. Updated systematic review of tonsillectomy and adenoidectomy for treatment of pediatric obstructive sleep apnea/hypopnea syndrome. *Otolaryngol Head Neck Surg.* 2009;140:800–808.

73. Bhattacharjee R, Kheirandish-Gozal L, Spruyt K, Mitchell RB, Promchiarak J, Simakajornboon N, Kaditis AG, Splaingard D, Splaingard M, Brooks LJ, Marcus CL, Sin S, Arens R, Verhulst SL, Gozal D. Adenotonsillectomy outcomes in treatment of obstructive sleep apnea in children: a multicenter retrospective study. *Am J Respir Crit Care Med.* 2010;182:676–683.

74. Nath A, Emani J, Suskind DL, Baroody FM. Predictors of persistent sleep apnea after surgery in children younger than 3 years. *JAMA Otolaryngol Head Neck Surg.* 2013;139(10):1002–1008.

75. Mitchell RB. Adenotonsillectomy for obstructive sleep apnea in children: Outcome evaluated by pre- and postoperative polysomnography. *Laryngoscope.* 2007;117(10):1844–1854.

76. O'Brien LM, Sitha S, Baur LA, Waters KA. Obesity increases the risk for persisting obstructive sleep apnea after treatment in children. *Int J Pediatr Otorhinolaryngol.* 2006;70(9):1555–1560.

77. Scheffler P, Wolter NE, Narang I, Amin R, Holler T, Ishman SL, Propst EJ. Surgery for obstructive sleep apnea in obese children: Literature review and meta-analysis. *Otolaryngol Head Neck Surg.* 2019;160(6):985–992.

78. Tauman R, Gulliver TE, Krishna J, Montgomery-Downs HE, Obrien LM, Ivanenko A, Gozal D. Persistence of obstructive sleep apnea syndrome in children after adenotonsillectomy. *J Pediatr.* 2006;149(6):803–808.

79. Coutras SW, Limjuco A, Davis KE, Carr MM. Sleep Endoscopy findings in children with persistent obstructive sleep apnea after

adenotonsillectomy. *Int J Pediatr Otorhinolaryngol.* 2018;107:190–193.

80. Abijay CA, Tomkies A, Rayasam S, Johnson RF, Mitchell RB. Children with Down syndrome and obstructive sleep apnea: Outcomes after tonsillectomy. *Otolaryngol Head Neck Surg.* 2021;166(3):557–564.

81. Maris M, Verhulst S, Wojciechowski M, Van de Heyning P, Boudewyns A. Outcome of adenotonsillectomy in children with Down syndrome and obstructive sleep apnoea. *Arch Dis Child.* 2016;102(4):331–336.

82. Moraleda-Cibrián M, Edwards SP, Kasten SJ, Buchman SR, Berger M, Obrien LM. Obstructive sleep apnea pretreatment and posttreatment in symptomatic children with congenital craniofacial malformations. *J Clin Sleep Med.* 2015;11(01):37–43.

83. Zandieh SO, Padwa BL, Katz ES. Adenotonsillectomy for obstructive sleep apnea in children with syndromic craniosynostosis. *Plast Reconst Surg.* 2013;131(4):847–852.

84. Imanguli M, Ulualp SO. Risk factors for residual obstructive sleep apnea after adenotonsillectomy in children. *Laryngoscope.* 2016;126(11):2624–2629.

85. Bluher AE, Ishman SL, Baldassari CM. Managing the child with persistent sleep apnea. *Otolaryngol Clin North Am.* 2019;52(5):891–901.

86. Manickam PV, Shott SR, Boss EF, Cohen AP, Meinzen-Derr JK, Amin RS, Ishman SL. Systematic review of site of obstruction identification and non-CPAP treatment options for children with persistent pediatric obstructive sleep apnea. *Laryngoscope.* 2015;126(2):491–500.

87. Croft CB, Pringle M. Sleep nasendoscopy: A technique of assessment in snoring and obstructive sleep apnoea. *Clin Otolaryngol Allied Sci.* 2009;16(5):504–509.

88. Kezirian EJ, Hohenhorst W, de Vries N. Drug-induced sleep endoscopy: The VOTE classification. *Eur Arch Otorhinolaryngol.* 2011;268(8):1233–1236.

89. Certal VF, Pratas R, Guimarães L, Lugo R, Tsou Y, Camacho M, Capasso R. Awake examination versus DISE for surgical decision making in patients with OSA: A systematic review. *Laryngoscope.* 2015;126(3):768–774.

90. Amos JM, Durr ML, Nardone HC, Baldassari CM, Duggins A, Ishman SL. Systematic review of drug-induced sleep endoscopy scoring systems. *Otolaryngol Head Neck Surg.* 2018;158(2):240–248.

91. Adler AC, Musso MF, Mehta DK, Chandrakantan A. Pediatric drug induced sleep endoscopy: A simple sedation recipe. *Ann Otol Rhinol Laryngol.* 2019;129(5):428–433.

92. Liu KA, Liu CC, Alex G, Szmuk P, Mitchell RB. Anesthetic management of children undergoing drug-induced sleep endoscopy: A retrospective review. *Int J Pediatr Otorhinolaryngol.* 2020;139:110440.

93. Baldassari CM, Lam DJ, Ishman SL, Chernobilsky B, Friedman NR, Giordano T, Lawlor C, Mitchell RB, Nardone H, Ruda J, Zalzal H, Deneal A, Dhepyasuwan N, Rosenfeld RM. Expert consensus statement: Pediatric drug-induced sleep endoscopy. *Otolaryngol Head Neck Surg.* 2021;165(4):578–591.

94. Wilcox LJ, Bergeron M, Reghunathan S, Ishman SL. An updated review of pediatric drug-induced sleep endoscopy. *Laryngoscope Investig Otolaryngol.* 2017;2(6):423–431.

95. Chen J, He S. Drug-induced sleep endoscopy-directed adenotonsillectomy in pediatric obstructive sleep apnea with small tonsils. *PLoS One.* 2019;14(2):e0212317.

96. Ulualp SO. Modified expansion sphincter pharyngoplasty for treatment of children with obstructive sleep apnea. *JAMA Otolaryngol Head Neck Surg.* 2014;140(9):817–822.

97. Ulualp SO, Szmuk P. Drug-induced sleep endoscopy for upper airway evaluation in children with obstructive sleep apnea. *Laryngoscope.* 2012;123(1):292–297.

98. Maniaci A, Di Luca M, Lechien JR, Iannella G, Grillo C, Grillo CM, Merlino F, Calvo-Henriquez C, De Vito A, Magliulo G, Pace A, Vicini C, Cocuzza S, Bannò V, Pollicina I, Stilo G, Bianchi A, La Mantia I. Lateral pharyngoplasty vs. traditional uvulopalatopharyngoplasty for patients with OSA: Systematic review and meta-analysis. *Sleep Breath.* 2022;26(4):1539–1550. https://doi.org/10.1007/s11325-021-02520-y.

99. Pinto JA, Balester Mello de Godoy L, Dos Santos Sobreira Nunes H, Abdo KE, Spinola Jahic G, Cavallini AF, Freitas GS, Ribeiro DK, Duarte C. Lateral-expansion pharyngoplasty: combined technique for the treatment of obstructive sleep apnea syndrome. *Int Arch Otorhinolaryngol.* 2019;24(01):e107–e111.

100. Cahali MB. Lateral pharyngoplasty: A new treatment for obstructive sleep apnea hypopnea syndrome. *Laryngoscope.* 2010;113(11):1961–1968.

101. Pang KP, Woodson BT. Expansion Sphincter Pharyngoplasty: A new technique for the treatment of obstructive sleep apnea. *Otolaryngol Head Neck Surg.* 2007;137(11):110–114.

102. Kerschner JE, Lynch JB, Kleiner H, Flanary VA, Rice TB. Uvulopalatopharyngoplasty with tonsillectomy and adenoidectomy as a treatment for obstructive sleep apnea in neurologically impaired children. *Int J Pediatr Otorhinolaryngol.* 2002 Feb 25;62(3):229–235.

103. Fehrm J, Nerfeldt P, Sundman J, Friberg D. Adenopharyngoplasty vs adenotonsillectomy in children with severe obstructive sleep apnea: A randomized clinical trial. *JAMA Otolaryngol Head Neck Surg.* 2018(7):580–586.

104. Durr ML, Meyer AK, Kezirian EJ, Rosbe KW. Drug-induced sleep endoscopy in persistent pediatric sleep-disordered breathing after adenotonsillectomy. *Arch Otolaryngol Head Neck Surg.* 2012;138(7):638–643.

105. Barakate M, Havas T. Lingual tonsillectomy: A review of 5 years experience and evolution of surgical technique. *Otolaryngol Head Neck Surg.* 2008;139(2):222–227.

106. Rivero A, Durr ML. Lingual tonsillectomy for pediatric persistent obstructive sleep apnea: A systematic review and meta-analysis. *Otolaryngol Head Neck Surg.* 2017;157(6):940–947.

107. Abdel-Aziz M, Ibrahim N, Ahmed A, El-Hamamsy M, Abdel-Khalik MI, El-Hoshy H. Lingual tonsils hypertrophy: A cause of obstructive sleep apnea in children after adenotonsillectomy: Operative problems and management. *Int J Pediatr Otorhinolaryngol.* 2011;75(9):1127–1131.

108. DeMarcantonio MA, Senser E, Meinzen-Derr J, Roetting N, Shott S, Ishman SL. The safety and efficacy of pediatric lingual tonsillectomy. *Int J Pediatr Otorhinolaryngol.* 2016;91:6–10.

109. Ulualp S. Outcomes of tongue base reduction and lingual tonsillectomy for residual pediatric obstructive sleep apnea after adenotonsillectomy. *Int Arch Otorhinolaryngol.* 2019;23(4):e415–e421.

110. Propst EJ, Amin R, Talwar N, Zaman M, Zweerink A, Blaser S, Zaarour C, Luginbuehl I, Karsli C, Aziza A, Forrest C, Drake J, Narang I. Midline posterior glossectomy and lingual tonsillectomy in obese and nonobese children with Down syndrome: Biomarkers for success. *Laryngoscope.* 2016;127(3):757–763.

111. Lin HS, Rowley JA, Badr MS, Folbe AJ, Yoo GH, Victor L, Mathog RH, Chen W. Transoral robotic surgery for treatment

112. Thottam PJ, Govil N, Duvvuri U, Mehta D. Transoral robotic surgery for sleep apnea in children: Is it effective? *Int J Pediatr Otorhinolaryngol.* 2015;79(12):2234–2237.

113. Montevecchi F, Bellini C, Meccariello G, Hoff PT, Dinelli E, Dallan I, Corso RM, Vicini C. Transoral robotic-assisted tongue base resection in pediatric obstructive sleep apnea syndrome: Case presentation, clinical and technical consideration. *Eur Arch Otorhinolaryngol.* 2016;274(2):1161–1166.

114. Camacho M, Noller MW, Zaghi S, Reckley LK, Fernandez-Salvador C, Ho E, Dunn B, Chan D. Tongue surgeries for pediatric obstructive sleep apnea: A systematic review and meta-analysis. *Eur Arch Otorhinolaryngol.* 2017;274(8):2981–2990.

115. Thevasagayam M, Rodger K, Cave D, Witmans M, El-Hakim H. Prevalence of laryngomalacia in children presenting with sleep-disordered breathing. *Laryngoscope.* 2010;120(8):1662–1666.

116. Digoy GP, Shukry M, Stoner JA. Sleep apnea in children with laryngomalacia: Diagnosis via sedated endoscopy and objective outcomes after supraglottoplasty. *Otolaryngol Head Neck Surg.* 2012;147(3):544–550.

117. Chan DK. Supraglottoplasty for occult laryngomalacia to improve obstructive sleep apnea syndrome. *Arch Otolaryngol Head Neck Surg.* 2012;138(1):50.

118. Camacho M, Dunn B, Torre C, Sasaki J, Gonzales R, Liu SYC, Chan DK, Certal V, Cable BB. Supraglottoplasty for laryngomalacia with obstructive sleep apnea: A systematic review and meta-analysis. *Laryngoscope.* 2015;126(5):1246–1255.

119. Farhood Z, Ong AA, Nguyen SA, Gillespie MB, Discolo CM, White DR. Objective outcomes of supraglottoplasty for children with laryngomalacia and obstructive sleep apnea: A meta-analysis. *JAMA Otolaryngol Head Neck Surg.* 2016;142(7):665–671.

120. Strollo Jr PJ, Soose RJ, Maurer JT, de Vries N, Cornelius J, Froymovich O, Hanson RD, Padhya TA, Steward DL, Gillespie MB, Woodson BT, Van de Heyning PH, Goetting MG, Vanderveken OM, Feldman N, Knaack L, Strohl KP, STAR Trial Group. Upper-airway stimulation for obstructive sleep apnea. *N Engl J Med.* 2014;370(2):139–149.

121. Diercks GR, Wentland C, Keamy D, Kinane TB, Skotko B, de Guzman V, Grealish E, Dobrowski J, Soose R, Hartnick CJ. Hypoglossal nerve stimulation in adolescents with Down syndrome and obstructive sleep apnea. *JAMA Otolaryngol Head Neck Surg.* 2017;144(1):37–42.

122. Caloway CL, Diercks GR, Keamy D, de Guzman V, Soose R, Raol N, Shott SR, Ishman SL, Hartnick CJ. Update on hypoglossal nerve stimulation in children with Down syndrome and obstructive sleep apnea. *Laryngoscope.* 2020;130(4):E263–E267.

123. Stenerson ME, Yu PK, Kinane TB, Skotko BG, Hartnick CJ. Long-term stability of hypoglossal nerve stimulation for the treatment of obstructive sleep apnea in children with Down syndrome. *Int J Pediatr Otorhinolaryngol.* 2021;149:110868.

124. Sidman JD, Sampson D, Templeton B. Distraction osteogenesis of the mandible for airway obstruction in children. *Laryngoscope.* 2001;111(7):1137–1146.

125. Breugem CC, Logjes RJH, Nolte JW, Flores RL. Advantages and disadvantages of mandibular distraction in Robin sequence. *Semin Fetal Neonatal Med.* 2021;26(6):101283.

126. Noller MW, Guilleminault C, Gouveia CJ, Mack D, Neighbors CL, Zaghi S, Camacho M. Mandibular advancement for

pediatric obstructive sleep apnea: A systematic review and meta-analysis. *J Craniomaxillofac Surg.* 2018;46(8):1296–1302.

127. Camacho M, Certal V, Brietzke SE, Holty JEC, Guilleminault C, Capasso R. Tracheostomy as treatment for adult obstructive sleep apnea. *Laryngoscope.* 2013;124(3):803–811.

128. Rizzi CJ, Amin JD, Isaiah A, Valdez TA, Jeyakumar A, Smart SE, Pereira KD. Tracheostomy for severe pediatric obstructive

sleep apnea: Indications and outcomes. *Otolaryngol Head Neck Surg.* 2017;157(2):309–313.

129. Fray S, Biello A, Kwan J, Kram YA, Lu K, Camacho M. Tracheostomy for paediatric obstructive sleep apnoea: A systematic review. *J Laryngol Otol.* 2018;132(8):680–684.

36

Sleep Disordered Breathing: A Dental Perspective

Kevin Lynn Boyd and Stephen H. Sheldon

CHAPTER HIGHLIGHTS

- Obstructive sleep apnea (OSA) is a chronic respiratory disorder that is linked to narrow and retrognathic skeletal malocclusions involving the hyoid bone, the base of the tongue, and its supporting musculature near the posterior pharynx.
- Anthropologists believe that the shrinking human craniofacial volume over the past 300 years or so predisposes to a higher likelihood of developing OSA.
- Pediatric dentistry and sleep clinicians collaborate in the management of children with extremely severe OSA, or with special health care needs who might be at even higher risk for developing OSA, such as patients diagnosed with Pierre Robin sequence, Down, Crouzon, Apert's, and Treacher Collins syndromes.
- For extremely severe cases of OSA, for which adenotonsillar surgery may not be sufficient treatment, a pediatric dentistry professional may get involved as maxillomandibular advancement surgery and/or tracheostomy placement may be considered as better surgical options.
- Recognition of known dentofacial risk indicators of OSA in early childhood can help pediatric healthcare professionals best collaborate on diagnosis and management

Introduction

In 1921 at the annual meeting of the American Academy of Dental Science held in Boston, Harvard orthodontist, Le Roy Johnson, DMD, ScD, delivered a paper titled "The Diagnosis of Malocclusion with Reference to Early Treatment." Therein Dr. Johnson opined, "The face has evolved with the functions of mastication and respiration. The perversion of either or both of these functions will result in some degree of modification of the structure of the jaws. This is the law of biology."[1] The dual facial responsibilities of chewing and breathing to which Dr. Johnson had referred as having *evolved* in *Homo sapiens* implies that each of these functions are essential survival, thriving and ability to pass on their genes (i.e., achieve evolutionary fitness). In the late 19th and early 20th centuries, discussions like this regarding biologic evolution, via the Darwinian-proposed mechanism of *natural selection*, were not uncommon in medical and dental circles as they helped explain not only how our species had evolved over deep geologic time, but also how and why we are still vulnerable to so many communicable and noncommunicable diseases (NCDs). With their 1981 publication *Western Diseases: Their Emergence and Prevention*,[1] authors Hugh Trowell and Denis Burkitt essentially launched a new paradigm in medical education now commonly referred to as *evolutionary medicine* (EM), also known as *Darwinian medicine*.[2] This new EM educational paradigm is clearly defining a novel and useful framework for allied health care professionals to better understand modern systemic diseases, also commonly referred to as *Western diseases*, *diseases of civilization*, or hereinafter referred to as *chronic and noncommunicable diseases* (CNCDs), from an *evolutionary* perspective; the EM framework has already led to several medical textbooks, peer-reviewed publications, didactic curriculum courses, and research investigations aimed at ultimately producing better health outcomes for patients.[3–6] Many CNCDs are best understood when viewed from an evolutionary perspective rather than from the more common vantage point of *proximate causality*. For example, the most likely proximate cause of a fever would be an assumed systemic invasion of bloodborne pathogens, whereas an evolutionary explanation of the fever mechanism per se would require a basic understanding of how the Darwinian framework of *natural selection* can enhance an organism's *evolutionary fitness* (ability to survive and reproduce) potential. As healthy circadian sleep cycling during childhood would have been necessary for achieving optimal *evolutionary fitness* for *Homo sapiens* over the vast time span of human evolutionary history,[7] severe sleep-disordered breathing (SDB) disorders such as obstructive sleep apnea (OSA), had likely not been a part of the human experience until fairly recently, and thus can be appropriately categorized as CNCDs.

Evolutionary oral medicine (EOM), or Darwinian dentistry, describes how EM principles can be applied to exploring the evolutionary basis of modern dental and craniofacial diseases, such as dental caries, periodontal disease, and malocclusion. For example, one proposed explanation by EM/EOM proponents for why humans have only *recently* begun to become vulnerable to many modern diseases, such as type 2 diabetes and dentofacial malocclusion (DFM), is the so-called *mismatch* hypothesis,[8] which postulates that current high prevalences of CNCDs in *culturally industrialized* populations are due, at least in part, to exposure to modernized feeding strategies that are increasingly reliant upon lifelong consumption of overly processed foods; and changed environmental conditions that are vastly dissimilar, or *mismatched* to the Paleolithic/preagricultural diets and environments to which the human genome has been best adapted.[9]

Pediatric SDB is a pathologic condition associated with a wide range of clinical symptoms, medical history data, dentofacial physical examination findings, environmental components, and genetic and epigenetic factors. Recently published controlled studies indicate a close association between pediatric SDB/OSA, neurocognitive impairments such as attention-deficit disorder, attention-deficit/hyperactivity disorder, and other behavioral disorders.[10,11] Certain DFM traits within the craniofacial complex, such as maxillary transverse deficiency, mandibular retrusion, and deep palatal vaults, can negatively affect optimal functioning of the hard and soft tissues of the intimately connected respiratory complex, which are collectively referred to as the craniofacial respiratory complex (CFRC; Fig. 36.1) and are

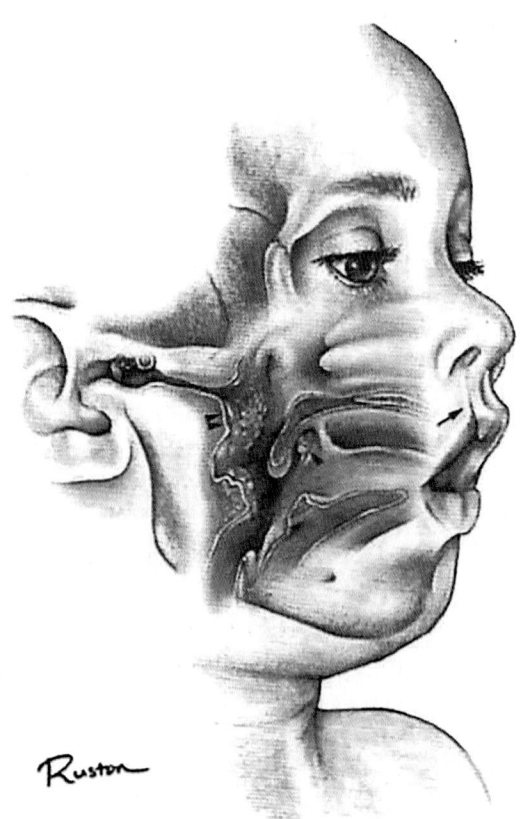

• **Fig. 36.1** The craniofacial and respiratory complex.

frequently associated with a high prevalence of pediatric SDB/OSA comorbidities. The comorbid association of various pediatric SDB/OSA behavioral traits and specific malocclusion phenotypes is also well described.[12,13]

Many CFRC characteristics are for the most part alterable during the early childhood stages of craniofacial and respiratory complex growth and development. As suboptimal development of the CFRC can often play an important role in the presence or absence of clinical symptoms associated with pediatric SDB/OSA and its associated clinical morbidities, dental professionals who provide services for infants, preschoolers, and young children (general dentists, pediatric dentists, dental hygienists, orofacial myofunctional therapists, and orthodontists) are absolutely essential in helping identify and treat these vulnerable children. Accordingly, the role of the child-focused dental professional as an integral member of every child's comprehensive health care team has never been more important.[14]

Etiology of Malocclusion

Anthropologic studies confirm that dentofacial malocclusion (poorly aligned jaws and teeth), a frequent comorbidity of SDB/OSA,[15] was infrequently suffered by our pre-*industrial* ancestors, and seldom occurs with frequency in extant non-*Westernized* aboriginal cultures.[16] In fact, skeletal malocclusion did not appear appreciably in humans until around the time of the *Industrial Revolution* of the mid-18th century in Great Britain, Western Europe, and North America,[17] and wherever occasionally observed before that era, it was usually confined to royalty, nobility, and other privileged-class individuals.[18]

To most efficiently address the health problems known to be associated with untreated and/or *inappropriately* treated DFM, it would first be helpful to have some idea about why our ancient, and also fairly recent, ancestors seldom suffered from these unpleasant dental, facial, and skeletal disharmonies. Anthropologists have long understood that human craniofacial volume has been steadily diminishing since around the time of the agricultural revolution some 10,000–12,000 years ago, and most rapidly over the past 350–400 years since the origins of global *cultural industrialization*. Although there seems to be a definite observable secular trend toward higher prevalences of DFM over the last three to four centuries, to date there is not yet firm consensus among dental anthropologists as to precisely *what happened;* but there does seem to be a growing body of evidence to suggest that feeding behaviors during infancy and early childhood are likely involved.[19] Specifically, *ancestral* patterns of breastfeeding and weaning are known to be protective against certain forms of malocclusion,[20] likely because of the physical challenges posed to the developing hard and soft tissues of the interconnected palatal and facial sutural complexes during infancy and early childhood; furthermore, the highly processed/soft baby foods and artificial infant formulas delivered through bottles with artificial nipples that are in so much use today were simply not readily available to children before the Industrial Revolution.

With ever accumulating physical evidence from anthropologic studies, combined with advances in the newly emerging scientific disciplines of sleep medicine, epigenetics, and EM, it can be stated with a reasonable degree of scientific certainty that DFM is *not* primarily a *genetically predetermined* disease entity, but rather, it would be better described as a Western diseases (WD) that is primarily modulated through a epigenetic (gene–environment) interaction that follows a fairly predictable pattern of pathologic progression: initially, most WDs are *preventable* so long as genetically predisposed individuals are identified before early expression of the disease is obvious, and where feasible, are allowed to thrive in a healthful nurturing environment; next, WDs can be *reversible*, but only in the very early stages of disease expression, and only when the precipitating environmental pressures (e.g., unhealthy eating, SDB) have been eliminated; subsequently, in cases where a WD has advanced beyond reversibility, it can still be *treated* with accurate diagnosis and appropriate therapeutic measures (e.g., dietary changes, pharmaceuticals, and medical interventions) if the disease state is not too far advanced; and finally, advanced end-stage WDs can be debilitating and sometimes even *fatal* if not accurately identified, reversed, and/or appropriately controlled.

Whereas a *causal* relationship between DFM and the pathophysiology of SDB/OSA has not yet been shown to be fully supportable,[21] a co-relationship does indeed appear to exist between the two disease entities. Similar to what is now understood about why diabetes and periodontal disease often coexist in the same host,[22] the underlying mechanism connecting SDB/OSA and DFM is more likely to be a *bidirectional* one rather than a unilateral *cause-and-effect* relationship. Simply stated, sometimes measures aimed at preventing the initiation and early progression of one disease entity might very well aid in preventing the initiation and early progression of another comorbid disease entity. Given that many DFM phenotypes might also sometimes portend increased risk for developing SDB/OSA behavioral traits, it seems fairly obvious that measures aimed at prevention, reversal, and/or adequate treatment of DFM might also help preclude the negative health outcomes that are often associated with SDB/OSA.

Pediatric Oral Health and Sleep

Dentists who treat children are uniquely positioned to identify patients who might be at increased risk for SDB/OSA. Due in part to the successful implementation of the American Academy of Pediatrics and American Academy of Pediatric Dentistry's (AAPD) joint effort to assure that all children establish a *dental home* by the age of 1 year,[23] pediatric dentists now have a higher frequency of patient encounters than do most other allied health professionals. Additionally, postgraduate specialty training programs in pediatric dentistry purposefully prepare clinicians for identifying and appropriately treating in earliest childhood when indicated, nonsyndromic patients with interferences

to normal dentofacial development, and children with special health care needs who might be at even higher risk for developing OSA, such as patients diagnosed with Pierre Robin sequence, Down, Crouzon, Apert's, and Treacher Collins syndromes.

During dental visits, many warning signs that a child might be experiencing sleep disturbances can be ascertained from both a thorough oral–medical health history interview with parents/primary caregivers and a comprehensive clinical dentofacial examination. To best assure a comfortable and safe dental visit, questions usually asked during a detailed pediatric oral–medical health history interview are designed not only to obtain information about the child's overall dental/medical health status, but also to acquire information about dietary/feeding history and previous dental and/or medical encounters that might impact a child's possible expectations about the dental appointment. A typical list of questions asked might include "Was your child breastfed, and if so, for how long?" and "What beverage does your child typically drink when thirsty?"

Although not necessarily a component of a *typical* pediatric medical–dental health history, it is certainly easy, useful, and appropriate for dentists who treat children to incorporate into the parent/caregiver interview a short series of questions specifically designed to gain valuable information about a child's possible risks for both worsening malocclusion and SDB/OSA comorbidity. Some examples from the validated Pediatric Sleep Questionnaire[24] might include "Does your child grind his/her teeth at night?", "Is your child a noisy open-mouth breather and/or snorer during sleep?", "Does your child occasionally wet the bed?", "Does your child ever wake up with either a sore jaw, headache, dry mouth and/or sore legs?", "Is your child at a healthy weight?", and "Does your child have night terrors or nightmares?"

In addition to the detailed medical–dental health history interview, a comprehensive dentofacial clinical examination might yield warning signs that a child might be suffering from the impaired ability to breathe properly during sleep.

Surgical Versus Nonsurgical Treatment Options for Pediatric SDB/OSA

It is well established that surgical removal of the tonsils and/or adenoids is the most common first-line treatment considered the gold standard intervention for pediatric OSA. For extremely severe cases of OSA for which adenotonsillar (A/T) surgery might not be indicated as the best treatment, maxillomandibular advancement surgery (MMA) and/or tracheostomy placement are on occasion considered as better surgical options. According to recently published guidelines by the American Academy of Otolaryngology,[25] craniofacial *abnormalities*, which are often comorbid with the aforementioned syndromic (i.e., genetically modulated) conditions, but are also frequently associated as maldevelopments of the maxilla and mandible in nonsyndromic children, are definite indications for recommending a polysomnographic (PSG) sleep study before A/T, MMA, or tracheostomy surgical procedure.

Constrictive maldevelopments (CMs; i.e., hypoplasias of the maxilla, mandible, and face) are common craniofacial abnormalities that can play an important role in the bidirectional relationship between malocclusion and OSA.[26] CMs that often are comorbid malocclusion phenotypes with SDB/OSA typically include narrow/deep-vaulted palate (Fig. 36.2), tapered dental arches, and retroposition of the mandible, maxilla, and/or mid-face relative to the anterior cranial base. Per the various comorbidities associated with various surgical interventions, wherever feasible, collaborative efforts aimed at preventing and treating pediatric OSA nonsurgically should be given the highest consideration.

Two commonly implemented *nonsurgical* medical interventions include inhaled nasal corticosteroids, usage of continuous (CPAP) and bi-level positive airway pressure (BPAP) devices and less invasive orofacial myofunctional therapy (OMT).[25,26] Although correctly classified as a nonsurgical treatment option, long-term usage of CPAP/BPAP facial masks can markedly reduce mid-facial development potential in growing children[27] in much the same manner as adult orthognathic surgical reduction procedures such as mandibular setback, and subapical anterior maxillary segmental osteotomy to treat so-called maxillary protrusion.

Silver and Bishara found in two separate studies[28,29] that when class II malocclusion is first detected within the deciduous dentition, as is also the case with deciduous maxillary transverse deficiency (MTD), it will always persist beyond if left untreated (i.e., it will not self-correct); furthermore, McNamara et al.[30] described class II malocclusion in the mixed dentition as most always a problem of mandibular retrusion and rarely as having a maxillary protrusive phenotype. Other common examples of nonsurgical prevention and treatment options for pediatric OSA include myofunctional training oral appliances (e.g., Infant Trainers, Myo-Munchees), adjunctive dietary counseling for overweight and obese OSA patients, functional orthodontic mandibular advancement appliances (e.g., Bionator, MARA, Twin Block and Herbst appliances), rapid maxillary expansion (RME) appliances (e.g., ALF, quad-helix appliances, bonded Schwartz Plate, Hyrax) with or without reverse pull maxillary protraction appliances (MPA) (e.g., Delaire face mask), and more recently, orthotropic postural appliances that are capable of nonsurgically increasing transverse and sagittal posterior airway dimensions through sequential advancement of both the mandible *and* maxilla with a series of removable acrylic mouthpieces.

Until the recognition of orthotropic strategies as a nonsurgical option for improving posterior airway volume in

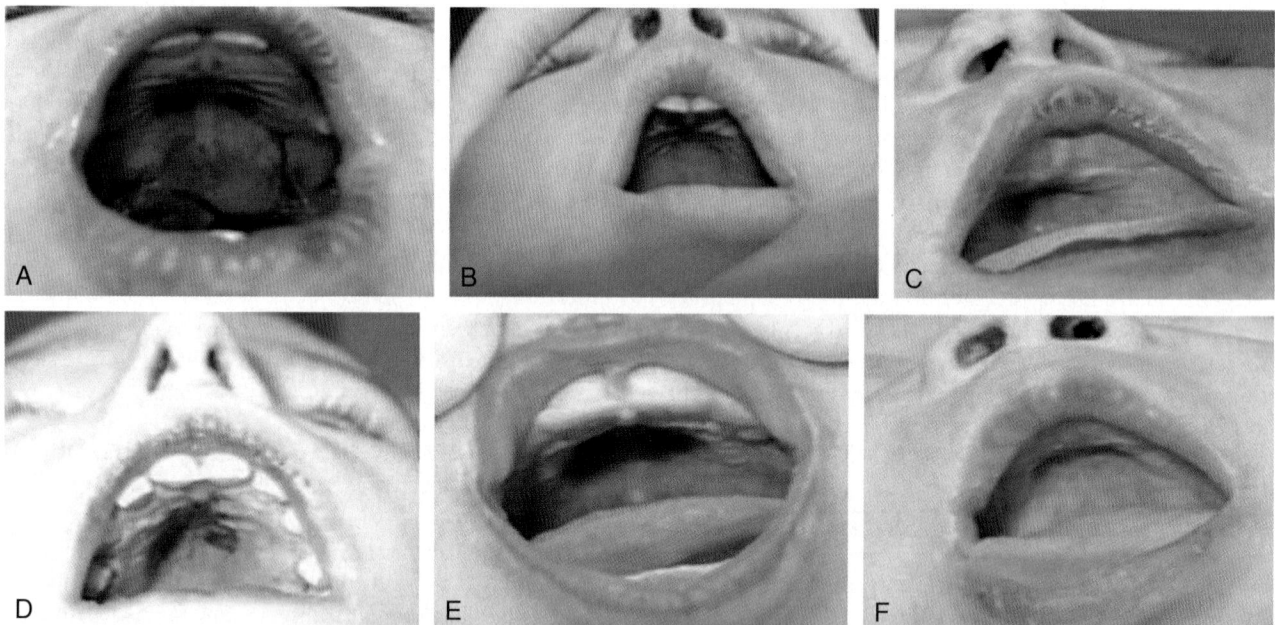

• **Fig. 36.2** Montage of abnormal high and narrow hard palate in Cases 1–6. Note that all children present a visually recognizable abnormal high and narrow hard palate that is related to the development of the nasomaxillary complex during embryonic development considering age of children. On the first row on the left, on the second row in both cases, and on the third row from the top on the right, note the abnormal noses presented by the patients. The asymmetry of the nostril may not be obvious at first investigation; using photographs taken below the nose may help performing better analyses. Asymmetrical opening is often associated with asymmetrical septum and change in nasal resistance. When associated with high palatal vault, they indicate presence of a higher upper airway resistance and greater risk of abnormal breathing during sleep with addition of infectious or inflammatory reaction. (From Rambaud C, Guilleminault C. Death, Nasomaxillary complex, and sleep in young children. *Eur J Pediatr.* 2012;171(9):1349-1358, with permission of Springer-Verlag 2012.)

actively growing children,[32] RME was considered the primary nonsurgical orthodontic/dentofacial orthopedic adjunctive treatment strategy of choice for treating SDB/OSA in children.[31]

RME is well established as an effective nonsurgical treatment option for decreasing upper airway resistance through increasing airway volumes within the nasomaxillary complex.[32,33] Depending on the age of the patient, by exerting orthopedic forces upon the entire maxillary suture complex, primarily with the use of fixed maxillary expansion appliances, RME orthopedic movement will occur when the relatively light forces applied to the teeth and the maxillary alveolar process eventually exceed the forces required for orthodontic tooth movement alone. After RME, there is usually a detectable decrease in nasal resistance, which is often best described as a treatment effect due to an increase in the transverse width of the nasal cavity and hard palate, most notably at the floor of the nose near the mid-palatal suture. However, there is increasing evidence that describes an additional nasorespiratory advantage often gained from transverse expansion of the maxilla in growing children; Linder-Aronson and Woodside[34] describe how the sagittal depth volume of the boney nasopharynx can often increase in conjunction with RME (Fig. 36.3). Whether or not this observed nasopharyngeal depth volume increase is indeed an RME treatment effect is somewhat controversial in that some argue, although indeed an observable phenomenon, quite possibly it could be attributable to inconsistencies due to non-standardization of patient positioning during acquisition of radiographic images (e.g., head inclination, tongue posture, breathing and swallowing movements, etc.).[35]

In cases where the narrow maxillary arch is also retrognathic (relative to the anterior cranial base and/or the mandible), RME can be assisted by reverse-pull headgear (e.g., Delaire face mask) to provide additional nasal airway volume through increasing the anterior dimension of the nasorespiratory space.[36]

A key participant at the 2012 NESCent Catalysis Conference, Professor Robert Corruccini, a dental anthropologist from Southern Illinois University, was recently cited in *Science*:[37] "As for malocclusion and jaw disorders, Corruccini noted that a branch of evolutionary dentistry has emerged in which children do mouth exercises and wear devices that put stronger force on their growing jaws." The branch that Professor Corruccini was referring to is called orthotropics. The orthotropic premise was originally developed in England in the late 1950s by Dr. John Mew, a dual-trained oral surgeon–orthodontist, as an alternative to the then and still commonly held belief that malocclusion is primarily a genetically predetermined inheritable condition. Mew, also a student of anthropology, studied ancient skulls at the Natural History Museum in London where he was further convinced that malocclusion is an environmentally influenced CNCD that had been brought about by factors related to environmental circumstances commonly associated with intensification of cultural industrialization. Specifically, the orthotropic premise implicitly states that improper resting and active tongue and head posture will invariably lead to malocclusion and other associated negative systemic health outcomes.

United by their common focus aimed at assuring optimal dentofacial growth potential and healthy wake–sleep nasorespiratory ability for their young and growing patients, the *supply* of pediatric health care professionals, (e.g., orthodontists, pediatric dentists, general dentists, OMTs, Sleep Medicine physicians, otolaryngologists, etc.) who are recommending earlier orthodontic and dentofacial orthopedic treatment interventions as a viable non-surgical intervention for patients, is unfortunately disproportional to the ever increasing *demand for these essential services*.

The orthotropic system uses a series of acrylic intraoral appliances to first develop the maxilla and mid-face to its optimal width and forward position underneath the anterior cranial base, after which the mandible is *postured* forward with a subsequent acrylic appliance to reunite both jaws to a

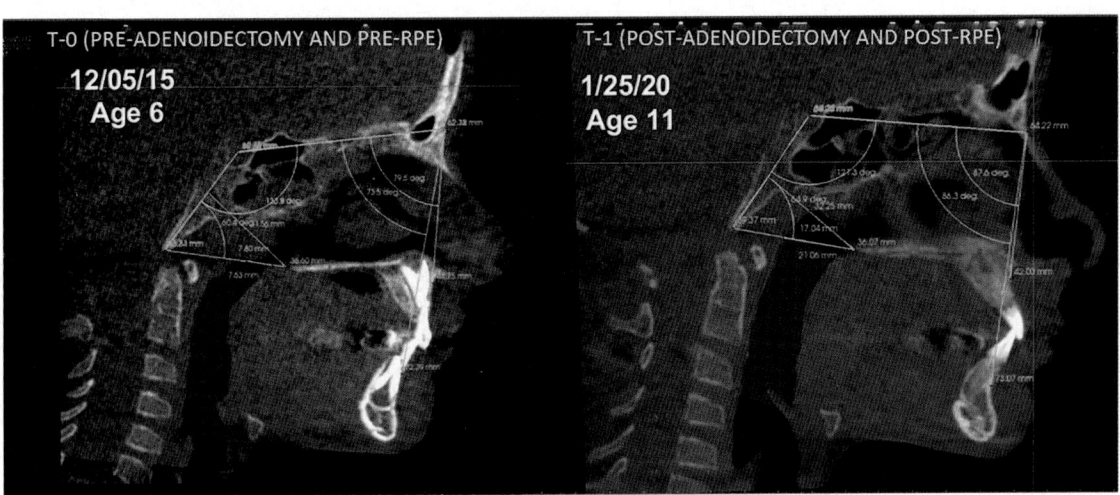

• **Fig. 36.3** pre tx (T-0 LEFT) Image of narrow saggittal depth of the bony nasopharynx (Ad-1 /Ad-2) post tx (T-1 RIGHT) Image of expanded saggittal depth of the bony nasopharynx (Ad-1 /Ad-2)

more forward post-treatment position. This maximally forwarded facial and jaw position provides not only for better esthetics and facial balance, but is also more conducive to development of increased posterior pharyngeal volume and less nasal airway resistance.

As previously mentioned, there are many other more traditional types of orthodontic/dentofacial orthopedic mandibular advancing-type appliances, such as Frankel's, Harvold Activators, Orthopedic Correctors, class II elastics, and others, all of which attempt to do the same thing, but most of these appliances are often only begun in the late-mixed to early adult dentition and can exert a retrusive (backward) force, or *headgear effect*, on the growing maxilla that can actually worsen esthetic appearance and/or an already compromised airway.

Orthotropic strategies differ mainly from conventional orthodontic treatment modalities in that they: (1) do not use treatment mechanics that place retrusive forces on the jaws, teeth, and face; (2) are usually begun in the primary or

early mixed dentition when maximum impact upon a child's nasorespiratory competence and neurologic, craniofacial, and somatic growth are most easily accomplished; and (3) often in conjunction with OMT regimens, which are chiefly designed to create a lifelong optimum oral environment for a properly postured and functioning tongue, which is also conducive to lifelong stable and well-aligned adult teeth.

Biobloc as an alternative to mandibular distraction surgery for severe OSA: case report. The case study described below is a good illustration of how Biobloc Orthotropic (BBO) can be used as a safe nonsurgical alternative to mandibular distraction osteogenesis for severe OSA. Note the improved cervical spine posture and posterior airway volume seen at the end of BBO Tx (Fig. 36.4) and the supportive PSG result. At baseline (Ba) (Fig. 36.5), the apnea-hypopnea index (AHI) was elevated at 12.4 events per hour of sleep, with the majority of events occurring during rapid eye movement (REM) sleep. Over the course of time, the AHI and REM AHI both decreased steadily, to a degree that at

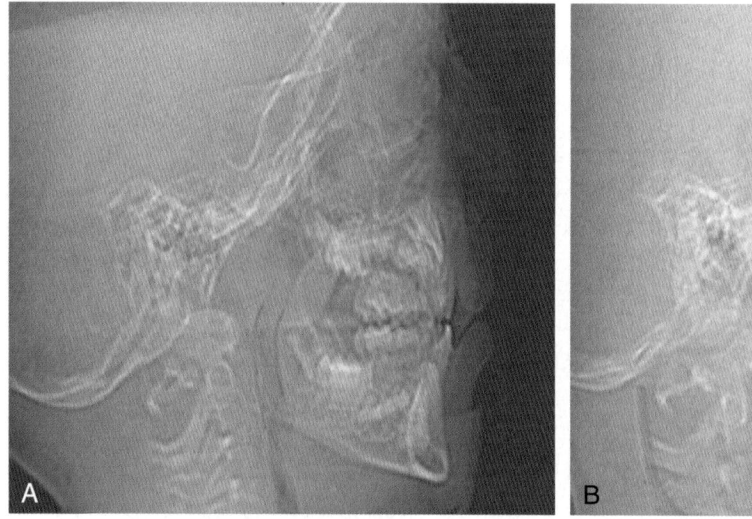
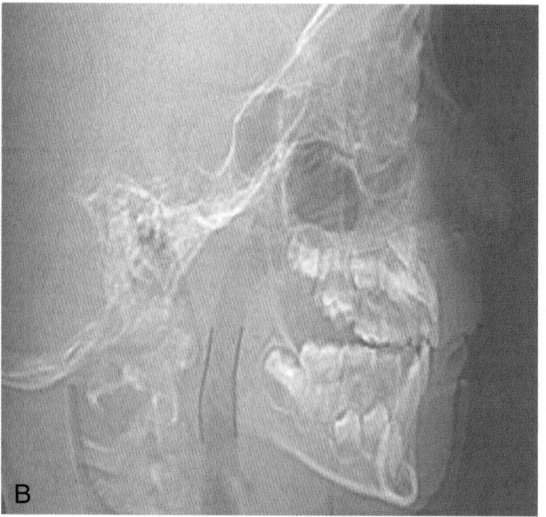

• **Fig. 36.4** Note differences in cervical spine erectness and posterior airway area in pre-BBO Tx image *(left)* vs. post-BBO Tx image *(right)*.

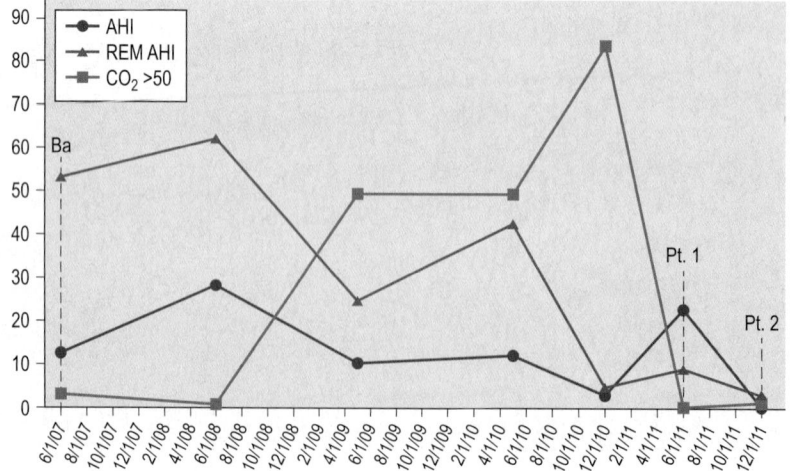

• **Fig. 36.5** Longitudinal polysomnograph assessment comparing the patient's AHI, REM AHI, and CO_2 levels as BBO treatment progresses.

point 1 on the graph the AHI was only 3 events per hour of sleep. Interestingly, as treatment continued from baseline and as the AHI fell, there was a concomitant increase in $ETCO_2$ with a peak when the AHI reached only 3 events per hour. Interpretation of these findings was initially difficult because there was numerical improvement in the frequency of occlusive and partially occlusive respiratory events, but apparent worsening of gas exchange exemplified by increasing obstructive hypoventilation. Etiology of elevation of CO_2 and presence of obstructive hypoventilation related to presumptive development of extremely prolonged partially occlusive respiratory events. For example, if each hypopnea lasted 20 minutes and they were continuously periodic, the

AHI will be only 3 events per hour of sleep despite persistence of partial upper airway obstruction. At point 2 at the end of the graph, AHI continued to fall to its nadir of 0.2 events per hour of sleep with concurrent decrease in CO_2 levels to normal and resolution of obstructive hypoventilation. At the same time, there was clear clinical evidence of improvement in symptoms with absence of snoring, resolution of restless sleep, and resolution of daytime sleepiness. At this point, based on both clinical resolution and polysomnographic evidence, SDB had resolved. Continued follow-up is still warranted and required to assure resolution. One final polysomnogram will be conducted to provide objective evidence.

Summary and Future Considerations

1. OSA is a chronic respiratory disorder that is clearly linked to narrow and retrognathic skeletal malocclusions that force the hyoid bone, base of the tongue, and its supporting musculature near to the posterior pharynx. Given what anthropologists have shown with regard to shrinking human craniofacial volume over the past 300 years or so, currently accepted cephalometric normative values are not completely reflective of our true genomic craniofacial growth potential. As a result of this disparity, many clinicians are currently being trained to diagnose, treat, and evaluate orthodontic treatment progress and final outcomes in accordance with cephalometric norms that are *anthropologically uniformed*, especially with regard to the baseline assessment of maxillary position relative to the anterior cranial base; this is potentially dangerous as this error can sometimes lead to diagnostic and treatment failures that in turn can have negative overall health implications related to inadequate posterior airway volume (e.g., cervical-pull headgear treatment and incisor retraction exacerbating already compromised posterior airway volume in class II retrognathic patients).[38,39] Cooperative efforts between anthropologists, dentists, and other concerned health care professionals should be undertaken to revise currently used cephalometric standards so as to better reflect the true forward growth potential of the human dentofacial complex.
2. Medical and dental educational programs should incorporate more cross-disciplinary/cross-curriculum activities and include evidence-based content into their teaching curriculums within the disciplines of EM, sleep medicine, orofacial myology, and nutrition and dietetics.
3. Overconsumption of sugar and other refined (fermentable) carbohydrates are clearly implicated in recent increases in nationwide prevalences of both early

childhood caries (ECC)[40] and childhood obesity.[41,42] Given that childhood obesity[43] and pain associated with untreated caries[44] are both known risk factors associated with fragmented sleep, it seems reasonable to suggest that medical and dental professionals should implement diet counseling as an adjunctive component to their existing preventive and therapeutic treatment protocols.
4. Orthodontists, pediatric dentists, general dentists, and orofacial myofunctional therapists should collaborate with other allied pediatric health care professionals efforts to raise awareness among themselves and their patients about the importance of early recognition of pediatric patients who might be at risk for SDB/OSA.
5. Guidelines for identifying SDB/OSA dentofacial risk indicators should be established and disseminated to all members of the allied pediatric health care team.

Future well-designed and controlled retrospective, observational, and prospective trials will be necessary to validate existing scientific and circumstantial evidence that early childhood feeding environments, dentofacial development, nasorespiratory competence, pediatric sleep hygiene, and neurocognitive development are interrelated. When indicated by the presence of multiple medical and/or dentofacial risk indicators for SDB/OSA, orthodontists, pediatric dentists, and general dentists will need to be properly trained to deliver effective nonsurgical modes of oral interventions and be willing and able to intervene or refer for appropriate screening (e.g., polysomnography) and/or treatment while children are still in their primary dentitions. Pediatric sleep medicine centers should have at least one dentist on their team who is experienced in dentofacial issues related to SDB/OSA. New methods for earlier detection of children at risk for SDB/OSA, such as in utero 3D ultrasonography facial imaging, should continually be explored.

CLINICAL PEARLS

- An increased emphasis on identifying malocclusion as more of a *symptom* rather than as a distinct disease entity can help medical and dental clinicians better understand and appreciate the interrelatedness between malocclusion and SDB/OSA. Evaluating SDB/OSA and malocclusion from an evolutionary perspective helps clarify that, similar to other *Western diseases* such as type 2 diabetes, susceptible individuals need not fully express the disease phenotype if environmental triggers are identified and eliminated early in a child's life.
- The ability to recognize known dentofacial risk indicators of SDB/OSA in early childhood can help dentists, physicians, and other allied health professionals better collaborate in providing comprehensive and coordinated care for their mutual patients.
- Both childhood obesity (CO) and pain from untreated early childhood caries (ECC) are known risk factors for SDB/OSA that can negatively impact sleep quality and quantity. As overconsumption of commercially processed fermentable carbohydrates in early childhood is a known etiologic component of both CO and ECC, dentists and physicians should discourage unhealthy snacking on simple sugars and starches as a component of their CO, ECC, and SDB/OSA prevention and treatment protocols.
- As breastfeeding is known to be protective against the development of SDB/OSA, adenotonsillar hypertrophy, and malocclusion, dentists and physicians should mutually provide consistent and accurate advice to parents regarding options for infant and early childhood feeding regimens.

References

1. Trowell HC, Burkitt DP. *Western Diseases: Their Emergence and Prevention.* Harvard University Press; 1981.
2. Nesse R, Williams GC. The dawn of Darwinian medicine. *Q Rev Biol.* 1991;66(1):1–22.
3. Gluckman P, Hanson M. *Mismatch: Why Our World No Longer Fits Our Bodies.* Oxford University Press; 2006.
4. Cordain L, Eaton SB, Sebastian A, et al. Origins and evolution of the Western diet: health implications for the 21st century. *Am J Clin Nutr.* 2005;81:341–354.
5. Beebe DW, Rausch J, Byars KC, et al. Persistent snoring in preschool children: predictors and behavioral and developmental correlates. *Pediatrics.* 2012;130:382–389.
6. Bonuck K, Freeman K, Chervin RD, et al. Sleep-disordered breathing in a population-based cohort: behavioral outcomes at 4 and 7 years. *Pediatrics.* 2012;129(4):1–9.
7. McNamara J. Influence of respiratory pattern on craniofacial growth. *Angle Orthodont.* 1981;51(4):269–300.
8. Zettergren-Wijk L, Linder-Aronson S, Nordlander B, et al. Longitudinal effect on facial growth after tonsillectomy in children with obstructive sleep apnea. *World J Orthodont.* 2002;3:67–72.
9. Hang W. Obstructive sleep apnea: dentistry's unique role in longevity enhancement. *J Am Orthod Assoc.* 2007;7(2):28–32.
10. Ruoff CM, Guilleminault C. Orthodontics and sleep-disordered breathing. *Sleep Breath.* 2012;16(2):271–273.
11. Flores-Mir C, Korayem M, Heo G, et al. Craniofacial morphological characteristics in children with obstructive sleep apnea syndrome: a systematic review and meta-analysis. *JADA.* 2013;144(3):269–277.
12. Price Weston A. Nutrition and Physical Degeneration; a Comparison of Primitive and Modern Diets and Their Effects. P.B. Hoeber; 1945.
13. Gilbert SF. Ecological developmental biology: developmental biology meets the real world. *Dev Biol.* 2001;2001(233):1–12.
14. Edelstein BL. Pediatric Dental-Focused Interprofessional Interventions: Rethinking Early Childhood Oral Health Management. *Dent Clin North Am.* 2017;61(3):589–606. https://doi.org/10.1016/j.cden.2017.02.005.
15. Boyd KL. Darwinian dentistry part 2: early childhood nutrition, dento-facial development and chronic disease. *J Am Orthodont Soc.* 2012;12(2):28–32.
16. Romero CC, Scavone-Junior H, Garib DG, et al. Breastfeeding and non-nutritive sucking patterns related to the prevalence of anterior open bite in primary dentition. *J Appl Oral Sci.* 2011;19(2):161–168.
17. Lavigne GJ. Dentofacial changes with orthopedic therapy. In: Lavigne GJ, Cistulli PA, Smith MT, eds. *Sleep Medicine for Dentists: A Practical Overview.* Quintessence Books; 2020:88–91.
18. Taylor GW. Bidirectional interrelationships between diabetes and periodontal diseases: an epidemiologic perspective. *Ann Periodontol.* 2001;6(1):99–112.
19. American Academy of Pediatrics Section on Pediatric Dentistry Oral health risk assessment timing and establishment of the dental home. *Pediatrics.* 2003;111(5):1113–1116.
20. Roland PS, Rosenfeld RM, Brooks LJ, et al. Clinical practice guideline: polysomnography for sleep-disordered breathing prior to tonsillectomy in children. *Otolaryngol Head Neck Surg.* 2012;145(1S):S1–S15.
21. Seto BH. Maxillary morphology in obstructive sleep apnoea syndrome. *Eur J Orthodont.* 2001;23(6):703–714.
22. Villa MP, Pagani J, Ambrosio R, et al. Mid-face hypoplasia after long-term nasal ventilation (LTE). *Am J Resp Crit Care Med.* 2002;166:1142.
23. Hang W, Singh D. Evaluation of the posterior airway space following bioblock therapy: geometric morphometrics. *J Craniomandib Pract.* 2002;25(2):84–89.
24. Timms DJ. The effect of rapid maxillary expansion of nasal airway resistance. *Br J Orthodont.* 1986;13:221–228.
25. Pirelli P, Saponara M, Guilleminault C. Rapid maxillary expansion in children with obstructive sleep apnea syndrome. *Sleep.* 2004;27(4):761–776.
26. Villa MP, Malagola C, Pagani J, et al. Rapid maxillary expansion in children with obstructive sleep apnea syndrome: 12-month follow-up. *Sleep Med.* 2007;8(2):128–134.
27. Yagci A, Uysal T, Usumez S, et al. Nonsurgical treatment of a class III malocclusion with maxillary skeletal retrusion using rapid maxillary expansion and reverse pull headgear. *Am J Orthod Dentofacial Orthop.* 1998;114(1):60–65.
28. SILVER EI. Forsyth orthodontic survey of untreated cases. *Am J Orthod Oral Surg.* 1944;42:103–127.

29. Bishara SE, Hoppens BJ, Jakobsen JR, Kohout FJ. Changes in the molar relationship between the deciduous and permanent dentitions: a longitudinal study. *Am J Orthod Dentofacial Orthop*. 1988;93(1):19–28. https://doi.org/10.1016/0889-5406(88)90189-8.

30. McNamara JA. Maxillary transverse deficiency. *Am J Orthod Dentofacial Orthop*. 2000;117(5):567–570. https://doi.org/10.1016/s0889-5406(00)70202-2.

31. Pirelli P, Saponara M, Guilleminault C. Rapid maxillary expansion in children with obstructive sleep apnea syndrome. *Sleep*. 2004;27(4):761–766. https://doi.org/10.1093/sleep/27.4.761.

32. Timms DJ. The Effect of Rapid Maxillary Expansion on Nasal Airway Resistance. *British Journal of Orthodontics*. 1986;13(4):221–228. https://doi:10.1179/bjo.13.4.221.

33. Yagci A, Uysal T, Usumez S, Orhan M. Effects of modified and conventional facemask therapies with expansion on dynamic measurement of natural head position in Class III patients. *Am J Orthod Dentofacial Orthop*. 2011;140(5):e223–e231. https://doi.org/10.1016/j.ajodo.2011.05.018.

34. Woodside DG, Linder-Aronson S, Lundstrom A, McWilliam J. Mandibular and maxillary growth after changed mode of breathing. *Am J Orthod Dentofacial Orthop*. 1991;100(1):1–18. https://doi.org/10.1016/0889-5406(91)70044-W.

35. Ribeiro AN, de Paiva JB, Rino-Neto J, Illipronti-Filho E, Trivino T, Fantini SM. Upper airway expansion after rapid maxillary expansion evaluated with cone beam computed tomography. *Angle Orthod*. 2012;82(3):458–463. https://doi.org/10.2319/030411-157.1.

36. Boyd KL, Sheldon SH. *Sleep Disorder Breathing: A Dental Perspective. Principles and Practice of Pediatric Sleep Medicine*. Second Edition. Elsevier Inc; 2012:275–280. https://doi.org/10.1016/B978-1-4557-0318-0.00034-6.

37. Gibbons A. Evolutionary biology. An evolutionary theory of dentistry. *Science*. 2012;336(6084):973–975. https://doi.org/10.1126/science.336.6084.973.

38. Savoldi F, Massetti F, Tsoi JKH, et al. Anteroposterior length of the maxillary complex and its relationship with the anterior cranial base. *Angle Orthod*. 2021;91(1):88–97. https://doi.org/10.2319/020520-82.1.

39. Wang Q, Jia P, Anderson NK, Wang L, Lin J. Changes of pharyngeal airway size and hyoid bone position following orthodontic treatment of Class I bimaxillary protrusion. *Angle Orthod*. 2012;82(1):115–121. https://doi.org/10.2319/011011-13.1.

40. Ludwig DS, Peterson KE, Gortmaker SL. Relation between consumption of sugar-sweetened drinks and childhood obesity: a prospective, observational analysis. *Lancet (London, England)*. 2001;357(9255):505–508. https://doi.org/10.1016/S0140-6736(00)04041-1.

41. Hujoel P. Dietary carbohydrates and dental-systemic diseases. *J Dent Res*. 2009;88(6):490–502. https://doi.org/10.1177/0022034509337700.

42. Lustig RH, Mulligan K, Noworolski SM, et al. Isocaloric fructose restriction and metabolic improvement in children with obesity and metabolic syndrome. *Obesity (Silver Spring)*. 2016;24(2):453–460. https://doi.org/10.1002/oby.21371.

43. Van Hoorenbeeck K, Verhulst SL. Metabolic complications and obstructive sleep apnea in obese children: time to wake up. *Am J Respir Crit Care Med*. 2014;189(1):13–15. https://doi.org/10.1164/rccm.201311-2079ED.

44. Low W, Tan S, Schwartz S. The effect of severe caries on the quality of life in young children. *Pediatr Dent*. 1999;21(6):325–326.

37

CPAP Therapy for OSA in Children

Irina Trosman, Allison Hayes Clarke, and Stephen H. Sheldon

CHAPTER HIGHLIGHTS

- CPAP is an excellent second-line option for children who are not candidates for or who have residual symptoms after adenotonsillectomy.
- CPAP is generally initiated with a titration study and less frequently by using an autoPAP option.
- Several social factors can predict CPAP adherence, however overall, CPAP compliance remains the major challenge to this treatment option, especially in adolescents.
- CPAP desensitization can improve adherence. Alternatively, high flow nasal cannula is an ideal alternative for those intolerant to CPAP.

Although obstructive sleep-disordered breathing (SDB)/obstructive sleep apnea syndrome (OSAS) has been described for centuries, obesity-related OSAS was described in the late 19th century and was termed *Pickwickian syndrome*. This first modern description of OSAS is credited to Burwell and colleagues.[1] However, obesity was not an essential feature for OSAS. Originally, tracheostomy appeared to be the treatment of choice for OSAS.[2,3] Because of the invasive nature of tracheostomy and patient reluctance, other methods of therapeutic intervention were required.

Nasal continuous positive airway pressure (CPAP) had been used for the treatment of respiratory distress syndrome (RDS) in neonates for decades.[4] However, use of nasal CPAP for management of OSAS was first described by Dr. Colin Sullivan. He applied a noninvasive treatment developed for dogs to pneumatically stent a collapsible upper airway to humans using masks specifically created for each patient.[2] Interestingly, one of the first five patients described by Sullivan in his seminal paper was a 13-year-old male who "Had been considered mentally retarded. However, a large component of this retardation was secondary to his inability to stay awake at school."[2] Nasal CPAP proved to be effective in management of upper airway obstruction and alleviated sequelae including, but not limited to, excessive daytime sleepiness in all five patients.

Clinical sleep medicine services gradually became available for adults in the mid-1970s, but few services were specifically designed for children.[5] Pediatric patients with OSAS were under the care of otolaryngologists, as surgical interventions were the only available treatment at that time.

Although adenotonsillectomy (AT) remained the first-line therapy for OSAS in children,[6,7] it became apparent that OSA did not always resolve after the surgery. Moreover, some children were not candidates for surgical interventions, and required positive air pressure (PAP) therapy.

Noninvasive therapeutic intervention methods became crucial. Careful modification of adult techniques was adapted by pediatricians specializing in pediatric sleep medicine. When utilizing PAP therapy for children, small adult masks were required because pediatric-specific nasal interfaces were not available. Currently, noninvasive pediatric interfaces and protocols have been developed and CPAP is available as an alternative therapy for the treatment of OSAS in children. Nevertheless, the U.S. Food and Drug Administration (FDA) has not approved utilization of CPAP therapy for children as a treatment for OSAS.

Treatment approaches to pediatric OSAS include AT, which is the recommended first-line treatment for pediatric OSAS[7] and is curative in the vast majority of non-obese, otherwise healthy patients.[8] Other treatment approaches include weight reduction; antiinflammatory agents; positional therapy; intranasal steroids; antihistamine medications; orthodontic/orthotropic interventions; surgeries beyond AT including, but not limited to, lingual tonsillectomy, supraglottoplasty, tongue base reduction surgery, uvulopalatopharyngoplasty; and other drug-induced endoscopy-guided surgical interventions.[9–11] PAP therapy is available for the patients who are not candidates for surgical intervention, patients waiting for surgical procedures, or those with persistent OSAS despite surgical treatment. Children at risk for persistent OSAS after AT include those with severe OSAS, obesity; concurrent asthma or allergic rhinitis; increased airway collapsibility; anatomic factors affecting cranial, oropharyngeal, or maxillomandibular anatomy; and patients with underlying medical conditions.[8,12] PAP therapy stents the airway by delivering intraluminal airway pressure that is greater than the critical closing pressure of the airway.[13,14] In addition to preserving airway patency, PAP enhances functional residual capacity, reduces the work of breathing associated with increased airway resistance,[15] lowers cardiac afterload, and may lead to a consequent increase in cardiac output.[16]

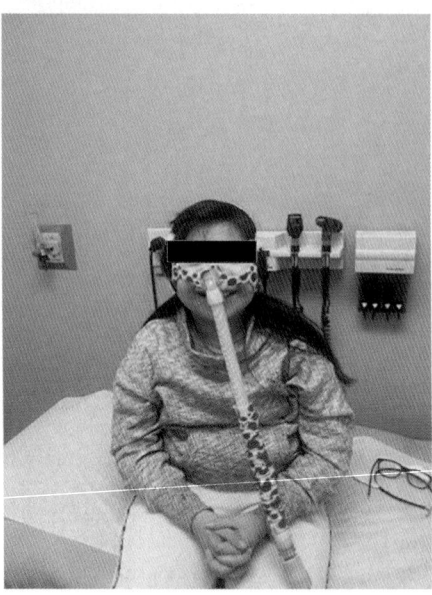

• **Fig. 37.1** A variety of nasal masks may be utilized to provide Positive Airway Pressure (PAP) for the pediatric Patient.

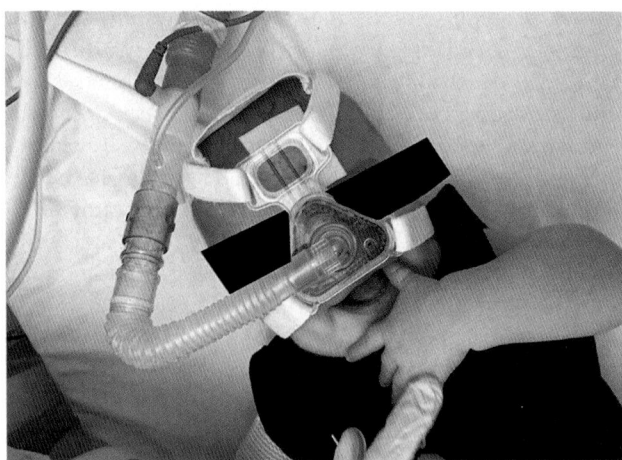

• **Fig. 37.2** Choice of the optimal mask is dependent upon the child's age, midface shape, and facial structure.

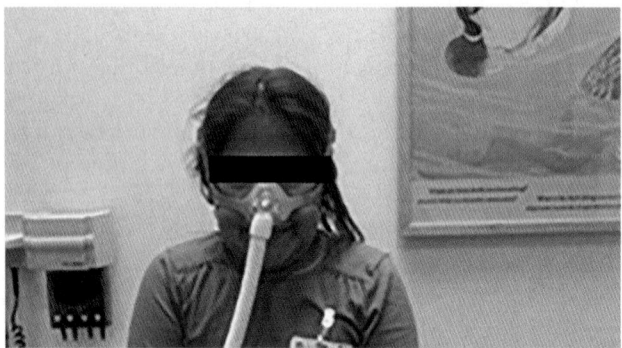

• **Fig. 37.3** Proper mask fit and mask desensitization are essential for the success of PAP therapy in infants and young children.

Understanding Positive Airway Pressure Therapy

PAP therapy is delivered by a device consisting of three main components: (1) a machine with an air compressor that delivers positive pressure, (2) a mask that fits over the nose or nose and mouth, and (3) tubing to connect the machine and the mask (Figs. 37.1–37.3).

An air compressor generates a positive pressure of 4–20 cm of water pressure (cwp) transmitted to the patient's upper airway through a single conduit that connects with the patient via a variety of interfaces. The device continually adjusts its output to the patient's breathing pattern to maintain a constant pressure. A fixed leak valve is positioned near the mask to prevent rebreathing of carbon dioxide. Most modern PAP devices are equipped with a heated humidifier to reduce airway dryness and data-storage capabilities for PAP compliance monitoring. Additionally, some PAP units also come with a timed pressure "ramp" setting that allows airflow to start at a low level and slowly raises the pressure to the set level within a period of time lasting up to 45 minutes. This feature may make it more comfortable to fall asleep at a lower pressure and facilitate adherence.

The two most common types of PAP therapy utilized in children are CPAP and bi-level positive airway pressure (BPAP). Despite widespread use of CPAP in children, it has not yet been approved by the FDA for patients ≤40 kg or children <7 years old. BPAP devices deliver preset inspiratory PAP during inspiration and expiratory PAP during expiration. Both CPAP and BPAP spontaneous mode (BPAP S) administration requires spontaneous (and effective) respiratory efforts. CPAP maintains the airway pressure constant throughout the respiratory cycle. This is achieved by a servo-controlled air compressor that maintains the airway pressure as closely to the prescribed pressure despite the pull (inspiration) and push (exhalation) of the patient. The maintenance of such pressure within an FDA-specified pressure range (for example, ±1.5 cm H_2O of the set pressure) is necessary as a quality-assurance measure that ensures the device maintains a certain prescription pressure. Such a prespecified error range is generally greater with larger tidal volume (V_T) or inspiratory effort from patient, at a faster respiratory rate, and at higher prescription pressure settings because the device would need to be more rapidly responsive to the perturbations in the airway pressure at such extremes to maintain the pressure at the prescribed level.[16] Although CPAP devices generally deliver constant pressure, newer features, such as expiratory pressure release (EPR) for ResMed devices and C-Flex (for Philips Respironics) allow a brief reduction in pressure during the expiratory phase to enhance the patient's comfort. These forms of EPR are based upon proprietary algorithms and can be used in CPAP, BPAP, or auto-titrating PAP devices. Although the studies looking at the compliance data of the adult patients using traditional PAP versus PAP devices with an expiratory relief option did not produce consistent results, EPR modification may be beneficial to the individual patient who is intolerant of PAP therapy.[17–19]

Bi-Level Positive Airway Pressure Therapy

BPAP therapy delivers a variable pressure between the inspiratory and expiratory cycles with the goal to decrease the amount of pressure against which the patient exhales, reduce abdominal muscle recruitment, unload respiratory muscles, and improve respiratory discomfort during the expiratory cycle.

The difference between the inspiratory airway pressure (IPAP) and expiratory positive airway pressure (EPAP) is considered as a pressure support level that could augment the inspired V_T. BPAP is available in various modes; however, only including BPAP-S and BPAP-ST (spontaneous timed) are practically used for the treatment of pediatric OSAS. The cycling of the device from the inspiratory (IPAP) to the expiratory phase (EPAP) and vice versa is triggered by the spontaneously breathing patient (spontaneous mode) or by a set respiratory rate programmed into the device (timed mode). Sensitivities or the triggering threshold for causing the device to cycle in the spontaneous mode may be based on pressure, flow contour, hardwired timing, or a proprietary combination of such measures.[16] The rate of pressurization from EPAP to IPAP level (the "rise time") can be adjusted for individual patient comfort. The administration of a backup rate (ST mode) during BPAP therapy may be considered under a few circumstances: OSAS associated with alveolar hypoventilation resulting in chronic respiratory insufficiency (elevated arterial PCO_2), OSAS and central sleep apnea, and treatment emergent central apneas in patients undergoing PAP therapy for OSA. The choice of the backup rate is probably arbitrary and best guided by polysomnography (PSG) resolution of central apneas or persistent hypoxemia due to alveolar hypoventilation. In general, a backup rate is set at two breaths below the patient's spontaneous rate during calm wakeful breathing and may be titrated upward at two-breath increments, if needed.[16]

BPAP therapy may be also indicated for the patients with morbid obesity and obesity hypoventilation syndrome, SDB, and neuromuscular weakness, or those who are unable to tolerate high positive end-expiratory pressures. Although it seems to be logical that BPAP therapy would be better tolerated, the studies so far failed to demonstrate better compliance with BPAP therapy. A prospective multicenter study of children randomly assigned to 6 months of CPAP or BPAP ventilation[20] revealed that 30% dropped out before the end of the study period, with no differences in adherence between CPAP and BPAP ventilation (mean use of 5.3 ± 2.5 hours/night).

Titration Studies and AutoPAP Therapy

Traditionally, children being considered for PAP therapy are scheduled for an overnight titration study in the sleep laboratory to determine the optimal PAP settings. There is consensus with regard to the end points of PAP titration studies that dictate the upward titration of CPAP level: obstructive apneas, obstructive hypopneas, severe flow limitation, or respiratory event–related arousals, and snoring.[21] Prior to the study, it is essential that children be fitted with an appropriately sized mask that maximizes comfort and minimizes air leak. The three types of masks typically used are nasal mask, nasal pillows, and oronasal or full-face masks (FFMs). The choice of the mask is mostly determined by the patient's facial features, nasal passage patency, presence of mouth breathing, and providers' and patients' preferences.

However, limited adult literature reported the need for higher CPAP pressure[22] and even paradoxical worsening of upper airway obstruction with FFM and an improvement in OSAS control with change to a nasal mask. The proposed mechanism is posterior tongue displacement caused by an FFM.[22]

Due to the potential for aspiration, children should be fit with FFMs only if they are developmentally and medically capable of removing the mask. During the overnight titration PSG, pressures are gradually increased until obstructive events and desaturations are reduced. An adequate titration study identifies the lowest pressure that eliminates obstruction in supine rapid eye movement (REM) sleep. Use of a chin strap, in addition to a nasal mask, may be appropriate for the children breathing through their mouth who are not candidates for an FFM.

Although titration studies are still considered to be a standard of care for children with OSAS, auto-titrating devices (APAP) are being used with increasing frequency in pediatric patients,[23] especially during the COVID-19 pandemic. The rationale for APAP is that the pressure required to treat OSAS may vary over the course of the night and between different nights, sleep stages, and body positions, with the variations not captured by a one-night titration study.[1,24]

Furthermore, APAP allows providers to initiate PAP therapy as soon as OSAS is diagnosed; thus it eliminates the delay in treatment that results from waiting for a formal titration study. However, an APAP eligibility and insurance reimbursement may vary across the states.

APAP's variable pressure response allows the device to adjust to situations such as upper airway congestion, sleeping positional change in pressure requirements, increased pressure needs during REM, and changes in weight. APAP's variable pressure delivery is based on the proprietary algorithms developed by the manufacturers based on adult respiratory physiology. Additionally, the algorithm's definition and detection of the respiratory events, such as obstructive apneas and obstructive hypopneas, vary among manufacturers.

APAP has the potential to improve compliance in children by achieving the same treatment efficacy with the lowest possible pressure. However, the majority of studies failed to demonstrate a clinically significant improvement in compliance and quality of life outcomes compared with fixed-pressure CPAP.[25]

APAP for the treatment of OSAS has been well documented and widely used in the adult population, particularly as a therapeutic option in the initiation phase of therapy.[26] However, only a few studies have assessed APAP for treatment of OSAS in children. Palombini and colleagues[23] investigated a single treatment night of APAP in 14 children aged 8 months to 18 years and demonstrated that auto-CPAP was sensitive and effective for children with obstructive sleep apnea in an attended setting. A study by Marshall and colleagues[27] investigated the use of APAP in the home for 6 weeks in 12 children with sickle cell anemia. Improvements in SDB were documented between baseline and titration PSG, and no adverse effects were reported by children using the APAP at home. Neither of these studies compared the auto-PAP pressure to the gold standard of manually titrated CPAP pressure, utilizing experienced sleep technologists. A handful of recent studies have examined APAP performance compared with the standard in-lab-attended PAP titration studies. In a small study of 26 children aged 4.5–18 years, APAP (Philips Respironics) was well tolerated and effective when used at home from the time of CPAP initiation. AutoMean and Auto90 pressures were usually below treatment pressure determined by titration PSG. The 90th percentile pressure derived from download of the APAP device was on average less <1 cm H_2O different from the pressure recommended following manual titration PSG leading authors to conclude that APAP therapy was likely to result in appropriate control of pediatric OSAS.[28] Another study looking at APAP devices use compared with PSG PAP titration in preteens and teens concluded that APAP-derived pressures correlated with the titration PSG-derived pressures, and that APAP could be successfully used in the pediatric population, as APAP pressures were close to the titration pressures.[29]

Safety and Benefits of Positive Airway Pressure Use for the Treatment of Childhood OSAS

An extensive clinical experience and numerous studies have demonstrated CPAP to be safe and efficacious in children of all ages, including infants.[30–33] PAP therapy in adults compliant with therapy showed improvement in daytime functioning, including improved alertness, quality of life, and at least some aspects of neurobehavioral functioning.[34,35] Nonetheless, only a handful of pediatric studies have examined the impact of PAP therapy on daytime functioning in children with OSAS. One study by Marcus and colleagues[20] had examined the impact of PAP therapy on the daytime functioning in 21 children with OSAS. This study demonstrated improved daytime sleepiness after 6 months of PAP treatment, but no change in other functional outcomes, including behavior, temperament, and school performance. However, the investigators did not differentiate participants who were adherent to treatment from those who were not and did not specifically assess attention. These methodologic factors may have impacted the findings and obscured changes in functioning for those individuals who were more adherent to PAP. Another study examined functional outcomes such as academic performance in a small sample of obese adolescents with OSAS compliant with PAP therapy compared with obese controls with OSAS not adhering to PAP therapy and obese controls without OSAS. The study found improvements in school performance, vigilance, and school-related quality of life in those who were adherent to PAP, similar to controls with obesity without OSAS, and worsening of the academic function in noncompliant CPAP users. However, the study had considerable limitations, as the patients' school performance and PAP compliance estimates were based on parent report of adherence and self-reported grades.[36] Nonetheless, study findings, despite small patient sample and the previously mentioned limitations, were significant, given the scarce evidence supporting PAP effectiveness in improving daytime functioning in adolescents. The findings may enable clinicians to convince already skeptical adolescents of the potential benefits of PAP therapy. Other studies of pediatric PAP adherence had larger samples, but most subjects had a heterogeneous mix of comorbid conditions, including neurodevelopmental conditions, which made standardized assessments of change in daytime functioning impossible.[37–39]

Positive Airway Pressure Side Effects

In general, PAP therapy rarely causes severe side effects. However, it can be associated with potential complications. As opposed to invasive ventilation, PAP uses single-lumen circuits; therefore the potential for CO_2 rebreathing exists, especially if flow settings are low. A minimum of 4 cwp is required to eliminate exhaled CO_2 to prevent rebreathing. PAP is applied to the oronasal pharynx that connects to the esophagus as well as the trachea. Aerophagia from high positive esophageal pressures may lead to gastric distention, emesis, and aspiration. Therefore, in our opinion, initiation of CPAP therapy in children, especially with significant comorbidities, should ideally occur in inpatient settings.

Furthermore, CPAP administration may reduce arterial PCO_2 below the apnea threshold and consequently lead to ventilatory instability leading to the emergence of central apneas and periodic breathing.[16] These treatment emergent central events are attributed to an active Hering-Breuer reflex,[40] and typically resolve with consistent PAP use.[41,42] However, they can lead to sleep disruption and subsequent therapy intolerance.[41,43] Switching from CPAP to BPAP with a backup rate (BPAP-ST) addresses this problem.[16]

PAP can have variable effects on cardiac function. It can help in patients with heart failure or fluid overload by reducing venous return, but it can also compromise cardiac output in others. PAP can also increase right ventricular afterload, but it can also reduce left ventricular afterload. A potential detrimental physiologic effect of PAP is an increase in alveolar distention and pneumothorax reported in adults;[44–47] nonetheless, the authors could not find reports of pneumothorax in otherwise healthy children with OSAS. PAP therapy in some patients may also trigger anxiety and insomnia. Less severe, but more common side effects include rhinorrhea, nasal congestion, epistaxis, and nasal and/or oral dryness.[48,49]

These symptoms can be ameliorated with a heated humidifier, intranasal steroids, saline, antihistamines, montelukast, use of nasal mask rather than nasal pillows, or appropriate mask fitting.[50–52] CPAP mask–related skin breakdowns seldomly associated with an infection and acne have been observed in our clinical practice. Skin irritation and even ulceration can occur from a tight-fitting mask or accumulation of skin oils and debris from poor mask maintenance; rarely, allergies to the mask may occur. Prolonged CPAP use might also lead to impaired growth of the facial bones, resulting in midfacial hypoplasia.[53,54]

Positive Airway Pressure Adherence and Factors Affecting Positive Airway Pressure Compliance

Adult Versus Pediatric Data

While PAP therapy is effective in treating OSAS in children,[38] widespread use is limited because of poor compliance.[20,39] Adult literature regarding CPAP adherence identified the following categories of factors that influence or predict adherence to CPAP use: disease characteristics, patient characteristics, treatment titration procedures, technologic device factors and side effects, and psychologic and social factors. Pediatric studies have produced variable results, mostly because of retrospective and observational study designs. In general, their findings identified somewhat different factors impacting CPAP adherence in children.[55-58] For instance, disease-specific factors such as OSAS severity, PAP pressure, presence of hypersomnolence, and nasal symptoms, which predict CPAP compliance in adults, did not appear to correlate with CPAP adherence in children.[55] In children or adolescent patients with OSAS, factors associated with better adherence included higher maternal education,[55,58] parental support,[59] and presence of a family member with PAP use.[58] Disease-specific factors such as PSG measures and symptoms of excessive daytime sleepiness did not significantly differ with CPAP use. Additionally, CPAP pressure did not appear to have a predictive value in the patient's compliance.[20,37,55,58,60-63] One pediatric study found that girls had a higher rate of CPAP adherence than boys.[57] This was in contrast to findings of no sex differences in adult CPAP use.[64] African American children, independent of socioeconomic status,[55] and older children, particularly adolescents, were less likely to be adherent to CPAP than children of other races and ages.[65-67] However, adolescents were more likely to use CPAP if the therapy was started before adolescence or they had a stable family structure with free communication between parents and patient.[68] Reduced PAP adherence also has been found in children with atopic illness, including eczema, allergic rhinosinusitis, and/or asthma.[57]

The largest cross-sectional analysis of PAP adherence in children ages 4–18 years using CPAP or APAP devices uploaded nightly evaluated PAP compliance based on the Centers for Medicare & Medicaid Services (CMS) criteria. Data revealed most children were actively using PAP therapy. A total of 61.8% of the cohort was still using their device after 90 days and did not have therapy terminated due to 30 consecutive nights of non-use. However, only 46% of the cohort met CMS criteria for adherence at 90 days. Average use per session was also highest in the age group of 6 years to <12 years, whereas the group aged 15 years to <18 years had the lowest use per session. Factors associated with poor adherence were increased residual apnea-hypopnea index (AHI), lower PAP pressure, and high mask leak, whereas improved compliance was found in patients enrolled in a patient engagement program.[53] Overall, these findings suggest that pediatric adherence to PAP therapy is worse than in adults.[53,69]

Positive Airway Pressure Adherence in Children with Developmental Delays

OSAS is common in children developmental delays (DDs) and genetic conditions including, but not limited to, trisomy 21, fragile X, Rett syndrome, Prader-Willi syndrome, and central nervous system abnormalities (e.g., congenital cytomegalovirus infection, stroke, hydrocephalus, cerebral palsy). For example, the prevalence of OSAS in children with Down syndrome has been reported to range from 30% to 50%.[70] There are limited data regarding PAP adherence in children with DD. Some studies, surprisingly, demonstrated a better adherence to PAP therapy in this patient population, although overall compliance was still low.[55,57,71] One large retrospective study[57] included[55] patients with various degree of OSAS severity with comorbid conditions such as DD (including trisomy 21), obesity, and atopy. The patients were typically desensitized to CPAP therapy through a mask fitting and air pressure trial in clinic by a respiratory therapist and had regular follow-up visits with a medical provider. CPAP CMS adherence criteria were used to determine the patient's PAP compliance. The study demonstrated children with DD were more likely to be adherent to CPAP therapy than youth with normal development. These results were similar to other reports of pediatric CPAP adherence in smaller samples.[20,39]

Nonetheless, these findings must be interpreted with caution given the broad spectrum of DD traits and severity (mild learning disability or speech delay to global DD or profound intellectual disability). Potential reasons why children with DD demonstrated better compliance may include medical providers closer attention to this high-risk population and CPAP desensitization, increased dependence upon caregiver support, and decreased ability to remove mask due to either physical or intellectual disability. Furthermore, parental perception of CPAP importance for a child with neurodevelopmental disabilities may be heightened. Alternatively, children without disabilities may be less adherent to PAP therapy due to increased independence or less parental supervision.

Device and Mask Factors

Studies in both children and adults comparing different types of pressure delivery, such as BPAP or C-Flex/Bi-Flex (which deliver a slight decrease in pressure during early expiration and/or inspiration), have had mixed results, but have generally not shown an improvement in adherence compared with standard CPAP.[20,72,73] There is paucity of data on interfaces and PAP compliance. One pediatric study showed that FFMs were associated with lower adherence than nasal masks.[39]

Positive Airway Pressure Device Compliance Monitoring and a Follow-Up

Most modern CPAP devices measure both "machine-on" and "mask-on" times, with the mask-on time used to measure compliance. Compliance data are downloaded onto electronic chips (SD cards) and transmitted to a cloud-based database that can be accessed by providers and patients. However, this PAP download information, especially in younger children, has to be interpreted with caution because the accuracy of PAP devices at assessing SDB in children has not been validated. Nevertheless, these reports provide useful feedback regarding the patient's consistency and duration of the device use.

Additionally, adherence to PAP therapy in a pediatric population is estimated by utilizing the CMS criteria for adherence.[74] These criteria (PAP use for 4 hours or more per night on at least 70% of the nights over a consecutive 30-day period during the initial 90 days of use) were developed for adults and were never validated for children. Unfortunately, it is not uncommon in our practice to see insurance companies discontinue reimbursing PAP therapy if children do not meet these strict compliance criteria while they are working with providers to adapt to their PAP devices.

It is worth mentioning that there is no optimal definition of PAP adherence in children. Given that total sleep time is longer in children than in adults, it is possible that more hours of PAP use are required to provide meaningful positive impact on health outcomes in children than in adults. Moreover, CMS criteria may not be applicable to pediatric population, and PAP adherence should be measured with consideration of the child's sleep requirements, developmental level, and comorbid conditions. In our practice, families of the medically complex patients who require nocturnal interventions (e.g., enteral feedings, respiratory care, positional changes, or medical intervention) may be overwhelmed and consider PAP therapy an additional burden. Some parents may be overwhelmed from a mere sleep disruption caused by the necessity to monitor the child's PAP use. To our knowledge, none of the previous studies focused on the caregivers' burden and its impact on the pediatric PAP adherence. Thus future studies and development of pediatric PAP adherence guidelines are warranted (Table 37.1).

Compliance data monitoring and patient support systems may vary depending on the available resources and sleep medicine program structure. However, a close follow-up is essential to identify problems and improve PAP adherence. Ideally, the team of providers caring for the patients prescribed with PAP therapy should include a respiratory and/or sleep technologist skilled at mask fittings, a specialist such as a behavioral psychologist who is able to provide PAP desensitization, a program coordinator, and a physician or a midlevel provider. This may be better achieved in a designated CPAP clinic space equipped with appropriate mask supplies, PAP devices, and a comfortable place for PAP desensitization and PAP naps. One study found that behavioral therapy, including PAP desensitization, may improve compliance in some pediatric patients.[75] Close communication with durable equipment companies with sufficient amount of pediatric expertise is essential for a successful CPAP program. Ideally, patients should be fitted with a CPAP mask and desensitized to PAP therapy prior to initiation of the PAP titration study and initiation of PAP therapy, especially in young children, children with DDs, anxiety, or other behavioral problems. They should be reevaluated within 30 days of initiating PAP therapy. Objective data regarding compliance should be obtained by downloading usage data. CPAP clinic staff should provide phone support to address any technical concerns or PAP side effects.[20] PAP compliance in the early stage or the first month of treatment was often indicative of whether the PAP treatment would be sustainable, suggesting that timely supervision and guidance with multidisciplinary comprehensive management may improve the overall adherence to PAP treatment in children.[76]

In summary, available pediatric data suggest that young children aged >4 years to <6 years and teenagers aged 15 to <18 years might need closer attention and support than other age groups. Furthermore, multidisciplinary PAP programs with an appropriate support, including age-specific behavioral interventions, are essential for PAP adherence in children with OSAS. Health education and family involvement are important components in promoting CPAP adherence. The support strategies should be tailored to the individual child and their developmental needs.

Positive Airway Pressure Desensitization

PAP desensitization and adherence is impacted by the complex interplay of numerous psychosocial, medical, and technical factors. Given poor adherence rates and difficulty adjusting to the PAP mask and equipment, a multidisciplinary team of medical (e.g., nurses, physicians), behavioral (e.g., psychologists, social workers), and respiratory therapists or sleep technicians is recommended to work together in assessing and intervening using their unique knowledge base and skill set.[77] Psychologists and social workers play an important role on the team at addressing psychologic, family, and behavioral factors that may increase adaptation. Research suggests that behavioral interventions can be effective at improving PAP tolerance and usage over time.[32,75,78,79]

After caregivers learn that PAP is a medical necessity for their child, they often work very hard to get their child to use the device. Without support and a plan for

TABLE 37.1 Representation of a Compliance Report

Compliance Information	12/5/2021–1/3/2022
Compliance Summary	
Date range	12/5/2021–1/3/2022 (30 days)
Days with device usage	30 days
Days without device usage	0 days
Percentage of days with device usage	100%
Cumulative usage	12 days, 12 hours, 47 minutes, 57 seconds
Maximum usage (1 day)	13 hour, 24 minutes, 4 seconds
Average usage (all days)	10 hours to 1 minute, 35 seconds
Average usage (days used)	1 hour, 1 minute, 35 seconds
Minimum usage (1 day)	6 hours, 32 minutes, 49 seconds
Percentage of days with usage ≥4 hours	100%
Percentage of days with usage <4 hours	0%
Total blower time	13 days, 21 hours, 39 minutes, 21 seconds
CPAP Summary	
Average time in large leak per day	14 seconds
Average AHI	1.4
CPAP	8.0 cm H_2O

AHI, apnea-hypopnea index; *CPAP*, continuous positive airway pressure.

As outlined by Harford and colleagues,[79] the initial assessment with the patient guides treatment goals and typically includes (1) patient and caregiver education regarding obstructive sleep apnea and rationale for PAP therapy, (2) identifying the best fitting mask/equipment, (3) assessing strengths and potential barriers to adherence, and (4) introducing desensitization and practicing first steps with the patient and family. To increase motivation, it is also important to talk about patient and caregiver PAP-related health beliefs, identify and address any misperceptions, and to allow children and their caregivers the opportunity to ask questions.[32]

For children who express discomfort in initially trying on their mask and tolerating the pressure, a systematic desensitization process can be used to help them get used to the equipment.[80] Using operant conditioning principles, the underlying goal of PAP desensitization is to help kids progressively get more and more used to the CPAP mask and machine through gradual and repeated exposures, leading to habituation.[79,81] Our objective is to move slow enough to avoid struggles and anxiety, while also using enjoyable activities, positive attention, praise, and rewards to increase positive associations with mask use. In practice, this takes significant time, effort, and patience both from providers and caregivers to be effective. By practicing repeatedly, gradually increasing length of exposures to the mask and use of air pressure, and praising and rewarding children for this practice, children begin to realize that they can tolerate the equipment and may become more motivated to continue mask practice and use going forward. Moreover, protests or complaints should be ignored, and caregivers can resume positive attention when the child returns to practice. Concurrently, classical conditioning[82] approaches may also be incorporated, pairing mask practice with pleasant activities, such as watching a favorite show, singing a favorite song, or caregivers giving the child desired sensory input (e.g., rubbing their arms or back). This serves to build positive associations with practice and is a means of distraction during the exposure to the equipment, which may help to reduce anxiety and increase tolerance of equipment.

The goal is to gradually shape the mask-wearing behavior, starting small and using verbal praise to reinforce each step. Where a child starts in the desensitization process depends on how they react to initially seeing and trying on the mask and knowledge of potential anxiety or sensory sensitivities, which may impact acclimation to the mask. We recommend that families practice mask use during the day to start. Sample steps in the desensitization process may include (1) holding and playing with the mask, (2) briefly placing the mask alone over the nose without straps over the head, (3) wearing the mask alone with straps over the head for increasingly longer periods of time, (4) playing with the PAP air tubing (e.g., blowing into the air and trying to speak into it), (5) feeling air pressure on different parts of the body and face, and (6) wearing the mask with air pressure on (starting with minimal pressure and, if appropriate, titrating to a recommended pressure). Once

desensitization, this can often result in child resistance and anxiety, and an unpleasant first experience with PAP has been demonstrated to impede progress and delay desensitization.[32,51] Therefore it is recommended that providers meet with children and their caregivers to discuss the gradual desensitization approach prior to their receiving PAP equipment. The ability to obtain PAP equipment from the durable medical equipment (DME) company prior to a titration sleep study varies by state, and one way we have found to help with desensitization is to request a practice blower be delivered to the family after our initial visit discussing PAP desensitization. Providers in other states may have the ability to order APAP for children to use prior to their titration studies.

children are confident with mask use during the day, it is recommended that families begin to incorporate their PAP device into the bedtime routine, reminding children in a manner consistent with their development, about how the device may help them sleep better. Children may easily tolerate some steps and need to move much more gradually through other steps. It is important to work with their sleep medicine team if they hit a point where progress stalls to try to identify barriers and alternate strategies that can be attempted.

For younger children and children with developmental disabilities, several additional techniques may help in managing discomfort or anxiety about mask usage. It is important to incorporate the children's own interests into the process and for adults and others they trust to model the desired behaviors. For instance, if children like dolls or stuffed animals, they can teach their stuffed animals to wear the mask. For those who demonstrate magical thinking, they could also think about their mask as a "super mask," similar to the masks that their favorite superheroes or firefighters wear. Even if they do not have a specific interest that aligns with the mask, the mask practice can be paired with favorite songs, games with caregivers, and/or a favorite show for older kids. Caregivers and siblings can model the desired behaviors, including using the mask themselves, having fun while wearing their mask. The goal is to make this practice as positive and enjoyable as possible. If developmentally appropriate, parents can dance around with the mask on or tickle children with the CPAP blower. Stickers or small rewards can be given after each practice and, depending on the child's age, a prespecified number of stickers could potentially be turned in for a larger reward. For children who benefit from visuals, the family can also draw or print out a list of desensitization steps and add stickers for completion of each step in the process. Last, children may also enjoy reading books about mask use and some children, especially those with autism or other developmental disabilities, may benefit from social stories about use of PAP devices and what they can expect as they practice.

Despite all these strategies, some children and adolescents continue to have anxiety about mask use or struggle significantly with using the mask overnight. For anxious children and adolescents, relaxation exercises prior to and during mask practice can help with their ability to engage in desensitization practice. In our experience, we observe that desensitization practice is most effective when it is incorporated into daily routines, so it does not get forgotten. Specifically, with adolescents who may be resistant to practice, sometimes only offering a desired activity (e.g., electronics use) after practice is completed, can boost motivation. When children and adolescents struggle to keep the mask on for the duration of the night, the use of a "PAP fairy" may help to remind them to replace the mask overnight. The fairy can visit and leave a small present under the child's pillow if the mask is on when they visit. For older kids, parents can simply describe that they will check on children intermittently overnight and leave a small reward if the mask is on when they visit. In extreme circumstances when outpatient PAP therapy teams are struggling to help the patient achieve desensitization, Harford and colleagues[78] found that desensitization was possible through intensive multidisciplinary inpatient hospital interventions. Finally, compared with care as usual, the development of multidisciplinary CPAP clinics has been shown to support improved PAP usage. As part of these specialized clinics, regular follow-up and phone calls from staff help to keep families engaged in treatment and identify barriers as they arise.[32,83]

High-Flow Nasal Cannula

Unfortunately, many children, particularly those with DD and craniofacial abnormalities, cannot tolerate or be appropriately fitted for masks required to deliver CPAP. Over the last decade, high-flow nasal cannula (HFNC) therapy has become an increasingly important and popular mode of noninvasive respiratory support for acute and chronic respiratory failure in adults. More recently, HFNC has been used as an alternative treatment to CPAP in some children and neonates with OSAS. HFNC is able to deliver very high flows (flow rates up to 60 L/min) of heated (30°C–32°C) and humidified air and gas mixture. HFNC is an open system that is not dependent on a tightly sealed nasal mask; thus a nasal cannula is used, which is less obtrusive and cumbersome than a nasal mask and should be better tolerated by children during sleep. The proposed mechanism of action of HFNC is 2-fold: reduction in dead space of the upper airways that are continuously flushed with pressurized humidified air and reduction in upper airway collapse, as the flow rate is greater than the normal inspiratory flow rate.[84–87]

Adult studies have supported this, demonstrating that the end-expiratory supraglottic pressure became less negative after the addition of high-flow therapy and inspiratory airflow no longer showed a flow-limited pattern.[88] Pressures have been measured by several authors at the nasopharynx or esophagus. Arora and coworkers[84] studied children with viral bronchiolitis and found a linear increase in pressure up to a flow of 6 L/min and a smaller gradient from 6–8 L/min, reaching a maximum of 5 cm H_2O. Similarly, Kubicka and colleagues[89] measured flow rates of up to 5 L/min in neonates over 1,500 g current weight and the highest pressure measured was 4.5 cm H_2O. Pressures achieved with mouth open were much smaller. Pressure generated by HFNC do not appear to exceed pressures used therapeutically in CPAP and may be sufficient to effectively stent the upper airway during sleep. A small prospective pediatric study utilizing HFNC at 20 L/min suggested that in the majority of children treatment with HFNC was comparable clinically to CPAP treatment.[88] A few other studies have demonstrated efficacy of HFNC therapy in pediatric patients with obstructive sleep apnea.[90-93]

The most commonly reported HFNC treatment complications were cannula dislodgement, skin irritation, dry mucus membranes, restlessness, oxygen desaturation, and increased central apneas.[92] Concerns for more significant complications, such as pneumothorax or pneumomediastinum, have been raised because HFNC airway pressure is not regulated. Sudden rise in pressure may lead to a rapid increase in the end-expiratory lung volume leading to pneumothorax or pneumomediastinum.[94] Although there have been few cases describing such incidences in children[95] who all had significant hyperinflation at the time of the development of air leak, the authors' institutional practice policy requires HFNC therapy initiation in a pediatric intensive care unit (PICU) setting, especially for the patients with an underlying chronic pulmonary disease or recovering from an acute respiratory illness. Alternatively, outpatient HFNC titration studies may be appropriate for otherwise healthy children with OSAS, as the risk of generating excessive pulmonary pressures is reduced when the patients are asleep, and breathing is shallower. Furthermore, heated, humidified air tends to prevent bronchospasm.[90] A second concern raised in the past was that the use of HFNC was associated with an increased incidence of gram-negative bacteremia, specifically due to *Ralstonia pickettii*. One brand of hospital-based devices was temporarily removed from the market in response to this risk. After appropriate methods of infection control were initiated, the devices were reapproved for public use.[96]

CLINICAL PEARLS

- Adenotonsillectomy is considered to be the first-line treatment; however, not all patients are surgical candidates, and some patients will continue to have symptoms after surgery.[7]
- Continuous positive airway pressure (CPAP) is a safe and effective treatment for children with obstructive sleep apnea syndrome (OSAS) who do not improve with surgery or who are not candidates for surgery.[38] The major limiting factor for successful treatment with CPAP is adherence.[20,39]
- Psychosocial factors and patient characteristics are the main predictors of poor adherence, with low maternal education being the strongest predictor.[55,58]
- Managing suboptimal adherence entails engaging and educating the child and parent about CPAP; this involves discussing preexisting attitudes, outcome expectations, and side effects, in addition to providing constant support from a dedicated team.
- More intensive cognitive behavioral interventions may prove useful in overcoming poor CPAP adherence in complex cases. Studies examining the barriers to PAP compliance have shown that age,[28] gender,[29] asthma,[28] family economic status,[30] level of family support, maternal education, strong caregiver self-efficacy,[31] and the use of humidification and warming are associated with adherence to PAP use in children.[32]
- The compliance with PAP use in the early stage or the first month of treatment is often indicative of whether the PAP treatment would be sustainable,[34,35] suggesting that timely supervision and guidance with multidisciplinary comprehensive management may improve the overall adherence to noninvasive ventilation treatment in children.
- High-flow nasal cannula seems to be a viable alternative therapy for children with severe OSAS for whom CPAP is not appropriate or the patient is intolerant.[88,90-93]

Summary

CPAP is a safe and effective treatment for children with OSAS who are not candidates for AT or who have persistent OSAS following surgical intervention. CPAP therapy provides many beneficial effects; however, adherence to therapy is the major limiting factor, especially in adolescents. Studies examining the barriers to PAP compliance have shown that age, gender, time of the therapy initiation, level of family support, higher maternal education level, strong caregiver self-efficacy, and the use of heated humidification are associated with better PAP therapy compliance in children. The compliance with PAP use in the early stage of treatment is often a predictor of the future adherence to PAP therapy. Thus timely supervision and guidance from a dedicated team may improve the overall adherence to PAP treatment in children.

More intensive cognitive-behavioral interventions may prove useful in overcoming poor CPAP adherence in complex cases. HFNC seems to be a viable alternative therapy for children with severe OSAS for whom CPAP is not appropriate or intolerant. However, larger randomized controlled trials are needed to determine whether HFNC could be considered as an established alternative for CPAP in OSAS.

References

1. Burwell CS, Robin ED, Whaley RD, Bickelmann AG. Extreme obesity associated with alveolar hypoventilation – a Pickwickian Syndrome. 1956. *Obes Res*. Jul 1994;2(4):390–397.
2. Sullivan CE, Issa FG, Berthon-Jones M, Eves L. Reversal of obstructive sleep apnoea by continuous positive airway pressure applied through the nares. *Lancet*. Apr 18 1981;1(8225):862–865.
3. Hormann K, Hirth K, Maurer JT. Surgical therapy of sleep-related respiratory disorders. *HNO*. Apr 1999;47(4):226–235.
4. Gregory GA, Kitterman JA, Phibbs RH, Tooley WH, Hamilton WK. Treatment of the idiopathic respiratory-distress syndrome with continuous positive airway pressure. *N Engl J Med*. Jun 17 1971;284(24):1333–1340.
5. Owens J, Kothare S, Sheldon S. "Not Just Little Adults": AASM Should Require Pediatric Accreditation for Integrated Sleep

Medicine Programs Serving Both Children (0–16 years) and Adults. *J Clin Sleep Med.* 2012;08(5):473–476.

6. Roland PS, Rosenfeld RM, Brooks LJ, et al. Clinical practice guideline: Polysomnography for sleep-disordered breathing prior to tonsillectomy in children. *Otolaryngol Head Neck Surg.* Jul 2011;145(1 Suppl):S1–S15.

7. Marcus CL, Brooks LJ, Draper KA, et al. Diagnosis and management of childhood obstructive sleep apnea syndrome. *Pediatrics.* Sep 2012;130(3):576–584.

8. Marcus CL, Moore RH, Rosen CL, et al. A randomized trial of adenotonsillectomy for childhood sleep apnea. *N Engl J Med.* Jun 20 2013;368(25):2366–2376.

9. Goldbart AD, Goldman JL, Veling MC, Gozal D. Leukotriene modifier therapy for mild sleep-disordered breathing in children. *Am J Respir Crit Care Med.* Aug 1 2005;172(3):364–370.

10. Kheirandish L, Goldbart AD, Gozal D. Intranasal steroids and oral leukotriene modifier therapy in residual sleep-disordered breathing after tonsillectomy and adenoidectomy in children. *Pediatrics.* Jan 2006;117(1):e61–e66.

11. Kheirandish-Gozal L, Bandla HP, Gozal D. Montelukast for children with obstructive sleep apnea: Results of a double-blind, randomized, placebo-controlled trial. *Ann Am Thorac Soc.* Oct 2016;13(10):1736–1741.

12. Shott SR. Evaluation and management of pediatric obstructive sleep apnea beyond tonsillectomy and adenoidectomy. *Curr Opin Otolaryngol Head Neck Surg.* Dec 2011;19(6):449–454.

13. Marcus CL, McColley SA, Carroll JL, Loughlin GM, Smith PL, Schwartz AR. Upper airway collapsibility in children with obstructive sleep apnea syndrome. *J Appl Physiol (1985).* Aug 1994;77(2):918–924.

14. Smith PL, Wise RA, Gold AR, Schwartz AR, Permutt S. Upper airway pressure-flow relationships in obstructive sleep apnea. *J Appl Physiol (1985).* Feb 1988;64(2):789–795.

15. Gozal D, Tan HL, Kheirandish-Gozal L. Treatment of obstructive sleep apnea in children: Handling the unknown with precision. *J Clin Med.* Mar 24 2020;9(3):888.

16. Antonescu-Turcu A, Parthasarathy S. CPAP and bi-level PAP therapy: New and established roles. *Respir Care.* Sep 2010;55(9):1216–1229.

17. Aloia MS, Stanchina M, Arnedt JT, Malhotra A, Millman RP. Treatment adherence and outcomes in flexible vs standard continuous positive airway pressure therapy. *Chest.* Jun 2005;127(6):2085–2093.

18. Dolan DC, Okonkwo R, Gfullner F, Hansbrough JR, Strobel RJ, Rosenthal L. Longitudinal comparison study of pressure relief (C-Flex) vs. CPAP in OSA patients. *Sleep Breath.* Mar 2009;13(1):73–77.

19. Pepin JL, Muir JF, Gentina T, et al. Pressure reduction during exhalation in sleep apnea patients treated by continuous positive airway pressure. *Chest.* Aug 2009;136(2):490–497.

20. Marcus CL, Rosen G, Ward SL, et al. Adherence to and effectiveness of positive airway pressure therapy in children with obstructive sleep apnea. *Pediatrics.* Mar 2006;117(3):e442–e451.

21. Kushida CA, Chediak A, Berry RB, et al. Clinical guidelines for the manual titration of positive airway pressure in patients with obstructive sleep apnea. *J Clin Sleep Med.* Apr 15 2008;4(2):157–171.

22. Ng JR, Aiyappan V, Mercer J, et al. Choosing an oronasal mask to deliver continuous positive airway pressure may cause more upper airway obstruction or lead to higher continuous positive airway pressure requirements than a nasal mask in some patients: A case series. *J Clin Sleep Med.* Sep 15 2016;12(9):1227–1232.

23. Palombini L, Pelayo R, Guilleminault C. Efficacy of automated continuous positive airway pressure in children with sleep-related breathing disorders in an attended setting. *Pediatrics.* May 2004;113(5):e412–e417.

24. Wickramasinghe H, Rowley JA. Obstructive Sleep Apnea (OSA) Treatment & Management. *MedScape.* 2020

25. Ayas NT, Patel SR, Malhotra A, et al. Auto-titrating versus standard continuous positive airway pressure for the treatment of obstructive sleep apnea: Results of a meta-analysis. *Sleep.* Mar 15 2004;27(2):249–253.

26. Rosen CL, Auckley D, Benca R, et al. A multisite randomized trial of portable sleep studies and positive airway pressure autotitration versus laboratory-based polysomnography for the diagnosis and treatment of obstructive sleep apnea: The HomePAP study. *Sleep.* Jun 1 2012;35(6):757–767.

27. Marshall MJ, Bucks RS, Hogan AM, et al. Auto-adjusting positive airway pressure in children with sickle cell anemia: Results of a phase I randomized controlled trial. *Haematologica.* Jul 2009;94(7):1006–1010.

28. Mihai R, Vandeleur M, Pecoraro S, Davey MJ, Nixon GM. Autotitrating CPAP as a Tool for CPAP Initiation for Children. *J Clin Sleep Med.* May 15 2017;13(5):713–719.

29. Khaytin I, Tapia IE, Xanthopoulos MS, et al. Auto-titrating CPAP for the treatment of obstructive sleep apnea in children. *J Clin Sleep Med.* Jun 15 2020;16(6):871–878.

30. Marcus CL, Ward SL, Mallory GB, et al. Use of nasal continuous positive airway pressure as treatment of childhood obstructive sleep apnea. *J Pediatr.* Jul 1995;127(1):88–94.

31. McNamara F, Sullivan CE. Obstructive sleep apnea in infants and its management with nasal continuous positive airway pressure. *Chest.* Jul 1999;116(1):10–16.

32. King MS, Xanthopoulos MS, Marcus CL. Improving positive airway pressure adherence in children. *Sleep Med Clin.* Jun 1 2014;9(2):219–234.

33. Downey R, 3rd, Perkin RM, MacQuarrie J. Nasal continuous positive airway pressure use in children with obstructive sleep apnea younger than 2 years of age. *Chest.* Jun 2000;117(6):1608–1612.

34. Gay P, Weaver T, Loube D, et al. Evaluation of positive airway pressure treatment for sleep related breathing disorders in adults. *Sleep.* Mar 2006;29(3):381–401.

35. Sanchez AI, Martinez P, Miro E, Bardwell WA, Buela-Casal G. CPAP and behavioral therapies in patients with obstructive sleep apnea: Effects on daytime sleepiness, mood, and cognitive function. *Sleep Med Rev.* Jun 2009;13(3):223–233.

36. Beebe DW, Byars KC. Adolescents with obstructive sleep apnea adhere poorly to positive airway pressure (PAP), but PAP users show improved attention and school performance. *PLoS One.* Mar 17 2011;6(3):e16924.

37. Uong EC, Epperson M, Bathon SA, Jeffe DB. Adherence to nasal positive airway pressure therapy among school-aged children and adolescents with obstructive sleep apnea syndrome. *Pediatrics.* Nov 2007;120(5):e1203–1211.

38. Marcus CL, Radcliffe J, Konstantinopoulou S, et al. Effects of positive airway pressure therapy on neurobehavioral outcomes in children with obstructive sleep apnea. *Am J Respir Crit Care Med.* May 1 2012;185(9):998–1003.

39. O'Donnell AR, Bjornson CL, Bohn SG, Kirk VG. Compliance rates in children using noninvasive continuous positive airway pressure. *Sleep.* May 2006;29(5):651–658.

40. Waters KA, Everett F, Bruderer J, MacNamara F, Sullivan CE. The use of nasal CPAP in children. *Pediatr Pulmonol Suppl.* 1995;11:91–93.

41. Javaheri S, Smith J, Chung E. The prevalence and natural history of complex sleep apnea. *J Clin Sleep Med.* Jun 15 2009;5(3):205–211.

42. Stanchina M, Robinson K, Corrao W, Donat W, Sands S, Malhotra A. Clinical Use of Loop Gain Measures to Determine Continuous Positive Airway Pressure Efficacy in Patients with Complex Sleep Apnea. A Pilot Study. *Ann Am Thorac Soc.* Sep 2015;12(9):1351–1357.

43. Mulgrew AT, Lawati NA, Ayas NT, et al. Residual sleep apnea on polysomnography after 3 months of CPAP therapy: Clinical implications, predictors and patterns. *Sleep Med.* Feb 2010;11(2):119–125.

44. Rajdev K, Idiculla PS, Sharma S, Von Essen SG, Murphy PJ, Bista S. Recurrent Pneumothorax with CPAP Therapy for Obstructive Sleep Apnea. *Case Rep Pulmonol.* 2020;2020:8898621.

45. Langner S, Kolditz M, Kleymann J, et al. Large Pneumothorax in a Sleep Apnea Patient with CPAP without Previously Known Lung and Thoracic Diseases - a Case Report. *Pneumologie.* Apr 2020;74(4):217–221.

46. Herrejón Silvestre A, Inchaurraga Alvarez I, Marín González M. Spontaneous pneumothorax associated with the use of nighttime BiPAP with a nasal mask. *Arch Bronconeumol.* Nov 1998;34(10):512.

47. Mao J, Bernabei A, Cutrufello N, Kern J. *Spontaneous pneumothorax caused by excessive positive airway pressure therapy for obstructive sleep apnea. D36. Pleural Disease: Case Reports II.* American Thoracic Society; 2018.A6682–A6682.

48. Pepin JL, Leger P, Veale D, Langevin B, Robert D, Levy P. Side effects of nasal continuous positive airway pressure in sleep apnea syndrome. Study of 193 patients in two French sleep centers. *Chest.* Feb 1995;107(2):375–381.

49. Constantinidis J, Knobber D, Steinhart H, Kuhn J, Iro H. Fine-structural investigations of the effect of nCPAP-mask application on the nasal mucosa. *Acta Otolaryngol.* Mar 2000;120(3):432–437.

50. Massie CA, Hart RW, Peralez K, Richards GN. Effects of humidification on nasal symptoms and compliance in sleep apnea patients using continuous positive airway pressure. *Chest.* Aug 1999;116(2):403–408.

51. Kirk VG, O'Donnell AR. Continuous positive airway pressure for children: A discussion on how to maximize compliance. *Sleep Med Rev.* Apr 2006;10(2):119–127.

52. Qureshi A, Ballard RD. Obstructive sleep apnea. *J Allergy Clin Immunol.* Oct 2003;112(4):643–651. quiz 652.

53. Bhattacharjee R, Benjafield AV, Armitstead J, et al. Adherence in children using positive airway pressure therapy: A big-data analysis. *Lancet Digit Health.* Feb 2020;2(2):e94–e101.

54. Li KK, Riley RW, Guilleminault C. An unreported risk in the use of home nasal continuous positive airway pressure and home nasal ventilation in children: Mid-face hypoplasia. *Chest.* Mar 2000;117(3):916–918.

55. DiFeo N, Meltzer LJ, Beck SE, et al. Predictors of positive airway pressure therapy adherence in children: A prospective study. *J Clin Sleep Med.* Jun 15 2012;8(3):279–286.

56. Simon SL, Duncan CL, Janicke DM, Wagner MH. Barriers to treatment of paediatric obstructive sleep apnoea: Development of the adherence barriers to continuous positive airway pressure (CPAP) questionnaire. *Sleep Med.* Feb 2012;13(2):172–177.

57. Hawkins SM, Jensen EL, Simon SL, Friedman NR. Correlates of Pediatric CPAP Adherence. *J Clin Sleep Med.* Jun 15 2016;12(6):879–884.

58. Puri P, Ross KR, Mehra R, et al. Pediatric Positive Airway Pressure Adherence in Obstructive Sleep Apnea Enhanced by Family Member Positive Airway Pressure Usage. *J Clin Sleep Med.* Jul 15 2016;12(7):959–963.

59. Sawunyavisuth B, Ngamjarus C, Sawanyawisuth K. Any Effective Intervention to Improve CPAP Adherence in Children with Obstructive Sleep Apnea: A Systematic Review. *Glob Pediatr Health.* 2021;82333794X211019884.

60. Machaalani R, Evans CA, Waters KA. Objective adherence to positive airway pressure therapy in an Australian paediatric cohort. *Sleep Breath.* Dec 2016;20(4):1327–1336.

61. Nixon GM, Mihai R, Verginis N, Davey MJ. Patterns of continuous positive airway pressure adherence during the first 3 months of treatment in children. *J Pediatr.* Nov 2011;159(5):802–807.

62. Ramirez A, Khirani S, Aloui S, et al. Continuous positive airway pressure and noninvasive ventilation adherence in children. *Sleep Med.* Dec 2013;14(12):1290–1294.

63. Perriol MP, Jullian-Desayes I, Joyeux-Faure M, et al. Long-term adherence to ambulatory initiated continuous positive airway pressure in non-syndromic OSA children. *Sleep Breath.* Jun 2019;23(2):575–578.

64. Budhiraja R, Parthasarathy S, Drake CL, et al. Early CPAP use identifies subsequent adherence to CPAP therapy. *Sleep.* Mar 2007;30(3):320–324.

65. Strunk RC, Bender B, Young DA, et al. Predictors of protocol adherence in a pediatric asthma clinical trial. *J Allergy Clin Immunol.* Oct 2002;110(4):596–602.

66. Smith BA, Shuchman M. Problem of nonadherence in chronically ill adolescents: Strategies for assessment and intervention. *Curr Opin Pediatr.* Oct 2005;17(5):613–618.

67. Khan M, Song X, Williams K, Bright K, Sill A, Rakhmanina N. Evaluating adherence to medication in children and adolescents with HIV. *Arch Dis Child.* Dec 2009;94(12):970–973.

68. Prashad PS, Marcus CL, Maggs J, et al. Investigating reasons for CPAP adherence in adolescents: A qualitative approach. *J Clin Sleep Med.* Dec 15 2013;9(12):1303–1313.

69. Cistulli PA, Armitstead J, Pepin JL, et al. Short-term CPAP adherence in obstructive sleep apnea: A big data analysis using real world data. *Sleep Med.* Jul 2019;59:114–116.

70. Lal C, White DR, Joseph JE, van Bakergem K, LaRosa A. Sleep-disordered breathing in Down syndrome. *Chest.* Feb 2015;147(2):570–579.

71. Brooks LJ, Olsen MN, Bacevice AM, Beebe A, Konstantinopoulou S, Taylor HG. Relationship between sleep, sleep apnea, and neuropsychological function in children with Down syndrome. *Sleep Breath.* Mar 2015;19(1):197–204.

72. Bakker J, Campbell A, Neill A. Randomized controlled trial comparing flexible and continuous positive airway pressure delivery: Effects on compliance, objective and subjective sleepiness and vigilance. *Sleep.* Apr 2010;33(4):523–529.

73. Chihara Y, Tsuboi T, Hitomi T, et al. Flexible positive airway pressure improves treatment adherence compared with auto-adjusting PAP. *Sleep.* Feb 1 2013;36(2):229–236.

74. Centers for Medicare & Medicaid Services (CMS). Decision memo for continuous positive airway pressure (CPAP) therapy for obstructive sleep apnea (OSA) (CAG-00093N). CMS; 2001.

75. Rains JC. Treatment of obstructive sleep apnea in pediatric patients. Behavioral intervention for compliance with nasal continuous positive airway pressure. *Clin Pediatr (Phila).* Oct 1995;34(10):535–541.

76. Soudorn C, Muntham D, Reutrakul S, Chirakalwasan N. Effect of heated humidification on CPAP therapy adherence in subjects with obstructive sleep apnea with nasopharyngeal symptoms. *Respir Care.* Sep 2016;61(9):1151–1159.

77. Xanthopoulos MS, Williamson AA, Tapia IE. Positive airway pressure for the treatment of the childhood obstructive sleep apnea syndrome. *Pediatr Pulmonol.* Aug 2022;57(8):1897–1093.

78. Harford KL, Jambhekar S, Com G, et al. An in-patient model for positive airway pressure desensitization: A report of 2 pediatric cases. *Respir Care.* May 2012;57(5):802–807.

79. Harford KL, Jambhekar S, Com G, et al. Behaviorally based adherence program for pediatric patients treated with positive airway pressure. *Clin Child Psychol Psychiatry.* Jan 2013;18(1):151–163.

80. Edinger JD, Radtke RA. Use of in vivo desensitization to treat a patient's claustrophobic response to nasal CPAP. *Sleep.* Oct 1993;16(7):678–680.

81. Skinner BF. Operant behavior. *Am Psychol.* 1963;18(8):503–515.

82. Pavlov IP, Anrep GV. *Conditioned Reflexes, an Investigation of the Physiological Activity of the Cerebral Cortex.* Dover Publications; 1960.

83. DeVries JK, Nation JJ, Nardone ZB, et al. Multidisciplinary clinic for care of children with complex obstructive sleep apnea. *Int J Pediatr Otorhinolaryngol.* Nov 2020;138:110384.

84. Arora B, Mahajan P, Zidan MA, Sethuraman U. Nasopharyngeal airway pressures in bronchiolitis patients treated with high-flow nasal cannula oxygen therapy. *Pediatr Emerg Care.* Nov 2012;28(11):1179–1184.

85. Frizzola M, Miller TL, Rodriguez ME, et al. High-flow nasal cannula: Impact on oxygenation and ventilation in an acute lung injury model. *Pediatr Pulmonol.* Jan 2011;46(1):67–74.

86. Spentzas T, Minarik M, Patters AB, Vinson B, Stidham G. Children with respiratory distress treated with high-flow nasal cannula. *J Intensive Care Med.* Sep-Oct 2009;24(5):323–328.

87. Dysart K, Miller TL, Wolfson MR, Shaffer TH. Research in high flow therapy: Mechanisms of action. *Respir Med.* Oct 2009;103(10):1400–1405.

88. McGinley BM, Patil SP, Kirkness JP, Smith PL, Schwartz AR, Schneider H. A nasal cannula can be used to treat obstructive sleep apnea. *Am J Respir Crit Care Med.* 2007;176(2):194–200.

89. Kubicka ZJ, Limauro J, Darnall RA. Heated, humidified high-flow nasal cannula therapy: Yet another way to deliver continuous positive airway pressure? *Pediatrics.* Jan 2008;121(1):82–88.

90. Joseph L, Goldberg S, Shitrit M, Picard E. High-flow nasal cannula therapy for obstructive sleep apnea in children. *J Clin Sleep Med.* Sep 15 2015;11(9):1007–1010.

91. Hawkins S, Huston S, Campbell K, Halbower A. High-flow, heated, humidified air via nasal cannula treats CPAP-intolerant children with obstructive sleep apnea. *J Clin Sleep Med.* Aug 15 2017;13(8):981–989.

92. Ignatiuk D, Schaer B, McGinley B. High flow nasal cannula treatment for obstructive sleep apnea in infants and young children. *Pediatr Pulmonol.* Oct 2020;55(10):2791–2798.

93. Gurbani N, Ehsan Z, Brockbank J, Simakajornboon N. Comparison of high-flow nasal cannula therapy to low-flow nasal oxygen as a treatment for obstructive sleep apnea in infants. *Am J Respir Crit Care Med.* 2020;201:A1165.

94. Hough JL, Pham TM, Schibler A. Physiologic effect of high-flow nasal cannula in infants with bronchiolitis. *Pediatr Crit Care Med.* Jun 2014;15(5):e214–e219.

95. Hegde S, Prodhan P. Serious air leak syndrome complicating high-flow nasal cannula therapy: A report of 3 cases. *Pediatrics.* Mar 2013;131(3):e939–e944.

96. Dani C, Pratesi S, Migliori C, Bertini G. High flow nasal cannula therapy as respiratory support in the preterm infant. *Pediatr Pulmonol.* Jul 2009;44(7):629–634.

38

Noninvasive Ventilation in Neuromuscular Disease

Lisa F. Wolfe

CHAPTER HIGHLIGHTS

- Neuromuscular disorders are a diverse group of acquired or inherited conditions that present with sleep-disordered breathing as restrictive lung disease than obstructive upper airway.
- Common symptoms of sleep-disordered breathing in patients with neuromuscular disease (NMD) are dyspnea, orthopnea, fatigue, and inattentiveness, which serve as harbingers to underlying hypopneas/hypoventilation.
- Polysomnography is not required for initiation of noninvasive ventilation (NIV) in NMD patients, and respiratory screening markers, including pulmonary function tests, laboratory measures of bicarbonate and/or $PaCO_2$, and/or overnight oximetry, are crucial in identifying sleep-disordered breathing in this specific population.
- The gold standard of treatment is bi-level spontaneous timed mode with many advanced settings including trigger, cycle, rise time, inspiratory time, and volume-assured pressure support (VAPS) technology.

Neuromuscular disorders are a diverse group of acquired or inherited conditions involving the nerves, muscles, or their connections. These disorders include but are not limited to spinal muscular atrophy (SMA), myotonic dystrophy, Duchenne muscular dystrophy, cerebral palsies, peripheral neuropathies, congenital myopathies, and myasthenia gravis, in addition to a multitude of gene duplications or deletions that may result in reduced diaphragmatic strength, neuromuscular weakness of upper airway dilators, or cardiomyopathy, which can contribute to the development of sleep-disordered breathing. The progression of neuromuscular disease (NMD) results in several sleep-disordered breathing events.[1]

The most common presentation of sleep-disordered breathing in NMD is hypopneas associated with hypoventilation. This is usually evident on polysomnography (PSG) with a sawtooth pattern of intermittent desaturation occurring during phasic rapid eye movement (REM) sleep (Fig. 38.1). As NMD progresses, hypoventilation develops initially during REM sleep from decreased accessory respiratory muscle activity compared with NREM sleep. Hypoventilation is most often due to a decrease in lung volumes in the supine position during sleep and a drop in ventilatory response to hypercarbia. This decrease in ventilatory response to hypercarbia can be due to neuromuscular weakness despite an intact central drive or from a decrease in chemosensitivity from chronic hypercapnia.[2] Nocturnal hypoventilation during sleep is defined for children when more than 25% of the sleep time is spent with an arterial $PaCO_2$ >50 mm Hg.[3] For adults nocturnal hypoventilation is defined as an increase in the arterial $PaCO_2$ to a value $\geq$ to 55 mm Hg for $\geq$10 minutes, or a $\geq$10 mm Hg increase in the arterial $PaCO_2$ relative to the awake supine value, to a value exceeding 50 mm Hg for $\geq$10 minutes.

Screening for respiratory weakness in patients with NMD is prudent as expiratory, inspiratory, or upper airway muscles can be compromised, ultimately leading to chronic respiratory failure. Accepted standards for assessing respiratory weakness are transdiaphragmatic pressure and esophageal pressure monitoring; however, these are impractical in a clinic setting. Surrogate markers for diaphragm weakness include maximum inspiratory pressure (P_{Imax}), supine and upright forced vital capacity (FVC), overnight oximetry, and $PaCO_2$. High serum bicarbonate $\geq$30 mEq/L, forced expiratory volume in 1 second (FEV_1) $\leq$40% of predicted value, FVC <80%, reduction in seated to supine vital capacity by 25% or greater, and significant reductions in maximal inspiratory pressure (MIP) or sniff nasal pressure (SNIP) have all been used in clinical settings to assess for progression of respiratory weakness.[4] Although these screening suggestions are based upon Medicare reimbursement for noninvasive ventilation (NIV) or respiratory assist devices in the adult population, they may be applied to pediatric patients when patients are able to tolerate screening tests.

Clinical signs and/or symptoms that may indicate the need for initiation of NIV include dyspnea, orthopnea, daytime fatigue, morning headaches, and progressive muscle weakness leading to diaphragm dysfunction and/or scoliosis. NIV has been used since the 1950s in the

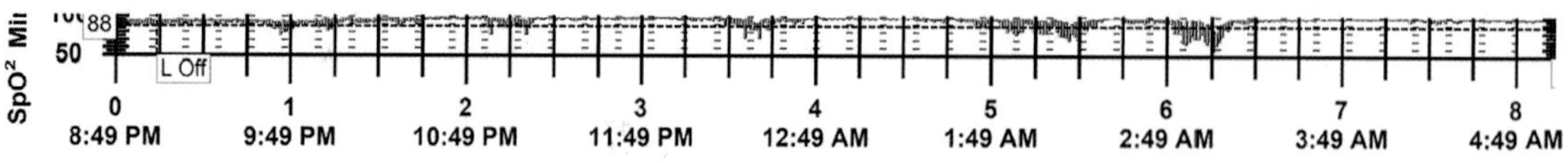

• **Fig. 38.1** Oxygen saturation showing sawtooth pattern during phasic rapid eye movement (REM) sleep suggesting hypoventilation.

polio epidemic; however, the development of modern bi-level positive airway pressure (BPAP) devices were not fully accepted for clinical use until the 1990s. NIV is widely used in hospitalized patients presenting with acute-on-chronic hypercapnic respiratory failure and can improve survival and quality of life of NMD patients. In a systematic review including 1,412 children across 36 different neuromuscular disorders, mortality has been shown to be lower for children using long-term NIV compared with supportive care across various NMD types. NIV utilization in patients with NMD had lower hospitalization rates, except for those with SMA type 1. Sleep study parameters improved from baseline by long-term NIV use.[5] NIV has been associated with an increase in survival rates among patients with Duchenne muscular dystrophy in Denmark with mortality falling between 1977 and 2021 due to a large increase in ventilator use.[6] NIV, along with nutritional support and cough-assist techniques, has shown to increase survival in infants with SMA type 1.[7] NIV associated with mechanical insufflation-exsufflation has been shown to prevent thoracic deformities and lung hypoplasia in children with NMD.[8]

NMDs are categorized as restrictive thoracic disorders for Medicare reimbursement for NIV or respiratory assist devices. Children with NMD represent the largest group of children requiring NIV.[9] Children with NMD often have weakness of the respiratory muscles resulting in the central drive increasing demand on respiratory muscles. However, the respiratory muscles are not able to cope with the respiratory load, and hypoventilation occurs as evidenced by hypercapnia and hypoxemia. NMD involving the motor neuron, peripheral nerve, neuromuscular junction, or the respiratory muscle complex may result in excessive weakness causing ineffective respiration and ventilation. Kyphoscoliosis, commonly found in children with NMD, may increase the respiratory load and result in a mechanical disadvantage of respiratory muscles leading to alveolar hypoventilation. The role of NIV in these patients is to assist weakened respiratory muscles to maintain a sufficient tidal volume and minute ventilation to correct alveolar hypoventilation.

Currently there are no validated criteria for when to start long-term NIV in children. Consensus conferences agree that the value of daytime hypercapnia and recurrent acute respiratory exacerbations are indications of established ventilatory failure.[10] In adults, the minimum requirement for initiation of NIV includes symptoms suggestive of hypoventilation (Fig. 38.2) and any of the following: awake arterial blood gas CO_2 levels ≥ 45 mm Hg or oxygen saturation of $\leq 88\%$ for at least 5 minutes of nocturnal recording, P_{Imax} -60 cm H_2O, or FVC <50% predicted performed in the

upright or supine position.[11] In children with NMD, the documentation of nocturnal hypoventilation by means of PSG is recommended but not mandatory prior to initiating NIV. NIV may be justified without a sleep study when the patient presents with acute respiratory failure triggered by a respiratory infection or an anesthesia event, which can serve as markers of an insufficient respiratory reserve.[12] It is recommended to screen with a minimum of overnight pulse oximetry to detect nocturnal hypoxemia and/or transcutaneous monitoring (TCM) for hypercapnia. When possible, obtaining a comprehensive polysomnogram should be a priority in children with any NMD that may be associated with nocturnal hypoventilation. Timing of such screening lacks validated recommendations as the heterogeneity of pediatric NMD, and variability of respiratory involvement varies significantly based on progression of disease specific to the neuromuscular etiology. It is important to note that the respiratory natural progression for many NMD patients starts with normal breathing that can be augmented with cough-assist techniques. The development of sleep-disordered breathing starting in REM sleep with progression to non–rapid eye movement (NREM) sleep as disease progresses necessitates the initiation of nocturnal NIV. As NMD progresses, daytime NIV may be required with invasive ventilation required at end-stage respiratory failure.

A thorough understanding of NIV modes and settings is essential in the initiation and management of NIV for NMD patients. In minimally monitored hospital areas and at home, the most common NIV device is the BPAP, which is designed to interact with a nasal or full-face interface mask. The device consists of a blower, a respiratory circuit, heated humidity, and a mask. Flow and pressure sensors within the device adjust the blower speed to reach a preset positive pressure output. NIV encompasses bi-level devices that are capable of separately adjusting inspiratory positive airway pressure (IPAP) and expiratory positive airway pressure (EPAP). The EPAP is set to maintain upper airway patency. IPAP and EPAP difference provides pressure support (PS) to augment the patient's tidal volume. The blower, depending on device manufacturer and mode, may provide a fixed bi-level or a bi-level that may be adjusted to support the patient's ventilation (volume-assured pressure support mode [VAPS]). VAPS devices can sense changes in the patient's respiratory flow over several breaths and adjust PS to reach a respiratory target. These respiratory targets are either expiratory tidal volume (for Respironics devices using average volume-assured pressure support [AVAPS]) or alveolar ventilation (for ResMed devices using intelligent volume-assured pressure support [iVAPS]). Bi-level devices

Symptoms	Signs
Dyspnea	Tachypnea
Morning headaches	Nocturnal hypoxemia
Impaired speech	Nocturnal hypoventilation
Recurrent infections	Weak sniff
Early satiety at meals	Ineffective cough
Daytime sleepiness	Thoracoabdominal paradox
Confusion/poor daytime concentration	
Disturbed sleep/frequent arousals	
Poor sleep quality	
Fatigue	
ADHD and learning difficulties	

• **Fig. 38.2** Symptoms and signs of neuromuscular diseases. ADHD, attention-deficit/hyperactivity disorder.

can be delivered in spontaneous mode (S), spontaneous timed (ST) mode, or pressure-assist control mode (PC). It is important to note that continuous positive airway pressure (CPAP) is not indicated for patients with NMD.

There are advanced settings in bi-level mode ST or PC mode that may be adjusted to achieve the goal of overcoming alveolar hypoventilation. Three advanced settings target main phase variables during the respiratory cycle: trigger sensitivity, target tidal volume, and cycle (Fig. 38.3). Trigger sensitivity sets the level of inspiratory flow change above when the device switches from EPAP (exhalation) to IPAP (inhalation). Trigger sensitivity applies to spontaneous breaths and is measured by pressure or flow changes detected by the device. The goal of trigger sensitivity is to decrease muscular effort and decrease the delay between a patient's initiation of breath and the start of the device's delivered breath. Rise time sets the time in the milliseconds that it takes for the device to transition from EPAP to IPAP. It is set to determine how quickly IPAP can be reached. Cycle sensitivity helps set the limit of when to switch from IPAP to EPAP. This limits the inhalation support by IPAP. The device detects the termination of a patient's breath by sensing flow reduction. When setting the cycle sensitivity, this allows the machine to detect the peak flow level below which the device would change from IPAP to EPAP.

The initiation of NIV in NMD patients results in subsequent decrease of respiratory system load, increase in minute ventilation, and decrease in physiologic dead space.[13] The first line of therapy is considered bi-level-ST; however, VAPS in ST or PC has been used as an acceptable alternative. Settings of NIV are individually adjusted for each patient. The goal is to deliver a physiologic tidal volume of 8–10 mL/kg.[14] For some NMD patients who have severe kyphoscoliosis, are under ideal body weight due to non-ambulatory status, or may have difficulty tolerating NIV, a physiologic tidal volume of 6–8 mL/kg is also appropriate. In young infants who have compliant lungs and chest wall, low inspiratory pressures may be used. Higher inspiratory

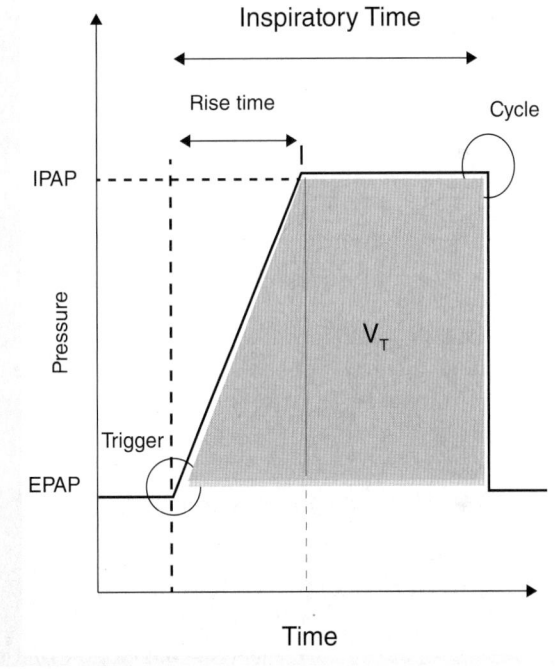

• **Fig. 38.3** Parameters for NIV for sleep-related hypoventilation. EPAP, expiratory positive pressure; IPAP, inspiratory positive pressure; V_T, ventricular tachycardia. (From Selim B, Wolfe L, Coleman J, et al. Initiation of noninvasive ventilation for sleep related hypoventilation disorders. *Chest.* 2018;153:251–265.)

pressures may be required for older children, especially in those with significant scoliosis and/or obesity. A backup rate close to the physiologic breathing rate during sleep is recommended to limit the inspiratory triggering of the ventilator by the patient. Many patients have difficulty with initiation of breaths due to their respiratory muscle weakness.

Advanced BPAP settings are frequently required for patients with NMD. Trigger setting decreases the delay between the patient's initiated breath and the start of device-delivered breathing. For NMD patients the goal is to have high trigger sensitivity to support weak respiratory muscle effort. A high trigger sensitivity requires less flow generation from the patient to initiate a device-generated breath. This can support NMD patients who have progressive respiratory muscle weakness. Sample settings include 1–3 L/min when using Respironics devices and high or very high in ResMed devices. The cycle sensitivity sets a level of peak flow detected that allows the flow generator to switch from IPAP to EPAP. Setting low to signal a late cycle provides longer inhalation time. For Respironics devices this is set to Auto-Trak, which is approximately 10–15% of peak flow. However, the use of Auto-Trak assumes normal diaphragmatic strength, which may result in premature cycling in patients with NMD. Sensitive Auto-Trak is a newer version of the software in Respironics devices that allows adults with weakness or children to more easily trigger breaths; at this time the function has not been developed or tested in patients with NMD.[13] In ResMed devices, the corresponding cycle is set at low or very low for NMD patients. The inspiratory time is the time that IPAP is maintained. In NMD patients, the goal of a long inspiratory time allows for maximal tidal volume and gas exchange. In Respironics devices, the inspiratory time is only applied to timed breaths and not spontaneous breaths. In ResMed devices, the inspiratory time is applied to timed and spontaneous breaths. Examples of NIV settings are referenced in Fig. 38.4.

Although benefits of NIV in NMD patients have been demonstrated, there are potential adverse effects. The most common is skin injury due to pressure from the mask interface, eye irritation from air leaks, and midface hypoplasia/dysplasia in young children.[14] Aerophagia, gastric distention, and gastric reflux may be observed in patients with high inspiratory pressures or patient-ventilator asynchrony.[15] Abdominal side effects may be minimized by decreasing inspiratory pressure or use of abdominal girdle. Unintentional leaks may be associated with discomfort, poor NIV tolerance, and poor sleep quality with arousal. They may be addressed with mask refitting, use of accessories such as masks pads/adhesive tape, or switching different mask interfaces from nasal to full-face mask or full-face mask to nasal mask.

Limitations of compliance, particularly in the pediatric NMD population, remains a significant issue. Mask desensitization, use of humidity and climate-controlled circuit, applying mask, and turning on device after a child has fallen asleep as well as close clinical follow-up are recommended.

Once NIV has been initiated, there are no validated guidelines for monitoring or long-term follow-up of children with NIV. Timing of follow-up visits depends on the age, medical condition, and availability of providers well versed in the management of NIV in NMD patients. Clinical practice varies greatly with some patients having an initial PSG followed by initiation of NIV. Other patients meet criteria without initial PSG and are followed 3–6 months after initiation of NIV. Management of NIV in NMD may be provided by pediatric pulmonologists, pediatric sleep medicine physicians, pediatric neurologists, or in a multidisciplinary team setting such as a muscular dystrophy association clinic. The increasing prevalence of telemedicine services since 2020 has also greatly increased patient and provider access.

In conclusion, NIV in NMD patients has provided an efficacious type of noninvasive respiratory support helping to avoid tracheotomies that has provided patients with support in a home environment that enhances quality of life for the patient and their family. Given the vast heterogeneity of neuromuscular disorders, disease progression timelines, prognosis and individual outcomes, management of NIV

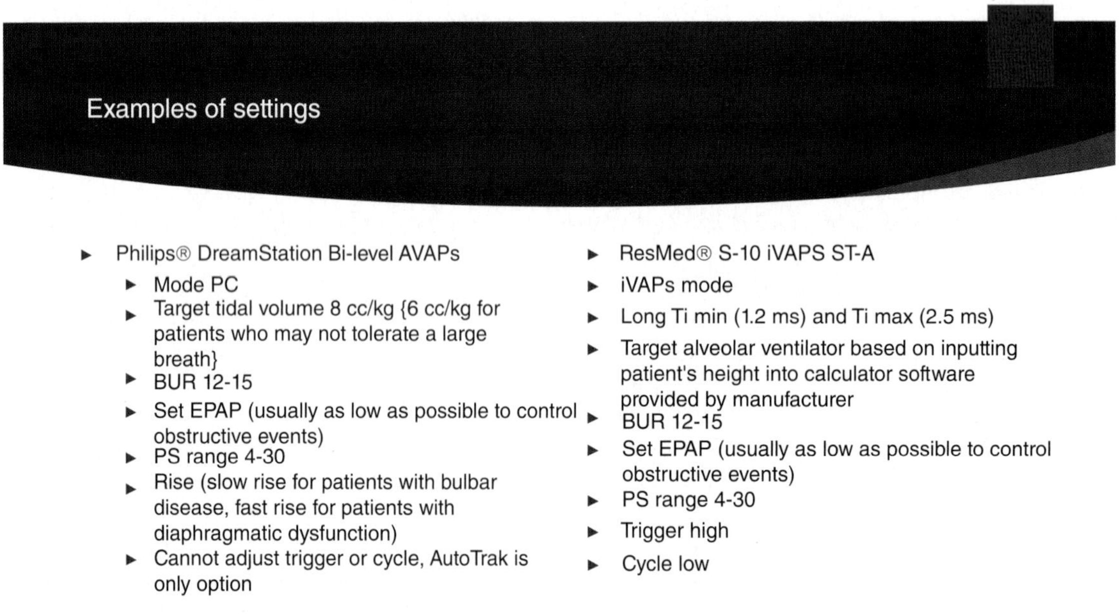

Examples of settings

- ▶ Philips® DreamStation Bi-level AVAPs
  - ▶ Mode PC
  - ▶ Target tidal volume 8 cc/kg {6 cc/kg for patients who may not tolerate a large breath}
  - ▶ BUR 12-15
  - ▶ Set EPAP (usually as low as possible to control obstructive events)
  - ▶ PS range 4-30
  - ▶ Rise (slow rise for patients with bulbar disease, fast rise for patients with diaphragmatic dysfunction)
  - ▶ Cannot adjust trigger or cycle, AutoTrak is only option

- ▶ ResMed® S-10 iVAPS ST-A
  - ▶ iVAPs mode
  - ▶ Long Ti min (1.2 ms) and Ti max (2.5 ms)
  - ▶ Target alveolar ventilator based on inputting patient's height into calculator software provided by manufacturer
  - ▶ BUR 12-15
  - ▶ Set EPAP (usually as low as possible to control obstructive events)
  - ▶ PS range 4-30
  - ▶ Trigger high
  - ▶ Cycle low

• **Fig. 38.4** Examples of settings. AVAPS, average volume-assured pressure support; EPAP, expiratory positive airway pressure; IVAPs, intelligent volume-assured pressures.

in NMD patients optimally requires an experienced and multidisciplinary pediatric team prepared to assess NMD patients as they progress from sleep-disordered breathing to end-stage respiratory failure. Proper management of NIV in NMD patients has demonstrated a dramatic decline in this progression.

CLINICAL PEARLS

- It is important to monitor respiratory function and overnight oximetry for hypoxemia/hypercapnia to determine whether NIV should be initiated.
- Recognize that NIV criteria for NMD patients does not require PSG.
- Consider bi-level in spontaneous timed mode, addition of VAPs mode and modifying inspiratory time, cycle, trigger, and rise to treat neuromuscular respiratory weakness and its progression
- CPAP is not indicated in the treatment of sleep-disordered breathing in NMD patients.

References

1. Aboussouan A. Sleep disordered breathing in neuromuscular disease. *Am J Respir Crit Care Med.* 2015;191:979–989.
2. Johnson DC, Kazemmi H. Central control of ventilation in neuromuscular disease. *Clin Chest Med.* 1994;15:607–617.
3. Berry RB, Brooks R, Gamaldo CE, Harding SM, Lloyd RM, Marcus CL, Vaughn BV, American Academy of Sleep Medicine. *The AASM Manual for the Scoring of Sleep and Associated Events: Rules, Terminology and Technical Specifications. Version 2.2.* Darien, IL: American Academy of Sleep Medicine; 2015. www.aasmnet.org.
4. Sahni AS, Wolfe L. Respiratory care in neuromuscular diseases. *Respir Care.* 2018;63:601–608.
5. Albalawi M, Castro-Codesal M, Featherstone R, et al. Outcomes of long-term non-invasive ventilation use in children with neuromuscular disease: systematic review and meta-analysis. *Ann Am Thorac Soc.* 2022;19:109–119.
6. Jeppesen J, Green A, Steffensen BF, et al. The Duchenne muscular dystrophy population in Denmark, 1977–2001: prevalence, incidence and survival in relation to the introduction of ventilator use. *Neuromuscul Disord.* 2003;13:804–812.
7. Bach Jr, Baird JS, Plosky D, et al. Spinal muscular atrophy type 1: management and outcomes. *Pediatr Pulmonol.* 2002;34:16–22.
8. Chatwin M, Bush A, Simonds AK. Outcome of goal-directed non-invasive ventilation and mechanical insufflation/exsufflation in spinal muscular atrophy type 1. *Arch Dis Child.* 2011;96:426–432.
9. Castro-Codesal ML, Dehann K, Featherstone R, et al. Long-term non-invasive ventilation therapies in children: a scoping review. *Sleep Med Rev.* 2018;37:138–158.
10. Hull J, Aniapravan R, Chan E, et al. Respiratory management of children with neuromuscular weakness guideline group on behalf of the British thoracic society standards of care committee. *Thorax.* 2012;57il–40.
11. Resmed. Respiratory assist device (RAD) coverage guidelines: Medicare revision effective date: January 1, 2019. 1010293_RAD_Guidelines.pdf. Accessed 12/23/2021. International Classification of Sleep Disorders. 3rd ed. Westchester, IL: American Academy of Sleep Medicine; 2014.
12. Amaddeo A, Moreau J, Frapin A, et al. Long term continuous positive airway pressure (CPAP) and non-invasive ventilation (NIV) in children: initiation criteria in real life. *Pediatr Pulmonol.* 2016;51:968–974.
13. Selim B, Wolfe L, Coleman J, et al. Initiation of noninvasive ventilation for sleep related hypoventilation disorders. *Chest.* 2018;153:251–265.
14. Schroth MK. Special considerations in the respiratory management of spinal muscular atrophy. *Pediatrics.* 2009;123(Suppl 4):S245–S249.
15. Fauroux B, Khirani S, Griffon L, et al. Non-invasive ventilation in children with neuromuscular disease. *Front Pediatr.* 2020;16(8):482.

39

Novel Pharmacologic Approaches for Treatment of Obstructive Sleep Apnea

Leila Kheirandish-Gozal and David Gozal

CHAPTER HIGHLIGHTS

- Adenotonsillar hypertrophy is the primary cause of upper airway obstruction in pediatric obstructive sleep apnea.
- Physiological compensatory mechanisms, including activation of upper airway muscles and increased central ventilatory drive, mitigate excessive upper airway collapsibility in childre.
- LT-dependent pathways contribute to intrinsic proliferative and inflammatory signaling pathways, playing a significant role in adenotonsillar hypertrophy in children.
- Leukotriene modifiers could serve as a direct therapeutic option for mild OSA, potentially as an alternative to adenotonsillectomy.
- Topical corticosteroids show promise as a therapy for mild obstructive sleep apnea in healthy children. Further research is needed to establish the optimal timing and efficacy of CS interventions in conjunction with other therapies for OSA.

Introduction

Adenotonsillar hypertrophy has been identified as the major pathophysiologic factor in the causation of upper airway obstruction in pediatric obstructive sleep apnea (OSA). Over the last few decades, novel immunologic techniques have enabled identification of some of the specific tonsillar cells underlying inflammatory immune responses in specific contextual settings; however, the exact mechanisms leading to the adenotonsillar cell proliferation are still not fully understood.[1] It is apparent that a combination of structural and neuromuscular abnormalities contributes to the occurrence of OSA in children.[2] Tonsils and adenoids continue to grow from birth to 12 years of age, with the greatest increase in size during the ages of 2 and 8 years, a process that is paralleled by the surrounding structures that constitute the upper airway. During this period of time, the gradual growth in the size of the skeletal boundaries of the upper airway

and the occurrence of disproportionate growth of adenoids and tonsils relative to the other upper airway structures will result in a relatively narrower upper airway, even if, as mentioned, the growth of all structures during this period is parallel to each other.[3] The relative physiologic narrowing of the upper airway space in children is, however, compensated by the activation of the upper airway muscles and through increased central ventilatory drive, preventing the excessive upper airway collapsibility when compared with adults.[4] As such, OSA only occurs when the interaction between the anatomical restriction and the neuromuscular reflexes fails to preserve airway patency, a state-dependent process, because it does not occur during wakefulness.

Nevertheless, the size of the adenoids and tonsils plays a significant role in the severity of OSA.[5,6] This excessive tissue enlargement can be induced by proliferation of specific cellular components and is due to various isolated or recurrent bacterial or viral infections as well as exposure to environmental irritants such as allergens, cigarette smoke, and air pollution.[7–11] The location of the adenoids and tonsils at the entrance of the respiratory and alimentary tracts positions them as the first site of contact with a variety of microorganisms and antigenic substances that are present in food and inhaled air, resulting in proliferation and growth in these organs.

Currently, surgical extirpation of these tissues is the first line of treatment for either recurrent infection or pediatric sleep apnea;[12] however, the efficacy of adenotonsillectomy (T&A) has recently been challenged, with informal assessments of highly variable reductions in estimated success rates ranging from 30–85% of cases,[13–29] further intensifying the need for developing non-surgical therapeutic options more than ever.[30–32]

Inflammation in Pediatric Obstructive Sleep Apnea

Because adenotonsillar hypertrophy and hyperplasia are the primary causes of OSA in children, the mechanisms leading

433

to the enlargement of these complex lymphoid structures has been a main focus of investigation among researchers in the field. The earlier studies were primarily focused on assessment of bacterial infections as the underlying cause of recurrent tonsillitis and as contributing factors to recurrent chronic otitis media and their epidemiologic links with adenotonsillar hypertrophy.[33–37] Since then, different theories have evolved, particularly in relation to the development of adenotonsillar hypertrophy that underlies OSA in children. Indeed, current opinion surmises that a low-grade systemic inflammation is present in addition to local upper inflammation in pediatric OSA. Multiple studies have investigated the cause and effect of mechanical vibration due to intermittent collapse and occlusion of the upper airway manifested by snoring as a potential primary source of inflammation in children with OSA. In this context, localized inflammation of the upper airway tissue would occur as a result of continuous and periodic mechanical insult due to tissue vibration and intraluminal pharyngeal pressure swings from the repeated upper airway obstructive events.[38,39] Thus, the initiation of mild snoring would promote inflammation that would progressively aggravate the snoring, leading to a vicious cycle of disease progression. Although this theory is definitely attractive, there is no available epidemiologic evidence supporting such a temporal trajectory of progressive worsening of OSA in children. Indeed, the time course of disease initiation and progression has yet to be investigated. Some investigators argue that snoring-related mechanical trauma to the soft palate and uvula may not be the sole factor underlying upper airway inflammation considering the fact that both nasal and oropharyngeal mucosal inflammation are also present in patients with OSA, and that the nasal mucosa is not subjected to repeated snoring-induced injury.[40–42] Conversely, the alternations between hypoxia and reoxygenation could produce excessive free radicals mediated through several intracellular pathways that potentially will lead to both local and systemic inflammation.[43] Another possible mechanism that has been advanced links early life infections with respiratory viruses as eliciting enduring immune cell-mediated amplificatory memory responses that will be triggered upon exposure to inhaled stimuli such as environmental pollution or recurrent viral infections.[44]

Thus, the mechanisms leading to the initiation, generation, and propagation of inflammatory processes within the upper airway among various age groups will definitely require more extensive investigation than simply just the evidence that was presented previously. A recent study identified an inflammatory protein, namely CHI3L1, that can promote the proliferation of tonsil lymphocytes via activation of ERK1/2-dependent pathways.[45] Thus, inhibition of CHI3L1 or ERK1/2 may be a potential therapeutic target for OSA by reducing the proliferative elements within tonsils and adenoids. Similar roles have been identified to other active putative pathways underlying tonsillar proliferation such as phosphatases, CD40, and indoleamine 2,3-dioxygenase.[46,47]

Evidence of Local Upper Airway and Systemic Inflammation in Pediatric Obstructive Sleep Apnea

In adults with OSA, increased concentrations of proinflammatory markers, such as interleukin (IL)-6 and 8-isopentane, and oxidative stress markers have been reported in the exhaled upper airway condensate.[48–50] Higher levels of nuclear factor κB-dependent genes such as tumor necrosis factor-alpha (TNF-α) and IL-6 are also present,[51] and treatment of OSA with continuous positive airway pressure was associated with reductions in serum levels of high-sensitivity C-reactive protein (hsCRP) and IL-6 concentrations,[52] while local airway inflammation was improved, as evidenced by reduced numbers of neutrophils.[53] Thus, adults with OSA present evidence of both local (i.e., upper airway) and systemic low-grade inflammatory changes.

What about children? Since the initial study by Tauman and colleagues, who reported increased plasma hsCRP levels in children with OSA compared to controls, multiple studies have corroborated such findings.[54] Interestingly, improved hsCRP levels and cardiovascular markers after effective treatment of OSA were also demonstrated.[54–57] Subsequent studies further suggested that variances in the hsCRP levels or in polymorphisms within the NADPH oxidase gene or its functional subunits such as p22phox, both of which reflect systemic inflammatory responses, appear to account for important components of the differences in cognitive function deficits associated with OSA in children.[55–58] Thus, the degree of systemic inflammation and oxidative stress may play a major contributor to the presence of morbidity in children with OSA and, as a result, targeting of such pathways may provide a viable therapeutic strategy toward prevention of end-organ morbidity.[56,58] We have recently systematically reviewed the evidence regarding two prototypic proinflammatory cytokines in the context of adult and pediatric OSA, illustrating the heterogeneity of findings in otherwise small cohorts.[59]

Another significant contributor to the pathophysiology of pediatric OSA and the treatment outcomes is obesity, which should be viewed as yet another systemic inflammatory condition. The rather accelerated increase over the last two decades in the prevalence of pediatric obesity has led to substantial changes in the cross-sectional demographic and anthropometric characteristics of the children who are referred for evaluation of suspected OSA.[60,61] Obesity is a proven and definitive risk factor that operates in a synergistic fashion among children at risk for OSA, and such interactions could, in fact, reflect augmented activation of inflammatory pathways.[62–64] Thus, considering the deleterious consequences of OSA in children if left untreated, the use of therapeutic agents toward reduction in inflammation or specific oxidative stress may yield to reverse or palliated morbidities.

The evidence of local inflammatory processes within the upper airway of children with OSA is not as well established and has not been as thoroughly investigated. Here, we will review the few selected pathways that have thus far gained attention in pediatric OSA, namely leukotriene and glucocorticoid pathways.

Leukotriene and Leukotriene Receptors

Cysteinyl leukotrienes are major mediators of inflammation in both humans and animals, and serve as potent neutrophil chemoattractants and activators.[65] The cysteinyl leukotriene receptors 1 and 2 are expressed on several tissues including the nasal mucosa and the lungs.[66,67] The leukotrienes B4 and the Cys LTs, C4, D4, and E4 can mediate inflammation in both the upper and lower airways by binding to Cys LT receptors, although LTB_4 has two cognate receptors that exhibit much higher affinity to this leukotriene. A considerable overlap and interdependency between asthma and OSA,[68–70] as well as compelling evidence of the favorable effect of CYS LT1-R antagonists in reducing inflammation in children with inflammatory conditions such as asthma and allergic rhinitis,[71,72] suggested a potential role for leukotriene modifiers in the management of pediatric OSA.

Assessment of the LT1-R and LT2-R expression in tonsils and adenoids of children with OSA compared with children with recurrent infectious tonsillitis without OSA revealed higher protein expression levels of LT1-R and LT2-R, along with a distinct topographical pattern of distribution, suggesting that different mechanisms promoting inflammation are operational in OSA versus infection-induced tonsillitis.[73] In this context, it would appear that leukotrienes may contribute to the higher proliferative pattern of upper airway lymphoid tissues than is present in the generation of adenotonsillar hypertrophy that characterizes the majority of children with OSA. Indeed, immunohistochemical characterization of germinal centers in tonsils of children with OSA showed a peripheral location of LT1-R (Fig. 39.1), which might be due to either its occurrence during late stages of maturation of lymphoid tissues or, as proposed by others, LT1-R-positive cells might have migrated from the vasculature to occupy sites within the tonsils, where their activation may be of functional importance.[74] The initial characterization of heightened expression of leukotrienes and their receptors in the adenoids and tonsils of OSA patients was subsequently confirmed by Kaditis and colleagues who showed that tonsils of children with OSA display an enhanced expression of cysteinyl leukotriene receptors in T lymphocytes without an associated increase in serum hsCRP concentrations.[75] Of note, an increased

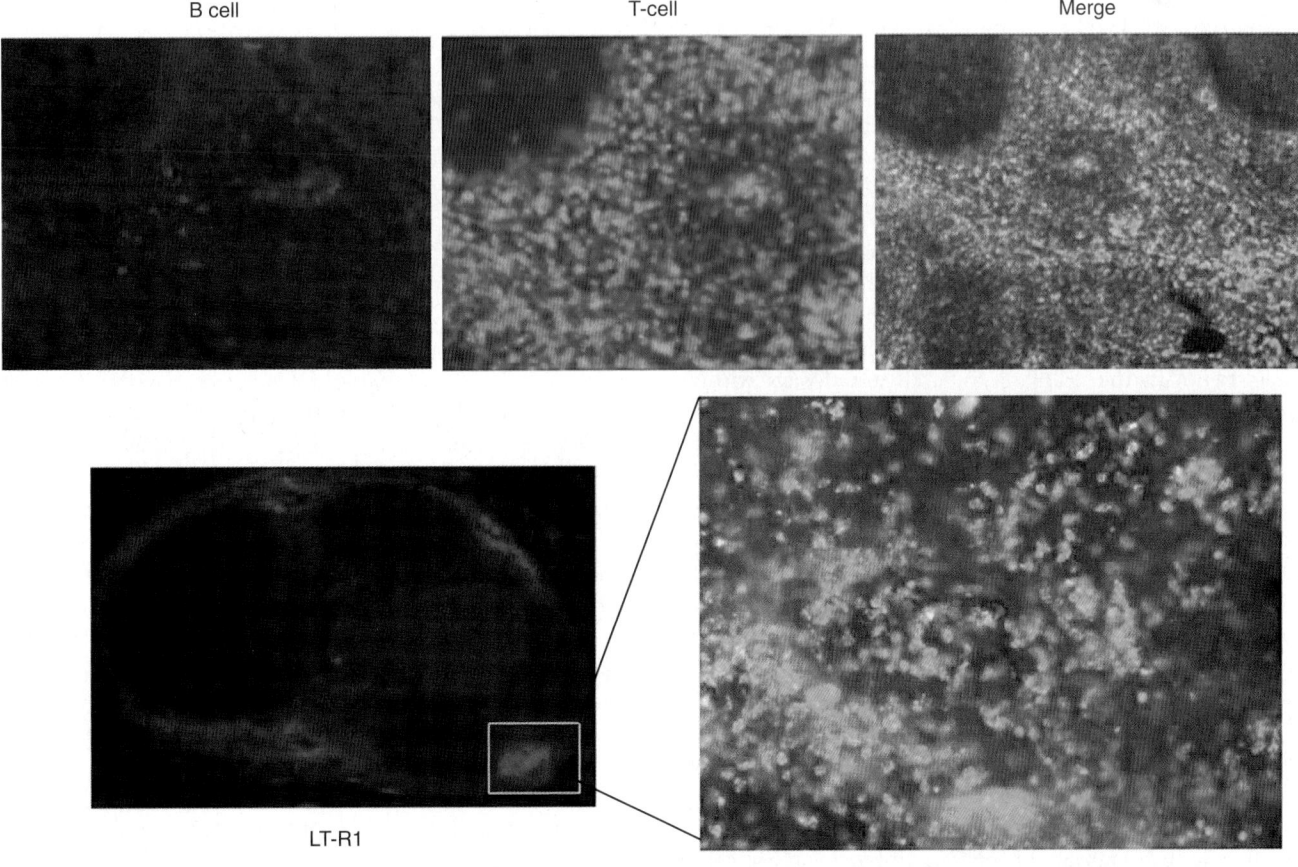

• **Fig. 39.1** Immunohistochemical stains of a tonsil from a child with obstructive sleep apnea (OSA) showing the disproportionate abundance of T-cell lymphocytes, particularly CD8+ lymphocytes, and the high level of expression of leukotriene receptors in the peripheral regions surrounding the germinal centers.

preponderance of CD8+ lymphocytes is present in tonsils of children with OSA (see Fig. 37.1). Increased concentrations of either LTB_4 or LTC4/LTD4/LTE4 in the adenotonsillar tissues of children with OSA could promote upper airway lymphoid hypertrophy/hyperplasia when compared with children with recurrent infectious tonsillitis.[76] Upregulation of LT1-R and LT2-R expression could potentially promote tonsillar enlargement in children with OSA by promoting the proliferation or the proinflammatory activity of T-cell lymphocytes within the tonsillar and adenoidal tissues.[77] Of note, increases in leukotriene concentrations LTB_4 and LTC4/LTD4/LTE4 are readily identified in the exhaled breath condensates of children with OSA.[78] Interestingly, and similar to children, LTB_4 concentrations were also found to be elevated in the exhaled condensates of adults with OSA and appear to be correlated with the severity of OSA.[79]

To further assess the effects of LTD4 and several LT receptor antagonists on lymphoid tissue proliferation, Gozal and colleagues developed a mixed-cell culture model using freshly dissociated tonsils or adenoids harvested during T&A from children with polysomnographically diagnosed OSA or recurrent tonsillitis. Cellular proliferation and release of inflammatory cytokines were assessed in cell culture supernatants using standard enzyme-linked immunosorbent assays.[80,81] In this ex vivo model, LTD4 elicited dose-dependent increases in adenotonsillar cell proliferation that were markedly enhanced in children with OSA.

On the other hand, LT antagonists exhibited dose-dependent reductions in adenotonsillar cellular proliferation rates, with montelukast showing superior potency compared with the other antagonists tested, suggesting that LT-dependent pathways underlie components of the intrinsic proliferative and inflammatory signaling pathways and play a significant role in adenotonsillar hypertrophy in children.[82] A more recent study has further confirmed the important role of leukotrienes in the cellular proliferative pathways within tonsillar tissues.[83]

Interestingly, the cell substrates mediating the hyperplastic responses of these tissues demonstrate a T-cell preponderance of proliferation of CD3+, CD4+, and CD8+ lymphocytes in OSA, while B-cell lymphocytes were more likely to be proliferative in recurrent infection (RI).[75,81] Circulating levels of LTB_4 and Cys LT were also found to be elevated in children with mild and moderate to severe OSA compared with controls, and decreased after treatment.[84]

Therefore, based on the previously mentioned studies, it is plausible to conclude that lipoxygenase-dependent pathways are involved in the pathophysiology of OSA in children, and may serve as targets for treatment of this condition, particularly in selected subgroups of children. Improving the severity of residual OSA after TA with leukotriene antagonists was shown as an effective approach, justifying the use of leukotriene receptor antagonists as potential adjuncts to pre and

to post T&A in pediatric OSA, in an effort to improve the outcomes associated with this surgery.[85] Leukotriene modifiers could also be considered as a direct therapeutic option in mild OSA as an alternative to T&A.[10] An initial randomized double-blind, placebo-controlled trial with oral montelukast in children with mild OSA showed significant improvements in apnea index and in adenoid size.[86] A subsequent randomized controlled trial (RCT) by our group further reiterated and confirmed such findings,[87] and additional studies in the last several years attest to the overall beneficial role and safety of montelukast in children with OSA.[88–92]

Glucocorticoid Receptors and Corticosteroids in Pediatric Obstructive Sleep Apnea

Corticosteroids (CS) are frequently used by pediatricians for clinical management of conditions such as asthma and allergic rhinitis; however, the favorable response is somewhat uneven in children with asthma, suggesting that some of these children may exhibit differential sensitivity to the activity of CS, a phenomenon that was initially ascribed to differences in glucocorticoid receptor (GCR) subtype expression (i.e., the expression of CS-sensitive GCRα expression was dominant as opposed to the presence of GCRβ expression). Furthermore, reduced ligand binding to CS, single nucleotide polymorphisms in the GCR gene, or defects in GCR translocation to the nucleus and binding to the glucocorticoid-binding response element account for a fraction of CS-resistant asthma.[93–98] Among other identified mechanisms for resistance to CS, a reduction in histone deacetylase (HDAC)-2 activity and expression, impaired GCR activity and increased proinflammatory signaling pathways could all be operational. Both GCRα and GCRβ are expressed in adenotonsillar tissues of children with OSA, are significantly abundant, and demonstrate specific topographic patterns within the germinal centers. In addition, the high GCRα:GCRβ ratios found in all tissues analyzed further indicate a favorable therapeutic response profile for topical CS therapy in snoring children with adenotonsillar hypertrophy.[99] Therefore, there is little if any reason to anticipate that upper airway lymphadenoid tissues exhibit resistance to treatment with CS. In a series of experiments, Kheirandish-Gozal and colleagues assessed the cellular proliferation rates and apoptotic rates using the previously mentioned mixed cell model of dissociated tonsils or adenoids harvested intraoperatively from children. In vitro treatments were conducted with three selected CS, namely dexamethasone (DEX), fluticasone (FLU), and budesonide (BUD). All three compounds reduced cellular proliferation rates and exhibited dose-dependent effects. In addition, increased apoptosis among T-cell lymphocytes and significant reduction in TNF-α, IL-8, and IL-6 concentrations in the supernatants was observed, suggesting the likelihood of successful treatment of pediatric OSA with CS topical application. Of note, the available cumulative experience with CS use in the treatment of pediatric OSA is quite limited, and will be reviewed in the following.[100]

In a very early study by Demain and Goetz, a small number of children with chronic obstructive nasal symptoms were randomly assigned to an 8-week, double-blind, placebo-controlled crossover study of standard-dose aqueous nasal beclomethasone followed by 16-week, open-label intranasal beclomethasone.[101] This trial resulted in significant improvements in obstructive symptom scores as well as in adenoidal hypertrophy, suggesting a favorable outcome for use of topical CS in children with OSA that was primarily due to adenotonsillar hypertrophy.[101] However, the latter study did not include sleep studies, and a pilot open-label study using short-term (5-day) oral prednisone in prepubertal children with OSA yielded no improvements in either clinical symptomatology or in adenotonsillar size.[102]

In a subsequent randomized triple-blind study, the efficacy of topical intranasal steroids in treating 25 children with polysomnographically proven moderately severe OSA who were scheduled for T&A was assessed. Although significant reduction in overall respiratory abnormalities was observed, the indices of adenoidal and tonsillar sizes remained unchanged, suggesting that inflammatory components are important contributors to upper airway collapsibility.[103] In addition, an open-label study of nasal BUD administered for 4 weeks reported sustained effect of intranasal steroids even months after discontinuation of CS therapy.[104]

Several subsequent studies have reported on the beneficial effect of another topical CS, i.e., mometasone furoate, on adenoid size; however, the authors in this study did not objectively evaluate breathing patterns during sleep.[105–107] In addition, reductions in cytokines were also reported.[108] In a recent randomized, double-blind controlled trial with a crossover design, intranasal BUD was administered at bedtime for a total of 6 weeks' duration, and was shown to substantially either reduce the severity of mild OSA or normalize sleep respiratory disturbance, as well as the size of the adenoids relative to the airway, and this beneficial effect persisted for at least 8 weeks after cessation of the therapy.[109] Such findings were substantiated using meta-analytical approaches that ultimately confirmed that long-term safety and efficacy data are unavailable.[110]

Therefore, the use of topical CS appears justified as a viable therapeutic option in otherwise healthy children with mild OSA, but larger and more pointed trials are needed to address issues such as efficacy in younger and older children, the usefulness of CS in obese children, and appropriate and optimal timing of such interventions in the context of other therapies. A real-life experience from our center involving more than 800 children with mild OSA revealed clinical improvements or resolution of the disease in >80% of the children,[111] further attesting to the importance of judicious treatment selection and long-term monitoring and follow-up of children suffering from OSA.

CLINICAL PEARLS

- Pediatric obstructive sleep apnea (OSA) is primarily the result of inflammatory processes in the upper airway that involve hyperplasia/hypertrophy of the adenoids and tonsils and is primarily treated by surgical removal of these tissues (adenotonsillectomy [T&A]).
- T&A is likely to reduce the severity of OSA in most cases but is rarely curative; furthermore, there is no consensus as to the apnea-hypopnea index (AHI) cutoff value that represents a clear-cut indication for T&A. Therefore, alternative non-surgical therapeutic options in milder cases of OSA should be considered.
- Increased expression of leukotrienes and their receptors is associated with increased proliferation of upper airway lymphoid tissues. Therefore, leukotriene modifiers are emerging as potentially useful agents in the treatment of mild pediatric OSA.
- The glucocorticoid receptor expression patterns in adenotonsillar tissues suggest a high likelihood for favorable responses to corticosteroid treatment of pediatric OSA, and this assumption has now been corroborated by a small number of randomized double-blind controlled trials.
- Although the effect of anti-inflammatory therapy in pediatric OSA has only been evaluated with randomized controlled trials (RCTs) in relatively small groups of patients, the overall encouraging results support the utilization of these approaches, particularly in mild OSA cases.

References

1. Heier I, Malmstrom K, Pelkonen AS, et al. Bronchial response pattern of antigen presenting cells and regulatory T cells in children less than 2 years of age. *Thorax*. 2008;63(8):703–709.
2. Marcus CL, McColley SA, Carroll JL, et al. Upper airway collapsibility in children with obstructive sleep apnea syndrome. *J Appl Physiol*. 1994;77(2):918–924.
3. Jeans WD, Fernando DC, Maw AR, et al. A longitudinal study of the growth of the nasopharynx and its contents in normal children. *Br J Radiol*. 1981;54(638):117–121.
4. Marcus CL, Lutz J, Hamer A, et al. Developmental changes in response to subatmospheric pressure loading of the upper airway. *J Appl Physiol*. 1999;87(2):626–633.
5. Brooks LJ, Stephens B, Bacevice AM. Adenoid size is related to severity but not the number of episodes of obstructive apnea in children. *J Pediatr*. 1998;132(4):682–686.
6. Li AM, Wong E, Kew J, et al. Use of tonsil size in the evaluation of obstructive sleep apnoea. *Arch Dis Child*. 2002;87(2):156–159.
7. Ersu R, Arman AR, Save D, et al. Prevalence of snoring and symptoms of sleep-disordered breathing in primary school children in Istanbul. *Chest*. 2004;126(1):19–24.
8. Snow A, Dayyat E, Montgomery-Downs HE, et al. Pediatric obstructive sleep apnea: A potential late consequence of respiratory syncytial virus bronchiolitis. *Pediatr Pulmonol*. 2009;44(12):1186–1191.
9. Goldbart AD, Mager E, Veling MC, et al. Neurotrophins and tonsillar hypertrophy in children with obstructive sleep apnea. *Pediatr Res*. 2007;62(4):489–494.
10. Kuhle S, Urschitz MS. Anti-inflammatory medications for obstructive sleep apnea in children. *Cochrane Database Syst Rev*. 2011;1CD007074.

11. Siegel G, Linse R, Macheleidt S. Factors of tonsillar involution: Age-dependent changes in B-cell activation and Langerhans' cell density. *Arch Otorhinolaryngol.* 1982;236(3):261–269.

12. Schechter MS. American Academy of Pediatrics, Section on Pediatrics Pulmonology, Subcommittee on Obstructive Sleep Apnea Syndrome. Technical Report: Diagnosis and Management of Childhood Obstructive Sleep Apnea Syndrome. *Pediatrics.* 2002;109(4):e69.

13. Lipton AJ, Gozal D. Treatment of obstructive sleep apnea in children: Do we really know how? *Sleep Med Rev.* 2003;7(1):61–80.

14. Bhattacharjee R, Kheirandish-Gozal L, Spruyt K, et al. Adenotonsillectomy outcomes in treatment of obstructive sleep apnea in children: A multicenter retrospective study. *Am J Respir Crit Care Med.* 2010;182(5):676–683.

15. Marcus CL, Moore RH, Rosen CL, et al. A randomized trial of adenotonsillectomy for childhood sleep apnea. *N Engl J Med.* 2013;368(25):2366–2376.

16. Liu CN, Kang KT, Yao CJ, et al. Changes in cone-beam computed tomography pediatric airway measurements after adenotonsillectomy in patients with OSA. *JAMA Otolaryngol Head Neck Surg.* 2022;148(7):621–629.

17. Abdel-Aziz M, Abdel-Naseer U, Elshahawy E, et al. Persistent obstructive sleep apnea in children with Down syndrome after adenotonsillectomy: Drug induced sleep endoscopy-directed treatment. *J Craniofac Surg.* 2022;33(2):e185–e187.

18. Rayasam SS, Abijay C, Johnson R, Mitchell RB. Outcomes of adenotonsillectomy for obstructive sleep apnea in children under 3 years of age. *Ear Nose Throat J.* 20221455613221086526.

19. Magnusdottir S, Hilmisson H, Raymann RJEM, Witmans M. Characteristics of children likely to have spontaneous resolution of obstructive sleep apnea: Results from the Childhood Adenotonsillectomy Trial (CHAT). *Children (Basel).* 2021;8(11):980.

20. Gourishetti SC, Hamburger E, Pereira KD, Mitchell RB, Isaiah A. Baseline apnea-hypopnea index threshold and adenotonsillectomy consideration in children with OSA. *Int J Pediatr Otorhinolaryngol.* 2021;151:110959.

21. Mills TG, Bhattacharjee R, Nation J, Ewing E, Lesser DJ. Management and outcome of extreme pediatric obstructive sleep apnea. *Sleep Med.* 2021;87:138–142.

22. Taniguchi K, Yoshitomi A, Kanemaru A, Baba S. Outcomes of adenoidectomy with and without tonsillectomy in patients younger than 2 years with moderate to severe upper airway obstruction. *Int J Pediatr Otorhinolaryngol.* 2021;149:110841.

23. Hines S, Pickett K, Tholen K, Handley E, Friedman NR. Tonsillectomy outcomes for children with severe obesity. *Laryngoscope.* 2022;132(2):461–469.

24. End C, Propst EJ, Cushing SL, et al. Risks and benefits of adenotonsillectomy in children with cerebral palsy with obstructive sleep apnea: A systematic review. *Laryngoscope.* 2022;132(3):687–694.

25. Van de Perck E, Van Hoorenbeeck K, Verhulst S, Saldien V, Vanderveken OM, Boudewyns A. Effect of body weight on upper airway findings and treatment outcome in children with obstructive sleep apnea. *Sleep Med.* 2021;79:19–28.

26. Øverland B, Berdal H, Akre H. Surgery for obstructive sleep apnea in young children: Outcome evaluated by polysomnography and quality of life. *Int J Pediatr Otorhinolaryngol.* 2021;142:110609.

27. Galluzzi F, Garavello W. Impact of adenotonsillectomy in children with severe obstructive sleep apnea: A systematic review. *Auris Nasus Larynx.* 2021;48(4):549–554.

28. Lee T, Wulfovich S, Kettler E, Nation J. Incidence of cure and residual obstructive sleep apnea in obese children after tonsillectomy and adenoidectomy stratified by age group *Int J Pediatr Otorhinolaryngol.* 2020;139:110394.

29. Billings KR, Somani SN, Lavin J, Bhushan B. Polysomnography variables associated with postoperative respiratory issues in children <3 Years of age undergoing adenotonsillectomy for obstructive sleep apnea. *Int J Pediatr Otorhinolaryngol.* 2020;137:110215.

30. Venekamp RP, Hearne BJ, Chandrasekharan D, Blackshaw H, Lim J, Schilder AG. Tonsillectomy or adenotonsillectomy versus non-surgical management for obstructive sleep-disordered breathing in children. *Cochrane Database Syst Rev.* 2015;2015(10):CD011165.

31. Schneuer FJ, Bell KJ, Dalton C, Elshaug A, Nassar N. Adenotonsillectomy and adenoidectomy in children: The impact of timing of surgery and post-operative outcomes. *J Paediatr Child Health.* 2022;58(9):1608–1615.

32. Suzuki M, Watanabe T, Mogi G. Clinical, bacteriological, and histological study of adenoids in children. *Am J Otolaryngol.* 1999;20(2):85–90.

33. Zuliani G, Carlisle M, Duberstein A, et al. Biofilm density in the pediatric nasopharynx: Recurrent acute otitis media versus obstructive sleep apnea. *Ann Otol Rhinol Laryngol.* 2009;118(7):519–524.

34. Nistico L, Kreft R, Gieseke A, et al. Adenoid reservoir for pathogenic biofilm bacteria. *J Clin Microbiol.* 2011;49(4):1411–1420.

35. Gozal D, Kheirandish-Gozal L, Capdevila OS, et al. Prevalence of recurrent otitis media in habitually snoring school-aged children. *Sleep Med.* 2008;9(5):549–554.

36. Tauman R, Derowe A, Ophir O, et al. Increased risk of snoring and adenotonsillectomy in children referred for tympanostomy tube insertion. *Sleep Med.* 2010;11(2):197–200.

37. Vuono IM, Zanoteli E, de Oliveira AS, et al. Histological analysis of palatopharyngeal muscle from children with snoring and obstructive sleep apnea syndrome. *Int J Pediatr Otorhinolaryngol.* 2007;71(2):283–290.

38. Boyd JH, Petrof BJ, Hamid Q, et al. Upper airway muscle inflammation and denervation changes in obstructive sleep apnea. *Am J Respir Crit Care Med.* 2004;170(5):541–546.

39. Rubinstein I. Nasal inflammation is present in patients with obstructive sleep apnea. *Laryngoscope.* 1995;105:175–177.

40. Müns G, Rubinstein I, Singer P. Phagocytosis and oxidative burst of granulocytes in the upper respiratory tract in chronic and acute inflammation. *J Otolaryngol.* 1995;24:105–110.

41. Sekosan M, Zakkar M, Wenig B, et al. Inflammation in the uvula mucosa of patients with obstructive sleep apnea. *Laryngoscope.* 1996;106:1018–1020.

42. Wang Y, Zhang SX, Gozal D. Reactive oxygen species and the brain in sleep apnea. *Respir Physiol Neurobiol.* 2010;174(3):307–316.

43. Goldbart AD, Mager E, Veling MC, et al. Neurotrophins and tonsillar hypertrophy in children with obstructive sleep apnea. *Pediatr Res.* 2007;62(4):489–494.

44. Carpagnano GE, Kharitonov SA, Resta O, et al. 8-Isoprostane, a marker of oxidative stress, is increased in exhaled breath condensate of patients with obstructive sleep apnea after night and is reduced by continuous positive airway pressure therapy. *Chest.* 2003;124(4):1386–1392.

45. Wang Y, Chen G, Lin C, Chen Y, Huang M, Ye S. Possible mechanism of CHI3L1 promoting tonsil lymphocytes proliferation

in children with obstructive sleep apnea syndrome. *Pediatr Res.* 2022;91(5):1099–1105.

46. Khalyfa A, Gharib SA, Kim J, Dayyat E, Snow AB, Bhattacharjee R, Kheirandish-Gozal L, Goldman JL, Gozal D. Transcriptomic analysis identifies phosphatases as novel targets for adenotonsillar hypertrophy of pediatric obstructive sleep apnea. *Am J Respir Crit Care Med.* 2010;181(10):1114–1120.

47. Lee HJ, Jung H, Kim DK. IDO and CD40 may be key molecules for immunomodulatory capacity of the primed tonsil-derived mesenchymal stem cells. *Int J Mol Sci.* 2021;22(11):5772.

48. Li Y, Chongsuvivatwong V, Geater A, et al. Exhaled breath condensate cytokine level as a diagnostic tool for obstructive sleep apnea syndrome. *Sleep Med.* 2009;10(1):95–103.

49. Carpagnano GE, Lacedonia D, Foschino-Barbaro MP. Non-invasive study of airways inflammation in sleep apnea patients. *Sleep Med Rev.* 2011;15(5):317–326.

50. Entzian P, Linnemann K, Schlaak M, et al. Obstructive sleep apnea syndrome and circadian rhythms of hormones and cytokines. *Am J Respir Crit Care Med.* 1996;153(3):1080–1086.

51. Yokoe T, Minoguchi K, Matsuo H, et al. Elevated levels of C-reactive protein and interleukin-6 in patients with obstructive sleep apnea syndrome are decreased by nasal continuous positive airway pressure. *Circulation.* 2003;107(8):1129–1134.

52. Shadan FF, Jalowayski AA, Fahrenholz J, et al. Nasal cytology: A marker of clinically silent inflammation in patients with obstructive sleep apnea and a predictor of noncompliance with nasal CPAP therapy. *J Clin Sleep Med.* 2005;1(3):266–270.

53. Tauman R, Ivanenko A, O'Brien LM, et al. Plasma C-reactive protein levels among children with sleep-disordered breathing. *Pediatrics.* 2004;113(6):e564–e569.

54. Gozal D, Capdevila OS, Kheirandish-Gozal L. Metabolic alterations and systemic inflammation in obstructive sleep apnea among nonobese and obese prepubertal children. *Am J Respir Crit Care Med.* 2008;177(10):1142–1149.

55. Kheirandish-Gozal L, Capdevila OS, Tauman R, et al. Plasma C-reactive protein in nonobese children with obstructive sleep apnea before and after adenotonsillectomy. *J Clin Sleep Med.* 2006;2(3):301–304.

56. Goldbart AD, Levitas A, Greenberg-Dotan S, et al. B-type natriuretic peptide and cardiovascular function in young children with obstructive sleep apnea. *Chest.* 2010;138(3):528–535.

57. Gozal D, Khalyfa A, Capdevila OS, et al. Cognitive function in prepubertal children with obstructive sleep apnea: A modifying role for NADPH oxidase p22 subunit gene polymorphisms? *Antioxid Redox Signal.* 2012;16(2):171–177.

58. Gozal D, Crabtree VM, Sans Capdevila O, et al. C-reactive protein, obstructive sleep apnea, and cognitive dysfunction in school-aged children. *Am J Respir Crit Care Med.* 2007;176(2):188–193.

59. Kheirandish-Gozal L, Gozal D. Obstructive sleep apnea and inflammation: Proof of concept based on two illustrative cytokines. *Int J Mol Sci.* 2019;20(3):459.

60. Tauman R, Gulliver TE, Krishna J, et al. Persistence of obstructive sleep apnea syndrome in children after adenotonsillectomy. *J Pediatr.* 2006;149(6):803–808.

61. Mitchell RB, Kelly J. Outcome of adenotonsillectomy for obstructive sleep apnea in obese and normal-weight children. *Otolaryngol Head Neck Surg.* 2007;137(1):43–48.

62. Bhattacharjee R, Kim J, Alotaibi WH, et al. Endothelial dysfunction in children without hypertension: Potential contributions of obesity and obstructive sleep apnea. *Chest.* 2012;141(3):682–691.

63. Bhattacharjee R, Kim J, Kheirandish-Gozal L, et al. Obesity and obstructive sleep apnea syndrome in children: A tale of inflammatory cascades. *Pediatr Pulmonol.* 2011;46(4):313–323.

64. Spruyt K, Gozal D. A mediation model linking body weight, cognition, and sleep-disordered breathing. *Am J Respir Crit Care Med.* 2012;185(2):199–205.

65. Peters-Golden M, Henderson Jr. WR. Leukotrienes. *N Engl J Med.* 2007;357(18):1841–1854.

66. Shirasaki H, Kanaizumi E, Watanabe K, et al. Expression and localization of the cysteinyl leukotriene 1 receptor in human nasal mucosa. *Clin Exp Allergy.* 2002;32(7):1007–1012.

67. Figueroa DJ, Breyer RM, Defoe SK, et al. Expression of the cysteinyl leukotriene 1 receptor in normal human lung and peripheral blood leukocytes. *Am J Respir Crit Care Med.* 2001;163(1):226–233.

68. Kheirandish-Gozal L, Dayyat EA, Eid NS, et al. Obstructive sleep apnea in poorly controlled asthmatic children: Effect of adenotonsillectomy. *Pediatr Pulmonol.* 2011;46(9):913–918.

69. Malakasioti G, Gourgoulianis K, et al. Interactions of obstructive sleep-disordered breathing with recurrent wheezing or asthma and their effects on sleep quality. *Pediatr Pulmonol.* 2011;46(11):1047–1054.

70. Ross KR, Storfer-Isser A, Hart MA, et al. Sleep-disordered breathing is associated with asthma severity in children. *J Pediatr.* 2012;160(5):736–742.

71. Bisgaard H, Loland L, Oj JA. NO in exhaled air of asthmatic children is reduced by the leukotriene receptor antagonist montelukast. *Am J Respir Crit Care Med.* 1999;160(4):1227–1231.

72. Chauhan BF, Ducharme FM. Anti-leukotriene agents compared to inhaled corticosteroids in the management of recurrent and/or chronic asthma in adults and children. *Cochrane Database Syst Rev.* 2012;(5):CD002314.

73. Goldbart AD, Goldman JL, Li RC, et al. Differential expression of cysteinyl leukotriene receptors 1 and 2 in tonsils of children with obstructive sleep apnea syndrome or recurrent infection. *Chest.* 2004;126(1):13–18.

74. Ebenfelt A, Ivarsson M. Neutrophil migration in tonsils. *J Anat.* 2001;198(Pt 4):497–500.

75. Kaditis AG, Ioannou MG, Chaidas K, et al. Cysteinyl leukotriene receptors are expressed by tonsillar T cells of children with obstructive sleep apnea. *Chest.* 2008;134(2):324–331.

76. Goldbart AD, Goldman JL, Veling MC, et al. Leukotriene modifier therapy for mild sleep-disordered breathing in children. *Am J Respir Crit Care Med.* 2005;172(3):364–370.

77. Tsaoussoglou M, Lianou L, Maragozidis P, et al. Cysteinyl leukotriene receptors in tonsillar B- and T-lymphocytes from children with obstructive sleep apnea. *Sleep Med.* 2012;13(7):879–885.

78. Goldbart AD, Krishna J, Li RC, et al. Inflammatory mediators in exhaled breath condensate of children with obstructive sleep apnea syndrome. *Chest.* 2006;130(1):143–148.

79. Petrosyan M, Perraki E, Simoes D, et al. Exhaled breath markers in patients with obstructive sleep apnoea. *Sleep Breath.* 2008;12(3):207–215.

80. Serpero LD, Kheirandish-Gozal L, Dayyat E, et al. A mixed cell culture model for assessment of proliferation in tonsillar tissues from children with obstructive sleep apnea or recurrent tonsillitis. *Laryngoscope.* 2009;119(5):1005–1010.

81. Kim J, Bhattacharjee R, Dayyat E, et al. Increased cellular proliferation and inflammatory cytokines in tonsils derived

from children with obstructive sleep apnea. *Pediatr Res.* 2009;66(4):423–428.

82. Dayyat E, Serpero LD, Kheirandish-Gozal L, et al. Leukotriene pathways and in vitro adenotonsillar cell proliferation in children with obstructive sleep apnea. *Chest.* 2009;135(5):1142–1149.

83. Shu Y, Yang DZ, Liang J, Zhang F, Wang B, Yao HB, Liu EM. Effects of leukotriene D4 on adenoidal T cells in children with obstructive sleep apnea syndrome. *Am J Transl Res.* 2016;8(10):4329–4337.

84. Abstract [519]: In: *Am J Respir Crit Care Med.* The American Thoracic Society International Conference. San Francisco, California, 2007;175:A15–1004.

85. Kheirandish L, Goldbart AD, Gozal D. Intranasal steroids and oral leukotriene modifier therapy in residual sleep-disordered breathing after tonsillectomy and adenoidectomy in children. *Pediatrics.* 2006;117(1):e61–e66.

86. Goldbart AD, Greenberg-Dotan S, Tal A. Montelukast for children with obstructive sleep apnea: A double-blind, placebo-controlled study. *Pediatrics.* 2012;130(3):e575–e580.

87. Kheirandish-Gozal L, Bandla HP, Gozal D. Montelukast for children with obstructive sleep apnea: Results of a double-blind, randomized, placebo-controlled trial. *Ann Am Thorac Soc.* 2016;13(10):1736–1741.

88. Kajiyama T, Komori M, Hiyama M, Kobayashi T, Hyodo M. Changes during medical treatments before adenotonsillectomy in children with obstructive sleep apnea. *Auris Nasus Larynx.* 2022;49(4):625–633.

89. Ji T, Lu T, Qiu Y, et al. The efficacy and safety of montelukast in children with obstructive sleep apnea: A systematic review and meta-analysis. *Sleep Med.* 2021;78:193–201.

90. Kuhle S, Urschitz MS. Anti-inflammatory medications for the treatment of pediatric obstructive sleep apnea. *Paediatr Respir Rev.* 2020;34:35–36.

91. Howard JJM, Sarber KM, Yu W, et al. Outcomes in children with down syndrome and mild obstructive sleep apnea treated non-surgically. *Laryngoscope.* 2020;130(7):1828–1835.

92. Sunkonkit K, Sritippayawan S, Veeravikrom M, Deerojanawong J, Prapphal N. Urinary cysteinyl leukotriene E4 level and therapeutic response to montelukast in children with mild obstructive sleep apnea. *Asian Pac J Allergy Immunol.* 2017;35(4):233–238.

93. Adcock IM, Lane SJ. Corticosteroid-insensitive asthma: Molecular mechanisms. *J Endocrinol.* 2003;178(3):347–355.

94. Adcock IM, Barnes PJ. Molecular mechanisms of corticosteroid resistance. *Chest.* 2008;134(2):394–401.

95. Barnes PJ, Adcock IM. Glucocorticoid resistance in inflammatory diseases. *Lancet.* 2009;373(9678):1905–1917.

96. De Iudicibus S, Franca R, Martelossi S, et al. Molecular mechanism of glucocorticoid resistance in inflammatory bowel disease. *World J Gastroenterol.* 2011;17(9):1095–1108.

97. Christodoulopoulos P, Leung DY, Elliott MW, et al. Increased number of glucocorticoid receptor-beta-expressing cells in the airways in fatal asthma. *J Allergy Clin Immunol.* 2000;106(3):479–484.

98. Gagliardo R, Chanez P, Vignola AM, et al. Glucocorticoid receptor alpha and beta in glucocorticoid dependent asthma. *Am J Respir Crit Care Med.* 2000;162(1):7–13.

99. Goldbart AD, Veling MC, Goldman JL, et al. Glucocorticoid receptor subunit expression in adenotonsillar tissue of children with obstructive sleep apnea. *Pediatr Res.* 2005;57(2):232–236.

100. Kheirandish-Gozal L, Serpero LD, Dayyat E, et al. Corticosteroids suppress in vitro tonsillar proliferation in children with obstructive sleep apnoea. *Eur Respir J.* 2009;33(5):1077–1084.

101. Demain G, Goetz DW. Pediatric adenoidal hypertrophy and nasal airway obstruction: Reduction with aqueous nasal beclomethasone. *Pediatrics.* 1995;95:355–364.

102. Al-Ghamdi SA, Manoukian JJ, Morielli A, et al. Do systemic corticosteroids effectively treat obstructive sleep apnea secondary to adenotonsillar hypertrophy? *Laryngoscope.* 1997;107:1382–1387.

103. Brouillette RT, Manoukian JJ, Ducharme FM, et al. Efficacy of fluticasone nasal spray for pediatric obstructive sleep apnea. *J Pediatr.* 2001;138:838–844.

104. Alexopoulos EI, Kaditis AG, Kalampouka E, et al. Nasal corticosteroids for children with snoring. *Pediatr Pulmonol.* 2004;38(2):161–167.

105. Berlucchi M, Valetti L, Parrinello G, et al. Long-term follow-up of children undergoing topical intranasal steroid therapy for adenoidal hypertrophy. *Int J Pediatr Otorhinolaryngol.* 2008;72:1171–1175.

106. Berlucchi M, Salsi D, Valetti L, et al. The role of mometasone furoate aqueous nasal spray in the treatment of adenoidal hypertrophy in the pediatric age group: Preliminary results of a prospective, randomized study. *Pediatrics.* 2007;119:e1392–e1397.

107. Rezende RM, Silveira F, Barbosa AP, et al. Objective reduction in adenoid tissue after mometasone furoate treatment. *Int J Pediatr Otorhinolaryngol.* 2012;76:829–831.

108. Esteitie R, Emani J, Sharma S, et al. Effect of fluticasone furoate on interleukin 6 secretion from adenoid tissues in children with obstructive sleep apnea. *Arch Otolaryngol Head Neck Surg.* 2011;137:576–582.

109. Kheirandish-Gozal L, Gozal D. Intranasal budesonide treatment for children with mild obstructive sleep apnea syndrome. *Pediatrics.* 2008;122:e149–e155.

110. Kuhle S, Urschitz MS. Anti-inflammatory medications for obstructive sleep apnea in children. *Cochrane Database Syst Rev.* 2011CD007074.

111. Kheirandish-Gozal L, Bhattacharjee R, Bandla HPR, Gozal D. Antiinflammatory therapy outcomes for mild OSA in children. *Chest.* 2014 Jul;146(1):88–95.

40

Congenital Central Hypoventilation Syndrome

Susan M. Slattery, Casey M. Rand, Ilya Khaytin, Tracey M. Stewart, Kai Lee Yap,
Elizabeth Berry-Kravis, and Debra E. Weese-Mayer

CHAPTER HIGHLIGHTS

- Congenital central hypoventilation syndrome (CCHS) is a disorder of respiratory control and autonomic nervous system (ANS) regulation resulting from a pathogenic *PHOX2B* gene variant. The type of *PHOX2B* variant (polyalanine repeat expansion mutations [PARMs] vs. non-PARMs [NPARMs]) and the PARM genotype as well as the NPARM location on the gene and its effect on the protein allow for anticipatory management related to disease phenotype.

- The hallmark feature of CCHS is hypoventilation during all sleep time and during intercurrent illness, though a subset of patients hypoventilate awake and asleep.

- As outlined in the American Thoracic Society Statement on CCHS and later-onset (LO-)CCHS, every 6 months for the first 3 years of life and then annually thereafter, comprehensive physiologic and autonomic testing awake and asleep and neurodevelopmental assessments are essential.

- Management includes a detailed respiratory care management and monitoring plan, to maintain normal gas exchange throughout various age-appropriate activities of daily living and needs over 24 hours/day. Longitudinal neurocognitive testing allows for early identification of need for targeted intervention. Screening for neural crest–derived tumors and Hirschsprung disease, as well as prolonged cardiac sinus pauses and other features of ANS dysregulation (ANSD), are key components of management, though incidence will vary by mutation type, PARM genotype, and NPARM location on the *PHOX2B* gene and its effect on the protein.

- Detailed management of patients' cardiorespiratory health improves cognitive outcomes for optimal quality of life.

Introduction

Congenital central hypoventilation syndrome (CCHS) is a rare disorder of respiratory control and autonomic nervous system (ANS) regulation. Patients with CCHS principally present with hypoventilation during all sleep time and with increased severity during intercurrent illness, though a subset of patients hypoventilate awake and asleep. The classic presentation for CCHS is in the first hours to days of life, with clinically apparent cyanosis consequent to shallow breathing or apnea, typically upon falling asleep and sustained throughout sleep.[1,2] Later-onset CCHS (LO-CCHS) indicates presentation over 1 month of age, in childhood and adulthood.[3] CCHS is caused by heterozygous pathogenic variants of the paired-like homeobox 2B (*PHOX2B*) gene, causing dysfunctional ANS differentiation during embryologic development.[4] The type of *PHOX2B* pathogenic variant (polyalanine repeat expansion mutations [PARMs] vs. non-PARMs [NPARMs]) and the PARM genotype as well as the NPARM location on the *PHOX2B* gene and its effect on the protein allow for anticipatory management relative to organ system phenotype.[4,5] Additional neural crest–derived features of CCHS include Hirschsprung disease, neural crest tumors,[4] abrupt and prolonged cardiac sinus pauses, and other signs and symptoms of physiologic ANS dysregulation (ANSD). The primary management of CCHS and LO-CCHS involves comprehensive age-appropriate physiologic and autonomic testing awake and asleep with aim to provide artificial respiratory support to maintain cardiorespiratory health and optimal cognitive outcomes, provided every 6 months for the first 3 years of life, then annually thereafter as recommended in the American Thoracic Society Statement on CCHS.[1,2]

Pathophysiology and Neuroanatomy

PHOX2B, located on chromosome 4 at 4p12, is the disease-defining gene for CCHS. It encodes a highly conserved 314–amino-acid transcription factor that determines neuronal cell fate/differentiation of sympathetic, parasympathetic, and enteric neurons of the ANS. *PHOX2B* is expressed in central autonomic neuronal circuits including neurons of the retrotrapezoid nucleus, which lies on the rostral surface of the medulla and contributes to central chemosensitivity, as well as additional areas of the medulla and the pons. Murine models and human functional magnetic resonance imaging studies show *PHOX2B* pathogenic variants are associated with abnormalities of the locus coeruleus, dorsal and parafacial respiratory groups, and nucleus ambiguous.[6–8] *PHOX2B* is also expressed peripherally in neural crest cells that develop into the main components of the peripheral ANS.[9]

Diagnosis

The diagnosis of CCHS is established by molecular genetic testing to identify a pathogenic heterozygous variant in *PHOX2B*. Stepwise *PHOX2B* testing is advised to identify the disease-causing pathologic variant (Fig. 40.1). Step 1 is the *PHOX2B* Fragment Analysis or Screening Test. This will identify all of the PARMs and a subset of the NPARMs including the larger deletions (35 and 38 base pair [bp] deletions), collectively accounting for variants responsible for approximately 95% of CCHS cases and is the only clinical test that will identify low-level mosaicism.[10] Additionally, fragment analysis is the first recommended test as sequencing can result in a false-negative test due to allele drop-out.[1] Step 2 is the *PHOX2B* Sequencing Test, performed in the event the step 1 testing is negative and the patient's phenotype is strongly suggestive of CCHS.[11] This test will identify all PARMs and NPARMs in a laboratory experienced in the technique but will not identify low level mosaicism. Step 3 is the *PHOX2B* multiplex ligation-dependent probe amplification (MLPA) test to identify loss of the entire exon 3 or the whole *PHOX2B* gene, and potentially neighboring genes.[12]

Unaffected individuals are homozygous for 20 alanines in the 20 alanine repeat region (genotype 20/20). Heterozygous expansion mutations in the 20 alanine repeat region are referred to as PARMs, with anywhere from 24 to 33 alanines on the affected allele (resulting genotypes are 20/24 to 20/33). *PHOX2B* PARMs account for 90–92% of the CCHS cases. The most common PARMs have genotypes 20/25, 20/26, and 20/27. NPARMs do not include an expansion mutation, rather they are missense, nonsense, stop codon, (likely) splice site, and frameshift variants, occurring anywhere in the *PHOX2B* gene, and accounting for 8–10% of the CCHS cases. The most common NPARMs are 35–38 bp deletions or duplications.[1,13]

PHOX2B partial and whole gene deletions account for less than 1% of CCHS cases and when present may additionally include several neighboring genes. Pathogenic variants of *PHOX2B* are most commonly de novo mutations, but 5–25% are inherited in an autosomal dominant manner from parents who are mosaic for the same mutation.[11]

Parental *PHOX2B* testing is recommended at the time their child is diagnosed with CCHS. In some cases, *PHOX2B*-causing CCHS variant alleles have been inherited from parents who may be mosaic carriers of the same *PHOX2B* variants, but without prior clinical detection. Parents of a child with either one of a small number of NPARMs or one of the smaller PARMs (20/24 or 20/25 genotype) may have absent or subclinical symptoms, indicating incomplete penetrance or variable expressivity.[4,14,15] It is imperative to test parents of patients with *PHOX2B* mutations for three reasons. First, parents may have subclinical symptoms that, if left unidentified, can lead to catastrophic consequences. There is growing evidence that in some of these cases, the mosaic parent may go unidentified until a stressor (e.g., respiratory infection or anesthesia during surgery) unmasks a potentially severe phenotype, with risk of mortality in the case of anesthesia. Second, it is critical for families to understand their genetic risk as they consider family planning for future pregnancies. Because these mutations have been identified in multigeneration families, tracing the origin of the inherited *PHOX2B* mutation may have implications for many family members.[16] And third, germline mosaicism may occur (with parental negative testing for somatic mosaicism), indicating the need to additionally offer chorionic villous sampling or amniocentesis for each pregnancy.[17] For parental testing, if the pathogenic variant causes an abnormal exon 3 allele size, as is the case with any PARMs and NPARM exon 3 frameshifts, deletions, and duplications, *PHOX2B* Fragment Analysis testing is recommended as it is the only clinically available test that will identify low-level somatic mosaicism.[12] For parents of children whose *PHOX2B* variants do not cause changes in the exon 3 allele size, the *PHOX2B* Sequencing Test is recommended. To note, for fetuses with a determined

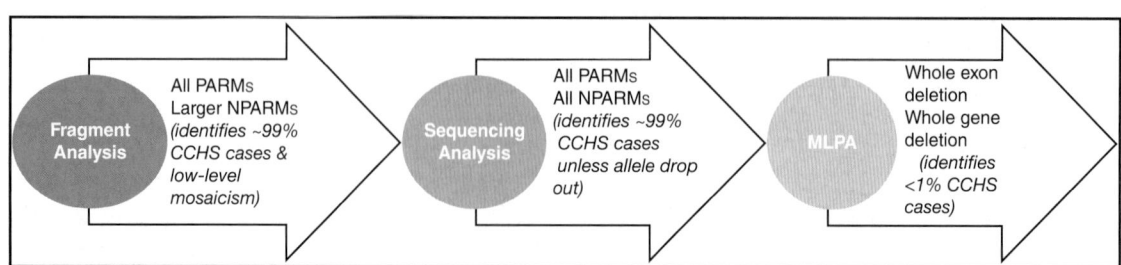

• **Fig. 40.1** *PHOX2B* genetic testing for CCHS and percentage of cases identified with each method. PARM (polyalanine repeat expansion mutation) with number of repeats on each allele (e.g., normal genotype is 20/20; range is 20/24–20/33); NPARM (non-polyalanine repeat expansion mutation). (Adapted from Jennings LJ, Yu M, Zhou L, Rand CM, Berry-Kravis EM, Weese-Mayer DE. Comparison of PHOX2B testing methods in the diagnosis of congenital central hypoventilation syndrome and mosaic carriers. *Diagn Mol Pathol.* 2010;19(4):224.)

PHOX2B disease-causing variant and with plans to sustain the pregnancy, delivery at a quaternary medical care facility is recommended for delivery and perinatal monitoring and intervention as needed with prompt transfer to the neonatal intensive care unit.[18] Preimplantation genetics has been successful in pregnancy planning to parents with *PHOX2B* mosaicism or who have *PHOX2B* mutation–confirmed CCHS.

Phenotype

CCHS phenotype may be anticipated based on the type of *PHOX2B* mutation (PARM vs. NPARM) and the PARM genotype and NPARM type (Table 40.1). Patients with longer PARMs have increased severity of hypoventilation (continuous vs. asleep only), risk of Hirschsprung disease, and number of systems and symptoms with ANSD.[10,14] Among the three most common PARMs (20/25, 20/26, 20/27), patients with the 20/27 genotype will have a more severe phenotype with risk for prolonged sinus pauses in more than 80% of cases and Hirschsprung disease in approximately 30% of cases. Only CCHS patients with PARM genotypes 20/30 to 20/33 are at risk (<5%) for neural crest tumors (screening is recommended for 20/28–20/33), and with one exception these have been reported to be ganglioneuromas or ganglioneuroblastomas.[19] Those with shorter polyalanine expansions with genotypes 20/24 and a subset with 20/25 may not manifest hypoventilation until older than 1 month of age at the time of an intercurrent illness such as pneumonia or when exposed to respiratory depressants such as sedation or anesthesia.[14] Less than 5% of patients with CCHS will be diagnosed after the first month of age

(LO-CCHS), though that is considered to be an underestimation of true disease prevalence. Patients with NPARMs, especially the larger variants with the 35 and 38 bp deletions/duplications, will require continuous artificial ventilation, have extensive Hirschsprung disease (usually colonic and part of small intestine), and a neural crest tumor (most often neuroblastoma).[5]

The CCHS facial features phenotype is immediately identifiable among patients with the more common heterozygous *PHOX2B* PARMs. Features include a boxy-shaped face, a flattened profile, and an overturned lateral one-third of the upper lip vermilion border such that it is flesh-colored instead of pink. Children with the NPARMs additionally may have epicanthal folds and reduced movement of the lower one-third of the face.[20]

Management

Overview

With a defined *PHOX2B* genotype, the American Thoracic Society (ATS) statement on CCHS outlines clear management recommendations that are based upon detailed physiologic assessments while awake (during varied age-appropriate activities of daily living including eating, physical exertion, and mental concentration) and asleep while optimizing artificial ventilatory management.[1,2,21] The comprehensive physiologic evaluations occur over a multiple-day hospital stay with all testing done in laboratory. Management involves the screening for additional features in CCHS (Table 40.1).[1,2] Surveillance and treatment occurs biannually under the age of 3 years old and annually thereafter.

TABLE 40.1   CCHS Phenotype by *PHOX2B* Categories

Feature[1] (percent risk, if known)	PARM*	NPARM^
Control of breathing[1,2]	~35–50% 24 hr ventilator support; severity increases with repeat size	~70% 24 hr ventilator support
Hirschsprung disease[1,2]	~19–30%; risk increases with repeat size	~90%
Neural crest tumor[1,3]	<5%; risk increases with repeat size (≥28)	~50%
Cardiac sinus pause[4,5,6]	~20–82%; risk increases with repeat size	Rare (one case reported)

[1]Weese-Mayer DE, Rand CM, Berry-Kravis EM, et al. Congenital central hypoventilation syndrome from past to future: model for translational and transitional autonomic medicine. *Pediatr Pulmonol.* 2009;44(6):521–535.
[2]Berry-Kravis EM, Zhou L, Rand CM, Weese-Mayer DE. Congenital central hypoventilation syndrome: PHOX2B mutations and phenotype. *Am J Respir Crit Care Med.* 2006;174(10):1139–1144.
[3]Matera I, Bachetti T, Puppo F, et al. PHOX2B mutations and polyalanine expansions correlate with the severity of the respiratory phenotype and associated symptoms in both congenital and late onset central hypoventilation syndrome. *J Med Genet.* 2004;41(5):373–380.
[4]Gronli JO, Santucci BA, Leurgans SE, Berry-Kravis EM, Weese-Mayer DE. Congenital central hypoventilation syndrome: PHOX2B genotype determines risk for sudden death. *Pediatr Pulmonol.* 2008;43(1):77–86.
[5]Laifman E, Keens TG, Bar-Cohen Y, Perez IA. Life-threatening cardiac arrhythmias in congenital central hypoventilation syndrome. *Eur J Pediatr.* 2020;179(5):821–825.
[6]Armstrong AE, Weese-Mayer DE, Mian A, et al. Treatment of neuroblastoma in congenital central hypoventilation syndrome with a PHOX2B polyalanine repeat expansion mutation: New twist on a neurocristopathy syndrome. *Pediatr Blood Cancer.* 2015;62(11):2007–2010.
*PARM ([polyalanine repeat expansion mutation]; normal genotype is 20/20 and PARM range is 20/24-20/33 with number of repeats on each allele [e.g., 20/24 is fewer alanines on the affected allele than 20/28]).
^NPARM (non-polyalanine repeat expansion mutation).

Respiratory Support

CCHS is a rare genetic condition and the expectation is for lifelong artificial ventilation as life support. Patients diagnosed in infancy require positive pressure mechanical ventilation via a tracheostomy tube (ideally cuffed, tight to the shaft to minimize air leak asleep and allow for voice awake). Invasive respiratory support is recommended for the first several years of life to maintain a stable airway with aim to optimize gas exchange for growth and neurodevelopment.[1,2] For those with a milder phenotype and older, other options for invasive and noninvasive support may be a consideration.[1,2,22] For instance, those children who require artificial ventilation during sleep only may be able to safely transition to mask ventilation via their home ventilator, practically best achieved when the child has mature facial development for best fit of the equipment and to avoid interfering/flattening bone maturation. Developmentally, transition from tracheostomy to mask is proposed when the patient can place the mask on themselves allowing for consistency in use and for routine events such as overnight bathroom trips. For patients requiring continuous artificial ventilation, phrenic nerve-diaphragm pacing allows for awake time mobility then ventilator use via tracheostomy during overnight sleep.[1,2,23] Diaphragm pacing during sleep does not provide any advantage in terms of mobility and may cause airway obstruction if used in a decannulated young child.[24,25]

Patients with shorter PARM *PHOX2B* variants (20/24 and 20/25) typically have milder hypoventilation and require only nighttime artificial ventilation versus those with the longer PARM and NPARM variants who require continuous artificial ventilation as life support.[1,2,15] Severity of hypoventilation is primarily determined by studies of spontaneous breathing awake and asleep including (at a minimum) continuous recording of respiratory inductance plethysmography of the chest and abdomen, peripheral pulse oximetry for oxygen saturation with pulse waveform, end-tidal carbon dioxide level with visible waveform, and electrocardiogram, as well as analyses of awake and asleep responses to exogenous and endogenous challenges of hypercarbia and/or hypoxemia. Patients with CCHS have shallow breathing without variation in respiratory rate or tidal volume even in the presence of gas derangements (hypercarbia and/or hypoxemia).

Each patient throughout their pediatric years and into adulthood requires a detailed and unique respiratory plan as their disease may vary with advancing age, puberty, facial and airway structural maturity, neurocognitive level, emotional and behavioral maturity, availability and quality of home health care, proximity of their home to a major medical facility with full pediatric expertise, school individualized educational plans, the patient and family goals of care, and many other factors.[1,2,15]

While prescribing awake and asleep breathing support for a patient with CCHS, the clinician must be aware of the patient's needs during wellness and intercurrent illness, because a severe upper respiratory infection may dramatically increase artificial ventilatory support needs.[1,2,21] The tether of the ventilator is perceptually lessened with the routine mild illnesses throughout early elementary school as the patient may be able to continue to attend school while receiving positive pressure support. With years of observed stability and understanding of the patient's disease severity, tracheal decannulation may be considered for those already transitioned to mask ventilation during sleep.[1,2,22] If this is the case, the patient and their family should understand that with severe intercurrent illness endotracheal intubation and continuous artificial ventilation may be required in the interim.

At-home care of the patient with CCHS includes maintaining the highest level of noninvasively monitoring gas exchange feasible. The patient must be monitored continuously during sleep and at recommended intervals awake, with pulse oximetry and capnography (both with visible waveforms, measures, and alarms).[1,2] These monitoring tools are crucial to care for patients with CCHS because, with attenuated or absent peripheral chemoreceptor responsiveness, there is no other indicator of oxygenation and ventilation to reflect optimal artificial ventilatory support asleep and awake. Family members, at-home nurses, and additional medical care providers must be fluent in the child's care and in their understanding of oximetry and capnography waveform interpretation and relationship of their values to a decided treatment plan. The plan includes custom ventilator management to adjust ventilator settings such as respiratory rate according to capnography values at home (called the "ventilator ladder") and clear indications when to contact a primary care doctor or pulmonologist and seek emergency medical care. An example of a customized ventilator ladder is provided in Fig. 40.2. This high level of personalized in-home care requires highly trained, experienced registered nurses to provide care when the patient is awake and asleep, attending to the continuously used oximetry and capnography monitors, making ventilator changes following the "ladder," and providing immediate intervention in acute and life-threatening situations. Patient providers must be trained and maintain certification in patient age-appropriate cardiopulmonary resuscitation.

Autonomic Nervous System Dysfunction and Comorbidities

The ANS regulates virtually all organ systems, and specific age-appropriate noninvasive testing for ANSD is invaluable among patients with CCHS. In addition to testing, administering a screening questionnaire of ANSD, by system and symptoms, is important for disease management and is now included in the International CCHS Registry at NIH.gov (https://clinicaltrials.gov/show/NCT03088020).[26,27] With increases in PARM repeat size, there is a positive correlation with the number of ANSD-involved systems and symptoms.[10,28] The prevalence of life-threatening components of the CCHS phenotype

Goal values for E_TCO_2 30-45 mm Hg and SpO_2 92% or higher.

E_TCO_2 below 25 mm Hg	Immediately decrease rate by 2 bpm
E_TCO_2 between 25-29 mm Hg	Wait 1 hour and then decrease rate by 2 bpm
E_TCO_2 between 46-55 mm Hg	Wait 1 hour and then increase rate by 2 bpm
E_TCO_2 above 55 mm Hg	Immediately increase rate by 2 bpm

Waiting 1 hour between each change until the minimum/maximum rate is reached on the Breath Rate "Ladder."

Breath Rate "Ladder"

34

32

30

28

26*   * Denotes starting point for asleep/sick

24

22

20^   ^ Denotes starting point for awake

18

DAILY DETAILS:
- ✓ Always be supported by the ventilator awake and asleep.
- ✓ When awake, the 3.5 mm ID Pediatric Bivona tight-to-shaft tracheostomy tube cuff should be deflated.
- ✓ Thirty minutes before bedtime and asleep, the 3.5 mm ID Pediatric Bivona tight-to-shaft tracheostomy tube cuff should be inflated with 1.5 mL of sterile water.
- ✓ If the "Ladder" top or bottom is reached or unable to achieve goal values, contact your Primary Care Physician or Pulmonologist immediately.
- ✓ Do not change ventilator parameters other than breath rate without a discussion with the Primary Care Physician or Pulmonologist.
- ✓ Please fax the last 7 days of the Flow Charts to your Primary Care Physician and Pulmonologist the 7th of each month for review.

• **Fig. 40.2** Example of a custom mechanical ventilator "ladder" for a patient with CCHS. The ladder provides a customized action plan to adjust ventilator settings at home based on end-tidal capnography measures during sleep, awake during sedentary activities and with varied exertion, and in the presence of an intercurrent illness. It also provides steps with acute changes when physiologic measures exceed this prescription.

also varies by genotype and include cardiac sinus pauses, Hirschsprung disease, and neural crest tumors.[4]

Cardiac function and electrophysiology constitute an important component of CCHS screening and management. The echocardiogram is recommended to identify early signs of right-sided heart dysfunction such as ventricular hypertrophy, pulmonary hypertension, and cor pulmonale and signifies inadequate respiratory support. An electrocardiogram and 72-hour Holter recording are recommended to identify abrupt, prolonged asystoles. Cardiac screening with Holter and echocardiogram is performed every 6 months under the age of 3 years and annually thereafter.[1,2] All patients with a *PHOX2B* disease-causing allele are at theoretical risk for abrupt sinus pauses, but the genotypes most commonly reported are those with 20/27 (83% of patients) and less frequently 20/26 (19% of patients).[29] In childhood, none of the patients with the 20/25 genotype have prolonged sinus pauses, though some adults with LO-CCHS have such reported pauses after decades of unrecognized nocturnal hypoventilation. Life-threatening sinus pause has been reported in one patient with an NPARM variant, though the authors note "not all pause-length data was available to review," suggesting the actual waveforms were not reviewed.[30] Prolonged sinus pauses of significant duration (≥ 3.0 seconds) warrant placement of a cardiac pacemaker to prevent sudden cardiac death and/or morbidity.[1,2,29,31] It is crucial to complete monthly cardiac pacemaker maintenance reviews to identify early pacer failure. Patients with CCHS are also noted to have decreased heart rate variability across a 24-hour period and an attenuated heart rate response to exercise.[31–34]

Cardiovascular measurements during in-hospital physiologic evaluations should also include serial blood pressure measurements and measures of cerebral regional blood flow/oxygenation in activities of daily living, as well as with orthostatic testing. Abnormalities are observed with attenuated circadian changes in blood pressure compared with what is expected in those without CCHS where blood pressure increases during the day and decreases overnight during sleep.[35] Furthermore, during orthostatic testing, those with CCHS may be asymptomatic amid profound orthostatic hypotension and measures of decreased cerebral regional blood flow.[36]

Interval screening for neural crest tumors including neuroblastoma, ganglioneuroblastoma, and ganglioneuroma is recommended for patients with NPARMs and longer PARM genotypes (20/28 to 20/33).[1,2] The overall tumor prevalence among patients with NPARMs is 40% or more and among patients with longer PARM genotype less than 5% (20/30 to 20/33).[21,37] Tumors of neural crest origin present at variable ages, but most often neuroblastoma is identified before the age of 2 years. Ganglioneuroma and ganglioneuroblastoma are usually not symptomatic until they become large enough to compromise surrounding tissue/organs.[13,37] Surgical removal of all CCHS-related tumors is recommended, even if benign, to prevent impingement on internal organs or vasculature.[1] Chemotherapy is indicated in neuroblastoma if advanced beyond stage 1. Tumor-related deaths are rare, but anticipatory management for early identification is essential.

In patients with PARM genotypes 20/28 to 20/33, tumor screening is performed biannually, then after age

10 years annually, to identify adrenal tumors primarily a ganglioneuroma or ganglioneuroblastoma, or exceedingly rarely a neuroblastoma (one case of metastatic neuroblastoma in a toddler with the 20/33 genotype).[1,2,19,38] Screening includes chest anteroposterior and lateral radiographs (for tumors along the sympathetic chain) and abdominal/pelvic ultrasound (for adrenal tumors). In patients with NPARMs, screening occurs at more frequent intervals primarily evaluating for neuroblastoma. In addition to the two-view chest x-ray, abdominal/pelvic ultrasound can be paired with urine catecholamines and obtained every 3 months until age 6 years, and then every 6 months through age 10 years.[1,2,38]

The *PHOX2B* mutation type and PARM genotype also correlates with the occurrence of Hirschsprung disease, with an overall prevalence of 20% of those with CCHS.[4,10,13,26] The degree of bowel involvement can vary from short segment to long segment affecting the entire length of colonic with even small bowel aganglionosis. Hirschsprung disease is more prevalent in patients with NPARMs (87–100%) than PARMs (13–30%) and more common in patients with longer (vs. shorter) PARM expansion genotypes.[37,39] Total aganglionosis of the intestine is rare, but extensive aganglionosis is not uncommon among children with the 35 and 38 bp deletion NPARMs. Hirschsprung disease typically presents in early infancy, but short segment disease has been diagnosed later into early childhood. For patients with constipation symptoms, a contrast study of the colon to evaluate for a transition zone and anal manometry may be performed. The condition is surgically confirmed by punch or full thickness rectal biopsy (depending upon the infant or child's age). When confirmed, the necessary treatment is resection of affected bowel with leveling to remove all aganglionic intestine with a clear margin identified by a leveling procedure.[40] Of note, patients with CCHS may also have altered esophageal and intestinal motility, even in the absence of Hirschsprung disease. Esophageal dysmotility often improves within the first year of life.[41]

Evaluation of patients with CCHS may also reveal altered thermoregulation and diaphoresis by the ANSD questionnaire and analyses with thermal stressors.[1,2,10] Individuals with CCHS may reveal sporadic diffuse sweating, a decrease in basal body temperatures, and attenuated circadian thermal patterning.[42] Patients with NPARMs have fewer ANSD symptoms than patients with PARMs. Furthermore, patients with PARMs demonstrate a positive correlation with repeat size and number of ANSD symptoms.[10,26] In addition, eye examination and quantification of findings with pupillometry most often reveals abnormal, asymmetric pupillary responses to light stimulus, including normal values in patients with the 20/25 genotype to nearly absent pupillary responses to light in patients with the 20/27 genotype. Patients with NPARMs also have markedly decreased pupillary response to light, but with larger baseline pupil diameter than those with 20/27 genotype.[43,44] Altered pupillary response to light stimulus is important to recognize allowing for changes in exposure to minimize discomfort in activities of daily living with bright sunlight, technology screen exposure, and nighttime driving. Autonomic ocular abnormalities including anisocoria and strabismus are common in CCHS.[1,2]

Neurocognition and Development

Detailed formal neurodevelopmental testing in patients with CCHS should be performed every 6 months under the age of 3 years and then annually older than 3 years, to assess for the impact of primary disease on growth and development, as well as to identify deficits and delays due to suboptimal ventilatory management and compliance.[1,2] School-age children with CCHS have reported reduced Full-Scale IQ with a mean score of 85 (normal population mean is 100) and standard deviation of 15, and without a *PHOX2B* genotype relationship.[45,46] Although, preschool age children with the 20/25 genotype are described to have normal IQs, whereas those with 20/26 and 20/27 genotypes have reduced IQs. CCHS-related cyanotic breath holding, prolonged sinus pauses, need for 24 hour/day artificial ventilation, and seizures negatively impact the neurodevelopmental testing scores in preschool-aged children.[47] However, children with conservative ventilatory management and excellent compliance often have very normal IQ test results. Taken together, these results raise concern for an intrinsic phenomenon affecting cognitive performance, which is magnified among children with suboptimal ventilatory management and with more severe phenotypic features that will impose recurrent intermittent hypoxemia and altered cerebral autoregulation.[36,45,46,48]

Outcomes

Identification of the disease-causing *PHOX2B* pathogenic variant/genotype to confirm diagnosis of CCHS allows for anticipatory management.[1,4,13] The aim is for prompt diagnosis, introduction of conservative ventilatory management, and an enriched learning environment for these high-risk patients. Paramount to the health of the child with CCHS is the day-to-day management and interventions needed to maintain normal gas exchange ultimately to optimize neurodevelopment and quality of life.[1,2,15] As the *PHOX2B* pathogenic variant imposes ANS maldevelopment, it is essential to support and maintain stable oxygenation and ventilation during wakefulness and sleep to minimize sequelae from the innate physiologic compromise, and in anticipation of future pharmacologic intervention that might decrease disease burden.

Recommended Resources

The National Institutes of Health ClinicalTrials.gov International Registry for CCHS can be accessed at https://clinicaltrials.gov/show/NCT03088020.

Information on current clinical trials supported by government funding and some privately funded studies are listed on www.clinicaltrials.gov. European clinical trials can be reviewed at www.clinicaltrialsregister.eu.

Further information and resources related to CCHS can be found online at the National Organization for Rare Disorders at https://rarediseases.org/rare-diseases/congenital-central-hypoventilation-syndrome.

CLINICAL PEARLS

- Congenital Central Hypoventilation Syndrome (CCHS) is a rare disorder caused by pathogenic variants of the *PHOX2B* gene.
- CCHS clinically presents most often in the neonatal period with hypoventilation during sleep, although a subset of patients will hypoventilate during wakefulness, too. Affected patients have a control of breathing deficit, and variable severity of autonomic nervous system dysregulation (ANSD), that may include Hirschsprung disease and tumors of neural crest origin. A later-onset presentation (>1month of age) involves asleep hypoventilation and milder ANSD.
- As described in the American Thoracic Society Statement on CCHS, management largely involves chronic mechanical ventilation via tracheostomy. Infrequently, older patients can be supported by full-face mask ventilation while asleep.
- Management is centered on a detailed respiratory care plan with varied support during awake activities and sleep and screening for additional symptoms of autonomic dysfunction, with aim to optimize long-term outcomes.

References

1. Weese-Mayer D.E., Berry-Kravis E.M., Ceccherini I., et al. An official ATS clinical policy statement: Congenital central hypoventilation syndrome: genetic basis, diagnosis, and management. *Am J Respir Crit Care Med.* 181(6):626-644. https://doi.org/10.1164/rccm.200807-1069ST.
2. Trang H, Samuels M, Ceccherini I, et al. Guidelines for diagnosis and management of congenital central hypoventilation syndrome. *Orphanet J Rare Dis.* 2020;15(1): https://doi.org/10.1186/s13023-020-01460-2. 252-252.
3. Antic NA, Malow BA, Lange N, et al. PHOX2B mutation-confirmed congenital central hypoventilation syndrome: presentation in adulthood. *Am J Respir Crit Care Med.* 2006;174(8):923–927. https://doi.org/10.1164/rccm.200605-607CR.
4. Bachetti T, Ceccherini I. Causative and common PHOX2B variants define a broad phenotypic spectrum. *Clin Genet.* 2020;97(1):103–113. https://doi.org/10.1111/cge.13633.
5. Zhou A., Rand C.M., Hockney S.M., et al. Paired-like homeobox gene (PHOX2B) nonpolyalanine repeat expansion mutations (NPARMs): genotype–phenotype correlation in congenital central hypoventilation syndrome (CCHS). *Genet Med.* Published online May 6, 2021. https://doi.org/10.1038/s41436-021-01178-x.
6. Takakura AC, Barna BF, Cruz JC, Colombari E, Moreira TS. Phox2b-expressing retrotrapezoid neurons and the integration of central and peripheral chemosensory control of breathing in conscious rats. *Exp Physiol.* 2014;99(3):571–585. https://doi.org/10.1113/expphysiol.2013.076752.
7. Rudzinski E, Kapur RP. PHOX2B immunolocalization of the candidate human retrotrapezoid nucleus. *Pediatr Dev Pathol Off J Soc Pediatr Pathol Paediatr Pathol Soc.* 2010;13(4):291–299. https://doi.org/10.2350/09-07-0682-OA.1.
8. Nobuta H., Cilio M.R., Danhaive O., et al. Dysregulation of locus coeruleus development in congenital central hypoventilation syndrome. *Acta Neuropathol (Berl).* 130(2):171-183. https://doi.org/10.1007/s00401-015-1441-0.
9. Pattyn A, Morin X, Cremer H, Goridis C, Brunet JF. The homeobox gene Phox2b is essential for the development of autonomic neural crest derivatives. *Nature.* 1999;399(6734):366–370. https://doi.org/10.1038/20700.
10. Weese-Mayer DE, Berry-Kravis EM, Zhou L, et al. Idiopathic congenital central hypoventilation syndrome: analysis of genes pertinent to early autonomic nervous system embryologic development and identification of mutations in PHOX2b. *Am J Med Genet A.* 2003;123A(3):267–278. https://doi.org/10.1002/ajmg.a.20527.
11. Jennings L.J., Yu M., Rand C.M., et al. Variable human phenotype associated with novel deletions of the PHOX2B gene. Pediatr Pulmonol. 47(2):153-161. https://doi.org/10.1002/ppul.21527.
12. Jennings LJ, Yu M, Zhou L, Rand CM, Berry-Kravis EM, Weese-Mayer DE. Comparison of PHOX2B testing methods in the diagnosis of congenital central hypoventilation syndrome and mosaic carriers. *Diagn Mol Pathol Am J Surg Pathol Part B.* 2010;19(4):224.
13. Berry-Kravis EM, Zhou L, Rand CM, Weese-Mayer DE. Congenital central hypoventilation syndrome: PHOX2B mutations and phenotype. *Am J Respir Crit Care Med.* 2006;174(10):1139–1144. https://doi.org/10.1164/rccm.200602-305OC.
14. Repetto GM, Corrales RJ, Abara SG, et al. Later-onset congenital central hypoventilation syndrome due to a heterozygous 24-polyalanine repeat expansion mutation in the PHOX2B gene. *Acta Paediatr.* 2009;98(1):192–195. https://doi.org/10.1111/j.1651-2227.2008.01039.x.
15. Kasi AS, Li H, Harford KL, et al. Congenital Central Hypoventilation Syndrome: Optimizing Care with a Multidisciplinary Approach. *J Multidiscip Healthc.* 2022;15:455–469. https://doi.org/10.2147/JMDH.S284782.
16. Doherty LS, Kiely JL, Deegan PC, et al. Late-onset central hypoventilation syndrome: a family genetic study. *Eur Respir J.* 2007;29(2):312–316. https://doi.org/10.1183/09031936.00001606.
17. Rand CM, Yu M, Jennings LJ, et al. Germline mosaicism of PHOX2B mutation accounts for familial recurrence of congenital central hypoventilation syndrome (CCHS. *Am J Med Genet A.* 2012;158(9):2297.
18. Yousif A., Chandler A., Ghandour M., Akinpeloye A. Congenital Central Hypoventilation Syndrome: What to Expect During Pregnancy. *Curēus Palo Alto CA.* Published online 2021. https://doi.org/10.7759/cureus.17827.
19. Armstrong AE, Weese-Mayer DE, Mian A, et al. Treatment of neuroblastoma in congenital central hypoventilation syndrome with a PHOX2B polyalanine repeat expansion mutation: New twist on a neurocristopathy syndrome. *Pediatr Blood Cancer.* 2015;62(11):2007–2010. https://doi.org/10.1002/pbc.25572.
20. Todd ES, Scott NM, Weese-Mayer DE, et al. Characterization of dermatoglyphics in PHOX2B-confirmed congenital central hypoventilation syndrome. *Pediatrics.* 2006;118(2):e408–414. https://doi.org/10.1542/peds.2005-3134.
21. Weese-Mayer D.E., Rand C.M., Khaytin I., et al. Congenital Central Hypoventilation Syndrome. In: Adam MP, Mirzaa GM, Pagon RA, et al., eds. *GeneReviews.* University of Washington, Seattle; 2021.

22. Porcaro F, Paglietti MG, Cherchi C, Schiavino A, Chiarini Testa MB, Cutrera R. How the Management of Children With Congenital Central Hypoventilation Syndrome Has Changed Over Time: Two Decades of Experience From an Italian Center. *Front Pediatr.* 2021;9 https://doi.org/10.3389/fped.2021.648927. 648927-648927.

23. Chin AC, Shaul DB, Patwari PP, Keens TG, Kenny AS, Weese-Mayer DE. Diaphragmatic pacing in infants and children with congenital central hypoventilation syndrome. In: Kheirandish-Gozal L, Gozal D, eds. *Sleep Disordered Breathing in Children: A Comprehensive Clinical Guide to Evaluation and Treatment.* Respiratory Medicine. Humana Press; 2012:553–573. https://doi.org/10.1007/978-1-60761-725-9_42.

24. Valika T, Chin AC, Thompson DM, et al. Airway obstruction during sleep due to diaphragm pacing precludes decannulation in young children with CCHS. *Respir Int Rev Thorac Dis.* 2019;98(3):263–267. https://doi.org/10.1159/000501172.

25. Diep B, Wang A, Kun S, et al. Diaphragm Pacing without Tracheostomy in Congenital Central Hypoventilation Syndrome Patients. *Respiration.* 2015;89(6):534–538. https://doi.org/10.1159/000381401.

26. Marazita ML, Maher BS, Cooper ME, et al. Genetic segregation analysis of autonomic nervous system dysfunction in families of probands with idiopathic congenital central hypoventilation syndrome. *Am J Med Genet.* 2001;100(3):229–236. https://doi.org/10.1002/ajmg.1284.

27. Weese-Mayer DE, Silvestri JM, Huffman AD, et al. Case/control family study of autonomic nervous system dysfunction in idiopathic congenital central hypoventilation syndrome. *Am J Med Genet.* 2001;100(3):237–245. https://doi.org/10.1002/ajmg.1249.

28. Matera I, Bachetti T, Puppo F, et al. PHOX2B mutations and polyalanine expansions correlate with the severity of the respiratory phenotype and associated symptoms in both congenital and late onset central hypoventilation syndrome. *J Med Genet.* 2004;41(5):373–380. https://doi.org/10.1136/jmg.2003.015412.

29. Gronli JO, Santucci BA, Leurgans SE, Berry-Kravis EM, Weese-Mayer DE. Congenital central hypoventilation syndrome: PHOX2B genotype determines risk for sudden death. *Pediatr Pulmonol.* 2008;43(1):77–86. https://doi.org/10.1002/ppul.20744.

30. Laifman E, Keens TG, Bar-Cohen Y, Perez IA. Life-threatening cardiac arrhythmias in congenital central hypoventilation syndrome. *Eur J Pediatr.* 2020;179(5):821–825. https://doi.org/10.1007/s00431-019-03568-5.

31. Silvestri JM, Hanna BD, Volgman AS, Jones PJ, Barnes SD, Weese-Mayer DE. Cardiac rhythm disturbances among children with idiopathic congenital central hypoventilation syndrome. *Pediatr Pulmonol.* 2000;29(5):351–358. https://doi.org/10.1002/(sici)1099-0496(200005)29:5<351::aid-ppul3>3.0.co;2-z.

32. Woo M.S., Woo M.A., Gozal D., Jansen M.T., Keens T.G., Harper R.M. Heart rate variability in congenital central hypoventilation syndrome. *Pediatr Res.* 31(3):291-296. https://doi.org/10.1203/00006450-199203000-00020.

33. Trang H, Girad A, Laude D, Elghozi JL. Short-term blood pressure and heart rate variability in congenital central hypoventilation syndrome (Ondine's curse. *Clin Sci.* 2005;108(3):225–230. https://doi.org/10.1042/CS20040282.

34. Silvestri JM, Weese-Mayer DE, Flanagan EA. Congenital central hypoventilation syndrome: cardiorespiratory responses to moderate exercise, simulating daily activity. *Pediatr Pulmonol.* 1995;20(2):89–93. https://doi.org/10.1002/ppul.1950200207.

35. Dudoignon B, Denjoy I, Patout M, et al. Heart rate variability in congenital central hypoventilation syndrome: relationships with hypertension and sinus pauses. *Pediatr Res. Published online.* July 26, 2022 https://doi.org/10.1038/s41390-022-02215-4.

36. Vu EL, Dunne EC, Bradley A, et al. Cerebral Autoregulation During Orthostatic Challenge in Congenital Central Hypoventilation Syndrome. *Am J Respir Crit Care Med.* 2021 https://doi.org/10.1164/rccm.202103-0732OC. Published online November 17, 2021.

37. Trochet D, O'Brien LM, Gozal D, et al. PHOX2B genotype allows for prediction of tumor risk in congenital central hypoventilation syndrome. *Am J Hum Genet.* 2005;76(3):421–426. https://doi.org/10.1086/428366.

38. Kamihara J, Bourdeaut F, Foulkes WD, et al. Retinoblastoma and Neuroblastoma Predisposition and Surveillance. *Clin Cancer Res.* 2017;23(13):e98–e106. https://doi.org/10.1158/1078-0432.Ccr-17-0652.

39. Amiel J, Sproat-Emison E, Garcia-Barcelo M, et al. Hirschsprung disease, associated syndromes and genetics: a review. *J Med Genet.* 2008;45(1):1–14. https://doi.org/10.1136/jmg.2007.053959.

40. Arshad A, Powell C, Tighe MP. Hirschsprung's disease. *BMJ Online.* 2012;345(oct01 2): https://doi.org/10.1136/bmj.e5521. e5521-e5521.

41. Balakrishnan K, Perez IA, Keens TG, Sicolo A, Punati J, Danialifar T. Hirschsprung disease and other gastrointestinal motility disorders in patients with CCHS. *Eur J Pediatr.* 2020;180(2):469–473. https://doi.org/10.1007/s00431-020-03848-5.

42. Saiyed R, Rand CM, Carroll MS, et al. Congenital central hypoventilation syndrome (CCHS): Circadian temperature variation. *Pediatr Pulmonol.* 2016;51(3):300–307. https://doi.org/10.1002/ppul.23236.

43. Patwari PP, Stewart TM, Rand CM, et al. Pupillometry in congenital central hypoventilation syndrome (CCHS): quantitative evidence of autonomic nervous system dysregulation. *Pediatr Res.* 2012;71(3):280–285. https://doi.org/10.1038/pr.2011.38.

44. Fadl-Alla A., Winston M., Rand C., et al. Pupillary Parasympathetic and Sympathetic Dysfunction in a Longitudinal Congenital Central Hypoventilation Syndrome (CCHS) Cohort from Infancy to Young Adulthood: Potential Biomarker for Intervention Trials. Published online May 2022. https://doi.org/10.1164/ajrccm-conference.2022.205.1_MeetingAbstracts.A4997.

45. Zelko F.A., Stewart T.M., Brogadir C.D., Rand C.M., Weese-Mayer D.E. Congenital central hypoventilation syndrome: Broader cognitive deficits revealed by parent controls. *Pediatr Pulmonol.* 53(4):492-497. https://doi.org/10.1002/ppul.23939.

46. Zelko FA, Nelson MN, Leurgans SE, Berry-Kravis EM, Weese-Mayer DE. Congenital central hypoventilation syndrome: neurocognitive functioning in school age children. *Pediatr Pulmonol.* 2010;45(1):92–98. https://doi.org/10.1002/ppul.21170.

47. Charnay AJ, Antisdel-Lomaglio JE, Zelko FA, et al. Congenital central hypoventilation syndrome: neurocognition already reduced in preschool-aged children. *Chest.* 2016;149(3):809. https://doi.org/10.1378/chest.15-0402.

48. Ogata T, Muramatsu K, Miyana K, Ozawa H, Iwasaki M, Arakawa H. Neurodevelopmental outcome and respiratory management of congenital central hypoventilation syndrome: a retrospective study. *BMC Pediatr.* 2020;20(1): https://doi.org/10.1186/s12887-020-02239-x. 342-342.

41

Rapid-Onset Obesity with Hypothalamic Dysfunction, Hypoventilation, and Autonomic Dysregulation Syndrome

Ilya Khaytin, Casey M. Rand, Susan M. Slattery, Tracey M. Stewart, Michael S. Carroll, and Debra E. Weese-Mayer

CHAPTER HIGHLIGHTS

- Rapid-onset obesity with hypothalamic dysfunction, hypoventilation, and autonomic dysregulation (ROHHAD) is a rare syndrome.
- The usual first symptom is rapid-onset obesity with weight gain of 20–30 pounds over 3–12 months in previously non-obese 2- to 7-year-old children.
- The evidence of hypothalamic abnormalities, then hypoventilation and autonomic dysregulation follow.
- There is a high rate of cardiorespiratory arrest in children with ROHHAD. Therefore, a high index of suspicion must be maintained.
- Management of ROHHAD necessitates comprehensive serial follow-up and addressing respiratory, cardiac, and endocrine abnormalities.
- As soon as hypoventilation is identified, ventilatory support should be initiated to avoid cardiac sequelae, including cor pulmonale, right ventricular hypertrophy, and cardiopulmonary arrest.
- Screening for neural crest tumors is necessary, because if found early, tumors can be excised.
- There is no identified genetic marker or cure for ROHHAD at present, but with aggressive management, morbidity and mortality can be avoided and neurocognition preserved.

Introduction

Rapid-onset obesity with hypothalamic dysfunction, hypoventilation, and autonomic dysregulation (ROHHAD) is a rare clinical disorder with a unique constellation of symptoms including altered respiratory control, endocrine function, and autonomic regulation. The initial report was in 1965 by Fishman and colleagues,[1] who described a 2.7-year-old boy with a dramatic weight gain of 10.4 kg over a 9-month span, accompanied by several cyanotic episodes. The authors named the syndrome "primary alveolar hypoventilation, 'Ondine's curse,'" introducing a literary misnomer. Just 5 years later, Mellins and coworkers[2] described a 12-day-old boy with cyanosis, polycythemia, and abnormal ventilatory response to hypercarbia, who they also diagnosed with "Ondine's curse.'" Both boys presented with central hypoventilation and autonomic abnormalities; however, there were significant differences in other aspects of their respective phenotypes, including age at presentation, presence/absence of obesity, and endocrine (dys)function. For more than two decades, both disorders were considered to potentially be part of the same spectrum as what we now call congenital central hypoventilation syndrome (CCHS), a rare neurocristopathy caused by mutations in the PHOX2B gene (see Chapter 40). As recently as 1996, del Carmen Sanchez and colleagues described two additional cases (ages 3 and 5 years),[3] diagnosed with "late onset central hypoventilation syndrome," but on careful review one of the children would meet the criteria for what we now call ROHHAD and the other child likely had CCHS. In 2000, Katz and coworkers[4] presented a single case and review of all 10 reported cases in the literature, called them "late-onset central hypoventilation with hypothalamic dysfunction," and postulated that this is an entity distinct from CCHS that is known to present in infancy, without obesity, and only rarely hypothalamic dysfunction. And finally, in 2007 Ize-Ludlow and colleagues[5] analyzed records from 23 children with rapid-onset weight gain in the first 10 years of life with hypothalamic dysfunction and then symptoms of autonomic dysregulation, offering the acronym ROHHAD for "rapid-onset obesity with hypothalamic dysfunction, hypoventilation, and autonomic dysregulation," inclusive of the neural crest tumors, with an aim to help pediatricians and subspecialists identify patients earlier in their course by recognizing an acronym describing the characteristic order of phenotype presentation. In 2008, Bougneres and colleagues[6] proposed the term ROHHADNET distinct from ROHHAD for those children with ROHHAD and neural crest tumors, though this term is less frequently used than ROHHAD.

Fewer than 200 cases of ROHHAD have been described in the literature or clinical care. Affected children with ROHHAD are seemingly normal until typically ages 2–7 years, when they present with the rapid-onset dramatic weight gain. Due to children becoming more independent during this age range, rapid-onset obesity is often attributed to overeating, though this is not typically the case among children with ROHHAD. The other phenotypic features, including hypothalamic dysfunction, hypoventilation, and autonomic dysfunction, appear later in the phenotype unfolding, over the next few months to years, making the initial diagnosis challenging. Unfortunately, delayed diagnosis may lead to suboptimal management, resulting in cardiorespiratory arrest as a frequent feature of ROHHAD. On the other hand, early recognition of ROHHAD and the introduction of appropriate artificial ventilatory support allow for normal neurodevelopment and dramatically reduced morbidity and mortality.

Unlike other obesity-related syndromes, such as Prader-Willi syndrome (PWS), Smith-Magenis syndrome, 16p11.2 microdeletion syndrome, and monogenetic obesity syndromes (e.g., leptin [LEP], proopiomelanocortin [POMC] mutations),[7] ROHHAD remains a clinical diagnosis without an identified genetic cause. Nevertheless, a high index of suspicion for ROHHAD together with appropriate physiologic testing allows for early identification of affected children. Once identified, all children with ROHHAD will eventually require some form of artificial ventilation with positive airway pressure support, leading in most cases to invasive ventilation via tracheostomy. With prompt identification and rigorous management of their ventilatory and endocrine needs, children with ROHHAD have good outcomes, and a subset shows some improvement with advancing age.

Pathophysiology

As the acronym implies, the most common presentation for a child with ROHHAD is rapid-onset obesity followed by hypothalamic dysfunction, hypoventilation, and autonomic dysregulation. However, the timing of each feature and the actual order of each symptom may vary from child to child (Fig. 41.1).[5] Rapid-onset obesity is almost invariably the first symptom, rarely preceded by autonomic dysregulation. Hypothalamic dysfunction usually presents next. Then hypoventilation, autonomic dysregulation, and tumors of neural crest origin usually follow. Because unfolding of the phenotype can occur over a few months to a few years, diagnosing ROHHAD represents a particular challenge. Unfortunately, it is also a dangerous time for the child as cardiorespiratory arrest is common if the hypoventilation and control of breathing deficit are unrecognized. It is still not clear what causes previously normally developing children to manifest the ROHHAD phenotype. Unlike CCHS, there is no known gene mutation that causes ROHHAD. In fact, finding a CCHS-related *PHOX2B* gene mutation

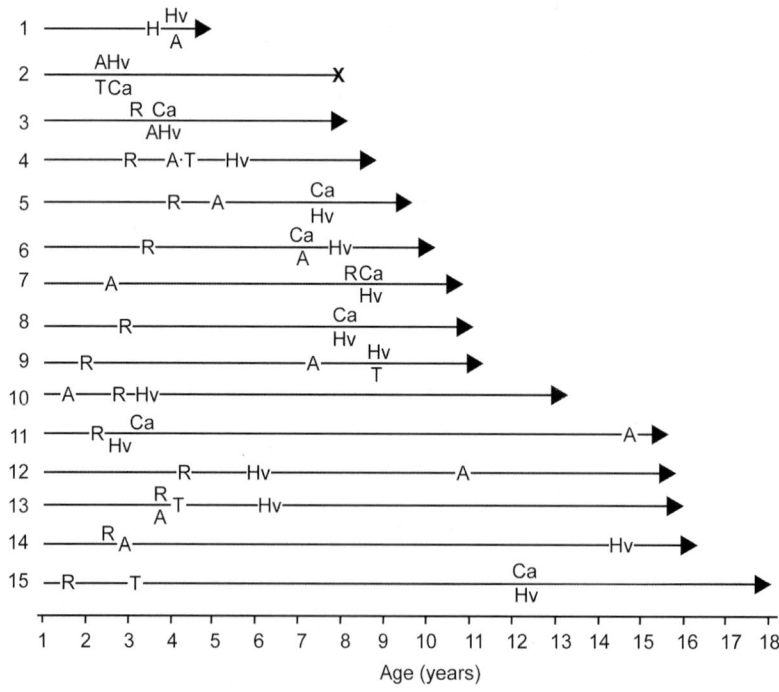

• **Fig. 41.1** Examples of 15 children with rapid-onset obesity with hypothalamic dysfunction, hypoventilation, and autonomic dysregulation (ROHHAD) demonstrating approximate timing of symptoms onset. The x-axis shows ages on patients in years. R, rapid-onset obesity; Hv, hypoventilation; A, autonomic dysfunction; T, neural crest tumor; Ca, cardiorespiratory arrest; X, death; H, hypothalamic manifestations (patient 1 developed obesity before 4 years of age, but no specific age at onset was available).[5]

excludes the diagnosis of ROHHAD.[5] Variants in several genes, including *BDNF, PICK3R3, SPTBN5, PCF11, SRMS, ZNF83, KMT2B*, and others, were reported in published ROHHAD cases, but none were identified as the disease-defining gene.[5,8–10] Because of the association with tumors of neural crest origin, an autoimmune cause of ROHHAD has been proposed. However, treatment with rituximab[11] and cyclophosphamide[12] had very limited success in three cases, and excision of the tumor did not abort the unfolding of the ROHHAD phenotype, as would have been anticipated in neuroimmune disorders associated with such tumors and opsoclonus-myoclonus. Cranial imaging has not provided guidance in ROHHAD, without consistent hypothalamic or pituitary pathology. Though several children with ROHHAD have succumbed to cardiorespiratory arrest, comprehensive autopsy and neuropathology examination of the nervous system has not yet revealed consistent abnormalities.[13,14]

Diagnosis and Presentation

Childhood obesity is a growing problem in the United States and worldwide. The Centers for Disease Control and Prevention (CDC) estimate that for children 2–19 years of age the prevalence of obesity is 18.5%, affecting more than 13.7 million children and adolescents in the United States. As described in the CDC report from 2015–2016,[15] among 2- to 5-year-olds the obesity prevalence is estimated as 13.9%, and among 6- to 11-year-olds it is 18.4%. Significant efforts have been dedicated to determining causes of obesity, and several genetic connections have been reported. Unfortunately, no genetic cause of ROHHAD has been identified to date despite a very focused investigation into a genetic cause. The herald in ROHHAD is the rapid weight gain between ages 2 and 7, overtly apparent on the child's growth chart completed at each well-child visit. The seemingly normal child, with typically non-obese family members and without food-seeking behavior, will gain up to 20–30 pounds of weight over 3–12 months. Often this rapid weight gain is either attributed to a change in diet or overlooked altogether until other symptoms in the ROHHAD phenotype emerge. Other early symptoms including behavioral problems such as irritability and aggression or hyperactivity have been reported in the early literature, but practice shows that with early detection and optimal management, these symptoms are not seen. It is important to stress that prior to the onset of rapid weight gain the children are developmentally normal as this distinguishes ROHHAD from most other syndromic causes of obesity.

Without comprehensive investigation, the rapid weight gain may appear to be the only abnormality for months or even years in a subset of patients who will later be diagnosed with ROHHAD. The initial weight gain is followed by hypothalamic dysfunction. Some children may develop secondary enuresis after being fully toilet trained. With the evaluation of electrolytes, hypernatremia is often identified, leading to a diagnosis of partial diabetes insipidus. Hyperprolactinemia

is frequently seen early in the development of the disease. As the phenotype unfolds, insulin-like growth factor (IGF)-1 and IGF-3 levels may be reduced, and the growth hormone stimulation test is abnormal (decreased response: <10 ng/ mL). A subset of children will develop precocious puberty and premature adrenarche. The rate of unfolding of these endocrine abnormalities can vary from child to child, necessitating the vigilance of the primary physician and pediatric endocrinologist monitoring with the entire panel of endocrine lab work (Box 41.1) every 2–3 months.

As the endocrine abnormalities unfold, features of the respiratory phenotype become apparent. If the physician is attentive and performs polysomnography (PSG), obstructive sleep apnea (OSA) may be identified. However, because obesity and OSA often co-occur, the physician may not consider ROHHAD or pursue more comprehensive physiologic testing for the child. If the child has adenotonsillar hypertrophy believed to cause the OSA and undergoes adenotonsillectomy, the hypoventilation during sleep becomes unmasked. Because exogenous ventilatory challenge[16] to evaluate central and peripheral chemoreceptor responsiveness is not widely available, it is not clear if control of breathing abnormalities precede the hypoventilation. All children with ROHHAD will develop hypoventilation during sleep, and in a subset during sleep and wakefulness, over the next months to years. Central hypoventilation becomes a major risk factor for cardiorespiratory arrest and requires intense monitoring and intervention with artificial ventilation, oximetry, capnography, and home nursing (to monitor the monitors and the artificial ventilation as well as to provide prompt intervention). Because a cardiorespiratory arrest is uncommon in obese children with OSA (likely because they have intact control of breathing), and an estimated 51–66% of obese children have residual OSA after adenotonsillectomy,[17,18] this is an important point to distinguish ROHHAD from other causes of OSA in obese children. Because traditional PSGs do not evaluate children with OSA during wakefulness in activities of daily living, the awake hypoventilation observed in many children with ROHHAD may not be identified until the child develops overt cyanosis with exertion. To characterize the hypoventilation phenotype, children with ROHHAD require comprehensive physiologic testing in varied activities of age-appropriate daily living and with varying levels of exertion to identify hypoxemia and hypercarbia, in addition to an attenuated heart rate and overheating in response to the exertion. Exogeneous ventilatory challenge testing of peripheral and central chemoreceptors reveals an attenuated ventilatory response[16] and absent perception or behavioral awareness to the levels of hypercarbia and hypoxemia that a child with ROHHAD might experience in daily living.

In addition to weight gain and endocrine abnormalities, children with ROHHAD develop autonomic nervous system dysregulation (Table 41.1), with insidious onset and variable presentation over months to years, sometimes delaying the definitive diagnosis of the ROHHAD syndrome. Altered peripheral vasomotor tone with ice-cold and

---

• BOX 41.1   **Suggested Evaluation of the Child with Suspected Rapid-Onset Obesity with Hypothalamic Dysfunction, Hypoventilation, and Autonomic Dysregulation**

Same laboratory evaluation should be conducted at each follow-up evaluation to guide management.

1. A detailed chronologic summary of your patient's medical history from birth to present. This annotated, chronologic summary of medical care should include growth charts from birth to the present time, polysomnograms (PSGs), awake physiologic cardiorespiratory recordings in activities of daily living, cranial and abdominal computerized tomography studies and magnetic resonance imaging studies (MRIs), ventilator settings, oxygen needs, history of neuroendocrine tumors, etc. Digital facial non-smiling photographs (frontal and both lateral views) should be reviewed.

2. The following is a list of labs for suspected rapid-onset obesity with hypothalamic dysfunction, hypoventilation, and autonomic dysregulation (ROHHAD) patients to be collected at the time of rapid weight gain and then every 2–3 months thereafter:
   - Complete blood count with differential
   - Reticulocytes, blood
   - Comprehensive metabolic profile
   - Osmolality, urine
   - Prolactin
   - Macroprolactin
   - Leptin
   - Thyroxine, free (FT4)
   - Thyroid-stimulating hormone-sensitive (s-TSH), serum
   - Insulin-like growth factor binding protein
   - Insulin-like growth factor-1, serum
   - Lipid, screen
   - Cortisol, free, urine
   - Cortisol, serum or plasma
   - Vitamin B$_{12}$, serum
   - Misc, CRANR—urine cortisol random
   - Vitamin D (25-hydroxy vitamin D$_2$ and D$_3$ serum)

3. If a suspected ROHHAD patient has precocious puberty, obtain the following labs:
   - Dehydroepiandrosterone sulfate (DHEA-s)
   - Luteinizing hormone (LH)
   - Follicle-stimulating hormone (FSH)
   If male, please also add the following labs:
   - Testosterone level
   - Gonadotropin-releasing hormone (GnRH)

4. If a suspected ROHHAD patient has iron deficiency, obtain the following labs:
   - Iron, total and total iron binding
   - Ferritin

---

swollen hands and feet are very evident as are decreased core temperature, aberrant sweating, and poikilotherm-like temperature regulation. Ophthalmologic manifestations with strabismus, light sensitivity, and variably altered pupillary response to light are also common. Children with ROHHAD often have an elevated pain threshold.[5] Constipation, diarrhea, and vomiting are commonly reported. Importantly, unlike children with CCHS, children with ROHHAD have not been reported to have Hirschsprung's disease (aganglionosis of the distal hindgut). Additionally, tumors of neural crest origin are found in 40–50% of children with ROHHAD.[5,6,19] In fact, along with rapid-onset weight gain, tumors of neural crest origin are among the early signs of ROHHAD in a subset of children. Ganglioneuromas and ganglioneuroblastomas are most common, occurring anywhere along the sympathetic chain (including a mediastinal presentation) or in either adrenal gland. A small subset of patients with ROHHAD will have a neuroblastoma.

Differential Diagnosis

It is important to distinguish ROHHAD from other obesity-related disorders. It is essential to emphasize that children with ROHHAD are usually normally developing and growing children prior to ROHHAD phenotype onset. Early developmental delay and cognitive impairment distinguish ROHHAD (usually no impairments unless there was an inadequate response to the cardiorespiratory arrest or the hypoventilation-related chronic intermittent hypoxemia and hypercarbia) from multiple causes of syndromic obesity, including PWS, Smith-Magenis syndrome, Carpenter

syndrome, and 16p11.2 deletion syndrome.[7] Probably the most common cause of obesity that can be confused with ROHHAD is PWS.[20] Unlike ROHHAD, PWS has a genetic marker on chromosome 15 (15q11.2-q13). Most children with PWS present in the neonatal period with hypotonia, feeding difficulties, and severe developmental delay. Their feeding difficulty usually transforms into obesity with hyperphagia by about 4–8 years of age. Unlike children with ROHHAD, children with PWS exhibit prominent food-seeking behaviors. Also, children with PWS usually have short stature, which responds well to growth hormone supplementation. Considering the high prevalence of obesity in the general population, it is important to do a thorough history and evaluation in children with obesity. Inquiring about a family history of obesity and any history of consanguinity is necessary. Discovery of neurodevelopmental and cognitive disabilities should lead to genetic evaluation including high-resolution karyotype, methylation study of chromosome 15, and obesity genetic panels (LEP, LEPR, POMC, PCSK1, etc.).

As noted earlier, ROHHAD shares several features with CCHS supporting a shared neural crest origin. However, most children with CCHS present during the first few days to weeks of life with overt hypoventilation or apnea necessitating artificial ventilation for life support. Though children with CCHS have related symptoms of autonomic dysregulation, they do not have related obesity. Later-onset CCHS (LO-CCHS) indicates presentation after 1 month of age, also with hypoventilation necessitating artificial ventilation during sleep, but is not associated with obesity. Individuals with neonatal-onset CCHS and LO-CCHS will have a

TABLE 41.1 Clinical Findings in the Children with Rapid-Onset Obesity with Hypothalamic Dysfunction, Hypoventilation, and Autonomic Dysregulation[5]

Clinical Findings	% of Patients	Clinical Findings	% of Patients
Hypothalamic Dysfunction		**Other Findings**	
Rapid-onset obesity	100.0	Abnormal brain MRI scans	46.7
Failed growth hormone stimulation test	60.0	Seizure	33.3
Hyperphagia	53.3	Enuresis	26.7
Polydipsia	53.3	Hypotonia	26.7
Hypernatremia	46.7	Asthma	20.0
Hyperprolactinemia	46.7	Hypercholesterolemia	20.0
Diabetes insipidus	33.3	Scoliosis	20.0
Hypothyroidism	33.3	Hypersomnolence	13.3
Adrenal insufficiency	26.7	Recurrent prior pneumonia	13.3
Hypodipsia	26.7	Deceased	6.7
Polyuria	26.7	Impaired glucose tolerance	6.7
Short stature	20.0	Type 2 diabetes mellitus	6.7
Delayed puberty	13.3	**Developmental Disorder**	
Hyponatremia	13.3	Developmental delay	20.0
Low IGF-1 and IGFBP-3 levels	13.3	Developmental regression	20.0
Precocious puberty	13.3	**Behavioral Disorders**	
Premature adrenarche	13.3	Depression	13.3
Transient SIADH	13.3	Flat affect	13.3
Amenorrhea	6.7	Psychosis	13.3
Hypogonadotropic hypogonadism	6.7	Behavioral outbursts	6.7
Irregular menses	6.7	Bipolar disorder	6.7
Transient diabetes insipidus	6.7	Emotional lability	6.7
Respiratory Manifestations		Obsessive-compulsive disorder	6.7
Alveolar hypoventilation	100.0	Oppositional-defiant disorder	6.7
Cardiorespiratory arrest	60.0	Tourette's syndrome	6.7
Reduced carbon dioxide ventilatory response	60.0	Hallucinations	6.7
Obstructive sleep apnea	53.3		
Cyanotic episodes	26.7		
Autonomic Dysregulation			
Ophthalmologic manifestations	86.7		
Thermal dysregulation	73.3		
Gastrointestinal dysmotility	66.7		
Altered perception of pain	53.3		

Abbreviations: SIADH, syndrome of inappropriate antidiuretic hormone secretion; IGF, insulin-like growth factor; IGFBP, insulin-like growth factor-binding protein; MRI, magnetic resonance imaging.

disease-causing mutation in the *PHOX2B* gene. ROHHAD is distinct from obesity hypoventilation in terms of age at the presentation, the weight gain trajectory, unfolding of the phenotype with advancing age, varied severity of hypothalamic dysfunction, and association of (typically) benign neural crest tumors. Also, children with ROHHAD usually have attenuated or absent peripheral and central chemoreceptor responsiveness in contrast to the blunted hypercarbia response in obesity hypoventilation.[21,22]

Management

Overview

Overall, diagnosing of ROHHAD relies on early recognition of the following: rapid-onset obesity after the age of 1.5–2 years with evidence of hypoventilation; evidence of hypothalamic dysfunction, including at least one of the following criteria, such as hyperprolactinemia, central hypothyroidism, disordered water balance, failed growth hormone stimulation test, corticotrophin deficiency, or altered onset of puberty (see Table 41.1); and absence of a CCHS-related *PHOX2B* gene mutation. Since at present there is no ROHHAD-related genetic or other diagnostic test, frequent in-laboratory physiologic and endocrine reevaluations are needed in all children suspected to have ROHHAD or diagnosed with ROHHAD. Optimized care and longitudinal outcomes come from cooperative partnerships among experts in pulmonology, autonomic medicine, endocrinology, oncology, sleep, psychiatry, cardiology, nutrition, and ROHHAD.

Diagnostic Testing

Since rapid-onset obesity is most often the first presenting sign in children with ROHHAD, a detailed growth chart from birth to the time of evaluation is essential to review. Growth charts often demonstrate a child who maintains a traditional growth trajectory in both height and weight until the dramatic increase in weight trajectory reaching a body mass index (BMI) frequently above the 95th percentile. A straightforward PSG including continuous breath-by-breath end-tidal carbon dioxide and beat-to-beat pulse oximetry and respiratory inductance plethysmography recording is necessary to determine the degree of OSA and possible hypoventilation. However, the lack of hypoventilation on the initial sleep study in such children does not rule out ROHHAD. As hypoventilation may develop abruptly within weeks of the weight gain or may develop more insidiously later, serial sleep studies, as frequently as every 2 months, and daytime physiologic evaluations in age-appropriate activities of daily living are required. Additionally, all children suspected of ROHHAD should have laboratory screening including the labwork listed in Box 41.1, including complete blood count (CBC) with differential, reticulocytes count, comprehensive metabolic panel (CMP), urine osmolality, prolactin and macroprolactin levels, leptin, free thyroxine (FT4), thyroid-stimulating hormone (TSH), IGF binding protein and IGF-1 levels, lipid screen, and

cortisol levels. Considering the frequency of cardiovascular arrest, electrocardiogram (ECG), echocardiography, and 72-hour Holter monitoring are necessary to identify potential arrhythmias. Magnetic resonance imaging (MRI) of the brain (hypothalamic-pituitary mode) to exclude hypothalamic-pituitary lesions is also recommended. Finally, imaging of chest and abdomen for evidence of neural crest tumors should be performed at the time of diagnosis then serially every 2–3 months thereafter (see Box 41.1).

Respiratory Support

Hypoventilation is not typically the presenting symptom of ROHHAD but is a cause for significant morbidity and mortality. Therefore, evaluation of spontaneous breathing asleep and awake in children with suspected ROHHAD is critically important. It is not unusual for children with ROHHAD to develop symptoms of OSA followed by central hypoventilation within a span of few months. Serial sleep studies with continuous end-tidal CO_2 monitoring before and after the introduction of artificial ventilation is a must. Optimally, a period of daytime spontaneous respiration should also be recorded in varied age-appropriate activities of daily living. Exogenous ventilatory challenge testing is also very useful for diagnosis and monitoring of control of breathing in children with ROHHAD. During exogenous ventilatory challenges in a wholly controlled in-lab, in-hospital setting, the child is presented serially with four different gas mixtures: 100% O_2, 95% O_2 with 5% CO_2, 14% O_2 with 7% CO_2, and five to seven breaths of 100% N_2. The challenges are designed to test the child's peripheral and central chemoreceptor responsiveness with physiologic compromise such as they might experience in age-appropriate daily activities. Unlike controls, children with ROHHAD have an attenuated response to hypoxia and hypercarbia (Figs. 41.2 and 41.3).[16]

All children with ROHHAD require artificial ventilatory support at least during sleep and most need artificial ventilatory support during both wakefulness and sleep. Many children with ROHHAD benefit from tracheostomy with mechanical ventilation. Optimally, a tight-to-the-shaft (TTS) cuffed tracheostomy tube should be used, allowing for cuff deflation when awake (to make voice) and inflation during sleep (minimization of air leak asleep). Some patients who only require nocturnal support may benefit from bi-level ventilation with mask interface, but the ventilation is less stable especially with severe obesity. However, it is important to evaluate each child with ROHHAD individually on the appropriateness of using mask ventilation. Unlike children with OSA, children with ROHHAD are at greater risk of cardiorespiratory arrest due to hypoventilation and the need for ventilation as life support. Therefore, younger children and children who are not yet mature enough to keep the mask on the face may not be good candidates for mask ventilation. Such children should be offered tracheostomy instead. A phrenic nerve stimulator may be considered for daytime use only in some children. However, due to increased adipose tissue, it may have

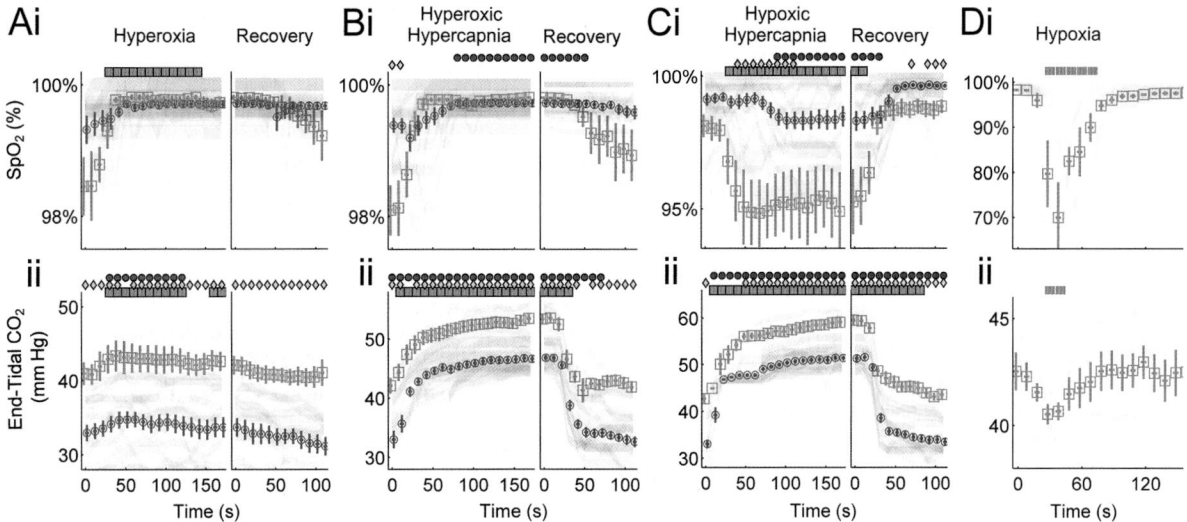

• **Fig. 41.2** Responses of children with rapid-onset obesity with hypothalamic dysfunction, hypoventilation, and autonomic dysregulation (ROHHAD) and controls to exogenous ventilatory challenges. Hemoglobin saturation (SpO_2; *subpanel i*) and end-tidal CO_2 *(subpanel ii)* values during ventilatory challenges and recovery for four different gas mixtures. (A) 100% O_2, (B) mix of 95% O_2 and 5% CO_2, (C) mix of 14% O_2 and 7% CO_2, (D) 5 or 7 tidal breaths of N_2. Values for ROHHAD cases are shown as *open squares* in blue at mean ± SEM, whereas controls are shown as *open circles* in pink. Significant excursions from baseline are indicated with *filled markers* above each data panel (*filled squares* for ROHHAD, *filled circles* for controls). Significant differences between ROHHAD and controls for each time bin are indicated by *diamonds*. Transparent background lines illustrate per subject raw data. Children with ROHHAD consistently demonstrated abnormal control of breathing as evidenced by elevated end-tidal CO_2 values with all challenges and a dramatic drop in oxygen saturation in hypoxic challenges.

limited success because of the adipose tissue-imposed distance between the external radiofrequency antennas and the surgically implanted receiver and because of the need to move significant added abdominal weight with each diaphragm excursion/breath. It is important to note that the phrenic nerve stimulator should never be used during the night in a decannulated patient due to a risk of very severe OSA not amenable to tonsillectomy and/or nasopharyngeal surgical procedures. However, no matter which mode of ventilation is most appropriate for a given child, oxygen saturation and end-tidal CO_2 should be monitored continuously in the home. Because children with ROHHAD do not have fully intact respiratory control, they are at risk for hypoxemia with hypercarbia and of hypocarbia, all of which may alter cerebral regional blood flow. The goal should be maintaining SpO_2 >92% and $ETCO_2$ in the 35–45 mm Hg range. Parents should be educated on how to administer cardiopulmonary resuscitation. Optimally, 24-hour care with a highly experienced registered nurse should be provided in the home to help keep the child with ROHHAD safe by monitoring the oximetry and capnography monitors and by intervening immediately as needed.

Children with ROHHAD should be evaluated every 2 months until their ventilatory needs and phenotype pattern is clear, then at least every 3–4 months during the first 2–3 years after diagnosis. Only after the child's ROHHAD phenotype has fully unfolded should evaluation every 6–12 months be considered. Each comprehensive evaluation in a wholly controlled attended in-laboratory in-hospital setting should include daytime and nighttime studies, with

continuous recording of the patient's hemoglobin saturation, $ETCO_2$, ECG, respiratory inductance plethysmography, blood pressure, temperature, and cerebral regional blood flow/oxygenation. The child should be evaluated during age-appropriate activities including quiet play, reading, watching an educational video, eating, walking, running, concentrational tasks, and any other activities that the child may experience at school or home. The evaluation should also include spontaneous breathing trials during both wakefulness and sleep to determine the child's innate response (or lack thereof) to an endogenous physiologic challenge. Exogenous ventilatory challenges should also be conducted to objectively characterize changes with advancing age in the child's response to hypoxia and hypercarbia. Anecdotal experience among children with ROHHAD suggests that at least some children will improve their awake breathing and begin to sense shortness of breath as they age. As a result, they may be able to have longer periods of spontaneous breathing during the day or may be considered for transitioning from tracheostomy to mask ventilation.

Hypothalamic Dysfunction

Rapid weight gain is the heralding feature of the ROHHAD phenotype, though it does not appear to be due to significantly increased appetite or food-seeking behavior. Instead, most likely this obesity is hypothalamic in origin. Therefore, early referral to a pediatric endocrinologist and a dietician to determine etiology and best approach to managing this obesity is advised. In a supportive family

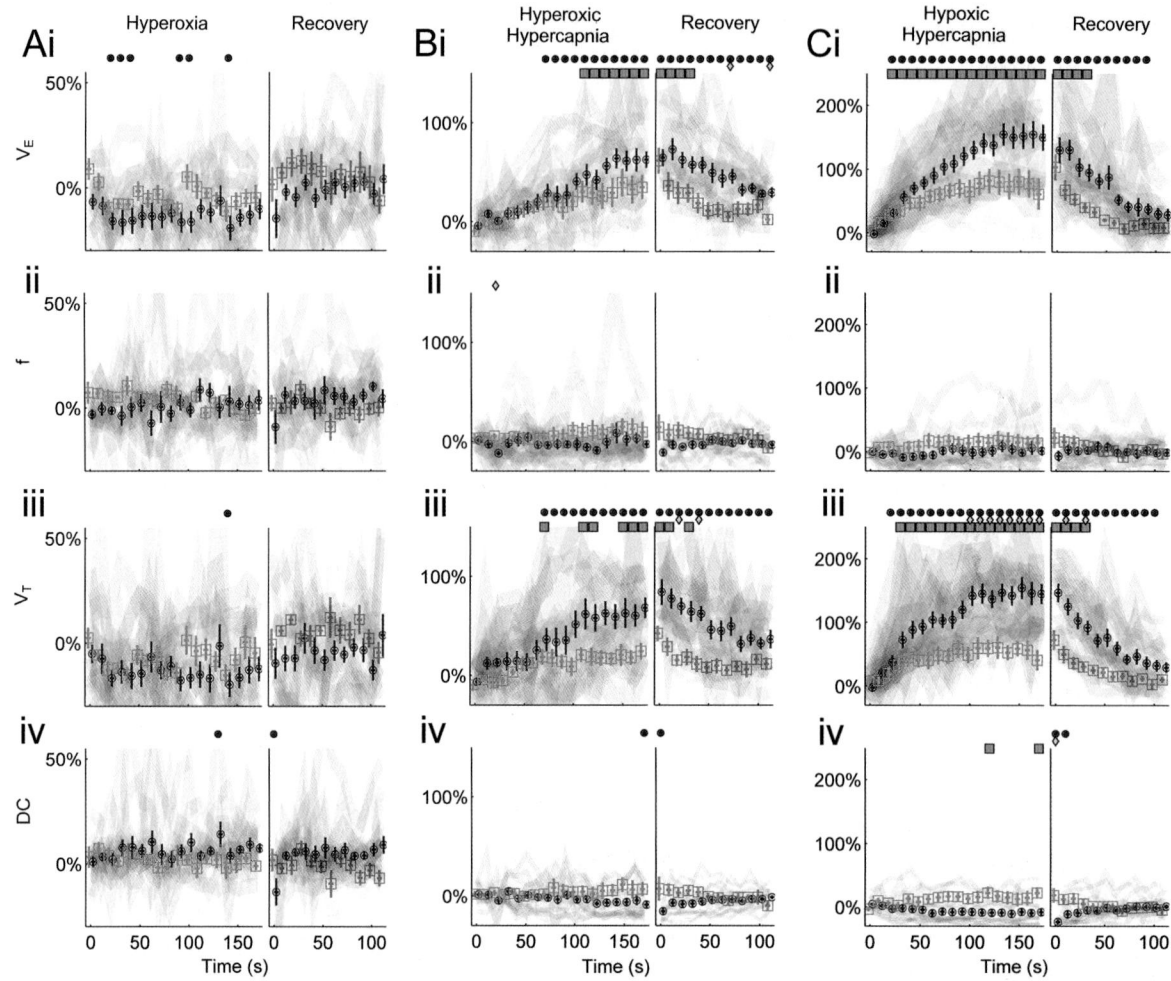

• **Fig. 41.3** Respiratory response to three distinct gas challenges, hyperoxia (10% FiO_2). (A) hyperoxic hypercapnia (95% FiO_2/5% $FiCO_2$), (B) and hypoxic hypercapnia (14% FiO_2/7% $FiCO_2$), (C) Percentage change from baseline is shown during gas exposure *(left)* and recovery *(right)*. Values are weight-normalized minute ventilation (V_E, row i), respiratory frequency *(f, row ii)*, weight-normalized tidal volume *(V_T, row iii)*, and inspiratory duty cycle *(DC, row iv)*. Rapid-onset obesity with hypothalamic dysfunction, hypoventilation, and autonomic dysregulation (ROHHAD) cases are shown as *open squares* in blue as mean ± SEM, whereas controls are shown as *open circles* in pink. Significant differences from baseline are indicated with *filled markers* above each data panel *(filled squares* for ROHHAD, *filled circles* for controls). Significant differences in mean values between ROHHAD and controls for each time point are indicated by *diamonds*. Transparent background lines represent per subject raw data.

setting, children with ROHHAD can slow weight gain and at times reverse BMI trajectory with meticulous attention to diet and exercise. Electrolyte abnormalities can be managed with tight regulation of salt and fluid intake and may necessitate desmopressin (DDAVP) in the event of diabetes insipidus. Cortisol deficiency and hypothyroidism can be managed with appropriate replacement therapies. Children with ROHHAD may require growth hormone therapy. Hormone replacement therapy may also be needed to help with pubertal development.

Autonomic Dysregulation

In addition to weight gain and endocrine abnormalities, autonomic dysregulation is a prominent feature of ROHHAD. Many children have an early presentation of

strabismus and variably altered pupillary response to light. Some children may even develop oculomotor apraxia, ptosis, and decreased tearing. Children with ROHHAD may have striking problems with peripheral and central thermoregulation. They may have reduced core temperature compared with normal controls and may have difficulty mounting an appropriate fever response. Due to inappropriate sweating response and dysfunctional peripheral vasomotor tone, it is not uncommon for children with ROHHAD to have the tips of the fingers and toes so cold as to be close to room temperature. Evaluation of a child with ROHHAD should include measurement of peripheral skin temperatures, QSWEAT test, and, if possible, a thermoregulatory sweat test, to objectively characterize the temperature and sweating regulation. The caregivers should always pay attention to appropriate clothing to avoid hypo- and hyperthermia. Children with ROHHAD may also have decreased pain response, observed with a decreased response to accidental trauma or phlebotomy. Constipation is common and should be managed with a healthy diet and, if necessary, pharmacologic intervention to improve motility under the guidance of a pediatric gastroenterologist familiar with ROHHAD.

Cardiac manifestation of ROHHAD includes decreased heart rate variability during both wakefulness and sleep at different stages of the unfolding of the phenotype. Though present, there may be decreased circadian and stages-of-sleep changes in heart rate. Due to intermittent hypoxia and hypercarbia, children with ROHHAD are at risk for cor pulmonale and/or right ventricular hypertrophy. Therefore, ECG and 72-hour Holter, and echocardiography annually are necessary. The exaggerated bradycardia during sleep is not associated with abrupt asystole, but an occasional patient has received an implanted cardiac pacemaker.

Neural Crest Tumors

All children with suspected ROHHAD should be monitored for tumors of neural crest origin. Ganglioneuromas and ganglioneuroblastomas are most common, though neuroblastoma has been occasionally reported; all potentially occurring anywhere along the sympathetic chain in the chest or in either adrenal gland. Up to 40% of children with ROHHAD have reported neural crest tumors.[5] Therefore, any child with rapid-onset obesity in the 1.5–7 year age range should have a chest X-ray and abdominal ultrasound at every 3–4 months' evaluation to look for a tumor of neural crest origin. Once identified the tumor should be surgically excised to prevent impingement on vital organs. It should be noted that surgical removal of the tumor does not prevent the unfolding of the ROHHAD phenotype or reversal of this syndrome. Also, even though no cases of recurrence have been documented to date, annual screening with chest X-ray, abdominal ultrasound, and urine catecholamines (vanillylmandelic acid [urine VMA]) and homovanillic acid (urine [HVA]) should be performed.

Neurocognition and Development

Although the American Academy of Sleep Medicine defines severe behavioral disturbances and developmental delay as part of ROHHAD syndrome, such abnormalities are not characteristic features of ROHHAD and more an outcome of poor management. Children whose ROHHAD diagnosis was established early demonstrate neurocognition scores at or above controls mean values for performance on Wechsler Intelligence Scales, Beery developmental test of visual-motor integration, and Woodcock-Johnson scale of achievement. However, a subgroup of children with ROHHAD have apparent developmental problems, thought to be related to delayed diagnosis, inadequate management of the hypoventilation, or inadequate intervention for cardiorespiratory arrest.

Outcomes

Due to the high prevalence of pediatric obesity in our society, it may be difficult to consider rare causes for obesity. ROHHAD is one of those causes for which early identification can save lives. Up to 40% of children with ROHHAD will experience a cardiorespiratory arrest if not diagnosed and managed properly. Therefore, any child who presents to their medical provider with dramatic weight gain between 1.5 and 7 years of age should be suspected of having ROHHAD, warranting a systematic evaluation and close follow-up. The acronym ROHHAD highlights features of the phenotype, though these features do not unfold simultaneously. Consequently, follow-up at 3- to 4-month intervals is warranted for prompt identification of changes to the phenotype. Discovering tumors of neural crest origin in a child who is rapidly gaining weight and who has hypernatremia must prompt full evaluation for ROHHAD, including daytime and nighttime cardiorespiratory evaluations. Once the diagnosis of ROHHAD is confirmed, children must receive appropriate ventilatory support to maintain stable oxygenation and ventilation. Tracheostomy should be offered early in the course to secure the airway as mask ventilation in markedly obese children may not be consistently effective. Publicly visible Internet alerts indicate that children with ROHHAD who have poor outcomes may have associated tracheostomy refusals and inadequate respiratory support during the day and during the night. With optimal support, children with ROHHAD can continue to participate in age-appropriate activities with mild to moderate exertion and have a normal developmental trajectory. Limited experience suggests that some children with ROHHAD may experience gradual improvement of symptoms after several years of disease, but only with aggressive management of their ventilatory support, endocrine abnormalities, autonomic abnormalities, and surgical removal of their tumor of neural crest origin.[23] Therefore, the best outcomes are associated with a team approach to management led by the pediatrician, with the patient followed by synchronized care from subspecialists including a pediatric pulmonologist, autonomic medicine specialist, endocrinologist, sleep specialist, cardiologist, gastroenterologist, nutritionist, and psychologist.

Additional Considerations

International ROHHAD Registry
https://clinicaltrials.gov/show/NCT03135730
ROHHAD Newsletter (ROHHAD Reader)
https://www.luriechildrens.org/en/specialties-conditions/
    rapid-onset-obesity-with-hypothalamic-dysfunction-
    hypoventilation-autonomic-dysregulation-rohhad/
ROHHAD Fight, Inc.
3 Surrey Lane
Hempstead NY 11550
Phone: 516-642-1177
Fax: 516-483-0566
Email: rohhadfight@aol.com
www.rohhadfight.org
ROHHAD Association

11 A Lomond Crescent
Alexandria, Scotland G83 0RJ
Phone: +44 7917-225-276
Email: rohhadassociation@gmail.com
ROHHAD Association Belgium
Rimière Street 22
B-4121
Neupré, Belgium
Phone: +32 (0)4 223 75 52
Email: association@rohhad.be

CLINICAL PEARLS

- ROHHAD (Rapid-onset obesity with hypothalamic dysfunction, hypoventilation, and autonomic dysregulation) is a rare disorder with a unique progression of symptom presentation.
- The child presents with rapid weight gain, hypothalamic abnormalities/autonomic dysregulation, and finally hypoventilation with no history of abnormalities of neurocognitive development.
- Tumors of neural crest origin and cardiorespiratory arrest may also occur.
- Management of ROHHAD requires close serial follow-up of sleep, respiratory, cardiac and endocrine function, including awake and sleep respiratory function (providing ventilatory support once hypoventilation is identified), electrocardiogram, 72-hour Holter, echocardiography, as well as abdominal and chest imaging.

References

1. Fishman LS, Samson JH, Sperling DR. Primary alveolar hypoventilation syndrome (Ondine's curse). *Am J Dis Child.* 1965;110:155–161.
2. Mellins RB, Balfour Jr. HH, Turino GM, Winters RW. Failure of automatic control of ventilation (Ondine's curse). Report of an infant born with this syndrome and review of the literature. *Medicine (Baltimore).* 1970;49(6):487–504.
3. del Carmen Sanchez M, Lopez-Herce J, Carrillo A, Moral R, Arias B, Rodriguez A, et al. Late onset central hypoventilation syndrome. *Pediatr Pulmonol.* 1996;21(3):189–191.
4. Katz ES, McGrath S, Marcus CL. Late-onset central hypoventilation with hypothalamic dysfunction: A distinct clinical syndrome. *Pediatr Pulmonol.* 2000;29(1):62–68.
5. Ize-Ludlow D, Gray JA, Sperling MA, Berry-Kravis EM, Milunsky JM, Farooqi IS, et al. Rapid-onset obesity with hypothalamic dysfunction, hypoventilation, and autonomic dysregulation presenting in childhood. *Pediatrics.* 2007;120(1):e179–e188.
6. Bougneres P, Pantalone L, Linglart A, Rothenbuhler A, Le Stunff C. Endocrine manifestations of the rapid-onset obesity with hypoventilation, hypothalamic, autonomic dysregulation, and neural tumor syndrome in childhood. *J Clin Endocrinol Metab.* 2008;93(10):3971–3980.
7. Thaker VV. Genetic and epigenetic causes of obesity. *Adolesc Med State Art Rev.* 2017;28(2):379–405.
8. Barclay SF, Rand CM, Borch LA, Nguyen L, Gray PA, Gibson WT, et al. Rapid-onset obesity with hypothalamic dysfunction, hypoventilation, and autonomic dysregulation (ROHHAD): Exome sequencing of trios, monozygotic twins and tumours. *Orphanet J Rare Dis.* 2015;10:103.
9. Barclay SF, Rand CM, Gray PA, Gibson WT, Wilson RJ, Berry-Kravis EM, et al. Absence of mutations in HCRT, HCRTR1 and HCRTR2 in patients with ROHHAD. *Respir Physiol Neurobiol.* 2016;221:59–63.
10. De Pontual L, Trochet D, Caillat-Zucman S, Abou Shenab OA, Bougneres P, Crow Y, et al. Delineation of late onset hypoventilation associated with hypothalamic dysfunction syndrome. *Pediatr Res.* 2008;64(6):689–694.
11. Ibanez-Mico S, Marcos Oltra AM, de Murcia Lemauviel S, Ruiz Pruneda R, Martinez Ferrandez C, Domingo Jimenez R. Rapid-onset obesity with hypothalamic dysregulation, hypoventilation, and autonomic dysregulation (ROHHAD syndrome): A case report and literature review. *Neurologia.* 2017;32(9):616–622.
12. Jacobson LA, Rane S, McReynolds LJ, Steppan DA, Chen AR, Paz-Priel I. Improved behavior and neuropsychological function in children with ROHHAD after high-dose cyclophosphamide. *Pediatrics.* 2016;138(1):e20151080.
13. Gharial J, Ganesh A, Curtis C, Pauranik A, Chan J, Kurek K, et al. Neuroimaging and pathology findings associated with rapid onset obesity, hypothalamic dysfunction, hypoventilation, and autonomic dysregulation (ROHHAD) syndrome. *J Pediatr Hematol Oncol.* 2021;43(4):e571–e576.
14. Chow C, Fortier MV, Das L, Menon AP, Vasanwala R, Lam JCM, et al. Rapid-onset obesity with hypothalamic dysfunction, hypoventilation, and autonomic dysregulation (ROHHAD) syndrome may have a hypothalamus-periaqueductal gray localization. *Pediatric Neurology.* 2015;52(5):521–525.
15. Hales CM, Carroll MD, Fryar CD, Ogden CL. Prevalence of obesity among adults and youth: United States, 2015–2016. *NCHS. Data Brief.* 2017;288:1–8.
16. Carroll MS, Patwari PP, Kenny AS, Brogadir CD, Stewart TM, Weese-Mayer DE. Rapid-onset obesity with hypothalamic dysfunction, hypoventilation, and autonomic dysregulation (ROHHAD): Response to ventilatory challenges. *Pediatr Pulmonol.* 2015;50(12):1336–1345.
17. Lee CH, Hsu WC, Chang WH, Lin MT, Kang KT. Polysomnographic findings after adenotonsillectomy for obstructive sleep apnoea in obese and non-obese children: A systematic review and meta-analysis. *Clin Otolaryngol.* 2016;41(5):498–510.
18. Scheffler P, Wolter NE, Narang I, Amin R, Holler T, Ishman SL, et al. Surgery for obstructive sleep apnea in obese children: Literature review and meta-analysis. *Otolaryngol Head Neck Surg.* 2019;160(6):985–992.
19. Harvengt J, Gernay C, Mastouri M, Farhat N, Lebrethon MC, Seghaye MC, et al. ROHHAD(NET) syndrome: Systematic review of the clinical timeline and recommendations for diagnosis and prognosis. *J Clin Endocrinol Metab.* 2020;105(7):dgaa247.
20. Barclay SF, Rand CM, Nguyen L, Wilson RJA, Wevrick R, Gibson WT, et al. ROHHAD and Prader-Willi syndrome (PWS): Clinical and genetic comparison. *Orphanet J Rare Dis.* 2018;13(1):124.
21. Masa JF, Pepin JL, Borel JC, Mokhlesi B, Murphy PB, Sanchez-Quiroga MA. Obesity hypoventilation syndrome. *Eur Respir Rev.* 2019;28(151):180097.
22. Mokhlesi B. Obesity hypoventilation syndrome: a state-of-the-art review. *Respir Care.* 2010;55(10):1347–1362; discussion 1363–1345.
23. Khaytin I, Khaytin I, Stewart TM, Zelko FA, et al. Evolution of physiologic and autonomic phenotype in rapid-onset obesity with hypothalamic dysfunction, hypoventilation, and autonomic dysregulation over a decade from age at diagnosis. *J Clin Sleep Med.* 2022;18(3):937–944.

42

Disorders of Arousal

Gerald M. Rosen

CHAPTER HIGHLIGHTS

- Disorders of arousal occur across a clinical spectrum from quietly sitting up in bed to a sudden bloodcurdling scream associated with frantic running and complete disregard for personal safety. These two very different types of arousal share a similar pathophysiology - an abrupt arousal from deep NREM sleep which accounts for the timing of these events , typically 1 1/2 hours after sleep onset.
- There is a strong familial predisposition to disorders of arousal.
- Confusional arousals are most prevalent among toddlers and preschoolers ; and sleepwalking is most prevalent among school age children. In both , the prevalence decreases with age after onset. Children who had confusional arousals as toddlers are more likely to have sleepwalking as they get older.
- Any problem that disrupts sleep quality or duration; or the synchronization of the homeostatic and circadian sleep processes can lead to disorders of arousal, especially in children who are predisposed.
- The treatment for disorders of arousal should include: education of the child and caregivers, safety, sleep extension, regularization of the sleep schedule, and the elimination of possible triggers, before consideration of pharmacotherapy.

Introduction

Parasomnias represent a broad group of sleep disorders that are defined as undesirable phenomena occurring predominantly during sleep, first described by Broughton.[1] These sleep disorders are of great interest to sleep specialists, primary care providers, and patients (and their parents) because this group comprises some of the most common and bizarre sleep problems seen in children. Disorders of arousal are the most common of the parasomnias seen in children. Disorders of arousal are defined similarly by the *Diagnostic and Statistical Manual of Mental Disorders*, 5th edition (DSM-5)[2] and the *International Classification of Sleep Disorders*, 3rd edition (ICSD-3).[3] Both classification schema define subtypes: sleepwalking, confusional arousals, and sleep terrors.

Clinical Description

The clinical features common to most children experiencing any of the disorders of arousal include the timing during the nighttime sleep cycle, misperception of and unresponsiveness to the environment, limited or no associated cognition or dream imagery, automatic behavior, a high arousal threshold, varying levels of autonomic arousal, and partial or complete amnesia on waking after an event or in the morning. The disorders of arousal typically occur during the first third of the night, beginning abruptly at the transition from the first period of the deepest phase of non–rapid eye movement (NREM) sleep (slow-wave sleep [SWS], stage N3) of the night (Figs. 42.1 and 42.2), which accounts for the typical timing 60 to 90 minutes after sleep onset at the end of the first sleep cycle. The duration of each event can vary from less than 1 minute to over 30 minutes. In most cases, the arousal terminates with the child returning to sleep without ever fully awakening. Although only a single event usually occurs on a given night, some children may have multiple events. When there are multiple events, they often will recur at 60- to 90-minute intervals during the night, corresponding to transitions out of SWS at the end of each subsequent ultradian sleep cycle, though the arousals may occur at any time during the night. Successive events on the same night tend to be progressively milder.

The ICSD-3 lists 5 diagnostic criteria for all disorders of arousal, all of which must be met: recurrent episodes of incomplete awakening from sleep; inappropriate or absent responsiveness to efforts of others to intervene or redirect the person during an episode; limited or no associated cognition or dream imagery; partial or complete amnesia for the episode; and the disturbance is not better explained by another sleep disorder, mental disorder, medical condition, medication, or substance use.[3]

Although the clinical manifestations of the disorders of arousal occur along a spectrum, for ease of description and to establish a common nomenclature, the DSM-5 and ICSD-3 have divided the spectrum of arousal disorders into three distinct entities: sleepwalking, confusional arousals, and sleep terrors. However, in the pediatric literature, no clear distinction is generally made between confusional arousals and sleep terrors. Confusional arousals are much more common in children, especially in young children. Sleep terrors occur much less frequently, are more violent, and typically occur in older children and adolescents. At the mildest end of the clinical spectrum,

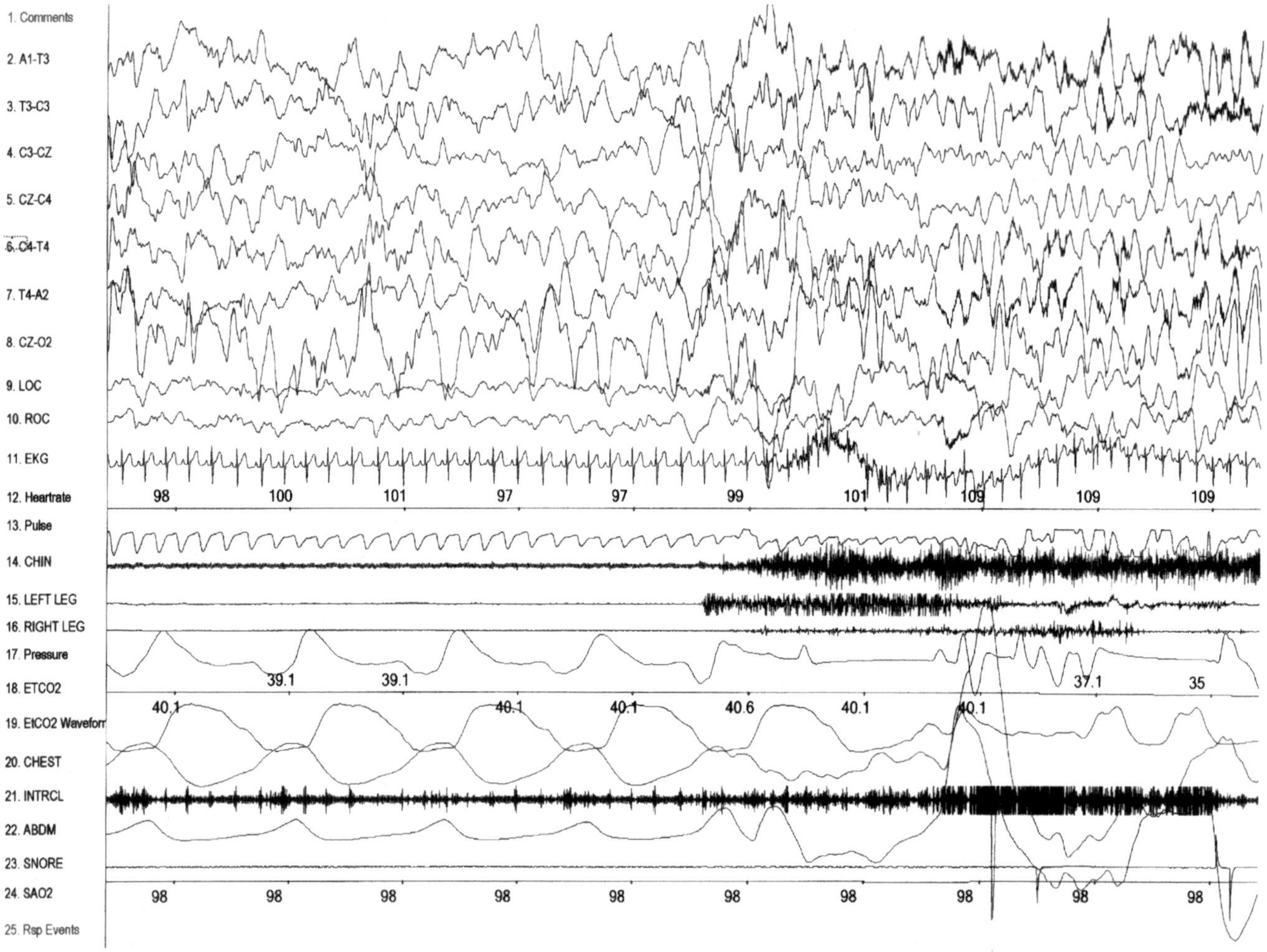

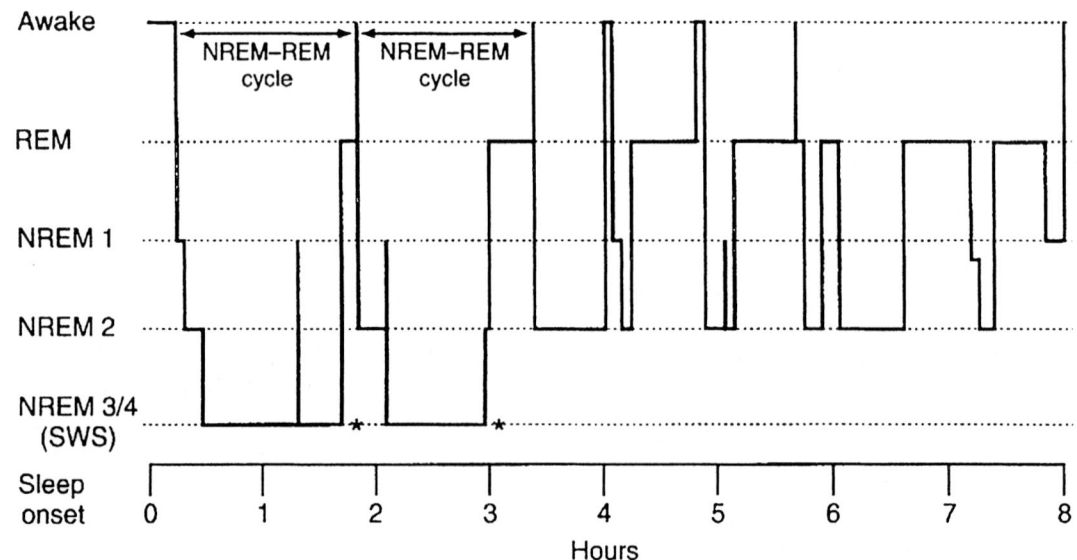

1. Comments	
2. A1-T3	
3. T3-C3	
4. C3-CZ	
5. CZ-C4	
6. C4-T4	
7. T4-A2	
8. CZ-O2	
9. LOC	
10. ROC	
11. EKG	
12. Heartrate	98 100 101 97 97 99 101 109 109 109
13. Pulse	
14. CHIN	
15. LEFT LEG	
16. RIGHT LEG	
17. Pressure	
18. ETCO2	39.1 39.1 37.1 35
19. EtCO2 Waveform	40.1 40.1 40.1 40.6 40.1 40.1
20. CHEST	
21. INTRCL	
22. ABDM	
23. SNORE	
24. SAO2	98 98 98 98 98 98 98 98 98 98
25. Rsp Events	

• **Fig. 42.1** Polysomnogram of a disorder of arousal that occurred precipitously out of slow-wave sleep (NREM 3).

• **Fig. 42.2** Idealized sleep hypnogram showing ultradian rhythm through the night. NREM–REM cycles are approximately 90 minutes; the majority of SWS occurs early in the sleep period, and the majority of REM sleep occurs late in the sleep period. Disorders of arousal generally occur during the transition out of SWS *(asterisks)*. *NREM,* Non-REM; *REM,* rapid eye movement; *SWS,* slow-wave sleep. (Rosen GM, Ferber R, Mahowald MW: Evaluation of parasomnias in children. *Child Adolesc Psychiatr Clin North Am.* 1996;5:601–616.)

a child will simply awaken from sleep, sit up in bed, look around briefly, lie back down, and return to sleep. These arousals are rarely noticed unless the child sleeps with a parent. Thus this type of arousal is usually not characterized as a problem by parents and is seldom brought to the attention of the child's physician. These arousals may be noted as an incidental finding in children who are studied by overnight polysomnography (PSG) for other reasons. At the other end of the spectrum are sleep terrors, which are the most dramatic and least common of the disorders of arousal. They are seen more often in older children and young adults. The events usually begin precipitously with the child bolting upright with a scream. There is generally a high level of autonomic arousal. The eyes are usually open, the heart is racing, and often there is diaphoresis and mydriasis. The facial expression is one of intense fear. A youngster may jump out of bed and run blindly as if to frantically avoid some unseen threat.

Sleepwalking

The presentation of sleepwalking is similar at all ages. There is a partial arousal from sleep that meets the diagnostic criteria for disorders of arousal listed above with some ambulation. The young child may simply awaken and crawl about in the crib before returning to sleep; such events may go unnoticed unless the child sleeps with another family member. An older child may get up and walk to the parents' room, or they may simply be found asleep at a location different from where they went to bed, with no recollection of having left their bed. Some inappropriate behavior, such as urinating in the closet or next to the toilet, is common. A sleepwalking child may be led back to bed easily, with little evidence of a complete awakening and no recall of the event the next day. Sleepwalking can be triggered in most children by simply standing them up within the first few hours of sleep onset. Because the child is unaware of their environment during a sleepwalking episode, they may be injured or put themselves into dangerous situations during a quiet sleepwalking episode.

Sleepwalking is common in children, as documented in two large, population-based studies by Klackenberg[4] in Sweden and by Laberge and Petit[5–7] in Québec. Klackenberg studied a group of 212 randomly selected children in Stockholm, longitudinally from ages 6 to 16 years. The prevalence of quiet sleepwalking (occurring at least once during the 10-year data collection period in this group) was 40%. The yearly incidence varied from 6% to 17%, although only 3% had more than one episode per month. In Klackenberg's study, the sleepwalking persisted for 5 years in 33% of children and for over 10 years in 12%.

The largest prospective longitudinal study of sleepwalking and confusional arousals/sleep terrors was conducted by Laberge[5] and Petit et al.[6,7] They studied 2675 randomly

selected children in Québec who were part of the Québec Longitudinal Study of Child Development conducted by the Québec Institute of Statistics. The parents completed a yearly sleep questionnaire regarding the presence of parasomnias in their children from 1.5 to 13 years of age. The overall prevalence of sleepwalking was 29.1%. The yearly prevalence of sleepwalking, shown in Table 42.1, varied from 2.6% to 13.4%. Table 42.2 describes the ages of onset and offset of sleepwalking and confusional arousals/night terrors. In the majority of these children, the sleepwalking began and ended between the ages of 3 and 13 years. There was no sex difference in sleepwalking prevalence. In the studies of Laberge, Petit, and Klackenberg, sleepwalking was frequently seen in those children who had confusional arousals/sleep terrors at a younger age.

Confusional Arousals/Sleep Terrors

Confusional arousal/sleep terrors seem bizarre and can be frightening for parents to see. The arousal usually starts with some movements and moaning, progressing to crying, often in association with intense thrashing about in the bed or crib. An infant may be described simply as crying inconsolably. These arousals are common in infants and toddlers. The child is typically described as appearing confused, with the eyes open or closed. These events can last anywhere from a few minutes to over 1 hour, with 5 to 15 minutes being typical. Even if the child calls for the parents, the child often does not recognize them. Even vigorous attempts to wake the child are often unsuccessful. Holding and cuddling

TABLE 42.1	Prevalence of Parasomnias at Various Ages in the Same Children	
Age	Sleepwalking (%)	CA&NT (%)
2.5	3.3	19.9
3.5	2.5	20.8
4.0	4.1	17.4
5.0	4.8	11.8
6.0	7.8	11.3
11	7.0	3.8
12	6.8	2.3
13	3.3	1.2
Overall	13.8	39.8

CA&NT, Confusional arousals and night terrors.

Modified with permission from Laberge L, Tremblay RE, Vitaro F, Montplaisir J: Development of parasomnias from childhood to early adolescence. Pediatrics 2000;106:67–74; Petit D, Touchette E, Tremblay R, Boivin M, Montplaisir J: Dysomnias and parasomnias in early childhood. *Pediatrics.* 2007;119:e1016–1025.

TABLE 42.2	Age of Onset and Disappearance of Parasomnias at Various Ages in the Same Children	
Age	Sleepwalking (%)	CA&NT (%)
2.5		
Onset	22.7	50.1
3.5		
Onset	13.3	25.8
Disappearance	12.7	15
4.0		
Onset	15.3	12.5
Disappearance	5.3	19
5.0		
Onset	20.7	6.3
Disappearance	13.3	20.2
6.0		
Onset	28.0	5.3
Disappearance	14.7	17.4
11		
Onset	17.2	9.4
Disappearance	18.1	14.8
12		
Onset	12.9	4.0
Disappearance	34.5	11.4
13		
Onset	3.5	2.0
Persisting	24.1	6.7

CA&NT, Confusional arousals and night terrors.
Modified with permission from Laberge L, Tremblay RE, Vitaro F, Montplasir J. Development of parasomnias from childhood to early adolescence. *Pediatrics*. 2000;106:67–74; Petit D, Touchette E, Tremblay R, Boivin M, Montplaisir J. Dyssomnias and parasomnias in early childhood. *Pediatrics*. 2007;119:e1016–1025.

usually do not provide reassurance; instead, the child often resists, twists, and pushes away and may become more agitated. It is the parents' inability to comfort their child, who appears to be in great distress, that is often of the greatest concern to them.

In the studies of Laberge[5] and Petit,[6,7] there was no distinction between confusional arousals, sleep terrors, and night terrors. However, from the age distribution and the description of the events, the current nomenclature would characterize these as confusional arousals. In the Laberge and Petit studies, the overall prevalence of confusional arousals between the ages of 1.5 and 13 years was 56.2% (see Table 42.1). The yearly incidence was 34.4% at age 1.5

years, 11.6% at age 6 years, 11.4% at 11 years of age, and 5.3% at 13 years of age. In 85% of the children the confusional arousals first appeared between the ages of 3 and 10 years, and in the majority of these children they disappeared before the age of 10 years (see Table 42.2). The confusional arousals persisted beyond 13 years of age in 6.7% of the children.

In the studies of Laberge, Petit, and Klackenberg, sleepwalking and confusional arousals were often seen in the same child at different ages. Thirty-six percent of the children with sleepwalking in the study of Laberge had confusional arousals as preschoolers, and all of the children with confusional arousals in Klackenberg's study had at least one episode of sleepwalking when they were older.

Pathophysiology of Disorders of Arousal

Disorders of arousal are best understood as a dissociated state during which elements of wakefulness and NREM sleep occur simultaneously, resulting in behavior that is neither fully awake nor fully asleep. This concept, first put forward by Mahowald,[8,9] is consistent with the current understanding of sleep neurophysiology. During the disorders of arousal, some facets of wakefulness appear during the transition out of SWS. This usually occurs at the end of the first sleep cycle. As a consequence, the transition out of SWS, which is usually behaviorally inapparent, can be dramatic. The child appears caught between deep NREM sleep and wakefulness. The child's behavior at this time has elements that we associate with wakefulness (walking, talking, crying, running complex motor behaviors) and sleeping (misperception of and unresponsiveness to the environment, high arousal threshold, amnesia, automatic behavior) occurring simultaneously. The EEG during these arousals from sleep is typically characterized by a mixture of waking and sleeping rhythms with the simultaneous occurrence of alpha, theta, and delta frequencies, and suggests that different areas of the brain are in different states simultaneously. This dissociated state is inherently unstable, and eventually one state is fully declared. In most cases, the child appears to simply return to quiet sleep. Alternatively, the child may awaken totally but will have no recall of the arousal and will usually rapidly return to sleep.

The causes of the disorders of arousal are multifactorial. Genetic predisposition, homeostatic drive, sleep–wake cycling and synchronization, and behavioral and emotional states all seem to play some role in the clinical appearance of the disorders of arousal. Of these factors, genetic predisposition is probably the most important, though the mechanism is unknown. Sleep–wake cycling and synchronization are affected by age, homeostatic factors, circadian factors, hormones, and drugs. Affective disorders, anxiety, and environmental stress have all been identified as important factors in the appearance of the disorders of arousal in clinical studies,[10,11] although the mechanisms by which these factors lead to the arousal is not known. Several lines of evidence suggest that the fundamental abnormality that underpins the disorders of arousal is the instability of SWS. This conclusion is supported by the clinical observation and experimental evidence that in individuals predisposed to the disorders of arousal, an event is much more likely to occur after a night of sleep deprivation[12] or after sleep fragmentation from sleep apnea[13–15] or periodic movements[16] of sleep that increases the homeostatic drive and would be expected to make an unstable homeostatic system more unstable.

Genetics of Disorders of Arousal

A familial predisposition toward the disorders of arousal has been recognized since these disorders were first described. The genetics of the disorders of arousal has been explored by Hublin et al.[17,18] and Nguyen et al.[19] (in population-based twin studies) and also by Lecendreux et al.[20] In Hublin's retrospective study of adults the phenotypic variance of sleepwalking was attributable to genetic factors at 65%, which he believed was the result of many genes, each with minor effects. In Nguyen's study, environmental information was gathered in an attempt to understand the relative contribution of genetic, shared environmental, and non-shared environmental factors leading to confusional arousals in children. They concluded that the best explanation was a two-component model with 44% of the variance explained by genetic factors and 56% of the variance explained by non-shared environmental factors. These results are consistent with the results of Lecendreux, who looked at human leukocyte antigens and sleepwalking. The familial predisposition to disorders of arousal may be at least in part secondary to the familial aggregation of restless legs syndrome (RLS), periodic limb movements (PLMs),[16] or sleep-disordered breathing (SDB), which are recognized as triggers for disorders of arousal.[13–15] A positive family history of a first-degree relative with a disorder of arousal is present in 60% of the children with a disorder of arousal compared with 30% in children without disorders of arousal. In the Québec Longitudinal Study,[7] the prevalence of sleepwalking in children correlated with the prevalence of sleepwalking in their parents. When neither parent experienced sleepwalking, 22% of the children walked in their sleep; when one parent experienced sleepwalking, 45% of the children walked in their sleep; when both parents experienced sleepwalking, 60% of the children walked in their sleep.

Sleep Homeostasis and Disorders of Arousal

There is good theoretical support and some experimental evidence that the familial predisposition toward the disorders of arousal is mediated by the genetic control of the sleep homeostatic process.[21] This process has been shown to be under strong genetic control in animal studies.[22] Studies in mice have demonstrated that sleep loss leads to an increase in homeostatic drive, with a change in slow-wave sleep activity

(SWA) as measured by delta power, in a dose–response fashion that varies with the duration of prior wakefulness and is different in different genotypes. A quantitative trait–loci analysis revealed that this trait is the product of multiple genes. Human electroencephalographic (EEG) studies have also shown that SWS and EEG SWA are markers for measuring homeostatic drive.[23–25] Increases in SWS and SWA occur after sleep deprivation and decline after sleep. The synchronization of the homeostatic and circadian processes optimizes the quality of sleep and wakefulness. This interaction is described in a comprehensive article by Dijk and Lockley.[24] Adequate sleep duration occurs only when the circadian and homeostatic systems are fully synchronized. The clinical implication of this observation is that a child with an irregular and/or chaotic sleep–wake schedule will simply not be able to have optimum synchronization of the homeostatic and circadian systems; this inevitably leads to sleep disruption and sleep deprivation, which may lead to a clinical event in a child who may be predisposed to the disorders of arousal.

Polysomnography in Disorders of Arousal

Polysomnographic studies have shown that individuals with the disorders of arousal, when compared with normal control subjects, have no consistent differences in sleep efficiency or sleep stage distribution.[26] However, there are subtle differences in the cyclic alternating patterns and arousal rates,[27] arousals from SWS,[27] and SWS activity delta counts between the sleep of patients with the disorders of arousal and that of control subjects.[26] These differences are the most prominent during the first sleep cycle, which is when the disorders of arousal usually occur. There were increased numbers of brief EEG arousals from SWS, decreases in SWS activity delta counts at the end of the first ultradian cycle, and increases in the cyclic alternating pattern cycles compared with control subjects. The subjects for these research studies were carefully screened for the presence of SDB, sleep deprivation, and RLS.

SDB[13–15] and RLS with PLMs[16] have both been identified as triggers for disorders of arousal. In children with SDB, often quite mild, the disorders of arousal disappeared after adenotonsillectomy.[13,14] In the children with restless legs/periodic movements of sleep,[16] who had iron deficiency diagnosed by serum ferritin level, 40% resolved after correction of the iron deficiency. However, the improvement came after 3–6 months of treatment in 58%, 25% after 6–12 months, and 12% after 1–2 years of treatment. These clinical responses suggests that these clinical causes of sleep disruption can unmask a disorder of arousal.

Clinical Evaluation of Children With Disorders of Arousal

The children described in this chapter will generally present with the complaint of unusual nocturnal awakenings. It is

• BOX 42.1   Sleep History

- Circadian
  - Sleep log for 2 weeks (time in bed, sleep onset, awakening time) (weekdays/weekends)
  - Vacation sleep schedule
  - 24-hour daily schedule of activities (school, work, meals, play)
  - Amount of light in room
  - Seasonal variations in sleep
  - Preferred sleep time and duration (present and at a younger age)
- Sleep Environment
  - Describe bedroom (What is in it? Who is there? How much natural light is there? Is there a television or radio?)
- Sleep Onset
  - How does the child fall asleep?
  - Who is present at sleep onset and what do they do?
  - Are there curtain calls, fears, hypnagogic hallucinations, sleep-onset paralysis, restless legs, head banging, body rocking?
- Arousals
  - Time of night, frequency
  - Triggers, association with injury
  - Description of the way in which the arousal terminates
  - Level of agitation/manner in which the ambulation child returns to sleep
  - Association with eating and drinking, recall the next day
  - Level of consciousness, age of onset
  - Duration
- Other Sleep Behavior
  - Seizures, enuresis, diaphoresis, restlessness, snoring, cough, choking, apnea, periodic movements of sleep, vomiting, nightmares, bruxism
- Waking Behavior
  - Hypnopompic hallucinations, paralysis, headaches

- Daytime Sleep
  - Naps, cataplexy, excessive daytime sleepiness, settings where sleep occurs
- Actigraphy can provide an objective measure of the sleep schedule, sleep duration, and fragmentation
- Medical
  - Neurologic: Migraine headaches, attention-deficit disorder, seizures, tics, mental retardation, narcolepsy, neuromuscular disease
  - Psychiatric: Depression, anxiety, dissociative disorders, conduct disorder, panic disorder, physical/sexual abuse, posttraumatic stress disorder, attention-deficit/hyperactivity disorder, substance use
  - Ear, Nose, Throat: Ear infections, ear effusions, nasal airway obstruction, sinusitis, streptococci infections
  - Cardiorespiratory: Asthma, cough, heart disease, pneumonia
  - Gastrointestinal: Vomiting, diarrhea, constipation, swallowing problems
  - Growth: Failure to thrive
  - Allergies: Milk, seasonal, asthma, eczema
  - Drug: Legal/illegal, prescription
  - School/behavior: School/developmental problems, behavioral problems
  - Acute medical illness
- Family History
  - Sleep apnea/snoring
  - Arousals (sleepwalking, confusional arousals, night terrors, restless legs/periodic movements)
  - Psychiatric condition (depression, anxiety)
  - Social issues (stress at home, divorce, family violence, drug/ethyl alcohol use)
  - Narcolepsy, hypersomnolence
  - Restless legs syndrome
  - Delayed/advanced sleep phase

---

important to recognize that there are many causes of unusual nocturnal awakenings in children. The most important tool for evaluating children with unusual nocturnal awakenings is a complete sleep and medical history. The sleep history will usually allow the clinician to distinguish between the different causes of unusual nocturnal arousals and to formulate an appropriate evaluation and treatment plan. The facets of the sleep history that are the most important in the evaluation of the disorders of arousal are listed in Box 42.1. Any problem that causes sleep disruption that results in awakenings or affects sleep duration or synchronization can lead to the appearance of the disorders of arousal in a child. It is important to keep in mind that the many causes of sleep disruption in a child are not mutually exclusive, and their effects are cumulative; thus all of the sources of sleep disruption need to be identified and treated to successfully manage this problem.

There are a number of distinguishing clinical characteristics in the histories of children with the disorders of arousal. The salient features are listed and discussed below.

- *Timing:* The first event generally (but not always) occurs about 60–90 minutes after sleep onset. If a second event occurs during the night, it typically occurs 90 minutes after the first, at the time of the transition out of SWS. Arousals occurring within 30 minutes of sleep onset, or

upon awakening from sleep in the morning, are more likely to represent unusual sleep-related seizures.

- *Description of the event:* The onset can be gradual, with sleepwalking and confusional arousals, or sudden, with sleep terrors. The behavior during an event is often bizarre and may be complex but is not stereotypical. The child is not normally responsive to the environment, although they may be partially responsive. A child will not typically recognize parents and often cannot be comforted by them. The events generally terminate with a return to sleep and without a complete awakening.
- *Frequency:* The frequency of occurrence is highly variable, from several times a night to once in a lifetime; multiple episodes in a single night may occur but are uncommon.
- *Level of consciousness:* The child is generally not arousable.
- *Memory of event:* Most children will have no recall the day after the event.
- *Daytime sleepiness:* Most children have no evidence of daytime sleepiness the next day.
- *Family history:* The family history is often positive in parents and siblings for any of the disorders of arousal.

Box 42.2 lists those conditions that mimic the disorders of arousal and those that may trigger them. The condition to recognize that may mimic the disorders of arousal are

• BOX 42-2 Conditions That Mimic or Trigger Disorders of Arousal

Neurologic
   *Seizures
   *Cluster headaches
Medical
   †Sleep-disordered breathing (even mild)
   †Gastroesophageal reflux
Behavioral/Psychiatric
   *Conditioned arousals
   *Posttraumatic stress disorder
   *Nocturnal dissociative state
   *Nocturnal panic
Sleep
   *Nightmares
   *Rhythmic movements of sleep
   *Rapid eye movement sleep behavior disorders
   †Periodic movements of sleep
   †Sleep deprivation
   †Irregular sleep–wake schedule
   *Conditions that mimic disorders of arousal.
   †Conditions that trigger disorders of arousal.

TABLE 42.3 Comparison of Disorders of Arousal and Seizures

Clinical Characteristics	Disorder of Arousal	Seizures
Age of onset (typical)	2–10 years	Any age
Timing of event	60–90 minutes after sleep onset	Any time of night, often multiple times during night, often at sleep onset or upon awakening
Sleep stage	Arises at end of stage N3	Arises out of stage N1, N2
Duration	2–60 minutes	1–2 minutes
Description of event	Variable, quiet-agitated	Stereotypical, repetitive
Family history	Positive	Positive for NFLE
EEG/PSG	Sudden arousal from stage N3, mixed alpha, theta, delta, OSA/PLMs	Normal, spikes may be present, focal, or generalized
Triggering events	OSA, PLMs, fever, sleep deprivation, irregular sleep	None
Amnesia	Yes	Yes
Daytime behavior	Normal, no EDS	Often EDS

EDS, Excessive daytime sleepiness; *EEG*, electroencephalography; *NFLE*, nocturnal frontal lobe epilepsy; *OSA*, obstructive sleep apnea; *PLM*, periodic limb movement; *PSG*, polysomnography.

sleep-related seizures, particularly nocturnal frontal lobe seizures.[28,29] Other, less common mimics are cluster headaches; psychiatric disorders such as nocturnal panic attacks, posttraumatic stress disorder, and nocturnal dissociative disorder; nightmares; REM sleep behavior disorder; and rhythmic movements of sleep. The most common conditions that may trigger disorders of arousal in a child are SDB, periodic movements of sleep, sleep deprivation, and an irregular sleep–wake schedule. The last two of these are the most common and most easily corrected triggers for the disorders of arousal. Other possible triggers are gastroesophageal reflux and behavioral or psychiatric disorders.

The distinction between disorders of arousal and sleep-related seizures is often difficult to make. The most consistent clinical difference between seizures and disorders of arousal are that seizures are usually stereotypical events, which can occur at any time throughout the night. Seizures occur exclusively during sleep 30% of the time and may not always have abnormal EEG correlates recorded from routine surface electrodes, especially in children with nocturnal frontal lobe epilepsy.[28,29] Evaluation in specialized centers is often necessary to establish the correct diagnosis and to develop an appropriate treatment. See Table 42.3 for comparison between disorders of arousal and seizures.

Polysomnography

The American Academy of Sleep Medicine has published a review of the non-respiratory indications for PSG in children.[29] PSG using an expanded EEG montage is indicated in children to confirm the diagnosis of an atypical or potentially injurious parasomnias, to differentiate a parasomnia from sleep-related epilepsy, or to identify when SDB or PLMD is believed to be contributing to frequent parasomnias or control of seizures. PSG was not indicated for the evaluation of children with typical parasomnias or confirmed sleep-related epilepsy.[29] The routine use of PSG in the evaluation of the disorders of arousal is limited because the sleep macroarchitecture in children with these disorders is generally normal. The primary role of PSG in the evaluation of children with suspected disorders of arousal is to rule out other sleep disorders and nocturnal seizures, which may either trigger or mimic the disorders of arousal.

If nocturnal seizures are suspected, based on the history of the stereotypical nature or the timing of the arousals throughout the sleep period or if there is an increased likelihood of seizures because of a concomitant neurologic problem, further diagnostic studies should be obtained. In most clinical settings, sleep-related seizures can be best evaluated with sleep-deprived EEG or an overnight study in an EEG telemetry unit. These children should be evaluated in a sleep lab only if the lab staff are experienced in the diagnosis and treatment of sleep-related seizures.

Treatment of Children With Disorders of Arousal

The most appropriate treatment for the child with a disorder of arousal will depend on the diagnosis. Before considering a treatment strategy, one must have completed a comprehensive medical, neurologic, and sleep evaluation such as the one described in this chapter. If the disorders of arousal are thought to be the most likely cause of the awakenings, the treatment may include some or all of the following recommendations, but one should start with the first five items listed, which represent essential components in any effective treatment plan for children with the disorders of arousal.

- *Education* of the parents and their children about the benign, self-limiting nature of the disorders of arousal. Discuss the pathophysiology of these disorders in a manner that is comprehendible to both the child and parents.
- *Child safety* is of paramount concern in managing children with the disorders of arousal. During an event, children can put themselves in danger such as by walking out of the house or by running into a glass door. In most cases, these concerns can be addressed using a simple, common-sense approach. The child should not sleep on the upper level of a bunk bed, obstructions should be removed from the room, double-cylinder locks may need to be installed on the doors of the house, or a security system (alerting the parents that a door or window has been opened) may need to be installed.
- *Demystification* of the disorders of arousal. The parents often misunderstand the problem and fear that the intensity of the arousal reflects severe psychological distress.
- *Sleep extension and schedule regularization* should always be considered. Sleep deprivation and an irregular sleep–wake schedule are very common problems for children and are often causally related to the appearance of these disorders.
- *Elimination of caffeine* if its use is identified.
- *Institution of a bedtime routine that is pleasant for both the parent and the child*, ideally one ending within 15 minutes of the transition to sleep. If there is conflict at bedtime, if sleep onset latency is prolonged, or if the child is fearful or requires close contact with a parent, these issues may need to be addressed.
- *Evaluation of iron nurriture* with a serum ferritin and C-reactive protein (CRP) should be a routine part of an evaluation of children with disorders of arousal. CRP is checked as a measure of inflammation, which can falsely elevate the serum ferritin level. If ferritin is < 50 ng/mL, treatment with iron supplementation, usually $FeSo_4$ 2–3 mg/kg + vitamin C. Correction of iron deficiency often can take at least 3–6 months, so other interventions are often necessary in addition to correcting iron deficiency.

- *Medication* may be a good short-term strategy in a child with frequent, disruptive, or potentially dangerous arousals while other nonpharmacologic modalities are initiated. If restless legs and/or PLMs are believed to be triggers for the disorders of arousal, consideration should be given as to whether pharmacologic treatment for these sleep disorders is warranted. Medication has been described as an effective treatment for the disorders of arousal in several case reports series, although it has not been the subject of well-controlled studies, and no medications are approved by the U.S. Food and Drug Administration for the treatment of disorders of arousal. Clonazepam[30,31] has been the most widely used off-label medication for the treatment of disorders of arousal. Clinicians should be cautious when beginning pharmacotherapy for these disorders in children because in most cases, the events are benign and self-limiting and have no direct, adverse impact on the child.[32] If medication is used, it should be given 1–1.5 hours before the anticipated sleep onset to ensure that there are adequate drug levels in the brain at the beginning of the night, when these disorders are most likely to occur. The beginning dose of clonazepam is generally 0.125 mg, gradually increasing until the arousals are eliminated or side effects are experienced. Once the arousals are eliminated, the medication should be continued for 4–6 weeks, during which time the family can work on sleep extension and regularization of the schedule. This allows everyone in the family to recover from the effects of the previous sleep disruption. Thereafter, the medication can be gradually tapered to ascertain if the arousals recur. If there is a recurrence of the arousals, there needs to be a discussion of the risks and benefits of longer-term use of medication. If medications are used long-term, an attempt at a medication taper and a reassessment of possible triggers and mimics should be done every 3–6 months.
- *In adolescents*, one should discuss the potential risks posed by the disorders of arousal when the teen moves out of the home, and the impact of alcohol use, sleep restriction, and an irregular sleep schedule.
- *Scheduled* awakening is a behavioral treatment for confusional arousals that has been described anecdotally in the literature first by Lask.[33] Although it is not clear why this intervention is helpful, several case reports have described its efficacy.[34,35] The recommended treatment is simple enough: the child is awakened 15 to 30 minutes before the usual time of the arousal and needs to open their eyes

and at least mumble a response before being allowed to return to sleep. The parents continue this intervention nightly for 1 month. In some cases this simple intervention has been effective. However, it should be noted that in some cases these scheduled awakenings actually trigger an arousal or cause one that usually occurs early in the night to occur later.

- *Relaxation and/or mental imagery and biofeedback* are behavioral approaches that have been described in case reports as being useful treatments for the disorders of arousal in school-aged children.[33,36–38]
- *Psychotherapy and counseling* are important interventions for any child who has evidence of significant psychological distress. However, a disorder of arousal is not a symptom of a psychologic problem.

> **CLINICAL PEARLS**
>
> - The timing of all of the disorders of arousal is most often 1–1.5 hours after sleep onset. This can be one of the most useful clinical signs for differentiating disorders of arousal from other causes of sudden arousals from sleep.
> - Disorders of arousal rarely have a stereotypical character.
> - SDB and/or periodic movements of sleep are treatable triggers for disorders of arousal.
> - Regularization and extension of nocturnal sleep are important interventions.
> - During any of the disorders of arousal, children can put themselves in harm's way, making a discussion of safety with the children (especially adolescents) and their parents a necessary part of the treatment plan.

Summary

To the casual observer, disorders of arousal represent a paradox during which an individual appears to engage in waking behavior while still asleep. With the understanding that sleep and wakefulness are not always mutually exclusive states of being, the paradox disappears. The concept of state dissociation provides an explanation for these events that is founded in the current understanding of the neurophysiology of sleep. The disorders of arousal are common problems, especially in young children, and can usually be fully evaluated and treated by a knowledgeable sleep clinician without the use of high technology.

References

1. Broughton RJ. Sleep disorders: disorders of arousal? *Science.* 1968;159:1070–1078.
2. American Psychiatric Association. *Diagnostic and Statistical Manual of Mental Disorders.* 5th ed. APA; 2013.
3. American Academy of Sleep Medicine. *International Classification of Sleep Disorders. Diagnostic and Coding Manual.* 3rd ed. American Academy of Sleep Medicine; 2014.
4. Klackenberg G. Somnambulism in childhood—prevalence, course and behavioral correlates: A prospective longitudinal study (6–16 years). *Acta Paediatr Scand.* 1982;71:495–499.
5. Laberge L, Tremblay RE, Vitaro F, et al. Development of parasomnias from childhood to early adolescence. *Pediatrics.* 2000;106:67–74.
6. Petit D, Touchette E, Tremblay R, et al. Dyssomnias and parasomnias in early childhood. *Pediatrics.* 2007;119:e1016–e1025.
7. Petit D, Pennestri H, Paquet J, et al. Childhood sleepwalking and sleep terrors a longitudinal study of prevalence and familial aggregation. *JAMA Pediatr.* 2015;169(7):653-8.
8. Mahowald MW, Schenck CH. Dissociated states of wakefulness and sleep. *Neurology.* 1992;42:44–52.
9. Mahowald M, Cramer Borneman C, Schenck C. State dissociation, human behavior, and consciousness. *Curr Topics Med Chem.* 2011;11:2392–2402.
10. Simonds JF, Parago H. Sleep behavior and disorders in children and adolescents evaluated at psychiatry clinics. *Dev Behav Pediatr.* 1984;6:6–10.
11. Dahl RE, Puig-Antich J. Sleep disturbance in children and adolescent psychiatric disorders. *Pediatrician.* 1990;167:32–37.
12. Joncas S, Zadra A, Paquet J, et al. The value of sleep deprivation as a diagnostic tool in adult sleepwalkers. *Neurology.* 2002;58:936–940.
13. Guilleminault C, Palombini L, Pelayo R, et al. Sleepwalking and sleep terrors in prepubertal children: What triggers them? *Pediatrics.* 2003;111:e17–e25.
14. Guilleminault C, Lee J, Chan A, et al. Non-REM sleep instability in recurrent sleepwalking in pre-pubertal children. *Sleep Med.* 2005;6:515–521.
15. Cao M, Guilleminault C. Families with sleepwalking. *Sleep Med.* 2010;11:726–734.
16. Gurbani N, Dye T. Dougherty. Improvement of parasomnias after treatment of restless leg syndrome/periodic limb movement disorder in children. *J Clin Sleep Med.* 2019;15(5):743–748.
17. Hublin C, Kaprio J, Partinen M, et al. Prevalence and genetics of sleepwalking: a population-based twin study. *Neurology.* 1997;48:177–181.
18. Hublin C, Kaprio J, Partinen M, et al. Parasomnias: co-occurrence and genetics. *Psychiatr Gen.* 2001;11:65–70.
19. Nguyen B, Perusse D, Paquet J, et al. Sleep terrors in children: a prospective study of twins. *Pediatrics.* 2008;122:e1164–e1167.
20. Lecendreux M, Bassetti C, Dauvilliers Y, et al. HLA and genetic susceptibility to sleepwalking. *Mol Psychiatry.* 2003;8:114–117.
21. Cao M, Guilleminault C. Families with sleepwalking. *Sleep Med.* 2010;11:726–734.
22. Franken P, Chollet D, Tafti M. The homeostatic regulation of sleep need is under genetic control. *J Neurosci.* 2001;21:2610–2621.
23. Dijk DJ, Czeisler CA. Contribution of the circadian pacemaker and the sleep homeostat to sleep propensity, sleep structure, electroencephalographic slow waves, and sleep spindle activity in humans. *J Neurosci.* 1995;15:3526–3538.

24. Dijk DJ, Lockley SW. Functional genomics of sleep and circadian rhythm: Integration of human sleep-wake regulation and circadian rhythmicity (invited lecture). *J Appl Physiol*. 2002;92:852–862.

25. Gaudreau H, Joncas S, Zadra A, et al. Dynamics of slow-wave activity during the NREM sleep of sleepwalkers and control subjects. *Sleep*. 2000;23:755–760.

26. Guilleminault C, Poyares D, Aftab FA, et al. Sleep and wakefulness in somnambulism: a spectral analysis study. *J Psychosom Res*. 2001;51:411–416.

27. Zuconi M, Oldani A. Arousal fluctuation in non-rapid eye movement parasomnias: the role of cyclic alternating pattern as a measure of sleep instability. *J Clin Neurophysiol*. 1995;12:147–154.

28. Smirne S, Ferini-Strambi L. Clinical applications of cyclic alternating pattern. In: Comi G, Lucking C, Kimura J, eds. *Clinical Neurophysiology: From Receptors to Perception*. Elsevier Science; 1999:109–112.

29. Tinuper P, Provini F, Bisulli F, et al. Movement disorders in sleep: guidelines for differentiating epileptic from non-epileptic motor phenomena arising from sleep. *Sleep Med Rev*. 2007;11:255–267.

30. Mallow BA. Paroxysmal events in sleep. *J Clin Neurophysiol*. 2002;19:522–534.

31. Kotagal S, Nichols C, Grigg-Danberger M, et al. Non-respiratory indications for polysomnography and related procedures in children: an evidenced-based review. *Sleep*. 2012;35:1451–1466.

32. Aurora R, Lamm C, Zak R, et al. Practice parameters for the non-respiratory indications for polysomnography and multiple sleep latency testing for children. *Sleep*. 2012;35:1467–1473.

33. Lask B. Novel and non-toxic treatment for night terrors. *BMJ*. 1988;297:592.

34. Mahowald M, Schenck C. NREM parasomnias. *Neurol Clin N Am*. 1996;14:675–696.

35. Dahl R. The pharmacologic treatment of sleep disorders. *Psych Clin North Am*. 1992;15:161–178.

36. Tobin J. Treatment of somnambulism with anticipatory awakening. *J Pediatr*. 1993;122:426–467.

37. Frank C, Spirito A. The use of scheduled awakenings to eliminate childhood sleepwalking. *J Pediatr Psychol*. 1997;22:345–353.

38. Kohen DP, Mahowald MW, Rosen GM. Sleep-terror disorder in children: the role of self-hypnosis in management. *Am J Clin Hypnosis*. 1991;4:233–244.

43

REM Sleep Parasomnia in Children

Allison Hayes Clarke, Thuan Dang, and Irina Trosman

CHAPTER HIGHLIGHTS

- Parasomnia may arise from non–rapid eye movement (NREM) and REM sleep.
- The most common REM parasomnia is nightmares.
- Nightmares and bad dreams are frequently observed in early childhood.
- Idiopathic nightmares frequency decreases with age.
- Post-trauma nightmares and frequent primary nightmares are frequently associated with other sleep problems such as insomnia, difficulties falling and staying asleep, and frequent awakenings.
- Treatment of nightmares usually focuses on anxiety-reducing techniques, psychologic counseling, cognitive-behavioral therapy (CBT) including image rehearsal therapy (IRT), and/or reduction in exposure to television, media, and video games.
- Prazosin and clonidine can be used for treatment of nightmares; however, little data is available on efficacy of this therapy in the pediatric population.
- REM behavior disorder (RBD) is rare in the pediatric population, and etiology does not suggest alpha synucleinopathies more commonly found in adult populations.
- RBD evaluation should include a sleep study and a consultation with pediatric neurologist and brain magnetic resonance imaging (MRI) should be considered to exclude structural brainstem lesions.

Introduction

Parasomnias are abnormal and undesirable behaviors that occur during sleep. The word parasomnia is derived from the Greek prefix "para" (meaning "alongside of") and the Latin noun "somnus" (meaning "sleep"). Parasomnias may arise from non–rapid eye movement (NREM) and REM sleep. Parasomnias are characterized by abnormal experiences, dreams, movements, and behavior during sleep. They may occur in the middle of the sleep during REM or NREM. REM sleep parasomnia is an umbrella term for nightmare disorders, REM sleep without atonia (RSWA), and REM behavior disorder (RBD). Most of the NREM parasomnias arise out of N3 NREM sleep.[1] REM parasomnias occur in REM sleep, which is characterized by

rapid eye movements, atonia of skeletal muscles, and vivid dream mentation. Muscle atonia is presumably generated by brainstem centers, the pedunculopontine nucleus, and locus coeruleus. Muscle atonia serves as a protective mechanism preventing dream enactment during REM sleep. REM parasomnias include two main group of disorders: nightmare disorder and RBD.

Nightmare disorder is classified by the International Classification of Sleep Disorders, 3rd edition (ICSD-3), as a parasomnia usually associated with REM sleep.[2] The diagnostic criteria are as follows: "recurrent episodes of awakenings from sleep with recall of intensely disturbing dream mentation, usually involving fear or anxiety, but also anger, sadness, disgust, and other dysphoric dysfunction.[2] There is a full alertness upon awakening, with little confusion or disorientation; recall of sleep mentation is immediate and clear. At least one of the following associated features is present: delayed return to sleep after the episodes and/or occurrence of episodes in the latter half of the habitual sleep period." In other words, nightmares are frightening dreams that awaken the dreamer from REM sleep with the individual typically being able to recall the dream content. Physiologic reactions to nightmares, albeit rare, can be quite disturbing and may include anticipatory anxiety around bedtime, panic attack symptoms on waking from a nightmare (e.g., racing heart, sweating, choking), and symptoms of sleep deprivation during daytime hours (e.g., confusion, memory loss, fatigue, excessive sleepiness, and emotional lability).[3] Nightmares are common in children with cross-sectional data demonstrating the highest prevalence rates between the ages of 5 and 10 years.[4–6] One study found a 75% prevalence of intermittent nightmares in school-aged children. Other studies found nightmares occur in about 10–20% of the general pediatric population, with higher prevalence among younger children than adolescents.[7,8] When young adults were surveyed, 70–90% reported that they experienced nightmares as children.[9,10] According to some studies, the rate of nightmares not related to traumatic events, also known as idiopathic nightmares, decreases with age. There is a reported close correlation between chronic nightmares and psychopathology with increased nightmare frequency associated with anxiety and stress.[10–12] However, some studies did not find such a relationship.[13–15] Specifically, some researchers found a positive trend between nightmares and frightening TV content rather than anxiety per se.[5,10] The relationship between nightmares and anxiety is complicated. It is unclear if anxiety is the cause of nightmares; it is feasible that children may perceive dreams differently and find them more frightening. It also possible that nightmares and anxiety may be associated with other behavioral or mental health problems.

Nightmares and sleep disturbances are definitely more common in children who have had severe traumatic experiences.[16–20] Post-trauma nightmares may occur during both REM and non-REM sleep as opposed to primary nightmares that generally occur during longest REM sleep periods in the second half of the night.[21] One study found 18.8% of adult patients with posttraumatic stress disorder (PTSD) reported nightmares, as opposed to the healthy comparison group, in which only 4.2% reported nightmares.[22] Several pediatric studies have documented similar, if not higher, rates of nightmares in children with a history of trauma, with some studies reporting prevalence rates as high as 50–80%.[23–25] The literature suggests that post-trauma–related nightmares may be long-lasting and cause significant impairment and distress. For instance, one study assessed sleep disturbance and fear of sleeping using the Revised Child Anxiety and Depression Scales in a sample of 202 children (aged 8 to 15 years) 24 months after they experienced trauma from Hurricane Katrina. Severity of sleep disturbance was associated with severity of PTSD symptoms and demonstrated the presence of sleep disturbances 24 months after the hurricane. This study also found positive correlation between the severity of PTSD symptoms 30 months after the hurricane and presence of sleep disturbances, suggesting that sleep disturbance after a trauma may be used as a biomarker for subsequent PTSD in children.[26]

Post-trauma nightmares and frequent primary nightmares are also associated with other sleep problems such as insomnia, difficulties falling and staying asleep, and frequent awakenings. As a result, children may develop maladaptive behaviors including reliance on melatonin or sedating antihistamines, watching television or other electronic devices in bed for distraction, and even substance abuse (in adolescents). Some children with PTSD and nightmares may try to avoid situations that are associated with nightmares and traumatic events and might even try to avoid sleep altogether because of fears of nightmares. Nightmares may also cause or exacerbate underlying psychiatric distress and illness.

Given the suspected correlation between anxiety and nightmares, treatment of nightmares usually focuses on anxiety-reducing techniques, psychologic counseling, Cognitive-behavioral treatment (CBT) including image rehearsal therapy (IRT), and/or reduction in exposure to television, media, and video games. CBTs have been mostly studied in adults and patients with PTSD. These include exposure, relaxation and rescripting therapy (ERRT); lucid dreaming therapy; systematic desensitization; progressive deep muscle relaxation training; and eye movement desensitization and reprocessing.[27,28] In rare cases of post-trauma

nightmares, pharmacologic treatment may be considered. Clonazepam in conjunction with CBT and/or ERRT has been used off-label for the most severe cases in adult patients, as well as children with PTSD.[29] However, its effectiveness has not been proven. In addition, benzodiazepine use may be associated with tolerance and addiction potential. Prazosin is an α_1-adrenergic receptor traditionally used to treat hypertension and benign prostatic hyperplasia. It reduces central nervous system sympathetic outflow throughout the brain. Prazosin has been shown to decrease the occurrence of trauma-related nightmares in both combat veterans and patients with non–combat-related PTSD.[30–32] Similar literature exists for adolescents with PTSD.[33] Clonidine is an α_2-adrenergic receptor agonist that suppresses sympathetic nervous system outflow throughout the brain. It is now frequently used in pediatric patients for the treatment of attention-deficit/hyperactivity disorder (ADHD) and insomnia associated with autistic spectrum disorders and ADHD. The rationale of using clonidine is similar to prazosin; however, little data is available regarding its use for nightmares. Low-dose clonidine (0.2–0.6 mg in divided doses) has been shown to increase REM sleep and decrease NREM sleep, whereas medium-dose clonidine decreases REM sleep and increases N2 sleep.[34,35] Thus a theoretical benefit of medium-dose clonidine therapy is suppression of REM sleep–related dream mentation. It is also worth mentioning clonidine therapy discontinuation may lead to significant rebound hypertension and cause rebound increase in REM sleep percentages.[34] The latter may lead to a potential worsening of nightmares. There is some sparse data on use of other medications. Some small studies in adults looked into the use of atypical antipsychotic medications, topiramate, low-dose cortisol, trazodone, gabapentin, cyproheptadine, and tricyclic antidepressants.[36] Unfortunately, pediatric data essentially does not exist.

REM Sleep Behavior Disorder

RBD is a sleep disorder associated with loss of REM-related muscle atonia associated with complex, vigorous, and frequently violent dream-enacting behavior during REM sleep. It is classified by the ICSD-3[2] as (1) repeated episodes of behavior or vocalization that are either documented by polysomnography (PSG) to arise from REM or are presumed to arise from REM based on reports of dream enactment, and (2) evidence of RSWA on PSG (as defined in the scoring manual). When RSWA is not observed, the diagnosis may be given on a provisional basis when other clinical findings are strongly suggestive. RBD in childhood is rare.

RBD is clinically characterized by dream-related abnormal motor behavior that is sometimes violent and aggressive. These aggressive behaviors may result in injury to self or others.

During REM sleep, RBD is characterized by polysomnographic evidence of intermittent loss of REM atonia, excessive sustained or phasic muscle twitch activity of the submental and/or limb electromyogram (EMG) during REM sleep. RSWA is defined by the American Academy of Sleep Medicine[37,38] as tonic segments of at least 50% of the duration of the epoch with the chin segment activity exceeding two times the lowest level background EMG amplitude. When assessing phasic muscle activity, RSWA can be scored when at least five mini-epochs with a duration of 3 seconds within a 30-second epoch of REM sleep are at least two times the lowest level EMG amplitude and 0.1–5.0 seconds in duration.

The animal equivalent of RBD was previously described by Jouvet's and Morrison's groups, dating back to 1965, when Jouvet's group firstly created experimentally lesioned cats (in the bilateral pontine tegmentum areas) presenting with "oneiric behaviors." RBD in adult patients was first reported by Schenck and his colleagues in 1986 and was subsequently incorporated as parasomnia in the International Classification of Sleep Disorders.[2,39] Studies on RBD in adults revealed that about half of RBD cases were associated with neurologic disorders, especially neurodegenerative diseases pathologically known as synucleinopathies (Parkinson's disease, dementia with Lewy bodies, and multiple system atrophy). A substantial number of idiopathic

RBD (iRBD) patients eventually developed parkinsonian diseases. In adults, in addition to a clear association of RBD with synucleinopathic degenerative disorders, it has also been associated with narcolepsy, antidepressant therapy, psychiatric diagnoses, and alcohol withdrawal onset.[40–42]

RSWA is not associated with dream-related motor behavior and may occur independent of RBD. However, RBD always requires the presence of RSWA.[43] In addition, RSWA can be found as an incidental finding during sleep studies (Fig. 43.1).

RBD is hypothesized to be caused by primary dysfunction of the pedunculopontine nucleus or other key brainstem structures associated with the basal ganglia pathway.[44] Neuroimaging data from human adult RBD cases have implicated the dorsal midbrain and pontine regions.[45,46]

From a sleep ontogenesis prospective, it has been postulated that RSWA and RBD represent regression to a more primitive, undifferentiated state of sleep.[43] Indeed, transitional sleep and REM sleep in infants comprises bursts of eye movements, intermittent bodily twitches, and tonic chin electromyographic sleep, resembling RSWA.

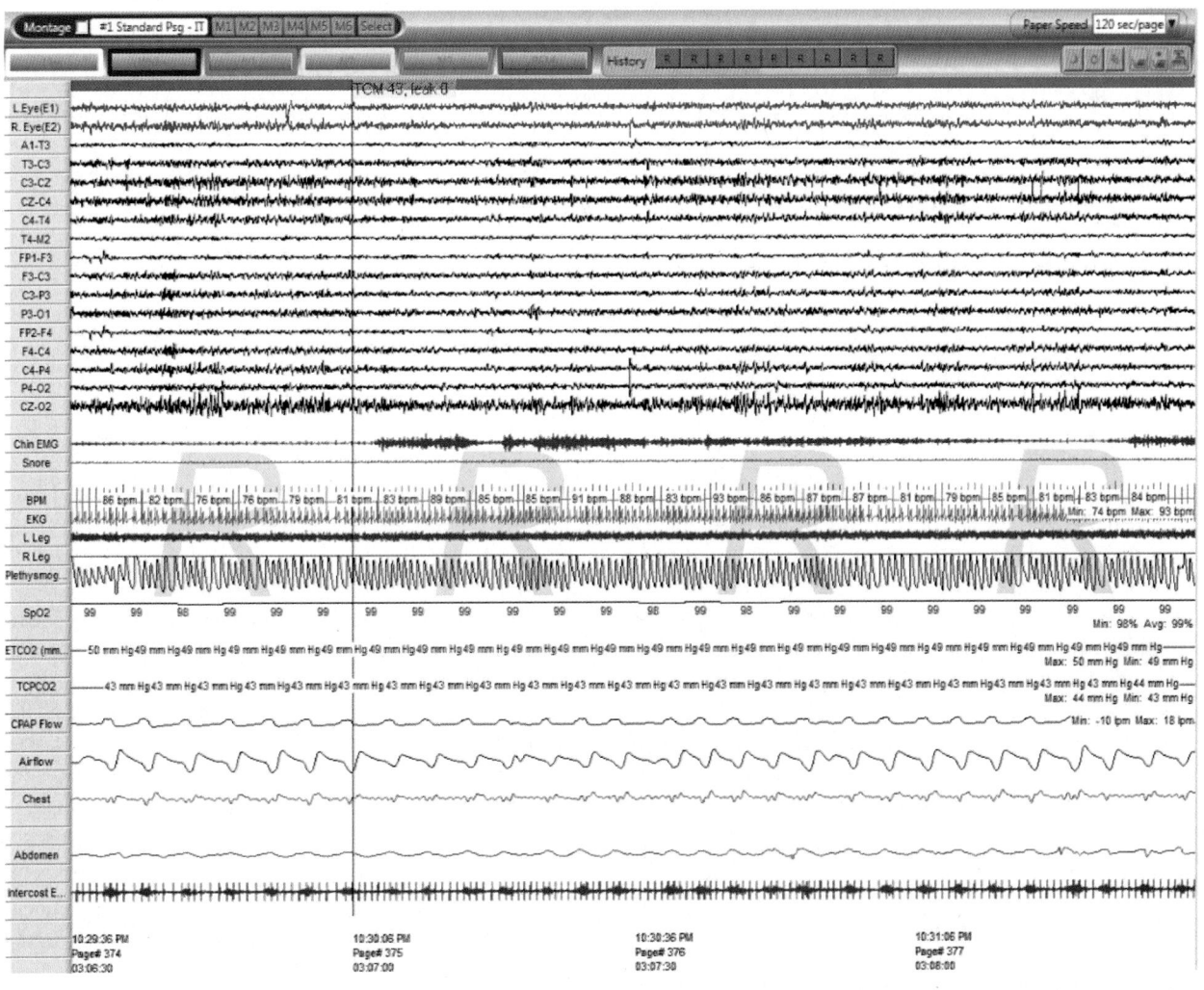

• **Fig. 43.1** Rapid eye movement sleep without atonia. A 12-year-old patient who presented for a sleep study because of concerns for sleep-disordered breathing; 120-second view.

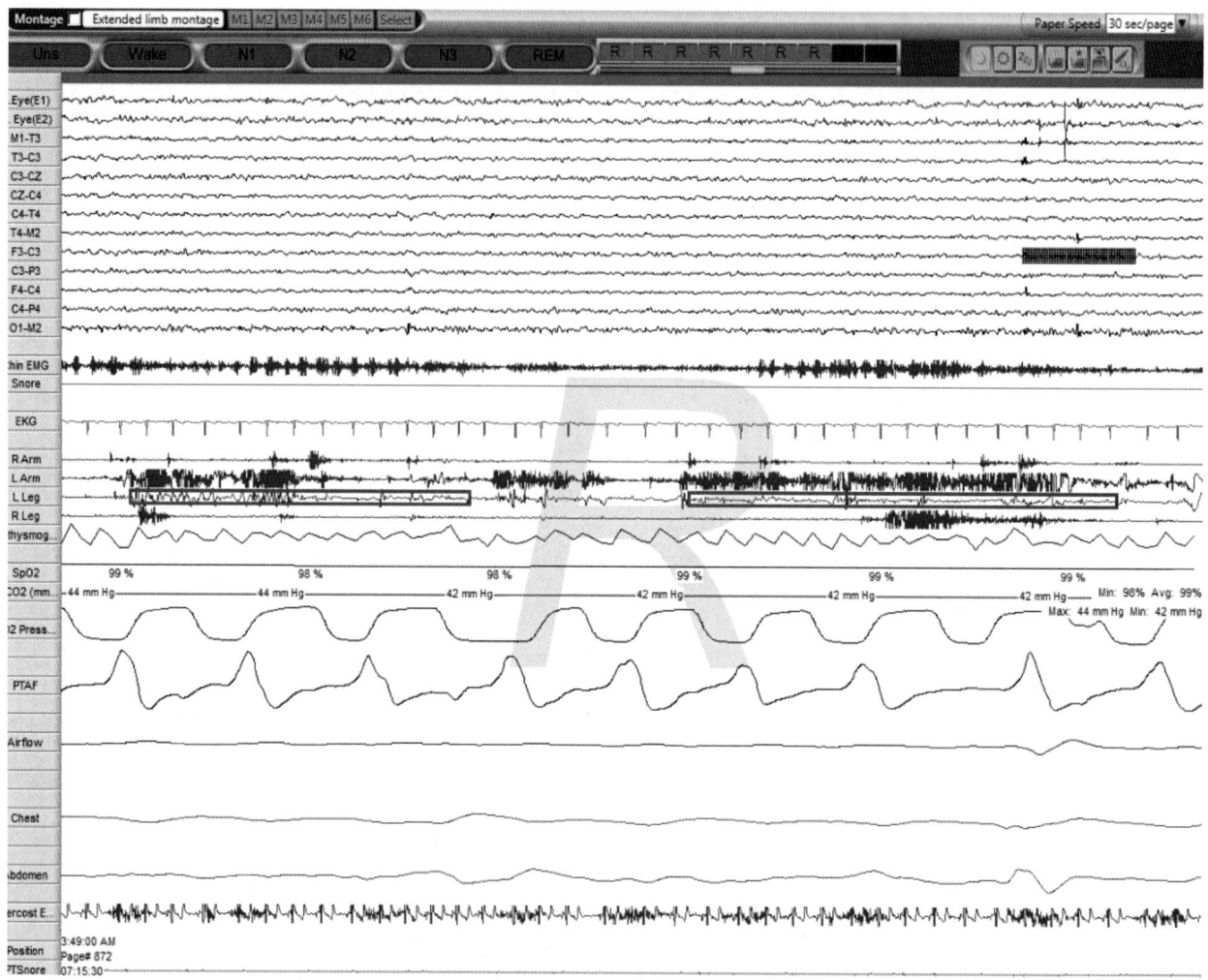

• **Fig. 43.2** Rapid eye movement sleep behavior disorder in a 7-year-old patient with nightmares and unusual behaviors during sleep such as sitting up on his knees, talking, flailing arms, and a full recall of dream mentation; 10-second epoch.

Pediatric RBD literature is sparse and composed of single case reports or small case series. RBD incidence in pediatrics is unknown as the diagnosis requires nocturnal PSG in the sleep laboratory environment. RBD semiology does have some resemblance to nightmares, because the child is experiencing a terrifying dream. Thus, it is feasible some reported nightmares in children may be underrecognized cases of RBD (Fig. 43.2).

Several childhood RBD cases have been associated with structural brainstem lesions such as neoplasms, juvenile Parkinson disease, Chiari type 1 malformation in combination with sleep-disordered breathing, autism, narcolepsy, Tourette's syndrome, the use of antidepressant medications (selective serotonin reuptake inhibitors [SSRIs], serotonin-norepinephrine reuptake inhibitors, tricyclics), and Smith-Magenis syndrome.[41,47–50]

RBD in children may be a completely different clinical entity. It most likely occurs more frequently in children and adolescents than previously recognized.[47]

RBD may lead to nocturnal awakenings and nightmares. Daytime symptoms may include daytime sleepiness, fatigue, and sleep initiation and maintenance difficulties.[47]

RBD evaluation requires detailed history and specific finding on nocturnal PSG. RBD management depends on the child's underlying medical problems. However, a consultation with a pediatric neurologist and brain MRI should be considered to exclude structural brainstem lesions such as Chiari malformation or brainstem tumor.[43] An evaluation by a psychiatrist or a developmental pediatrician may be required in case of suspected psychiatric comorbidities or developmental disorder. Genetic workup should be considered for children with suspected Smith-Magenis syndrome or other genetic disorders.

REM Sleep Behavior Disorder Management

RSWA does not require intervention.[43] Treatment should be considered for children with RBD-associated sleep disruption resulting in self-injurious behavior, non-refreshing sleep, and/or daytime symptoms including inattentiveness, excessive sleepiness, or behavioral problems. Discontinuation of antidepressant therapy when possible and pharmacologic treatment with melatonin 3–5 mg and/or low-dose clonazepam (0.125–0.5 mg) at bedtime may be considered.[47] However, the safety and efficacy data for pediatric RBD has not been established. In addition, melatonin therapy may be associated with an increase in nightmares, and clonazepam therapy may cause daytime drowsiness, cognitive impairment, and dependence.

Conclusions

RBD in children is rare but most likely occurs more frequently in children than has been identified. In children, RBD is not associated with synucleinopathies. It may be associated with neurodevelopmental disabilities, narcolepsy, or SSRI use. RBD seems to be modestly responsive to benzodiazepines or melatonin. Further studies assessing for RSWA, particularly in children with reported sleep disruptions, such as nightmares, may be beneficial in determining the prevalence and incidence of RBD in the pediatric population. This would help to identify children whose sleep disruptions may be due to underdiagnosed RBD and who may benefit from treatment to increase safety at night and reduce daytime symptoms that are impacting optimal growth and development.

CLINICAL PEARLS

- RBD can occur in childhood, although infrequently.
- History and PSG are required for RBD diagnosis confirmation.
- Neurodevelopmental disorders, narcolepsy, structural brainstem lesions, and medication effect are common etiologies.
- In contrast to adults, RBD in children is not associated with synucleinopathies.
- RBD in children seems to be modestly responsive to benzodiazepines or melatonin.

References

1. Espa F, Ondze B, Deglise P, Billiard M, Besset A. Sleep architecture, slow wave activity, and sleep spindles in adult patients with sleepwalking and sleep terrors. *Clin Neurophysiol.* 2000; 111(5):929–939.
2. American Academy of Sleep Medicine. *International Classification of Sleep Disorders.* 2014.
3. Fernandez S, Demarni Cromer L, Borntrager C, Swopes R, Hanson RF, Davis JL. A case series: cognitive-behavioral treatment (exposure, relaxation, and rescripting therapy) of trauma-related nightmares experienced by children. *Clin Case Stud.* 2013;12(1):39.
4. Hawkins C, Williams TI. Nightmares, life events and behaviour problems in preschool children. *Child: Care, Health Dev.* 1992;18(2):117.
5. Fisher BE, Wilson AE. Selected sleep disturbances in school children reported by parents: prevalence, interrelationships, behavioral correlates and parental attributions. *Percept Mot Skills.* 1987;64(3 Pt 2):1147.
6. Simonds JF, Parraga H. Prevalence of sleep disorders and sleep behaviors in children and adolescents. *J Am Acad Child Psychiatry.* 1982;21(4):383.
7. Yang L, Zuo C, Eaton LF. Research note: sleep problems of normal Chinese adolescents. *J Child Psychol Psychiatry.* 1987;28(1): 167–172.
8. Vignau J, Bailly D, Duhamel A, Vervaecke P, Beuscart R, Collinet C. Epidemiologic study of sleep quality and troubles in French secondary school adolescents. *J Adolesc Health.* 1997;21(5):343–350.
9. Englehart RJ, Hale DB. Punishment, nail-biting, and nightmares: a cross-cultural study. *J Multicult Couns Dev.* 1990;18(3):126.
10. Mindell JA, Barrett KM. Nightmares and anxiety in elementary-aged children: is there a relationship. *Child Care Health Dev.* 2002;28(4):317–322.
11. Nielsen TA, Laberge L, Paquet J, Tremblay R, Vitaro F, Montplaisir J. Development of disturbing dreams during adolescence and their relation to anxiety symptoms. *Sleep.* 2000;23(6):727.
12. Schredl M, Fricke-Oerkermann L, Mitschke A, Wiater A, Lehmkuhl G. Longitudinal study of nightmares in children: stability and effect of emotional symptoms. *Child Psychiatry Hum Dev.* 2009;40(3):439.
13. Dunn KK, Barrett D. Characteristics of nightmare subjects and their nightmares. *Psychiatr J Univ Otta.* 1988;13(2):91–93.
14. Levin R. Relations among nightmare frequency and ego strength, death anxiety, and sex of college students. *Percept Mot Skills.* 1989;69(3_suppl):1107.
15. Wood JM, Bootzin RR. The prevalence of nightmares and their independence from anxiety. *J Abnorm Psychol.* 1990; 99(1):64.
16. Connolly D, McClowry S, Hayman L, Mahony L, Artman M. Posttraumatic stress disorder in children after cardiac surgery. *J Pediatr.* 2004;144(4):480.
17. Dollinger SJ, Molina BS, Monteiro JMC. Sleep and anxieties in Brazilian children: the role of cultural and environmental factors in child sleep disturbance. *Am J Orthopsychiatry.* 1996;66(2):252.
18. Finkelhor DQD. *A Sourcebook on Child Sexual Abuse.* Sage; 1986.
19. Terr LC. Chowchilla revisited: the effects of psychic trauma four years after a school-bus kidnapping. *Am J Psychiatry.* 1983;140(12): 1543–1550.
20. Wittmann L, Zehnder D, Schredl M, Jenni OG, Landolt MA. Posttraumatic nightmares and psychopathology in children after road traffic accidents. *J Trauma Stress.* 2010;23(2):232.
21. Nader K. *Children's traumatic dreams. In: Trauma and Dreams.* Harvard University Press; 1996:9–24.
22. Ohayon MM, Shapiro CM. Sleep disturbances and psychiatric disorders associated with posttraumatic stress disorder in the general population. *Compr Psychiatry.* 2000;41(6):469.
23. Carrion VG, Weems CF, Ray R, Reiss AL. Toward an empirical definition of pediatric PTSD: the phenomenology of PTSD symptoms in youth. *J Am Acad Child Adolesc Psychiatry.* 2002;41(2):166.
24. Pynoos RS, Frederick C, Nader K, et al. Life threat and posttraumatic stress in school-age children. *Arch Gen Psychiatry.* 1987;44(12):1057.

25. Thabet AA, Ibraheem AN, Shivram R, Winter EA, Vostanis P. Parenting support and PTSD in children of a war zone. *Int J Soc Psychiatry*. 2009;55(3):226.

26. Brown TH, Mellman TA, Alfano CA, Weems CF. Sleep fears, sleep disturbance, and PTSD symptoms in minority youth exposed to Hurricane Katrina. *J Trauma Stress*. 2011;24(5):575.

27. Simard V, Nielsen T. Adaptation of imagery rehearsal therapy for nightmares in children: a brief report. *Psychotherapy (Chic)*. 2009;46(4):492.

28. Davis JL. *Treating Post-trauma Nightmares: A Cognitive Behavioral Approach*. Springer; 2009.

29. Keeshin B, Presson A, Berkowitz S, Strawn JR. 1.38 Prazosin in children and adolescents with posttraumatic stress disorder and nightmares: a retrospective chart review of 34 cases. *J Am Acad Child Adolesc Psychiatry*. 2016;55(10):S112.

30. Boynton L, Bentley J, Strachan E, Barbato A, Raskind M. Preliminary findings concerning the use of prazosin for the treatment of posttraumatic nightmares in a refugee population. *J Psychiatr Pract*. 2009;15(6):454.

31. Miller LJ. Prazosin for the treatment of posttraumatic stress disorder sleep disturbances. *Pharmacotherapy*. 2008;28(5):656.

32. Dierks MR, Jordan JK, Sheehan AH. Prazosin treatment of nightmares related to posttraumatic stress disorder. *Ann Pharmacother*. 2007;41(6):1013.

33. Keeshin B, Ding Q, Presson A, Berkowitz S, Strawn J. Use of prazosin for pediatric PTSD-associated nightmares and sleep disturbances: a retrospective chart review. *Neurol Ther*. 2017;6(2):247.

34. Cates ME, Bishop MH, Davis LL, Lowe JS, Woolley TW. Clonazepam for treatment of sleep disturbances associated with combat-related posttraumatic stress disorder. *Ann Pharmacother*. 2004;38(9):1395.

35. Miyazaki S, Uchida S, Mukai J, Nishihara K. Clonidine effects on all-night human sleep: Opposite action of low- and medium-dose clonidine on human NREM–REM sleep proportion. *Psychiatry Clin Neurosci*. 2004;58(2):138.

36. Aurora RN, Zak RS, Auerbach SH, et al. Best practice guide for the treatment of nightmare disorder in adults. *J Clin Sleep Med*. 2010;6(4):389.

37. Berry RB, Brooks R, Gamaldo C, et al. AASM Scoring Manual Updates for 2017 (Version 2.4). *J Clin Sleep Med*. 2017;13(5):665–666.

38. Iber C, Ancoli-Israel S, Chesson AL, Quan S. The AASM Manual for the Scoring of Sleep and Associated Events: Rules, Terminology and Technical Specifications. *Am Acad Sleep Med*. 2007

39. Tachibana N. [Historical overview of REM sleep behavior disorder in relation to its pathophysiology]. *Brain Nerve*. 2009;61(5):558–568.

40. Postuma RB, Gagnon JF, Vendette M, Fantini ML, Massicotte-Marquez J, Montplaisir J. Quantifying the risk of neurodegenerative disease in idiopathic REM sleep behavior disorder. *Neurology*. 2009;72(15):1296.

41. Teman PT, Tippmann-Peikert M, Silber MH, Slocumb NL, Auger RR. Idiopathic rapid-eye-movement sleep disorder: associations with antidepressants, psychiatric diagnoses, and other factors, in relation to age of onset. *Sleep Med*. 2009;10(1):60–65.

42. Schenck CH, Mahowald MW, Kim SW, Connor KA, Hurwitz TD. Prominent eye movements during NREM sleep and REM sleep behavior disorder associated with fluoxetine treatment of depression and obsessive-compulsive disorder. *Sleep*. 1992;15(3):226.

43. Kotagal S. Rapid eye movement sleep behavior disorder during childhood. *Sleep Med Clin*. 2015;10(2):163.

44. Abad V, Guilleminault C. Review of rapid eye movement behavior sleep disorders. *Curr Neurol Neurosci Rep*. 2004;4(2):157.

45. Shirakawa S, Takeuchi N, Uchimura N, et al. Study of image findings in rapid eye movement sleep behavioural disorder. *Psychiatry Clin Neurosci*. 2002;56(3):291–292.

46. Culebras A, Moore JT. Magnetic resonance findings in REM sleep behavior disorder. *Neurology*. 1989;39(11):1519–1523.

47. Lloyd R, Tippmann-Peikert M, Slocumb N, Kotagal S. Characteristics of REM sleep behavior disorder in childhood. *J Clin Sleep Med*. 2012;8(2):127–131.

48. Trajanovic NN, Voloh I, Shapiro CM, Sandor P. REM sleep behaviour disorder in a child with Tourette's syndrome. *Can J Neurol Sci*. 2004;31(4):572–575.

49. Gropman AL, Duncan WC, Smith AC. Neurologic and developmental features of the Smith-Magenis syndrome (del 17p11.2). *Pediatr Neurol*. 2006;34(5):337–350.

50. Nevsimalova S, Prihodova I, Kemlink D, Lin L, Mignot E. REM behavior disorder (RBD) can be one of the first symptoms of childhood narcolepsy. *Sleep Med*. 2007;8(7):784–786.

Movement Disorders

44

Restless Legs Syndrome, Periodic Leg Movements, and Periodic Limb Movement Disorder

Jeffrey S. Durmer

CHAPTER HIGHLIGHTS

- RLS and periodic limb movement disorder (PLMD) are common sleep disorders in children that often present with a family history and non-specific sleep complaints such as bedtime resistance, difficulty falling asleep, and excessive movement during sleep.
- Periodic leg movements, periodic limb movement disorder, and "growing pains" may present years before the sensori-motor symptoms of RLS develop.
- RLS often presents with other comorbid conditions including ADHD, iron deficiency, anxiety, depression, autism spectrum disorder, and other neurodevelopmental conditions.
- The diagnosis of RLS in children involves not only identifying the traditional symptoms of RLS but also a clear description of symptoms by the child in words, drawings, or other representations.
- While there are no FDA approved treatments for RLS or PLMD in children, clinical studies support oral and iv iron supplementation for relative iron storage deficits and behavioral interventions as first line treatments. Pharmaceutical therapies utilized in adult RLS and PLMD including alpha-2-delta ligands, dopamine agonists, L-dopa, melatonin, opioids, benzodiazepines, and other agents may have utility in cases of pediatric RLS; however, side effects must be considered along with comorbid conditions, and potential developmental risks.

Introduction

A feeling of restlessness can describe both a physical and a psychologic sensation that prompts movement or the urge to move. This ubiquitous human experience is at once recognizable as normal yet, in genetically susceptible individuals, an exaggeration of these (sometimes painful) sensations results in intrusive compensatory movements and the degradation of rest, sleep, performance, and health. It is in these instances, when feelings of internal restlessness and the urge

to move interfere with routine activities, that we use the term restless legs syndrome (RLS) or Willis-Ekbom disease.[1] The characteristic symptoms of RLS have been known for hundreds of years and were first reported in the 1600s. The Swedish neurologist Karl Ekbom formally described the clinical, epidemiologic, and pathophysiologic correlates of the condition in 1945.[2]

The syndrome has four well-known clinical criteria: (1) an uncomfortable sensation or unexplainable urge to move the legs or other affected body part, (2) increasing symptoms with rest or inactivity, (3) a reduction of symptoms with movement, and (4) a circadian enhancement of symptoms in the evening or night. Ekbom reported all aspects of RLS occurring in children, but it was not until the mid-1990s that the first case reports of children with RLS were published and research began to focus on the potential genetic causes for this familial disorder.[3,4]

Much has been discovered with regards to the genetics, potential pathophysiology, and epidemiology of RLS in the past 30 years, but advances have included very little specific information about children. The recognition of significant correlations between RLS and select pediatric conditions, such as attention-deficit/hyperactivity disorder (ADHD) and iron deficiency, has helped generate new perspectives with regards to pathophysiology. Because pediatric-specific information concerning RLS is limited, age-adjusted adult criteria have been adopted for the diagnosis of this condition in children. Although additional pediatric criteria were included to increase selectivity, having to rely on verbal descriptions in a linguistically developing population to diagnose a largely subjective disorder increases the clinical complexity. Still, an accurate diagnosis of RLS is the single most important aspect of treating children with this condition. Clinicians must consider potential mimics as well as comorbid and associated conditions. More objective findings, such as of periodic leg movements in sleep (PLMS) and of a family history of RLS, can increase diagnostic certainty.

Periodic limb movement disorder (PLMD), which is clinically defined as a disorder distinct from RLS, is noted in children as well as adults. The diagnostic criteria for PLMD include increased PLMS for age (>5/hr) and a clinical sleep disturbance that is not accounted for by another sleep disorder, including RLS. Clinical case studies suggest that children may manifest PLMD before developing RLS later in childhood.[5] Observations such as these help our understanding of the biologic relationships between the sensory and motor components of these seemingly distinct but related disorders. Due to the limited available pediatric research, this chapter provides consensus opinion-based, as well as current evidence-based, information on the subject of childhood RLS and PLMD. In addition, new studies of prevalence, pathophysiology, diagnosis, treatment, and clinical associations with these conditions are also discussed.

Symptoms and Prevalence of Restless Legs Syndrome and Periodic Limb Movement Disorder in Children

RLS and PLMD are very common in northern European populations and are believed to be among the most common inherited conditions known. Surveys show that between 4% and 15% of adults in the United States and Western Europe have symptoms consistent with RLS.[6–8] In addition, there is evidence that up to 40% of adult RLS sufferers may have had the onset of symptoms in childhood or adolescence.[9]

Validated RLS inventories, such as the *International Restless Legs Syndrome Study Group Rating Scale* (IRLS) *International Restless Legs Syndrome Study Group Rating Scale (IRLS)*,[10] have allowed investigators to utilize common tools in adult studies. The occurrence of RLS is increased in women compared with men (3:2 female:male). In younger populations the female:male ratio is closer to 2:1. Studies of adults over the age of 65 years show RLS prevalence increasing up to 10–20%.[11] Approximately 8–20% of adults fulfill standard RLS criteria,[12,13] but only 2.7–3.9% of adults meet criteria for moderate to severe RLS (episodes twice or more per week with moderate to severe distress).[12,14] Not all people with RLS symptoms require medical attention.

Picchietti and colleagues, using the National Institutes of Health (NIH) consensus criteria for the diagnosis of *definite* RLS in children, performed the most comprehensive prevalence survey to date of RLS in children from the United States and United Kingdom.[15] They demonstrated that 1.9% of 8- to 11-year-olds and 2% of 12- to 17-year-olds fulfilled these criteria. The prevalence of moderately severe RLS was 0.5% and 1% in 8- to 11-year-olds and 12- to 17-year-olds, respectively. There was no gender preference noted, unlike in adult RLS. In addition, the data showed a potentially strong genetic predisposition for RLS with 71–80% of children having at least one affected parent.[15] In 2010, an RLS symptom severity scale for children and adolescents was developed,[16] although large-scale validation studies have yet to be performed.

Periodic Limb Movement Disorder and Periodic Leg Movements

PLMD is delineated as a separate sleep-related movement disorder,[17] although many experts in the field consider PLMD to exist on a continuum with RLS. Both disorders are associated with low ferritin levels, respond to dopaminergic medications, share similar genetics, and are more common in Caucasian children than in other racial groups (odds ratio [OR] = 9.5).[18] The supposition of a continuum from PLMD to RLS is further bolstered by clinical evidence that some children manifest PLMD or PLMS years before the symptoms of RLS develop.[5] In a retrospective longitudinal study, Picchietti and Stevens identified PLMD or probable/possible RLS in 18 children (mean age = 10.3 years) and subsequently diagnosed these children with definite RLS an average of 11.6 years later. In addition, these children had many of the comorbidities commonly associated with RLS such as ADHD, parasomnias, and a low serum ferritin level.[5]

With the recent discovery of a dose-dependent association between the *BTBD9* gene (on chromosome 6p) and the findings in RLS of both PLMS and low serum ferritin, there remains no doubt that the motor and sensory features of RLS are related.[19] In addition, given that the vast majority of RLS sufferers have PLMS on polysomnography (PSG) testing (reports vary from 80–100%), the presence of a common neural mechanism for both sensory and motor symptoms is suggested. In contrast, PLMS is noted in a number of other disorders (such as Parkinson's disease and Tourette's syndrome), in association with certain medical conditions (such as pregnancy), in association with other sleep disorders (such as narcolepsy, sleep deprivation, and obstructive sleep apnea [OSA]), as a result of OSA treatment with continuous positive airway pressure),[20] and as a result of certain medications (such as selective serotonin reuptake inhibitors [SSRIs] and tricyclic antidepressants [TCAs]).[21–27]

Counter to the argument that PLMS represents normal motor activity are data that demonstrate the impact of PLMS and RLS on both health and psychologic well-being. Sympathetic overactivation may explain the association between PLMS and chronic cardiovascular conditions in adults;[28] in RLS sufferers, this relationship is thought to elevate the risk for stroke and even the risk for insulin resistance and type 2 diabetes.[29] The natural state of sympathetic *hyperactivity* associated with youth may actually place children and younger adults at an even higher risk.[30] A number of adult and pediatric studies demonstrate a strong relationship with ADHD, behavioral disorders, and cognitive deficits as well as with depression and anxiety in RLS populations.[31–34] Recently, a study of 412 adolescents with ADHD associated with the Penn State Child Cohort demonstrated that PLMS was associated with a dose-dependent increase in ADHD severity (self-control, elevated internalizing and externalizing behaviors) and worse neurobehavioral functioning (executive deficits, anxiety, and mood dysfunction).[35] In addition, a recent retrospective review of all cases

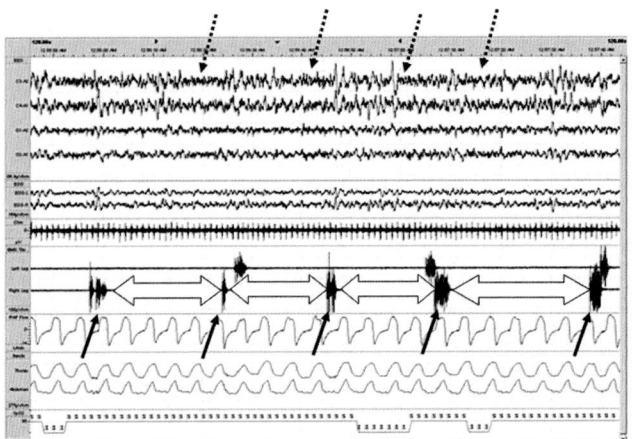

• **Fig. 44.1** Periodic leg movements during sleep (PLMS) depicted on 2-minute polysomnography (PSG) recording page. Each *solid arrow* demonstrates an individual PLM in a sequence of PLMS recorded with right and left anterior tibialis electromyography (EMG). *Block arrows* denote the intermovement interval, which is very consistent as noted in restless legs syndrome (RLS). Also, note cortical arousals *(dashed arrows)* associated with PLMS that are thought to confer excessive autonomic activity and sleep fragmentation. *(From Durmer JS and Quraishi GH. Restless legs syndrome, periodic leg movements and periodic leg movement disorder in children. Pediatr Clin N Am. 2011;58:591–620.)*

requiring a PSG at Seattle Children's Sleep Disorders Center between 2017 and 2019 showed that children with PLMD had a wide array of comorbidities including insomnia, mood disorders, behavioral problems, morning headaches, kidney disease, epilepsy, and heart disease.[36] Adults with RLS carry a 4- to 5-fold increased risk for depression and self-harm and a 13-fold increased risk for panic disorder.[37–41] Patient-reported outcome measures demonstrate a significant impact of RLS in adults.[12,42–45] Studies demonstrating that RLS causes clinical morbidity in pediatric populations, however, are lacking (Fig. 44.1).

Measuring Periodic Leg Movements in Sleep

PLMS in children is not uncommon, especially in children with RLS; studies suggested that between 8.4% and 11.9% of children may have PLMD.[46] Normative pediatric data from studies that record PLMS via PSG and/or accelerometry (also referred to as actigraphy and actometry) demonstrate that most children and adolescents exhibit a periodic leg movement index (PLMi) no greater than 5/hr.[46–50] By contrast, up to 74% of children with definite RLS have a PLMi in excess of 5/hr.[51] When PLMi is noted in children, clinicians should consider further investigation into the possibility of RLS.

Standardized criteria commonly utilized to score PLMS recorded via bilateral anterior tibialis electromyography (EMG)[52] have been modified in the past 5 years. These criteria allow for significant variability in the expression and periodicity of PLMS. Using a Markov-based stochastic mathematical process to measure intermovement intervals and characterize the periodicity of PLMS,[53] researchers have demonstrated that subjects with RLS-related PLMS (and

likely PLMD) have less intermovement interval variability (with intervals clustering between 24 and 28 seconds) than is seen in PLMS due to other conditions (such as narcolepsy and ADHD).[54–56] There has been speculation that this particular frequency range is caused by neural pattern generators in the spinal cord and/or diencephalon.

PLMS demonstrates marked night-to-night variability, in children as well as in adults, and multiple nights of testing may be required to accurately quantify and diagnose PLMS.[57] Ambulatory or home-based PLMS measurements made using accelerometry in adults correlate with PLMS measured by PSG, and the same technique may be useful in the clinical evaluation of a child.[58,59]

Pathophysiology of Restless Legs Syndrome/Periodic Limb Movement Disorder

The neurobiologic mechanisms leading to the motor and sensory symptoms of RLS/PLMD remain the topic of scientific inquiry. Clinical observations demonstrate that most primary cases of RLS respond to dopaminergic treatments, which suggests that monoaminergic neurotransmitter systems within the central nervous system play a pivotal role in the expression of RLS/PLMD symptoms. Neuroanatomic and physiologic models of diencephalic and spinal cord dopaminergic systems support an intriguing hypothesis related to the sole source of dopamine innervation in the spinal cord, namely the bilateral A-11 hypothalamic cell groups. These cells project to all levels of the spinal cord and provide dorsal (sensory), ventral (motor), and mediolateral (sympathetic) dopaminergic activity. This important neuroanatomic property suggests that the A-11 dopaminergic cell groups may be major contributors to the development of RLS.[60] Animal models using dopamine receptor (D2-like) knock-out mice suggest that the loss of spinal cord gating via D2-like receptors may precipitate the sensory and motor symptoms of RLS/PLMD (Fig. 44.2).[61]

An association between iron deficiency and RLS was first noted by Nordlander in 1954.[62] Serum iron indices, such as total iron, hemoglobin levels, and hematocrit, are usually within the normal ranges in RLS patients. Nevertheless, brain iron deficiency (BID) has been implicated using cerebrospinal fluid analysis of iron and ferritin,[63,64] magnetic resonance imaging (MRI) and ultrasound of the substantia nigra,[65–67] and autopsy examination of brain tissue from RLS subjects.[68,69] The link between iron deficiency and dysfunction of central dopaminergic systems is based on evidence that iron is a cofactor for the rate-limiting enzyme in dopamine synthesis, tyrosine hydroxylase, and is required for postsynaptic D2 receptor function. Iron deficiency results in downregulation of striatum and nucleus accumbens dopamine receptors as well as dysregulation of dopamine vesicular release.[70–72] Correlations between peripheral serum ferritin levels and cerebrospinal ferritin levels in RLS patients demonstrate that serum ferritin levels <50 ng/mL correlate with relative body iron storage deficiency.[63,64]

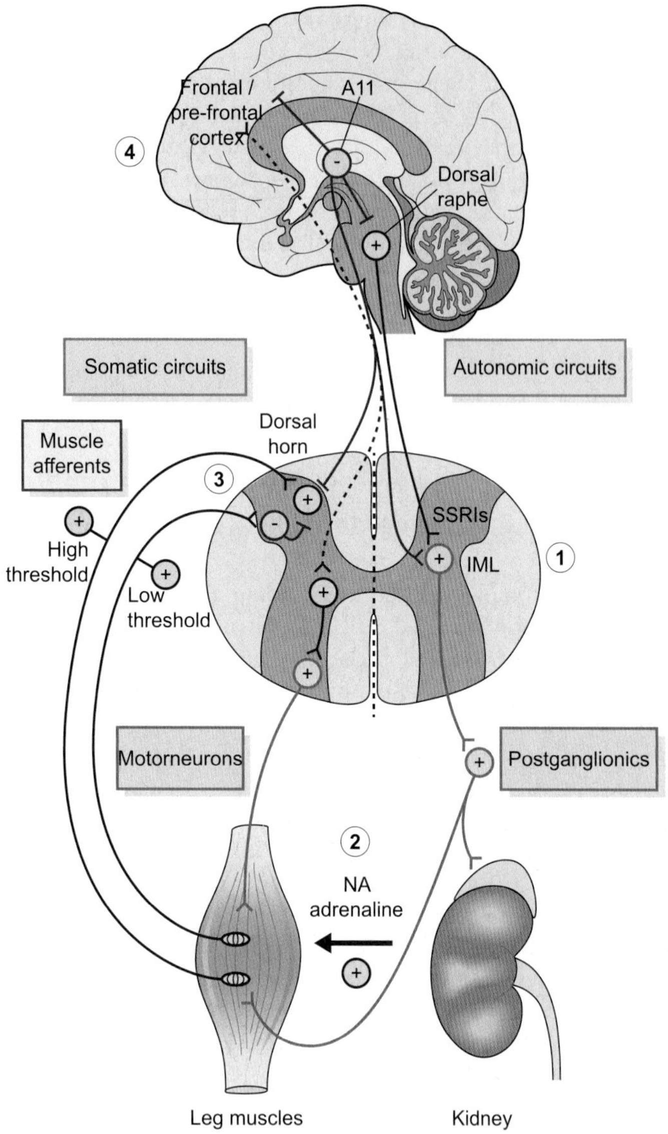

• **Fig. 44.2** The proposed role of the diencephalic dopaminergic cell group A-11 in the pathophysiology of restless legs syndrome (RLS). A-11 neurons project caudally to inhibit the dorsal raphe nucleus. This results in less sympathetic excitation via the spinal cord intermediolateral cell column (*IML*). A-11 neurons also project to all levels of the spinal cord and inhibit dorsal horn sensory transmission as well as the afferent projections of the IML (1). As proposed in RLS, a loss of A-11 dopaminergic inhibition results in increased sensory input to cortex (uncomfortable sensations or urge to move), increased sensory activation of the spinal cord reflex arc (3) (causing periodic leg movements during sleep [PLMS]), and increased sympathetic activity (2) (accentuating PLMS and associated medical conditions such as hypertension and proinflammatory states). The loss of rostral A-11 projections would also enhance cortically mediated sensory discomfort associated with RLS (4).[61] NA, noradrenaline; SSRI, selective serotonin reuptake inhibitor.

Recent evidence suggests that lower ferritin status in RLS may not only correlate with alterations in dopamine metabolism and neural transmission but may also be associated with an inability to retain intracellular ferritin.[73] Thus patients with RLS seem to have an intracellular need for iron; yet, the proteins responsible for regulating cellular iron content create a situation tantamount to a *leaky bucket*.

Continued investigations into BID and its association with RLS symptomology in animal models indicate that alterations in the adenosine system may be involved in upstream modulation of dopamine systems.[74–76] In the presence of BID, adenosine 1 receptors (A1Rs) become downregulated, resulting in both an increase in striatal glutamate and dopamine. The adenosine-dependent hyperexcitability associated with glutamate release increases activation of arousal systems in the brain, resulting in hyperarousal, which is a noted feature during sleep in RLS patients. Simultaneously, the adenosine-dependent increase in central dopamine activity results in many of the typical features of RLS including akathisia and PLMS. Additionally, in these animal models, the administration of dipyridamole, which corrects the BID-induced hypoadenosinergic state, has been shown to reduce locomotor activity (hyperarousal) in a dose-dependent manner.

The Genetics of Restless Legs Syndrome/Periodic Limb Movement Disorder

Genetic investigations over the past two decades using twin concordance, family association, familial linkage, and genomic association methods have created a more complex picture. Twin studies suggest a heritability of approximately 54% for RLS.[77] Ten different genetic loci for RLS have been identified (on multiple chromosomes) using familial linkage analysis, and these findings suggest that RLS/PLMD is a complex genetic trait that interacts with environmental factors.[78–91]

Genomic association studies of RLS phenotypes using single nucleotide polymorphisms (SNPs) have been performed since 2007. An Icelandic/U.S. investigation of 306 RLS cases and 15,664 controls identified three genes (*BTBD9, GLO1,* and *DNAH8*) on chromosome 6p that were associated with RLS patients with PLMS as a major component of their phenotype.[19] This study demonstrated dose-dependent associations among the BTBD9 allele, PLMS, and serum ferritin levels. Heterozygous individuals for this allele showed twice the risk for RLS with PLMS, whereas those homozygous for this variant had four times the risk. Serum ferritin levels were also lower in those with the additional BTBD9 allele. In a second genomic study performed in a German cohort of 401 familial RLS sufferers and 1,644 controls, four genes (MEIS1 – ch2p, BTBD9 – ch6p, MAP2K5 – ch15q, and LBXCOR1 – ch15q) were found in association with RLS.[92] In both the German and Icelandic/U.S. investigations, the BTBD9 allele, which is widely distributed in the brain and body, was found to be associated with RLS. The contribution of genetics to RLS is still being actively investigated.[93]

The complexity of gene-environment interactions suggests that the currently accepted view of primary RLS being due to a primarily genetic trait versus secondary RLS as primarily related to an environmental exposure is an oversimplification. In a systematic review of the literature, Trenkwalder and colleagues identified that RLS was

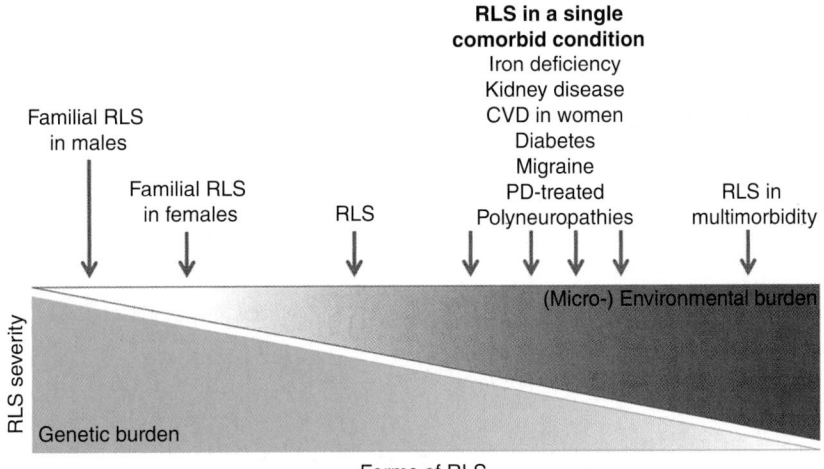

CVD = cardiovascular disease; PD = Parkinson's disease.

• **Fig. 44.3** Theoretic model of genetic and environmental factors leading to the manifestation of restless legs syndrome (RLS) and comorbid diseases. CVD, cardiovascular disease; PD, Parkinson's disease.

more prevalent in only kidney disease and iron deficiency.[94] Although there was significant evidence to suggest associations with cardiovascular disease, hypertension, diabetes, migraine, and Parkinson's disease, the authors concluded that the methodologies of these studies were poor.

In relation to these findings, the authors suggest a new concept related to the expression of RLS that underscores the complex nature of the interaction between noted genetic and environmental factors. In this conceptual framework, RLS expression occurs on a spectrum that depends on a ratio of genetic factors and a multitude of environmental factors including the multitude of comorbid diseases associated with RLS (Fig. 44.3) Presumably, because most children with RLS also have a family history of the same, one would expect that they would lie to the left of the diagram given a higher burden of genetic factors.

Replication studies of the familial and genomic findings from adult studies have proven inconclusive in children. One study assessed gene variants in 23 children and found an 87% positive family history of RLS and a trend toward association with MEIS1 and MAP2K/LBX-COR1 variants, but no association was found with BTBD9.[95] Another study of 386 children with ADHD and RLS did not find a genetic association.[96] Most recently, a reassessment of previously published single-variant candidate genes for idiopathic RLS using a genome-wide association study dataset demonstrated no variant was significantly associated with RLS. Thus larger sample sizes with more stringent significance thresholds were suggested for future studies.[93]

The Diagnosis of Restless Legs Syndrome/ Periodic Limb Movement Disorder in Children

As stated previously, the diagnosis of PLMD in children and adolescents formally requires the following: (1) PLMS

documented by PSG and exceeding a PLMi of 5/hr, (2) clinical sleep disturbance, and (3) the absence of another primary sleep disorder or reason for the PLMS (including RLS). In 1995, the *International RLS Study Group* developed standardized criteria for the diagnosis of RLS in adults.[97] In addition to the four essential features (noted earlier), five additional clinical features of RLS were included: (1) sleep disturbance, or daytime results of sleep disturbance; (2) involuntary movements during sleep (PLMS) and during wake (periodic leg movements during wakefulness [PLMW])); (3) neurological examination findings consistent with RLS; (4) typical clinical course and exacerbating factors; and (5) positive family history. Idiopathic or primary RLS was also distinguished from reactive or secondary RLS (which may be caused by conditions such as uremia, neuropathy, medications, and anemia).

In 2003, an NIH workshop produced expert consensus criteria for the diagnosis of RLS in children and special populations.[98] Categories of diagnostic certainty for RLS in children aged 2–12 years old were established based on varying levels of clinical evidence (Box 44.1). The essential four adult criteria were retained for the diagnosis of *definite* RLS in adolescents (13–18 years old). In addition, categories of *possible* and *probable* RLS were established, suggesting that individuals with incomplete RLS should be followed for progression of symptoms.

In 2013, the International RLS Study Group reviewed and updated the 2003 NIH criteria for pediatric RLS and PLMD, which further delineated the four essential clinical criteria for the diagnosis of pediatric RLS and the noted clinical criteria for PLMD.[100] In addition, supporting clinical features, including a family history of RLS or PLMD among first-degree relatives and a personal or family history of PLMS >5/hr were added. The group published criteria proposed for "probable" and "possible" RLS to support further investigation.

• BOX 44.1   Definite Restless Legs Syndrome Criteria for Pediatrics[99]

National Institutes of Health Workshop Diagnostic Criteria for Restless Legs Syndrome in Children and Adolescents

For definite restless legs syndrome (RLS), children (ages 2–12 years) must meet ALL of the following adult criteria:

- An urge to move the legs, usually accompanied or caused by uncomfortable and unpleasant sensations in the legs. (Sometimes the urge to move is present without the uncomfortable sensations and sometimes the arms or other body parts are involved in addition to the legs.)
- The urge to move or unpleasant sensations begin or worsen during periods of rest or inactivity such as lying or sitting.
- The urge to move or unpleasant sensations are partially or totally relieved by movement, such as walking or stretching, at least as long as the activity continues.

- The urge to move or unpleasant sensations are worse in the evening or night than during the day or only occur in the evening or night. (When symptoms are very severe, the worsening at night may not be noticeable but must have been previously present.)

AND

- A description of the leg discomfort in the child's own words using terms that are age-appropriate.

OR

- Demonstrate at least two of the three following supportive criteria:
- Sleep disturbance for age (e.g., sleep-onset/maintenance insomnia).
- A biologic parent or sibling with definite RLS.
- The child has documented PLMS index of ≥5/hour.

PLMS, periodic leg movements of sleep.
For definite RLS, adolescents (ages 13–18 years) must meet ALL of the four adult criteria as shown.

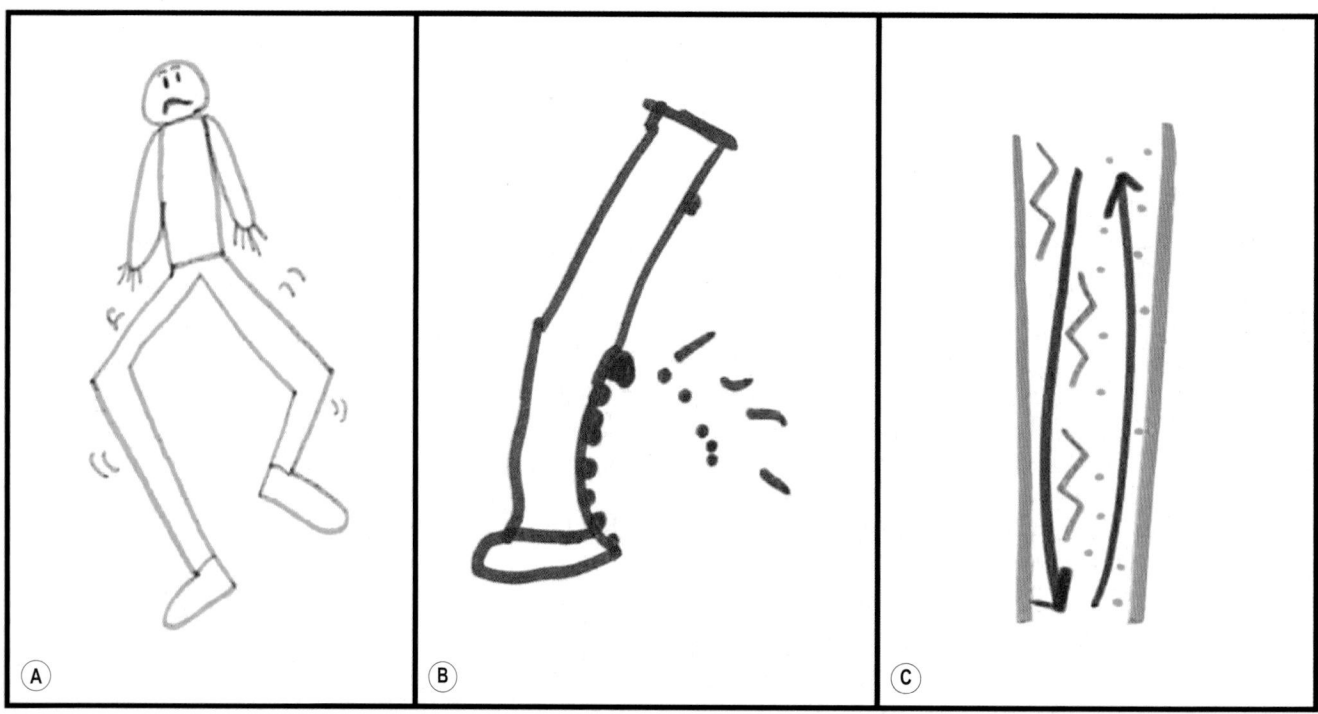

• **Fig. 44.4** Children's drawings of RLS symptoms: (A) From an 8-year-old boy: "It's like my legs are wiggly." (B) From an 11-year-old girl: "Well this picture shows like, see like it's ant bites that's kind of showing you that it's really hurting me like in those areas." (C) From a 14-year-old girl: "I feel stuff going up and down my legs where it just tingles. And that's more when it starts feeling like a little numb and then these represent my tingles. And then the red would be just when it hurts."[101]

In 2010, a multidimensional, self-administered, patient-reported outcome questionnaire (the *Pediatric Restless Legs Syndrome Severity Scale* [P-RLS-SS]) was published to assess pediatric RLS symptom severity and impact.[16] In addition to establishing a metric, this study demonstrated that children experience RLS symptoms during both daytime and nighttime. Many children provided nonverbal descriptions of their symptoms using a visual analog scale and free-hand drawings of their experiences.[101] Despite variations of interpretation, such visual approaches may be more appropriate for diagnosing RLS in younger or less fluent children, especially when one is searching for a starting point in the diagnostic process (Fig. 44.4).

Children provide imaginative descriptions of RLS symptoms: "soda bubbles in my legs," "ants biting my leg," "just want to move," or "got to kick."[5,15,102] Although it is not common for children to use the term "urge to move" in relationship to their description of RLS symptoms, it is

---

• BOX 44.2   Conditions that May Result in Secondary (or Reactive) Restless Legs Syndrome in Children

- Endocrine
  - Diabetes
  - Thyroid disease
- Musculoskeletal
  - Osgood-Schlatter
  - Muscle soreness
  - Injury (e.g., sprain, bruise, strain)
  - Cramps
  - Arthritis
  - Connective tissue disorders (e.g., plantar fasciitis)
  - Myopathy (congenital or acquired)
- Neurovascular
  - Positional discomfort (e.g., "pins-and-needles")
  - Peripheral neuropathy
  - Radiculopathy
  - Myelopathy
  - Sickle cell disease
  - Multiple sclerosis
- Neoplasm
- Skin
  - Dermatitis
  - Dry skin substances
- Antidopaminergic medications
  - SSRI medications
  - Tricyclic medications
  - Caffeine
- Other
  - ADHD
  - Iron deficiency
  - Oppositional defiant disorder
  - Pregnancy
  - Celiac disease
  - Uremia

ADHD, Attention-deficit/hyperactivity disorder; *SSRI*, selective serotonin reuptake inhibitor.

---

helpful to allow them to physically demonstrate compensatory maneuvers such as wiggling, rubbing, kicking, hitting, and even constantly moving "to find the cool spot." After exhausting one's direct inquiry with a child it is sometimes helpful to incorporate the parent into the discussion to remind the child of bedtime rituals and activities that may provide some recall. During the day, it is common to note some degree of classroom difficulty, and the child's teacher or parent may be helpful in this regard. Difficulty sitting quietly at a desk and paying attention, irritability, and hyperactivity may be notable symptoms of children with RLS. The overlap with ADHD-like symptoms is often brought up in this context. To distinguish between these two sets of *restlessness* symptoms, it is helpful to remember that in RLS the hyperactivity is caused by an *internal* sensory discomfort, whereas in ADHD it is related to an interaction with the *external* environment.

Age-associated causes of secondary RLS include joint pain and arthritis, Osgood-Schlatter disease, dysesthesias related to peripheral neuropathy or radiculopathy, akathisia related to antidopaminergic medications, and cutaneous pain related to dermatitis or rashes (Box 44.2). Identification of one of these entities or RLS should prompt clinicians to ask for symptoms of the other. Another condition commonly associated with, and often possibly identical to, RLS is that of *growing pains*. Children diagnosed with growing pains unrelated to any other identifiable disorder commonly demonstrate a strong family history of RLS and, in many cases, fulfill the diagnostic criteria for RLS.[103] The prevalence of growing pains in children ages 4–6 years measured with validated instruments is as high as 37%.[104] And, the presence of typical growing pains in children with either a family history of growing pains or RLS should prompt clinicians to consider a diagnosis of RLS.

Irritability, depression, anxiety, and hyperactivity are noted in children with RLS and often are associated with sleep deprivation and comorbid conditions such as panic disorder, generalized anxiety disorder, ADHD, oppositional defiant disorder (ODD), and depression. Parasomnias, sleep-related movement disorders, and insomnias also may be the presenting symptoms in some cases of childhood RLS.[5,102,105]

Although RLS is a clinical diagnosis that does not require testing, it is not possible to determine the presence or effect of PLMS on a child's sleep without a test. Parental reports and even clinical evaluation by trained sleep clinicians are not adequate predictors of PLMS.[106,107] Sleep testing is also required when symptoms suggest other sleep disorders.

Restless Legs Syndrome and Attention-Deficit/Hyperactivity Disorder

From the mid-1990s to the present, an increased prevalence of RLS and PLMD has been noted in children with symptoms consistent with ADHD.[4,31] Despite limited sample sizes, estimates for RLS in the ADHD pediatric population range between 10.5% and 44%, and the estimated prevalence of ADHD in the RLS population is similarly increased (18–30%).[15,99,108–112] The relationship between RLS and attention-deficit disorder (ADD)/ADHD is complex because sleep deprivation in children may mimic the hyperactivity and inattention noted in ADD and ADHD.

Objective sleep measures demonstrate increased sleep disruption in children with ADHD (with findings of PLMS, sleep-disordered breathing [SDB], increased sleep-onset latency, and increased number of stage shifts per hour of sleep).[113,114] Theories concerning the high correlation between RLS/PLMD and ADHD often focus on sleep deprivation as a cause for the symptoms of hyperactivity and inattention in ADHD. ADHD, like RLS, is a complex neurodevelopmental disorder with multiple subtypes that likely represent dysfunction within several neural systems. A relationship with RLS is supported by the observation that the most effective treatments for ADHD are stimulants (which block dopamine transport), neural imaging findings in ADHD demonstrate neuroanatomical and physiologic dysfunction of the frontostriatal system, and executive function deficits noted in ADHD are secondary to dopaminergic transmission abnormalities. Initial investigations using several of the previously identified RLS-linked SNPs (MEIS1, BTBD9, and MAP2K5) demonstrated no significant associations with ADHD, although BTBD9 SNPs show nominal significance.[115]

Both RLS and ADHD demonstrate an association with iron deficiency. Studies of children with RLS, ADHD, or both show a relationship with relatively low serum ferritin measures when compared to age- and gender-matched controls.[114,116–118] Treatment for relative iron deficiency using oral iron repletion in children with ADHD has been studied in a small randomized, double-blind, placebo-controlled trial.[119] Iron treatment demonstrated benefits in both Clinical Global Impression scales and ADHD rating scales.

For additional discussion, also see Chapter 15.

Restless Legs Syndrome and Restless Sleep Disorder in Children

In 2018, DelRosso and colleagues described a group of children with restless sleep who did not fulfill criteria for RLS or PLMD.[120] PSG metrics demonstrated a similar decreased sleep efficiency in the restless sleep group versus an RLS group when compared with controls, without evidence of PLMS that was noted in the RLS group. Serum iron testing showed an association with a relatively more severe iron deficiency in the restless sleep group versus the RLS group. Both parental reports and PSG data suggested that the "restlessness" in the restless sleep group was due to large body movements, whereas in the RLS group restlessness was due to leg discomfort, and an urge to move the legs along with PLMS. Movement analysis indicated that the number of total body movements (head, trunk, four limbs, legs, and entire body) per hour was significantly higher in the restless sleep group (7.34/hr ± 1.3) versus the RLS group (3.38/hr ± 1.1) or controls (2.25/hr ± 0.6).

From these data, the authors specified a total body movement index of 5/hr or more as a threshold for the diagnosis of a potentially novel pediatric sleep disorder, restless sleep disorder (RSD).

In addition to having a higher total body movement index, children fulfilling these criteria do not show the periodicity of movements, unlike the periodicity of leg movements in children with RLS, and their body movements occur throughout the night without regard to sleep stage or circadian time. In a separate retrospective analysis of 300 consecutive children evaluated for sleep problems in a single center (252 with PSG data), the RSD criteria set by DelRosso's group were applied and an estimated prevalence of 7.7% was observed.[121]

Additional large-scale studies are needed to corroborate these findings; however, these observations are of particular interest in relation to RLS, because many children with restless sleep who do not fulfill standard RLS and/or PLMD criteria, may in fact be suffering with a separate disorder that includes features of RLS such as iron deficiency, reduced sleep efficiency, and daytime neurocognitive symptoms.

Treatment and Management of Restless Legs Syndrome/Periodic Limb Movement Disorder

The Behavioral Approach

Sleep-onset association and limit-setting behavioral sleep disorders, inadequate sleep hygiene, and insufficient sleep can all result in symptomatic worsening and render even the best medical therapies ineffective (see Chapters 8 and 14). For this reason, the initial approach to RLS/PLMD treatment is education to establish proper bedtime behaviors, ensure a nonstimulating environment, avoid exercise and excitement before bed, and control access to food and drink during the night. The use of cognitive and physical countermeasures for RLS symptoms, such as physical relaxation techniques, warm baths, and cognitive restructuring, may be helpful during the sleep-onset routine in children suffering from RLS. It is also critical to consider activators of RLS symptoms such as sleep deprivation and certain drugs and medications (caffeine, nicotine, SSRIs, TCAs, antiemetics, and antihistamines). Recently, studies in adults using cognitive behavioral therapy (CBT) approaches typically applied to patients suffering with insomnia demonstrate significant benefits in sleep efficiency, total sleep time, latency to sleep onset, wake after sleep onset, and anxiety for RLS patients.[122] Additional research is needed to understand if traditional CBT approaches may be applied in children with RLS as well.

The Pharmacologic Approach

Iron Supplementation

Initial studies in children with comorbid RLS and ADHD showed that they had lower ferritin levels than children with ADHD alone, and they also had more severe symptoms of ADHD.[118] More recently, a retrospective analysis of children with RLS treated with oral iron therapy showed a clear benefit that was noted on average 3 months after starting therapy.[123] Symptom resolution occurred in 57% of children, and improvement in 33%; only 10% were nonresponders.

Given the evidence of relative iron body storage deficits in children with RLS, it is now recommended to obtain serum levels before embarking on any therapy. At a minimum, a

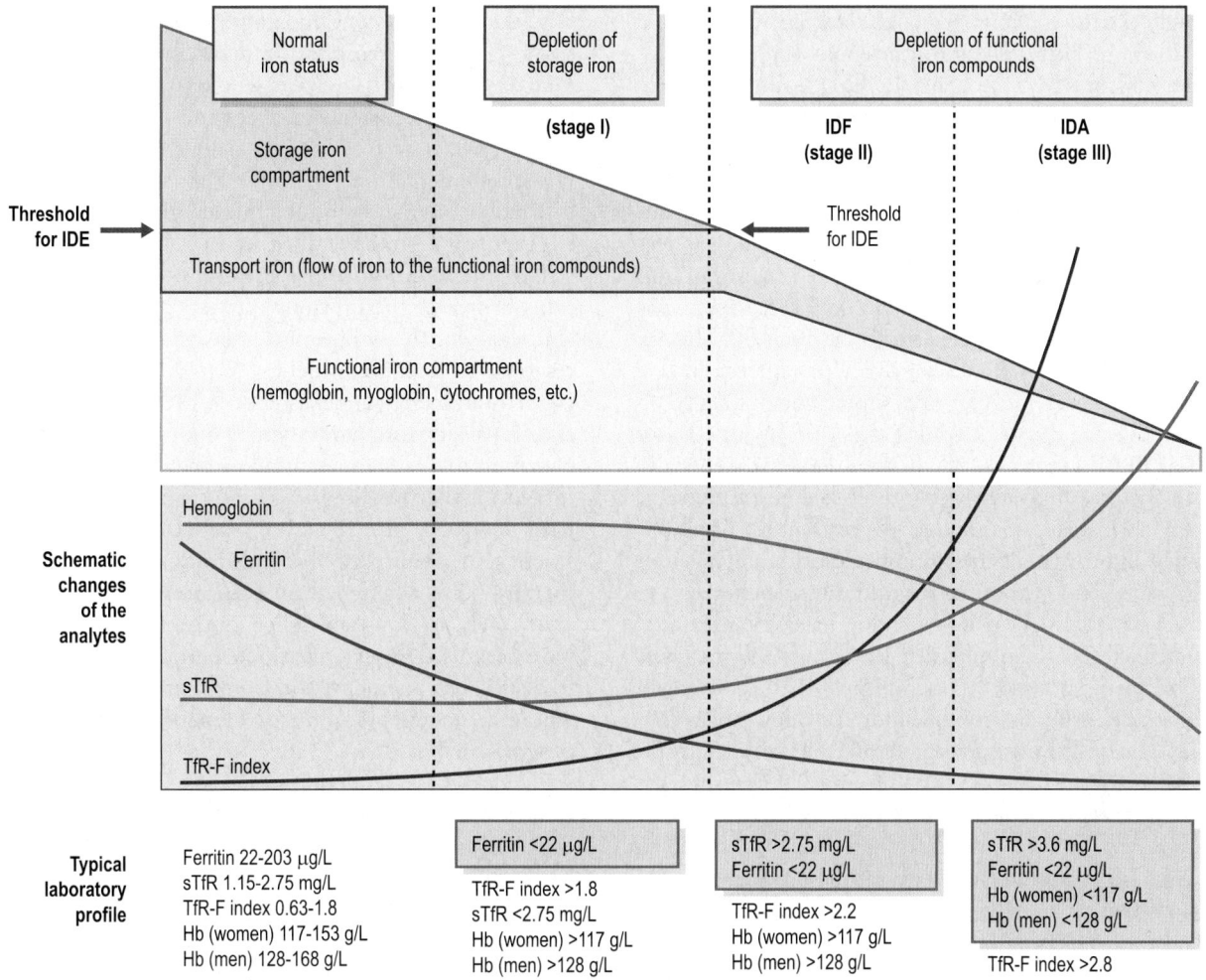

• **Fig. 44.5** Stages of iron deficiency (ID) in the body correlated with typical laboratory values. From left to right, as body iron stores become depleted, storage becomes increasingly reduced as reflected by falling serum ferritin levels. As the stages of ID progress (defined by laboratory values within the boxes at the bottom of the figure), transport and functional iron compartments become impacted resulting in iron-deficient erythropoiesis (*IDE*) and iron-deficiency anemia (*IDA*). Of note, hemoglobin *(Hb)* values do not reflect iron depletion until the last stages of iron deficiency. IDF, iron-deficient functional component. (*From Suominen P, Punnonen K, Rajamaki A, Irjala K. Serum transferrin receptor and transferrin receptor-ferritin index identify healthy subjects with subclinical iron deficits. Blood. 1998;92(8):2934–2939.*)

serum ferritin and a complete blood count (CBC) should be obtained, although total iron-binding capacities, transferrin, and transferrin receptor (TfR) are often included. It is important to remember that infection, liver disease, cancer, or significant stress can elevate ferritin levels and lead to inaccurate conclusions about iron status. Serum ferritin levels (and iron stores) may also be decreased without overt iron-deficiency anemia (i.e., without low hemoglobin or hematocrit levels). It is particularly important to understand the physiology of body iron compartmentalization when testing RLS patients (Fig. 44.5). Functional iron constituents such as hemoglobin, generally used as surrogates for body iron levels, are preserved at the expense of stored iron. Thus just knowing that hemoglobin levels are normal is incomplete information; it is important to also note the relative ferritin and transferrin levels to complete the iron metabolism picture.

Current recommendations for iron supplementation in children with RLS symptoms suggest treatment when the serum ferritin is <50 ng/mL.[124] This recommendation is partially based on the finding that in adult RLS patients a serum ferritin <50 ng/mL is associated with increased symptoms.[125,126] Also, subjects with ferritin levels below that level are significantly more responsive to iron repletion therapy. The goal of therapy is to achieve a ferritin level of 80–100 ng/mL because saturation of peripheral iron stores typically occurs in this range.

Deficits in serum ferritin often go unrecognized, even with testing, because the lower end of the normal reference ranges typically are listed as well below the 50 ng/mL level, i.e., below the level where RLS and PLMD symptoms may emerge.

The literature supports the use of iron repletion therapy to treat both RLS and PLMS symptoms in children.[105,123,127,128]

Although extensive clinical data are lacking with regards to this therapy, both oral and intravenous (IV) iron repletion methods for RLS are available. Oral dosing is usually 3–6 mg/kg/day and supplements should be taken on an empty stomach with vitamin C for improved absorption. To help reduce common gastrointestinal side effects and to maximize absorption, supplements should be taken without calcium-containing foods or drinks. Repeat testing is recommended within 2–3 months to confirm a change in iron levels and also to ensure that levels do not exceed the therapeutic range. Once serum ferritin levels reach 80–100 ng/mL, iron therapy may be discontinued or tapered. In one retrospective 2-year study of iron supplementation in 105 children (average age 10.2 years ± 5.3 years) with RLS (n = 41) or PLMD (n = 64), all children demonstrated a significant increase in average ferritin levels and a significant decrease in PLMi at 3–6 months, 1–2 years, and >2 years.[129] Sustained improvement in symptoms and underlying iron storage were noted without any significant side effects.

In adults, trials of IV iron therapy have demonstrated significant effects on serum ferritin levels and, in some cases, complete amelioration of RLS symptoms.[130–132] There are no similar studies using IV iron in children. Following IV iron therapy, serum ferritin retesting should be considered if a child reports a return of RLS symptoms or to ensure that ferritin levels remain >50 ng/mL. Clinically, the use of low-molecular-weight IV iron dextran compounds is noted to result in a superior outcomes without the previously noted hypersensitivity and allergic reactions related to higher-molecular-weight formulations.[133,134]

Other Forms of Pharmacotherapy

In addition to iron repletion, other forms of pharmacotherapy may be required if symptoms impact sleep or daytime activities on a regular basis, although no current U.S. Food and Drug Administration (FDA)-approved options are available for children. Occasional symptoms, occurring less than once a week, may be treated on an as-needed basis rather than with daily prophylactic treatment. When moderately severe RLS symptoms are present in adults (symptoms 2 days per week or more), daily drug therapy is suggested. Painful, intrusive nighttime symptoms, or those that cause daytime dysfunction, are more likely to engender a medical response.

The five general categories of medications most commonly used to treat RLS symptoms are dopaminergic agents, antiadrenergics, opioids, anticonvulsants (including alpha-2-delta ligands), and benzodiazepines.

Dopaminergics

Treatment with dopamine therapy may control both sensory and motor symptoms. Dopaminergic medications have also proven successful in case reports and small open-label studies of children with RLS with and without ADHD;[5,135–143] but there have been no large-scale, double-blind, placebo-controlled trials using dopaminergic medications in children with RLS or PLMD.

L-dopa was the first dopamine agent shown to be effective for both the sensory and motor symptoms of RLS.[144] Due to its short half-life (1.5–2 hours), it is usually reserved as an abortive or diagnostic agent and is not routinely used for prophylaxis.[12] In addition, L-dopa has a high reported rate of augmentation (up to 60–73% of adult users).[145,146] The rate of augmentation in children has not been studied.

Augmentation, as defined by the Max Planck Institute Criteria, includes three basic features: (1) increased symptoms in five of the previous 7 days, (2) no other identifiable cause for the symptom change, and (3) a prior positive response to dopamine therapy. Two additional features of augmentation are (1) persistence or paradoxical response to additional dopaminergic therapy and (2) an earlier return of symptoms.[147] Augmentation causes a shift of RLS symptoms to earlier in the day, it leads to an increase in body parts involved, and it may be associated with change in severity or quality of discomfort during pharmacologic therapy. Also, augmentation is increased when serum ferritin levels are low and when dopaminergic medications have been used for extended time periods.[148] It is important to distinguish augmentation from tolerance, early morning rebound, neuroleptic-induced akathisia, and RLS disease progression.[148]

Tolerance is a reduction in medication effectiveness over time, often necessitating an increase in dose. It is unclear if this is related to the development of augmentation, but it has been reported to precede some cases of augmentation in adults.

Neuroleptic-induced akathisia is distinguished from augmentation by its non-circadian pattern as well as the inner *sense* of overall body restlessness rather than discrete limb restlessness.

If augmentation is noted, the first course of action is to test serum ferritin levels and treat the patient accordingly. Following this, an immediate reduction of dopaminergic therapy to the lowest tolerated dose should both result in symptomatic improvement and serve to confirm the diagnosis of augmentation. If augmentation persists, the dopaminergic agent should be discontinued and alternative medical therapy (such as described next) may be instituted.[148]

Dopaminergic agents that are approved by the FDA to treat moderate to severe RLS in adults include the nonergot selective D2, D3, D4 agonists ropinirole, pramipexole, and rotigotine. The longer half-lives of the first two of these (oral) agents (6–8 hours for ropinirole and 8–10 hours for pramipexole) and the lower total daily dose and lower augmentation rate (3.5–30%) favors them for prophylactic therapy in moderate to severe RLS.[149] In 2012, a transdermal dopamine agonist delivery system with rotigotine was approved by the FDA for moderate to severe RLS. Initial studies conducted with this delivery system demonstrate significant benefit for adult RLS patients with less augmentation and side effects when compared with oral treatments.[150] The risk/benefit of dopamine agonist therapies in children should be addressed on a case-by-case basis.

The common side effects of dopamine agonists in adults include nausea, vomiting, nasal congestion, headaches, insomnia, hypersomnia, fluid retention, and augmentation. The neurodevelopmental effects of dopamine agonists on humans are unknown. Given the plasticity of the central nervous system's dopaminergic pathways, it is difficult to predict the rates of side effects, augmentation, and any potential detrimental effects in children. In some cases, particularly with co-occurring ADHD or obsessive-compulsive disorder (OCD), children may manifest increased impulsive behaviors and even obsessive thinking with dopaminergic therapy. The long-term effects of childhood dopamine agonist therapy on the symptomatic progression of RLS are also unknown, and longitudinal research is required to understand the complex interaction between therapy and the course of disease progression from childhood into adulthood.

Antiadrenergics

Clonidine is sometimes employed in the treatment of RLS and comorbid ADHD-related insomnia, although it is generally used as an antihypertensive or anxiolytic (due to its alpha-2-receptor agonist properties).[151,152] In a small randomized, double-blind, placebo-controlled trial, clonidine was shown to effectively treat RLS sensory symptoms in adults without significant side effects.[153] Clonidine is commonly used as a pediatric sleep aid[154] (even though not approved by the FDA for this purpose) and has pharmacologic attributes that make it particularly useful for treating hyperactivity-related symptoms in children. For RLS sufferers, it may also aid in reducing overactive sympathetic nervous system outflow that is theorized to contribute to PLMS and the exacerbation of associated medical conditions such as hypertension and cardiovascular disease. The most common side effects are sedation and hypotension.

Opioids

Opioids are not often prescribed as prophylactic therapy but usually are reserved for treatment of painful refractory RLS or cases of dopaminergic augmentation. In adults with RLS, the efficacy of oral and intrathecal opioids, such as methadone, morphine, and oxycodone, has been demonstrated in double-blind, placebo-controlled trials and case reports.[155–159] The pharmacologic action of opioids with regards to RLS is thought to be mediated through interactions with the dopamine system.[160] In 2011, a 10-year retrospective analysis compared adults who were treated for moderate to severe RLS with dopamine agonists (pergolide and pramipexole) with those treated with methadone and demonstrated some important outcomes favoring opioid therapy.[161] Treatment with low-dose methadone (median of 10 mg), for example, demonstrated none of the discontinuation or augmentation that is seen with dopamine agonists. In addition, the successful use of opioids as a bridging agent after withdrawal from dopaminergic therapy (partly due to

an indirect dopaminergic mechanism) suggests that opioids may be safely implemented in specific RLS populations. The effective control of refractory pain-related symptoms (that can occur in severe RLS or as a result of augmentation) is a primary reason to consider opioid therapy. Polysomnographic studies also demonstrate that opioids do not consistently reduce PLMS but do reduce associated arousals.[156]

The centrally acting, non-narcotic analgesic, tramadol, is an alternative to opioid use in children, given its lower abuse potential and fewer adverse side effects. Small open-label studies have demonstrated the effectiveness of this medication in treating the subjective complaints associated with RLS in adults;[162] however, similar studies have not been conducted in children.

Anticonvulsants

In adults, studies demonstrate the acute and long-term benefits of the alpha-2-delta agonist gabapentin[163–165] and the prodrug gabapentin enacarbil[166–168] in the management of RLS-related symptoms. Data suggest that the major effect of this class of agents in the treatment of RLS is amelioration of sensory symptoms; however, a significant reduction in PLMS has been noted as well.[163,164] In addition, it is now thought that alpha-2-delta ligands may act by reducing excitatory glutamate neurotransmission associated with BID adenosinergic-mediated hyperarousal.[169] Gabapentin is often considered a first choice for children experiencing sleep-onset difficulty and RLS symptoms because this drug is known to enhance slow-wave sleep and reduce pain. There are few adverse side effects (emotional lability and edema are most notable). Because there is no appreciable metabolism of gabapentin in humans, resulting in circulatory renal excretion, it is safe to use in combination with many other medications. In 2011, gabapentin enacarbil was approved by the FDA for the treatment of moderate to severe RLS in adults.[170] A single dose of 600 mg was suggested. However, there is no evidence to support this treatment in children. One study investigating gabapentin for insomnia in children used doses at bedtime starting at 5 mg/kg/dose up to 15 mg/kg/dose.[171] Gabapentin is excreted in human breast milk and both gabapentin and gabapentin enacarbil are classified as pregnancy category C, which means they should only be used in pregnancy if the potential benefits justify the potential risks to the fetus.

Benzodiazepines

In the past, clonazepam was the most commonly used medication for RLS.[172,173] Double-blind, placebo-controlled trials demonstrated significant benefits in objective sleep efficiency and subjective sleep quality despite an absence of effects on PLMS.[174] Clonazepam has a very long half-life of 18–50 hours, which may be useful in children due to prolonged sleeping times. When it has been used to treat children with RLS and ADHD, hyperactivity has been aggravated in some children. In adults with RLS, the benefits

CLINICAL PEARLS

- Childhood RLS is usually familial.
- Periodic leg/limb movement disorder may be present before sensory symptoms of RLS appear.
- Children with restless sleep, who do not fulfill RLS or PLMD criteria, may have a newly described sleep disorder, restless sleep disorder (RSD).
- RLS incidence is increased in children with ADHD, depression, iron deficiency, or central nervous system disorders; it is also increased in those taking medications that impact dopamine function.
- Low iron stores, and iron-dependent adenosine and dopamine impairment, are likely factors in the development of RLS.
- Low iron stores are detected by measurement of ferritin (not simply iron, hemoglobin, or hematocrit).
- Patients with low iron stores, as determined by findings of ferritin levels below 50 ng/mL, may benefit from iron therapy.
- Although there are no FDA-approved medications for childhood RLS, there are several medical and behavioral therapies available that provide symptomatic relief with limited side effects.

of other benzodiazepines, such as temazepam, and non-benzodiazepine sedative hypnotics in the imidazopyridine class, such as zolpidem, are documented in the literature.[175,176]

Other Agents

Pharmacotherapies that alter dopaminergic and/or other monoaminergic pathways have demonstrated benefits for RLS sufferers. Bupropion inhibits dopamine and noradrenaline reuptake and is typically used as an antidepressant. A number of small studies in the adult literature demonstrate the beneficial effects of bupropion use for RLS sensory symptoms and sleep quality outcomes.[177,178] Research in adults also supports the use of bupropion for treating PLMS and PLMD.[177,178] Of note, bupropion is often a treatment of choice for cases of co-occurring RLS and depression. It may be especially useful when antidepressant-induced RLS exacerbation occurs and as an alternative to traditional SSRI and TCA treatments. The side effects of bupropion include potentiating seizures (in epilepsy patients) and hypomania (in genetically susceptible individuals) due to heightened dopaminergic function. In children and adolescents, an increased risk for suicide has also been reported with the use of some antidepressants. For these reasons, clinicians should discuss the potential risks with parents prior to prescription.

References

1. DelRosso LM, Mogavero MP, Baroni A, Bruni O, Ferri R. Restless Legs Syndrome in Children and Adolescents. *Psychiatr Clin North Am.* 2024;47(1):147–161.
2. Ekbom KA. Restless legs syndrome. *Acta Med Scand Supp.* 1945;158:1–122.
3. Walters AS, Picchietti DL, Ehrenberg BL, et al. Restless legs syndrome in childhood and adolescence. *Pediatr Neurol.* 1994;11(3):241–245.
4. Picchietti DL, Walters AS. Restless legs syndrome and periodic limb movement disorder in children and adolescents: Comorbidity with attention-deficit hyperactivity disorder. *Child Adolesc Psychiatr Clin N Am.* 1996;5:729–740.
5. Picchietti DL, Stevens HE. Early manifestations of restless legs syndrome in childhood and adolescence. *Sleep Med.* 2008;9(7):770–781.
6. Lavigne GJ, Montplaisir JY. Restless legs syndrome and sleep bruxism: Prevalence and association among Canadians. *Sleep.* 1994;17:739–743.
7. Berger K, Luedemann J, Trenkwalder C, et al. Sex and the risk of restless legs syndrome in the general population. *Arch Intern Med.* 2004;164:196–202.
8. Ulfberg J, Nystrom B, Carter N, et al. Prevalence of restless legs syndrome among men aged 18 to 64 years: An association with somatic disease and neuropsychiatric symptoms. *Mov Disord.* 2001;16:1159–1163.
9. Walters AS, Hickey K, Maltzman J, et al. A questionnaire study of 138 patients with restless legs syndrome: The "Night-Walkers" survey. *Neurology.* 1996;46(1):92–95.
10. The International RLS Study Group. Validation of the International Restless Legs Syndrome Study Group rating scale for restless legs syndrome. *Sleep Med.* 2003;4:121–132.
11. Zucconi M, Ferini-Strambi L. Epidemiology and clinical findings of restless legs syndrome. *Sleep Med.* 2004;5:293–299.
12. Allen RP, Walters AS, Montplaisir J, et al. Restless legs syndrome prevalence and impact: REST general population study. *Arch Intern Med.* 2005;165(11):1286–1292.
13. Juuti AK, Laara E, Rajala U, et al. Prevalence and associated factors of restless legs in a 57-year-old urban population in northern Finland. *Acta Neurol Scand.* 2010;122(1):63–69.
14. Henning W, Walters AS, Allen RP, et al. Impact, diagnosis and treatment of restless legs syndrome (RLS) in a primary care population: The REST (RLS epidemiology, symptoms and treatment) primary care study. *Sleep Med.* 2004;5(3):237–246.
15. Picchietti D, Allen RP, Walters AS, et al. Restless legs syndrome: Prevalence and impact in children and adolescents – the Peds REST study. *Pediatrics.* 2007;120(2):253–266.
16. Arbuckle R, Abetz L, Durmer JS, et al. Development of the pediatric restless legs syndrome severity scale (P-RLS-SS): A patient-reported outcome measure of pediatric RLS symptoms and impact. *Sleep Med.* 2010;11:897–906.
17. American Academy of Sleep Medicine. International Classification of Sleep Disorders. 2nd ed. Diagnostic and Coding Manual. American Academy of Sleep Medicine; 2005.
18. O'Brien LM, Holbrook CR, Jones F, et al. Ethnic difference in periodic limb movements in children. *Sleep Med.* 2007;8(3):240–246.
19. Stefansson H, Rye DB, Hicks A, et al. A genetic risk factor for periodic limb movements in sleep. *N Eng J Med.* 2007;357(7):639–647.
20. Walters AS, Lavigne G, Hening The scoring of movements in sleep. *J Clin Sleep Med.* 2007;3(2):155–167.
21. Gamaldo CE, Earley CJ. Restless legs syndrome: A clinical update. *Chest.* 2006;130(5):1596–1604.
22. Benes H, Walters AS, Allen RP, et al. Definition of restless legs syndrome, how to diagnose it, and how to differentiate it from

RLS mimics. *Mov Disord.* 2007;22(Suppl. 18):S401–S408. Review. Erratum in *Mov Disord.* 2008;23(8):1200.

23. Yang C, White DP, Winkelman JW. Antidepressants and periodic leg movements of sleep. *Biol Psychiatry.* 2005;58:510–514.

24. Hoque R, Chesson AL. Pharmacologically induced/exacerbated restless legs syndrome, periodic limb movements of sleep, and REM behavior disorder/REM sleep without atonia: Literature review, qualitative scoring, and comparative analysis. *J Clin Sleep Med.* 2010;6(1):79–83.

25. Shraf SM, Tubman A, Smale P. Prevalence of concomitant sleep disorders in patients with obstructive sleep apnea. *Sleep Breath.* 2005;9:50–56.

26. Al-Alawi A, Mulgrew A, Tench E, et al. Prevalence, risk factors and impact on daytime sleepiness and hypertension of periodic leg movements with arousals in patients with obstructive sleep apnea. *J Clin Sleep Med.* 2006;2(3):281–287.

27. Baran AS, Richert AC, Douglass AB, et al. Change in periodic limb movement index during treatment of obstructive sleep apnea with continuous positive airway pressure. *Sleep.* 2003;26(6):717–720.

28. Sforza E, Pichot V, Barthelemy JC, et al. Cardiovascular variability during periodic leg movements: A spectral analysis approach. *Clin Neurophysiol.* 2005;116:1096–1104.

29. Walters AS. ad Rye DB. Review of the relationship of restless legs syndrome and periodic limb movements in sleep to hypertension, heart disease and stroke. *Sleep.* 2009;32(5):589–597.

30. Gosselin N, Lanfranchi P, Michaud M, et al. Age and gender effects on heart rate activation associated with periodic leg movements in patients with restless legs syndrome. *Clin Neurophysiol.* 2003;114:2188–2195.

31. Picchietti DL, England SJ, Walters AS, et al. Periodic limb movement disorder and restless legs syndrome in children with attention-deficit hyperactivity disorder. *J Child Neurol.* 1998;13(12):588–594.

32. Chervin RD, Archbold KH, Dillon JE, et al. Associations between symptoms of inattention, hyperactivity, restless legs and periodic leg movements. *Sleep.* 2002;25(2):213–218.

33. Chervin RD, Dillon JE, Archbald KH, et al. Conduct problems and symptoms of sleep disorders in children. *J Am Acad Child Adolesc Psychiatry.* 2003;42(2):201–208.

34. Pearson VE, Allen RP, Dean T, et al. Cognitive deficits associated with restless legs syndrome (RLS). *Sleep Med.* 2006;7:25–30.

35. Frye SS, Fernandez-Mendoza J, Calhoun SL, et al. Neurocognitive and behavioral significance of periodic limb movements during sleep in adolescents with attention-deficit/hyperactivity disorder. *Sleep.* 2018;41(10):zsy129.

36. DelRosso LM, Lockhart C, Wrede JE, et al. Comorbidities in children with elevated periodic limb movement index during sleep. *Sleep.* 2020;13(2):zsz221.

37. Sevim S, Dogu O, Kaleagasi H, et al. Correlation of anxiety and depression symptoms in patients with restless legs syndrome: A population based survey. *J Neurol Neurosurg Psychiatry.* 2004;75(2):226–230.

38. Picchietti D, Winkelman JW. Restless legs syndrome, periodic limb movements in sleep, and depression. *Sleep.* 2005;28(7):891–898.

39. Winkelmann J, Prager M, Lieb R, et al. "Anxietas tibiarum." Depression and anxiety disorders in patients with restless legs syndrome. *J Neurol.* 2005;252(1):67–71.

40. Lee HB, Hening WA, Allen RP, et al. Restless legs syndrome is associated with DSM-IV major depressive disorder and panic disorder in the community. *J Neuropsychiatry Clin Neurosci.* 2008;20(1):101–105.

41. Zhuang S, Na M, Winkelman JW, et al. Association of restless legs syndrome with risk of suicide and self-harm. *JAMA Netw Open.* 2019;2(8):e199966.

42. Winkelman JW, Redline S, Baldwin CM, et al. Polysomnographic and health-related quality of life correlates of restless legs syndrome in the sleep heart health study. *Sleep.* 2009;32(6):772–778.

43. Happe S, Reese JP, Stiasny-Kolster K, et al. Assessing health-related quality of life in patients with restless legs syndrome. *Sleep Med.* 2009;10(3):295–305.

44. Allen RP, Burchell BJ, MacDonald B, et al. Validation of the self-completed Cambridge–Hopkins questionnaire (CH-RLSq) for ascertainment of restless legs syndrome (RLS) in a population survey. *Sleep Med.* 2009;10(10):1097–1100.

45. Rothdach AJ, Trenkwalder C, Haberstock J, et al. Prevalence and risk factors of RLS in an elderly population: The MEMO study. Memory and morbidity in Augsburg elderly. *Neurology.* 2000;54(5):1064–1068.

46. Crabtree VM, Ivanenko A, O'Brien LM, et al. Periodic limb movement disorder of sleep in children. *J Sleep Res.* 2003;12:73–81.

47. O'Brien LM, Holbrook CR, Faye Jones V, et al. Ethnic difference in periodic limb movements in children. *Sleep Med.* 2007;8:240–246.

48. Montgomery-Downs HE, O'Brien LM, Gulliver TE, et al. Polysomnographic characteristics in normal preschool and early school-aged children. *Pediatrics.* 2006;117(3):741–753.

49. Pennestri MH, Whittom S, Adam B, et al. PLMS and PLMW in healthy subjects as a function of age: Prevalence and interval distribution. *Sleep.* 2006;29(9):1183–1187.

50. Traeger N, Schultz B, Pollock AN, et al. Polysomnographic values in children 2–9 years old: Additional data and review of the literature. *Pediatr Pulmonol.* 2005;40(1):22–30.

51. Picchietti DL, Picchietti MA. Pediatric restless legs syndrome and periodic limb movement disorder: Parent–child pairs. *Sleep Med.* 2009;10:925–931.

52. Walters AS, Lavigne G, Hening W, et al. The scoring of movements in sleep. *J Clin Sleep Med.* 2007;3(2):155–167.

53. Ferri R, Zucconi M, Manconi M, et al. New approaches to the study of periodic leg movements during sleep in restless legs syndrome. *Sleep.* 2006;29(6):759–769.

54. Ferri R, Manconi M, Lanuzza B, et al. Age-related changes in periodic leg movements during sleep in patients with restless legs syndrome. *Sleep.* 2008;9(7):790–798.

55. Ferri R, Franceschini C, Zucconi M, et al. Sleep polygraphic study of children and adolescents with narcolepsy/cataplexy. *Dev Neuropsychol.* 2009;34(5):523–538.

56. Bruni O, Ferri R, Verrillo E, et al. New approaches to the study of leg movements during sleep in ADHD children. In Proceedings of the 20th meeting of the Associated Sleep Societies. *Sleep.* 2006;29(Suppl. 2006):259.

57. Trotti LM, Bliwise DL, Greer SA, et al. Correlates of PLMs variability over multiple nights and impact upon RLS diagnosis. *Sleep Med.* 2009;10:668–671.

58. Sforza E, Johannes M, Bassetti C. The PAM-RL ambulatory device for detection of periodic leg movements: A validation study. *Sleep Med.* 2005;6:407–413.

59. Morrish E, King MA, Pilsworth SN, et al. Periodic limb movement in a community population detected by a new actigraphy technique. *Sleep Med.* 2002;3:489–495.

60. Rye DB. Parkinson's disease and RLS: The dopaminergic bridge. *Sleep Med.* 2004;5:317–328.

61. Clemens S, Rye D, Hochman S. RLS revisiting the dopamine hypothesis from the spinal cord perspective. *Neurology.* 2006;67:125–130.

62. Nordlander NB. Restless legs. *Br J Phys Med*. 1954;17:160–162.

63. Earley CJ, Connor JR, Beard JL, et al. Abnormalities in CSF concentrations of ferritin and transferrin in restless legs syndrome. *Neurology*. 2000;54(8):1698–1700.

64. Mizuno S, Mihara T, Miyaoka T, et al. CSF iron, ferritin and transferrin levels in restless legs syndrome. *J Sleep Res*. 2005;14(1):43–47.

65. Earley CJ, Barker PB, Horska A, et al. MRI-determined regional brain iron concentrations in early- and late-onset restless legs syndrome. *Sleep Med*. 2006;7:459–461.

66. Allen RP, Barker PB, Wehrl F, et al. MRI measurement of brain iron in patients with restless legs syndrome. *Neurology*. 2001;56(2):263–265.

67. Schmidauer C, Sojer M, Seppi K, et al. Transcranial ultrasound shows nigral hypoechogenicity in restless legs syndrome. *Ann Neurol*. 2005;58(4):630–634.

68. Connor JR, Boyer PJ, Menzies SL, et al. Neuropathological examination suggests impaired brain iron acquisition in restless legs syndrome. *Neurology*. 2003;61(3):304–309.

69. Connor JR, Wang XS, Patton SM, et al. Decreased transferrin receptor expression by neuromelanin cells in restless legs syndrome. *Neurology*. 2004;62(9):1563–1567.

70. Erikson KM, Jones BC, Beard JL. Iron deficiency alters dopamine transporter functioning in rat striatum. *J Nutr*. 2000;130:831–837.

71. Erikson KM, Jones BC, Hess EJ, et al. Iron deficiency decreases dopamine D1 and D2 receptors in rat brain. *Pharmacol Biochem Behav*. 2001;69:409–418.

72. Wang X, Wiesinger J, Beard J, et al. Thy1 expression in the brain is affected by iron and is decreased in restless legs syndrome. *J Neurol Sci*. 2004;220(1–2):59–66.

73. Earley CJ, Ponnuru P, Wang X, et al. Altered iron metabolism in lymphocytes from subjects with restless legs syndrome. *Sleep*. 2008;31(6):847–852.

74. Quiroz C, Gulyani S, Ruiqian W, et al. Adenosine receptors as markers of brain iron deficiency: Implications for restless legs syndrome. *Neuropharmacology*. 2016;111:160–168.

75. Ferre S, Quiroz C, Guitart X, et al. Pivotal role of adenosine neurotransmission in restless legs syndrome. *Front Neurosci*. 2018;11:722.

76. Ferre S, Garcia-Borreguero D, Allen RP, Earley CJ. New insights into the neurobiology of restless legs syndrome. *Neuroscientist*. 2019;25(2):113–125.

77. Desai AV, Cherkas LF, Spector TD, et al. Genetic influences in self-reported symptoms of obstructive sleep apnoea and restless legs: A twin study. *Twin Res*. 2004;7(6):589–595.

78. Desautels A, Turecki G, Montplaisir J, et al. Identification of a major susceptibility locus for restless legs syndrome on chromosome 12q. *Am J Hum Genet*. 2001;69(6):1266–1270.

79. Desautels A, Tuercki G, Montplaisir J, et al. Restless legs syndrome: Confirmation of linkage to chromosome 12q, genetic heterogeneity, and evidence of complexity. *Arch Neurol*. 2005;62(4):591–596.

80. Bonati MT, Ferini-Strambi L, Aridon P, et al. Autosomal dominant restless legs syndrome maps on chromosome 14q. *Brain*. 2003;126(Pt 6):1485–1492.

81. Chen S, Ondo WG, Rao S, et al. Genomewide linkage scan identifies a novel susceptibility locus for restless legs syndrome on chromosome 9p. *Am J Hum Genet*. 2004;74(5):876–885.

82. Winkelmann J, Lichtner P, Putz B, et al. Evidence for further genetic locus heterogeneity and confirmation of RLS-1 in restless legs syndrome. *Mov Disord*. 2006;21(1):28–33.

83. Pichler I, Marroni F, Volpato CB, et al. Linkage analysis identifies a novel locus for restless legs syndrome on chromosome 2q in a South Tyrolean population isolate. *Am J Hum Genet*. 2006;79(4):716–723.

84. Levchenko A, Provost S, Montplaisir J, et al. A novel autosomal dominant restless legs syndrome locus maps to chromosome 20p13. *Neurology*. 2006;67(5):900–901.

85. Levchenko A, Montplaisir JY, Asselin G, et al. Autosomal dominant locus for restless legs syndrome in French-Canadians on chromosome 16p.12.1. *Mov Disord*. 2009;24(1):40–50.

86. Kemlink D, Plazzi G, Vetrugno R, et al. Suggestive evidence for linkage for restless legs syndrome on chromosome 19p13. *Neurogenetics*. 2008;9:75–82.

87. Winkelmann J, Czamara D, Schormair B, et al. Genome-wide association study identifies novel restless legs syndrome susceptibility loci on 2p14 and 16q12.1. *PLoS Genet*. 2011;7(7):e1002171.

88. Desaultes A, Turecki G, Montplaisir J, et al. Dopaminergic neurotransmission and restless legs syndrome: A genetic association analysis. *Neurology*. 2001;57:1304–1306.

89. Schormair B, Kemlink D, Roeske D, et al. PTPRD (protein tyrosine phosphatase receptor type delta) is associated with restless legs syndrome. *Nat Genet*. 2008;40:946–948.

90. Winkelmann J, Lichtner P, Schormair B, et al. Variants in the neuronal nitric oxide synthase (nNOS, NOS1) gene are associated with restless legs syndrome. *Mov Disord*. 2008;23:350–358.

91. Oexle K, Schormair B, Ried JS, et al. Dilution of candidates: The case of iron-related genes in restless legs syndrome. *Eur J Hum Genet*. 2012;21(4):410–414.

92. Winkelmann J, Schormair B, Lichtner P, et al. Genome-wide association study of restless legs syndrome identifies common variants in three genomic regions. *Nat Genet*. 2007;39(8):1000–1006.

93. Schormair B, Zhao C, Salminen AV, Oexle K, Winkelmann J. International EU-RLS-GENE Consortium. Reassessment of candidate gene studies for idiopathic restless legs syndrome in a large GWAS dataset of European ancestry. *Sleep*. 2022;45(8):zsac098.

94. Trenkwalder CM, Allen R, Hogel B, et al. Restless legs syndrome associated with major diseases–a systematic review and new concept. *Neurology*. 2016;86:1336–1343.

95. Muhle H, Neumann A, Lohmann-Hedrich K, et al. Childhood-onset restless legs syndrome: Clinical and genetic features of 22 families. *Mov Disord*. 2008;23(8):1113–1121.

96. Young JE, Vilariño-Güell C, Lin SC, et al. Clinical and genetic description of a family with a high prevalence of autosomal dominant restless legs syndrome. *Mayo Clin Proc*. 2009;84(2):134–188.

97. The International Restless Legs Syndrome Study Group. Toward a better definition of the restless legs syndrome. *Mov Disord*. 1995;10:634–642.

98. Allen RP, Picchietti DL, Henning WA, et al. Restless legs syndrome: Diagnostic criteria, special considerations, and epidemiology. A report from the RLS diagnosis and epidemiology workshop at the NIH. *Sleep Med*. 2003;4:101–119.

99. Cortese S, Konofal E, Lecendreux M, et al. Restless legs syndrome and attention-deficit/hyperactivity disorder: A review of the literature. *Sleep*. 2005;28(8):1007–1013.

100. Picchietti DL, Bruni O, Weer A, et al. Pediatric restless legs syndrome diagnostic criteria: An update by the International RLS Study Group. *Sleep Med*. 2013;14:1253–1259.

101. Picchietti DL, Arbuckle RA, Abetz L, et al. Pediatric restless legs syndrome: Analysis of symptom descriptions and drawings. *J Child Neurol*. 2011;26(11):1365–1376.

102. Mohri I, Kato-Nishimura K, Tachibana N, et al. RLS: An unrecognized cause for bedtime problems and insomnia in children. *Sleep Med*. 2008;9:701–702.

103. Rajaram A, Walters AS, England SJ, et al. Some children with growing pains may actually have restless legs syndrome. *Sleep*. 2004;27(4):767–773.

104. Evans AM, Scutter SD. Prevalence of growing pains in young children. *J Pediatr*. 2004;145:255–258.

105. Kryger MH, Otake K, Foerster J. Low body stores of iron and restless legs syndrome: A correctable cause of insomnia in adolescents and teenagers. *Sleep Med*. 2002;3:127–132.

106. Martin BT, Williamson BD, Edwards N, et al. Parental symptom report and periodic limb movements of sleep in children. *J Clin Sleep Med*. 2008;4(1):57–61.

107. Chervin RD, Hedger KM. Clinical prediction of periodic leg movements during sleep in children. *Sleep Med*. 2001;2:501–510.

108. Oner P, Dirik EB, Taner Y, et al. Association between low serum ferritin and restless legs syndrome in patients with attention deficit hyperactivity disorder. *Tohoku J Exp Med*. 2007;213(3):269–276.

109. Silvestri R, Gagliano A, Arico I, et al. Sleep disorders in children with attention-deficit/hyperactivity disorder (ADHD) recorded overnight by video-polysomnography. *Sleep Med*. 2009;10(10):1132–1138.

110. Wagner ML, Walters AS, Fisher BC. Symptoms of attention-deficit/hyperactivity disorder in adults with restless legs syndrome. *Sleep*. 2004;27(8):1499–1504.

111. Wiggs L, Montgomery P, Stores G. Actigraphic and parent reports of sleep patterns and sleep disorders in children with subtypes of attention-deficit hyperactivity disorder. *Sleep*. 2005;28(11):1437–1445.

112. Picchietti D, Allen RP, Walters AS, et al. Restless legs syndrome: Prevalence and impact in children and adolescents – the Peds REST study. *Pediatrics*. 2007;120(2):253–266.

113. Silvestri R, Gagliano A, Arico I, et al. Sleep disorders in children with ADHD recorded overnight by video-polysomnography. *Sleep Med*. 2009;10:1132–1138.

114. Konofal E, Lecendreux M, Cortese S. Sleep and ADHD. *Sleep Med*. 2010;11:652–658.

115. Schimmelmann BG, Friedel S, Nquyen TT, et al. Exploring the genetic link between RLS and ADHD. *J Psychiatr Res*. 2009;43(10):941–945.

116. Oner P, Dirik EB, Taner Y, et al. Association between low serum ferritin and restless legs syndrome in patients with attention deficit hyperactivity disorder. *Tohoku J Exp Med*. 2007;213:269–276.

117. Konofal E, Lecendreux M, Arnulf I, et al. Iron deficiency in children with attention-deficit/hyperactivity disorder. *Arch Pediatr Adolesc Med*. 2004;158:1113–1115.

118. Konofal E, Cortese S, Marchand M, et al. Impact of restless legs syndrome and iron deficiency on attention-deficit/hyperactivity disorder in children. *Sleep Med*. 2007;8:711–715.

119. Konofal E, Lecendreux M, Deron J, et al. Effects of iron supplementation on attention deficit hyperactivity disorder in children. *Pediatr Neurol*. 2008;38:20–26.

120. DelRosso LM, Bruni O, Ferri R. Restless sleep disorder in children: A pilot study on a tentative new diagnostic category. *Sleep*. 2018;41(8).

121. DelRosso LM, Ferri R. The prevalence of restless sleep disorder among a clinical sample of children and adolescents referred to a sleep centre. *J Sleep Res*. 2019;00:e12870.

122. Song ML, Park KM, Motamedi GK, Cho YW. Cognitive behavioral therapy for insomnia in restless legs syndrome patients. *Sleep Med*. 2020;74:227–234.

123. Mohri I, Kato-Nishimura K, Kagitani-Shimono K, et al. Evaluation of oral iron treatment in pediatric restless legs syndrome (RLS). *Sleep Med*. 2012;13(4):429–432.

124. Earley CJ. Restless legs syndrome. *N Engl J Med*. 2003;348(21):2103–2109.

125. Sun ER, Chen CA, Ho G, et al. Iron and the restless legs syndrome. *Sleep*. 1998;21:371–377.

126. O'Keeffe ST, Gavin K, Lavan JN. Iron status and restless legs syndrome in the elderly. *Age Ageing*. 1994;23(3):200–203.

127. Simakajornboon N, Gozal D, Vlasic V, et al. PLMS and iron status in children. *Sleep*. 2006;26(6):735–738.

128. Davis BJ, Rajput A, Rajput ML, et al. A randomized double-blind placebo-controlled trail of iron in restless legs syndrome. *Eur Neurol*. 2000;43:70–75.

129. Dye TJ, Jain SV, Simakajornboon N. Outcomes of long-term iron supplementation in pediatric restless legs syndrome/periodic limb movement disorder. *Sleep Med*. 2017;32:213–219.

130. Early CJ, Heckler D, Allen RP. Repeated IV doses of iron provide effective supplemental treatment of restless legs syndrome. *Sleep Med*. 2005;6(4):301–305.

131. Ondo IV WG. iron dextran for severe refractory RLS. *Sleep Med*. 2010;11:494–496.

132. Grote L, Leissner L, Hedner J, et al. A randomized, double-blind, placebo controlled, multi-center study of intravenous iron sucrose and placebo in the treatment of restless legs syndrome. *Mov Disord*. 2009;24(10):1445–1452.

133. Vaage-Nilsen O. Acute, severe and anaphylactoid reactions are very rare with low-molecular-weight iron dextran, CosmoFer. *Nephrol Dial Transplant*. 2008;23(10):3372 author reply 3372.

134. Auerbach M, Al Talib K. Low-molecular weight iron dextran and iron sucrose have similar comparative safety profiles in chronic kidney disease. *Kidney Int*. 2008;73(5):528–530.

135. Walters AS, Mandelbaum DE, Lewin DS, et al. Dopaminergic therapy in children with restless legs/periodic limb movements in sleep and ADHD. Dopaminergic Study Group. *Pediatr Neurol*. 2000;22:182–186.

136. Konofal E, Arnulf I, Lecendreux M, et al. Ropinirole in a child with ADHD and RLS. *Pediatr Neurol*. 2005;32:350–351.

137. Kotagal S, Silber MH. Childhood-onset restless legs syndrome. *Ann Neurol*. 2004;56(6):803–807.

138. Muhle H, Neumann A, Lohmann-Hedrich K, et al. Childhood-onset restless legs syndrome: Clinical and genetic features of 22 families. *Mov Disord*. 2008;23(8):1113–1121.

139. Starn AL, Udall JN Jr. Iron deficiency anemia, pica, and restless legs syndrome in a teenage girl. *Clin Pediatr (Phila)*. 2008;47(1):83–85.

140. Cortese S, Konofal E, Lecendreux M. Effectiveness of ropinirole for RLS and depressive symptoms in an 11-year-old girl. *Sleep Med*. 2009;10(2):259–261.

141. Picchietti DL, Walters AS. Moderate to severe periodic limb movement disorder in childhood and adolescence. *Sleep*. 1999;22(3):297–300.

142. Guilleminault C, Palombini L, Pelayo R, et al. Sleepwalking and sleep terrors in prepubertal children: What triggers them? *Pediatrics*. 2003;111(1):e17–e25.

143. Martinez S, Guilleminault C. Periodic leg movements in prepubertal children with sleep disturbance. *Dev Med Child Neurol.* 2004;46(11):765–770.

144. Conti CF, de Oliveira MM, Andriolo RB, et al. Levodopa for idiopathic restless legs syndrome: Evidence-based review. *Mov Disord.* 2007;22(13):1943–1951.

145. Allen RP, Earley CJ. Augmentation of the restless legs syndrome with carbidopa/levodopa. *Sleep.* 1996;19:205–213.

146. Garcia-Borreguero D, Williams A. Dopamine augmentation of restless legs syndrome. *Sleep Med Rev.* 2010;14:339–346.

147. Garcia-Borrequero D, Hogl B, Ferini-Strambi L, et al. Systemic evaluation of augmentation during treatment with ropinirole in restless legs syndrome (Willis–Ekbom disease): Results from a prospective, multicenter study over 66 weeks. *Mov Disord.* 2012;27(2):277–283.

148. Paulus W, Trenkwalder C. Less is more: Pathophysiology of dopaminergic related augmentation in restless legs syndrome. *Lancet Neurol.* 2006;5:878–886.

149. Trenkwalder C, Benes H, Poewe W. and the SP790 study group. Efficacy of rotigotine for treatment of moderate to severe restless legs syndrome: A randomized, double-blind, placebo-controlled trial. *Lancet Neurol.* 2008;7:595–604.

150. Newcorn JH, Schulz K, Harrison M, et al. Alpha 2 adrenergic agonists. Neurochemistry, efficacy, and clinical guidelines for use in children. *Pediatr Clin North Am.* 1998;45(5):1022–1099. [viii].

151. Prince JB, Wilens TE, Biederman J, et al. Clonidine for sleep disturbances associated with attention-deficit hyperactivity disorder: A systematic chart review of 62 cases. *J Am Acad Child Adolesc Psychiatry.* 1996;35(5):599–605.

152. Wager ML, Walters AS, Coleman RG, et al. Randomized double-blind placebo-controlled study of clonidine in restless legs syndrome. *Sleep.* 1996;19(1):52–58.

153. Owens JA, Rosen CL, Mindell JA. Medication use in the treatment of pediatric insomnia: Results of a survey of community-based pediatricians. *Pediatrics.* 2003;111(5 Pt 1):e628–e635.

154. Walters AS, Wagner ML, Hening WA, et al. Successful treatment of the idiopathic restless legs syndrome in a randomized double-blind trial of oxycodone versus placebo. *Sleep.* 1993;16:327–332.

155. Kaplan PW, Allen RP, Buchholz DW, et al. A double-blind, placebo-controlled study of the treatment of periodic limb movements in sleep using carbidopa/levodopa and propoxyphene. *Sleep.* 1993;16:717–723.

156. Ross DA, Narus MS, Nutt JG. Control of medically refractory RLS with intrathecal morphine:case report. *Neurosurgery.* 2008;62(1):e263.

157. Jakobsson B, Ruuth K. Successful treatment of RLS with an implanted pump for intrathecal drug delivery. *Acta Anaesthsiol Scand.* 2002;46:114–117.

158. Ondo WG. Methadone for refractory RLS. *Mov Disord.* 2005;20(3):345–348.

159. Walters AS. Review of receptor agonist and antagonist studies relevant to the opiate system in restless legs syndrome. *Sleep Med.* 2002;3:301–330.

160. Silver N, Allen RP, Senerth J, et al. A 10-year longitudinal assessment of dopamine agonists and methadone in the treatment of restless legs syndrome. *Sleep Med.* 2011;12:440–444.

161. Laurma H, Markkula J. Treatment of restless legs syndrome with tramadol: An open study. *J Clin Psychiatry.* 1999;60:241–244.

162. Garcia-Borreguero D, Larrosa O, de la Llave Y, et al. Treatment of restless legs syndrome with gabapentin: A double-blind, cross-over study. *Neurology.* 2002;59(10):1573–1579.

163. Happe S, Klosch G, Saletu B, et al. Treatment of idiopathic restless legs syndrome (RLS) with gabapentin. *Neurology.* 2001;57(9):1717–1719.

164. Happe S, Sauter C, Klosch G, et al. Gabapentin versus ropinirole in the treatment of idiopathic restless legs syndrome. *Neuropsychobiology.* 2003;48(2):82–86.

165. Cundy KC, Sastry S, Luo W, et al. Clinical pharmacokinetics of XP13512, a novel transported prodrug of gabapentin. *J Clin Pharmacol.* 2008;48(12):1378–1388.

166. Kushida CA, Becker PM, Ellenbogan AL, et al. XP052 Study Group. A randomized, double-blind, placebo-controlled trial of XP13512/GSK1838262 in patients with RLS. *Neurology.* 2009;72(5):439–446.

167. Bogan R, Bornemann MA, Kushida CA, et al. XP060 Study Group. Long-term maintenance treatment of RLS with gabapentin enacarbil: A randomized control study. *Mayo Clinic Proc.* 2010;85(7):693–694.

168. Lee DO, Zinman RB, Perkins AT, et al. XP053 Study Group. A randomized, double-blind, placebo-controlled study to assess the efficacy and tolerability of gabapentin enacarbil in subjects with restless legs syndrome. *J Clin Sleep Med.* 2011;7(3):282–292.

169. Ferre S, Earley C, Gulyani S, et al. In search of alternatives to dopaminergic ligands for the treatment of restless legs syndrome: Iron, glutamate and adenosine. *Sleep Med.* 2017;31:86–92.

170. Matthews WB. Treatment of restless legs syndrome with clonazepam. *BMJ.* 1979;1:751.

171. Robinson AA, Malow BA. Gabapentin shows promise in treating refractory insomnia in children. *J Child Neurol.* 2013;28(12):1618–1621.

172. Oshtory MA, Vijayan N. Clonazepam treatment of insomnia due to sleep myoclonus. *Arch Neurol.* 1980;37:119–120.

173. Saletu M, Ander P, Prause W, et al. RLS and PLMD acute placebo-controlled sleep laboratory studies with clonazepam. *Eur Neuropsychopharmacol.* 2001;11:153–161.

174. Silber MH, Ehrenberg BL, Allen RP, et al. An algorithm for the management of restless legs syndrome. *Mayo Clin Proc.* 2004;79(7):916–922.

175. Hening W, Allen R, Earley C, et al. The treatment of restless legs syndrome and periodic limb movement disorder. An American academy of sleep medicine review. *Sleep.* 1999;22(7):970–999.

176. Kim SW, Shin IS, Kim JM, et al. Bupropion may improve restless legs syndrome. A report of three cases. *Clin Neuropharmacol.* 2005;28:298–301.

177. Lee JJ, Erdos J, Wilkosz MF, et al. Bupropion as a possible treatment option for restless legs syndrome. *Ann Pharmacother.* 2009;43:370–374.

178. Nofzinger EA, Fasiczka A, Berman S, et al. Bupropion SR reduces periodic limb movements associated with arousals from sleep in depressed patients with periodic limb movement disorder. *J Clin Psychiatry.* 2000;61:858–862.

45

Sleep-Related Movement Disorders

Stephen H. Sheldon and Brittany Nance

CHAPTER HIGHLIGHTS

- Sleep-related movement disorders are relatively common in childhood. Diagnosis can generally be achieved through a thorough history and physical examination; however, polysomnogram may be necessary with consideration to expanded encephalography (EEG) to rule out seizure.
- As many sleep-related movement disorders are largely behavioral in nature, it is essential to reassure and educate families that these simple, non-purposeful, and usually stereotyped movements are benign and generally self-limited.
- Restless sleep disorder has been identified as a relatively new sleep-related movement disorder with pediatric research ongoing regarding long-term complications.
- Treatment should also focus on ensuring the safety of the child and easing the transition between wakefulness and sleep, often achieved by establishing consistent bedtime routines consisting of progressively more relaxing activities and strengthening positive associations between the sleep environment and relaxation.

Introduction

Sleep-related movement disorders (SRMDs) present a unique challenge to practitioners caring for children, as they can cause significant distress in parents and families. This class of clinical conditions is characterized by relatively simple, non-purposeful, and usually stereotyped movements that occur in sleep, primarily during sleep–wake transitions. These generally benign movements can represent self-soothing mechanisms, but at times are associated with physical injury, interfere with the sleep of the child and family, and may cause excessive daytime sleepiness. Typically, these movement disorders resolve spontaneously and do not have significant long-term consequences. Although the International Classification of Sleep Disorders (ICSD-3) lists restless legs syndrome (RLS) and periodic limb movements of sleep (PLMS) as SRMDs,[1]

these conditions will only be covered briefly, as they are described elsewhere in this book.

Assessment of Rhythmic Movements Surrounding the Sleep Period

When considering the diagnosis of a SRMD, it is essential to have a systematic and thorough approach (Box 45.1).[1] To differentiate SRMD from neurologic conditions with variable persistence during sleep such as a seizure disorder, dystonia, or Tourette's syndrome, one must first determine whether the movement disorder occurs only during sleep or if it also occurs during periods of wakefulness. If the movements occur only during sleep–wake transitions, then one must next decide if the movements are simple or complex. Complex, purposeful, and goal-directed movements, such as those represented by sleepwalking or confusional

---

• BOX 45.1 Diagnostic Criteria for Sleep-Related Rhythmic Movement Disorder[1]

Alternate names: body rocking, head banging, head rolling, body rolling, jactatio capitis nocturna, jactatio corporis nocturna, rhythmie du sommeil

Diagnostic Criteria

Criteria A–D must be met
A. The patient exhibits repetitive, stereotyped, and rhythmic motor behaviors involving large muscle groups.
B. The movements are predominantly sleep related, occurring near naptime or bedtime, or when the individual appears drowsy or asleep.
C. The behaviors result in a significant complaint as manifest by at least one of the following:
1. Interference with normal sleep.
2. Significant impairment in daytime function.
3. Self-inflicted bodily injury or likelihood of injury if preventive measures are not used.
D. The rhythmic movements are not better explained by another movement disorder or epilepsy.

TABLE 45.1	Clinical and Pathophysiological Subtypes of Sleep-Related Movement Disorder
Body rocking type	The whole body is rocked while on the hands and knees
Head banging type (*jactatio capitis nocturna*)	The head is forcibly moved, striking an object
Head rolling type	The head is moved laterally, typically while in the supine position
Other type	Includes body rolling, leg rolling, and leg banging
Combined type	Includes two or more of the individual types

arousals, are considered parasomnias and are not included in this category. If the movement occurs only during wake–sleep transitions and appears to be relatively simple and stereotypic, the SRMD diagnosis can be initially assessed by comprehensive history, physical examination, neurological examination, and if necessary, a polysomnogram (PSG). If a PSG is required, an expanded electroencephalography (EEG) electrode array is usually needed to rule out seizure. A dedicated sleep-deprived EEG may be warranted if clearly indicated by clinical signs or symptoms or if abnormal findings are noted on the EEG montage performed with the PSG.[2]

Sleep-Related Movement Disorders

Rhythmic Movement Disorder

Rhythmic movement disorder (RMD) is defined as a group of stereotyped, repetitive movements most often involving large muscles, which typically begins prior to sleep onset and may be sustained into transitional sleep. The most frequent forms of RMD are head banging (often referred to as *jactatio capitis nocturna*), body rocking, and body rolling, whereas leg rolling and leg banging are less common (see Table 45.1).[1] These movements can range in intensity from subtle to violent, and treatment is not usually required unless daytime consequences related to sleep quality are present, sleep-related injury occurs, or there are significant life-threatening issues for other family members.[1] The duration of these movements can last from several minutes to several hours. The movement frequency can vary, but the rate is usually between 0.5 and 2 per second, with duration of the individual cluster of movements generally <15 minutes.[1] In contrast to sleep-related epilepsy, children with RMD usually can voluntarily stop the movements upon request. Movements can be manifest at sleep onset, after nocturnal arousals, or in combination. Patients in whom frequent episodes of RMD are noted during the night should be clinically evaluated for causes of sleep fragmentation, such as obstructive sleep apnea or PLMS. In patients

with head banging, physical examination can demonstrate bruising, callus formation, or discrete patches of hair loss at the point of contact with the object they are striking with their head. Patients with leg rolling or body rolling may demonstrate bruising at sites of impact with furniture or the wall. PSG is rarely needed to make the diagnosis but will generally demonstrate rhythmic movements during wakefulness and extending into transitional sleep.[2]

Rhythmic head banging, body rocking, and head rolling are very common in childhood, with up to 59% of infants displaying the characteristic signs and symptoms by 9 months of age.[1] RMD prevalence decreases with age, and is only seen in 5% of 5-year-old children.[1] Gogo et al. found an estimated total prevalence of RMD between 0.3% and 2.9%.[3] This disorder is thought to be more common in males. Prihodova et al. noted an association with RMD and "prematurity, surgical delivery for intrauterine hypoxia, and neonatal jaundice requiring phototherapy," as well as attention-deficit/hyperactivity disorder (ADHD), and learning disabilities such as dyslexia. They found when excluding patients >15 years old that the prevalence of RMD associated with ADHD increased from 35.6% to 54.1%.[4]

Assessment of sleep-related movements can be difficult and can easily be misinterpreted, because parents/caretakers are often asleep when symptoms begin. Errors of perception are common and can lead to diagnosis of seizure disorder.[5]

Various management and treatment strategies have been suggested. The key aspect of RMD management is helping prevent injury to the child and providing parental education about the nature of this condition. In a typical child with RMD who has no apparent daytime behavioral or social issues, parents should be reassured that the condition is common and almost always self-limiting. Parents should be instructed to place the child in an environment where injury from these repetitive and sometimes violent movements can be avoided. Cribs and beds should be in good repair and inspected regularly. If falling off the bed is a concern, safe bedrails might be considered. Parents can also move the bed away from the wall or have the child sleep on a mattress on the floor to ensure their safety.[2]

Interventions to control the movements generally seek to provide the child with alternative means of self-soothing. The establishment of a bedtime routine made up of consistent and progressively less stimulating activities focused on helping the child decelerate can be a sufficient intervention to help the child fall asleep without needing to engage in rhythmic movements. Fixing a wake-up time and manipulating naps can also be effective in helping the child fall asleep without relying on repetitive motions to relax. A more comprehensive review of these behavioral approaches is included in Chapter 6.

Other behavioral and psychological approaches have given attention to replacing the rhythmic movements with alternate means of soothing. The use of a metronome as a stimulus substitution demonstrated some success in one study,[6] as has holding the child while patting or rocking the child at the same rate as their rhythmic movements. Etzioni and colleagues used a 3-week controlled sleep restriction regimen, and found that the combination of mild sleep deprivation along with usage of hypnotics at treatment initiation abolished rhythmic movements and treat the disorder.[7] This study suggests that RMD may represent a learned behavior that the child uses to help transition from wakefulness to sleep. In severe cases, or in cases in which the patient's rhythmic movements are a threat to the child's safety, pharmacologic treatment can be considered. A small dose of clonazepam has been shown to be effective in up to 50% of cases.[6] Antidepressants have also been tried with limited success.

Benign Sleep Myoclonus of Infancy

This SRMD occurs solely in infants and consists of repetitive myoclonic jerks involving the whole body, limbs, or trunk. These movements usually disappear by 6 months of age and occur only during sleep. As soon as the child is aroused or awakened from sleep, the movements abruptly and consistently stop. This disorder can sometimes be difficult to distinguish from sleep-related epilepsy and infantile spasms. If focal findings are present on examination, developmental issues are present, or clinical concern is heightened for a seizure disorder, an EEG may be ordered. The prevalence and etiology of this sleep-related condition are unknown. Rare, occasional myoclonic jerks often greatly worry parents of infants who may quickly seek out their pediatrician for a consultation. Parents can be reassured that this condition is benign without sequelae, and that symptoms will disappear after a few months of life.[2]

Sleep-Related Bruxism

Sleep-related bruxism (SB) is a stereotyped movement disorder characterized by grinding or clenching of the teeth during sleep. These rhythmic movements are the result of involuntary, repetitive contractions of the masseter, temporalis, and pterygoid muscles.[2] The child or adolescent may report jaw muscle discomfort, jaw lock, or headaches upon awakening in the morning. According to the ICSD-3 (Box 45.2), a diagnosis of SB requires that one or more of the following must be present: (1) abnormal wear of the teeth; (2) jaw muscle discomfort, fatigue, or pain and jaw lock upon awakening; and (3) regular sound of teeth grinding during sleep. Poor sleep can also be seen in severe cases. There can be significant negative impact on quality of life.[8] The exact prevalence of this condition is unclear, although a large literature review by Manfredini et al. found SB had an estimated prevalence of 12.8% ± 3.1%.[9] There appears to be an equal sex distribution, a familial pattern without clear genetic transmission has been observed, and the condition decreases with age.

SB can occur during all stages of sleep but is most common in non–rapid eye movement (NREM) stages 1 and 2.[1] In children, bruxism can be associated with obstructive sleep apnea. This is thought to represent an attempt to

---

• BOX 45.2 Consensus Diagnostic Criteria for Restless Sleep Disorder[10]

Criteria A–H must be met
A. Complaint of "restless sleep" as reported by the patient's parent, caregiver, or bedpartner, or by the patient.
B. Restless sleep movements involve large muscle groups of the whole body, all four limbs, arms, legs, or head.
C. The movements occur during sleep or when the individual appears to be asleep.
D. Video-polysomnography shows a total movement index (by video analysis) of 5 or more per hour of sleep.
E. Restless sleep occurs at least three times per week.
F. Restless sleep has been present for at least 3 months.
G. Restless sleep causes clinically significant impairment in behavioral, educational, academic, social, occupational, or other important areas of functioning as reported by the patient's parent, caregiver, or bedpartner, or by the patient (e.g., daytime sleepiness, irritability, fatigue, mood disturbance, impaired concentration, or impulsivity).
H. The condition is no better explained by another sleep disorder, medical disorder, mental disorder, behavior disorder, environmental factor (e.g., sleep-disordered breathing, restless legs syndrome, periodic limb movement disorder, sleep-related rhythmic movement disorder, insomnia disorder, atopic dermatitis, seizure disorder, etc.), or the physiological effects of a substance (e.g., caffeine).

---

open the airway during obstructive events by advancing the mandible and is usually noted during arousals at the termination of respiratory events. Khoury et al. demonstrated that SB is linked to transient sleep arousal, higher sleep-time sympathetic-cardiac activity, and a rise in respiration prior to and during the rhythmic masticatory muscle activity that typifies bruxism.[11] Although the relevance of these findings is still unclear, these physiologic changes during sleep may contribute to the morning orofacial pain and headaches seen in patients with this movement disorder.

Although SB can be a sign of an underlying sleep disorder (e.g., obstructive sleep apnea or periodic limb movement disorder [PLMD]) or dental disorders (e.g., malocclusion, poor oral habits, or temporomandibular disorders), it can also represent emotional conditions such as high stress or anxiety.[12] Tonsillar hypertrophy, restricted tongue mobility, and nasal obstruction may have a synergistic association on the presentation of SB.[13] Dental treatment focuses on preventing tooth destruction, reducing pain, and improving overall sleep quality. In many cases these goals can be achieved through the use of a mouth guard. Treatment strategies focused on addressing emotional concerns rely primarily on behavioral approaches designed to teach the child about relaxation[14] and establishing a consistent and relaxing bedtime routine to reduce stress or anxiety. Benzodiazepines and muscle relaxants have been shown to improve SB, and other medications (e.g., propranolol, clonidine, levodopa) are currently being looked at in an attempt to decrease SB events. Given the complex nature of treatment plans for SB, consultation between sleep medicine physicians, dentists, psychologists, and psychiatrists is often required.[2]

Faciomandibular myoclonus is similar to SB, but is considered to be more benign (Table 45.2). Compared with the more sustained jaw closure seen in SB, faciomandibular myoclonus is associated with rapid jaw jerks or twitches. Children and adolescents with this movement disorder, in contrast to SB, show no tooth wear, temporomandibular dysfunction, or masseter muscle hypertrophy. Although rarely required clinically, a PSG can differentiate between these two disorders.

Restless Legs Syndrome

RLS is an SRMD with several cardinal features, including an urge to move the legs, typically accompanied by an uncomfortable sensation in the lower extremities. These urges usually begin or worsen on lying down to go to sleep, and can interfere with the onset of sleep. Patients describe the sensations as "restless," "uncomfortable," "twitchy," "need to stretch," "urge to move," and "legs want to move on their own,"[1] which are partially or completely relieved with leg movement. Younger children may report these symptoms as pain due to their limited vocabulary. In severe cases, other parts of the body, including the arms, can also be affected.[15] These symptoms may last from a few minutes to several hours, but even the most severely affected patients can still sleep for several hours each night. Diagnosis generally can be made based on clinical features; however, PSG and actigraphy can be performed if diagnosis is in doubt. Both of these diagnostic modalities are very sensitive and specific in detecting and diagnosing RLS by monitoring the activity of the anterior tibialis muscle.[16]

A relatively new movement disorder termed restless sleep disorder (RSD) has been identified and described by DelRosso et al. RSD involves frequent nocturnal large body movements involving limbs, head, and trunk, and restless sleep and perception of sleep disruption without nocturnal waking.[17] The International RLS Study Group developed a task force to establish diagnostic criteria for pediatric patients age 6–18 (see Box 45.2).[10] A total movement index obtained by the sum of all types of movements divided by the total sleep time is prominent in children with RSD in all sleep stages. Calculation of five movements per hour of sleep using video-PSG accurately separates RSD from control subjects with 100% accuracy. It may also differentiate RSD from RLS with 90% accuracy.[18] Another differentiating factor between RSD and RLS is the absence of sleep-onset insomnia in RSD (Table 45.3).[19] It has also been shown that children with RSD have increased sympathetic activation during sleep as demonstrated by heart rate variability in N3 sleep and REM sleep.[20] Although restless sleep is a very common complaint from parents of children with ADHD, less than 10% of children with ADHD can be identified with RSD.[21] Most are secondary and associated with other sleep disorders, psychiatric comorbidities, or medications.[21] Further research into pediatric RSD has found iron deficiency with serum ferritin <20 ng/dL, sleep instability, and sympathetic activation to be possible contributors to the pathophysiology of RSD.[19] Long-term implications of RSD have yet to be determined, but given the increased sympathetic activation with heart rate variability cardiovascular effects may be considered. At this time, only oral or intravenous (IV) iron has been identified as a potential treatment.

Periodic Limb Movement Disorder

PLMD is characterized by periodic episodes of stereotyped, repetitive limb movements that manifest during

TABLE 45.2	Sleep-Related Bruxism versus Faciomandibular Myoclonus[2]	
	Sleep-Related Bruxism	Faciomandibular Myoclonus
Tooth destruction	Yes	No
Temporomandibular dysfunction	Yes	No
Masseter muscle hypertrophy	Yes	No

TABLE 45.3	Clinical Differentiation of RSD, RLS, and PLMD (DelRosso, et al, 2021)[19]		
	RSD	RLS	PLMD
Clinical presentation	Restless sleep Daytime impairment	Urge to move legs Sleep-onset insomnia Daytime impairment	Periodic limb movements of sleep Daytime impairment
Diagnosis	Clinical + PSG	Clinical	Clinical + PSG
PSG findings	Body movement >5/hr	May or may not have elevated PLMI	PLMI >5
Pathophysiology	Sleep instability Iron deficiency Sympathetic activation	Dopamine dysfunction Iron deficiency	Unknown (probably shared with RLS)

Abbreviations: *RSD*, restless sleep disorder; *RLS*, restless legs syndrome; *PLMD*, periodic limb movement disorder; *PSG*, polysomnography; *PLMI*, periodic leg movement index.

sleep. In contrast to RLS, PLMD does not occur prior to sleep onset, but only when the child or adolescent is asleep. Polysomnographic monitoring demonstrates repetitive episodes of muscle contraction and intermittent arousals or awakenings. However, recent studies have questioned the correlation between severity of PLMD and excessive daytime sleepiness, including one in which several surveys investigating this link did not show any association between PLMD and sleep–wake complaints.[12,14,22]

Care must be taken when diagnosing RLS and PLMD in the pediatric population because other disorders such as atopic dermatitis have been shown to be associated with increased episodic and/or periodic limb movements during sleep.[23]

Sleep-Related Leg Cramps

Sleep-related or nocturnal leg cramps are painful sensations of muscular hardness, tightness, or tension that occur in the calf or foot during sleep (Box 45.3). These leg cramps can last for a few seconds and remit spontaneously, or in some cases persist for up to 15–30 minutes. These painful sensations can result in arousals or awakenings from sleep, and may occur many times each night and up to several times a week. Polysomnographic monitoring reveals increased electromyographic activity in the affected leg with associated arousal or awakening. The exact prevalence of this condition is unknown, but sleep-related leg cramps can occur at any age, with the highest frequency found in the elderly (Box 45.4). Patients affected by neurological conditions (e.g., peripheral neuropathies) and metabolic disturbances (e.g., hypokalemia, hypothyroidism, or dehydration) may be at increased risk for sleep-related leg cramps. If these illnesses are contributing to this movement disorder, first-line treatment should clearly be to effectively manage the underlying condition. Otherwise, nocturnal leg cramps can usually be relieved by local massage, application of heat, stretching, or movement of the affected limb. Treatment with vitamin E or quinine can sometimes be effective,[15] but no one pharmacologic approach has been shown to be effective in every case.

Isolated Symptoms/Normal Variants

These symptoms/normal variants include sleep starts/hypnic jerks, hypnagogic foot tremor (HFT)/alternating leg muscle activation (ALMA), and excessive fragmentary myoclonus (EFM). Sleep starts, known also as hypnic or hypnagogic jerks, are sudden, single, brief contractions of the legs and occasionally the arms or head that occur at sleep onset. This disorder is a transition problem from wakefulness; it is extremely common and has been experienced by almost everyone at one time or another. Often, these movements are associated with a subjective impression of falling or a visual hypnagogic dream or hallucination. It has been hypothesized that sleep starts represent aberrant muscle contractions triggered as a result of instability of the brainstem

> **• BOX 45.3 Diagnostic Criteria for Sleep-Related Bruxism[1]**
>
> Alternate Names: nocturnal bruxism, nocturnal tooth grinding, tooth clenching
>
> **Diagnostic Criteria**
> Criteria A and B must be met
> A. The presence of regular or frequent tooth grinding sounds occurring during sleep.
> B. The presence of one of more of the following clinic signs:
>   1. Abnormal tooth wear consistent with reports of tooth grinding during sleep.
>   2. Transient morning jaw muscle pain or fatigue; and/or temporal headache; and/or jaw locking upon awakening consistent with reports of tooth grinding during sleep.

> **• BOX 45.4 Diagnostic Criteria for Sleep-Related Leg Cramps[1]**
>
> Alternate Names: leg cramps, "charley horse," nocturnal leg cramps
>
> **Diagnostic Criteria**
> Criteria A–C must be met
> A. A painful sensation in the leg or foot associated with sudden, involuntary muscle hardness or tightness, indicating a strong muscle contractions.
> B. The painful muscle contractions occur during the time in bed, although they may arise from either wakefulness or sleep.
> C. The pain is relieved by forceful stretching of the affected muscles, thus releasing the contraction.

reticular formation at the transition between wakefulness and sleep.[15] These movements can be frightening for parents, especially when they are accompanied by vocalization or crying. Parents should be reassured that sleep starts are a normal phenomenon and have no sequelae for the growing child. No treatment is necessary unless the movements result in injuries from kicking hard surfaces such as the crib railings, wall, or a bedpost. In these cases, treatment modalities similar to those used in RMD could be considered.

HFTs occur at the transition between wake and sleep or during light sleep, and consist of rhythmic foot movements occurring every second or so for several minutes. This SRMD may represent a variant of RMD; polysomnographic monitoring typically demonstrates recurrent electromyography (EMG) potentials or foot movements at the 0.5- to 3-Hz range in one or both feet as well as burst potential longer than the myoclonic range (>250 ms).[1] The prevalence in childhood is unknown, but one study estimated the adult prevalence at 7.5%.[24] HFTs are considered a benign entity with no known sequelae, and no treatment has been found to be effective.

ALMA is used to describe brief contractions of the lower leg alternating with activation of the muscle in the other leg. This sleep-related condition may represent the same disorder as HFT, except for the alternating nature seen clinically. PSG shows the characteristic anterior tibialis activation in one leg alternating with similar activation in the other leg. Both HFT and ALMA have been seen in one series in patients who were taking antidepressants; many patients with ALMA have been found concurrently to have obstructive sleep apnea syndrome or PLMD.[25] Although no treatment has been successful in reducing symptoms associated with HFT, dopamine agonists have been shown to be of benefit in patients with ALMA who report disrupted sleep.[26]

EFM is characterized by brief, involuntary "twitch-like" local contractions involving various areas of both sides of the body. These contractions are asymmetric and asynchronous, and occur during sleep. In many cases, this movement disorder is diagnosed strictly as an incidental finding of PSG. Involved areas may include muscles from the face, arms, legs, fingers, or toes. The EMG findings in EFM are similar to REM twitches that are a normal finding in REM sleep, except that these twitches also occur in other, NREM stages of sleep.[15] Although, often an incidental finding during PSG, there is suggestion that EFM may represent peripheral nerve pathology such as polyneuropathy, nerve root lesions, and/or benign fasciculations, in which further electrophysiology workup may be indicated.[27] PSG findings demonstrate a considerable correlation with advancing age, and have been found to be more frequent during REM sleep, although can be seen in other stages of sleep.[28] There are no current definitive treatments for EFM.

A variety of movement disorders may be associated with pediatric anti-N-methyl-D-receptor (NMDAR) encephalitis.[29] This is the most common autoimmune encephalitis in the pediatric age group. Clinical presentation varies, but all seem to present with prominent neurological symptoms of complex motor symptoms and orofacial dyskinesias that persist during sleep.

Non-epileptic myoclonus occurs in 40% of individuals with Angelman syndrome over 10 years, and prevalence appears to increase with age. Myoclonic episodes can last from seconds to hours, always occurring in the hands and spreading to the face and all extremities in some. With non-epileptic myoclonic activity, there is a discrete beginning and end, there is no postictal period, and they are not associated with significant alteration in consciousness.[30]

CLINICAL PEARLS

- Sleep-related movement disorders (SRMD) are characterized by relatively simple, non-purposeful, and usually stereotyped movements that occur in sleep, primarily during sleep–wake transitions.
- SRMDs are common, generally benign, and often self-soothing. Occasionally, physical injury may occur in association with these repetitive movements.
- SRMDs often resolve spontaneously and do not require pharmacological treatment. However, behavioral modification treatment focusing on safety should be considered in the setting of severe physical injury.

References

1. American Sleep Disorders Association Diagnostic Classification Steering Committee. *International Classification of Sleep Disorders, Revised: Diagnostic and Coding Manual.* American Academy of Sleep Medicine; 2014.
2. Sheldon SH, Ferber R, Kryger MH,, Gozal D. *Principles and Practice of Pediatric Sleep Medicine.* 2nd ed. Elsevier; 2014.
3. Gogo E, van Sluijs RM, Cheung T, et al. Objectively confirmed prevalence of sleep-related rhythmic movement disorder in preschool children. *Sleep Med.* 2019;53:16–21.
4. Prihodova I, Skibova J, Nevsimalova S. Sleep-related rhythmic movements and rhythmic movement disorder beyond early childhood. *Sleep Med.* 2019;64:112–115.
5. Frenette E, Guilleminault C. Nonepileptic paroxysmal sleep disorders. *Handb Clin Neurol.* 2013;112:857–860.
6. Haywood PM. Rhythmic movement disorder: Managing the child who head-bangs to get to sleep. *Paediatrics and Child Health.* 2012;22(5):207–210.
7. Etzioni T, Katz N, Hering E, Ravid S, Pillar G. Controlled sleep restriction for rhythmic movement disorder. *J Pediatr.* 2005;147(3):393–395.
8. Suguna S, Gurunathan D. Quality of life of children with sleep bruxism. *J Family Med Prim Care.* 2020;9(1):332–336.
9. Manfredini D, Winocur E, Guarda-Nardini L, Paesani D, Lobbezoo F. Epidemiology of bruxism in adults: A systematic review of the literature. *J Orofac Pain.* 2013;27(2):99–110.
10. DelRosso LM, Ferri R, Allen RP, et al. Consensus diagnostic criteria for a newly defined pediatric sleep disorder: Restless sleep disorder (RSD). *Sleep Med.* 2020;75:335–340.
11. Khoury S, Rouleau GA, Rompre PH, Mayer P, Montplaisir JY, Lavigne GJ. A significant increase in breathing amplitude precedes sleep bruxism. *Chest.* 2008;134(2):332–337.
12. Hornyak M, Feige B, Riemann D, Voderholzer U. Periodic leg movements in sleep and periodic limb movement disorder: Prevalence, clinical significance and treatment. *Sleep Med Rev.* 2006;10(3):169–177.
13. Oh JS, Zaghi S, Ghodousi N, et al. Determinants of probable sleep bruxism in a pediatric mixed dentition population: A multivariate analysis of mouth vs. nasal breathing, tongue mobility, and tonsil size. *Sleep Med.* 2021;77:7–13.
14. Monaco A, Ciammella NM, Marci MC, Pirro R, Giannoni M. The anxiety in bruxer child. A case-control study. *Minerva Stomatol.* 2002;51(6):247–250.
15. Walters AS. Clinical identification of the simple sleep-related movement disorders. *Chest.* 2007;131(4):1260–1266.
16. Merlino G, Gigli GL. Sleep-related movement disorders. *Neurol Sci.* 2012;33(3):491–513.
17. DelRosso LM, Bruni O, Ferri R. Restless sleep disorder in children: A pilot study on a tentative new diagnostic category. *Sleep.* 2018;41(8).
18. DelRosso LM, Jackson CV, Trotter K, Bruni O, Ferri R. Video-polysomnographic characterization of sleep movements in children with restless sleep disorder. *Sleep.* 2019;42(4).
19. DelRosso LM, Mogavero MP, Ferri R. Restless sleep disorder, restless legs syndrome, and periodic limb movement disorder–Sleep in motion! *Pediatr Pulmonol.* 2021;57(8):1879–1886.
20. DelRosso LM, Bruni O, Ferri R. Heart rate variability during sleep in children and adolescents with restless sleep disorder: A comparison with restless legs syndrome and normal controls. *J Clin Sleep Med.* 2020;16(11):1883–1890.

21. Kapoor V, Ferri R, Stein MA, Ruth C, Reed J, DelRosso LM. Restless sleep disorder in children with attention-deficit/hyperactivity disorder. *J Clin Sleep Med.* 2021;17(4):639–643.

22. Chervin RD. Periodic leg movements and sleepiness in patients evaluated for sleep-disordered breathing. *Am J Respir Crit Care Med.* 2001;164(8 Pt 1):1454–1458.

23. Treister AD, Stefek H, Grimaldi D, et al. Sleep and limb movement characteristics of children with atopic dermatitis coincidentally undergoing clinical polysomnography. *J Clin Sleep Med.* 2019;15(8):1107–1113.

24. Wichniak A, Tracik F, Geisler P, Ebersbach G, Morrissey SP, Zulley J. Rhythmic feet movements while falling asleep. *Mov Disord.* 2001;16(6):1164–1170.

25. Chervin RD, Consens FB, Kutluay E. Alternating leg muscle activation during sleep and arousals: A new sleep-related motor phenomenon? *Mov Disord.* 2003;18(5):551–559.

26. Cosentino FI, Iero I, Lanuzza B, Tripodi M, Ferri R. The neurophysiology of the alternating leg muscle activation (ALMA) during sleep: Study of one patient before and after treatment with pramipexole. *Sleep Med.* 2006;7(1):63–71.

27. Raccagni C, Loscher WN, Stefani A, et al. Peripheral nerve function in patients with excessive fragmentary myoclonus during sleep. *Sleep Med.* 2016;22:61–64.

28. Frauscher B, Gabelia D, Mitterling T, et al. Motor events during healthy sleep: A quantitative polysomnographic study. *Sleep.* 2014;37(4):763–773. 773A–773B.

29. Granata T, Matricardi S, Ragona F, et al. Pediatric NMDAR encephalitis: A single center observation study with a closer look at movement disorders. *Eur J Paediatr Neurol.* 2018;22(2):301–307.

30. Pollack SF, Grocott OR, Parkin KA, Larson AM, Thibert RL. Myoclonus in Angelman syndrome. *Epilepsy Behav.* 2018;82:170–174.

Sleep in Medical Disorders and Special Populations

46

Sleep and Sleep Disorders in Children with Epilepsy

Madeleine Marie Grigg-Damberger

CHAPTER HIGHLIGHTS

- Children with epilepsy are much more likely to have parasomnias, nocturnal awakenings, shorter sleep duration, daytime sleepiness, sleep-onset delay, and bedtime resistance than controls.
- Sleep problems in children with epilepsy increase the likelihood of inattention, hyperactivity, impulsivity, and oppositional defiant disorder than in their siblings or controls.
- Abnormalities in sleep architecture seen in some children with epilepsy include reduced sleep efficiency, decreased sleep time, increased non–rapid eye movement (NREM) 1, increased arousals and awakenings, and reduced REM sleep time.
- Video-polysomnography (PSG) with expanded electroencephalogram (EEG) is indicated in children with epilepsy for suspected obstructive sleep apnea to identify primary sleep disorders contributing to complaints of sleepiness, fragmented sleep and/or poorly controlled seizures, and/or to confirm whether nocturnal events are epileptic.

Introduction

Sleep problems are common in children with epilepsy (CWE) and in those who care for them.[1-15] The etiology of sleep disruption in CWE may be multifactorial including epilepsy per se, frequent nocturnal seizures disrupting nocturnal sleep organization, effects of anti-seizure medications (ASMs) on daytime alertness and nighttime sleep, and treatable primary sleep disorders. Comorbidities such as physical disability,[8] intellectual disability,[2,16,17] neurodevelopmental syndromes,[18,19] autism spectrum disorder (ASD),[20] and behavioral disorders[1,7-9,21] increase the likelihood of sleep disorders in CWE.[22] The presence of them in CWE has been associated with behavior problems and impaired academic performance.[23-25] Recognition of these relationships has led to increasing numbers of children or adolescents referred to pediatric sleep specialists to evaluate whether undiagnosed sleep disorders are contributing to their seizures.

Questionnaire-Based Studies on the Prevalence of Sleep Disorders in Children with Epilepsy

Several large prospective questionnaire-based studies have found sleep disorders are much more prevalent in CWE than the general pediatric population.[1,5-7,17,22,26-30] A case-control study found sleep problems were 2-fold higher (mean 4 ± 3 sleep problems vs. 2 ± 2) in 79 CWE (mean age 10 ± 3 years) compared with 73 age- and gender-matched controls.[7] Other questionnaire-based studies have demonstrated: (1) symptoms of obstructive sleep apnea (OSA) were 15 times more likely to be reported by the parents of 26 CWE (mean age 15 years) than a similar number of healthy controls (65% vs. 4%);[6] (2) CWE compared with control subjects had more daytime sleepiness, less on-task behavior, and less attention;[17] and (3) children with self-limited epilepsy with centrotemporal spikes (previously called benign rolandic epilepsy) had significantly shorter sleep duration, more frequent parasomnias, and daytime sleepiness than a reference sample of children.[28]

Another study found even children with idiopathic focal- or generalized-onset epilepsy in whom seizures were more often well controlled and not associated with comorbidities were significantly more likely to have more sleep problems than their siblings or age-matched healthy controls.[1] Post ad hoc comparisons found the CWE had significantly more excessive daytime sleepiness (EDS), bedtime difficulties, sleep fragmentation, and parasomnias than their siblings or controls. Multiple regression analyses showed (1) sleep complaints, longer sleep latencies, and shorter sleep times were much likely to be found in the children whose seizures were poorly controlled; (2) daytime seizures and high nighttime interictal epileptiform discharge (IED) rates predicted daytime drowsiness, and explained 15% of its variance; (3) sleep problems in CWE greatly increased the likelihood they would have far more behavior problems (inattention, hyperactivity, impulsivity, oppositional defiant disorder

[ODD]) than their siblings or controls; and (4) age, higher IED rates during sleep, and length of freedom from seizures accounted for 24% of the variance identifying which CWE were at greatest risk for sleep problems.[1]

A third study explored the relationships between the effect of pediatric epilepsy on child sleep, parental sleep and fatigue, and household sleeping arrangements on 105 households with a CWE and 79 controls.[26] Using multiple different validated pediatric sleep questionnaires, the authors found CWE compared with healthy controls had increased rates of parent–child room-sharing and co-sleeping and more sleep disturbances especially parasomnias, nocturnal awakenings, sleep duration, daytime sleepiness, sleep-onset delay, and bedtime resistance.[26] Further findings are worthy of mention: (1) severity of a child's epilepsy correlated with the severity of child and parent sleep dysfunction and parental fatigue; (2) ASM polypharmacy predicted greater childhood sleep disturbances would be reported; (3) sleep problems in CWE were associated with room-sharing and co-sleeping; (4) 62% of parents described decreased quantity and/or quality of sleep when co-sleeping; and (5) 42% of parents reported never/rarely feeling rested because they were concerned about their children having seizures during sleep.[26]

Poor sleep hygiene may contribute to sleep problems in CWE.[2,26] A prospective case-control study including 121 CWE found poor sleep habits were more common in those whose seizures were poorly controlled, especially those whose seizures primarily occurred during sleep.[2] Higher rates of parent and child room-sharing and co-sleeping have been observed especially when the child's seizures are nocturnal.[26] Sleep problems and poor quality sleep are frequently reported by parents when the child's seizures are nocturnal.[26]

Sleep disorders in CWE are more likely (and then more severe and even persistent) in CWE with comorbidities, especially neurodevelopmental disorders (NDDs), attention-deficit/hyperactivity disorder (ADHD), ASDs, and behavioral disorders. Using the Children's Sleep Habits Questionnaire (CSHQ), a 2021 study found 82% of 164 children with West syndrome had problematic sleep, which contributed to reduced quality of life (QoL).[29]

A 2020 study harvested a wealth of data from national health registers in Denmark evaluating the risk for sleep problems in children with ADHD, ASD, ODD/compulsive disorder (CD), and epilepsy.[22] They found the 5-year risk for developing sleep problems was 34% in children with ADHD, 17% ASD, 15% ODD/CD, and 6% epilepsy compared with 1% in the general population. Of note, the risk for sleep problems in CWE and children with ASD and ODD/CD was driven largely by comorbid ADHD.[22]

Non–Rapid Eye Movement Activator and Rapid Eye Movement Neuroprotective of Interictal Epileptiform Activity and Seizures

IEDs and seizures are activated by non–rapid eye movement (NREM) sleep and inhibited by (rapid eye movement) REM sleep.[31] IEDs increase in frequency as the depth of NREM sleep increases, with the highest in NREM 3 (N3) and lowest during REM sleep. A meta-analysis (including 42 studies and 1,458 patients) found that the focal IED discharge rate was 1.11-fold higher in wakefulness (W), 1.8-fold N1, 1.7-fold N2, and 2.5-fold N3 compared with REM (R) sleep.[31] Generalized IED rates were even greater: 6.6-fold greater in N3 and 3.1-fold in N1 and N2 compared with IED rates in REM sleep. A recent study found generalized IED rates were highest in the first hour of sleep in 39 adults with genetic generalized epilepsies (calling this a "sleep surge").[32] Recording 24-hour ambulatory electroencephalogram (EEG), they found the mean generalized IED rate was 4-fold higher in the first hour after sleep onset and significantly dropped (0.4) in the second hour compared with the last hour before sleep offset.[32] The sleep surge was not influenced by epilepsy syndrome, duration of epilepsy/seizure freedom, ASMs, or age.

Whereas epileptic seizures occur most frequently during N1 and N2 rather than N3,[33] frontal lobe seizures are more likely to occur in sleep than those that emanate from the temporal lobe.[34] However, when temporal lobe seizures occur during sleep they are more likely to spread and generalize than those that occur awake. Seizures are least likely to occur in REM sleep.[31] The meta-analysis mentioned earlier found 7.8-fold fewer focal and 3.25-fold fewer generalized seizures occurred during REM sleep compared with W.[31]

The spatial extent (also called epileptic field) of focal IED often becomes more widespread during N3 sleep.[35-38] New foci not seen in W may appear in NREM sleep.[37] The epileptic field of focal IEDs is often most circumscribed during REM sleep (especially phasic REM when rapid eye movements are present).[35]

Wider propagation of epileptic fields of focal IEDs in N2 and N3 are probably best explained by EEG synchronization during NREM sleep (and perhaps specifically by phase coupling with slow oscillations),[35,36,39] whereas neurons tend to discharge asynchronously during REM sleep promoting cortical desynchronization and restricting propagation of IEDs. A 2020 study using a high-density EEG source analysis confirmed focal IEDs when present in REM sleep tend to be shorter in duration, more spatially restricted, and had a higher concordance with the clinical ictal-onset zone compared with NREM.[40] Some use these data to help localize the epileptogenic zone for epilepsy surgery and neurostimulation therapies.

Sleep-Related Epilepsies

Sleep-related epilepsies (SRE) include three main categories of epilepsies or epilepsy syndromes: (1) seizures occur exclusively or almost exclusively in sleep (sleep-associated epilepsies), (2) EEG marked activation of epileptiform activity during sleep (sleep-accentuated epilepsies), and (3) seizures typically occur after awakening from sleep (arousal-related epilepsies).[41,42]

In 10–15% of all people with epilepsy, seizures occur exclusively or predominantly during sleep (sleep-associated epilepsies). *Sleep-associated epilepsies* most often begin in childhood (benign focal epilepsies of childhood with either central-midtemporal or occipital spikes) or adolescence (sleep-related hypermotor epilepsy [SHE]). All of the *sleep-accentuated epilepsies* begin in childhood and are drug-resistant epileptic encephalopathies as seen in West, Lennox-Gastaut, Landau-Kleffner, and Dravet syndromes, and electrical status epilepticus in sleep (ESES). Tonic seizures are activated during sleep in Lennox-Gastaut syndrome; tonic or tonic-vibratory seizures in Dravet syndrome.[43] *Awakening epilepsies* most often first develop in late childhood or adolescence and include juvenile myoclonic epilepsy (JME) and generalized tonic-clonic (GTC) seizures upon awakening. JME accounts for 25–30% of genetic generalized epilepsies and up to 10% of all epilepsies.

Is Sleep Architecture Abnormal in Children with Epilepsy?

Perhaps the single consistent finding across multiple studies recording polysomnography (PSG) in CWE is the percentage of sleep time spent in REM sleep is reduced in CWE compared with age-matched controls.[44] Two such studies found the percentage of REM sleep time was significantly lower in children with self-limited benign focal epilepsies (mean 15.5 and 17%) compared with 21% in healthy age-matched controls.[45,46] Another study found REM sleep time was even lower in children with drug-resistant focal lesional epilepsies (5.5 ± 5%) compared with self-limited epilepsy with centrotemporal spikes (9 ± 10%) versus controls (23 ± 5%).[47] This study also found the percentage of NREM 3 sleep was significantly lower in children with lesional epilepsies (7 ± 8%) versus controls (24 ± 5%).[47]

A 2020 prospective cross-sectional study recorded overnight PSG in 35 children with drug-resistant epilepsy (DRE), 35 with well-controlled epilepsy (WCE), and 17 typically developing children (TDC).[48] They found the children with DRE compared with WCE and TDC had significantly reduced sleep efficiency of median 86% vs. 92–93% in other groups, a median <57 minutes of NREM 3, and 22 minutes less of REM sleep.[48] On multiple logistic regression, only frequency of seizures and number of ASMs independently predicted poor sleep efficiency.

PSG findings in other studies of note showed (1) children who had focal-onset seizure(s) during an overnight video-PSG had significantly less sleep time compared with CWE who did not have seizures during the study or normal controls;[49] (2) children with genetic generalized epilepsy whose seizures were well controlled still had significantly more NREM 1 and longer REM sleep latency than normal controls;[50] (3) reduced percentages of N2, N3, and REM sleep in children with Lennox-Gastaut syndrome;[51] (4) significantly decreased total sleep time, increased N1, lower percentage of REM sleep time in children in intractable epileptic encephalopathy;[52] (5) CWE whose seizures were poorly controlled had significantly lower sleep efficiency, a higher arousal index, and a higher percentage of REM sleep compared with children who were seizure free or exhibited good seizure control;[53] (6) children with intellectual disability and epilepsy had longer sleep latency, higher percentage of wake after sleep onset (WASO) and N3, lower sleep efficiency, more awakenings and stage shifts, a higher cyclic alternating pattern (CAP) with increased A1 index, and long and less numerous CAP sequences;[54] but (7) sleep architecture on overnight PSG was normal in children with absence epilepsy whose seizures typically occur awake.[55,56] Larger prospective studies are needed to confirm these observations collected in children with varying seizure types and epilepsies often accompanied by comorbidities.

Prevalence of Sleep Apnea on Sleep Studies in Children with Epilepsy

A prospective cross-sectional study found OSA on overnight PSG in 35% of 40 children with idiopathic epilepsy compared with 7% of 27 healthy controls.[57] The odds ratio (OR) of an obstructive apnea index (OAI) ≥1 in the epilepsy group was 10.6 compared with the control group. Of note, the mean obstructive apnea–hypopnea index (OAHI) was 2.5 ± 1.2/hr of sleep in the CWE compared with 1.2 ± 0.8/hr) in the controls (modestly elevated values at best). Longest apnea duration was significantly higher in the group of poor seizure control.

A retrospective study compared 40 CWE referred for suspected OSA with 11 children who had moderate pediatric OSA (mean OAHI 7/hr of sleep).[53] Twenty percent of the CWE had OSA (OAHI) >1, mean 3/hr), 33% obstructive hypoventilation, 18% primary snoring and 10% periodic limb movements >5/hr. CWE with OSA compared with uncomplicated OSA controls (1) had higher body mass index (BMI) and were more likely to be obese (BMI >95th percentile in 62% vs. 18%) and (2) had longer sleep latencies (51 vs. 16 min), higher arousal indexes, and lower nadir arterial oxygen saturation (SpO$_2$) (86% vs. 90%).[53]

Not particularly surprising OSA is more likely to occur in CWE who also have cerebral palsy.[58,59] A prospective cross-sectional questionnaire-based study found children with cerebral palsy of greater severity or comorbid epilepsy were at greater risk of OSA.[58] Another study found OSA was more likely in CWE on ASM polytherapy and whose seizures were poorly controlled.[60] Eighty percent of the CWE whose epilepsy was uncontrolled had OSA compared with 47% in those with primary snoring. Based on these findings, the investigators recommended screening for OSA in children with uncontrolled seizures and/or ASM polypharmacy.

Even fewer studies have examined the effects of treating OSA in CWE. A retrospective 2012 analysis found a 53% median reduction in seizure frequency in 27 CWE (median age 5 years) 3 months following adenotonsillectomy.[61] Thirty-seven percent became seizure free, 11% had a >50% reduction in seizure frequency, 22% had lesser degrees of improvement. In 7% seizure frequency was unchanged and worse in 22%. Multivariate analysis demonstrated a trend toward seizure freedom with each percentile increase in BMI and early age of surgery.

Sleep/Wake and Circadian Patterns and Types of Seizures in Children

Growing evidence suggests epileptic seizures often cluster at specific times following a diurnal and nocturnal distribution with an overall peak of seizures in most patients during the day and least at night.[62-64] However, patients preferentially referred to pediatric sleep specialists are often those whose confirmed or suspected seizures are exclusively or most often during sleep (and few more upon awakening from sleep).

Frontal lobe seizures occur most often during sleep with an early morning peak and mesial temporal lobe seizures have two circadian peaks during the morning and late afternoon, whereas occipital seizures peak early evening and rarely occur in sleep.[33,65-68] Nocturnal or sleep-related seizures are more likely to emanate from the frontal rather than temporal region. However, while two-thirds of SHE seizures emanate from the frontal regions, about one-third are from the temporal lobe and a few from the insula or posterior parietal region.

A series of retrospective analyses from the same research found only tonic seizures in children were more frequently seen in sleep.[69-71] All other seizures preferentially occur awake. Clonic seizures exhibited two peaks (6 a.m. to 9 a.m. and noon to 3 p.m.) as did absence (9 a.m. to noon and 6 p.m. to midnight). GTC seizures peaked during 9–12 p.m., atonic seizures noon to 6 p.m., and myoclonic seizures 6 a.m. to noon. The clock timing of epileptic spasms varies with age with two peak times for seizures for children younger than 3 years of age (9 a.m. to noon and 3–6 p.m.) but only one peak (6 a.m. to 9 a.m.) in children older than 3 years.[69-71] Another retrospective analysis evaluated the clock timing and sleep/wake in CWE undergoing inpatient video-EEG monitoring and found tonic, clonic, and hypermotor seizures in children occurred more often asleep and frontal lobe seizures occurred in sleep between midnight and 3 a.m.[72]

Knowing the circadian and sleep/wake timing of particular seizures and seizure types can be helpful prompting adjustment of timing and dosing of antiseizure therapies, and safety planning. In a small retrospective case series adjusting the dosing of twice daily ASMs giving two-thirds of the total daily dose in the evening and one-third in the morning markedly improved seizure control in 17 children with nocturnal or early morning seizures (11 became seizure free, 4 experienced 75–90% reductions in seizure frequency).[73]

Indications for Video-Polysomnography in Children with Suspected or Known Epilepsy

Comprehensive video-PSG is most often done in CWE for suspected OSA or to identify primary sleep disorders contributing to complaints of sleepiness, fragmented sleep, and/or poorly controlled seizures. When symptoms suggest this, a PSG is warranted.[74] Sometimes we are asked to confirm whether paroxysmal nocturnal behaviors are epileptic or not in children with or without known epilepsy. The

majority referred for parasomnias have NREM sleep disorders of arousal (DOA). This is not surprising as a recently published longitudinal study of child development reported an overall prevalence of 40% for sleep terrors and 15% for sleepwalking in children 6 years or younger.[75]

The American Academy of Sleep Medicine (AASM) practice parameters indications for PSG advise that a PSG is unnecessary if the nocturnal events are typical, infrequent, non-injurious, and nondisruptive to the patient and/or family.[76] In 2012, the AASM published practice parameters for non-respiratory indications for PSG in children write that video-PSG can help differentiate atypical paroxysmal nocturnal behaviors from nocturnal seizures and/or identify when sleep-disordered breathing or other sleep disorders contribute to frequent parasomnias, enuresis, or affect control of seizures.[77,78] Box 46.1 summarizes the differential diagnosis of nocturnal behavioral events in children. Box 46.2 provides a summary of the clinical features that are typical for an NREM arousal disorder. Box 46.3 summarizes red flags for atypical parasomnias that warrant consideration of video-PSG.

Common, uncomplicated, non-injurious parasomnias (such as typical DOA, nightmares, enuresis, sleep talking, and bruxism) can usually be diagnosed by a clinical history. However, unusually frequent sleep terrors/sleepwalking events occurring ≥2–3 times per week warrant PSG to identify whether another sleep disorder is precipitating them (most often OSA, occasionally periodic limb movement disorder [PLMD]). One study found OSA on overnight PSG in 58% of 84 prepubertal children who had sleep terrors and/or sleepwalking;[79] OSA and parasomnias were eliminated in 43 who had tonsillectomy. Two had restless legs syndrome (RLS) and treatment of it with pramipexole eliminated the confusional arousals, restless legs, and periodic leg movements in sleep [PLMS].

Sleep-Related Hypermotor Epilepsy (Formerly Called Nocturnal Frontal Lobe Epilepsy)

Most CWE referred to sleep specialists already have a diagnosis of epilepsy. Most often we are asked to evaluate them for primary sleep disorders, but occasionally the question

---

• BOX 46.1   Differential Diagnosis of Nocturnal Behavioral Events in a Child

- Non–rapid eye movement (NREM) partial arousal disorder (confusional arousal; sleep walking; sleep terror)
- Sleep-related epilepsy
- REM sleep-behavior disorder (RBD)
- Nightmare disorder
- Sleep-related dissociative disorder
- Sleep-related panic disorder
- Sleep-related choking, laryngospasm or gastroesophageal reflux
- Sleep-related rhythmic movement disorder with vocalization
- Sleep-related expiratory groaning (catathrenia)

BOX 46.2 "Typical" Non–Rapid Eye Movement Arousal Disorders Usually Do Not Need a Sleep Study

- Occur first third of night when non–rapid eye movement (NREM) 3 sleep predominates
- Appear confused and disoriented
- Usually cannot be fully aroused from event
- If aroused, dream imagery recall only fragmentary
- Exhibit automatic motor behaviors and autonomic disturbances suggesting sympathetic activation
- Cannot console; may resist intervention
- Little or no responsiveness to external environment
- Positive family history
- Moderate to high likelihood of injury in agitated sleepwalking or sleep terrors

BOX 46.3 Red Flags for Atypical Parasomnias

- Spells are stereotyped
- Spells occur just after sleep onset
- Spells frequently occur second half of the night
- Behaviors potentially injurious or have caused injury to child or others
- Multiple episodes per night, not just ≤3 hours after sleep onset
- More than two to three spells per week
- Excessive daytime sleepiness
- Impaired daytime functioning
- Symptoms suggestive of sleep apnea or periodic limb movements
- Failure of conventional therapy

is are recurring paroxysmal events focal-onset SHE versus NREM arousal parasomnias (DOA)? SHE seizures in children are often initially misdiagnosed as sleepwalking, sleep terrors, nightmares, or even a psychiatric problem.[80,81] Because children with SHE often have multiple seizures a night (granted some minor), sleep specialists can record events suspicious for SHE prompting confirmation of the diagnosis.

The term SHE is now preferred over the previous name nocturnal frontal lobe epilepsy (NFLE) because (1) seizures occur from anytime sleep including daytime naps; (2) while the majority (70%) originate in the frontal lobe, 30% are "extrafrontal" emanating from a temporal (30%), and a few from the insular or posterior parietal regions;[82,83] and (3) hypermotor characterizes their ictal motor behaviors.[84]

SHE are brief stereotyped seizures that begin from N2 (less often within a few seconds after an arousal from N2) characterized by asymmetric tonic-dystonic posturing and/or complex hyperkinetic behaviors and usually associated with explosive vocalizations.[84,85] The complex motor behaviors accompanying SHE vary between patients but are often fairly stereotyped for the individual patient and include hand and foot automatisms, rocking body movements, distal stereotypies, bicycling of limbs, or abrupt rotation

(supine to prone).[83,85,86] Untreated, patients often have one or more overt seizures a night (hence why a single night of PSG can lead to the diagnosis). Most patients with SHE also have more subtle stereotyped "minor motor" seizures characterized by sudden head elevation, eye opening, downward turn of their lips (ictal pouting), abrupt movements of trunk and upper limbs, and brief arousals.[87]

A case series of 22 children with NFLE found seizures occurred exclusively from sleep in 77%, were brief (30 seconds to 2 minutes), frequent (3–22 per night), and characterized by a sudden arousal from N2 sleep accompanied by screaming, agitation, dystonic posturing, kicking or bicycling of the legs, and/or urinary incontinence.[80] Scalp-recorded ictal EEG activity was observed in some of their seizures in 95% but IEDs only seen in 14%. Ictal EEG activity was often not observed in patients with SHE because the seizures are short, obscured by muscle and movement artifact, and not associated with postictal confusion or EEG slowing. The absence of scalp-recorded ictal EEG activity does not preclude a diagnosis of SHE.

Adding to the diagnostic challenge, NREM DOA and sleep bruxism are significantly more common in patients and their relatives with NFLE.[88] A retrospective study found the lifetime prevalence of DOA was 6-fold greater and bruxism 5-fold higher in patients with NFLE compared with controls.[88] The lifetime prevalence of DOA was 4.7-fold higher and nightmares 2.6-fold greater in relatives of NFLE patients compared with relatives of controls.

A recent retrospective analysis sought to identify the particular discriminating video-PSG features between SHE seizures and DOA events in 59 patients with DOA and 30 with SHE.[89] The total number of motor events (major and minor) was significantly lower in those with DOA (3 ± 2) than in SHE (7 ± 8). DOA emerged mostly from N3 in patients with DOA and N2 in those with SHE. The occurrence of at least one major event outside N3 was highly suggestive for SHE (sensitivity 79%, specificity 95%). The occurrence of at least one minor event during N3 was highly suggestive for DOA (73% sensitivity, 72% specificity).

The estimated prevalence of SHE is 1.8 per 100,000 persons.[87] Seizures often respond to ASM, but 10% of drug-resistant focal-onset epilepsies referred for epilepsy surgery evaluation have SHE.[83,85] Quite often, a structural lesion is found to cause SHE and surgical resection of it can be curative. Most often, the lesion is a Taylor type 2b focal cortical dysplasia (FCD2). Sometimes the FCD is microscopic and not found until resection.

Recent studies have sought to identify video-PSG features that distinguish frontal from extrafrontal SHE, especially when the brain magnetic resonance imaging (MRI) shows no obvious lesion. SHE seizures that originate from the frontal lobe are more likely to occur from N2, whereas those that emanate from extrafrontal foci begin shortly after arousal from N2 sleep.[90] The mean duration of electrographic seizures and ictal behaviors are significantly shorter in frontal SHE seizures than those originating from extrafrontal foci.[91] A delay of >5 seconds between the first

TABLE 46.1	**Four Patterns of Clusters of Clinical Seizure Semiology in Sleep-Related Hypermotor Epilepsy**		
Early Elementary Motor (SP1)	**Unnatural Hypermotor Movements (SP2)**	**Natural or Integrated Hypermotor Movements (SP3)**	**Gestural Behaviors with High Emotions (SP4)**
• Proximal/distal contralateral tonic posturing • Contralateral version • Asymmetric tonic posturing • Early clonic signs	• Unnatural hypermotor behaviors • Proximal/distal contralateral tonic posturing • Rotation/version of trunk • Ictal pouting (chapeau de gendarme sign)	• Integrated/natural hypermotor behaviors (e.g., kicking, rocking, pedaling) • Distal stereotypies • Manipulation or utilization behaviors	• Integrated gestural behaviors with negative emotional/affective facial expressions • Feelings of fear/anxiety/rage • Speech production • Epileptic wandering

video-detectable ictal behavior (eye opening or a minor motor event) and onset of hypermotor behaviors suggests the focus is extrafrontal (sensitivity 75% and specificity 90%).[91] Gestural behaviors with high emotional content are more frequently seen in temporal SHE but are absent in parietal and insular SHE.[83] Postictal confusion when seen is more common in temporal SHE.[83] As many as 70% of patients with SHE report auras and the character of these may help to localize the seizure-onset zone.[83] Table 46.1 summarizes four clusters of clinical seizure semiology in SHE epilepsies that may help predict localization of the seizure focus in the frontal lobe or extrafocal regions.

Perhaps as many as 30% of cases of SHE have a familial basis, and there were predisposing genetic mutations identified in 9% of familial cases, 7% sporadic.[92] The first genetic mutation identified was a gain-of-function mutation in the alpha 4 subunit of the neuronal nicotinic acetylcholine receptor *(CHRNA4)* gene and was associated with autosomal dominant NFLE.[93] As of 2020, 103 pathogenic variants have been associated with SHE; most are related to the cholinergic system including *CHRNA2, CHRNB2, CRH, KCNT1, DEPDC 5,* and *GATOR-1* complex genes.[92] Genetic testing in patients with sporadic drug-resistant SHE (especially those with FCD on neuroimaging) is warranted.[92]

Patients with SHE often respond to carbamazepine, but 30% require add-on ASMs for drug resistance. When SHE seizures are not controlled by carbamazepine (or oxcarbamazepine), consider lacosamide or topiramate as add-ons.[94-96] A 2018 case series of 8 SHE patients found lacosamide (mean doses 400 mg, range 300–600 mg/day) reduced seizures >50% in 5.93, topiramate reduced seizure frequency >50% in 24 patients with SHE using a mean dose of 100 mg before bed.[95]

Transdermal nicotine (7 mg/24 hr in two 10-year-olds and 3.5 mg/24 hr in one 6-year-old) improved SHE control with three children with SHE due to a *CHRNA4*.[97] Neuroimaging is necessary in all patients with SHE. Patients who fail two appropriate drugs should be referred for epilepsy surgery evaluation. Some who are not readily surgical candidates (lesion in insula or eloquent cortex) may be treated with neurostimulation therapies such as responsive neurostimulator system (RNS) or vagal nerve stimulation (VNS).

Many childhood-onset epilepsies remit with adulthood but not SHE. A retrospective analysis of 139 patients with SHE followed for a median of 16 years (86% sporadic, 14% familial, 16% structural) found only 20% had terminal remission (≥5 years seizure free) at 10 years, 28% at 30 years.[86]

Diagnosing Sleep-Related Epilepsy

In 2021, consensus-based guidelines were published by the European Academy of Neurology, the European Sleep Research Society, and the International League Against Epilepsy Europe for diagnosing SRE.[42] Diagnosis as usual begins with a detailed history of the clinical seizure semiology, precipitants, timing of events (day and/or night; sleep/wakefulness; time during the night), and frequency of events (across the night, clusters).

A validated questionnaire fairly useful for distinguishing SHE from NREM sleep arousal parasomnias is the Frontal Lobe Epilepsy and Parasomnias (FLEP) scale.[98] Maytum and colleagues published a pilot study using the FLEP scale modified for children.[99] They found it correctly identified the four children with SHE (score >2, sensitivity 100%), but only 5 of 12 children with DOA were accurately identified as unlikely to have SHE (score <2, specificity 58%).

Patient diaries are more useful in tracking SRE (or DOA) when the diagnosis is established.[100] However, underreporting of seizures is common, especially in SRE if the patient sleeps alone or seizures are subtle.[101,102]

It is worthwhile to ask caregivers to obtain a smartphone video recording of paroxysmal nocturnal events but often the crucial onset of the event is not captured (parent sleeping).[103] More elaborate motion-detection video camera systems have been used when recurring nocturnal events were missed by in-laboratory or in-hospital recordings.[103,104]

Diagnosis of Sleep-Related Epilepsy Best Confirmed by Video-Electroencephalography

A diagnosis of SRE is best confirmed by video-EEG during sleep recorded for sufficient time to capture distinctive epileptiform discharges and ictal events cognizant that some patients may have both SRE and parasomnias. Clinical features that warrant concern for SRE seizures are (1) events occur any time in the night, just after falling asleep, or shortly before awakening in the morning; (2) multiple events a night; and (3) occasional occurrence of these events awake or during a brief nap. If you suspect the parasomnia may be sleep-related seizures and the child has not had an EEG with sleep, request one first.

A prospective study of EEGs done on 534 children referred for possible epilepsy reported epileptiform activity was found in 37% of the children with definite epilepsy, and 13% of clinically suspected cases.[105] However, the initial routine EEG will be normal in approximately one-half of children *with* clinically diagnosed epilepsy.[106,107]

Is sleep deprivation needed for the first EEG to confirm a diagnosis of epilepsy in children? A prospective study of 820 EEGs specifically examining the diagnostic utility of sleep or varying degrees of sleep deprivation for finding IEDs in a child's EEG showed the following: (1) NREM sleep was observed in 57% of sleep-deprived, 44% of partially sleep-deprived, and 21% of non–sleep-deprived pediatric EEGs; (2) a 6-fold increased yield of recording NREM 2 sleep with sleep deprivation and a 2.8-fold increase with partial sleep deprivation; (3) the OR that IEDs would be found was not increased by the presence of sleep, nor the use of total or partial sleep deprivation; and (4) the only significant effect of sleep deprivation was to increase the odds sleep would occur.[108] Sleep is likely to occur with only partial sleep deprivation and more stringent sleep deprivation will not increase the yield.[109] The better mix of sleep yield and cost containment is to order an EEG with partial sleep deprivation asking that a child >2 years of age stay awake 2 hours later than usual the night before the EEG and performing sleep-deprived EEGs in the morning, and no naps the day of the EEG for those <2 years.

It is useful to record video during *routine* or sleep-deprived outpatient pediatric EEGs. A study found adding video when recording routine EEGs (average duration 26 minutes) helped confirm the diagnosis in 45% of children referred for frequent paroxysmal events, and in 55% of the children with cognitive impairment.[110] Types of paroxysmal nonepileptic events confirmed by video in these children included staring spells, tics, stereotypies, tremor, paroxysmal eye movements, breath holding, or cyanotic spells.

If the child's paroxysmal events are daily (and only in sleep), a day of recording in the laboratory (with partial sleep deprivation or sleep deprivation the night before) can be diagnostic.[111,112] A retrospective study of prolonged video-EEG monitoring in 230 children found outpatient in-laboratory daytime recordings (4–8 hours) captured and confirmed the nature of the paroxysmal events in 80% of children whose events occurred on a daily basis.[111] Ordering 1 day of video-EEG done as an outpatient in-laboratory is best reserved for children whose events occur daily.[111,112]

If the first (or second) routine EEG with sleep is normal and your clinical suspicion for an SRE remains, request continuous inpatient video-EEG monitoring (long-term

epilepsy monitoring [LTM]) for 2–5 days when (1) the nocturnal behaviors do not occur nightly or every other night, (2) a primary sleep disorder (e.g., OSA or childhood restless legs syndrome [RLS]) is unlikely, (3) a history exists of postictal agitation or wandering, and/or (4) cooperation of the patient is questionable. Typical spells will be recorded in prolonged LTM in 45–80% of patients who have one or more event per week.[111,113,114]

Characteristic events were captured in 53% of 444 children with suspected epileptic seizures by recording 1–5 days of inpatient video-EEG, confirming the diagnosis of epilepsy in 34%.[114] The likelihood of capturing an event was greater if a patient had an event frequency of at least one per week. long-term epilepsy monitoring (LTM) can help confirm other nonepileptic paroxysmal behavior. One study of the diagnostic yield of LTM in 666 children (ages 2 weeks to 17 years) found they were able to confirm events in 96% of cases, such as staring in 34%, sleep-related arousals in 13%, benign infant sleep myoclonus in 15%, motor tics 11%, and shuddering in 7%.[113]

If a patient's spells occur only at night and are frequent, consider ordering a video-PSG with expanded EEG before prolonged inpatient video-EEG monitoring, especially if concomitant OSA or REM sleep behavior disorder is suspected. If the typical events are not captured on a single night of video-PSG consider recording a second or order LTM. Prolonged inpatient video-EEG monitoring from the beginning is often a better choice in patients with undiagnosed paroxysmal nocturnal events when (1) the nocturnal behaviors do not occur nightly or every other night, (2) a primary sleep disorder (e.g., OSA) is unlikely, (3) a history exists of postictal agitation or wandering, and/or (4) cooperation of the patient is questionable.

Technical Considerations When Recording Video-Polysomnography in Children with Epilepsy

The AASM practice parameters recommend that video-PSGs done to diagnose parasomnias need (1) "additional EEG derivations in an expanded bilateral montage" to diagnose paroxysmal arousals or other sleep disruptions thought to be seizure related when the initial clinical evaluation and results of a standard EEG are inconclusive, (2) recording surface electromyography (EMG) activity from the left and right anterior tibialis and extensor digitorum muscles, (3) obtaining good audiovisual recording, (4) having a sleep technologist present throughout the study to observe and document events, and (5) sleep specialists who are not experienced or trained in recognizing and interpreting both PSG and EEG abnormalities should seek appropriate consultation or should refer patients to a center where this expertise is available.[76]

Regarding how many additional EEG derivations should be recorded in a PSG in a person with epilepsy, a study by Foldvary and colleagues found that recording an 18-channel EEG during video-PSG did not improve the ability to recognize frontal lobe seizures.[115] To recognize frontal lobe seizures by EEG alone was not helped by either more EEG channels, slower screen times, or midline electrodes. When seizures are suspected or known it warrants recording an 18-channel EEG during a video-PSG, particularly if seizures, electrographic seizure activity, or IEDs are thought to contribute to the sleep/wake complaints. However, a recent retrospective analysis found clinical utility for ordering video-PSG with an 18- or 24-channel EEG in 240 children.[116] The EEG was abnormal in 53% and events or seizures were recorded in 40% of the studies.

Unfortunately, the habitual nocturnal event may not be captured by one night of in-laboratory video-PSG (unless the child has NFLE). One to two consecutive nights of video-PSG provided valuable diagnostic information in 69% of 41 patients whose paroxysmal motor behaviors were "prominent," 41% of 11 patients referred for minor motor activity in sleep, and 78% of 36 patients with known epilepsy.[117] Another study found video-PSG was diagnostic in 65% and "helpful" in another 26% of 100 consecutive adults referred for frequent sleep-related injuries; video-PSG identified DOA in 54, REM sleep-behavior disorder (RBD) in 36, sleep-related dissociative disorders in 7, nocturnal seizures in 2, and OSA in 1.[118] Unfortunately, only a third of patients with paroxysmal nocturnal events will have a typical spell a single night of video-PSG.[117,119]

Sleep researchers have found they were able to increase the diagnostic yield of one night of video-PSG for recording NREM DOAs by recording in-laboratory PSG after 25 hours of total sleep deprivation then ringing loud auditory stimuli. Patients arrive at their customary bedtime, remained awake the entire night, then are permitted to fall asleep 1 hour later than their usual wake time (i.e., 25 hours of prior wakefulness). To further provoke DOA events, patients are subjected to auditory stimuli delivered via earphones inserted in both ears. The auditory stimulus was a pure sound lasting 3 seconds. Most often 40–90 dB was needed to arouse both sleepwalkers and healthy controls from NREM 3. Using this technique, the investigators found they could trigger one to three sleepwalking events in 30% of 10 patients with DOA by sounding a 40–70 dB buzzer during NREM 3 sleep. After 25 hours of total sleep deprivation, the buzzer technique provoked NREM arousal disorder behaviors in 100% of their subjects (and none of their controls). Sleep deprivation nearly tripled the percentage of auditory stimulus trials that induced a behavioral event (57% vs. 20%).

Scoring sleep studies in patients with epilepsy can be difficult especially when IEDs are frequent, even more difficult when their sleep spindles are dysmorphic or low in amplitude, or if they have inappropriate alpha intrusions in their sleep EEG.[120] Almost continuous generalized spike-wave discharges first appearing during NREM sleep in a child warrant consideration of continuous electrographic status epilepticus in NREM sleep.[121,122] Fig. 46.1 A and B show an example of this and how the discharges are easier to identify in a 15-second epoch compared with a 30-second epoch.

Electrographic seizures and IEDs in video-PSG are best identified by increasing the high-frequency filter of the EEG derivations to 70 Hz; remapping the frontal, central, and occipital channels to the ipsilateral mastoid to more easily recognize laterality of the discharges; and reviewing portions of the recording using vertical screen times (epochs) of 10 seconds or 15 seconds.[78,123] Fig. 46.2 A–C shows focal spike-wave discharges emanating from the midline central (Cz)-left central (C3) region. These were activated by NREM sleep. Note how these are least frequent during REM sleep. Figs. 46.3 and 46.4 show an electrographic seizure from NREM 2 sleep in two different patients. Both had SHE and in one the seizures were primarily hypermotor, in the other they were asymmetric tonic.

Effects of Vagal Nerve Stimulation on Respiration During Sleep

VNS, a treatment for medically refractory epilepsy, often alters the rate and amplitude of breathing when it "activates" during sleep.[124-129] VNS has been approved by the U.S. Food and Drug Administration as an adjunctive treatment for drug-resistant focal epilepsy since 1997.

The VNS neurostimulator (Cyberonics, Inc) is a compact generator that is implanted subcutaneously by a neurosurgeon or otolaryngologist in the left thorax or anterior axillary region with two platinum helical bipolar electrodes wires and the anchor tether wrapped around the left vagus nerve distal to the superior laryngeal nerve and superior and inferior cervical cardiac branches.[130] The left vagus is preferred because it has proportionally fewer cardiac efferent fibers than the right.

Sleep specialists need to know about the programmable VNS settings (stimulation ON time, stimulation OFF time, output current, frequency and pulse width). The generator typically produces a 0.5-ms pulse that is repeated at 10–30 Hz for 30 seconds every 150–300 seconds. The current output is typically increased every 2–4 weeks by 0.25–0.50 mA to control seizures and minimize side effects. The patient (or parent/caregiver) can initiate the stimulator to deliver a burst of vagal stimulation when a seizure is felt; this can shorten or abort the seizure. The VNS can be "turned off" by taping the magnet over the generator.

The most common adverse events reported with VNS include dyspnea (OR 2.45), voice alteration and hoarseness (OR 2.17), and cough (OR 1.09), all of which occur during the ON phase. Most adverse events remit after 1 year of continued treatment. Far less reported is VNS precipitation or exacerbation of obstructive and/or central sleep apnea, inspiratory stridor, and left vocal cord paresis.[124,131-133]

The VNS can decrease the amplitude of respiratory effort and cause oxygen saturations and airflow obstruction when the device activates during sleep.[130] The typical pattern observed is sustained tachypnea and fall in the tidal volume during the ON period, which lasts during the ON time. VNS activation may cause oxygen desaturations but usually does

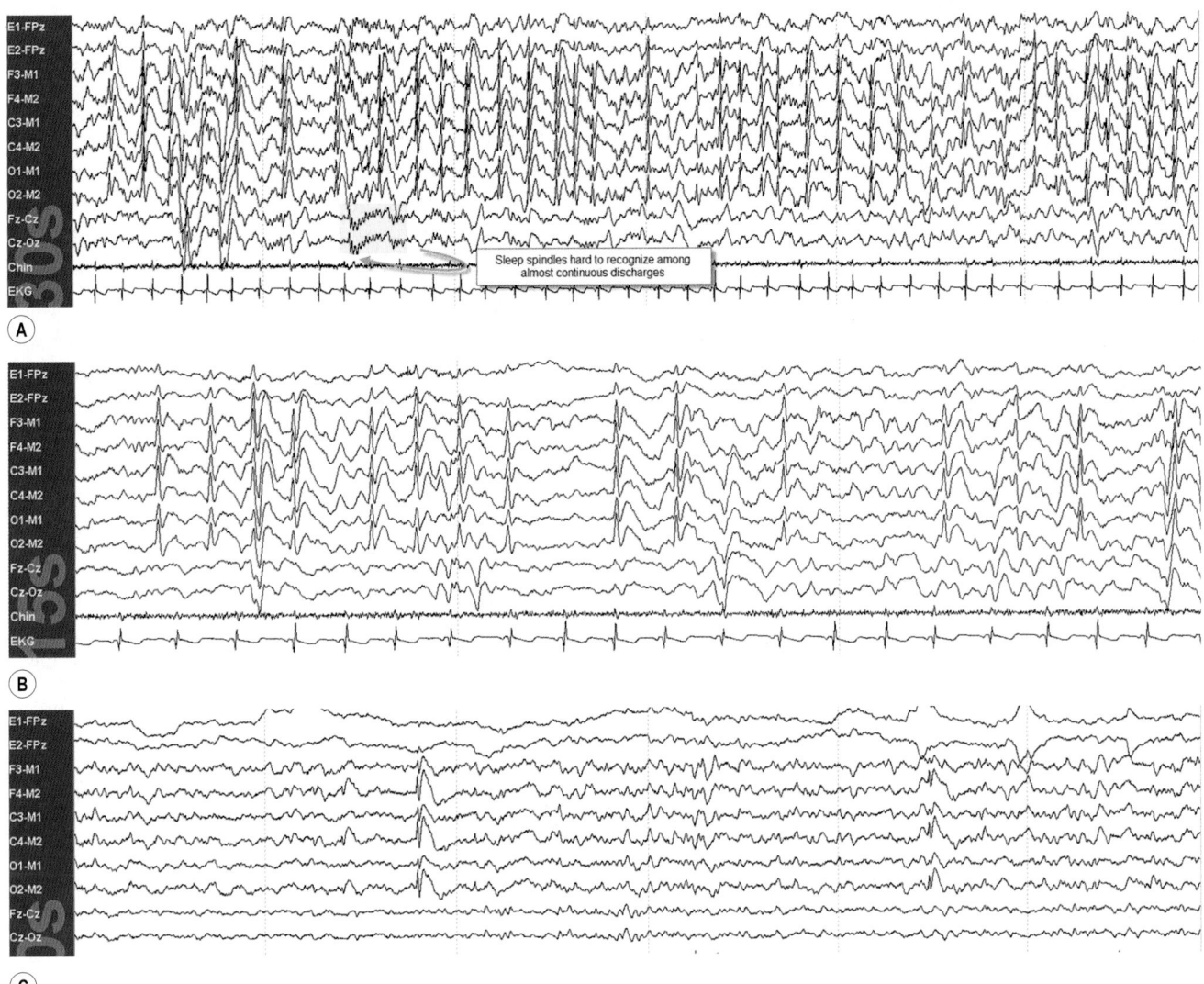

• **Fig. 46.1** (A) Staging sleep challenging when interictal epileptiform discharges are almost continuous. (B) Discharges are easier to recognize if reviewed in 15-second epochs. (C) Note how much fewer discharges are seen in rapid eye movement (REM) sleep.

not cause arousals, nor changes in heart rate or blood pressure.[130] Some patients have an increase in their apnea-hypopnea index (AHI; perhaps because of airflow obstruction induced by the electrical stimulation). Patients with VNS can have central apneas, obstructive hypopneas, and obstructive apneas. Reports of VNS-induced sleep-related inspiratory stridor has been reported in two children.[132] However, changes in sleep-related respiration when the VNS activates, which do not cause significant desaturations and/or arousals, probably have no clinical significance.

Should VNS therapy appear to cause or worsen sleep-disordered breathing (SDB), adjustments in the VNS settings are the first best step. The medical literature suggests that respiratory events observed during VNS ON time can usually be reduced or eliminated by lengthening the duration of OFF time (increasing the cycling time to 300 seconds), reducing the stimulation intensity from 30 to 20 Hz (and if needed 10 Hz). Some observe the VNS effect on

sleep apnea is positional and avoiding the supine position effective. Sometimes, continuous positive airway pressure (CPAP) is tried for scorable apneas and hypopneas, but is only sometimes effective. As a last resort, the device can be turned off when sleeping by taping the magnet over it.

Why this occurs is not fully understood. Experimental stimulation of the vagus nerve in humans has been shown to produce partial or complete inhibition of inspiration, prolongation of expiratory time, and modest changes in arterial pressure and bradycardia.[134]

Treating Sleep Disorders in Children with Epilepsy

Identifying and treating sleep disturbances in CWE can lead to improvements in daytime functioning and seizure control. If a CWE has EDS or impaired daytime functioning,

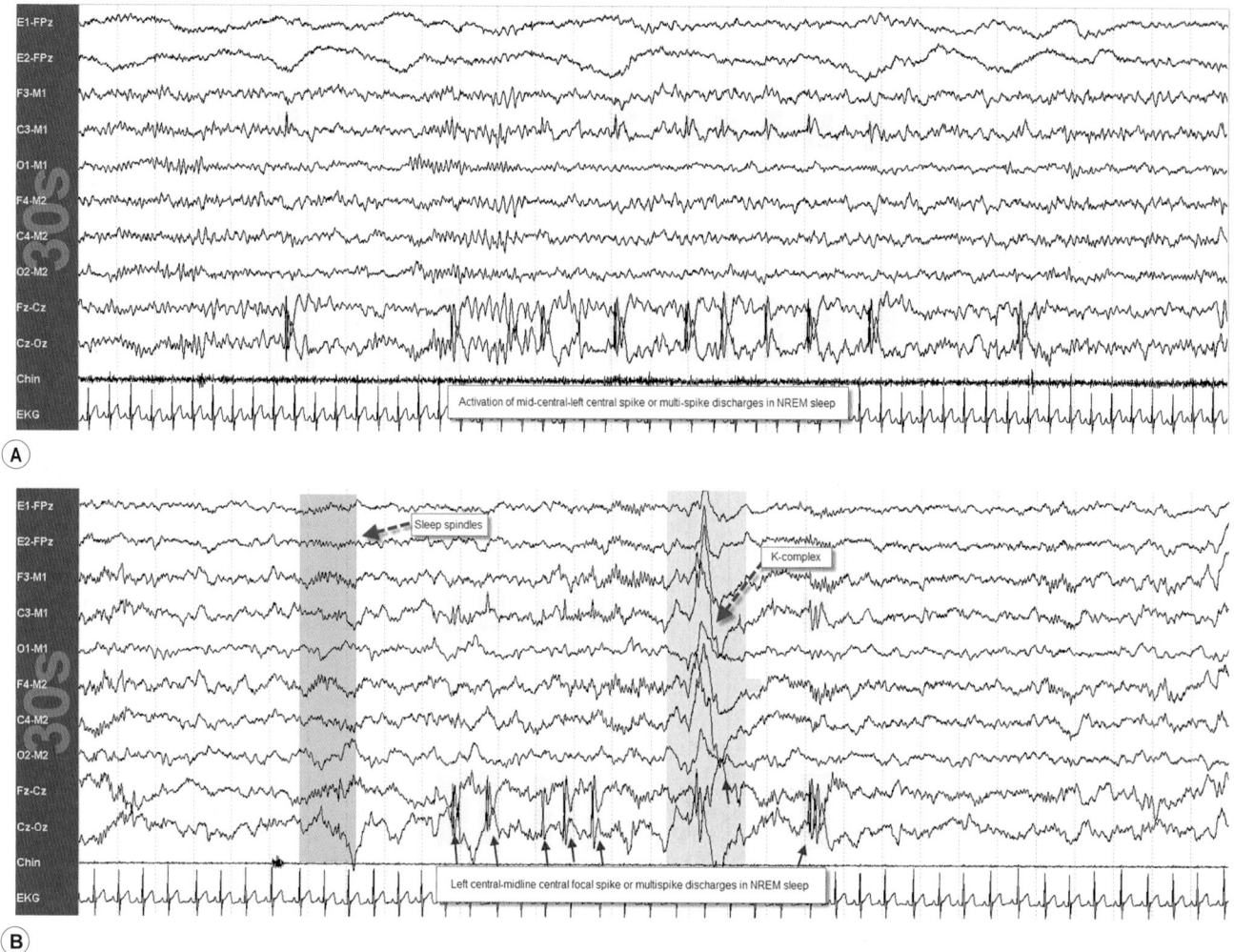

• **Fig. 46.2** (A) Activation of focal spike or multispike discharges midline central–left central in non–rapid eye movement (NREM) 1 sleep in a 3-year-old girl. (B) Midline central–left central spike-wave discharges during NREM 2 (*Yellow: activation of left central and midline central spike or multispike wave discharges in NREM 2 sleep*).

assess for (1) insufficient/irregular/excessive sleep (confirmed by sleep log and actigraphy); (2) sleep hygiene; (3) effects of ASMs; (4) poor seizure control and its impact on sleep, wakefulness, and daytime functioning; (4) primary sleep disorders (snoring, OSA, periodic limb movements, parasomnias).

Use of Melatonin to Treat Sleep Disorders in Children with Epilepsy

Alterations in the circadian rhythm secretion of melatonin and lower nocturnal melatonin levels have been reported in CWE, especially those with medically intractable epilepsy.[135-137] The anticonvulsant effects of melatonin have been demonstrated in many different animal models of epilepsy.[138]

Mechanisms by which melatonin may improve seizure control include its ability to reduce the electrical activity of neurons secreting glutamate (the primary central nervous system [CNS] excitatory neurotransmitter) while enhancing neuronal release of neurons that secrete γ-aminobutyric acid (GABA; the primary CNS inhibitory neurotransmitter).

Moreover, melatonin is metabolized to kynurenic acid (an endogenous anticonvulsant).

Last, melatonin and its metabolites may have neuroprotective effects in that they can act as a free radical scavenger and antioxidant. However, relatively high doses of melatonin are needed to inhibit experimental seizures and such doses are much more likely to have undesirable adverse effects of decreased body temperature, and even cognitive and motor impairment.

Five small, randomized, double-blind, placebo-controlled crossover studies of bedtime oral melatonin in CWE have shown positive effects on sleep.[4,139-142] One study found sustained-release melatonin (9 mg) decreased the mean sleep latency by 11 minutes and WASO by 22 minutes compared with placebo in 11 prepubertal developmental normal ages 6–11 CWE treated for 4 weeks followed by a 1-week washout period and a 4-week crossover condition. Another reported nightly oral melatonin in 23 children with medically refractory epilepsy for 3 months compared with controls not treated with melatonin resulted in significant improvements in bedtime

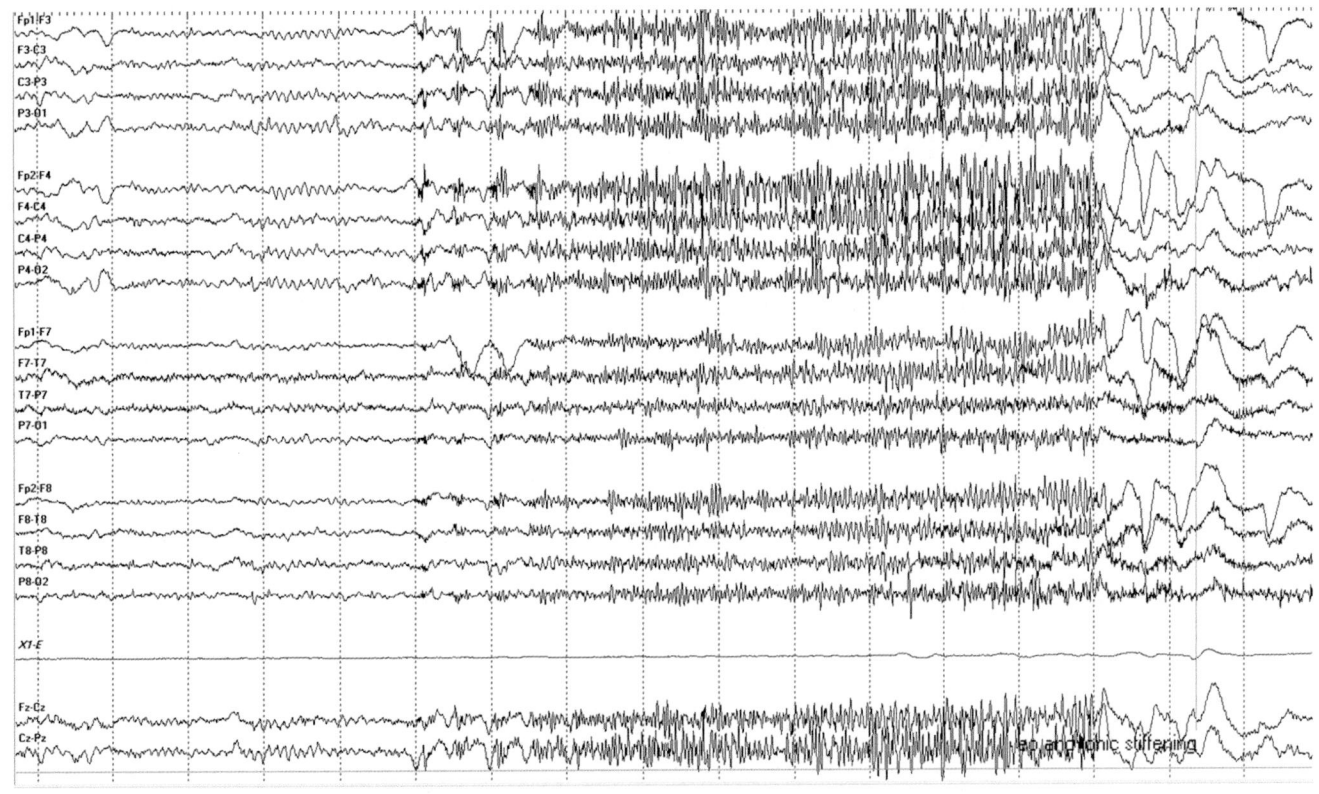

• **Fig. 46.3** Brief frontal lobe seizure from non–rapid eye movement (NREM) 2 sleep.

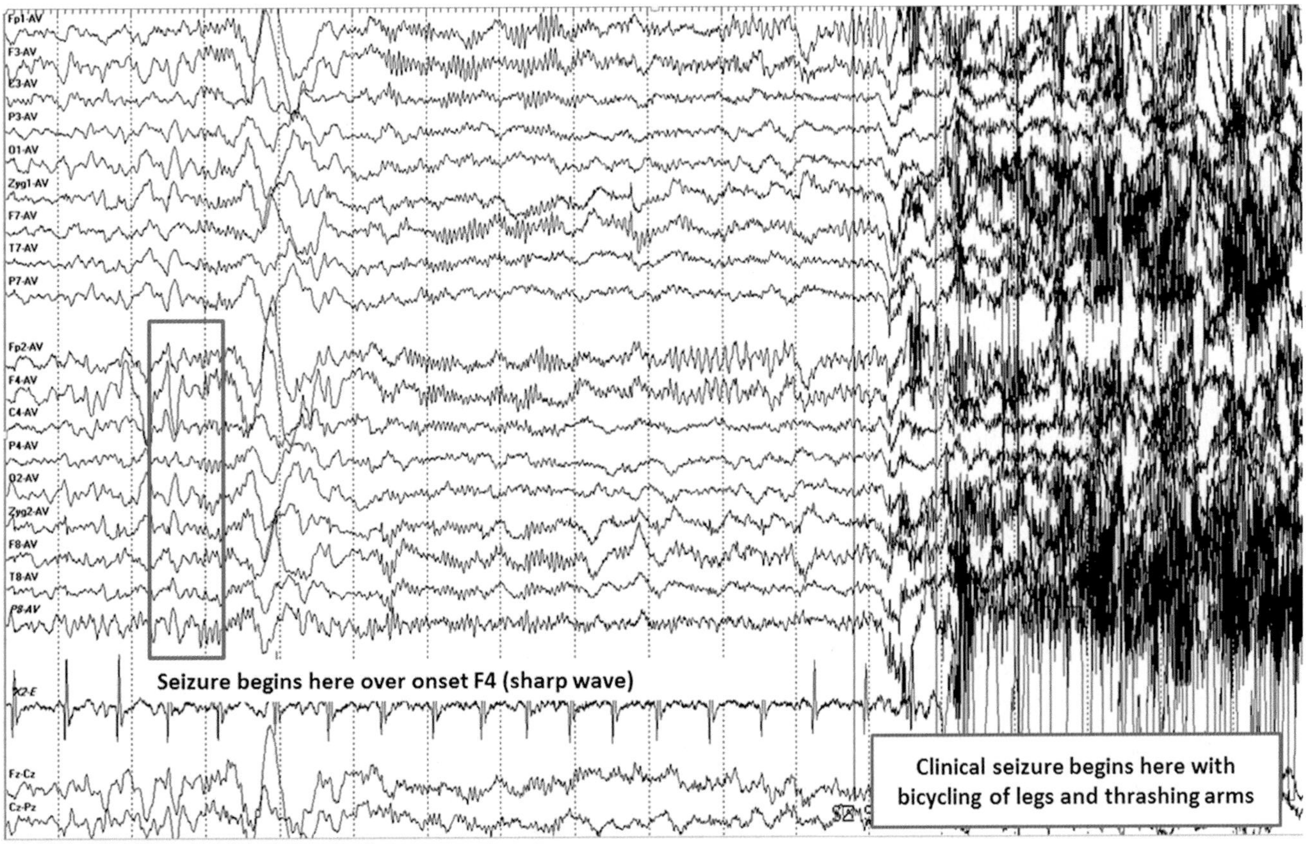

Seizure begins here over onset F4 (sharp wave)

Clinical seizure begins here with bicycling of legs and thrashing arms

• **Fig. 46.4** Nocturnal frontal lobe hypermotor seizure (*Red box: seizure begins here with a focal sharp wave maximal right frontal [F4] electrode*).

resistance, sleep duration, sleep latency, nocturnal arousals, sleepwalking, nocturnal enuresis, daytime sleepiness, and even seizure frequency.[4] Melatonin with doses ranging from 3 to 9 mg were associated with subjective improvements in sleep quality and were reported in 25 CWE with intellectual disability.[141] There were significantly fewer nocturnal awakenings and better control of convulsions in 10 children with severe medically intractable epilepsy given 3 mg of oral melatonin before bed nightly for 3 months followed by placebo for 3 months.[142]

In humans, melatonin has relatively low toxicity with only rare reports of nightmares, hypotension, and daytime sleepiness. A Cochrane database review found there were too few studies and of poor methodological quality to draw any conclusions about the role of melatonin in reducing seizure frequency or improving QoL in patients with epilepsy.[143]

Conclusion

The relationship between sleep and epilepsy is a fruitful and rewarding area for research. Much more research and knowledge is needed to better understand (1) why sleep macro- and microarchitecture are altered in patients with epilepsy, (2) whether treating OSA in patients with epilepsy improves seizure control, (3) the influence of circadian rhythms and chronotypes on different epilepsy syndromes, and (4) whether frequent IEDs during sleep without few or no seizures should be treated. Better understanding of the link among particular epilepsies, nonepileptic parasomnias, sleep fragmentation, and arousal is needed to understand how to best improve overall function and that a multidisciplinary model will best serve patients with these disorders.

CLINICAL PEARLS

- Children with epilepsy are much more likely to have parasomnias, nocturnal awakenings, shorter sleep duration, daytime sleepiness, sleep-onset delay, and bedtime resistance than controls.
- Even children with epilepsy whose seizures were controlled were more likely to have sleep problems than their siblings or controls.
- Sleep problems in children with epilepsy increase the likelihood of inattention, hyperactivity, impulsivity, and oppositional defiant disorder than in their siblings or controls.
- Poor sleep hygiene may contribute to sleep problems in children with epilepsy, especially in those whose seizures occur primarily during sleep and/or are poorly controlled.
- Abnormalities in sleep architecture seen in some children with epilepsy include reduced sleep efficiency, decreased sleep time, increased non–rapid eye movement (NREM) 1, increased arousals and awakenings, and reduced REM sleep time.
- Obstructive sleep apnea is more likely to be found in children with epilepsy who are on multiple antiepileptic medications and whose seizures are poorly controlled; children with uncontrolled seizures on multiple antiepileptics should be screened for obstructive sleep apnea.
- Tonic and hypermotor seizures more often occur during sleep; clonic and absence seizures while awake.

- Nocturnal frontal lobe seizures are often initially misdiagnosed as sleepwalking, sleep terrors, nightmares, or a psychiatric problem.
- The lifetime risk of NREM arousal disorders is 6 fold higher in individuals with nocturnal frontal lobe epilepsy (NFLE).
- Video-polysomnography (PSG) with expanded electroencephalography (EEG) is indicated in children with epilepsy for suspected obstructive sleep apnea, to identify primary sleep disorders contributing to complaints of sleepiness, fragmented sleep and/or poorly controlled seizures, and/or to confirm whether nocturnal events are epileptic.
- Sleep deprivation the night before a sleep study may increase the likelihood of an NREM arousal disorder occurs during a single night of in-laboratory video-PSG.
- When a vagal nerve stimulator fires for 30 seconds during sleep, it most often causes an increase in respiratory rate and fall in respiratory amplitude for the time the stimulator fires. This usually does not cause an arousal or desaturation. On occasion, obstructive apneas occur during and when the vagal nerve stimulator fires; reducing the stimulator current from 1 to 2 mA often lessens this effect.
- Melatonin may have anticonvulsive effects and can have positive effects on sleep in children with epilepsy, especially those with other neurological comorbidities.

References

1. Cortesi F, Giannotti F, Ottaviano S. Sleep problems and daytime behavior in childhood idiopathic epilepsy. *Epilepsia*. Nov 1999;40(11):1557–1565.
2. Batista BH, Nunes ML. Evaluation of sleep habits in children with epilepsy. *Epilepsy Behav*. Aug 2007;11(1):60–64. https://doi.org/10.1016/j.yebeh.2007.03.016.
3. Ong LC, Yang WW, Wong SW, alSiddiq F, Khu YS. Sleep habits and disturbances in Malaysian children with epilepsy. *J Paediatr Child Health*. Mar 2010;46(3):80–84. https://doi.org/10.1111/j.1440-1754.2009.01642.x.
4. Elkhayat HA, Hassanein SM, Tomoum HY, Abd-Elhamid IA, Asaad T, Elwakkad AS. Melatonin and sleep-related problems in children with intractable epilepsy. *Pediatr Neurol*. Apr 2010;42(4):249–254. https://doi.org/10.1016/j.pediatrneurol.2009.11.002.
5. Tang SS, Clarke T, Owens J, Pal DK. Sleep behaviour disturbances in rolandic epilepsy. *J Child Neurol*. Feb 2011;26(2):239–243. doi:0883073810381925 [pii] 10.1177/0883073810381925.
6. Maganti R, Hausman N, Koehn M, Sandok E, Glurich I, Mukesh BN. Excessive daytime sleepiness and sleep complaints among children with epilepsy. *Epilepsy Behav*. Feb 2006;8(1):272–277. https://doi.org/10.1016/j.yebeh.2005.11.002.

7. Stores G, Wiggs L, Campling G. Sleep disorders and their relationship to psychological disturbance in children with epilepsy. *Child Care Health Dev*. Jan 1998;24(1):5–19.

8. Wirrell E, Blackman M, Barlow K, Mah J, Hamiwka L. Sleep disturbances in children with epilepsy compared with their nearest-aged siblings. *Dev Med Child Neurol*. Nov 2005;47(11):754–759. https://doi.org/10.1017/S001216220 5001581.

9. Byars AW, Byars KC, Johnson CS, et al. The relationship between sleep problems and neuropsychological functioning in children with first recognized seizures. *Epilepsy Behav*. Nov 2008;13(4):607–613. doi:S1525-5050(08)00215-1 [pii] 10.1016/j.yebeh.2008.07.009.

10. Williams J, Lange B, Sharp G, et al. Altered sleeping arrangements in pediatric patients with epilepsy. *Clin Pediatr (Phila)*. Nov 2000;39(11):635–642.

11. de Weerd A, de Haas S, Otte A, et al. Subjective sleep disturbance in patients with partial epilepsy: A questionnaire-based study on prevalence and impact on quality of life. *Epilepsia*. Nov 2004;45(11):1397–1404. https://doi.org/10.1111/j.0013-9580.2004.46703.x.

12. Khatami R, Zutter D, Siegel A, Mathis J, Donati F, Bassetti CL. Sleep-wake habits and disorders in a series of 100 adult epilepsy patients–a prospective study. *Seizure*. Jul 2006;15(5):299–306. https://doi.org/10.1016/j.seizure.2006.02.018.

13. Piperidou C, Karlovasitou A, Triantafyllou N, et al. Influence of sleep disturbance on quality of life of patients with epilepsy. *Seizure*. Oct 2008;17(7):588–594. https://doi.org/10.1016/j.seizure.2008.02.005.

14. Jenssen S, Gracely E, Mahmood T, Tracy JI, Sperling MR. Subjective somnolence relates mainly to depression among patients in a tertiary care epilepsy center. *Epilepsy Behav*. Dec 2006;9(4):632–635. https://doi.org/10.1016/j.yebeh.2006.08.010.

15. Tsai SY, Tsai HY, Lin YY, Chen SR, Kuo SY, Lou MF. Sleep and its disturbance in parents of children and adolescents with epilepsy: A systematic review and meta-analysis. *Nat Sci Sleep*. 2023;15:1139–1152. https://doi.org/10.2147/NSS.S437349.

16. Didden R, Korzilius H, van Aperlo B, van Overloop C, de Vries M. Sleep problems and daytime problem behaviours in children with intellectual disability. *J Intellect Disabil Res*. Oct 2002;46(Pt 7):537–547. doi:404 [pii].

17. Didden R, de Moor JM, Korzilius H. Sleepiness, on-task behavior and attention in children with epilepsy who visited a school for special education: A comparative study. *Res Dev Disabil*. Nov-Dec 2009;30(6):1428–1434. https://doi.org/10.1016/j.ridd.2009.07.003.

18. Conant KD, Thibert RL, Thiele EA. Epilepsy and the sleep-wake patterns found in Angelman syndrome. *Epilepsia*. Nov 2009;50(11):2497–2500. https://doi.org/10.1111/j.1528-1167.2009.02109.x.

19. Segawa M, Nomura Y. Polysomnography in the Rett syndrome. *Brain Dev*. May 1992;14(Suppl.):S46–S54.

20. Liu X, Hubbard JA, Fabes RA, Adam JB. Sleep disturbances and correlates of children with autism spectrum disorders. *Child Psychiatry Hum Dev*. Winter 2006;37(2):179–191.

21. Becker DA, Fennell EB, Carney PR. Daytime behavior and sleep disturbance in childhood epilepsy. *Epilepsy Behav*. Oct 2004;5(5):708–715. https://doi.org/10.1016/j.yebeh.2004.06.004.

22. Hvolby A, Christensen J, Gasse C, Dalsgaard S, Dreier JW. Cumulative incidence and relative risk of sleep problems among children and adolescents with newly diagnosed neurodevelopmental disorders: A nationwide register-based study. *J Sleep Res*. Jun 21 2020:e13122. https://doi.org/10.1111/jsr.13122.

23. Chan S, Baldeweg T, Cross JH. A role for sleep disruption in cognitive impairment in children with epilepsy. Research Support, Non-U.S. Gov't Review. *Epilepsy Behav*. Mar 2011;20(3):435–440. https://doi.org/10.1016/j.yebeh.2010.12.047.

24. Parisi P, Bruni O, Pia Villa M, et al. The relationship between sleep and epilepsy: The effect on cognitive functioning in children. Review. *Dev Med Child Neurol*. Sep 2010;52(9):805–810. https://doi.org/10.1111/j.1469-8749.2010.03662.x.

25. Manni R, Terzaghi M. Comorbidity between epilepsy and sleep disorders. Review. *Epilepsy Res*. Aug 2010;90(3):171–177. https://doi.org/10.1016/j.eplepsyres.2010.05.006.

26. Larson AM, Ryther RC, Jennesson M, et al. Impact of pediatric epilepsy on sleep patterns and behaviors in children and parents. *Epilepsia*. Jul 2012;53(7):1162–1169. https://doi.org/10.1111/j.15281167.2012.03515.x.

27. Tang SS, Clarke T, Owens J, Pal DK. Sleep behavior disturbances in rolandic epilepsy. Research Support, N.I.H., Extramural Research Support, Non-U.S. Gov't. *J Child Neurol*. Feb 2011;26(2):239–243. https://doi.org/10.1177/0883073810381925.

28. Tang SS, Clarke T, Owens J, Pal DK. Sleep behavior disturbances in rolandic epilepsy. *J Child Neurol*. Feb 2011;26(2):239–243. https://doi.org/10.1177/0883073810381925.

29. Bhanudeep S, Madaan P, Sankhyan N, et al. Long-term epilepsy control, motor function, cognition, sleep and quality of life in children with West syndrome. *Epilepsy Research*. 2021;173:106629. https://doi.org/10.1016/j.eplepsyres.2021.106629.

30. Zambrelli E, Turner K, Peron A, et al. Sleep and behavior in children and adolescents with tuberous sclerosis complex. *Am J Med Genet A*. May 2021;185(5):1421–1429. https://doi.org/10.1002/ajmg.a.62123.

31. Ng M, Pavlova M. Why are seizures rare in rapid eye movement sleep? Review of the frequency of seizures in different sleep stages. *Epilepsy Res Treat*. 2013;2013:932790. https://doi.org/10.1155/2013/932790.

32. Seneviratne U, Lai A, Cook M, D'Souza W, Boston RC. "Sleep surge": The impact of sleep onset and offset on epileptiform discharges in idiopathic generalized epilepsies. *Clin Neurophysiol*. May 2020;131(5):1044–1050. https://doi.org/10.1016/j.clinph.2020.01.021.

33. Herman ST, Walczak TS, Bazil CW. Distribution of partial seizures during the sleep--wake cycle: Differences by seizure onset site. *Neurology*. Jun 12 2001;56(11):1453–1459.

34. Crespel A, Coubes P, Baldy-Moulinier M. Sleep influence on seizures and epilepsy effects on sleep in partial frontal and temporal lobe epilepsies. *Clin Neurophysiol*. Sep 2000;111(Suppl 2):S54–S59.

35. Frauscher B, von Ellenrieder N, Dubeau F, Gotman J. EEG desynchronization during phasic REM sleep suppresses interictal epileptic activity in humans. *Epilepsia*. Jun 2016;57(6):879–888. https://doi.org/10.1111/epi.13389.

36. Frauscher B, Gotman J. Sleep, oscillations, interictal discharges, and seizures in human focal epilepsy. *Neurobiol Dis*. Jul 2019;127:545–553. https://doi.org/10.1016/j.nbd.2019.04.007.

37. Sammaritano M, Gigli GL, Gotman J. Interictal spiking during wakefulness and sleep and the localization of foci in temporal lobe epilepsy. *Neurology*. Feb 1991;41(2 (Pt 1)):290–297.

38. Montplaisir J, Laverdière M, Saint-Hilaire JM, Rouleau I. Nocturnal sleep recording in partial epilepsy: A study with

depth electrodes. *J Clin Neurophysiol.* Oct 1987;4(4):383–388. https://doi.org/10.1097/00004691-198710000-00003.

39. Frauscher B. Localizing the epileptogenic zone. *Curr Opin Neurol.* Apr 2020;33(2):198–206. https://doi.org/10.1097/wco.0000000000000790.

40. Kang X, Boly M, Findlay G, et al. Quantitative spatio-temporal characterization of epileptic spikes using high density EEG: Differences between NREM sleep and REM sleep. *Sci Rep.* Feb 3 2020;10(1):1673. https://doi.org/10.1038/s41598-020-58612-4.

41. Nobili L, de Weerd A, Rubboli G, et al. Standard procedures for the diagnostic pathway of sleep-related epilepsies and comorbid sleep disorders: A European Academy of Neurology, European Sleep Research Society and International League against Epilepsy-Europe consensus review. *J Sleep Res.* Dec 2020;29(6):e13184. https://doi.org/10.1111/jsr.13184.

42. Nobili L, de Weerd A, Rubboli G, et al. Standard procedures for the diagnostic pathway of sleep-related epilepsies and comorbid sleep disorders: An EAN, ESRS and ILAE-Europe consensus review. *Eur J Neurol.* Jan 2021;28(1):15–32. https://doi.org/10.1111/ene.14468.

43. Losito E, Kuchenbuch M, Chemaly N, et al. Age-related "Sleep/nocturnal" tonic and tonic clonic seizure clusters are underdiagnosed in patients with Dravet Syndrome. *Epilepsy Behav.* Sep 2017;74:33–40. https://doi.org/10.1016/j.yebeh.2017.05.037.

44. Chan SY. Sleep architecture and homeostasis in children with epilepsy: A neurodevelopmental perspective. *Dev Med Child Neurol.* Apr 2020;62(4):426–433. https://doi.org/10.1111/dmcn.14437.

45. Bruni O, Novelli L, Luchetti A, et al. Reduced NREM sleep instability in benign childhood epilepsy with centro-temporal spikes. *Clin Neurophysiol.* May 2010;121(5):665–671. https://doi.org/10.1016/j.clinph.2009.12.027.

46. Gogou M, Haidopoulou K, Eboriadou M, Pavlou E. Sleep disturbances in children with rolandic epilepsy. *Neuropediatrics.* Feb 2017;48(1):30–35. https://doi.org/10.1055/s-0036-1593611.

47. Pereira AM, Bruni O, Ferri R, Palmini A, Nunes ML. The impact of epilepsy on sleep architecture during childhood. *Epilepsia.* Sep 2012;53(9):1519–1525. https://doi.org/10.1111/j.1528-1167.2012.03558.x.

48. Manokaran RK, Tripathi M, Chakrabarty B, Pandey RM, Gulati S. Sleep abnormalities and polysomnographic profile in children with drug-resistant epilepsy. *Seizure.* 2020;82:59–64. https://doi.org/10.1016/j.seizure.2020.09.016.

49. Nunes ML, Ferri R, Arzimanoglou A, Curzi L, Appel CC, Costa da Costa J. Sleep organization in children with partial refractory epilepsy. *J Child Neurol.* Nov 2003;18(11):763–766. https://doi.org/10.1177/08830738030180110601.

50. Maganti R, Sheth RD, Hermann BP, Weber S, Gidal BE, Fine J. Sleep architecture in children with idiopathic generalized epilepsy. *Epilepsia.* Jan 2005;46(1):104–109. https://doi.org/10.1111/j.0013-9580.2005.06804.x.

51. Eisensehr I, Parrino L, Noachtar S, Smerieri A, Terzano MG. Sleep in Lennox-Gastaut syndrome: The role of the cyclic alternating pattern (CAP) in the gate control of clinical seizures and generalized polyspikes. Comparative Study Research Support, Non-U.S. Gov't. *Epilepsy Res.* Sep 2001;46(3):241–250.

52. Nenadic-Baranasic N, Gjergja-Juraski R, Lehman I, Turkalj M, Nogalo B, Barisic N. Overnight video-polysomnographic studies in children with intractable epileptic encephalopathies. *Med Sci Monit.* Aug 4 2018;24:5405–5411. https://doi.org/10.12659/msm.908911.

53. Kaleyias J, Cruz M, Goraya JS, et al. Spectrum of polysomnographic abnormalities in children with epilepsy. *Pediatr Neurol.* Sep 2008;39(3):170–176. doi:S0887-8994(08)00265-8 [pii] 10.1016/j.pediatrneurol.2008.06.002.

54. Miano S, Bruni O, Arico D, Elia M, Ferri R. Polysomnographic assessment of sleep disturbances in children with developmental disabilities and seizures. *Neurol Sci.* Oct 2010;31(5):575–583. https://doi.org/10.1007/s10072-010-0291-8.

55. Sato S, Dreifuss FE, Penry JK. The effect of sleep on spike-wave discharges in absence seizures. *Neurology.* Dec 1973;23(12):1335–1345.

56. Terzano MG, Parrino L, Anelli S, Boselli M, Clemens B. Effects of generalized interictal EEG discharges on sleep stability: Assessment by means of cyclic alternating pattern. Comparative Study Research Support, Non-U.S. Gov't. *Epilepsia.* Mar-Apr 1992;33(2):317–326.

57. Gogou M, Haidopoulou K, Eboriadou M, Pavlidou E, Hatzistylianou M, Pavlou E. Sleep respiratory parameters in children with idiopathic epilepsy: A cross-sectional study. *Epilepsy Res.* Oct 2016;126:10–15. https://doi.org/10.1016/j.eplepsyres.2016.06.015.

58. Garcia J, Wical B, Wical W, et al. Obstructive sleep apnea in children with cerebral palsy and epilepsy. *Dev Med Child Neurol.* Oct 2016;58(10):1057–1062. https://doi.org/10.1111/dmcn.13091.

59. Koyuncu E, Türkkani MH, Sarikaya FG, Özgirgin N. Sleep disordered breathing in children with cerebral palsy. *Sleep Med.* Feb 2017;30:146–150. https://doi.org/10.1016/j.sleep.2016.01.020.

60. Jain SV, Horn PS, Simakajornboon N, Glauser TA. Obstructive sleep apnea and primary snoring in children with epilepsy. *J Child Neurol.* May 10 2012;28(1):77–82. https://doi.org/10.1177/0883073812440326.

61. Segal E, Vendrame M, Gregas M, Loddenkemper T, Kothare SV. Effect of treatment of obstructive sleep apnea on seizure outcomes in children with epilepsy. *Pediatr Neurol.* Jun 2012;46(6):359–362. https://doi.org/10.1016/j.pediatrneurol.2012.03.005.

62. Sánchez Fernández I, Gaínza-Lein M, Abend NS, et al. The onset of pediatric refractory status epilepticus is not distributed uniformly during the day. *Seizure.* Aug 2019;70:90–96. https://doi.org/10.1016/j.seizure.2019.06.017.

63. Hofstra WA, Grootemarsink BE, Dieker R, van der Palen J, de Weerd AW. Temporal distribution of clinical seizures over the 24-h day: A retrospective observational study in a tertiary epilepsy clinic. *Epilepsia.* Sep 2009;50(9):2019–2026. https://doi.org/10.1111/j.1528-1167.2009.02044.x.

64. Quigg M, Straume M, Menaker M, Bertram 3rd EH. Temporal distribution of partial seizures: Comparison of an animal model with human partial epilepsy. *Ann Neurol.* Jun 1998;43(6):748–755. https://doi.org/10.1002/ana.410430609.

65. Durazzo TS, Spencer SS, Duckrow RB, Novotny EJ, Spencer DD, Zaveri HP. Temporal distributions of seizure occurrence from various epileptogenic regions. *Neurology.* Apr 8 2008;70(15):1265–1271. https://doi.org/10.1212/01.wnl.0000308938.84918.3f.

66. Karafin M, St Louis EK, Zimmerman MB, Sparks JD, Granner MA. Bimodal ultradian seizure periodicity in human mesial temporal lobe epilepsy. *Seizure.* Jul 2010;19(6):347–351. https://doi.org/10.1016/j.seizure.2010.05.005.

67. Nzwalo H, Menezes Cordeiro I, Santos AC, Peralta R, Paiva T, Bentes C. 24-hour rhythmicity of seizures in refractory

focal epilepsy. *Epilepsy Behav.* Feb 2016;55:75–78. https://doi.org/10.1016/j.yebeh.2015.12.005.

68. Mirzoev A, Bercovici E, Stewart LS, Cortez MA, Snead 3rd OC, Desrocher M. Circadian profiles of focal epileptic seizures: A need for reappraisal. *Seizure.* Jul 2012;21(6):412–416. https://doi.org/10.1016/j.seizure.2012.03.014.

69. Zarowski M, Loddenkemper T, Vendrame M, Alexopoulos AV, Wyllie E, Kothare SV. Circadian distribution and sleep/wake patterns of generalized seizures in children. Comparative Study. *Epilepsia.* Jun 2011;52(6):1076–1083. https://doi.org/10.1111/j.1528-1167.2011.03023.x.

70. Ramgopal S, Vendrame M, Shah A, et al. Circadian patterns of generalized tonic-clonic evolutions in pediatric epilepsy patients. Research Support, Non-U.S. Gov't. *Seizure.* Sep 2012;21(7):535–539. https://doi.org/10.1016/j.seizure.2012.05.011.

71. Ramgopal S, Shah A, Zarowski M, et al. Diurnal and sleep/wake patterns of epileptic spasms in different age groups. *Epilepsia.* Jul 2012;53(7):1170–1177. https://doi.org/10.1111/j.1528-1167.2012.03499.x.

72. Gurkas E, Serdaroglu A, Hirfanoglu T, Kartal A, Yilmaz U, Bilir E. Sleep-wake distribution and circadian patterns of epileptic seizures in children. *Eur J Paediatr Neurol.* Jul 2016;20(4):549–554. https://doi.org/10.1016/j.ejpn.2016.04.004.

73. Guilhoto LM, Loddenkemper T, Vendrame M, Bergin A, Bourgeois BF, Kothare SV. Higher evening antiepileptic drug dose for nocturnal and early-morning seizures. *Epilepsy Behav.* Feb 2011;20(2):334–337. https://doi.org/10.1016/j.yebeh.2010.11.017.

74. Aurora RN, Zak RS, Karippot A, et al. Practice parameters for the respiratory indications for polysomnography in children. *Practice Guideline Research Support, U.S. Gov't, Non-P.H.S. Sleep.* Mar 2011;34(3):379–388.

75. Petit D, Touchette E, Tremblay RE, Boivin M, Montplaisir J. Dyssomnias and parasomnias in early childhood. *Pediatrics.* May 2007;119(5):e1016–e10125.

76. Kushida CA, Littner MR, Morgenthaler T, et al. Practice parameters for the indications for polysomnography and related procedures: An update for 2005. *Sleep.* Apr 1 2005;28(4):499–521.

77. Aurora RN, Lamm CI, Zak RS, Kristo DA, Bista SR, Rowley JA, Casey KR. Practice parameters for the non-respiratory indications for polysomnography and multiple sleep latency testing for children. *Sleep.* 2012;35(11):1467–1473.

78. Kotagal SNC, Grigg-Damberger MM, et al. Non-respiratory indications for polysomnography and related procedures in children: An evidence-based review. *Sleep.* 2012;35(11):1451–1466.

79. Guilleminault C, Palombini L, Pelayo R, Chervin RD. Sleepwalking and sleep terrors in prepubertal children: What triggers them? Research Support, U.S. Gov't, P.H.S. *Pediatrics.* Jan 2003;111(1):e17–e25.

80. Sinclair DB, Wheatley M, Snyder T. Frontal lobe epilepsy in childhood. *Pediatr Neurol.* Mar 2004;30(3):169–176.

81. Oldani A, Zucconi M, Asselta R, et al. Autosomal dominant nocturnal frontal lobe epilepsy. A video-polysomnographic and genetic appraisal of 40 patients and delineation of the epileptic syndrome. *Brain.* Feb 1998;121(Pt 2):205–223.

82. Ryvlin P, Minotti L, Demarquay G, et al. Nocturnal hypermotor seizures, suggesting frontal lobe epilepsy, can originate in the insula. *Epilepsia.* Apr 2006;47(4):755–765. https://doi.org/10.1111/j.1528-1167.2006.00510.x.

83. Gibbs SA, Proserpio P, Francione S, et al. Clinical features of sleep-related hypermotor epilepsy in relation to the seizure-onset zone: A review of 135 surgically treated cases. *Epilepsia.* Apr 2019;60(4):707–717. https://doi.org/10.1111/epi.14690.

84. Tinuper P, Bisulli F, Cross JH, et al. Definition and diagnostic criteria of sleep-related hypermotor epilepsy. *Neurology.* May 10 2016;86(19):1834–1842. https://doi.org/10.1212/WNL.0000000000002666.

85. Menghi V, Bisulli F, Tinuper P, Nobili L. Sleep-related hypermotor epilepsy: Prevalence, impact and management strategies. *Nat Sci Sleep.* 2018;10:317–326. https://doi.org/10.2147/nss.S152624.

86. Licchetta L, Bisulli F, Vignatelli L, et al. Sleep-related hypermotor epilepsy: Long-term outcome in a large cohort. *Neurology.* Jan 03 2017;88(1):70–77. https://doi.org/10.1212/WNL.0000000000003459.

87. Tinuper P, Bisulli F. From nocturnal frontal lobe epilepsy to sleep-related hypermotor epilepsy: A 35-year diagnostic challenge. *Seizure.* Jan 2017;44:87–92. https://doi.org/10.1016/j.seizure.2016.11.023.

88. Bisulli F, Vignatelli L, Naldi I, et al. Increased frequency of arousal parasomnias in families with nocturnal frontal lobe epilepsy: A common mechanism? *Epilepsia.* Apr 30 2010;51(9):1852–1860. doi:EPI2581 [pii] 10.1111/j.1528-1167.2010.02581.x.

89. Proserpio P, Loddo G, Zubler F, et al. Polysomnographic features differentiating disorder of arousals from sleep-related hypermotor epilepsy. *Sleep.* Dec 24 2019;42(12):zsz166. https://doi.org/10.1093/sleep/zsz166.

90. Eltze CM, Landre E, Soufflet C, Chassoux F. Sleep related epilepsy in focal cortical dysplasia type 2: Insights from sleep recordings in presurgical evaluation. *Clin Neurophysiol.* Mar 2020;131(3):609–615. https://doi.org/10.1016/j.clinph.2019.11.055.

91. Gibbs SA, Proserpio P, Francione S, et al. Seizure duration and latency of hypermotor manifestations distinguish frontal from extrafrontal onset in sleep-related hypermotor epilepsy. *Epilepsia.* Sep 2018;59(9):e130–e134. https://doi.org/10.1111/epi.14517.

92. Licchetta L, Pippucci T, Baldassari S, et al. Sleep-related hypermotor epilepsy (SHE): Contribution of known genes in 103 patients. *Seizure.* Jan 2020;74:60–64. https://doi.org/10.1016/j.seizure.2019.11.009.

93. Steinlein OK, Mulley JC, Propping P, et al. A missense mutation in the neuronal nicotinic acetylcholine receptor alpha 4 subunit is associated with autosomal dominant nocturnal frontal lobe epilepsy. *Nat Genet.* Oct 1995;11(2):201–203. https://doi.org/10.1038/ng1095-201.

94. Samarasekera SR, Berkovic SF, Scheffer IE. A case series of lacosamide as adjunctive therapy in refractory sleep-related hypermotor epilepsy (previously nocturnal frontal lobe epilepsy). *J Sleep Res.* Oct 2018;27(5):e12669. https://doi.org/10.1111/jsr.12669.

95. Oldani A, Manconi M, Zucconi M, Martinelli C, Ferini-Strambi L. Topiramate treatment for nocturnal frontal lobe epilepsy. *Seizure.* Dec 2006;15(8):649–652. https://doi.org/10.1016/j.seizure.2006.07.002.

96. Asioli GM, Rossi S, Bisulli F, Licchetta L, Tinuper P, Provini F. Therapy in sleep-related hypermotor epilepsy (SHE). *Curr Treat Options Neurol.* Jan 30 2020;22(1):1. https://doi.org/10.1007/s11940-020-0610-1.

97. Lossius K, de Saint Martin A, Myren-Svelstad S, et al. Remarkable effect of transdermal nicotine in children with CHRNA4-related autosomal dominant sleep-related hypermotor epilepsy. *Epilepsy Behav.* Apr 2020;105:106944. https://doi.org/10.1016/j.yebeh.2020.106944.

98. Derry C. Nocturnal frontal lobe epilepsy vs parasomnias. *Curr Treat Options Neurol.* Oct 2012;14(5):451–463. https://doi.org/10.1007/s11940-012-0191-8.

99. Maytum J, Garcia J, Leighty D, Belew J. Utility of the Frontal Lobe Epilepsy Parasomnia Scale in evaluation of children with nocturnal events. *J Neurosci Nurs.* Feb 1 2021;53(1):34–38. https://doi.org/10.1097/jnn.0000000000000567.

100. Aghaei-Lasboo A, Fisher RS. Methods for measuring seizure frequency and severity. *Neurol Clin.* May 2016;34(2):383–394. https://doi.org/10.1016/j.ncl.2015.11.001. viii.

101. Elger CE, Hoppe C. Diagnostic challenges in epilepsy: Seizure under-reporting and seizure detection. *Lancet Neurol.* Mar 2018;17(3):279–288. https://doi.org/10.1016/S1474-4422(18)30038-3.

102. Provini F, Plazzi G, Tinuper P, Vandi S, Lugaresi E, Montagna P. Nocturnal frontal lobe epilepsy. A clinical and polygraphic overview of 100 consecutive cases. *Brain.* Jun 1999;122(Pt 6):1017–1031. https://doi.org/10.1093/brain/122.6.1017.

103. Ricci L, Boscarino M, Assenza G, et al. Clinical utility of home videos for diagnosing epileptic seizures: A systematic review and practical recommendations for optimal and safe recording. *Neurological Sciences.* 2021;42(4):1301–1309. https://doi.org/10.1007/s10072-021-05040-5.

104. Van de Vel A, Milosevic M, Bonroy B, et al. Long-term accelerometry-triggered video monitoring and detection of tonic-clonic and clonic seizures in a home environment: Pilot study. *Epilepsy Behav Case Rep.* 2016;5:66–71. https://doi.org/10.1016/j.ebcr.2016.03.005.

105. Aydin K, Okuyaz C, Serdaroglu A, Gucuyener K. Utility of electroencephalography in the evaluation of common neurologic conditions in children. *J Child Neurol.* Jun 2003;18(6):394–396.

106. Camfield P, Gordon K, Camfield C, Tibbles J, Dooley J, Smith B. EEG results are rarely the same if repeated within six months in childhood epilepsy. *Can J Neurol Sci.* Nov 1995;22(4):297–300.

107. Gilbert DL, Gartside PS. Factors affecting the yield of pediatric EEGs in clinical practice. *Clin Pediatr (Phila). Jan-.* Feb 2002;41(1):25–32.

108. Gilbert DL. Interobserver reliability of visual interpretation of electroencephalograms in children with newly diagnosed seizures. *Dev Med Child Neurol.* Dec 2006;48(12):1009–1010. author reply 1010-1.

109. Gilbert DL, DeRoos S, Bare MA. Does sleep or sleep deprivation increase epileptiform discharges in pediatric electroencephalograms? *Pediatrics.* Sep 2004;114(3):658–662.

110. Watemberg N, Tziperman B, Dabby R, Hasan M, Zehavi L, Lerman-Sagie T. Adding video recording increases the diagnostic yield of routine electroencephalograms in children with frequent paroxysmal events. *Epilepsia.* May 2005;46(5):716–719.

111. Chen LS, Mitchell WG, Horton EJ, Snead 3rd OC. Clinical utility of video-EEG monitoring. *Pediatr Neurol.* Apr 1995;12(3):220–224.

112. Valente KD, Freitas A, Fiore LA, Gronich G, Negrao N. The diagnostic role of short duration outpatient V-EEG monitoring in children. *Pediatr Neurol.* Apr 2003;28(4):285–291.

113. Bye AM, Kok DJ, Ferenschild FT, Vles JS. Paroxysmal non-epileptic events in children: A retrospective study over a period of 10 years. *J Paediatr Child Health.* Jun 2000;36(3):244–248.

114. Mohan KK, Markand ON, Salanova V. Diagnostic utility of video EEG monitoring in paroxysmal events. *Acta Neurol Scand.* Nov 1996;94(5):320–325.

115. Foldvary-Schaefer N, De Ocampo J, Mascha E, Burgess R, Dinner D, Morris H. Accuracy of seizure detection using abbreviated EEG during polysomnography. *J Clin Neurophysiol.* Feb 2006;23(1):68–71. https://doi.org/10.1097/01.WNP.0000174544.86406.8D.

116. Jain SV, Dye T, Kedia P. Value of combined video EEG and polysomnography in clinical management of children with epilepsy and daytime or nocturnal spells. *Seizure.* Feb 2019;65:1–5. https://doi.org/10.1016/j.seizure.2018.12.009.

117. Aldrich MS, Jahnke B. Diagnostic value of video-EEG polysomnography. *Neurology.* Jul 1991;41(7):1060–1066.

118. Schenck CH, Milner DM, Hurwitz TD, Bundlie SR, Mahowald MW. A polysomnographic and clinical report on sleep-related injury in 100 adult patients. *Am J Psychiatry.* Sep 1989;146(9):1166–1173.

119. Blatt I, Peled R, Gadoth N, Lavie P. The value of sleep recording in evaluating somnambulism in young adults. *Electroencephalogr Clin Neurophysiol.* Jun 1991;78(6):407–412.

120. Marzec ML, Malow BA. Approaches to staging sleep in polysomnographic studies with epileptic activity. *Sleep Med.* Sep 2003;4(5):409–417.

121. Brazzo D, Pera MC, Fasce M, Papalia G, Balottin U, Veggiotti P. Epileptic encephalopathies with status epilepticus during sleep: New techniques for understanding pathophysiology and therapeutic options. *Epilepsy Res Treat.* 2012;2012:642725. https://doi.org/10.1155/2012/642725.

122. Loddenkemper T, Fernandez IS, Peters JM. Continuous spike and waves during sleep and electrical status epilepticus in sleep. Review. *J Clin Neurophysiol.* Apr 2011;28(2):154–164. https://doi.org/10.1097/WNP.0b013e31821213eb.

123. Grigg-Damberger M, Ralls F. Primary sleep disorders and paroxysmal nocturnal nonepileptic events in adults with epilepsy from the perspective of sleep specialists. Review. *J Clin Neurophysiol.* Apr 2011;28(2):120–140. https://doi.org/10.1097/WNP.0b013e3182120fed.

124. Nagarajan L, Walsh P, Gregory P, Stick S, Maul J, Ghosh S. Respiratory pattern changes in sleep in children on vagal nerve stimulation for refractory epilepsy. *Can J Neurol Sci.* Aug 2003;30(3):224–227.

125. Hsieh T, Chen M, McAfee A, Kifle Y. Sleep-related breathing disorder in children with vagal nerve stimulators. *Pediatr Neurol.* Feb 2008;38(2):99–103. doi:S0887-8994(07)00492-4 [pii] 10.1016/j.pediatrneurol.2007.09.014.

126. Pruvost M, Zaaimi B, Grebe R, Wallois F, Berquin P, Perlitz V. Cardiorespiratory effects induced by vagus nerve stimulation in epileptic children. *Med Biol Eng Comput.* Apr 2006;44(4):338–347. https://doi.org/10.1007/s11517-006-0041-5.

127. Zaaimi B, Heberle C, Berquin P, Pruvost M, Grebe R, Wallois F. Vagus nerve stimulation induces concomitant respiratory alterations and a decrease in SaO_2 in children. *Epilepsia.* Nov 2005;46(11):1802–1809. https://doi.org/10.1111/j.1528-1167.2005.00283.x.

128. Khurana DS, Reumann M, Hobdell EF, et al. Vagus nerve stimulation in children with refractory epilepsy: Unusual complications and relationship to sleep-disordered breathing. *Childs Nerv Syst.* Nov 2007;23(11):1309–1312. https://doi.org/10.1007/s00381-007-0404-8.

129. Zaaimi B, Grebe R, Berquin P, Wallois F. Vagus nerve stimulation induces changes in respiratory sinus arrhythmia of epileptic children during sleep. *Epilepsia.* Nov 2009;50(11):2473–2480. https://doi.org/10.1111/j.1528-1167.2009.02190.x.

130. Parhizgar F, Nugent K, Raj R. Obstructive sleep apnea and respiratory complications associated with vagus nerve stimulators. *J Clin Sleep Med.* Aug 15 2011;7(4):401–407. https://doi.org/10.5664/jcsm.1204.

131. Aron M, Vlachos-Mayer H, Dorion D. Vocal cord adduction causing obstructive sleep apnea from vagal nerve stimulation: Case report. *Journal Pediatr.* May 2012;160(5):868–870. https://doi.org/10.1016/j.jpeds.2012.01.045.

132. Kelts G, O'Connor PD, Hussey RW, Maturo S. An electrical cause of stridor: Pediatric vagal nerve stimulators. *Int J Pediatr Otorhinolaryngol.* Feb 2015;79(2):251–253. https://doi.org/10.1016/j.ijporl.2014.10.037.

133. Zambrelli E, Saibene AM, Furia F, et al. Laryngeal motility alteration: A missing link between sleep apnea and vagus nerve stimulation for epilepsy. *Epilepsia.* Jan 2016;57(1):e24–e27. https://doi.org/10.1111/epi.13252.

134. Banzett RB, Guz A, Paydarfar D, Shea SA, Schachter SC, Lansing RW. Cardiorespiratory variables and sensation during stimulation of the left vagus in patients with epilepsy. *Epilepsy Res.* May 1999;35(1):1–11.

135. Tarcin G, Aksu Uzunhan T, Kacar A, Kucur M, Saltik S. The relationship between epileptic seizure and melatonin in children. *Epilepsy Behav.* Aug 27 2020;112:107345. https://doi.org/10.1016/j.yebeh.2020.107345.

136. Paprocka J, Dec R, Jamroz E, Marszal E. Melatonin and childhood refractory epilepsy–a pilot study. *Med Sci Monit.* Aug 7 2010;16(9):CR389–CR396. doi:881124 [pii].

137. Ardura J, Andres J, Garmendia JR, Ardura F. Melatonin in epilepsy and febrile seizures. *J Child Neurol.* Jul 2010;25(7):888–891. doi:0883073809351315 [pii] 10.1177/0883073809351315.

138. Banach M, Gurdziel E, Jędrych M, Borowicz KK. Melatonin in experimental seizures and epilepsy. *Pharmacol Rep.* 2011;63(1):1–11. https://doi.org/10.1016/s1734-1140(11)70393-0.

139. Jain SV, Horn PS, Simakajornboon N, et al. Melatonin improves sleep in children with epilepsy: A randomized, double-blind, crossover study. *Sleep Med.* May 2015;16(5):637–644. https://doi.org/10.1016/j.sleep.2015.01.005.

140. Gupta M, Aneja S, Kohli K. Add-on melatonin improves sleep behavior in children with epilepsy: Randomized, double-blind, placebo-controlled trial. *J Child Neurol.* Feb 2005;20(2):112–115. https://doi.org/10.1177/08830738050200020501.

141. Coppola G, Iervolino G, Mastrosimone M, La Torre G, Ruiu F, Pascotto A. Melatonin in wake-sleep disorders in children, adolescents and young adults with mental retardation with or without epilepsy: A double-blind, cross-over, placebo-controlled trial. *Brain Dev.* Sep 2004;26(6):373–376. https://doi.org/10.1016/S0387-7604(03)00197-9.

142. Uberos J, Augustin-Morales MC, Molina Carballo A, Florido J, Narbona E, Munoz-Hoyos A. Normalization of the sleep-wake pattern and melatonin and 6-sulphatoxy-melatonin levels after a therapeutic trial with melatonin in children with severe epilepsy. *J Pineal Res.* 2011;50(2):92–196. https://doi.org/10.1111/j.1600-079X.2010.00828.x.

143. Brigo F, Del Felice A. Melatonin as add-on treatment for epilepsy. Review. *Cochrane Database Syst Rev.* 2012;6:CD006967. https://doi.org/10.1002/14651858.CD006967.pub2.

47

Neoplasms and Sleep: Impact and Implications

Valerie McLaughlin Crabtree, Kayla N. LaRosa, and Merrill S. Wise

CHAPTER HIGHLIGHTS

- Youth with cancer and pediatric cancer survivors are at increased risk for sleep disturbances including insomnia and excessive daytime sleepiness.
- Cancer-related fatigue is a burdensome symptom that appears to be distinct from disrupted sleep.
- Sleep difficulties seen most commonly in pediatric oncology patients and survivors are multifactorial and are likely caused by a combination of physiologic effects of cancer and its treatment, changes in routine, stress, and environmental disruptions within hospital units.
- Nonpharmacologic and pharmacologic interventions should be tailored to the specific symptoms experienced and the needs of the youth.
- Although more specific research within samples of youth with cancer and childhood cancer survivors is necessary, tailored interventions have shown promise in improving nighttime symptoms and daytime function.

Introduction

Approximately 210 per 1 million children were diagnosed with cancer from 2013 to 2017,[1] with 5-year survival rates of nearly 85%.[2] Survival rate varies based on cancer diagnosis and treatment, as well as age at diagnosis.[2] With improved survival, there is an increased need to reduce symptom burden and improve quality of life during and after cancer treatment.[3] Sleep and circadian rhythm disruptions, as well as cancer-related fatigue (CRF), are frequently reported as distressing symptoms throughout the cancer continuum and are negatively associated with survivorship rates, quality of life, activities of daily living, learning and cognition, and psychosocial well-being.[3–5]

Between 25% and 40% of healthy children are affected by sleep problems, and 50–60% of pediatric oncology patients endorse fatigue and/or sleep disturbance.[6–8] However, the prevalence of sleep difficulties increases to 80% in children with brain tumors where the hypothalamic-pituitary-adrenal (HPA) axis is often affected by the impact of the tumor

and treatment on sleep–wake modulation.[6,8] Common sleep concerns include excessive daytime sleepiness (EDS) and behavioral insomnia, which may exacerbate CRF and interfere with day-to-day functioning.[8]

Mechanisms of Sleep Disturbance

Youth with cancer may have preexisting sleep problems, and cancer itself can create sleep disruption and/or fatigue because of the direct effect of the tumor on the body's major sleep centers (e.g., HPA axis). Also, cancer may have a negative impact on metabolism and endocrine function, leading to sleep problems.[6] Sleep disruption may occur as a product of cancer treatment (e.g., radiation, chemotherapy[9]) or medication side effects (e.g., corticosteroids), or sleep fragmentation may accompany pain, nausea, or anemia.[10]

Environmental changes may also negatively impact sleep and contribute to fatigue. Hospitalization during cancer treatment is associated with frequent sleep interruptions for medical care (e.g., taking vital signs, nighttime medication administration), resulting in decreased nighttime sleep duration and increased levels of fatigue that persist post-discharge. Shorter nighttime sleep duration is associated with greater mood disturbance and increased daytime napping. Limited mobility and diminished daytime activity, as well as decreased light exposure, increases the risk for circadian rhythm disruption.[10] In addition, increased stress, anxiety, and mood problems resulting from a cancer diagnosis and disrupted routine can exacerbate sleep difficulties.[11,12] Youth with cancer have been found to have inconsistent sleep habits as well as later bedtimes and waketimes.[11,13] Common sleep difficulties in pediatric cancer including EDS, insomnia, and fatigue are described further below.

Excessive Daytime Sleepiness

EDS is defined as "the inability to maintain wakefulness and alertness throughout the day, with sleep occurring unintentionally or during inappropriate times of the day for at least three months."[14] Individuals with EDS may have trouble waking and experience sleepiness despite obtaining sufficient nighttime sleep. In addition, engagement in physical, social, and academic functioning may be limited. EDS is associated with inattention, impaired concentration, hyperactivity, irritability, and mood disturbance.[15,16]

EDS is common in youth with neoplasms of the central nervous system (CNS) due to involvement of the hypothalamus, thalamus, and brainstem, with studies citing EDS prevalence rates between 30% and 80%.[17–21] EDS likely results from multiple factors, including damage to the HPA axis, which can directly impact sleep–wake regulation, and increased risk for obesity, which can lead to obstructive sleep apnea (OSA).[17,22–25] The location of the brain tumor may have more impact on the development of EDS than the type of tumor. Specifically, in youth with craniopharyngioma, hypothalamic involvement (tumor involving both the anterior and posterior hypothalamus, including the mammillary bodies) was associated with increased risk for narcolepsy. In one study, in youth who were overweight or obese, the risk of EDS was significantly higher (present in 100%) when documented objectively.[26] Children currently receiving treatment for brain tumors are more likely to have EDS if their tumor is centrally located,[17] but among pediatric brain tumor *survivors*, the location of the tumor has not been shown to be significantly associated with EDS symptoms.[18] Therefore, in the survivorship period additional risks, such as ongoing disrupted sleep, psychosocial challenges associated with brain tumor survivorship, and other complex medical and behavioral factors, also appear to influence daytime functioning.[17,18,20,21]

Insomnia

Insomnia is defined as delayed sleep onset or nocturnal awakenings and must occur at least three times per week for 3 months to meet criteria for a diagnosis of chronic insomnia. Conditions associated with insomnia include depression, risk-taking behavior, and suicidal ideation in healthy populations. Insomnia may also lead to difficulty concentrating and maintaining attention due to insufficient sleep.[27] For children diagnosed with cancer, psychosocial distress and difficulty initiating sleep are likely exacerbated by disrupted routines, frequent hospitalizations, and physical symptoms such as recurrent pain.[27]

Children with acute lymphoblastic leukemia (ALL), the most common childhood cancer, have sleep disruption during cancer treatment (prevalence of 87% in one study), including difficulty initiating and maintaining sleep, bedtime resistance, recurrent nightmares, and changing their sleep location throughout the night. Parenting practices around sleep may also change as a result of a cancer diagnosis and because of being in an unfamiliar setting (e.g., inpatient room), which could exacerbate sleep difficulties during and after cancer treatment. Co-sleeping was associated with sleep problems in young children with ALL, and parents were more likely to be lenient with typical rules around bedtime or sleep hygiene during cancer-directed therapy.[9,10]

Up to one-third of childhood cancer survivors experience insomnia-related difficulties post-treatment, with one out of every four pediatric brain tumor survivors reporting their sleep efficiency was low enough to warrant intervention for clinical insomnia. In addition, 31% of adolescents and young adults diagnosed with cancer exhibited a sleep efficiency <85% within 1 year of completing cancer treatment, indicating a clinical concern for insomnia.[27–29]

Fatigue

Unlike typical fatigue, CRF is greater in magnitude and includes physical, cognitive, and emotional tiredness that is persistent, not relieved by rest, and disproportionate to the level of energy exerted.[11,30] It is consistently reported as one of the most distressing symptoms for pediatric oncology patients because of the negative effect on global distress, physical and psychosocial well-being, and treatment adherence.[8]

Fatigue is reported in up to 80% of youth receiving chemotherapy, and it persists for newly diagnosed youth for at least 8 weeks of treatment. Of the 87% of children diagnosed with ALL experiencing sleep disruption described above, problematic sleep and fatigue were highly correlated.[6,31] This suggests that nocturnal sleep disruption can affect entrainment, or the alignment of the internal biologic clock with external cues, therefore exacerbating fatigue. Maintaining a consistent sleep schedule supports circadian rhythm entrainment, which in turn should lead to reductions in fatigue. Although fatigue is known to cause difficulties in youth undergoing cancer treatment, it has been demonstrated to persist after the end of cancer-directed therapy.[11,32–34]

The mechanisms of CRF are multifactorial and may include disrupted nighttime sleep (associated with EDS and insomnia), circadian rhythm disturbances, cytokine dysregulation, HPA axis dysfunction, and serotonin dysregulation.[35] Although the relationship between circadian rhythm disturbance and CRF has not been widely studied in pediatric oncology, adults with cancer are at elevated risk for circadian dysregulation, with increased symptom burden and reduced survival that is purported to be a result of the disrupted circadian rhythm.[36–41] Circadian rhythms are likely to be disrupted during cancer treatment because of treatment-related changes in lifestyle behaviors such as poor sleep hygiene or other sleep disturbance, lowered mobility and physical activity, and reduced natural light exposure related to increased time in bed, daytime napping, extended school absences, and/or fewer outdoor activities.[12,42,43] Furthermore, these lifestyle behaviors may create a negative feedback loop whereby they persist after treatment has ended, further exacerbating disrupted circadian rhythm and fatigue into the cancer survivorship period.

Demographic and Treatment Variables Related to Differences in Sleep Problems

There is some evidence that sex and age may contribute to sleep disturbance and fatigue. For example, in a study examining sleep disruption in children with ALL in the maintenance phase of treatment, girls were found to nap more and had more consolidated nighttime sleep than did boys, even after controlling for differences in age, treatment, and risk group.[44] Another study examining changes in fatigue over the course of cancer treatment found that girls reported more fatigue than boys.[45] However, this finding is not consistent, because other studies of pediatric oncology patients have found no sex differences.[42,46,47]

Research related to age differences has demonstrated that adolescents are at greater risk for fatigue than younger or older patients with cancer.[9,48–51] Further, children report that they experience a decrease in fatigue over the course of treatment, whereas adolescents experience no improvement.[42,52] Age-related findings in sleep disturbance among pediatric oncology patients, on the other hand, have been more equivocal. In a study comparing children with ALL to their healthy same-age peers, van Litsenburg and colleagues[53] found that only children younger than 5 years with ALL had parent-reported significantly worse total sleep quality. Conversely, a study of children successfully treated for CNS tumors found that patients aged 8–12 years exhibited significantly more sleep disturbances than older or younger pediatric oncology patients.[54]

Cancer diagnosis and treatment variables have also been related to sleep disruption and fatigue. Whereas most children with cancer have been found to have significant fatigue around the time of diagnosis, those with leukemia have significant reductions in fatigue, and those with solid or CNS tumors have relatively stable reports of fatigue over the first 8 weeks of treatment.[11] Long-term survivors of hematopoietic stem cell transplant continue to have both self- and parent-reported fatigue at significantly higher rates than the general population, and as would be expected, those with EDS are significantly more likely to report co-occurring fatigue.[55] Further, 44% of adult survivors of childhood cancer have been found to report short sleep duration (≤ 6 hr/night). Pulmonary, endocrine, and gastrointestinal chronic conditions were significantly related to the risk of short sleep duration, and those with shorter sleep related to prolonged sleep onset latency reported the greatest burden from chronic health conditions.[56]

Corticosteroids, a backbone of many pediatric cancer treatments, particularly for ALL, have long been demonstrated to have a negative impact on sleep. Dexamethasone has been associated with less stable sleep–wake rhythms and more fatigue.[57] Compared with prednisone, dexamethasone has a significantly greater negative impact on sleep, with poorer sleep quality, more night awakenings, and higher rates of fatigue.[32] These sleep and fatigue symptoms demonstrated overlap, with pediatric oncology patients who demonstrate sleep–wake disturbance also having higher rates of fatigue.[58]

Impact of Sleep Disturbance

Sleep disturbances have been associated with poorer health, mood, behavior regulation, academic performance,

neurocognitive function, immune function, and overall quality of life.[16,59–64] In children with cancer, it is crucial to address sleep needs because sleep is critical for neural recovery and tissue healing and renewal. As a result, disrupted sleep may hinder the child's recovery.[19,65,66] In animal models and epidemiologic studies, sleep and circadian disturbances and disorders (e.g., OSA) have been found to be linked with increased cancer incidence, accelerated tumor growth, and lower survival rates.[3] Similarly, the consequences of sleep disruption on the child's psychologic well-being should be recognized. More specifically, poorer social functioning, physical and mental health, and more emotional distress, anxiety, pain, and behavioral and mood problems have been associated with sleep disturbances and fatigue.[13,47,48,67–69]

Cognitive and Academic Functioning. Disrupted sleep has been found to negatively impact cognitive and academic functioning in children without cancer, particularly those with obesity.[63,70] Whereas the relationship between sleep, cancer, and cognitive/academic performance has not been explicitly studied, the impact of sleep disturbances on cognitive performance has been studied in subpopulations within pediatric oncology. In particular, when youth with craniopharyngioma were studied with functional magnetic resonance imaging, those with EDS demonstrated greater activation in frontal brain regions, supporting a compensatory activation. This is important, as it provides some evidence that sustained attention may be more effortful for those children with daytime sleepiness, which in turn may directly impact academic performance.[71] Further, parents of pediatric brain tumor survivors have been more likely to describe poorer executive functioning for those with sleep difficulties.[72] In adults who are pediatric cancer survivors, those with poor sleep, daytime sleepiness, and fatigue have demonstrated poor task efficiency, organization, and memory.[73]

Whereas some data are available regarding relationships between sleep and cognitive performance in pediatric oncology patients, less is known about academic functioning. Observations of school performance in children with sleep-disordered breathing indicate that OSA in early childhood may impair future school performance.[74] Children with pediatric cancer are already at risk for poor school performance because of extended school absences and neurocognitive late effects of cancer treatments.[75,76] Thus it is likely that problematic sleep and fatigue may only compound this risk,[75] and this area warrants further investigation.[3]

Mood and Behavior. Both sleep disruption and fatigue can have significant impact on youths' ability to regulate behavior, emotions, and attention.[77] In adolescent oncology patients, those with significant fatigue have higher rates of depression and negative affect with lower rates of positive affect.[78] Among hospitalized pediatric brain tumor patients completing daily mood diaries, those with poorer mood during the day demonstrated longer actigraphically documented sleep onset latency and less sleep duration at night.[79] In youth undergoing chemotherapy (primarily on an inpatient unit), the combination of sleep disturbances and fatigue negatively influenced interpersonal relations, anxiety, and depressive symptoms in adolescents, whereas fatigue alone was associated with depressive symptoms and behavioral changes in children.[48]

In survivors of pediatric hematopoietic stem cell transplants, excessive sleepiness was found to be associated with more internalizing problems, and fatigue was related to more behavioral and emotional regulation difficulties and internalizing symptoms.[55] Within a broader group of pediatric cancer survivors, those with poor sleep efficiency, lower total sleep time, and more daytime sleepiness and fatigue were more likely to report emotional distress.[67] Taken together, it is clear that youth with a variety of cancer diagnoses and disrupted sleep and/or daytime fatigue demonstrate more behavioral and emotional regulation difficulties than are observed in healthy youth.

Health-Related Quality of Life (HRQoL). HRQoL has been defined in multiple ways across the literature. Of importance is the role of health within global quality of life, thus the concept of HRQoL must focus on the utility of health in impacting overall well-being.[80] A robust literature has identified poorer HRQoL in youth with cancer and in pediatric cancer survivors; higher-risk disease and extended, aggressive treatment was associated with lower quality of life.[81–83]

Both sleep and fatigue are important contributors to HRQoL in pediatric and adolescent patients with cancer.[84] Pediatric and adolescent patients with cancer who report high levels of fatigue are more likely to engage in less physical activity and to report poorer HRQoL.[47,52] It is important to consider that the symptom cluster of disrupted sleep, EDS, and the physical and social-emotional consequences of pediatric cancer may result in greater detriment to HRQoL than any one symptom alone.[30,78] Thus, interventions targeted toward improving sleep and fatigue may have the potential to improve HRQoL in pediatric oncology patients and survivors.

Interventions

Interventions that facilitate efficient sleep and developmentally appropriate activities of daily living despite CRF should be explored.[3,84] Both parents and oncologists have expressed a desire for interventions that promote healthy sleep in pediatric oncology patients.[85] Unfortunately, research on the efficacy of interventions to improve sleep quality in children and adolescents with pediatric cancer is limited, potentially because few formalized interventions have been developed specifically for this population. However, interventions for facilitating healthy sleep that have been used to address the antecedents to sleep disruptions, such as bedtime refusal, anxiety, and problematic sleep–wake cycles, may be effective. Because sleep involves both biologic and psychologic components,[23] a variety of potential interventions are possible. Similarly, the cause of the child's sleep disruption, such as cancer treatment, hospitalization, or behavioral disruptions, should be identified to better tailor sleep interventions.[84]

Nonpharmacologic interventions. Behavioral and cognitive-behavioral strategies may facilitate and maintain development of healthy sleep habits in youth with cancer and in cancer survivors. Establishing and maintaining adequate sleep hygiene is the backbone of most sleep interventions. Caregivers of children with cancer may pay less attention to sleep hygiene and routine as a result of increased attention on the child's health status, as well as increased caregiver distress, overprotectiveness, or disrupted routines as a result of medication schedules or hospitalizations.[9] Thus establishing a daily schedule with specific periods of rest and activity is likely to be beneficial.[9,84] Enforcing a consistent bedtime and wake time, developing or maintaining a bedtime routine, eliminating stimulating activities before sleep, decreasing caffeine intake, and providing a cool and quiet sleep environment are strategies recommended for pediatric oncology patients, just as for healthy children.[86] Graduated extinction methods have also demonstrated effectiveness in case reports for children with comorbid medical conditions and sleep problems,[87] as well as for young children preparing for stem cell transplantation.[88] This gradual approach may be more acceptable to caregivers of children with cancer, as it is less likely than traditional extinction methods to induce aversive extinction bursts in which the negative behavior temporarily worsens prior to extinguishing.[89]

Both yoga and massage have shown promise in improving sleep for pediatric oncology inpatients.[90,91] Exercise may also serve as a beneficial intervention, as pediatric oncology patients who engage in higher levels of activity have been found to have healthier sleep.[49] For treatment of fatigue, bright light therapy (BLT) used for 30 minutes each morning has been shown to improve fatigue in adults with cancer and has shown promise in adolescents and young adults receiving and after cancer-directed therapy.[92–96] Finally, support exists for both in-person and internet-delivered cognitive-behavioral therapy for insomnia to address sleep problems in adolescent and young adult cancer survivors.[97,98]

Hospital-Based Interventions. Changes made within the hospital environment may serve to protect children's sleep while they are admitted for cancer-directed treatment and in turn potentially improve sleep after discharge. During an inpatient stay, children with cancer have an average of 11 room entries/exits by staff during the nighttime period, with a mean of 12–16 nighttime awakenings each night of the admission, and 66% have inadequate sleep duration.[10,99] Not surprisingly, over the course of the hospital admission, children's reported fatigue steadily increased, which was associated with the number of nighttime awakenings.[10] Environmental interventions should include family-oriented psychoeducation, increased physical activity, and protected time for sleep.[3] To protect sleep times, changes in nursing practices are important to consider. This includes measures such as "bundled care" whereby all necessary, scheduled care occurs simultaneously during the night, with the remainder of room entries confined to unexpected needs that arise. A nighttime nursing bundle and protected sleep environment for children undergoing high-dose chemotherapy and stem cell rescue resulted in youth in the intervention condition having more extended sleep than those in the control condition. Unfortunately, because of the significant nighttime care needs, sleep remained quite disrupted even in the intervention group.[100]

Pharmacological Interventions. Pharmacological interventions may be required to address nocturnal sleep issues such as acute or chronic insomnia, circadian rhythm sleep–wake disorders (often of the delayed sleep phase type), and EDS in children with cancer. As with any treatment plan, the clinician should develop a clear understanding of the underlying cause(s) of the sleep disturbance. For example, acute or chronic insomnia caused by pain should be addressed using behavioral and, in many cases, pharmacological approaches to alleviate pain. Insomnia caused by anxiety or mood disorders may require a different approach, often involving the combined use of behavioral and pharmacological interventions. Insomnia associated with suspected OSA syndrome should be assessed with nocturnal polysomnography whenever possible and managed according to commonly used treatment pathways including medical and surgical approaches, or continuous positive airway pressure.[101] Restless legs syndrome (RLS), which may be associated with certain chemotherapy agents, peripheral neuropathy, and anemia, should be addressed with assessment of iron status, reduced exposure to caffeine, and in some cases, medications.[102–104] Circadian rhythm sleep–wake disorders should be addressed with behavioral interventions and, in some cases, melatonin.[105,106]

Clear and well-defined treatment goals should be established in advance. Dosing of medication should begin at the lowest level that is likely to be effective followed by titration as necessary. It is important for the clinician to monitor the child's response, to inquire about adverse side effects, and to reevaluate periodically to ascertain whether therapeutic goals are being met. Drug-drug interactions are an important consideration in this population given the high likelihood that the child is receiving other medications concurrently.

Pharmacological approaches to insomnia in childhood are covered in a comprehensive fashion in this text (Chapter 5). There are no medications approved by the U.S. Food and Drug Administration for use in children with insomnia other than an old indication for chloral hydrate. However, medications such as antihistamines and α-agonists such as clonidine are commonly used in children with insomnia.[107] Antidepressants such as selective serotonin reuptake inhibitors and tricyclic antidepressants are sometimes used in children, particularly when anxiety or mood disorders are present.[108] Benzodiazepines and nonbenzodiazepine receptor agonists are seldom used for treatment of insomnia in children because of the potential risk of tolerance and addiction.

Pharmacological approaches to restless legs syndrome in children are covered in this text Chapter 44). Supplementation of iron can be helpful when the child's serum ferritin is depressed.[102] Pharmacological treatment options for RLS include dopaminergic agents, but

further investigation of these medications in children is needed, including assessment of adverse side effects such as sedation and long-term outcome. The development of augmentation (worsening of symptom intensity or appearance of symptoms earlier in the day) is well-known to occur in adults who are treated for RLS with dopaminergic agents. Benzodiazepines such as clonazepam, α-agonists such as clonidine, anticonvulsants such as gabapentin, and opioids (typically used only for cases refractory to standard measures) represent other treatment options.[103,104]

The circadian rhythm sleep–wake disorder, delayed sleep phase type, is typically managed with a combination of behavioral interventions and melatonin administered 3–4 hours in advance of the desired bedtime. BLT provided as soon as possible after awakening for 30–45 minutes represents another option. The recent development of wearable technology (such as LED lights within a visor or special glasses) has improved the acceptance of BLT.

Children with brain tumors may experience EDS, particularly when the tumor involves the diencephalon or brainstem region. Hypersomnia can occur because of direct involvement of the tumor or due to surgical intervention.[18,19,109,110] These children require comprehensive evaluation including nocturnal polysomnography followed by a multiple sleep latency test for characterization of sleepiness and propensity for entry into stage REM sleep. Children with pathological sleepiness may respond to traditional stimulants, modafinil, or other agents.[109,110] Management by a pediatric sleep specialist with expertise in this area is typically required because of the complexity of these cases.

In summary, pharmacological intervention may play an important role in managing children with sleep problems and cancer. However, nonpharmacological approaches should be considered initially, and medications alone are rarely effective. There is a pressing need for more systematic investigation into the optimal pharmacological approaches for sleep problems in children with cancer.

CLINICAL PEARLS

- Children, adolescents, and young adults with cancer as well as survivors of pediatric cancer are at increased risk for sleep disturbances including insomnia and excessive daytime sleepiness.
- The most commonly seen sleep difficulties in pediatric oncology patients and survivors are multifactorial and are likely caused by a combination of physiological effects of cancer and its treatment, changes in routine, stress, and environmental disruptions within inpatient hospital environments.
- Although more specific research within samples of youth with cancer and childhood cancer survivors is necessary, tailored interventions have shown promise in improving nighttime symptoms and daytime function.

Summary

It is becoming increasingly clear that children and adolescents receiving cancer-directed treatment are at elevated risk for sleep disturbances that contribute to fatigue and EDS. These sleep disturbances are multifactorial and include difficulty initiating and maintaining sleep and restless sleep, likely caused by a combination of direct physiological effects of cancer and medications, changes in routine, stress, and environmental disruptions on the inpatient unit. Resulting fatigue and sleepiness may be related not only to sleep disruptions but also to the physiological effects of cancer-directed therapy such as pain and anemia. After completion of cancer-directed therapy, pediatric cancer survivors have risks for insomnia as well as ongoing fatigue and EDS. Interventions should target symptoms during cancer treatment and survivorship periods and should include a combination of both nonpharmacologic and pharmacologic interventions targeted to specific symptoms. Although more research is necessary, targeted interventions should demonstrate a positive impact on patients' HRQoL.

References

1. Institute NC. Surveillance, Epidemiology, and End Results Program. Accessed November 29, 2023. https://seer.cancer.gov/csr/1975_2017/results_merged/sect_29_childhood_cancer_iccc.pdf#search=pediatric%20cancer%20incidence.
2. Institute NC. Cancer in Children and Adolescents. Accessed November 29, 2023. https://www.cancer.gov/types/childhood-cancers/child-adolescent-cancers-fact-sheet#how-common-is-cancer-in-children.
3. Daniel LC, van Litsenburg RRL, Rogers VE, et al. A call to action for expanded sleep research in pediatric oncology: a position paper on behalf of the International Psycho-Oncology Society Pediatrics Special Interest Group. *Psychooncology.* 2020;29(3):465–474.
4. Howlader N, Noone AM, Krapcho M, et al. SEER Cancer Statistics Review, 1975-2016. National Cancer Institute. Updated April 9, 2020. Accessed November 19, 2023. https://seer.cancer.gov/csr/1975_2016/.
5. Siegel R, DeSantis C, Virgo K, et al. Cancer treatment and survivorship statistics, 2012. *CA Cancer J Clin.* 2012;62(4):220–241.
6. Kaleyias J, Manley P, Kothare SV. Sleep disorders in children with cancer. *Semin Pediatr Neurol.* 2012;19(1):25–34.
7. Mindell JA, Owens JA. *A Clinical Guide to Pediatric. Sleep: Diagnosis and Management of Sleep Problems.* 2nd ed. Lippincott Williams & Wilkins; 2010.
8. Spathis A, Booth S, Grove S, Hatcher H, Kuhn I, Barclay S. Teenage and young adult cancer-related fatigue is prevalent, distressing, and neglected: it is time to intervene. a systematic literature review and narrative synthesis. *J Adolesc Young Adult Oncol.* 2015;4(1):3–17.
9. Zupanec S, Jones H, Stremler R. Sleep habits and fatigue of children receiving maintenance chemotherapy for ALL and their parents. *J Pediatr Oncol Nurs.* 2010;27(4):217–228.
10. Hinds PS, Hockenberry MJ, Gattuso JS, et al. Dexamethasone alters sleep and fatigue in pediatric patients with acute lymphoblastic leukemia. *Cancer.* 2007;110(10):2321–2330.
11. Crabtree VM, Rach AM, Schellinger KB, Russell KM, Hammarback T, Mandrell BN. Changes in sleep and fatigue in newly treated pediatric oncology patients. *Support Care Cancer.* 2015;23(2):393–401.
12. Walker AJ, Johnson KP, Miaskowski C, Lee KA, Gedaly-Duff V. Sleep quality and sleep hygiene behaviors of adolescents during chemotherapy. *J Clin Sleep Med.* 2010;6(5):439–444.
13. Daniel LC, Meltzer LJ, Gross JY, Flannery JL, Forrest CB, Barakat LP. Sleep practices in pediatric cancer patients: indirect effects on sleep disturbances and symptom burden. *Psychooncology.* 2021.
14. Medicine AAoS. *International Classification of Sleep Disorders.* 3rd ed. American Academy of Sleep Medicine; 2014.
15. Paavonen EJ, Raikkonen K, Pesonen AK, et al. Sleep quality and cognitive performance in 8-year-old children. *Sleep Med.* 2010;11(4):386–392.
16. Astill RG, Van der Heijden KB, Van IJzendoorn MH, Van Someren EJ. Sleep, cognition, and behavioral problems in school-age children: a century of research meta-analyzed. *Psychol Bull.* 2012;138(6):1109–1138.
17. Rosen G, Brand SR. Sleep in children with cancer: case review of 70 children evaluated in a comprehensive pediatric sleep center. *Support Care Cancer.* 2011;19(7):985–994.
18. Brimeyer C, Adams L, Zhu L, et al. Sleep complaints in survivors of pediatric brain tumors. *Support Care Cancer.* 2016;24(1):23–31.
19. Mandrell BN, Wise M, Schoumacher RA, et al. Excessive daytime sleepiness and sleep-disordered breathing disturbances in survivors of childhood central nervous system tumors. *Pediatr Blood Cancer.* 2012;58(5):746–751.
20. Muller HL, Muller-Stover S, Gebhardt U, Kolb R, Sorensen N, Handwerker G. Secondary narcolepsy may be a causative factor of increased daytime sleepiness in obese childhood craniopharyngioma patients. *J Pediatr Endocrinol Metab.* 2006;19(Suppl 1):423–429.
21. Olson K. Sleep-related disturbances among adolescents with cancer: a systematic review. *Sleep Med.* 2014;15(5):496–501.
22. O'Gorman CS, Simoneau-Roy J, Pencharz P, et al. Sleep-disordered breathing is increased in obese adolescents with craniopharyngioma compared with obese controls. *J Clin Endocrinol Metab.* 2010;95(5):2211–2218.
23. Rosen GM, Shor AC, Geller TJ. Sleep in children with cancer. *Curr Opin Pediatr.* 2008;20(6):676–681.
24. Marcus CL, Trescher WH, Halbower AC, Lutz J. Secondary narcolepsy in children with brain tumors. *Sleep.* 2002;25(4):435–439.
25. Lipton J, Megerian JT, Kothare SV, et al. Melatonin deficiency and disrupted circadian rhythms in pediatric survivors of craniopharyngioma. *Neurology.* 2009;73(4):323–325.
26. Mandrell BN, LaRosa K, Hancock D, et al. Predictors of narcolepsy and hypersomnia due to medical disorder in pediatric craniopharyngioma. *J Neurooncol.* 2020;148(2):307–316.
27. Daniel LC, Aggarwal R, Schwartz LA. Sleep in adolescents and young adults in the year after cancer treatment. *J Adolesc Young Adult Oncol.* 2017;6(4):560–567.

28. Yusufov M, Zhou ES, Recklitis CJ. Psychometric properties of the Insomnia Severity Index in cancer survivors. *Psychooncology.* 2019;28(3):540–546.
29. Zhou ES, Manley PE, Marcus KJ, Recklitis CJ. Medical and psychosocial correlates of insomnia symptoms in adult survivors of pediatric brain tumors. *J Pediatr Psychol.* 2016;41(6):623–630.
30. Berger AM, Mooney K, Alvarez-Perez A, et al. Cancer-Related Fatigue, Version 2.2015. *J Natl Compr Canc Netw.* 2015;13(8):1012–1039.
31. Dupuis LL, Milne-Wren C, Cassidy M, et al. Symptom assessment in children receiving cancer therapy: the parents' perspective. *Support Care Cancer.* 2010;18(3):281–299.
32. Daniel LC, Li Y, Kloss JD, Reilly AF, Barakat LP. The impact of dexamethasone and prednisone on sleep in children with acute lymphoblastic leukemia. *Support Care Cancer.* 2016;24(9):3897–3906.
33. Nap-van der Vlist MM, Dalmeijer GW, Grootenhuis MA, et al. Fatigue in childhood chronic disease. *Arch Dis Child.* 2019;104(11):1090–1095.
34. Poort H, Kaal SEJ, Knoop H, et al. Prevalence and impact of severe fatigue in adolescent and young adult cancer patients in comparison with population-based controls. *Support Care Cancer.* 2017;25(9):2911–2918.
35. O'Higgins CM, Brady B, O'Connor B, Walsh D, Reilly RB. The pathophysiology of cancer-related fatigue: current controversies. *Support Care Cancer.* 2018;26(10):3353–3364.
36. Innominato PF, Giacchetti S, Bjarnason GA, et al. Prediction of overall survival through circadian rest-activity monitoring during chemotherapy for metastatic colorectal cancer. *Int J Cancer.* 2012;131(11):2684–2692.
37. Innominato PF, Mormont MC, Rich TA, Waterhouse J, Levi FA, Bjarnason GA. Circadian disruption, fatigue, and anorexia clustering in advanced cancer patients: implications for innovative therapeutic approaches. *Integr Cancer Ther.* 2009;8(4):361–370.
38. Innominato PF, Roche VP, Palesh OG, Ulusakarya A, Spiegel D, Levi FA. The circadian timing system in clinical oncology. *Ann Med.* 2014;46(4):191–207.
39. Levi F, Dugue PA, Innominato P, et al. Wrist actimetry circadian rhythm as a robust predictor of colorectal cancer patients survival. *Chronobiol Int.* 2014;31(8):891–900.
40. Levi F, Okyar A, Dulong S, Innominato PF, Clairambault J. Circadian timing in cancer treatments. *Annu Rev Pharmacol Toxicol.* 2010;50:377–421.
41. Sephton SE, Lush E, Dedert EA, et al. Diurnal cortisol rhythm as a predictor of lung cancer survival. *Brain Behav Immun.* 2013;30(Suppl):S163–170.
42. Hooke MC, Garwick AW, Gross CR. Fatigue and physical performance in children and adolescents receiving chemotherapy. *Oncol Nurs Forum.* 2011;38(6):649–657.
43. Sun JL, Wu SC, Chang LI, Chiou JF, Chou PL, Lin CC. The relationship between light exposure and sleep, fatigue, and depression in cancer outpatients: test of the mediating effect. *Cancer Nurs.* 2014;37(5):382–390.
44. Sanford SD, Okuma JO, Pan J, et al. Gender differences in sleep, fatigue, and daytime activity in a pediatric oncology sample receiving dexamethasone. *J Pediatr Psychol.* 2008;33(3):298–306.
45. Perdikaris P, Merkouris A, Patiraki E, Papadatou D, Vasilatou-Kosmidis H, Matziou V. Changes in children's fatigue during
the course of treatment for paediatric cancer. *Int Nurs Rev.* 2008;55(4):412–419.
46. Ince D, Demirag B, Karapinar TH, et al. Assessment of sleep in pediatric cancer patients. *Turk J Pediatr.* 2017;59(4):379–386.
47. Nunes MDR, Jacob E, Bomfim EO, et al. Fatigue and health related quality of life in children and adolescents with cancer. *Eur J Oncol Nurs.* 2017;29:39–46.
48. Hockenberry MJ, Hooke MC, Gregurich M, McCarthy K, Sambuco G, Krull K. Symptom clusters in children and adolescents receiving cisplatin, doxorubicin, or ifosfamide. *Oncol Nurs Forum.* 2010;37(1):E16–27.
49. Orsey AD, Wakefield DB, Cloutier MM. Physical activity (PA) and sleep among children and adolescents with cancer. *Pediatr Blood Cancer.* 2013;60(11):1908–1913.
50. Ream E, Gibson F, Edwards J, Seption B, Mulhall A, Richardson A. Experience of fatigue in adolescents living with cancer. *Cancer Nurs.* 2006;29(4):317–326.
51. Singer S, Kuhnt S, Zwerenz R, et al. Age- and sex-standardised prevalence rates of fatigue in a large hospital-based sample of cancer patients. *Br J Cancer.* 2011;105(3):445–451.
52. Van Dijk-Lokkart EM, Steur LMH, Braam KI, et al. Longitudinal development of cancer-related fatigue and physical activity in childhood cancer patients. *Pediatr Blood Cancer.* 2019;66(12):e27949.
53. van Litsenburg RR, Huisman J, Hoogerbrugge PM, Egeler RM, Kaspers GJ, Gemke RJ. Impaired sleep affects quality of life in children during maintenance treatment for acute lymphoblastic leukemia: an exploratory study. *Health Qual Life Outcomes.* 2011;9:25.
54. Greenfeld M, Constantini S, Tauman R, Sivan Y. Sleep disturbances in children recovered from central nervous system neoplasms. *J Pediatr.* 2011;159(2):268–272. e261.
55. Graef DM, Phipps S, Parris KR, et al. Sleepiness, fatigue, behavioral functioning, and quality of life in survivors of childhood hematopoietic stem cell transplant. *J Pediatr Psychol.* 2016;41(6):600–609.
56. Lubas MM, Mandrell BN, Ness KK, et al. Short sleep duration and physical and psychological health outcomes among adult survivors of childhood cancer. *Pediatr Blood Cancer.* 2021:e28988.
57. Steur LMH, Kaspers GJL, van Someren EJW, et al. The impact of maintenance therapy on sleep-wake rhythms and cancer-related fatigue in pediatric acute lymphoblastic leukemia. *Support Care Cancer.* 2020;28(12):5983–5993.
58. Steur LMH, Kaspers GJL, Van Someren EJW, et al. Sleep-wake rhythm disruption is associated with cancer-related fatigue in pediatric acute lymphoblastic leukemia. *Sleep.* 2020;43(6).
59. Palmer CA, Alfano CA. Sleep and emotion regulation: an organizing, integrative review. *Sleep Med Rev.* 2017;31:6–16.
60. Li L, Zhang S, Huang Y, Chen K. Sleep duration and obesity in children: a systematic review and meta-analysis of prospective cohort studies. *J Paediatr Child Health.* 2017;53(4):378–385.
61. Magee CA, Robinson L, Keane C. Sleep quality subtypes predict health-related quality of life in children. *Sleep Med.* 2017;35:67–73.
62. Moldofsky H. Sleep and the immune system. *Int J Immunopharmacol.* 1995;17(8):649–654.
63. Beebe DW, Lewin D, Zeller M, et al. Sleep in overweight adolescents: shorter sleep, poorer sleep quality, sleepiness, and sleep-disordered breathing. *J Pediatr Psychol.* 2007;32(1):69–79.
64. Buckhalt JA, El-Sheikh M, Keller P. Children's sleep and cognitive functioning: race and socioeconomic status as moderators of effects. *Child Dev.* 2007;78(1):213–231.

65. Fleming MK, Smejka T, Henderson Slater D, et al. Sleep disruption after brain injury is associated with worse motor outcomes and slower functional recovery. *Neurorehabil Neural Repair.* 2020;34(7):661–671.

66. Walker MP. Cognitive consequences of sleep and sleep loss. *Sleep Med.* 2008;9(Suppl 1):S29–34.

67. Daniel LC, Wang M, Mulrooney DA, et al. Sleep, emotional distress, and physical health in survivors of childhood cancer: a report from the Childhood Cancer Survivor Study. *Psychooncology.* 2019;28(4):903–912.

68. Kim S, Han J, Lee MY, Jang MK. The experience of cancer-related fatigue, exercise and exercise adherence among women breast cancer survivors: Insights from focus group interviews. *J Clin Nurs.* 2020;29(5-6):758–769.

69. Schulte FSM, Chalifour K, Eaton G, Garland SN. Quality of life among survivors of adolescent and young adult cancer in Canada: a Young Adults With Cancer in Their Prime (YACPRIME) study. *Cancer.* 2021;127(8):1325–1333.

70. Chaput JP, Brunet M, Tremblay A. Relationship between short sleeping hours and childhood overweight/obesity: results from the "Quebec en Forme" Project. *Int J Obes (Lond).* 2006;30(7):1080–1085.

71. Jacola LM, Conklin HM, Scoggins MA, et al. Investigating the role of hypothalamic tumor involvement in sleep and cognitive outcomes among children treated for craniopharyngioma. *J Pediatr Psychol.* 2016;41(6):610–622.

72. van Kooten J, Maurice-Stam H, Schouten AYN, et al. High occurrence of sleep problems in survivors of a childhood brain tumor with neurocognitive complaints: the association with psychosocial and behavioral executive functioning. *Pediatr Blood Cancer.* 2019;66(11):e27947.

73. Clanton NR, Klosky JL, Li C, et al. Fatigue, vitality, sleep, and neurocognitive functioning in adult survivors of childhood cancer: a report from the Childhood Cancer Survivor Study. *Cancer.* 2011;117(11):2559–2568.

74. Gozal D, Pope DWJr. Snoring during early childhood and academic performance at ages thirteen to fourteen years. *Pediatrics.* 2001;107(6):1394–1399.

75. Krull KR, Hardy KK, Kahalley LS, Schuitema I, Kesler SR. neurocognitive outcomes and interventions in long-term survivors of childhood cancer. *J Clin Oncol.* 2018;36(21):2181–2189.

76. Moore 3rd BD. Neurocognitive outcomes in survivors of childhood cancer. *J Pediatr Psychol.* 2005;30(1):51–63.

77. Dahl RE, Lewin DS. Pathways to adolescent health sleep regulation and behavior. *J Adolesc Health.* 2002;31(6 Suppl):175–184.

78. Daniel LC, Brumley LD, Schwartz LA. Fatigue in adolescents with cancer compared to healthy adolescents. *Pediatr Blood Cancer.* 2013;60(11):1902–1907.

79. Graef DM, Crabtree VM, Srivastava DK, et al. Sleep and mood during hospitalization for high-dose chemotherapy and hematopoietic rescue in pediatric medulloblastoma. *Psychooncology.* 2018;27(7):1847–1853.

80. Karimi M, Brazier J. Health, health-related quality of life, and quality of life: what is the difference? *Pharmacoeconomics.* 2016;34(7):645–649.

81. Fardell JE, Vetsch J, Trahair T, et al. Health-related quality of life of children on treatment for acute lymphoblastic leukemia: a systematic review. *Pediatr Blood Cancer.* 2017;64(9).

82. Speechley KN, Barrera M, Shaw AK, Morrison HI, Maunsell E. Health-related quality of life among child and adolescent survivors of childhood cancer. *J Clin Oncol.* 2006;24(16):2536–2543.

83. Bhat SR, Goodwin TL, Burwinkle TM, et al. Profile of daily life in children with brain tumors: an assessment of health-related quality of life. *J Clin Oncol.* 2005;23(24):5493–5500.

84. Erickson JM, Beck SL, Christian BR, et al. Fatigue, sleep-wake disturbances, and quality of life in adolescents receiving chemotherapy. *J Pediatr Hematol Oncol.* 2011;33(1):e17–25.

85. Daniel LC, Schwartz LA, Mindell JA, Tucker CA, Barakat LP. Initial validation of the sleep disturbances in pediatric cancer model. *J Pediatr Psychol.* 2016;41(6):588–599.

86. Meltzer LJ, Crabtree VM. *Pediatric Sleep Problems: A Clinician's Guide to Behavioral Interventions.* APA Books; 2015.

87. Wiggs L, France K. Behavioural treatments for sleep problems in children and adolescents with physical illness, psychological problems or intellectual disabilities. *Sleep Med Rev.* 2000;4(3):299–314.

88. LaRosa KN, Crabtree VM, Jurbergs N, Harman J. Behavioral sleep intervention to reduce bedsharing prior to stem cell transplant. *J Clin Sleep Med.* 2021;17(2):333–335.

89. Etherton H, Blunden S, Hauck Y. Discussion of extinction-based behavioral sleep interventions for young children and reasons why parents may find them difficult. *J Clin Sleep Med.* 2016;12(11):1535–1543.

90. Diorio C, Schechter T, Lee M, et al. A pilot study to evaluate the feasibility of individualized yoga for inpatient children receiving intensive chemotherapy. *BMC Complement Altern Med.* 2015;152

91. Jacobs S, Mowbray C, Cates LM, et al. Pilot study of massage to improve sleep and fatigue in hospitalized adolescents with cancer. *Pediatr Blood Cancer.* 2016;63(5):880–886.

92. Liu L, Marler MR, Parker BA, et al. The relationship between fatigue and light exposure during chemotherapy. *Support Care Cancer.* 2005;13(12):1010–1017.

93. Rogers VE, Mowbray C, Rahmaty Z, Hinds PS. A morning bright light therapy intervention to improve circadian health in adolescent cancer survivors: methods and preliminary feasibility. *J Pediatr Oncol Nurs.* 2021;38(2):70–81.

94. Ancoli-Israel S, Rissling M, Neikrug A, et al. Light treatment prevents fatigue in women undergoing chemotherapy for breast cancer. *Support Care Cancer.* 2012;20(6):1211–1219.

95. Crabtree VM, LaRosa KN, MacArthur E, et al. Feasibility and acceptability of light therapy to reduce fatigue in adolescents and young adults receiving cancer-directed therapy. *Behav Sleep Med.* 2020:1–13.

96. Neikrug AB, Rissling M, Trofimenko V, et al. Bright light therapy protects women from circadian rhythm desynchronization during chemotherapy for breast cancer. *Behav Sleep Med.* 2012;10(3):202–216.

97. Zhou ES, Recklitis CJ. Internet-delivered insomnia intervention improves sleep and quality of life for adolescent and young adult cancer survivors. *Pediatr Blood Cancer.* 2020;67(9).e28506.

98. Zhou ES, Vrooman LM, Manley PE, Crabtree VM, Recklitis CJ. Adapted delivery of cognitive-behavioral treatment for insomnia in adolescent and young adult cancer survivors: a pilot study. *Behav Sleep Med.* 2017;15(4):288–301.

99. Traube C, Rosenberg L, Thau F, et al. Sleep in hospitalized children with cancer: a cross-sectional study. *Hosp Pediatr.* 2020;10(11):969–976.

100. Rogers VE, Zhu S, Ancoli-Israel S, Liu L, Mandrell BN, Hinds PS. A pilot randomized controlled trial to improve sleep and fatigue in children with central nervous system tumors hospitalized for high-dose chemotherapy. *Pediatr Blood Cancer.* 2019;66(8):e27814.

101. Pereira KD, Jon CK, Szmuk P, Lazar RH, Mitchell RB. Management of obstructive sleep apnea in children: a practical approach. *Ear Nose Throat J.* 2016;95(7):E14–22.

102. Allen RP, Picchietti DL, Auerbach M, et al. Evidence-based and consensus clinical practice guidelines for the iron treatment of restless legs syndrome/Willis-Ekbom disease in adults and children: an IRLSSG task force report. *Sleep Med.* 2018;41:27–44.

103. DelRosso L, Bruni O. Treatment of pediatric restless legs syndrome. *Adv Pharmacol.* 2019;84:237–253.

104. Rulong G, Dye T, Simakajornboon N. Pharmacological management of restless legs syndrome and periodic limb movement disorder in children. *Paediatr Drugs.* 2018;20(1):9–17.

105. Auger RR, Burgess HJ, Emens JS, Deriy LV, Thomas SM, Sharkey KM. Clinical practice guideline for the treatment of intrinsic circadian rhythm sleep-wake disorders: advanced sleep-wake phase disorder (ASWPD), delayed sleep-wake phase disorder (DSWPD), non-24-hour sleep-wake rhythm disorder (N24SWD), and irregular sleep-wake rhythm disorder (ISWRD). an update for 2015: an American Academy of Sleep Medicine clinical practice guideline. *J Clin Sleep Med.* 2015;11(10):1199–1236.

106. Culnan E, McCullough LM, Wyatt JK. Circadian rhythm sleep-wake phase disorders. *Neurol Clin.* 2019;37(3):527–543.

107. Owens JA, Rosen CL, Mindell JA. Medication use in the treatment of pediatric insomnia: results of a survey of community-based pediatricians. *Pediatrics.* 2003;111(5 Pt 1):e628–635.

108. Owens JA, Rosen CL, Mindell JA, Kirchner HL. Use of pharmacotherapy for insomnia in child psychiatry practice: A national survey. *Sleep Med.* 2010;11(7):692–700.

109. Rosen GM, Bendel AE, Neglia JP, Moertel CL, Mahowald M. Sleep in children with neoplasms of the central nervous system: case review of 14 children. *Pediatrics.* 2003;112(1 Pt 1):e46–54.

110. Weil AG, Muir K, Hukin J, Desautels A, Martel V, Perreault S. Narcolepsy and hypothalamic region tumors: presentation and evolution. *Pediatr Neurol.* 2018;84:27–31.

48

Sleep in Psychiatric Disorders

Christine J. So, Candice A. Alfano, and Anna Ivanenko

CHAPTER HIGHLIGHTS

- Children and adolescents who exhibit mental health symptoms are particularly vulnerable to the adverse consequences associated with insufficient sleep.
- This chapter reviews the research to date describing sleep problems associated with mood disorders and anxiety and related disorders, as well as risk factors including developmental stage.
- Sleep disturbance may manifest differently depending on psychiatric and other symptoms present, highlighting the importance of comprehensive sleep assessments among youth.
- Research on psychosocial and pharmacologic interventions for treating sleep in this population is discussed.

Introduction

Behavioral and emotional development in children and adolescents is closely linked to the maturation of sleep–wake regulatory systems. Early disruptions in the organization of sleep states may contribute to dysregulation of affect and behavior and subsequently lead to the development of psychopathology. Alternatively, psychiatric disorders can contribute to the development of sleep disturbances that are long-lasting and require specific interventions to prevent further deterioration of the neurobehavioral functions.

Sleep problems are pervasive among children and adolescents with virtually all types of psychiatric disorders. Epidemiologic and clinical studies uniformly describe a high prevalence of sleep-related disorders among clinical samples of youth that include insomnia, bedtime refusal, nightmares, night terrors, delayed sleep phase, and restless sleep.[1] Long sleep latencies, short sleep durations, frequent nocturnal awakenings, and restless sleep have all been shown to correlate with the severity of psychiatric symptoms in a diverse cohort of children with psychiatric disorders.[1,2] However, even in nonclinical samples, strong associations exist between sleep complaints and symptoms of emotional distress, depression, and anxiety in children.[3–5] For example, in a large community-based prospective study of 6-year-old children, 13% of those with trouble sleeping were found to have clinically elevated anxiety and depressive

scores compared with just 3% of children without problems sleeping; at age 11, the percentage of children with anxiety or depressive symptoms increased to 29% and 4%, respectively.[6]

Adolescents are particularly vulnerable to both types of problems, which likely act synergistically to elevate overall risk during this developmental stage.[7] Specifically, just as sleep disturbances are ubiquitous among teens with psychiatric disorders, inadequate sleep is known to independently elevate the risk for depression, anxiety, low self-esteem, excessive worry, and irritability, as well as an increased likelihood of using alcohol, nicotine, and caffeine.[4,5,8] A cross-sectional and prospective study of 12- to 18-year-olds found that 54% of adolescents with insomnia reported depressive symptoms, 26% had suicidal ideation, and 10% indicated a history of suicide attempts, with all frequencies higher than those found in a non-insomnia group (which were 32%, 12%, and 3%, respectively).[9] A host of adolescent experimental studies published in recent years further confirm inadequate sleep to produce emotional and behavioral disturbances.[4,10,11]

Subjective Sleep in Early-Onset Major Depression

Major depressive disorder (MDD) is a severe and debilitating clinical condition that is often recurrent and associated with poor psychosocial, academic, and occupational outcomes. Approximately 2% of children and 8% of adolescents are affected by MDD with a male-to-female ratio of 1:1 in children and 1:2 in adolescents.[12] Suicide is the most dramatic outcome of MDD and the second leading cause of death for people aged 10–34.[13]

Early studies of sleep complaints in clinically depressed preadolescent children revealed that two-thirds of children with depression reported sleep-onset problems and sleep maintenance problems and half suffered from terminal insomnia (i.e., awakening earlier than desired). Furthermore, their sleep complaints continued throughout the depressive episode with 10% of children experiencing insomnia after remission.[14,15] More recent investigations have observed sleep complaints in up to 83% of children and adolescents diagnosed with MDD via structured diagnostic interviews.[16,17] Children and adolescents with sleep disturbances also had more severe depression with higher rates of concurrent anxiety. The most common forms of sleep disturbance in depressed youth were nonrestorative sleep (69%) and insomnia (between 51% and 54%). Report of multiple sleep disturbances was also associated with not only an increased risk of depression,[18] but also more severe forms of depression.[16,17]

Sleep disturbances, especially insomnia and nightmares, have also been associated with increased rates of reported suicidal ideation and suicide attempts in youth.[19] In the only known study that examined sleep disturbances in 15- to 19-year-old suicide completers, insomnia was 10 times more likely to have been reported in that group than it was in community controls. Furthermore, adolescents who completed suicide were five times more likely than controls to have exhibited insomnia in the week preceding death.[20]

Associations between suicidality and sleep duration among adolescents were examined in a recent meta-analysis of 12 cross-sectional reports. A curvilinear dose–response was observed, such that adolescents who reported a total sleep time (TST) of 8–9 hours per night had the lowest risk for suicidal ideation and attempts.[21] Further, there was an 11% decrease in risk of suicide plans for each hour increase in TST.[21] Findings collectively suggest that disordered sleep is strongly associated with suicidal behavior, with insufficient sleep duration as the most salient risk factor.

In a 2012 prospective study of nationally represented U.S. adolescents, Wong and Brower examined 6,504 adolescents across three waves spanning 6 years. They found that reports of difficulty falling or staying asleep at an initial time point predicted suicidal thoughts and attempts at a later time point, even when controlling for other variables such as gender, depression, and alcohol problems.[22] In another prospective study, Sivertsen and colleagues found that toddlers who experienced short sleep duration and frequent nightly awakenings were at increased risk of developing depressive symptoms as children.[23] This study emphasized the importance of sleep assessment when screening for risk factors of depression and suicidal behaviors in youth of all ages.

Objective Sleep Measures in Early-Onset Major Depression

Polysomnographic (PSG) characteristics of sleep in prepubertal children with major depression have yielded inconsistent results. The early work by Puig-Antich and colleagues[14] failed to reveal significant differences in any sleep variables between children with major depression and normal controls. Their findings were later supported by other studies that demonstrated no differences in PSG characteristics between children with MDD and healthy controls.[24,25] However, when depressed children were recruited from inpatient facilities, reduced rapid eye movement (REM)-onset latencies, increased REM time, and increased sleep-onset latencies were found in a subset of prepubertal children with MDD.[24,26] Based on these findings, it was suggested that

inpatient status, severity of MDD, and presence of other psychiatric comorbidities may influence sleep characteristics in preadolescent depressives. Over the years of PSG research, a prolonged latency to sleep onset has emerged as one of the more stable characteristics of sleep dysregulation associated with early-onset MDD.[27]

PSG characteristics have been examined much more extensively in adolescents with MDD. A 2014 meta-analysis examined sleep macro- and microarchitecture among children and adolescents with MDD; in a comparison of 28 studies, modest changes in macro- and microarchitecture were observed, though increased sleep-onset latency was the strongest marker of depression collectively among youth.[28] However, significant heterogeneity was noted among studies with regards to macroarchitectural features of REM sleep (e.g., latency and density), as well as microarchitectural features (PSG-detected frequencies).[28] The discrepancies between studies may be explained by subtypes of depression, the severity of clinical state (e.g., inpatient vs. outpatient samples), gender, age range of participants, and presence of comorbid anxiety, attention-deficit/hyperactivity disorder (ADHD), and/or other psychiatric symptoms.[28]

Based on the available research data, there seems to be a stronger association between subjective sleep complaints and depression in adolescents than for objective measures of sleep and MDD. When both subjective and electroencephalographic (EEG) sleep characteristics were examined in young people with MDD, there was no evidence of EEG sleep disruptions in children with depression compared with healthy controls, even in the presence of significant sleep-related complaints. Perhaps even more interesting is that children with the highest rating of insomnia showed the highest sleep efficiencies according to PSG reports.[29] Sleep–wake state discrepancy[30] thus seems to be more prominent in depressed individuals compared with healthy controls.

Given its relative ease of administration compared with PSG, actigraphy has also been used to estimate objective sleep parameters in depressed youth, such as sleep-onset latency, sleep efficiency, frequency and duration of nocturnal awakenings, nocturnal and diurnal activity levels, and circadian rhythmicity in patients with MDD. Sadeh and colleagues[31] examined actigraphy-estimated sleep patterns among inpatient youth (ages 7–14) hospitalized in a psychiatric unit, and found that depressive symptoms and emotionality were positively associated with interruptions in nightly sleep; furthermore, youth with a history of physical abuse exhibited less TST than sexually abused or nonabused youth.[31] In another investigation comparing children with depression with and without a history of abuse found that children who had been abused showed both the highest levels of nocturnal activity and the longest sleep-onset latencies.[32] The authors concluded that abuse has a more profound effect on sleep regulation than does depression alone.

Abnormal circadian rhythms were also described in children and adolescents with depression compared with controls; these were characterized by blunted activity levels with diurnal variations that did not peak until early evening.[33,34]

Armitage and colleagues found that among children (as opposed to adolescents) with MDD, there were sex differences noted with dampened circadian amplitudes seen only in girls,[33] suggestive of weaker circadian entrainment in this subsample.

Sleep in Early-Onset Bipolar Disorder

Bipolar disorder is a chronic severe psychiatric illness with a prevalence rate in the pediatric population of 5%. There are seven types of bipolar spectrum disorders currently defined in the *Diagnostic and Statistical Manual of Mental Disorders, 5th Edition (DSM-5):* bipolar I disorder, bipolar II disorder, cyclothymic disorder, substance/medication-induced bipolar and related disorder, bipolar and related disorder due to another medical condition, other specified bipolar and related disorder, and unspecified bipolar and related disorder.[35] Research studies in adults with bipolar disorders show sleep problems to be associated with every phase of their illness and usually include insomnia with reduced need for sleep during the manic phase, and insomnia or hypersomnia during the depressed phase.[36,37] Circadian and social rhythm dysfunction has been proposed as one of the pathophysiologic mechanisms of bipolar disorder in adults.[38] Although research on circadian rhythms in pediatric bipolar disorder is limited, some evidence exists that interpersonal and social rhythm therapy is beneficial to adolescents with bipolar illness,[39] as well as high-risk youth.[40] Interpersonal and social rhythm therapy is based on the belief that sleep deprivation, and disruptions of our circadian rhythms, may provoke or exacerbate symptoms commonly associated with bipolar disorder. This form of therapy uses methods from both interpersonal psychotherapy and cognitive-behavioral therapy to teach patients the importance of, and help them maintain in a regular fashion, their daily circadian rhythms and activity routines such as eating and sleeping.

Subjective Sleep in Early-Onset Bipolar Disorder

Examinations of sleep complaints among different samples of children and adolescents with bipolar I disorder, bipolar II disorder, and cyclothymic disorder revealed a weighted average of 72% of patients reporting a decreased need for sleep with symptoms of mania.[41] In a recent study characterizing sleep complaints during bipolar phases among children and adolescents, Lopes and colleagues found that the vast majority of participants reported sleep complaints during manic episodes (66.4%) and during depressive episodes (52.3%), though specific characteristics of sleep disturbance differed based on phase.[42] Specifically, increased time spent in bed and enuresis were more common for depressive episodes, while unrestful sleep was more prevalent in manic episodes.

Baroni and colleagues evaluated sleep complaints in youth with bipolar I and bipolar not otherwise specified (NOS) via DSM-5 criteria[43] using a structured diagnostic interview during both manic and depressive episodes.[44] At least one sleep symptom was reported by 84.3% of subjects: 71.4% of patients had insomnia during depressive episodes, 51.4% experienced a decreased need for sleep during hypomania/mania, 22% of subjects reported circadian reversal, and 27% reported nocturnal enuresis. Decreased need for sleep correlated significantly with measures of global functioning, suggesting that manic symptoms, perhaps, have a more profound impact on global functioning in youth with bipolar disorder. There were no significant differences found in sleep characteristics between bipolar I and bipolar NOS, according to this study.

Diurnal variations of mood have been described in youth with bipolar disorder, particularly evening acceleration of mood and energy and of delayed sleep onset with difficulty waking up in the morning. Nearly 30% of children exhibited elevated mood during the day switching into depression overnight.[45] Longitudinal studies have also established strong associations between sleep disturbance and mood, such that various facets of sleep disturbance (including instability in sleep duration and variability in sleep timing) were positively correlated with concurrent manic and depressive symptoms in diagnosed youth,[46] and were predictive of future psychiatric symptoms in high-risk youth.[47]

Objective Sleep Measures in Early-Onset Bipolar Disorder

Studies using PSG or actigraphic assessment of sleep in youth with bipolar spectrum disorders are notably limited. In the first such study, published by Rao and colleagues in 2002, EEG characteristics of sleep were compared among three groups: adolescents with unipolar depression, those with bipolar disorder, and normal healthy controls.[48] There were no differences in REM sleep found among the groups; however, those with bipolar disorder demonstrated increased amounts of stage 1 sleep and reduced percentages of stage 4 sleep.

In a study by Mehl and colleagues, PSGs of children, whose results on the Child Behavior Checklist (CBCL) were suggestive of bipolar disorder, were compared with normal controls.[49] Sleep measures of children with a *bipolar profile* revealed reduced sleep efficiencies, reduced amounts of REM sleep, and increased numbers of nocturnal awakenings. This study, however, was limited by the lack of validated clinical assessment of bipolar disorder in children participating in the study.

In a 2011 preliminary study, sleep was assessed in a small sample of adolescents with bipolar disorder who were between mood episodes, and compared both to children with ADHD and to normal controls.[50] Patients with bipolar disorder experienced their sleep as more fragmented and less restorative than their peers. However, actigraphy indicated the reverse, namely longer periods of sleep and fewer interruptions compared with their peers. In a more recent study with a larger sample in the same comparison groups, youth with bipolar disorder (ages 5–18) exhibited less TST, as well as increased nocturnal activity via actigraphy compared with the ADHD group and healthy controls, though no subjective measure of sleep was assessed.[51] Although this sample was also neither depressed nor manic at the time of the assessment, the bipolar group's presentation was described as "mixed or ultrarapidly cycling" in mood.[51] Further research is needed to understand clinical characteristics that may contribute to objectively measurable alterations in sleep, as well as potential discrepancies between self-perception of sleep and objective sleep in this population.

Sleep in Childhood Anxiety and Related Disorders

The presence and frequency of sleep disruption in children with anxiety and related disorders are among the highest seen in any form of child psychopathology. For example, in addition to rates of sleep problems >90% in samples of anxious youth,[52–54] group-based comparisons have found anxious youth experience more frequent and more varied types of sleep problems than their counterparts with ADHD.[55] Conversely, children presenting with insomnia complaints were most likely to have co-occurring anxiety disorders.[2,56] Problems with sleep initiation, nighttime awakenings, nightmares, and bedtime resistance are among the problems most commonly reported by anxious youth.[52,53,57]

Retrospective reports of sleep are nonetheless subject to a range of potential limitations including reporter and recall biases. Far fewer studies have investigated the sleep of anxious youth prospectively. In one of the first studies to examine at-home sleep patterns, anxiety-disordered and healthy control children completed prospective 1-week sleep diaries. Later bedtimes, less sleep on weekdays, and more variable weekend sleep patterns were found among those with anxiety.[58] Conversely, another study reported that nightmares were significantly more common among anxious youth based on retrospective reports but prospective examination across 1 week revealed a similar low frequency in both groups.[59] Certain forms of sleep disturbance, such as parasomnias, may therefore be more susceptible to overreporting among anxious youth due to increased perception of severity.

Reports of sleep also have been found to vary based on the informant. In particular, and in contrast to community samples where parents tend to underestimate child sleep problems,[60,61] anxious youth have been shown to report fewer sleep problems than their parents.[53,62] Differential findings may be explained by greater parental awareness of sleep problems in clinically anxious youth due to the frequency of such complaints, the severity of these problems, and/or their impact on parents' sleep patterns (e.g., nighttime fears, requests to co-sleep, night terrors).

In one of the first studies to examine PSG sleep patterns in children with anxiety disorders (with and without comorbid depression), Forbes and colleagues used two nights of laboratory-based PSG to compare the EEG sleep patterns of three groups of children, all aged 7–17 years: those with anxiety disorders (including generalized anxiety disorder [GAD], panic disorder, separation anxiety disorder [SAD], or social phobia), those with depression, and those comprising a group of healthy controls.[63] On both nights the anxiety group had more awakenings than did the depressed group, as well as less slow-wave (deep) sleep than depressed and control children. On the second PSG night, anxious youth exhibited a prolonged sleep-onset latency, whereas the latency to REM sleep decreased in both other groups. A greater percentage of missing data from night two was also reported in the anxious group. Thus, in addition to alterations in sleep architecture, results suggested that anxious children experience greater difficulty adapting to the sleep lab environment. Such data underscore a need for research examining objective sleep patterns in the home environment.

There is also evidence to suggest that rates and types of sleep problems differ among the various forms of anxiety, as well as other related disorders. DSM-5 has reclassified obsessive-compulsive disorder (OCD) and posttraumatic stress disorder (PTSD) from anxiety disorders to their respective categories. However, we include OCD and PTSD in this chapter for two reasons: first, the majority of past research has used DSM-5 criteria and therefore categorize them as anxiety disorders, and second, extensive overlap exists in the features of anxiety disorders, obsessive-compulsive and related disorders, and trauma- and stressor-related disorders.[35] The following sections provide a review of available findings across specific diagnoses most closely associated with sleep disruption.

Generalized Anxiety Disorder

Diagnostic criteria and empirical data indicate that sleep plays an important role in pediatric GAD. First, in addition to excessive and uncontrollable worry, DSM-5 criteria specifically include "difficulty falling or staying asleep, or restless, unsatisfying sleep" as one of six possible physiologic symptoms.[35] Similar to rates in adults with GAD,[64] a majority of youth experience difficulty sleeping, with rates as high as 94%.[52–54] Other common sleep-related problems include nightmares and daytime sleepiness. Although a majority of research is based on parent report, one study found 87% of youth with a primary GAD diagnosis self-report difficulty sleeping and difficulty awakening in the morning, a greater proportion than seen in children with other primary anxiety disorders.[53]

Whether subjective complaints of sleep disturbance are corroborated by objective measurement appears to be mixed. In a study of EEG-based sleep patterns, Alfano and colleagues found that prepubertal children with GAD (without depression) exhibited significantly longer sleep-onset latency and reduced latency to REM sleep compared with matched healthy controls.[65] A marginally significant increase in REM sleep and a decrease in sleep efficiency were also observed in the GAD group. However, no differences in sleep architecture were found when these same groups (i.e., nondepressed GAD vs. control) were studied overnight in the home environment.[66,67] Other research has found that irrespective of differences in sleep architecture, lower percentages of slow-wave sleep relate to greater negative affect among youth with GAD, and higher percentages of REM sleep relate to more somatic complaints.[67] Thus, even when children with GAD do not meet the criteria for comorbid depressive diagnoses, objective sleep parameters observed among youth with generalized anxiety appear to be similar to those with depression.[68–70] A shared genetic basis for GAD and depression, with overlapping of clinical features (i.e., negative affectivity) and/or of other neurobiologic markers of risk, may serve to explain a similar overlap in sleep parameters.[71]

Separation Anxiety Disorder

SAD is characterized by developmentally inappropriate and excessive anxiety surrounding separation from major attachment figures.[35] Two possible diagnostic symptoms of SAD are specific to sleep: persistent reluctance or refusal to sleep alone, and repeated nightmares involving themes of separation. Refusing to sleep alone is among the most common reasons for referral to an anxiety specialty clinic.[72] Although empirical studies examining sleep problems in children with SAD specifically are limited, two studies, based on parent and clinician reports, found that a diagnosis of SAD was strongly linked to concurrent sleep problems, which was more than that seen in children with social anxiety disorder (but not more than seen in children with GAD).[52,57] Parents of children with primary SAD also reported that their children exhibited more parasomnias (including sleepwalking, bed-wetting, and night terrors) than did parents of youth with social anxiety disorder.[53,57] This last finding agrees with other results that children diagnosed with SAD were most likely to have concurrent sleep terror disorder.[73] Based on child reports, 60% of children with SAD reported difficulty sleeping,[53] with the most frequently listed sleep problems being insomnia, reluctance or refusal to sleep alone, and nightmares.[52,57] Another study examining young children found that internalizing symptoms predicted nighttime fear, which in turn predicted co-sleeping.[74] The authors also found that separation anxiety specifically was inversely associated with number of nights slept alone.[74] Although the American Academy of Pediatrics recommends against bed-sharing with infants to mitigate risk for sleep-related infant deaths or unintentional injury,[75] no specific recommendations are made for youth above the age of 1. However, co-sleeping that occurs in response to sleep difficulties, anxiety, or nighttime fear can reinforce the fears and avoidance behaviors (i.e., sleeping alone) in the long run.

Obsessive-Compulsive Disorder

Although sleep-related difficulties are not explicitly listed in the DSM-5 diagnostic criteria for pediatric OCD, it has been posited that obsessions and compulsions may interfere with

nightly sleep duration, which in turn exacerbates symptoms of OCD.[76] A recent literature review of 20 empirical studies reported the prevalence of subjective sleep disturbance to range from 28.8% to 92%.[77] Another study using parental report compared sleep duration among youth with OCD, youth from outpatient psychiatry units, and youth from the general population, and noted that those with OCD were reported to have shorter sleep duration.[78] Storch and colleagues also found that less sleep also was associated with greater OCD severity, though a limitation of this study was that the majority of youth were taking medication for their OCD at the time of the assessment.[62] Thus heterogeneity in prevalence rates may be attributable to variations in certain demographic and clinical (e.g., medication status) characteristics, given that sleep may be particularly problematic for younger children and females with OCD.[62]

In the only published OCD study to utilize PSG, Rapoport and colleagues compared the sleep of nine adolescents with OCD to a matched healthy control group.[79] Adolescents with OCD exhibited less TST, longer sleep-onset latency, and shortened latency to REM sleep than did controls. However, because a majority of subjects had a current or previous depressive disorder, the extent to which these sleep patterns were reflective of other forms of psychopathology is unclear.

Among the few studies that utilized actigraphy to compare sleep patterns among youth with OCD and matched healthy controls, parents of children with OCD reported greater sleep problems, and in line with this, actigraphic data revealed greater sleep fragmentation in children with OCD, as exhibited by longer sleep-onset latency[80] and nightly awakenings.[80,81] A negative association between TST and severity of compulsive behaviors was also found, such that as sleep duration decreased, OC symptom severity increased.[81] Interestingly, neither study showed differences in bedtime between groups. This observation contrasts previous assertions that compulsive rituals delay bedtimes in pediatric patients,[82] as noted in adult patients.[83] Given the consistent finding of reduced TST in youth with OCD and the profound effects that sleep deprivation has on behavioral and emotional inhibition,[84,85] research appears to support the hypothesis that insufficient sleep in children and adolescents with OCD adversely affects their ability to inhibit obsessions and compulsions.[81] Further work is needed to investigate the specific mechanisms by which OCD symptoms may lead to decreased sleep duration among youth.

Posttraumatic Stress Disorder and Trauma

In general, children who have been exposed to one or more traumatic events/experiences exhibit significantly higher rates of sleep problems than children without these experiences.[86] The most common forms of trauma-related sleep disturbances in youth include problems initiating or maintaining sleep, short sleep duration, nightmares, and nighttime fears.[87] Evidence for unique relationships between specific types of trauma and sleep disruption across development is also beginning to emerge. For example, using data from the National Child Traumatic Stress Network, Hall Brown and colleagues found that sexual abuse was independently predictive of sleep disturbance in children ages 7–12 years, whereas community violence was predictive of sleep disturbance in adolescents ages 13–18 years.[88] Other data provide evidence of a dose–response effect between the number of traumatic events experienced and the risk of insomnia in youth.[89]

A proportion of children exposed to trauma will develop PTSD, characterized by four distinct symptom clusters including reexperiencing a traumatic event, avoidance of reminders of the trauma, negative changes in cognitions and mood, and alterations in arousal and reactivity associated with the traumatic event.[35] Sleep disturbances, including distressing nightmares and difficulty initiating or maintaining sleep, are core features of PTSD and encompass two of the four symptom clusters required for diagnosis.[35] Although there are many studies focused on the relationship between trauma exposure and sleep disruption in adults, research in pediatric samples is limited. Sleep-onset insomnia and maintenance insomnia, nightmares, and night terrors nonetheless appear to be common in the aftermath of trauma, with prevalence rates ranging from 13% to nearly 80%.[86] In a study of children and adolescents exposed to Hurricane Hugo, bad dreams showed a strong diagnostic correlation to a subsequent PTSD diagnosis.[90] Longitudinal studies of youth who experienced natural disasters also demonstrated that severity of sleep disturbance following the traumatic events was not only associated with more severe concurrent PTSD symptoms but predicted the development and persistence of future psychopathology.[91,92]

In an actigraphy-based study of a sample of inpatient youth in a psychiatric unit, Sadeh and colleagues found that children who were physically abused spent less time asleep in bed compared with children who were sexually abused and non-abused children.[31] These data converge with more recent studies[88] to suggest that certain types of trauma exposure, irrespective of a PTSD diagnosis, have robust effects on children's sleep patterns. Similarly, in a sample of trauma-exposed children, Glod and colleagues reported that abused children demonstrated significantly longer sleep-onset latency than did both a sample of depressed youth and a group of controls.[32] A lower sleep efficiency was also seen in the abused group compared with controls, and in those with a history of physical as opposed to sexual abuse. Differences in sleep patterns as a function of a PTSD diagnosis were not found. In contrast, Jones and colleagues compared sleep macroarchitecture in children with and without PTSD following an affective memory task, and found that the PTSD group exhibited decreased slow-wave activity, suggesting that this group had impaired sleep depth and worse sleep quality.[93]

Other research, too, suggests that the negative impact of early trauma on sleep may persist into the adult years. For example, Bader and colleagues found childhood trauma to be the strongest predictor of values of sleep-onset latency, sleep efficiency, and nocturnal activity in adulthood, even after controlling for levels of stress and depression.[94] Similarly, females who experienced sexual abuse as children were more likely to experience sleep problems as adults irrespective of depressive symptoms.[95] Overall, available research suggests that trauma exposure, more so than a PTSD diagnosis per se, is closely associated with persistent sleep disruption, and that heterogeneity in types of trauma may be reflective of variations in the trajectory of sleep disturbance.

Shared Factors and Mechanisms of Interest for Anxiety and Related Disorders

At a basic level an increased state of arousal, which is a central feature of all anxiety and related disorders, is incompatible with quiescence and sleep.[96] Similarly, insufficient sleep produces increases in arousal systems, mood disturbance, anxiety, and tension.[84,85,97] At a more complex level, the pervasive overlap between symptoms of sleep and these disorders appears rooted in a variety of potentially mediating and synergistic factors including biologic factors, cognitive style, and environmental influences. For example, genetics alone have been found to account for 74% of the covariance in the association between early sleep and anxiety symptoms.[98] Certain circadian clock–related genes, specifically *BCL2, DRD2,* and *PAWR* are also associated with anxiety disorders.[99] The latter set of genes belongs to the signaling pathway connecting circadian rhythmicity and anxiety-related behavior, thus suggesting a possible shared genetic predisposition for problems in both domains. However, a specific link with anxiety, as opposed to a broader range of psychiatric symptoms and disorders, has not been established. For example, results from a large study of 8-year-old twin pairs reported that the genes influencing sleep problems are more closely associated with depression than anxiety.[60] Also, the serotonin transporter gene *(5-HTTLPR)* has been implicated in sleep disturbance[100] and depression[101] as well as in anxiety.[102,103]

Problems sleeping are also consistently associated with a range of cognitive factors and styles shared by anxious individuals. *Catastrophizing,* which is a negative, iterative thought process similar to rumination or worry, is hypothesized to play a critical role in the development and maintenance of insomnia.[104] In support of this theory, Barclay and Gregory found that poor sleepers are more likely than good sleepers to catastrophize about the consequences of sleeplessness as well as other topics, though findings were largely mediated by anxiety and worry.[105] Further, *anxiety sensitivity* (i.e., the belief that anxiety-related symptoms are uncontrollable, harmful, or otherwise negative) is uniquely associated with sleep-onset latency, rather than sleep problems as a whole, in clinically anxious youth.[106] An association between decreased total sleep duration and greater levels of pre-sleep cognitive arousal has also been documented in children with various anxiety disorders,[53] suggesting that anxiety-related arousal before bedtime may inadvertently make sleep onset more challenging.

Receiving insufficient sleep may also exacerbate existing maladaptive cognitions in those with anxiety disorders. One study found that although sleep restriction did not result in increased worries or longer catastrophizing sequences, catastrophizing following sleep restriction produced more anxiety and increased estimation of the likelihood that "catastrophes" might occur.[97] Furthermore, an early adolescent subgroup (aged 10–13 years) rated their most threatening worry as significantly more threatening when they were sleep deprived than when rested.

In addition to evolving interest in biologic and cognitive factors, the sleep environment in which problems develop remains a critically important area of investigation. Research examining specific familial characteristics of, and parenting behaviors within, the early sleep environment interestingly revealed that both under- or over-involvement in behaviors related to sleep impacted sleep negatively. For example, in a manner consistent with findings that the regularity of children's sleep schedules is essential for optimal daytime functioning,[107] familial disorganization (e.g., lacking structure and routines in the home) was found to account for a significant portion of the variance in childhood sleep problems and anxiety.[108] Although the precise pathways through which *familial disorganization* impacts children's sleep remain to be delineated, it is known that lack of parental rules concerning sleep is associated with shorter sleep duration in school-aged children.[109]

Conversely, parental over-involvement in their children's sleep may be problematic, particularly for at-risk and anxious children.[110] Such parental behaviors might function as moderators, such that at-risk children who do not adequately learn how to negotiate sleep onset independently may similarly struggle with managing their anxiety in other contexts. Sleep disruption that results from prolonged sleep onset or nighttime awakenings related to a need for parental support could further exacerbate daytime anxiety.[111] Overall, the broad range of intraindividual and interindividual factors impacting both sleep and anxiety dictate a need for investigations aimed at understanding how multiple levels of factors interact to create these commonly co-occurring problems.

COVID-19 Considerations

In late 2019 and early 2020, unprecedented safety measures were enforced across the globe in response to the public health threat posed by the novel coronavirus disease 2019 (COVID-19). Measures aimed at promoting social distancing included limiting in-person gatherings, keeping a physical distance of at least 6 feet from others not in the same household, and shifting academic obligations to a "distance learning" model. These disruptions in normal, daily schedules (e.g., schooling, extracurricular activities, and peer socialization) hold potential implications for child development, sleep patterns, and emotional well-being.

Several studies have examined the effects of the COVID-19 pandemic on various mental health and sleep-related

outcomes in youth. Ma and colleagues[112] conducted a meta-analysis of 23 studies, and reported pooled prevalence rates of depression, anxiety, sleep disorders, and posttraumatic stress symptoms to be 29%, 26%, 44%, and 48%, respectively. They also found adolescents and females exhibited higher rates of depression and anxiety. These prevalence rates for depression and sleep disorders are higher than those previously reported in children from the same population.[113,114] However, the broad categorization of "sleep disorders" examined makes it difficult to determine the occurrence of specific types of sleep disturbances during the pandemic. Prospective studies have also observed changes in mental and sleep from before the pandemic/"lockdown," though inconsistencies are notable. For instance, some studies reported adverse changes in sleep (e.g., decreased sleep duration, greater sleep difficulties)[115,116] and mental health symptoms[115] during the lockdown, whereas others have noted increased sleep duration[117] and reduced mental health symptom severity.[118] Certain risk factors for the development or exacerbation of mental health and/or sleep problems have also been identified, including older child age, parental depression, and household discord (e.g., caregiving strain, income loss).[115] In light of potential for similar stressful circumstances (i.e., pandemics) in the future, parents should ensure that youth receive sufficient sleep and maintain regularity in daily schedules to foster adaptive coping and mitigate risk for psychopathology.

Psychosocial Treatment

Although sleep disturbances commonly co-occur with psychiatric disorders (particularly those of mood and anxiety) in both children and adults,[119,120] understanding of optimal methods for, and ideal timing of, treatment targeting sleep problems in this context is limited.[52] Lack of understanding is directly linked to the fact that empirically supported treatments for anxiety and mood disorders do not typically address sleep problems directly, and behavioral interventions for childhood sleep problems do not specifically measure changes in anxiety or mood.[121] A growing body of evidence nonetheless suggests that addressing sleep in anxious and depressed youth is likely important for positive long-term outcomes.

As in anxious and depressed adults, the most common sleep problems in youth relate to difficulty initiating and/or maintaining sleep.[52,111,122] Like adult-based interventions, effective child-focused treatments consider behavioral, somatic, and cognitive symptoms, as each may have relevance for sleep disruption. Behavioral aspects of treatment target maladaptive sleep-related behaviors such as bedtime avoidance, inconsistent sleep schedules and routines, interfering sleep-onset associations (e.g., parental presence), and poor sleep hygiene.[123,124] However, because sleep problems may be more disruptive to parents than to children, the child's lack of motivation for change can be a barrier to treatment success. For youth initially hesitant or unwilling to address maladaptive sleep behaviors, intangible and tangible rewards may be used with success. In other cases, setting firmer parental limits surrounding sleep may be necessary.[125]

As previously discussed, cognitive factors that often prolong sleep onset can be particularly problematic during the pre-sleep period.[36,53] Reduction of problematic nighttime cognitive activity through the provision of corrective information about sleep and the effects of sleep loss, positive imagery techniques, and scheduled *worry periods* during afternoon hours can be effective.[126] Pre-sleep cognitive activity also may result in increased somatic arousal at night, for which progressive muscle relaxation techniques are commonly used. Importantly, increased levels of arousal and wakefulness at bedtime can also contribute to feelings of frustration at bedtime, thereby undermining the development of positive sleep-onset associations. Temporarily delaying a child's bedtime may serve to increase the homeostatic sleep drive and better align the sleep–wake schedule.

At present, it is not fully understood the extent to which sleep is impacted by interventions aimed at treating psychologic disorders, and vice versa (i.e., psychologic functioning impacted by sleep interventions). Results from the Treatment for Adolescents with Depression Study (TADS)[127] indicate sleep problems were the most common residual symptoms in youth who responded to mood-focused treatment (either cognitive behavioral therapy [CBT], fluoxetine, or their combination),[128] whereas another study found that adolescents treated for depression with a longer sleep-onset latency were more likely to relapse within 12 months.[129] In a pilot trial, Clarke and colleagues examined the effects of CBT for insomnia (CBT-I) combined with CBT for depression (CBT-D) in adolescents diagnosed with concurrent insomnia and unipolar depression.[130] They observed improvements in some sleep (e.g., actigraphy-derived TST) and mood (e.g., faster recovery time) outcomes, though the study was likely limited by small sample sizes.

Several studies have examined the efficacy of anxiety-focused treatments on sleep outcomes among youth. Overall, findings indicate that interventions for anxiety provide some (albeit not clinically meaningful) improvement in sleep-related problems, particularly those associated with bedtime difficulties (e.g., bedtime resistance, sleep anxiety).[131–133] Another study noted improvements in sleep in children only, as opposed to adolescents,[134] indicating that teenage patients may be more treatment resistant. Studies investigating sleep-focused treatments in youth with emotional problems are more ubiquitous. Recent studies utilized "multicomponent" sleep interventions that integrated components of different treatment approaches; while the treatments had profound effects in improving subjective[135–137] and objective[136,137] sleep parameters, effects on emotional outcomes were small to none. However, a recent study that compared an integrated anxiety-sleep intervention with "gold standard" CBT for childhood GAD found similar sleep (and anxiety) improvements in both groups based on both subjective and objective sleep measures.[138] McMakin and colleagues examined the effects of an anxiety treatment and a subsequent sleep intervention on sleep in anxious children and found small improvements in subjective sleep following the anxiety treatment, and large, clinically meaningful improvements in subjective sleep following the sleep treatment.[133] Collectively, research highlighting a bidirectional relationship between sleep and emotional functioning in youth underscores the potential importance of addressing functioning in both domains.[111]

Pharmacologic Treatment

There is limited evidence-based research for the pharmacologic treatment of depression and anxiety-related sleep problems in children and adolescents. Common psychotropic medications, such as selective serotonin reuptake inhibitors (SSRIs), are effective in reducing symptoms in youth with a range of psychologic disorders, including GAD,[52] OCD,[139] and depression. However, some antidepressants may cause changes in sleep characteristics when used in the pediatric population. For example, imipramine (a tricyclic antidepressant [TCA]) can increase stage 2 sleep and wakefulness and decrease stage 4 sleep, and it also appears to decrease sleep efficiency and cause REM suppression.[140,141] Similarly, fluoxetine (an SSRI) was found to increase stage 1 sleep and REM density. However, REM suppression was not evident in this sample of children. Fluoxetine may also cause oculomotor abnormalities, increased myoclonic activity, and subjectively reported lower-quality sleep and more awakenings.[142] Adverse effects of antidepressants on sleep appear to be inconsistent, however, and may be differentially observed. In one comparison study, the SSRI fluvoxamine was shown to be effective in reducing sleep-related problems (specifically insomnia symptoms and reluctance to sleep alone) among clinically anxious children versus placebo.[52]

Pharmacologic treatments for sleep disorders among youth have increased in recent years, particularly among those with emotional disorders. In a study of treatment-resistant depression in adolescents, depressed adolescents who previously had an inadequate response to an SSRI were randomly assigned another SSRI, venlafaxine (a serotonin-norepinephrine reuptake inhibitor [SNRI]), another SSRI + CBT, or venlafaxine + CBT. Augmentation with sleep medication was used as clinically indicated. Results demonstrated that adolescents who received trazodone were six times less likely to respond than those with no sleep medication and were three times more likely to experience self-harm, even after adjusting for baseline differences associated with trazodone use. The authors of the study warned that the findings should be interpreted with caution because sleep agents were not assigned randomly, but at clinician discretion. Nevertheless, the very low response rate of patients cotreated with trazodone and an SSRI could be due to inhibition of CYP2D6 by these antidepressants.[143] Future research is needed to explore safe and effective treatment algorithms for youth with mood and anxiety disorders and comorbid insomnia.

Concurrent treatment of insomnia and psychopathology should be considered in youth, with careful selection of sedative-hypnotic agents based on knowledge of the drugs' pharmacologic properties and individual patient characteristics.

CLINICAL PEARLS

- Sleep assessment is an essential part of the comprehensive evaluation of children and adolescents with mood and anxiety disorders.
- Increased sleep-onset latency is the most consistent finding in the sleep of children and adolescents with early depression.
- In adolescents, there is an apparent relationship between the presence of sleep disturbances and an increased risk for suicide.
- Decreased need for sleep is a characteristic feature of mania in youth with bipolar disorder.
- Children presenting with insomnia complaints also have an increased likelihood of currently or subsequently meeting criteria for an anxiety disorder.
- Irrespective of trauma-related diagnosis, children exposed to traumatic events commonly suffer from significant sleep disturbances.
- Childhood sleep and anxiety disorders are linked by a range of genetic, behavioral, cognitive, and environmental influences.
- Effective psychosocial interventions target child behaviors and cognitions, physiologic tensions, and parenting and environmental influences that maintain hyperarousal at night.

References

1. Shahid A, Khairandish A, Gladanac B, Shapiro C. Peeking into the minds of troubled adolescents: The utility of polysomnography sleep studies in an inpatient psychiatric unit. *J Affect Disord.* 2012;139(1):66–74.
2. Ivanenko A, Crabtree VM, Obrien LM, Gozal D. Sleep complaints and psychiatric symptoms in children evaluated at a pediatric mental health clinic. *J Clin Sleep Med.* 2006;2(1):42–48.
3. Armstrong JM, Ruttle PL, Klein MH, Essex MJ, Benca RM. Associations of child insomnia, sleep movement, and their persistence with mental health symptoms in childhood and adolescence. *Sleep.* 2014;37(5):901–909.
4. Baum KT, Desai A, Field J, Miller LE, Rausch J, Beebe DW. Sleep restriction worsens mood and emotion regulation in adolescents. *J Child Psychol Psychiatry.* 2014;55(2):180–190.
5. Ojio Y, Nishida A, Shimodera S, Togo F, Sasaki T. Sleep duration associated with the lowest risk of depression/anxiety in adolescents. *Sleep.* 2016;39(8):1555–1562.
6. Johnson EO, Chilcoat HD, Breslau N. Trouble sleeping and anxiety/depression in childhood. *Psychiatry Res.* 2000;94(2):93–102.
7. McMakin DL, Alfano CA. Sleep and anxiety in late childhood and early adolescence. *Curr Opin Psychiatry.* 2015;28(6):483–489.
8. Kenney SR, Lac A, Labrie JW, Hummer JF, Pham A. Mental health, sleep quality, drinking motives, and alcohol-related consequences: A path-analytic model. *J Stud Alcohol Drugs.* 2013;74(6):841–851.
9. Roane BM, Taylor DJ. Adolescent insomnia as a risk factor for early adult depression and substance abuse. *Sleep.* 2008;31(10):1351–1356.
10. McMakin DL, Dahl RE, Buysse DJ, et al. The impact of experimental sleep restriction on affective functioning in social and nonsocial contexts among adolescents. *J Child Psychol Psychiatry.* 2016;57(9):1027–1037.
11. Reddy R, Palmer CA, Jackson C, Farris SG, Alfano CA. Impact of sleep restriction versus idealized sleep on emotional experience, reactivity and regulation in healthy adolescents. *J Sleep Res.* 2017;26(4):516–525.
12. Birmaher B, Brent D. AACAP Work Group on Quality Issues, et al. Practice parameter for the assessment and treatment of children and adolescents with depressive disorders. *J Am Acad Child Adolesc Psychiatry.* 2007;46(11):1503–1526.
13. Centers for Disease Control and Prevention. Preventing Suicide Factsheet. 2019.
14. Puig-Antich J, Goetz R, Hanlon C, et al. Sleep architecture and REM sleep measures in prepubertal children with major depression: A controlled study. *Arch Gen Psychiatry.* 1982;39(8):932–939.
15. Puig-Antich J, Goetz R, Hanlon C, Tabrizi MA, Davies M, Weitzman ED. Sleep architecture and REM sleep measures in prepubertal major depressives. Studies during recovery from the depressive episode in a drug-free state. *Arch Gen Psychiatry.* 1983;40(2):187–192.
16. Liu X, Buysse DJ, Gentzler AL, et al. Insomnia and hypersomnia associated with depressive phenomenology and comorbidity in childhood depression. *Sleep.* 2007;30(1):83–90.
17. Urrila AS, Karlsson L, Kiviruusu O, Pelkonen M, Strandholm T, Marttunen M. Sleep complaints among adolescent outpatients with major depressive disorder. *Sleep Med.* 2012;13(7):816–823.
18. Koo DL, Yang KI, Kim JH, et al. Association between morningness-eveningness, sleep duration, weekend catch-up sleep and depression among Korean high-school students. *J Sleep Res.* 2021;30(1):e13063.
19. Lopes MC, Boronat AC, Wang YP, Fu IL. Sleep complaints as risk factor for suicidal behavior in severely depressed children and adolescents. *CNS Neurosci Ther.* 2016;22(11):915–920.
20. Goldstein TR, Bridge JA, Brent DA. Sleep disturbance preceding completed suicide in adolescents. *J Consult Clin Psychol.* 2008;76(1):84–91.
21. Chiu HY, Lee HC, Chen PY, Lai YF, Tu YK. Associations between sleep duration and suicidality in adolescents: A systematic review and dose-response meta-analysis. *Sleep Med Rev.* 2018;42:119–126.
22. Wong MM, Brower KJ. The prospective relationship between sleep problems and suicidal behavior in the National Longitudinal Study of Adolescent Health. *J Psychiatr Res.* 2012;46(7):953–959.
23. Sivertsen B, Harvey AG, Reichborn-Kjennerud T, Ystrom E, Hysing M. Sleep problems and depressive symptoms in toddlers and 8-year-old children: A longitudinal study. *J Sleep Res.* 2021;30(1):e13150.
24. Dahl RE, Ryan ND, Birmaher B, et al. Electroencephalographic sleep measures in prepubertal depression. *Psychiatry Res.* 1991;38(2):201–214.
25. Young W, Knowles JB, MacLean AW, Boag L, McConville BJ. The sleep of childhood depressives: Comparison with age-matched controls. *Biol Psychiatry.* 1982;17(10):1163–1168.
26. Emslie GJ, Rush AJ, Weinberg WA, Rintelmann JW, Roffwarg HP. Children with major depression show reduced rapid eye movement latencies. *Arch Gen Psychiatry.* 1990;47(2):119–124.

27. Dahl RE, Ryan ND, Matty MK, et al. Sleep onset abnormalities in depressed adolescents. *Biol Psychiatry*. 1996;39(6):400–410.

28. Augustinavicius JL, Zanjani A, Zakzanis KK, Shapiro CM. Polysomnographic features of early-onset depression: A meta-analysis. *J Affect Disord*. 2014;158:11–18.

29. Bertocci MA, Dahl RE, Williamson DE, et al. Subjective sleep complaints in pediatric depression: A controlled study and comparison with EEG measures of sleep and waking. *J Am Acad Child Adolesc Psychiatry*. 2005;44(11):1158–1166.

30. Bensen-Boakes DB, Lovato N, Meaklim H, Bei B, Scott H. "Sleep-wake state discrepancy": Toward a common understanding and standardized nomenclature. *Sleep*. 2022;45(10):zsac187. https://doi.org/10.1093/sleep/zsac187

31. Sadeh A, McGuire JP, Sachs H, et al. Sleep and psychological characteristics of children on a psychiatric inpatient unit. *J Am Acad Child Adolesc Psychiatry*. 1995;34(6):813–819.

32. Glod CA, Teicher MH, Hartman CR, Harakal T. Increased nocturnal activity and impaired sleep maintenance in abused children. *J Am Acad Child Adolesc Psychiatry*. 1997;36(9):1236–1243.

33. Armitage R, Hoffmann R, Emslie G, Rintelman J, Moore J, Lewis K. Rest-activity cycles in childhood and adolescent depression. *J Am Acad Child Adolesc Psychiatry*. 2004;43(6):761–769.

34. Teicher MH, Glod CA, Harper D, et al. Locomotor activity in depressed children and adolescents: I. Circadian dysregulation. *J Am Acad Child Adolesc Psychiatry*. 1993;32(4):760–769.

35. American Psychiatric Association. *Diagnostic and Statistical Manual of Mental Disorders*. 5th ed. American Psychiatric Association; 2013.

36. Harvey AG, Schmidt DA, Scarna A, Semler CN, Goodwin GM. Sleep-related functioning in euthymic patients with bipolar disorder, patients with insomnia, and subjects without sleep problems. *Am J Psychiatry*. 2005;162(1):50–57.

37. Wehr TA, Sack DA, Rosenthal NE. Sleep reduction as a final common pathway in the genesis of mania. *Am J Psychiatry*. 1987;144(2):201–204.

38. Goodwin FK, Jamison KR. *Manic-Depressive Illness: Bipolar Disorder and Recurrent. Depression*. 2nd ed. Oxford University Press; 2007.

39. Hlastala SA, Frank E. Adapting interpersonal and social rhythm therapy to the developmental needs of adolescents with bipolar disorder. *Dev Psychopathol*. 2006;18(4):1267–1288.

40. Goldstein TR, Merranko J, Krantz M, et al. Early intervention for adolescents at-risk for bipolar disorder: A pilot randomized trial of Interpersonal and Social Rhythm Therapy (IPSRT). *J Affect Disord*. 2018;235:348–356.

41. Kowatch RA, Youngstrom EA, Danielyan A, Findling RL. Review and meta-analysis of the phenomenology and clinical characteristics of mania in children and adolescents. *Bipolar Disord*. 2005;7(6):483–496.

42. Lopes MC, Boarati MA, Fu IL. Sleep and daytime complaints during manic and depressive episodes in children and adolescents with bipolar disorder. *Front Psychiatry*. 2019;10:1021.

43. American Psychiatric Association. *Diagnostic and Statistical Manual of Mental Disorders*. IV-TR ed. American Psychiatric Association; 2000.

44. Baroni A, Hernandez M, Grant MC, Faedda GL. Sleep disturbances in pediatric bipolar disorder: A comparison between bipolar I and bipolar NOS. *Front Psychiatry*. 2012;3:22.

45. Staton D, Volness LJ, Beatty WW. Diagnosis and classification of pediatric bipolar disorder. *J Affect Disord*. 2008;105(1–3):205–212.

46. Gershon A, Singh MK. Sleep in adolescents with bipolar I disorder: Stability and relation to symptom change. *J Clin Child Adolesc Psychol*. 2017;46(2):247–257.

47. Soehner AM, Bertocci MA, Levenson JC, et al. Longitudinal associations between sleep patterns and psychiatric symptom severity in high-risk and community comparison youth. *J Am Acad Child Adolesc Psychiatry*. 2019;58(6):608–617.

48. Rao U, Dahl RE, Ryan ND, et al. Heterogeneity in EEG sleep findings in adolescent depression: Unipolar versus bipolar clinical course. *J Affect Disord*. 2002;70(3):273–280.

49. Mehl RC, O'Brien LM, Jones JH, Dreisbach JK, Mervis CB, Gozal D. Correlates of sleep and pediatric bipolar disorder. *Sleep*. 2006;29(2):193–197.

50. Mullin BC, Harvey AG, Hinshaw SP. A preliminary study of sleep in adolescents with bipolar disorder, ADHD, and non-patient controls. *Bipolar Disord*. 2011;13(4):425–432.

51. Faedda GL, Ohashi K, Hernandez M, et al. Actigraph measures discriminate pediatric bipolar disorder from attention-deficit/hyperactivity disorder and typically developing controls. *J Child Psychol Psychiatry*. 2016;57(6):706–716.

52. Alfano CA, Ginsburg GS, Kingery JN. Sleep-related problems among children and adolescents with anxiety disorders. *J Am Acad Child Adolesc Psychiatry*. 2007;46(2):224–232.

53. Alfano CA, Pina AA, Zerr AA, Villalta IK. Pre-sleep arousal and sleep problems of anxiety-disordered youth. *Child Psychiatry Hum Dev*. 2010;41(2):156–167.

54. Mullin BC, Pyle L, Haraden D, et al. A Preliminary multi-method comparison of sleep among adolescents with and without generalized anxiety disorder. *J Clin Child Adolesc Psychol*. 2017;46(2):198–210.

55. Beriault M, Turgeon L, Labrosse M, et al. Comorbidity of ADHD and anxiety disorders in school-age children: Impact on sleep and response to a cognitive-behavioral treatment. *J Atten Disord*. 2018;22(5):414–424.

56. Chase RM, Pincus DB. Sleep-related problems in children and adolescents with anxiety disorders. *Behav Sleep Med*. 2011;9(4):224–236.

57. Shanahan L, Copeland WE, Angold A, Bondy CL, Costello EJ. Sleep problems predict and are predicted by generalized anxiety/depression and oppositional defiant disorder. *J Am Acad Child Adolesc Psychiatry*. 2014;53(5):550–558.

58. Hudson JL, Gradisar M, Gamble A, Schniering CA, Rebelo I. The sleep patterns and problems of clinically anxious children. *Behav Res Ther*. 2009;47(4):339–344.

59. Reynolds KC, Alfano CA. Things that go bump in the night: Frequency and predictors of nightmares in anxious and nonanxious children. *Behav Sleep Med*. 2016;14(4):442–456.

60. Gregory AM, Rijsdijk FV, Dahl RE, McGuffin P, Eley TC. Associations between sleep problems, anxiety, and depression in twins at 8 years of age. *Pediatrics*. 2006;118(3):1124–1132.

61. Schreck KA, Mulick JA, Rojahn J. Parent perception of elementary school aged children's sleep problems. *J Child Fam Stud*. 2005;14(1):101–109.

62. Storch EA, Murphy TK, Lack CW, Geffken GR, Jacob ML, Goodman WK. Sleep-related problems in pediatric obsessive-compulsive disorder. *J Anxiety Disord*. 2008;22(5):877–885.

63. Forbes EE, Bertocci MA, Gregory AM, et al. Objective sleep in pediatric anxiety disorders and major depressive disorder. *J Am Acad Child Adolesc Psychiatry*. 2008;47(2):148–155.

64. Monti JM, Monti D. Sleep disturbance in generalized anxiety disorder and its treatment. *Sleep Med Rev*. 2000;4(3):263–276.

65. Alfano CA, Reynolds K, Scott N, Dahl RE, Mellman TA. Polysomnographic sleep patterns of non-depressed, non-medicated children with generalized anxiety disorder. *J Affect Disord.* 2013;147(1-3):379–384.

66. Palmer CA, Alfano CA. Sleep architecture relates to daytime affect and somatic complaints in clinically anxious but not healthy children. *J Clin Child Adolesc Psychol.* 2017;46(2):175–187.

67. Patriquin MA, Mellman TA, Glaze DG, Alfano CA. Polysomnographic sleep characteristics of generally-anxious and healthy children assessed in the home environment. *J Affect Disord.* 2014;161:79–83.

68. Giles DE, Kupfer DJ, Roffwarg HP, Rush AJ, Biggs MM, Etzel BA. Polysomnographic parameters in first-degree relatives of unipolar probands. *Psychiatry Res.* 1989;27(2):127–136.

69. Giles DE, Kupfer DJ, Rush AJ, Roffwarg HP. Controlled comparison of electrophysiological sleep in families of probands with unipolar depression. *Am J Psychiatry.* 1998;155(2):192–199.

70. Reynolds 3rd CF, Kupfer DJ. Sleep research in affective illness: State of the art circa 1987. *Sleep.* 1987;10(3):199–215.

71. Lind MJ, Hawn SE, Sheerin CM, et al. An examination of the etiologic overlap between the genetic and environmental influences on insomnia and common psychopathology. *Depress Anxiety.* 2017;34(5):453–462.

72. Eisen AR, Schaefer CE. *Separation Anxiety in Children and Adolescents: An Individualized Approach to Assessment and Treatment.* The Guilford Press; 2005.

73. Verduin TL, Kendall PC. Differential occurrence of comorbidity within childhood anxiety disorders. *J Clin Child Adolesc Psychol.* 2003;32(2):290–295.

74. El Rafihi-Ferreira R, Lewis KM, McFayden T, Ollendick TH. Predictors of nighttime fears and sleep problems in young children. *J Child Fam Stud.* 2019;28(4):941–949.

75. Moon RY, Carlin RF, Hand I. Task Force on Sudden Infant Death Syndrome, The Committee on Fetus and Newborn. Sleep-related infant deaths: Updated 2022 recommendations for reducing infant deaths in the sleep environment. *Pediatrics.* 2022;150(1):e2022057990.

76. Reynolds KC, Gradisar M, Alfano CA. Sleep in children and adolescents with obsessive-compulsive disorder. *Sleep Med Clin.* 2015;10(2):133–141.

77. Segal SC, Carmona NE. A systematic review of sleep problems in children and adolescents with obsessive compulsive disorder. *J Anxiety Disord.* 2022;90:102591.

78. Ivarsson T, Larsson B. Sleep problems as reported by parents in Swedish children and adolescents with obsessive-compulsive disorder (OCD), child psychiatric outpatients and school children. *Nord J Psychiatry.* 2009;63(6):480–484.

79. Rapoport J, Elkins R, Langer DH, et al. Childhood obsessive-compulsive disorder. *Am J Psychiatry.* 1981;138(12):1545–1554.

80. Jaspers-Fayer F, Lin SY, Belschner L, et al. A case-control study of sleep disturbances in pediatric obsessive-compulsive disorder. *J Anxiety Disord.* 2018;55:1–7.

81. Alfano CA, Kim KL. Objective sleep patterns and severity of symptoms in pediatric obsessive compulsive disorder: A pilot investigation. *J Anxiety Disord.* 2011;25(6):835–839.

82. Stewart SE, Hu YP, Leung A, et al. A multisite study of family functioning impairment in pediatric obsessive-compulsive disorder. *J Am Acad Child Adolesc Psychiatry.* 2017;56(3):241–249. e243.

83. Coles ME, Sharkey KM. Compulsion or chronobiology? A case of severe obsessive-compulsive disorder treated with cognitive-behavioral therapy augmented with chronotherapy. *J Clin Sleep Med.* 2011;7(3):307–309.

84. Dinges DF, Pack F, Williams K, et al. Cumulative sleepiness, mood disturbance, and psychomotor vigilance performance decrements during a week of sleep restricted to 4–5 hours per night. *Sleep.* 1997;20(4):267–277.

85. Yoo SS, Gujar N, Hu P, Jolesz FA, Walker MP. The human emotional brain without sleep–a prefrontal amygdala disconnect. *Curr Biol.* 2007;17(20):R877–R878.

86. Kovachy B, O'Hara R, Hawkins N, et al. Sleep disturbance in pediatric PTSD: Current findings and future directions. *J Clin Sleep Med.* 2013;9(5):501–510.

87. Hall Brown T, Garcia E. Trauma-related sleep disturbance in youth. *Curr Opin Psychol.* 2020;34:128–132.

88. Hall Brown TS, Belcher HME, Accardo J, Minhas R, Briggs EC. Trauma exposure and sleep disturbance in a sample of youth from the National Child Traumatic Stress Network Core Data Set. *Sleep Health.* 2016;2(2):123–128.

89. Wang Y, Raffeld MR, Slopen N, Hale L, Dunn EC. Childhood adversity and insomnia in adolescence. *Sleep Med.* 2016;21:12–18.

90. Lonigan CJ, Phillips BM, Richey JA. Posttraumatic stress disorder in children: Diagnosis, assessment, and associated features. *Child Adolesc Psychiatr Clin N Am.* 2003;12(2):171–194.

91. Brown TH, Mellman TA, Alfano CA, Weems CF. Sleep fears, sleep disturbance, and PTSD symptoms in minority youth exposed to Hurricane Katrina. *J Trauma Stress.* 2011;24(5):575–580.

92. Fan F, Zhou Y, Liu X. Sleep disturbance predicts posttraumatic stress disorder and depressive symptoms: A cohort study of Chinese adolescents. *J Clin Psychiatry.* 2017;78(7):882–888.

93. Jones S, Castelnovo A, Riedner B, et al. Sleep and emotion processing in paediatric posttraumatic stress disorder: A pilot investigation. *J Sleep Res.* 2021:e13261.

94. Bader K, Schafer V, Schenkel M, Nissen L, Schwander J. Adverse childhood experiences associated with sleep in primary insomnia. *J Sleep Res.* 2007;16(3):285–296.

95. Noll JG, Trickett PK, Susman EJ, Putnam FW. Sleep disturbances and childhood sexual abuse. *J Pediatr Psychol.* 2006;31(5):469–480.

96. Dahl RE. The regulation of sleep and arousal: Development and psychopathology. *Dev Psychopathol.* 1996;8(1):3–27.

97. Talbot LS, McGlinchey EL, Kaplan KA, Dahl RE, Harvey AG. Sleep deprivation in adolescents and adults: Changes in affect. *Emotion.* 2010;10(6):831–841.

98. Gregory AM, Buysse DJ, Willis TA, et al. Associations between sleep quality and anxiety and depression symptoms in a sample of young adult twins and siblings. *J Psychosom Res.* 2011;71(4):250–255.

99. Sipila T, Kananen L, Greco D, et al. An association analysis of circadian genes in anxiety disorders. *Biol Psychiatry.* 2010;67(12):1163–1170.

100. Barclay NL, Eley TC, Mill J, et al. Sleep quality and diurnal preference in a sample of young adults: Associations with 5HTTLPR, PER3, and CLOCK 3111. *Am J Med Genet B Neuropsychiatr Genet.* 2011;156B(6):681–690.

101. Stockmeier CA. Involvement of serotonin in depression: Evidence from postmortem and imaging studies of serotonin receptors and the serotonin transporter. *J Psychiatr Res.* 2003;37(5):357–373.

102. Gunthert KC, Conner TS, Armeli S, Tennen H, Covault J, Kranzler HR. Serotonin transporter gene polymorphism (5-HTTLPR) and anxiety reactivity in daily life: A daily process approach to gene-environment interaction. *Psychosom Med.* 2007;69(8):762–768.

103. Jorm AF, Prior M, Sanson A, Smart D, Zhang Y, Easteal S. Association of a functional polymorphism of the serotonin transporter gene with anxiety-related temperament and behavior problems in children: A longitudinal study from infancy to the mid-teens. *Mol Psychiatry.* 2000;5(5):542–547.

104. Harvey AG, Greenall E. Catastrophic worry in primary insomnia. *J Behav Ther Exp Psychiatry.* 2003;34(1):11–23.

105. Barclay NL, Gregory AM. The presence of a perseverative iterative style in poor vs. good sleepers. *J Behav Ther Exp Psychiatry.* 2010;41(1):18–23.

106. Weiner CL, Meredith Elkins R, Pincus D, Comer J. Anxiety sensitivity and sleep-related problems in anxious youth. *J Anxiety Disord.* 2015;32:66–72.

107. Bates JE, Viken RJ, Alexander DB, Beyers J, Stockton L. Sleep and adjustment in preschool children: Sleep diary reports by mothers relate to behavior reports by teachers. *Child Dev.* 2002;73(1):62–74.

108. Gregory AM, Eley TC, O'Connor TG, Plomin R. Etiologies of associations between childhood sleep and behavioral problems in a large twin sample. *J Am Acad Child Adolesc Psychiatry.* 2004;43(6):744–751.

109. Meijer AM, Habekothe RT, van den Wittenboer GL. Mental health, parental rules and sleep in pre-adolescents. *J Sleep Res.* 2001;10(4):297–302.

110. Warren SL, Gunnar MR, Kagan J, et al. Maternal panic disorder: Infant temperament, neurophysiology, and parenting behaviors. *J Am Acad Child Adolesc Psychiatry.* 2003;42(7):814–825.

111. Cousins JC, Whalen DJ, Dahl RE, et al. The bidirectional association between daytime affect and nighttime sleep in youth with anxiety and depression. *J Pediatr Psychol.* 2011;36(9):969–979.

112. Ma L, Mazidi M, Li K, et al. Prevalence of mental health problems among children and adolescents during the COVID-19 pandemic: A systematic review and meta-analysis. *J Affect Disord.* 2021;293:78–89.

113. Rao WW, Xu DD, Cao XL, et al. Prevalence of depressive symptoms in children and adolescents in China: A meta-analysis of observational studies. *Psychiatry Res.* 2019;272:790–796.

114. Xiao D, Guo L, Zhao M, et al. Effect of sex on the association between nonmedical use of opioids and sleep disturbance among Chinese adolescents: A cross-sectional study. *Int J Environ Res Public Health.* 2019;16(22):4339.

115. Dayton L, Kong X, Powell TW, et al. Child mental health and sleep disturbances during the early months of the COVID-19 pandemic in the United States. *Fam Community Health.* 2022;45(4):288–298.

116. Dellagiulia A, Lionetti F, Fasolo M, Verderame C, Sperati A, Alessandri G. Early impact of COVID-19 lockdown on children's sleep: A 4-week longitudinal study. *J Clin Sleep Med.* 2020;16(9):1639–1640.

117. Zhao J, Xu J, He Y, Xiang M. Children and adolescents' sleep patterns and their associations with mental health during the COVID-19 pandemic in Shanghai, China. *J Affect Disord.* 2022;301:337–344.

118. Penner F, Hernandez Ortiz J, Sharp C. Change in youth mental health during the COVID-19 pandemic in a majority Hispanic/Latinx US sample. *J Am Acad Child Adolesc Psychiatry.* 2021;60(4):513–523.

119. Benca RM, Obermeyer WH, Thisted RA, Gillin JC. Sleep and psychiatric disorders. A meta-analysis. *Arch Gen Psychiatry.* 1992;49(8):651–668. discussion 669–670.

120. Harvey AG. A transdiagnostic approach to treating sleep disturbance in psychiatric disorders. *Cogn Behav Ther.* 2009;38(Suppl 1):35–42.

121. Belleville G, Cousineau H, Levrier K, St-Pierre-Delorme ME, Marchand A. The impact of cognitive-behavior therapy for anxiety disorders on concomitant sleep disturbances: A meta-analysis. *J Anxiety Disord.* 2010;24(4):379–386.

122. Clarke G, Harvey AG. The complex role of sleep in adolescent depression. *Child Adolesc Psychiatr Clin N Am.* 2012;21(2):385–400.

123. Sadeh A. Cognitive-behavioral treatment for childhood sleep disorders. *Clin Psychol Rev.* 2005;25(5):612–628.

124. Tikotzky L, Sadeh A. The role of cognitive-behavioral therapy in behavioral childhood insomnia. *Sleep Med.* 2010;11(7):686–691.

125. Kuhn BR, Elliott AJ. Treatment efficacy in behavioral pediatric sleep medicine. *J Psychosom Res.* 2003;54(6):587–597.

126. Harvey AG, Payne S. The management of unwanted pre-sleep thoughts in insomnia: Distraction with imagery versus general distraction. *Behav Res Ther.* 2002;40(3):267–277.

127. March J, Silva S, Petrycki S, et al. Fluoxetine, cognitive-behavioral therapy, and their combination for adolescents with depression: Treatment for Adolescents With Depression Study (TADS) randomized controlled trial. *JAMA.* 2004;292(7):807–820.

128. Kennard B, Silva S, Vitiello B, et al. Remission and residual symptoms after short-term treatment in the Treatment of Adolescents with Depression Study (TADS). *J Am Acad Child Adolesc Psychiatry.* 2006;45(12):1404–1411.

129. Emslie GJ, Armitage R, Weinberg WA, Rush AJ, Mayes TL, Hoffmann RF. Sleep polysomnography as a predictor of recurrence in children and adolescents with major depressive disorder. *Int J Neuropsychopharmacol.* 2001;4(2):159–168.

130. Clarke G, McGlinchey EL, Hein K, et al. Cognitive-behavioral treatment of insomnia and depression in adolescents: A pilot randomized trial. *Behav Res Ther.* 2015;69:111–118.

131. Clementi MA, Alfano CA, Holly LE, Pina AA. Sleep-related outcomes following early intervention for childhood anxiety. *J Child Fam Stud.* 2016;25(11):3270–3277.

132. Peterman JS, Carper MM, Elkins RM, Comer JS, Pincus DB, Kendall PC. The effects of cognitive-behavioral therapy for youth anxiety on sleep problems. *J Anxiety Disord.* 2016;37:78–88.

133. McMakin DL, Ricketts EJ, Forbes EE, et al. Anxiety treatment and targeted sleep enhancement to address sleep disturbance in pre/early adolescents with anxiety. *J Clin Child Adolesc Psychol.* 2019;48(Supp 1):S284–S297.

134. Donovan CL, Spence SH, March S. Does an online CBT program for anxiety impact upon sleep problems in anxious youth? *J Clin Child Adolesc Psychol.* 2017;46(2):211–221.

135. Schlarb AA, Liddle CC, Hautzinger M. JuSt – a multimodal program for treatment of insomnia in adolescents: A pilot study. *Nat Sci Sleep.* 2011;3:13–20.

136. Bei B, Byrne ML, Ivens C, et al. Pilot study of a mindfulness-based, multi-component, in-school group sleep intervention in adolescent girls. *Early Interv Psychiatry.* 2013;7(2):213–220.

137. Blake M, Waloszek JM, Schwartz O, et al. The SENSE study: Post intervention effects of a randomized controlled trial of a cognitive-behavioral and mindfulness-based group sleep improvement intervention among at-risk adolescents. *J Consult Clin Psychol.* 2016;84(12):1039–1051.

138. Clementi MA, Alfano CA. An integrated sleep and anxiety intervention for anxious children: A pilot randomized controlled trial. *Clin Child Psychol Psychiatry*. 2020;25(4):945–957. https://doi.org/10.1177/1359104520933936

139. March JS, Biederman J, Wolkow R, et al. Sertraline in children and adolescents with obsessive-compulsive disorder: A multicenter randomized controlled trial. *JAMA*. 1998;280(20):1752–1756.

140. Kupfer DJ, Coble P, Kane J, Petti T, Conners CK. Imipramine and EEG sleep in children with depressive symptoms. *Psychopharmacology (Berl)*. 1979;60(2):117–123.

141. Shain BN, Naylor M, Shipley JE, Alessi N. Imipramine effects on sleep in depressed adolescents: A preliminary report. *Biol Psychiatry*. 1990;28(5):459–462.

142. Armitage R, Emslie G, Rintelmann J. The effect of fluoxetine on sleep EEG in childhood depression: A preliminary report. *Neuropsychopharmacology*. 1997;17(4):241–245.

143. Shamseddeen W, Clarke G, Keller MB, et al. Adjunctive sleep medications and depression outcome in the treatment of serotonin-selective reuptake inhibitor resistant depression in adolescents study. *J Child Adolesc Psychopharmacol*. 2012;22(1):29–36.

49

School Start Times

Rafael Pelayo, Kyla L. Wahlstrom, and Amy Ruth Wolfson

CHAPTER HIGHLIGHTS

- Middle school and high school starting times of 8:30 a.m. or later can significantly reduce deficit sleep in adolescents and allow greater alignment between their circadian timing and their daily schedules and functioning. Positive outcomes for adolescents obtaining consistently more sleep are numerous, with the body of research overwhelmingly concluding that this type of policy intervention is a public health success initiative for adolescent well-being.
- Shifting secondary schools to a later start time has been deliberated and slowly implemented in hundreds of high schools across the United States in the past 20+ years. The history of the movement includes collaboration between medical and educational research communities. Although pushback has been strong in some schools and districts, coalitions that formed in successful support of the change include education and health care professionals, associations such as the American Academy of Pediatrics, and the non-profit organization Start School Later (https://www.startschoollater.net/). Media coverage has also played a significant role by sharing research findings and educating the public about the importance of the biology and circadian timing shift of the adolescent brain.
- California (2019) became the first state in the nation to enact legislation that mandates later start times for both high schools and middle schools statewide (i.e., 8 a.m. for middle schools and 8:30 a.m. for high schools). The path to passing this legislation was years in the making. Ultimately, the evidence for creating a public health policy with the potential to improve the health and well-being of adolescents became the impetus for the change. This chapter concludes with the details of how the legislation evolved in California.

Introduction

In the field of pediatric sleep medicine, it would be difficult to find another example of how such a simple idea as delaying school start times has had such a profound effect on the lives of so many people and that it launched an international public health effort with ensuing legislative ramifications.[1–4] For decades it has been recognized that adolescents are usually sleep deficient. In the 1970s,

early work validating the Multiple Sleep Latency Test, Drs. Carskadon and Dement showed that the adolescents they tested were so sleep deprived they could not sleep satiate them with their initial protocol.[5,6] The description in the 1980s of delayed sleep phase syndrome brought awareness of the clinical importance of the circadian system in adolescents and further heightened concerns of the widespread consequences of adolescents and emerging adults obtaining insufficient sleep.[7,8] The sleep debt carried by these young people was felt to be such a complicated, multifactorial problem that little progress was made other than to simply ask parents and teenagers to try get more sleep.[9,10]

Early Years of School Start Time Research

This fundamentally started to change in 1990s when researcher Dr. Kyla Wahlstrom, a former Minnesota elementary school teacher and principal, working along Dr. Mark Mahowald, tested the hypothesis that starting school later would allow these teenagers to sleep more.[1] Dr. Carskadon had already called for this school schedule change based on her earlier work that included a finding that with puberty there was a delay in the preferred bedtime, in particular in girls. These results supported the involvement of a biologic factor in the adolescent phase preference delay and requiring a "revision" of prior understanding of adolescent sleep patterns.[11] The educational journal *Clearing House* published a paper on adolescent chronobiology in 1995 foreshadowing the necessary future convergence of education policy and medical researchers in improving adolescent sleep health.[12] However, up until the mid-1990s the emerging knowledge of adolescent sleep science was not routinely crossing over into the realm of education policy makers. In 1993, the Minneapolis Psychiatric Society initiated a resolution with the Minnesota Medical Association that led the association to contact more than 450 school districts in the state asking superintendents not to start school before 8 a.m., while also explaining the new science at that time about adolescent circadian rhythms. None of the superintendents agreed with the suggestion. The next year, the Minnesota Medical Association partnered with the American Academy of Sleep Medicine (AASM) to work with the state superintendents. It is historically important to point out that the AASM was based in Minnesota at the time. Finally, in 1995 the school district in Edina, Minnesota, agreed to delay their school start time from 7:20 a.m. to 8:30 a.m. in a high school (grades 9–12) in its next school year. That school district's superintendent, Kenneth Dragseth, contacted Kyla Wahlstrom, at the University of Minnesota's Center for Applied Research and Educational Improvement (CAREI), to study the impact of this schedule change with regard to learning, as well as students' health and well-being.

Dr. Wahlstrom recalls being very skeptical that changing the school schedule would make a difference for these adolescents (personal communication). Nevertheless, a comprehensive system-wide research plan was developed that included surveying the students, teachers, parents, and administrators, along with also measuring transportation effects, athletic performance of the school's sports teams, after-school employment, and participation in extracurricular activities. They also simultaneously studied the impact on custodians, cafeteria workers, and teacher contracts. The CAREI center issued a report of this work in 1998.[13] The results appeared to be too good to true. The prevailing cynicism at that time among members of the community when delaying the school start time was proposed that, if school started later, the students would simply stay up later. The same cynical argument is still echoed to this day when local communities are debating starting school at a later time. In retrospect, that argument was analogous to saying you would not feed a starving teenager because they would waste the food. In fact, the students in Minnesota reported going to bed around the same time and getting significantly more sleep with a later start time. In addition, both students and teachers reported increased alertness in the morning, along with better grades. Also, the students reported they were less likely to fall asleep doing homework. School officials including the nurses reported overall improvements in mental health and general wellness among these students. The custodians reported less trash, which they attributed to the students snacking less between classes. Finally, an overwhelming majority of parents reported that their children were easier to live with. This latter finding may be due to the known effect of lack of sleep on attentiveness and irritability.[14,15] The most significant adverse effect of making the school time change in this community was a change in traffic patterns around the school that required attention of government officials to ameliorate. Overall, this early work concluded that a later school start time appeared to be related to better achievement, less sleepiness, and fewer reports of depressive feelings and behaviors. Once this local story and other school start time outcome studies were popularized by the media, a national movement began to emerge.

Promptly after the initial success of a single high school in Minnesota, in 1997 the Minneapolis School District changed the start time of all seven high schools from 7:15 a.m. to 8:40 a.m. Unlike the first public high school in Edina, Minnesota, which was in a suburban and relatively affluent community, these Minneapolis high schools were in urban areas with over 83% of the students receiving nutrition assistance. The schools were studied for 5 years, and once again, improvements in academic and overall health were found among the students. In addition, improvements in school attendance and reduced tardiness were found, and an 8% improvement in the dropout rates was reported.[1] It is interesting that early on researchers had the foresight to consider the impact of delaying school start time on diverse communities and found it was particularly beneficial in lower socioeconomic populations. Despite this data, as we shall discuss in this chapter, 18 years later opponents of delaying school start times in California launched a publicity campaign saying that delaying start times in the state would hurt working families in the state.

Emergence of a National Dialogue and Movement

As the findings from these studies was reported in the local press, increasingly more national media outlets publicized the research findings. This in turn pushed sleep experts and educators throughout the country to comment to their local media about these reports, as well as address this innovation with other parents and school boards. Even though the research that led to the initial trial of delaying school start time was several years old, the findings were not appreciated until widespread news coverage of the implementation findings in Minnesota reached national and, later, international audiences.

It was not just the media that helped popularize the findings on delayed school start times. Professional societies stepped up to share this information and provide a forum for researchers to share their findings and plan future investigations. For example, the National Academy of Sciences convened a meeting in 1999 to bring together researchers in sleep health, educators, policy makers, and key stakeholders to review and discuss adolescent sleep patterns and difficulties. In addition, the Associated Professional Sleep Societies (APSS) annual meetings included early opportunities to share this emerging research at an international level with the entire sleep scientific community. The National Sleep Foundation sponsored similar events as early as 2005 via their Sleep and Teens Task Force, bringing together adolescent sleep experts and education researchers to help school districts learn the importance of providing their students with healthier sleep. Despite this increased awareness in the medical and health care community, the information transfer and application were suboptimal in the school districts around the country. Many communities argued that scientific research findings might not apply to their own communities (e.g., "our kids are different") or that the implementation may be too onerous.

As the value of delaying school start was being debated nationally and heatedly at the local level, more research on the dangers of adolescent sleep deprivation emerged. Sleep-deprived adolescents were reported to be more likely to be involved in automobile accidents, which is one of their most common causes of death.[16] Of particular interest were studies from two different states showing links between school start time and teenage driver safety.[17–19] The first article, published by Danner and Phillips, studied a community in Kentucky. They reported for the first time that decreased automobile accidents were associated with delayed school start times[17] 2 years after the school start time had been delayed by 1 hour. Of particular note, the rate of adolescents' accidents in the surrounding communities that did not change the school schedule actually increased. Other studies were conducted in Virginia where they compared the crash rates between schools with earlier start times and found higher crash rates in the schools that started earlier and that the accidents clustered around the time of school starting and letting out. As a control, there was no difference in the adult crash rates between these communities. They further found significantly more run-off road crashes to the right, which were thought to be potentially sleep related.[18,19] The authors showed great vision to study the convergence of driving safety, school start time, and adolescent sleep deprivation.

More recently, the RAND Corporation published a report on the economic impact of delaying school start times, finding that billions of dollars would be saved with delaying school start times. It is important to note that decreased car crash rates played an important role in the analysis.[20] These crash studies, plus the studies showing reduced drug, cigarette, alcohol use, and reduced depression, have been repeatedly quoted in local school districts throughout the country when they have debated changing school start times. When California became the first state in the nation to pass a law promoting healthy sleep for adolescents, these research findings were quoted in every public hearing.

In addition to sleep researchers and clinicians' concerns about the health benefits of delaying school start times to help adolescents get sufficient and regular sleep, parents who could obviously see that their teenagers were sleep deprived were frustrated with the schedules imposed by their local schools. In fact, in late 2011, the U.S. government launched the online petitioning portal *We the People* within https://WhiteHouse.gov, which promised petitions that reached a certain threshold of signatures would get a response from the government. Dr. Terra Ziporyn Snider launched one of those petitions, and thousands of people signed on. This led to a national grassroots movement bringing together parents, educators, and the medical community for the first time. This coalition created the non-profit organization Start School Later, which provided and continues to develop educational materials and resources to help local groups change their own schools' schedules. In 2017, they partnered with leading start time researchers to create the first-ever national conference on delaying school start times for adolescents, held in Washington, DC.[21]

As the reports of the benefits of delaying school start times increased, the Centers for Disease Control and Prevention (CDC) awarded a 3-year grant to Dr. Wahlstrom to conduct a larger comprehensive study with over 9000 students in eight public high schools in three states. The study found that high schools that started at 8:30 a.m. or later allow for more than 60% of students to obtain at least 8 hours of sleep per school night.[22] Adolescents obtaining less than 8 hours of sleep reported significantly higher depression symptoms, greater use of caffeine, and were at increased risk for making poor choices regarding substance use. Academic performance outcomes, including grades earned in core subject areas of math, English, science, and social studies, plus performance on state and national achievement tests, attendance rates, and reduced tardiness showed significantly positive improvement with the start times of 8:35 a.m. or later. Finally, the number of car crashes for teen drivers from 16 to 18 years of age was significantly reduced by 70% in one of the districts in the study when their high school shifted start times from 7:35 a.m. to 8:55 a.m.[22] This latter finding further supporting the prior studies on teen drivers from Kentucky and Virginia.

The American Academy of Pediatrics 2014 Report

With the release of Wahlstrom's CDC study findings, the American Academy of Pediatrics (AAP) convened a working group to review the literature school start times. A landmark review was published in 2014 in which the AAP came out in full support of delaying school start times to improve adolescent health. In their summary statement, they reported:

Insufficient sleep in adolescents as an important public health issue that significantly affects the health and safety, as well as the academic success, of our nation's middle and high school students. Although a number of factors, including biological changes in sleep associated with puberty, lifestyle choices, and academic demands, negatively affect middle and high school students' ability to obtain sufficient sleep, the evidence strongly implicates earlier school start times (i.e., before 8:30 am) as a key modifiable contributor to insufficient sleep, as well as circadian rhythm disruption, in this population. Furthermore, a substantial body of research has now demonstrated that delaying school start times is an effective countermeasure to chronic sleep loss and has a wide range of potential benefits to students with regard to physical and mental health, safety, and academic achievement. The American Academy of Pediatrics strongly supports the efforts of school districts to optimize sleep in students and urges high schools and middle schools to aim for start times that allow students the opportunity to achieve optimal levels of sleep (8.5–9.5 hours) and to improve physical (e.g., reduced obesity risk) and mental health (e.g., lower rates of depression) safety (e.g., drowsy driving crashes), academic performance, and quality of life.[23]

The release of the AAP review strongly called for recognition that the early school start time was a "modifiable" cause of adolescent sleep health problems that could not be easily ignored, although many had tried. Soon other national health organizations also called for delaying school start times to help adolescents get more sleep, such as the National Association of School Nurses. The AASM (2017) released a position statement "calling on communities, school boards, and educational institutions to implement start times of 8:30 am or later for middle schools and high schools to ensure that every student arrives at school healthy, awake, alert, and ready to learn."[24] Other organizations that released statements in support of delaying school start time include American Academy of Child & Adolescent Psychiatry, American Association of Sleep Technologists, American Medical Association, American Psychological Association, American Sleep Association, American Thoracic Society, Centers for Disease Control and Prevention, National Association of School Nurses, Society of Behavioral Medicine, National Parent Teacher Association, and numerous regional health and civic organizations.

As pediatricians, psychologists, and sleep and public health professionals increasingly called for greater attention in the media to the potential benefits of delaying school start times, more school districts started to consider making the change. This was met with resistance from several segments of the various communities who were opposed to making the necessary changes. Decisions about a school schedule are determined at the individual school or district level. There are over 26,000 secondary schools in the United States, with each one of them having to decide if the published data could be applied to their own school. Discussions have often turned into debates, wondering if the potential benefits could outweigh the opposition arguments and logistical issues involved in making the school schedule change. It would seem obvious that an individual community would want to make local decisions about how to operate a school, yet when these decisions involve public health, such as the dangers of chronic sleep deprivation in adolescents, then leaving these health decisions to be made in an ad hoc or piecemeal basis seems suboptimal. Delaying school start times would be inconvenient to those accustomed to their current schedules. If one school made the change, it would be out of sync with neighboring schools with regard to interscholastic activities such as sporting events. It is not surprising that local debates can be heated, and maintaining the status quo is often easier. For example, a 2017 national survey was conducted of how parental knowledge about adolescent sleep needs, and other beliefs inform their support for or objection to later school start times.[25] The study found that the majority (88%) of the parents had adolescents attending schools with start times before 8:30 a.m. Just over half of the parents (51%) expressed support for later school start times. Support was strongest among parents whose school started before 7:30 a.m. and had a favorable opinion of the AAP recommendations about school start times. Support also was associated with anticipation of improved school performance and increased sleep duration. Parents who were opposed were concerned about reduced time for after-school activities and the impact on school

transportation plans. The authors concluded that parental education about healthy sleep needs and anticipated health benefits increases their support for later school start times. The study also noted that 77% of the parents in the study did not recall discussing their adolescent child's sleep with their pediatrician. The authors go on to stress the need for discussions about sleep health and sleep hygiene as a part of a child's well-visit care with their primary physician.[25]

State Legislation to Delay School Start Times: California SB-328

In 1997, U.S. Representative Zoe Lofgren (D–Calif.) introduced the "ZZZ's to A's Act" to examine the relationship between school start times and adolescent health, well-being, and performance. Although to date this bill has not become law, it has been repeatedly brought up for consideration ever since. Rep. Lofgren became the first congressional sponsor of the House's Sleep Health Caucus and was awarded the Mark Hatfield Public Policy or Advocacy Award by the AASM in 2020.

Aside from this notable exception, up until 2016 attempts to change school start times were mostly limited to individual school districts. Over 80% of public middle and highs schools across the United States were starting before 8:30 a.m.[26] Progress beyond some states and schools agreeing to study the issue proved difficult despite education and health experts writing to support the AAP position statement.[27–29] Although there were numerous existing newspaper articles and editorials throughout the country on adolescent sleep and the benefits of delaying school start times, attention to the issue changed with Lisa Lewis's (freelance journalist) op-ed in the *Los Angeles Times* (September 2016). She called attention to the problems of adolescent sleep deprivation and benefits of delaying school start times. The op-ed was read by California State Senator Anthony Portantino, leading him to draft a short bill calling for public schools in California to follow the AAP position and delay the start of public middle and high schools to start no earlier than 8:30 a.m. The bill was titled *Senate Bill 328 Pupil Attendance: School Start Time* and was henceforth referred to as SB-328.[30] The bill was promptly opposed by school board administrators and the largest teacher's union in the state, which asserted school start times should be left up to the local control of individual school administrators. Supporters of charter schools also were opposed to statewide mandates that were considered to potentially limit their autonomy. The opposition argued that any individual school district could change its starting time, so a new law was not needed. Supporters of the bill pointed out that because schools interact with each other, it was very difficult for them to change their schedule without the cooperation of their neighboring schools. This was demonstrated by how few schools changed their schedules even though studies clearly demonstrated the benefits of providing greater time for adolescents' sleep.

SB-328 initially did not advance through the legislative process. When it was brought up again in 2018, opponents and supporters were more organized. Many leading national and regional health care and education organizations supported the bill including the California Sleep Society, AASM, and the AAP, as well as—very importantly—the Parent Teacher Association of California. Without doing any fundraising, volunteers walked the halls of the state capitol to meet with elected officials and explained the science behind SB-328. Sen. Portantino's office compiled the literature and circulated it throughout the legislature. This author (RP) testified at the hearings in addition to many other adolescent sleep advocates. Surprisingly, the bill made it through the California Assembly and Senate by one vote, making it to Governor Jerry Brown's desk for him to sign it into law. This was the furthest any prior legislative actions had ever reached in support of adolescent sleep health. The opposition launched a campaign calling for the governor to veto the bill that included radio ads saying that the bill would be harmful to working families. Governor Brown vetoed the bill in 2018; however, Sen. Portantino agreed to try again to pass SB-328 the next legislative year.[31]

In 2019, Governor Gavin Newsom was elected governor of California. Because SB-328 had been vetoed by the prior governor, the entire legislative process had to be restarted. Sen. Portantino rewrote the bill with the following changes to increase its likelihood of passing: the bill still called for public high schools to not have mandated start times before 8:30 a.m. but allowed for middle schools to start as early as 8 a.m. It also included an exception for rural districts because they may have different transportation problems. The bill also respected existing union collective bargaining agreements. The bill allowed for optional elective activity to start before 8:30 a.m. Perhaps most importantly, the bill created a 3-year implementation schedule so local schools could have logistical flexibility and time to work with their school district communities. At this time there were even greater lobbying efforts to thwart the bill in the legislature by its opponents. Many powerful interest groups in the state were opposed to the bill. Yet, at the same time, not only had the prior version of the bill brought greater awareness of circadian and sleep science to legislators, but more parents, teachers, and students joined in support. Supporters from California and around the country were mostly limited to writing letters, sharing PDF copies of published literature on the topic and, when possible, speaking directly to elected officials and staff. Several more national health and civic organizations including law enforcement joined in support. Perhaps the report that seemed to help sway elected officials was the circulation of data linking adolescent sleep deprivation and suicide.[32] The RAND Corporation analysis that California would ultimately save funds if it delayed school start times was important, because opponents feared that the measure would add to immediate transportation costs.[20] This time SB-328 passed the legislative chambers by a wider margin. Governor Newsom, however, did not make any public statements in favor of or against the bill, so it was not clear whether he would sign it into law. On October 13, 2019, which was the last day of the bill's eligibility, Governor Newsom signed SB-328 into law (!). This bill became the first state law ever passed focusing on improving adolescent sleep health.

Not surprisingly, the passing of the law made national and international headline news. Other states took notice and also started debating more the merits of applying this change to their own schools. Moreover, delaying school start times on a national level is included in the AASM's legislative agenda. The successful or failed implementation of this law in California will undoubtedly influence how delaying school start times is carried out in other places. Efforts to monitor the longitudinal outcomes of this law are underway with the support of the National Sleep Foundation, the AASM, Sleep Research Society (SRS), World Sleep Society, and other organizations. Public schools are at a crossroads for many elements of society. Monitoring the forthcoming research of this new law will bring together sleep scientists and education policy researchers to work alongside parents and students and school officials. What began as a local effort in Minnesota, spurred on by an opinion piece in a local newspaper, evolved into a national movement to correct what has been described as a public health and social justice problem.[33]

International and Ongoing Research

As evidence accumulates, beginning with studies in the mid-1990s, on the benefits of delaying middle and high school start times as a way of providing all adolescents more time to sleep, later school start times were associated with greater psychologic health.[34] A study in an all-girls' school in Singapore found that delaying its start time from 7:30 a.m. to 8:15 a.m. resulted in an actigraphy-estimated increase in 23 minutes of time in bed, which was sustained throughout the school year. Participants also reported lower levels of subjective sleepiness and improvement in well-being at both follow-ups. Notably, increased sleep duration on school nights was associated with improved alertness and well-being. The authors concluded that delaying school start time could result in "sustained benefits on sleep duration, daytime alertness, and mental well-being even within a culture where trading sleep for academic success is widespread."[35] The importance of this work showing a sustained effect in an international setting was lauded in an accompanying editorial.[36] On the other hand, a study in the UK attempted to apply a randomized controlled trial approach to delaying school start times. They had difficulty recruiting schools and described using a randomized controlled trial as "unfeasible."[37] Larger studies using actigraphy have been researching adolescents from different backgrounds and are taking into account health care disparities. They find that later school start times are associated with later wake times and that teens starting school at 8:30 a.m. or later are the only group with an average time in bed permitting 8 hours of sleep.[38–40]

The early studies on school start times were criticized for relying on self-report; however, it is challenging to use actigraphy in large community samples. Using actigraphy to provide a more objective estimate of sleep was introduced. In a study of 383 adolescents from different cities and with different school starting times, the authors found that adolescents starting school at 8:30 a.m. or later exhibited significantly longer actigraphically measured sleep.[39] This finding helps put to bed the cynical argument that if school starts later, teenagers will just stay up later and not get more sleep.

A longitudinal study conducted in Canada also found that a later school start time could "ameliorate sleep debt" among adolescents.[41] Similarly, a study carried out in Fairfax County, Virginia, found that a 50-minute delay in school start time in high schools and middle schools was associated with a "decreased prevalence of low mood, drowsy driving, and skipping breakfast," but was not seen in comparison schools that had students start only 30 minutes earlier.[42,43]

Throughout this chapter, we have been focusing on the role of delaying school start time in adolescents, but what about younger children? Clara and Gomes, researchers in Portugal, assessed children aged 4–11 years. They found that as the children grew older, their schools started increasingly earlier and the children started sleeping in more on weekends. This resulted in "a progressive reduction in the amount of sleep on school nights as grade level increased." They concluded the "social jet lag" in adolescents may be starting at a relatively young age.[44]

Studies have also examined relatively short delays in school start time. For example, a Switzerland study investigated a 20-minute school start time delay (7:40 a.m. to 8:00 a.m.) in comparison with no change in school start for eighth and ninth graders. Using self-report data, they found that the students with the 20-minute delay shifted their bed and wake times, but ultimately did not differ from the other group with regard to behavioral outcomes. They concluded that the 20-minute delay in school start times may have been too small to have a significant effect on daytime sleepiness and other outcome measures.[45] Moreover, a common strategy in some districts has been to have staggered or alternating schedules. In Croatia, researchers assessed adolescents attending school on alternating weekly morning (SST = 8 a.m.) and afternoon schedules (SST = 2 p.m.). Students slept over an hour more per night on the afternoon schedule, which resulted in less sleepiness, depressed mood, and substance use.[46]

Early critics faulted the studies for the lack of control groups, absence of long-term results, and no objective measures of sleep. As the field has matured, these limitations have been addressed and robust effects of delaying sleep have been demonstrated. Recently, Widome and colleagues studied a cohort from 5 public high schools in the metropolitan area of Minneapolis and St. Paul, Minnesota. Baseline data was collected from 455 students. Two of the schools delayed their starting time by 50 and 65 minutes, whereas the other schools kept the same schedule. Actigraphy was used to provide objective sleep data and students were followed for

2 years. Students who attended delayed-start schools had sustained more than 40 minutes of sleep per night during the 2-year follow-up study. They also decreased the amount of time they slept in on weekends by about half an hour. This study found that delaying high school start times was a "durable strategy" to extend adolescent school night sleep duration and lessen their need for catch-up sleep on weekends.[47] The editorial in *JAMA Pediatrics* that accompanied the Widome study concurred with the need for school districts to change their high school start times, based on the overwhelming public health benefit for adolescents.[48]

Two examples of how far the field of adolescent sleep and school start times has reached in less than 30 years include *Sleep Health*'s special issue on adolescent sleep and school start times (2018) and the international journal *Current Opinion in Physiology*'s (2020) special issue on the physiology of sleep. Among the articles describing cellular mechanisms of sleep in laboratory animals, the editors included two review articles on adolescent sleep and school start times.[49,50] Fontanellaz-Castiglione and colleagues reviewed the maturation changes that occur in the adolescent brain. In both humans and mice, "adolescence is accompanied by increased risk-taking, novelty-seeking and peer-directed social interaction in both species. Biologically, a period of rapid synaptic pruning is seen, wherein the number of synaptic connections undergoes marked decline. Generally speaking, in both species this pruning commences around the time of puberty and continues to the end of the adolescence" (p. 167). This pruning may explain the decrease of slow wave sleep across adolescence.[49] Sharman and Illingworth review the circadian physiology causing adolescents to shift to later bedtimes, with the ensuing sleep deprivation imposed by the school start time, and describe the global reach of this situation.[50]

Conclusion

The confluence of medical and behavioral science and public policy with regard to adolescent sleep and the time school starts raises the question of whether a public institution such as a school district, unintentionally or not, mandates an unhealthy requirement for a child. When I (RP) started to first hear of the reports coming out of Minnesota, I recall also being skeptical and thinking, "This can't be that easy." Scientific skepticism should not be equated with cynicism. Certainly, delaying school start times is not a panacea for all that ails adolescents in our society. However, those early studies of improved adolescent health led to wider studies in different populations throughout the country and the world with consistently positive outcomes. Insufficient, misaligned, and irregular sleep is one of the most common and potentially remediable health risks in teens. Critics of this effort will often cite "local control" as a dogmatic philosophy as to why the children in their own communities should continue to be sleep deprived by the educational system. It is important to realize that this all began at the local level with physicians and researchers working through their regional societies to share, at the time, the new information about adolescent sleep physiology and health. Researchers and health care providers then partnered with local education experts to implement the necessary changes. The resulting data was publicized widely in the press, which allowed more people to ask why their children were still being sleep deprived by the school system. When an adolescent is systematically awakened too early, we are depriving them of REM sleep time. We need to allow these children an opportunity to get sufficient REM time if we ever expect them to be healthy and follow their dreams.

CLINICAL PEARLS

- The combination of a delayed sleep phase and early school start times may lead to pathological sleepiness and poor academic performance.
- The clinician should interact with the patient, family, and school system to mitigate the negative impact of early school start times.
- Providing more time to sleep during the school week is a successful public health policy for adolescent well-being based on decades of research.
- Collaboration between medical, parent, and educational organizations and resources along with interest from the media have facilitated implementation of healthier school schedules despite frequent initial resistance to make the scheduling changes required by some members of the local community.
- Policies are focused on middle and high school schedules because this coincides with adolescent's brain biology development and in particular their shifting circadian timing.
- Synchronized scheduling policies across multiple school districts, entire states or countries will facilitate the implementation of public health policies to promote healthier sleep for all.

References

1. Wahlstrom K. Changing Times; Findings from the first longitudinal study of later high school start times. *NASSP Bulletin.* 2002;86(633):18.
2. Wahlstrom K. School start time and sleepy teens. *Arch Pediatr Adolesc Med.* 2010;164(7):676–677.
3. Skeldon AC, Dijk DJ. School start times and daylight saving time confuse California lawmakers. *Curr Biol.* 2019;29(8):R278–R279.
4. Bryan CS, Weingart R, Lindsey A, Hale L, Johnson DA, Gazmararian JA Impact of school start time delays and learning modality on sleep timing and duration during COVID-19. *Behav Sleep Med.* 2024;22(2):206–216. https://doi.org/10.1080/15402002.2023.2217974.
5. Anders TF, Carskadon MA, Dement WC. Sleep and sleepiness in children and adolescents. *Pediatr Clin North Am.* 1980;27(1):29–43.
6. Anders TF, Carskadon MA, Dement WC, Harvey K. Sleep habits of children and the identification of pathologically sleepy children. *Child Psychiatry Hum Dev.* 1978;9(1):56–63.
7. Thorpy MJ, Korman E, Spielman AJ, Glovinsky PB. Delayed sleep phase syndrome in adolescents. *J Adolesc Health Care.* 1988;9(1):22–27.
8. Weitzman ED, Czeisler CA, Coleman RM, et al. Delayed sleep phase syndrome. A chronobiological disorder with sleep-onset insomnia. *Arch Gen Psychiatry.* 1981;38(7):737–746.
9. Crowley SJ, Wolfson AR, Tarokh L, Carskadon MA. An update on adolescent sleep. *new evidence informing the perfect storm model. J Adolesc.* 2018;67:55–65.
10. Carskadon MA. Sleep in adolescents: the perfect storm. *Pediatr Clin North Am.* 2011;58(3):637–647.
11. Carskadon MA, Vieira C, Acebo C. Association between puberty and delayed phase preference. *Sleep.* 1993;16(3):258–262.
12. Callan R. Early morning challenge: the potential effects of chronobiology on taking the scholastic aptitude test. *Clearing House.* 1995;68(3):174–176.
13. Wahlstrom K.L. School start time study final report, volume 2: analysis of student survey data. University of Minnesota, Center for Applied Research and Educational Improvement. (1998). Digital Conservancy. Accessed November 19,2023. http://hdl.handle.net/11299/4249.
14. Yeo SC, Jos AM, Erwin C, et al. Associations of sleep duration on school nights with self-rated health, overweight, and depression symptoms in adolescents: problems and possible solutions. *Sleep Med.* 2019;60:96–108.
15. Baum KT, Desai A, Field J, Miller LE, Rausch J, Beebe DW. Sleep restriction worsens mood and emotion regulation in adolescents. *J Child Psychol Psychiatry.* 2014;55(2):180–190.
16. Martiniuk AL, Senserrick T, Lo S, Williamson A, Du W, Grunstein RR, et al. Sleep-deprived young drivers and the risk for crash: the DRIVE prospective cohort study. *JAMA Pediatr.* 2013;167(7):647–655.
17. Danner F, Phillips B. Adolescent sleep, school start times, and teen motor vehicle crashes. *J Clin Sleep Med.* 2008;4(6):533–535.
18. Vorona RD, Szklo-Coxe M, Wu A, Dubik M, Zhao Y, Ware JC. Dissimilar teen crash rates in two neighboring southeastern Virginia cities with different high school start times. *J Clin Sleep Med.* 2011;7(2):145–151.
19. Vorona RD, Szklo-Coxe M, Lamichhane R, Ware JC, McNallen A, Leszczyszyn D. Adolescent crash rates and school start times in two central Virginia counties, 2009-2011: a follow-up study to a southeastern Virginia study, 2007-2008. *J Clin Sleep Med.* 2014;10(11):1169–1177.
20. Hafner M, Stepanek M, Troxel WM. The economic implications of later school start times in the United States. *Sleep Health.* 2017;3(6):451–457.
21. Wikipedia. Start school later movement. [Available from: https://en.wikipedia.org/wiki/Start_school_later_movement.
22. Wahlstrom K.D.B., Gordon M., Peterson K., Edwards K., Gdula J. Examining the Impact of later high school start times on the health and academic performance of high school students: a multi-site study. 2014. Accessed November 19, 2023. http://conservancy.umn.edu/handle/11299/162769.
23. Adolescent Sleep Working G, Committee on A, Council on School H. School start times for adolescents. *Pediatrics.* 2014;134(3):642–649.
24. Watson NF, Martin JL, Wise MS, et al. Delaying Middle school and high school start times promotes student health and performance: an American Academy of Sleep Medicine position statement. *J Clin Sleep Med.* 2017;13(4):623–625.

25. Dunietz GL, Matos-Moreno A, Singer DC, Davis MM, O'Brien LM, Chervin RD. Later School start times: what informs parent support or opposition? *J Clin Sleep Med.* 2017;13(7):889–897.

26. Wheaton AG, Ferro GA, Croft JB. School Start times for middle school and high school students—United States, 2011–12 school year. *MMWR Morb Mortal Wkly Rep.* 2015;64(30):809–813.

27. Barnes M, Davis K, Mancini M, Ruffin J, Simpson T, Casazza K. Setting adolescents up for success: promoting a policy to delay high school start times. *J Sch Health.* 2016;86(7):552–557.

28. Temkin DA, Princiotta D, Ryberg R, Lewin DS. Later start, longer sleep: implications of middle school start times. *J Sch Health.* 2018;88(5):370–378.

29. Wheaton AG, Chapman DP, Croft JB. School start times, sleep, behavioral, health, and academic outcomes: a review of the literature. *J Sch Health.* 2016;86(5):363–381.

30. Portantino A. California Legislative Information. October 14, 2019. Accessed November 19, 2023. https://leginfo.legislature.ca.gov/faces/billTextClient.xhtml?bill_id=201920200SB328

31. Huber J. https://news.stanford.edu/thedish/2018/09/25/defeat-of-bill-for-later-school-start-times-wont-deter-sleep-specialist/ 2018 [Available from: https://news.stanford.edu/thedish/2018/09/25/defeat-of-bill-for-later-school-start-times-wont-deter-sleep-specialist/.]

32. Chiu HY, Lee HC, Chen PY, Lai YF, Tu YK. Associations between sleep duration and suicidality in adolescents: a systematic review and dose-response meta-analysis. *Sleep Med Rev.* 2018;42:119–126.

33. Hale L, Troxel W. Embracing the school start later movement: adolescent sleep deprivation as a public health and social justice problem. *Am J Public Health.* 2018;108(5):599–600.

34. Berger AT, Widome R, Troxel WM. School start time and psychological health in adolescents. *Curr Sleep Med Rep.* 2018;4(2):110–117.

35. Lo JC, Lee SM, Lee XK, et al. Sustained benefits of delaying school start time on adolescent sleep and well-being. *Sleep.* 2018;41(6):1–8.

36. Wolfson AR. Current scholarship and future questions on delayed school start times for adolescents' sleep and well-being. *Sleep.* 2018;41(6):1–3.

37. Illingworth G, Sharman R, Jowett A, Harvey CJ, Foster RG, Espie CA. Challenges in implementing and assessing outcomes of school start time change in the UK: experience of the Oxford Teensleep study. *Sleep Med.* 2019;60:89–95.

38. James S, Chang AM, Buxton OM, Hale L. Disparities in adolescent sleep health by sex and ethnoracial group. *SSM Popul Health.* 2020;11:100581.

39. Nahmod NG, Lee S, Master L, Chang AM, Hale L, Buxton OM. Later high school start times associated with longer actigraphic sleep duration in adolescents. *Sleep.* 2019;42(2):1–10.

40. Nahmod NG, Lee S, Buxton OM, Chang AM, Hale L. High school start times after 8:30 am are associated with later wake times and longer time in bed among teens in a national urban cohort study. *Sleep Health.* 2017;3(6):444–450.

41. Patte KA, Qian W, Cole AG, et al. School start time changes in the COMPASS study: associations with youth sleep duration, physical activity, and screen time. *Sleep Med.* 2019;56:16–22.

42. Whitaker RC, Dearth-Wesley T, Herman AN, Oakes JM, Owens JA. A quasi-experimental study of the impact of school start time changes on adolescents' mood, self-regulation, safety, and health. *Sleep Health.* 2019;5(5):466–469.

43. Owens JA, Dearth-Wesley T, Herman AN, Oakes JM, Whitaker RC. A quasi-experimental study of the impact of school start time changes on adolescent sleep. *Sleep Health.* 2017;3(6):437–443.

44. Clara MI, Allen Gomes A. An epidemiological study of sleep-wake timings in school children from 4 to 11 years old: insights on the sleep phase shift and implications for the school starting times' debate. *Sleep Med.* 2020;66:51–60.

45. Das-Friebel A, Gkiouleka A, Grob A, Lemola S. Effects of a 20 minutes delay in school start time on bed and wake up times, daytime tiredness, behavioral persistence, and positive attitude towards life in adolescents. *Sleep Med.* 2020;66:103–109.

46. Koscec Bjelajac A, Bakotic M, Ross B. Weekly alternation of morning and afternoon school start times: implications for sleep and daytime functioning of adolescents. *Sleep.* 2020;43(8):1–11.

47. Widome R, Berger AT, Iber C, Wahlstrom K, Laska MN, Kilian G, et al. Association of Delaying school start time with sleep duration, timing, and quality among adolescents. *JAMA Pediatr.* 2020;174(7):697–704.

48. Cheng E. Delaying school start times to improve population health. *JAMA Pediatr.* 2020;174(7):641–643.

49. Fontanellaz-Castiglione CEM, Markovic A, Tarokh L. Sleep and the adolescent brain. *Curr Opin Physiol.* 2020;15:167–171.

50. Sharman R, Illingworth G. Adolescent sleep and school performance—the problem of sleepy teenagers. *Curr Opin Physiol.* 2020;15:23–28.

Scoring and Assessment of Sleep and Related Physiological Events

50

Polysomnography and Multiple Sleep Latency Test

Jyoti Krishna

CHAPTER HIGHLIGHTS

- A variety of physical and physiologic phenomena associated with sleep may be recorded and analyzed by means of a sleep study. Such studies may be ordered for diagnostic or therapeutic purposes.
- Modern equipment and software provides flexibility to run tests in the sleep laboratory or in the hospital at the patient's bedside. Abbreviated screening tests for sleep apnea are increasingly being performed at home, especially in the adult setting.
- In this chapter, we present the indications and techniques pertaining to in-lab polysomnography (PSG) and multiple sleep latency test (MSLT), with special emphasis on infants and children. We describe features that are unique to pediatric sleep testing and present an overview of the layout of a typical sleep laboratory, day-to-day logistics and triage operations, preparation of the family, equipment setup and patient hookup in a pediatric-friendly setting.
- The reader will gain insight into the complexity and scope of sleep testing in children. Nuances of data acquisition, interpretation, and reporting are also discussed.

Introduction

Clichéd as it may sound, the wisdom in the art of medical evaluation of the sick lies primarily in a thorough history and clinical examination. The preceding chapters have aptly illustrated the complexities of evaluating the child with sleep disorders in this regard. Thus the reader will have appreciated that several medical and non-medical conditions can lead to, or, even masquerade as, a sleep disorder. The reverse is certainly true as well. For instance, excessive daytime sleepiness (EDS) may present with depressive symptoms and obstructive sleep apnea syndrome (OSAS) as attention-deficit disorder. As in all other branches of medicine, recourse to diagnostic testing is helpful to clarify clinical suspicions and confirm diagnoses. It is now clearly established by several studies that no combination of clinical history and physical examination will reliably distinguish the presence or absence of

OSAS in a snoring child.[1-3] This observation illustrates the need for confirmatory diagnostic testing, specifically polysomnography (PSG). Similarly, PSG is required for the diagnosis of rapid eye movement (REM) sleep behavior disorder (RBD) where the absence of the skeletal muscle atonia normally present during REM sleep is useful to confirm clinical suspicion. Furthermore, the multiple sleep latency test (MSLT) is a standard tool to objectively ascertain the propensity of daytime sleepiness in patients with symptoms suggestive of EDS.

Alternate tools for the evaluation of the child with a sleep disorder do exist. For instance, with respect to the child with suspected OSAS (the most common indication for PSG), it has been felt that due to a shortage of pediatric sleep testing centers in the United States or for financial reasons, substitute diagnostic tests such as home video monitoring, daytime nap testing, and abbreviated sleep studies (such as overnight oximetry and portable home recordings) may be useful.[4] However, the relatively lower predictive values of these tests make them less desirable when compared with the "gold standard" PSG.[3] Other tools often used in sleep clinics include a variety of sleep logs and questionnaires for sleep habit screening and to evaluate daytime sleepiness or circadian preferences.[5] Actigraphs, which are wristwatch-sized devices housing accelerometers, sense motion or lack thereof as a measure of rest and activity levels. These activity-reporting data are then useful as surrogate indicators of wake and sleep. Less commonly, human leukocyte antigen (HLA) markers and cerebrospinal fluid hypocretin levels are used in the evaluation of patients with EDS who are suspected to have narcolepsy.[6,7]

In this chapter, we will discuss the indications and techniques pertaining to PSG and MSLT, with special emphasis on infants and children. Technical details relative to the standards of clinical practice and laboratory space, laboratory protocols, instrumentation, and specific scoring rules are not discussed in detail in this chapter. The reader is directed to the official guidelines set forth in publications by the American Academy of Sleep Medicine (AASM).[8-10] Excellent information on the requirements for maintaining accreditation of sleep diagnostic facilities is also available at the AASM's website (https://aasm.org/accreditation/). Furthermore, while the merits and standards of studying childhood sleep disorders in integrated adult and pediatric laboratories versus pediatric-specific accredited laboratories continues to be debated,[11,12] this chapter will concern itself with traditional "attended in-lab" types of sleep studies in a child-friendly setting.

Indications for Polysomnography

By far, the most common reason for ordering a sleep study is to confirm the suspected diagnosis of OSAS and other types of sleep-related breathing disorders (SRBDs) or provide a therapeutic intervention. In recent statements, the American Academy of Pediatrics and the AASM have outlined their positions on the diagnosis and management of OSAS and emphasized that follow-up PSG should be additionally performed after an intervention such as

tonsillectomy and adenoidectomy (T&A) in children with persisting symptoms and those at high risk for incomplete resolution of OSAS after T&A. Such children include those with severe OSAS, obesity, craniofacial anomalies impacting the upper airway, certain neurologic conditions (e.g., meningomyelocele), and genetic disorders (e.g., Down syndrome). If OSA remains unresolved after T&A, these children may require additional interventions such as positive airway pressure (PAP) therapy.[3,13] Evidence is less robust for the use of PSG for suspected SRBD accompanying chronic lower airway diseases such as asthma, cystic fibrosis, pulmonary hypertension, bronchopulmonary dysplasia, chest wall abnormality such as kyphoscoliosis, or brief resolved unexplained events (BRUE; formerly known as apparent life-threatening events [ALTEs]).[14] Non-respiratory indications for PSG include evaluation of narcolepsy, periodic limb movement disorder (PLMD), RBD, and selected cases of childhood restless legs syndrome (RLS)[15] (Table 50.1).

TABLE 50.1 Respiratory and Non-Respiratory Indications For and Against Polysomnography in Children[13,15]

	Respiratory	Non-Respiratory
Standard indications	• To confirm clinically suspected OSAS • After T&A in children with mild OSAS preoperatively only if suspicion of non-resolution remains on clinical follow-up • To confirm resolution of OSAS after T&A in children with high preoperative risk of non-resolution of OSAS following T&A • For PAP titration for treatment of OSAS	• To confirm clinical suspicion of PLMD • For evaluation of narcolepsy (in conjunction with MSLT)
Guideline indications	• For suspected hypoventilation due to congenital central hypoventilation, neuromuscular, or chest wall disease • For selected cases of primary sleep apnea of infancy or ALTE/BRUE • In children being considered for T&A for suspected OSA • To monitor for changes in PAP support requirement in growing children, in those with recurrence of symptoms, or those treated with other methods for OSAS	• For evaluation of nocturnal phenomena such as non-REM parasomnia, epilepsy, or enuresis when there is clinical suspicion of comorbid OSAS or PLMD
Optional indications	• To assess response of OSAS to rapid maxillary expansion or oral appliance • To titrate noninvasive positive pressure ventilation in breathing disorders other than OSAS • To adjust mechanical ventilator settings • To assess readiness for decannulation of tracheostomy for sleep-related breathing disorder • To assess suspected sleep-related breathing disorder in certain chronic pulmonary airway, parenchymal, vascular, or chest wall conditions	• In conjunction with MSLT for hypersomnia other than narcolepsy • Utilizing an expanded montage EEG to investigate atypical or dangerous parasomnia behaviors (including RBD) or to distinguish these from suspected seizures • To support clinical suspicion of RLS
PSG not recommended	• For diagnosis of OSAS using abbreviated duration PSG (nap study) • For titration of oxygen therapy	• Sleep-related bruxism

Standard, guideline, and optional categories reflect patient-care strategy with high, moderate, and conflicting degrees of clinical certainty based on expert opinion or available evidence.

Abbreviations: OSAS, obstructive sleep apnea syndrome; T&A, tonsillectomy and adenoidectomy; PAP, positive airway pressure; PLMD, periodic limb movement disorder; MSLT, multiple sleep latency test; ALTE, apparent life-threatening events; BRUE, brief resolved unexplained events; REM, rapid eye movement; PSG, polysomnography; EEG, electroencephalography; RBD, REM sleep behavior disorder; RLS, restless legs syndrome.

Organization of Sleep Services in the Context of the Sleep Study

Equipment and Study Timing

While the pediatric sleep study is broadly very similar to its adult counterpart in the scope of the sleep disorders tested,[16] several key differences are worthy of emphasis. Pediatric populations are diverse in age, and any sleep laboratory catering to childhood sleep disorders needs to be equally adept in monitoring a newborn infant as well as an older teenager. It is therefore essential to maintain the equipment inventory to cater to these diverse age groups. This applies to the bed (e.g., crib), sensors (e.g., small-size nasal cannula), and therapy (e.g., pediatric interfaces to deliver PAP).

The study may need to be timed to match the variable sleep times of children at different levels of maturity. Newborns will sleep for substantial periods in the day and planning of daytime PSGs may free up beds at night for the laboratory. Conversely, a delayed testing schedule may be needed to match the teenager likely to present with a circadian phase delay.[17]

Location

While the physical location of the sleep laboratory is typically in an outpatient setting for adults, many pediatric centers do cater to medically complex children within the hospital setting. For example, "ventilator checks" and tracheostomy decannulation protocols may be safer to run in an inpatient setting. As a result, many exclusively pediatric sleep laboratories are located within the floor space of a pediatric ward. In other instances, mobile equipment capable of running a complete attended sleep study is utilized at bedside within the hospital, whereas the bulk of the sleep studies are run in an outpatient laboratory setting (Fig. 50.1A and B). Although the clear advantage of in-hospital PSG is the availability of trained on-call staff to respond to emergencies should such a need arise for the complex medically unstable child, this scenario has the distinct potential disadvantage of poor sound and electrical insulation from the ambient hospital environment. Nonetheless, creative ways of ensuring an uninterrupted night (e.g., private room) may be utilized because safety and reassurance of trained backup is usually the priority driving a bedside study in such cases.

Friendliness Factor

Perhaps the single most important factor that makes a sleep laboratory worthy of qualifying as a *pediatric* sleep laboratory is its "child friendliness factor." This applies not only to the physical space itself, but also extends most vitally to the friendliness of the technical and non-technical staff. Zaremba and colleagues have described the ingredients of such a setting very well.[18] As soon as they enter the door,

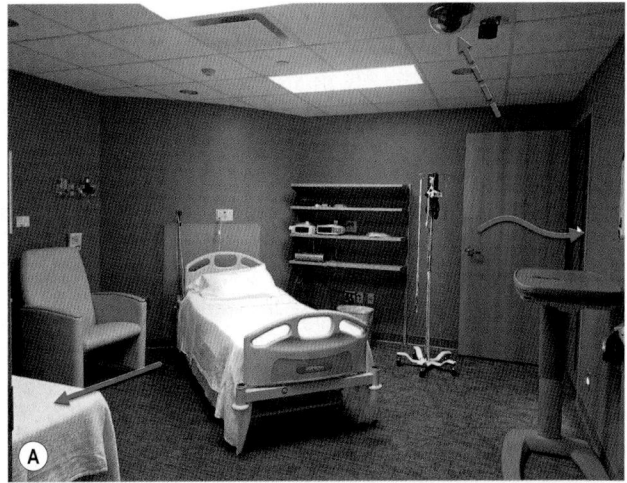

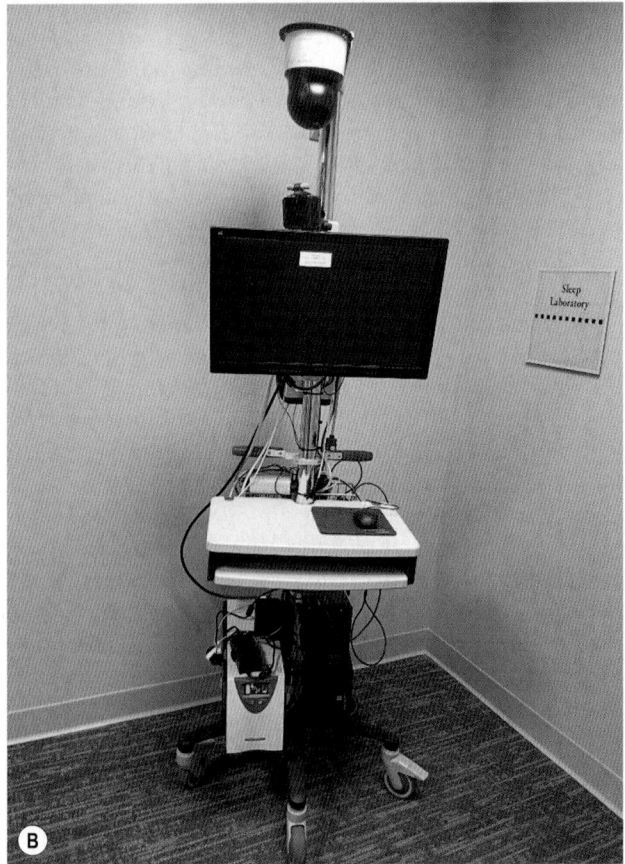

• **Fig. 50.1** (A) A typical bedroom in the author's sleep laboratory. Note the extra bed for the parent *(solid arrow)* and the overhead high-definition low light camera *(broken arrow)*. The bedroom may be reconfigured by rolling out the main bed and replacing it with a crib for younger patients. Should they wish, an attached full bath *(curved arrow)* allows for the patient to shower and be ready for school the morning after the sleep test. (B) A mobile unit at the author's sleep laboratory is used to run attended multichannel polysomnograms at the patient's bedside within the children's hospital. It is equipped with high-definition camera, oximetry, capnometry, and positive airway pressure treatment capabilities. Even though the main sleep laboratory is housed within the hospital complex, a mobile unit is useful for patients who are not stable enough to be transported there.

the child's experience often begins to shape the likelihood of cooperation. The decor, the friendliness of the reception area, and reassuring words all go a long way in setting the stage. While teens should not be talked down to or patronized, the younger children may need repeated reassurance and gentle handling. Simple language should be used to describe the plan for the night. A "show and tell" attitude for equipment needs to be borne in mind before the hookup. The child should understand that the hookup will be painless ("no ouchies," "no needlesticks") and the technologist must not neglect to assure the young patient that all equipment will come off painlessly the next morning. A quick little demonstration with an electroencephalogram (EEG) sticker application on a parent (with the child's permission!) may be very reassuring to reinforce this fact and to enlist the child's active participation in the process. Younger girls may be excited about wearing "shiny hair jewelry," whereas boys may like to hear they will look "like a space cadet" once they are all hooked up with the EEG electrodes. Asking families to bring their cameras along to take "cool looking" pictures adds to the excitement of "camping out at the sleep center!"; TV, DVD, and other diversions help. The child may need reassurance that their parent will be in the room and that their favorite teddy bear can accompany them to bed (Fig. 50.2A and B).

The beds used in the pediatric sleep laboratory have to be configurable enough to allow a parent to room-in with the child in their own separate bed. Ability to roll in a crib or toddler bed for the younger patient or substitute these with a full-size bed for the teenager requires adequate planning and storage space for extra beds. Furthermore, beds have to have safety rails for the appropriate cases, and other safety cautions may have to be modified for the child.[19] Finally, easy access to restroom facilities, odor-sealing diaper disposals, and accommodations for wheelchairs or special equipment for the medically challenged child all need to be considered while planning and designing the sleep center.

Preplanning the Logistics of the Study

Given the foregoing description, the reader will have appreciated the complexity of the task involved in running a sleep laboratory smoothly. Both equipment and personnel must work together in a situation where the patient may be fearful, anxious, or simply unwilling for the procedure. It is perhaps safe to say that every pediatric sleep laboratory will have a few "failed studies" for one reason or another from time to time. Barring illness on the day of study, which can rarely be predicted, there are many things that can be preempted to increase the likelihood of an optimal outcome.

First, the clinical encounter must clarify if a study is needed at all and articulate the exact clinical question to be answered during the study. This becomes especially important if the laboratory accepts direct referrals from non-sleep physicians. Tailoring the study to the child is highly desirable to prevent or minimize chance of failure. To this end, information on the child's age, baseline state of health, and nature of sleep issues must be available to the testing

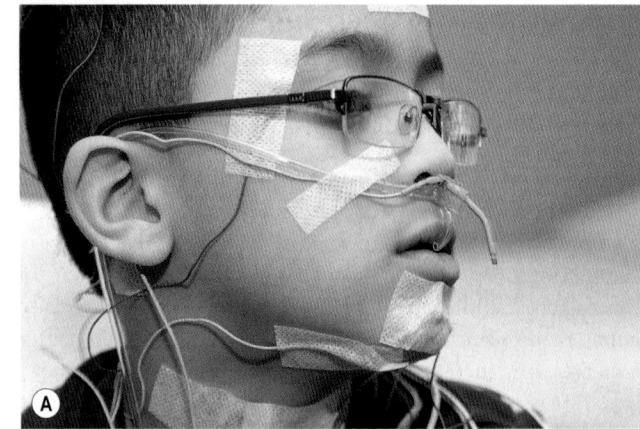

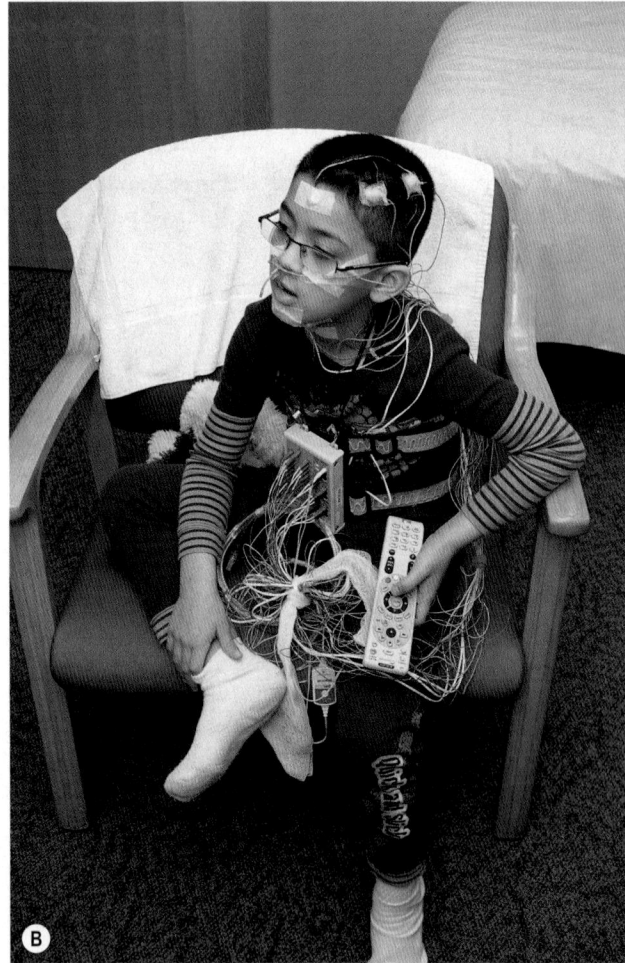

• **Fig. 50.2** (A) This child has been hooked up for a polysomnogram (PSG). This close-up shows the placement of oronasal thermistor and transducer to capture airflow as well as measure $ETCO_2$. Right ocular and chin electrodes covered with tape can be seen. The referential right mastoid lead can be seen behind the right pinna. A snore microphone is attached to the neck. *Reprinted with permission, Cleveland Clinic Center for Medical Art & Photography © 2013. All Rights Reserved.* (B) The nonthreatening environment of this child-friendly sleep center is apparent. This young child feels right at home and is able to watch his favorite DVD during and after his PSG hookup. Visible scalp electrodes include ground (mid-forehead), left frontal, and central electrodes. Notice the stuffed toy animal by his side for comfort. The jack box hanging around his neck accepts all the electrodes allowing mobility. The jack box will be finally connected to the control room computers once the child is in bed. (Reprinted with permission, Cleveland Clinic Center for Medical Art & Photography © 2013. All Rights Reserved).

laboratory. Usually, accredited laboratories have standardized sleep order sets that ask the appropriate screening questions from ordering physicians.

All orders ideally should be carefully scrutinized by a knowledgeable person in the laboratory to ascertain that the study can be run as directed. For instance, usually one PSG technologist runs two studies at night in most adult settings. This is commonly referred to as 1:2 staffing. In the pediatric setting, however, for children with special needs or for the younger child, a ratio of 1:1 is often required. Timing of the start of the PSG ("lights out") will be very different for a toddler versus a teenager who sleeps late, or a patient who is traveling multiple time zones to a referral center. Furthermore, sleep technologists often come with prior training in other fields. The laboratory manager will use this knowledge to ensure that the sleep technologist assigned to run any particular study is matched to the clinical need. Thus a technologist with a respiratory therapy background may be more suited to run a "ventilator check" while the child with complex parasomnia and suspected seizure disorder may be the forte of the EEG-trained technologist. For 1:2 staffing too, the anticipated "easy hookup" may be paired with a "tough hookup," or the early lights out study be matched with a late sleeper to allow the technologist time to accomplish the studies on both patients more comfortably.

Preparing the Family for the Sleep Study

Any visit to the doctor is an anxiety-provoking experience for the child and the family. For most, the sleep study is a novel experience. Therefore seeds for a successful study are best planted during the clinical visit. Careful explanation of the reason for the study and the types of sensors and their importance are crucial to enlist patient and parental cooperation during the PSG. An informed parent is the technologist's best ally when struggling with an uncooperative child at night. For instance, while most children dislike the nasal cannula, a partnership with the parents helps provide reassurance to the child and transmits the expectation to keep the device on. Similar considerations apply to the other sensors as well. With rare exception, the use of sedation to accomplish the PSG is generally not recommended, and adverse events have been reported in children with OSA.[20]

Accordingly, the patient's family may benefit from touring the laboratory a few days prior to the test night. This approach not only reduces anxiety, but also helps the parents and child to plan what clothing, medications, personal effects, or entertainment items to bring along in their overnight bags to make the child comfortable at night. Also, they get an opportunity to see the sleeping options for the accompanying parent. As part of standard instructions at the author's center, parents are reminded to bring any special home equipment such as for G-tube feedings, tracheostomy supplies, or vagal nerve stimulator (VNS) magnet. Online educational videos are a great tool for providing the

patient and their family with a guided tour of the laboratory if they are not physically able to tour in advance.

The importance of maintaining a stable age-appropriate sleep schedule leading up to the sleep study should be discussed and avoiding, for instance, that late-night party on Friday and consequently a non-representative study night on Saturday. Similarly, a late afternoon nap or caffeinated beverage may delay sleep onset at night significantly. Parents should also be advised to reschedule the PSG if the child is sick. An acute upper airway infection may compromise the accuracy of OSAS diagnosis. Discontinuation of medications that may affect the sleep study should be discussed and, if necessary and safely possible, an adequate wash-out period should be planned prior to the sleep study. This is especially true if an MSLT study is to follow the next day, as several medications are known to compromise the quality of the MSLT by direct or withdrawal–rebound effect on the sleep architecture.[9]

Running the Polysomnogram

The Polysomnography Montage

The standard overnight PSG measures sleep parameters utilizing limited EEG, electrooculogram (EOG), chin and leg electromyogram (EMG), electrocardiogram (ECG), respiratory effort at the chest and abdomen via respiratory inductance plethysmography (RIP) belts, pulse oximetry, capnometry via end-tidal or transcutaneous measurement ($ETCO_2$, $TcpCO_2$), and oronasal airflow via pressure transducer and thermistor (see Fig. 50.2A and B).

The EEG electrode placement is based on an imaginary grid on the head measured in a standard fashion using the widely accepted 10–20 system.[21] While specialized sleep centers may occasionally utilize the more extensive EEG montage essential for seizure diagnosis, only frontal (F), central (C), occipital (O), and eye (E) exploring electrodes are used to capture EEG and EOG data during the standard PSG. These are referenced to the contralateral mastoid (M) electrode on either side. Standardized numbering of these electrodes is based on location (e.g., C3, C4) with odd numbers represented on the left side by convention (Fig. 50.3). EOG leads help monitor REM of dream sleep (Fig. 50.4). When combined with EMG data from chin leads, these channels allow for the scoring of sleep and wake into several stages (Fig. 50.5). Each stage has several key characteristics that are described in greater detail elsewhere.[8] Briefly, stage Wake shows some eye movements, persistent EMG tone in the chin, and age-appropriate dominant posterior rhythm in the occipital leads when the eyes are closed. Stage N1 is characterized by slow rolling eye movements and vertex sharp waves in the central leads. This usually gives way to sleep spindles and K-complexes characteristic of stage N2 as sleep progresses. Stage N3 is the deepest stage of sleep and comprises abundant delta waves that are 0.5–2 Hz in frequency and 75 µV in amplitude. Stage REM is scored when rapid eye movements are seen alongside

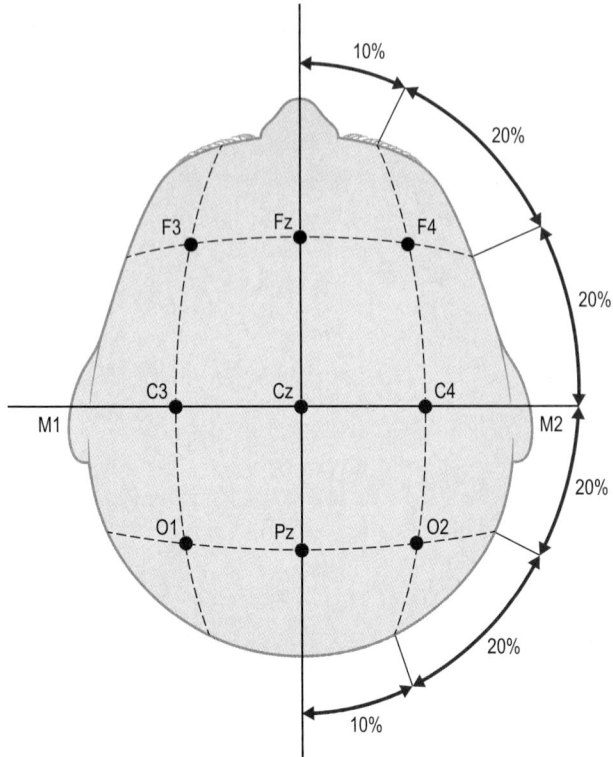

• **Fig. 50.3** The International 10–20 system of electrode placement utilizes bony landmarks on the skull to delineate an imaginary grid that is numbered using standard nomenclature as shown. Measurements are made as a fraction of the total head circumference. See text for details. (Reprinted with permission, Cleveland Clinic Center for Medical Art & Photography © 2013. All Rights Reserved).

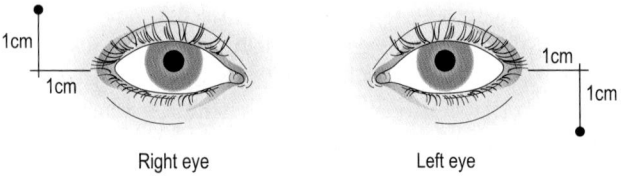

Right eye | Left eye

• **Fig. 50.4** Recommended placement of ocular leads. The distances may be halved for younger children. (Reprinted with permission, Cleveland Clinic Center for Medical Art & Photography © 2013. All Rights Reserved).

mixed-frequency low-voltage EEG and importantly, a low EMG tone. Sawtooth waves are characteristic of this stage as well. Thus Wake, N1, N2, N3, and REM sleep stages can be scored throughout the sleep record. The EEG and EMG are also used to score arousals that are defined as 3-second long EEG frequency shifts in any sleep stage. There needs to be an accompanying EMG increase in REM stage, however. Arousals in turn are also of importance in the scoring of hypopneas.[22]

A special case is made for stage scoring of very young infants. Here, due to the normal maturational delay of several months in the evolution of sleep spindles and K-complexes, the scoring is simplified to comprise wakefulness (stage W), transitional sleep (stage T), REM sleep (stage R), and non-REM sleep (stage N).[8] This has replaced the older nomenclature of Active (equivalent of REM sleep), Quiet (equivalent of NREM sleep), and Indeterminate sleep.[23]

Measuring Breathing

Sensors useful for the measurement of respiratory status during PSG include the chest and abdominal effort belts, nasal pressure transducer and thermistor (which both measure oronasal airflow), as well as instruments to measure gas exchange. Reliability and validity of respiratory event measurement and scoring has been recently reviewed and forms the basis for the current recommendations by the AASM.[24]

Respiratory effort implies that there is a signal from the central neuronal control centers to the motor neurons targeting muscles of respiration to fire. In the normal circumstance, this results in abdominal and thoracic excursion and alternating ingress and egress of air from the upper airway. The absence of airflow from the nose or mouth over a specified duration is termed apnea. It is "central" in nature if there are no respiratory efforts associated with absent airflow; it is "obstructive" if there is lack of airflow in the face of continuing efforts to respire.

RIP belts are now the instrument of choice for measuring respiratory effort. Mercury strain gauges and piezoelectric sensor-equipped belts are no longer used. The RIP belts are

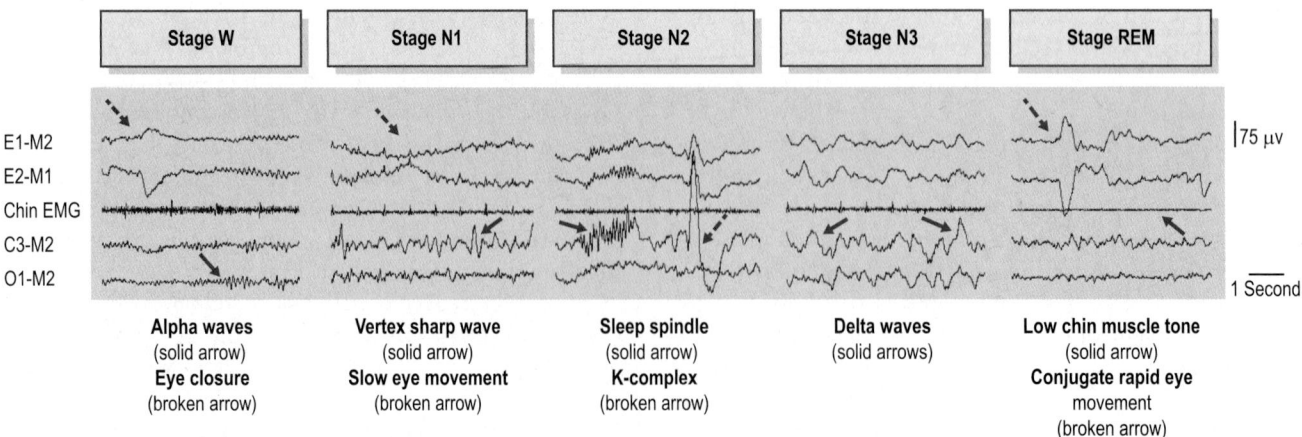

• **Fig. 50.5** This composite illustrates key features of various sleep stages using standard polysomnography (PSG) electrodes. See text for details. REM, rapid eye movement. (From Krishna J, Foldvary-Schaefer N, Budur K. Introduction to the sleep laboratory. In Foldvary-Schaefer N, Krishna J, Budur K, eds. *A Case A Week – Sleep disorders from the Cleveland Clinic*; pp. 19; Fig. 12.4. By permission of Oxford University Press; 2010.)

essentially elastic belts that go around the patient's chest and abdomen. They have a wire woven into the fabric that reliably measures the cross-sectional expansion and contraction of the thorax and abdomen due to the change in self-inductance that the instrument creates. While RIP belts may be calibrated against a known measure of pulmonary volume such as a pneumotachometer, uncalibrated RIP belts are most commonly used in pediatric settings. The direction of these signals can be used to distinguish thoracoabdominal paradoxing, which may be a sign of increased respiratory effort, particularly beyond the age of 3 years after which physiologically normal paradoxical breathing that is common in normal infants (due to a pliant rib cage) becomes increasingly uncommon with maturity.[25] Another technology for measuring respiratory effort is the esophageal pressure (Pes) catheter. This is considered the most reliable of all in recognizing respiratory effort by detecting intrathoracic respiratory pressure swings. Pes values become negative with inspiration and increasing negativity is expectedly seen with increased upper airway resistance.[26] However, the invasive nature of Pes limits its popularity. Intercostal EMG applied to the lower intercostal region may also be used by some laboratories to capture diaphragmatic and intercostal muscle firing.[8,27] Airflow is measured by the nasal pressure cannula and the thermistor. The advent of the nasal pressure transducer has provided a reasonable alternative to Pes as well. The nasal pressure cannula is essentially hollow plastic tubing that captures airflow at the nose and mouth. It looks very much like the ubiquitous oxygen cannula used in hospitals. It is connected to a pressure transducer at the other end to generate a signal that is unique in two respects. First, the amplitude of the signal correlates with the size of the breath. Second, the flattened shape of the waveform correlates with airflow resistance.[24] It is the recommended sensor for hypopnea detection, whereas the thermistor is the recommended sensor for apnea detection.

Most cannulas are able to sample $ETCO_2$ as well from one of the nasal ports. $TcpCO_2$ is an alternative. The author's laboratory utilizes both in most studies. Both instruments need to be calibrated against a standard. Capnometry is useful in assessing congenital and acquired causes of hypoventilation from a multitude of causes such as neuromuscular and chest wall disorders, spinal dysraphism, and obesity, among others. Thus this assessment is crucial in guiding therapeutic options. It is notable that pediatric OSA may at times present predominantly with alveolar hypoventilation, which has been termed obstructive hypoventilation.[28,29] In general, alveolar hypoventilation is deemed to be present if more than 25% of the total sleep time is spent with $ETCO_2$ >50 mm Hg.[8,10]

The pulse oximeter is a vital part of the PSG. The finger, toe, and the earlobe in the older child, or the lateral aspect of the young baby's foot, are useful sites for application of the sensor. It is essential that the averaging time of the instrument is relatively short (e.g., 3 seconds) to improve responsiveness to changes in oxygenation with each breath.[30] Accuracy of readings may be compromised by a loosely applied sensor, interference from ambient light, motion of the finger or toes, nail polish, artificial nails, hemoglobinopathies (e.g., sickle cell anemia), and peripheral vasoconstriction.[24]

Thus using the previously mentioned respiratory sensors, hypopneas, apneas, desaturations, and hypoventilation may be scored (Fig. 50.6). Criteria for scoring are set forth and recently updated.[8,10] Although a detailed discussion is not within the scope of this chapter, it should be noted that there is a critical difference in the duration criteria for these events between adults and children. By definition, apneas manifest as a total or near complete (≥90%) fall of discernable airflow from pre-event baseline breathing, whereas hypopneas require that the flow be reduced by ≥30% from baseline and temporally associated with an event such as an EEG arousal or a ≥3% desaturation that should follow such a reduction. In accordance with the faster respiratory rates in childhood, apneas and hypopneas need to be only the equivalent of "two breaths" in duration before being counted (unlike the 10-second duration for adults). This duration criteria increases to 20 seconds in the case of central apneas unless accompanied by EEG arousals and/ or ≥3% desaturations (and/or bradycardia in infants), in which case the two breaths rule holds.

Ancillary Channels

Snoring, limb EMG, ECG, video, body position, VNS channel, and pH probe are additional channels utilized in the PSG. Of these, the last two are only used in special circumstances.

Snoring is the hallmark of OSA and its presence implies at least some increased upper airway resistance. It is usually recorded via a microphone attached to the patient's neck and displayed as a separate channel in the PSG (see Figs. 50.2 and 50.6). Piezoelectric sensors to detect snore vibration in the neck have been used as well.[10] As such, snoring often serves to differentiate central from obstructive events, especially when the effort belts may be compromised or equivocal. It is also a criterion used to score respiratory effort–related arousals (RERAs), where the reduction in airflow is accompanied by an EEG arousal but falls short of meeting the previously mentioned amplitude reduction criteria for scoring an apnea or hypopnea.[10]

Leg EMG is useful to score a host of abnormalities of leg movements of sleep including periodic leg movements, hypnagogic foot tremor, and alternating leg muscle activation.[8] Periodic limb movements (PLMs), for instance, are scored in accordance with very specific rules. Each component limb movement begins with an initial EMG amplitude rise of at least 8 μV above the resting baseline. The limb movement is deemed to start at the point where such an increase occurs and ends at a point where the EMG is less than 2 μV above resting baseline. The duration between the start and end points must be at least 0.5 seconds but no more than 10 seconds to be counted as a limb movement. To be counted as a PLM series, there need to be four such

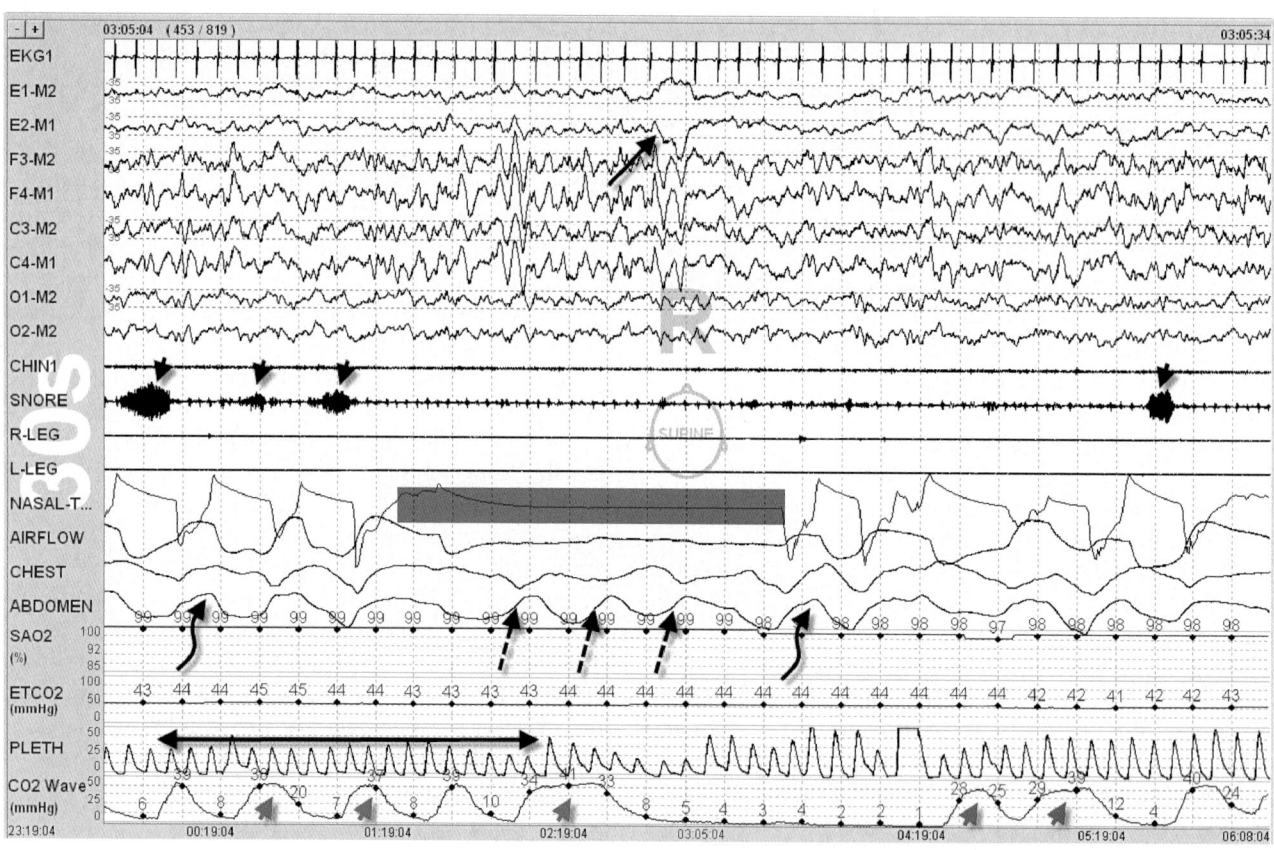

• **Fig. 50.6** This is a 30-second epoch of a child in rapid eye movement (REM) sleep showing an obstructive apnea *(red bar)* with absent flow in both the nasal transducer *(Nasal-T)* and thermistor *(Airflow)* channels. Snoring disappears with the onset of the apnea and reappears a few breaths after offset of apnea *(black arrowheads)*. A REM *(black arrow)* is seen in the eye channels. The chest and abdominal respiratory inductance plethysmography (RIP) belts show paradoxical out-of-phase respirations *(broken black arrows)* during the apnea, indicating distress. Before and after the apnea the belts are in phase *(curved arrows)*. Of note, unlike hypopneas, apnea scoring does not require the presence of arousals or desaturations. The oximeter shows a good plethysmographic signal *(double-headed arrow)*, and there is a good plateau in the ETCO$_2$ wave channel *(red arrowheads)*. Both of these features provide reassurance of reliable readings.

movements in succession with 5–90 seconds between each individual limb movement. Such PLM scoring may be supportive of the diagnosis of PLMD or corroborate a clinical suspicion of pediatric RLS.[31] Typically, the anterior tibialis muscle is used to obtain the leg EMG. Rarely, in children, if there is clinical suspicion of absence of the normal REM sleep-related atonia, such as in disorders of dream enactment (RBD), additional limb leads may be useful in the upper limb as well.[32,33]

The ECG is a standard single-channel recording (lead II). It is useful to correlate cardiac dysrhythmia with respiratory events. Sleep-related normative data are available.[34,35] Because ECG artifact can sometimes contaminate the EEG trace, an ECG channel is useful to distinguish this EEG artifact with certainty from true EEG abnormalities such as sharp or spike activity.

Body position is best scored using real-time video, although body position sensors are available as well. Most laboratories have low-light or infrared cameras, which are additionally useful in observing motor phenomena such as parasomnia, bruxing, rhythmic movements of sleep, restless

legs, or seizures. OSA is often positional (e.g., worse when supine) and this may be useful information to plan intervention in certain cases.[36] Indeed, occasional insights into sleep-related behaviors such as sleep-onset association disorder, or the use of television or cellular phone during the sleep period may be apparent. In the case of neonates where eye closure is important in differentiating sleep from quiet wakefulness, a high-definition camera with zoom-in capability is very useful to score sleep stages.[23]

Children with VNS implants are not uncommonly encountered in the pediatric sleep setting in tertiary care centers. It is known that intermittent VNS discharge can cause changes in respirations and heart rate and may result in OSA (Fig. 50.7). These changes are distinguished by their cadence, which is in tune with the setting (firing interval and duration) of the VNS device. Thus the current VNS setting is useful information to have when interpreting the study in such patients.[37]

Esophageal pH probes are used in some centers to test for gastroesophageal reflux (GER) associated with SRBD.[27] In general, however, the pH probe is not commonly utilized

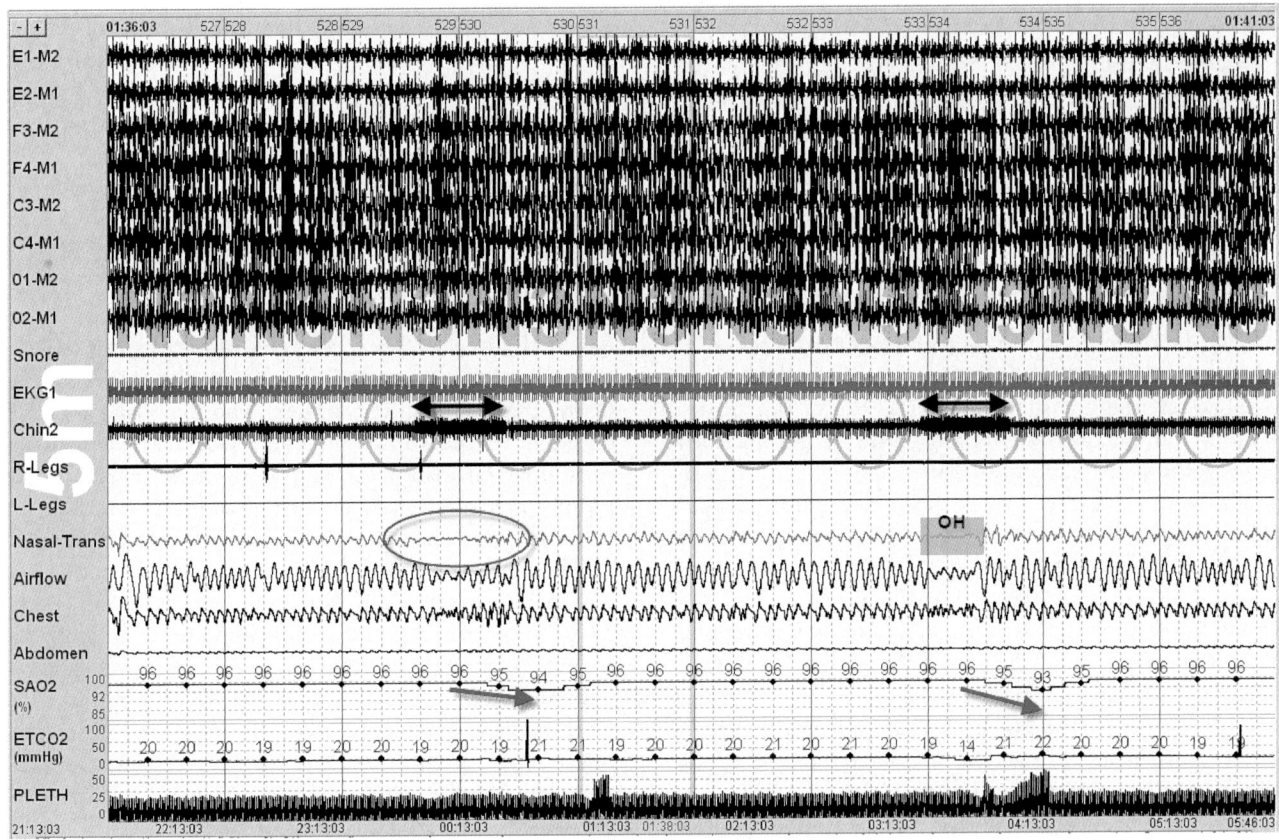

• **Fig. 50.7** This child had difficult-to-control epilepsy and had a vagal nerve stimulator (VNS) in place. A polysomnography (PSG) was done to screen for a breathing disorder associated with her condition. This 5-minute epoch shows VNS discharges occurring every 2 minutes for about 20 seconds each. These are captured on the chin electrode *(double-headed arrows)*. Concomitant reduction in oronasal airflow is seen *(red oval)*. The chest belt shows continued respiratory efforts. The abdominal belt is not working. The second event *(green bar)* meets scoring criteria for obstructive hypopnea *(OH)* due to an associated 3% fall in oxygen saturation (compare *red arrows*). The end-tidal CO_2 reading is unreliable but the plethysmographic signal from the pulse oximeter is robust. The electroencephalogram (EEG) showed florid spikes that are not apparent in this view.

due to its invasive nature. It is to be further noted that a temporal relationship has not been proven between SRBD and GER episodes.[38] Thus the AASM does not consider it an essential part of the standard PSG setup.

Positive Airway Pressure Titration Study

Because T&A does not cure OSA in a significant number of cases, an alternative therapeutic recourse often used is PAP therapy.[3,39] Continuous or bi-level PAP (continuous PAP [CPAP]; BPAP) is the most common mode of delivering this therapy. Before titration can be attempted, however, the child and the family ought to have been educated and prepared to accept the treatment. This implies that, unlike adult studies, PAP titration in children is generally not initiated during a "split-night" protocol (which refers to initial part-night PSG and subsequent part-night PAP titration). Instead, low pressure, say 5 cm H_2O PAP, is initially empirically chosen after careful mask fitting to habituate the child to the device for several nights at home. Finally, the PAP study is run in a

laboratory setting where the goal is to titrate the pressure in various sleep stages and body positions to optimally control the respiratory events.[40] A final prescription pressure is thus obtained.

The montage for PAP titration is very similar to the standard PSG, with the flow measurements obtained from the mask interface rather than nasal cannula or thermistor, and $TcpCO_2$ measured in lieu of $ETCO_2$.[10] Other variations to the standard PSG studies described earlier include testing for readiness of tracheostomy decannulation and checking for adequacy of ventilator management.[13,41,42] (see Table 50.1).

The Multiple Sleep Latency Test

EDS is a common presenting complaint in the pediatric sleep center. Generally speaking, abnormal daytime sleepiness implies the inability to stay alert during the expected waking period and may be accompanied by unanticipated or unintentional periods of sleep.[16] Various disorders may lead to this complaint. Although screening instruments may serve to raise the index of suspicion,[43,44] a comprehensive history and detailed physical examination are the cornerstone of such diagnoses. The MSLT is frequently employed to confirm clinical suspicion by objectively quantifying and characterizing daytime sleepiness.[9,45]

The MSLT is mainly indicated for the diagnosis of narcolepsy and idiopathic hypersomnia. It essentially comprises a series of daytime nap tests and is used in conjunction with a PSG performed on the prior night. Strict guidelines of conduct including restrictions on stimulants such as caffeine, smoking, and exercise need to be followed to maintain the validity of the test. Specific rules are also described for the environment of the study, light exposure, and timing of meals. Furthermore, it is prescribed that certain REM-suppressing medications and stimulants be stopped at least 2 weeks prior to the test to avoid REM rebound or REM suppression. Careful planning is required to avoid sleep deprivation in the several days leading up to the test. This may be documented by sleep logs or actigraphy. Ideally sleep laboratories will require urine drug screening on the day of the test to corroborate adherence to a medication weaning plan and to ensure substance abuse is not a potential confounder. The AASM has put forth detailed practice parameters describing the indications for this test and its format.[9]

The MSLT typically comprises five nap opportunities given 2 hours apart during the day. The first nap begins 2 hours after the patient rises in the morning following the overnight PSG. Following this awakening, most of the sensors that were used during the PSG are discontinued barring those essential for scoring sleep stages. Thus the EEG, EOG, chin EMG, and ECG sensors are kept on for the rest of the day until all five naps are done. Each nap opportunity usually lasts for 20 minutes. However, multiple pediatric laboratories have debated the use of 30-minute nap opportunities due to the longer normative sleep latency in young prepubertal children.[46,47] At the start of each nap the patient is asked to lie quietly in a comfortable position with eyes closed and instructed to try and fall sleep. The underlying premise is that the sleepier the person, the more likely they are to fall asleep given the chance and conditions to do so. If sleep onset occurs within the assigned 20 minutes, the nap opportunity is extended for an additional 15 minutes to allow other stages of sleep to emerge. Of special interest is the emergence of REM sleep during daytime nap testing. Narcoleptics classically show two or more REM episodes during the five-nap test. Such REM episodes occurring soon (within 15 minutes) after sleep onset are termed sleep-onset REM periods (SOREMPs). If no sleep occurs within the assigned 20 minutes, the test is terminated. The mean sleep latency is calculated as an arithmetic average of the sleep-onset latencies of five naps. SOREMPs are reported as well.

It should be readily evident to the reader that this test has a high likelihood of being confounded by sleep debt,

use of medications and drugs, or any disruption of the protocol including extraneous noise in the sleep-testing environment. Sleep logs and actigraph recordings are generally very useful to ensure pretest sleep–wake routines have been adhered to and documented. Patient motivation may also impact the mean sleep latency.[48] At the risk of being repetitious, it cannot be overemphasized that strict protocol needs to be followed. Given appropriate testing conditions, the MSLT is known to have high test–retest reliability among normal healthy subjects.[9] Uncertainties arise in using this test in children <6 years of age or outside of the standard 8 a.m. to 6 p.m. hours.[16] Challenges may arise in the case of children (especially teenagers) who may have abnormal circadian rhythms in conjunction with a suspicion for an additional intrinsic hypersomnia disorder. Further, compromises are often needed when discontinuation of certain medications is contraindicated or medically problematic.

There are varying opinions about the normative values of the mean sleep latency. There is evidence that mean sleep latency is longer in prepubertal children and reduces by several minutes with advancing Tanner stages.[49] Sometimes, serial MSLT studies may be required in childhood because narcolepsy may still be an evolving pathology not as yet fully established.[50] Nevertheless, a mean sleep latency of 8 minutes or less and the presence of two SOREMPs support a diagnosis of narcolepsy. A SOREMP on the prior night PSG may be used to satisfy the criteria of two SOREMPs.[16]

A cautionary note in the interpretation of the adequately run MSLT remains the fact that the mean sleep latency by itself does not distinguish well between clinical and control populations but rather lends support to clinical suspicion. Extensive data for children are lacking and recent research suggests criteria different from standard adult data may be more applicable to children with suspected narcolepsy.[51]

Scoring and Interpreting the Data

Once the sleep study has been completed, typically a trained technologist will be assigned to analyze the raw data in 30-second intervals (epochs) using standard AASM criteria for scoring of sleep and associated events.[8–10] It is then the sleep specialist's task to examine the study in its entirety to accurately and judiciously interpret the data presented. To do this skillfully, the physician has to be knowledgeable in several areas. To begin with, it is very important to understand the clinical context within which the study was ordered. This will allow the final report to be tailored to the question at hand. Next, attention needs to be turned to any changes in the child's clinical status, including changes in medications or sleep habits since the time of ordering the study until its execution. For example, an inadvertently taken nap or caffeinated beverage just prior to the sleep study may skew the findings of the test. Similarly, the start and stop of certain medications may alter sleep architecture by suppressing REM or other sleep stages or conversely causing a rebound of certain sleep stages.[52] It is also useful to know if the parents thought the recorded sleep period represented a typical night for the child or not. To help with this, most sleep centers use pre-study and post-study questionnaires that not only record pertinent clinical status immediately prior to the study, but also allow the patient and/or the parent to provide feedback on the conditions of the study itself.

Much information is also gathered from the attending technologist's log and this needs to be reviewed by the interpreting sleep expert as well. Problematic environmental and technical conditions that may have interfered with the study are noted. As an example, such notes may be useful in distinguishing whether the noise on the microphone is patient-related snoring, wheezing, stertor, or parental snoring artifact. Similarly, semiology of nocturnal events such as parasomnia or seizures may be crucial, as can notes such as "has a cold, thick nasal discharge" or "was on cell phone for 1 hour after lights out."

Having acquired this background information, the sleep expert needs to bring to bear knowledge of developmental neurology and respiratory physiology while reviewing the data. A fair depth of knowledge is required to be able to interpret the rapidly evolving EEG in the growing infant, for example. The pediatric expert will need to keep in mind that periodic breathing may be normal in infants and that babies may regularly exhibit paradoxical respiration, the frequency of which reduces over the first few years of life, as mentioned previously. A frequent problem in the interpretation of pediatric sleep studies is the presence of artifact from parental intervention such as feeding, holding, patting, or rocking, or from technologist intervention to replace sensors. The use of pacifiers is a common cause for dislodgment of nasal or oral airflow sensors. Occasionally, the parent may need to co-sleep with the anxious child and this itself may induce either movement or snore artifact into the child's recording. It is therefore important to have a plethysmographic signal to lend support to the reliability of pulse oximetry. Similarly, visualization of a plateau in the $ETCO_2$ waveform is reassuring that *end-tidal* CO_2 is indeed being measured (see Fig. 50.6). Accordingly, capnometry, and pulse oximetry trends need to be reviewed carefully lest such artifact be erroneously used to score events in the night. Review of the video in real time is additionally very helpful in these circumstances. The video is also vital to

confirm rhythmic movement disorder and characterize parasomnias or seizures. Often, reviewing portions of the record at 10-, 60-, or 120-second epoch lengths is useful to clarify certain observations.

While attention to minute details during epoch-by-epoch review of the study is critical, a careful perusal of the hypnogram is essential prior to formulating a report. This bird's-eye view of the full study period is very useful for analyzing sleep architecture and discerning patterns that may not be evident during event scoring (Fig. 50.8). Based upon a detailed review of the sleep study, a report is generated that not only contains a descriptive summary of the numeric data from the PSG/MSLT, but also attempts to correlate this data to the clinical question at hand.

In the end, it is the interpretive portion of the report that is most crucial for further therapeutic interventions. Therefore, despite the fact that normative PSG data have been published,[53–58] and diagnostic criteria for various sleep disorders have been refined over time,[16] the final analysis and interpretation of complex data from the sleep study remains as much art as it is science.

CLINICAL PEARLS

- A thorough clinical evaluation and formulation of a testing hypothesis is essential before ordering a sleep study so that a well-defined clinical query may be addressed.
- The utility of adequate pretest education cannot be overstated. This serves to reduce patient and parent anxiety and enlist their cooperation.
- Essential preplanning for the sleep study also includes attention to behavioral and developmental needs, age-appropriate sleep requirements, unique sleep habits (including circadian timing), comorbid conditions (including acute illnesses), and medication effects (both at time of initiation and withdrawal).
- The pediatric-friendly sleep lab lives up to its name less because of its ambient decor and available toys, but more importantly by the patience, kindness, knowledge, and skills exhibited by its technologic personnel and medical providers.
- The sleep test data must be interpreted by a clinician with sound knowledge of developmental aspects of child physiology, including EEG and respiratory physiology. Such a clinician must also be up-to-date on the evolving criteria of pediatric sleep diagnosis and be mindful of gaps in the existing normative data as distinct from adult norms.

Summary

The study of children in the sleep laboratory poses unique challenges that many adult laboratories may not be equipped to handle. The requirements and the rules of scoring and interpreting pediatric sleep studies are significantly different from those in adults. Indeed, many physiologic parameters change even within the pediatric age group as the infant matures into a teenager. The pediatric sleep laboratory should therefore be able to cater to children from birth through adulthood with equal ease. This requires expertise at all levels, beginning with technologists and ending with the sleep specialist.

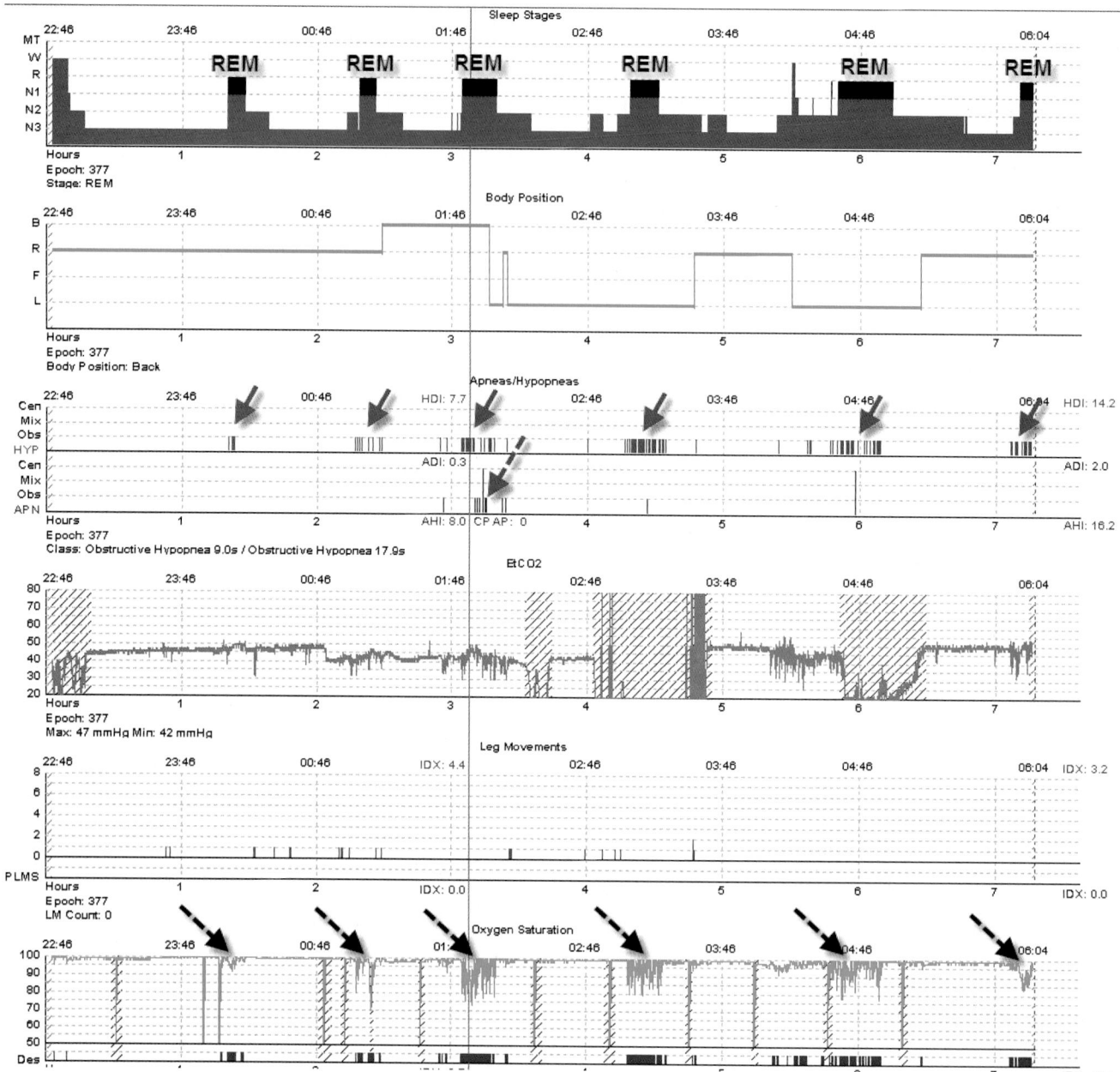

• **Fig. 50.8** This is an overnight hypnogram showing sleep architecture with six rapid eye movement (REM) cycles *(top channel)* separated by non-REM periods. From top to bottom, the remaining channels are body position *(B, back or supine; R, right; L, left; F, front or prone)*, apneas and hypopneas, ETCO$_2$, leg movements, and oxygen saturation. Notice the clustering of hypopneas *(solid red arrows)* and apneas *(broken red arrow)* in temporal conjunction with desaturations *(broken black arrows)* and REM. For the sake of accuracy in generating cumulative data for the final report, "bad data" in the ETCO$_2$ and oxygen channels has been manually "artifacted out" *(crosshatches).*

References

1. Carroll JL, McColley SA, Marcus CL, et al. Inability of clinical history to distinguish primary snoring from obstructive sleep apnea syndrome in children. *Chest.* 1995;108(3):610–618.
2. Wang RC, Elkins TP, Keech D, et al. Accuracy of clinical evaluation in pediatric obstructive sleep apnea. *Otolaryngol Head Neck Surg.* 1998;118(1):69–73.
3. Marcus CL, Brooks LJ, Draper KA, et al. Diagnosis and management of childhood obstructive sleep apnea syndrome. American Academy of Pediatrics. *Pediatrics.* 2012;130(3):576–584.
4. American Academy of Pediatrics Section on Pediatric Pulmonology, Subcommittee on obstructive sleep apnea syndrome. Clinical practice guidelines: Diagnosis and management of childhood obstructive sleep apnea syndrome. *Pediatrics.* 2002;109:704–712.
5. Spruyt K, Gozal D. Pediatric sleep questionnaires as diagnostic or epidemiological tools: A review of currently available instruments. *Sleep Med Rev.* 2011;15(1):19–32.
6. Mignot E, Young T, Lin L, et al. Nocturnal sleep and daytime sleepiness in normal subjects with HLA-DQB1*0602. *Sleep.* 1999;22(3):347–352.

7. Nishino S, Ripley B, Overeem S, et al. Hypocretin (orexin) deficiency in human narcolepsy. *Lancet*. 2000;355(9197):39–40.

8. Troester MM, Quan SF, Berry RB, et al., for the American Academy of Sleep Medicine. The AASM manual for the scoring of sleep and associated events: Rules, terminology and technical specifications. Version 3. American Academy of Sleep Medicine; 2023.

9. Maski KP, Amos LB, Carter JC, et al. Recommended protocols for the Multiple Sleep Latency Test and Maintenance of Wakefulness Test in children: guidance from the American Academy of Sleep Medicine. *J Clin Sleep Med*. 2024;20(4):631–641.

10. Berry RB, Budhiraja R, Gottlieb DJ, et al. Rules for scoring respiratory events in sleep: Update of the 2007 AASM Manual for the Scoring of Sleep and Associated Events. Deliberations of the Sleep Apnea Definitions Task Force of the American Academy of Sleep Medicine. *J Clin Sleep Med*. 2012;8(5):597–619.

11. Owens J, Kothare S, Sheldon S. PRO: "Not just little adults": AASM should require pediatric accreditation for integrated sleep medicine programs serving both children (0–16 years) and adults. *J Clin Sleep Med*. 2012;8(5):473–476.

12. Gozal D. CON: Specific pediatric accreditation is not critical for integrated pediatric and adult sleep medicine programs. *J Clin Sleep Med*. 2012;8(5):477–479.

13. Aurora RN, Zak RS, Karippot A, et al. American Academy of Sleep Medicine. Practice parameters for the respiratory indications for polysomnography in children. *Sleep*. 2011;34(3):379–388.

14. Tieder JS, Bonkowsky JL, Etzel RA, et al. Brief resolved unexplained events (formerly apparent life-threatening events) and evaluation of lower-risk infants. *Pediatrics*. 2016;137(5): e20160590.

15. Aurora RN, Lamm CI, Zak RS, et al. Practice parameters for the non-respiratory indications for polysomnography and multiple sleep latency testing for children. *Sleep*. 2012;35(11):1467–1473.

16. American Academy of Sleep Medicine. *International Classification of Sleep Disorders*. 3rd ed. Text Revision. American Academy of Sleep Medicine; 2023.

17. Wolfson AR, Carskadon MA. Sleep schedules and daytime functioning in adolescents. *Child Dev*. 1998;69:875–887.

18. Zaremba EK, Barkey ME, Mesa C, et al. Making polysomnography more child friendly: A family-centered care approach. *J Clin Sleep Med*. 2005;1:189–198.

19. Kothare SV, Vendrame M, Sant JL, et al. Fall-prevention policies in pediatric sleep laboratories. *J Clin Sleep Med*. 2011;7(1):9–10.

20. Biban P, Baraldi E, Pettennazzo A, et al. Adverse effect of chloral hydrate in two young children with obstructive sleep apnea. *Pediatrics*. 1993;92:461–463.

21. Jasper HH. The ten-twenty electrode system of the International Federation. *Electroencephalogr Clin Neurophysiol*. 1958;10:371–375.

22. Grigg-Damberger M, Gozal D, Marcus CL, et al. The visual scoring of sleep and arousals in infants and children: Development of polygraphic features, reliability, validity, and alternative methods. *J Clin Sleep Med*. 2007;3:201–240.

23. Anders T, Emde R, Parmelee A, eds. *A Manual of Standardized Terminology, Techniques and Criteria for Scoring of States of Sleep and Wakefulness in Newborn Infants*. UCLA Brain Information Service: NINDS Neurological Information Network; 1971.

24. Redline S, Budhiraja R, Kapur V, et al. Reliability and validity of respiratory event measurement and scoring. *J Clin Sleep Med*. 2007;3:169–200.

25. Glautier C, Praud JP, Canet E, et al. Paradoxical inward ribcage motion during rapid eye movement sleep in infants and young children. *J Dev Physiol*. 1987;9:391–397.

26. Guilleminault Stoohs R, Clerk A, et al. A cause of excessive daytime sleepiness. *The upper airway resistance syndrome*. *Chest*. 1993;104:781–787.

27. Spriggs WH. Instrumentation. In: Spriggs WH, ed. *Principles of Polysomnography*. 1st ed. Sleep Ed. LLC; 2002:50–121.

28. American Thoracic Society Standards and indications for cardiopulmonary sleep studies in children. *Am J Resp Crit Care Med*. 1996;153:866–878.

29. Brouillette RT, Fernbach SK, Hunt CE. Obstructive sleep apnea in infants and children. *J Pediatr*. 1982;100:31–40.

30. Farre R, Montserrat JM, Ballester E, et al. Importance of the pulse oximeter averaging time when measuring oxygen desaturation in sleep apnea. *Sleep*. 1998;21:386–390.

31. Simakajornboon N, Kheirandish-Gozal L, Gozal D. Diagnosis and management of restless legs syndrome in children. *Sleep Med Rev*. 2009;13(2):149–156.

32. Stores G. Rapid eye movement sleep behaviour disorder in children and adolescents. *Dev Med Child Neur*. 2008;50: 728–732.

33. Boeve BF. REM sleep behavior disorder: Updated review of the core features, the RBD-neurodegenerative disease association, evolving concepts, controversies, and future directions. *Ann NY Acad Sci*. 2010;1184:15–54.

34. Caples SM, Rosen CL, Shen WK, et al. The scoring of cardiac events during sleep. *J Clin Sleep Med*. 2007;3:147–154.

35. Archbold KH, Johnson NL, Goodwin JL, et al. Normative heart rate parameters during sleep for children aged 6 to 11 years. *J Clin Sleep Med*. 2010;6:47–50.

36. Pereira KD, Roebuck JC, Howell L. The effect of body position on sleep apnea in children younger than 3 years. *Arch Otolaryngol Head Neck Surg*. 2005;131(11):1014–1016.

37. Hsieh T, Chen M, McAfee A, et al. Sleep-related breathing disorder in children with vagal nerve stimulators. *Pediatr Neurol*. 2008;38:99–103.

38. Noronha AC, de Bruin VM, Nobre e Souza MA, et al. Gastroesophageal reflux and obstructive sleep apnea in childhood. *Int J Pediatr Otorhinolaryngol*. 2009;73(3):383–389.

39. Bhattacharjee R, Kheirandish-Gozal L, Spruyt K, et al. Adenotonsillectomy outcomes in treatment of obstructive sleep apnea in children – A multicenter retrospective study. *Am J Respir Crit Care Med*. 2010;182(5):676–683.

40. Kushida CA, Chediak A, Berry RB, et al. Positive airway pressure titration task force of the American Academy of Sleep Medicine. Clinical guidelines for the manual titration of positive airway pressure in patients with obstructive sleep apnea. *J Clin Sleep Med*. 2008;4:157–171.

41. Tunkel DE, McColley SA, Baroody FM, et al. Polysomnography in the evaluation of readiness for decannulation in children. *Arch Otolaryngol Head Neck Surg*. 1996;122(7):721–724.

42. Mukherjee B, Bais AS, Bajaj Y. Role of polysomnography in tracheostomy decannulation in the paediatric patient. *J Laryngol Otol*. 1999;113(5):442–445.

43. Drake C, Nickel C, Burduvali E, et al. The pediatric daytime sleepiness scale (PDSS): Sleep habits and school outcomes in middle-school children. *Sleep*. 2003;26:455–458.

44. Spilsbury JC, Drotar D, Rosen CL, et al. The Cleveland adolescent sleepiness questionnaire: A new measure to assess excessive daytime sleepiness in adolescents. *J Clin Sleep Med*. 2007;3:603–612.

45. Carskadon MA, Dement WC, Mitler MM, et al. Guidelines for the multiple sleep latency test (MSLT): A standard measure of sleepiness. *Sleep*. 1986;9:519–524.

46. Gozal D, Wang M, Pope DW Jr. Objective sleepiness measures in pediatric obstructive sleep apnea. *Pediatrics.* 2001;108(3):693–697.

47. Gozal D, Kheirandish-Gozal L. Obesity and excessive daytime sleepiness in prepubertal children with obstructive sleep apnea. *Pediatrics.* 2009;123(1):13–18.

48. Bonnet MH, Arand DL. Impact of motivation on multiple sleep latency test and maintenance of wakefulness test measurements. *J Clin Sleep Med.* 2005;1(4):386–390.

49. Carskadon MA, Dement WC. Sleepiness in the normal adolescent. In: Guilleminault C, ed. *Sleep and Its Disorders in Children.* Raven Press; 1987:53–66.

50. Kotagal S, Goulding PM. The laboratory assessment of daytime sleepiness in children. *J Clin Neurophysiol.* 1996;13:208–218.

51. Pizza F, Barateau L, Jaussent I, et al. Validation of multiple sleep latency test for the diagnosis of pediatric narcolepsy type 1. *Neurology.* 2019;93(11):e1034–e1044.

52. Schweitzer PK. Effects of drugs on sleep. In: Barkoukis TJ, Avidan AY, eds. *Review of Sleep Medicine.* 2nd ed. Butterworth-Heinemann; 2007:169–184.

53. Montgomery-Downs HE, O'Brien LM, Gulliver TE, et al. Polysomnographic characteristics in normal preschool and early school-aged children. *Pediatrics.* 2006;117:741–753.

54. Uliel S, Tauman R, Greenfield M, et al. Normal polysomnographic respiratory values in children and adolescents. *Chest.* 2004;125:872–878.

55. Traeger N, Schultz B, Pollock AN, et al. Polysomnographic values in children 2–9 years old: Additional data and review of the literature. *Pediatr Pulmonol.* 2005;40:22–30.

56. Daftary AS, Jalou HE, Shively RN, et al. Polysomnography reference values in healthy newborns. *J Clin Sleep Med.* 2019; 15:437–443.

57. Brockmann PE, Poets A, Poets CF. Reference values for respiratory events in overnight polygraphy from infants aged 1 and 3 months. *Sleep Med.* 2013;14:1323–1327.

58. Scholle S, Wiater A, Scholle HC. Normative values of polysomnographic parameters in childhood and adolescence: Cardiorespiratory parameters. *Sleep Med.* 2011;12(10):988–996.

Normal Development

51

The Premature Infant

Stephen H. Sheldon

Introduction

Although it may be trite to say that children are not just small adults, they are extraordinarily different and require approaches and technologies designed to meet their unique needs. Importance of neuroanatomical, neurophysiologic, and developmental biology on understanding sleep as a neurodevelopmental landmark cannot be overstated. Just as development of an infant's ability to roll from back to front, front to back, sit, stand, walk, and talk, attention to maturation of sleep from the newborn through adolescence provides significant insight into health and well-being.

Just as the practice of pediatrics grew from internal medicine, pediatric sleep medicine grew from adult sleep medicine. In 2007, the American Board of Medical Specialists (ABMS) certified the first Diplomates in Sleep Medicine and the Accreditation Council for Graduate Medical Education (ACGME) provided certification of one year fellowships in Sleep Medicine following completion of an ACGME accredited residency program in a variety of specialties including but not limited to pediatrics, internal medicine, otolaryngology, family medicine, neurology, and psychiatry. There is much to learn in one year. Most accredited fellowships are located in Departments of Neurology, Pulmonary Medicine, and Psychiatry. Few are housed in Departments of Pediatrics. Due to a paucity of Pediatric Sleep Medicine Fellowship positions, few pediatricians and child health care practitioners are becoming certified as competent in caring for children with pediatric sleep disorders, leaving most adult-oriented sleep medicine specialists required to care for children (if they choose). In 2012, an online survey of all sleep centers accredited by the American Academy of Sleep Medicine (AASM) was conducted to determine access to sleep health care for children.[1] It was determined that only 47% of all accredited sleep centers accepted children <5 years of age and only about 20% of the centers accepted children <3 years of age. Of all the accredited sleep centers surveyed, only 1.5% were identified as accredited pediatric sleep centers.

Indeed, pediatric sleep medicine and the understanding of sleep in infants, children, and adolescents have progressed significantly over the past two decades. The impact of disturbed sleep on growth and development is beginning to be understood. There have been significant advances in comprehension of sleep (particularly REM sleep) on learning and memory.[2,3] Nevertheless, what is currently understood is likely only the "tip of the iceberg" with the majority of what is to be known well ahead.

The comprehensive evaluation of sleep in infants, children, and adolescents begins with a complete medical and sleep history and physical examination followed by establishing a focused differential diagnosis. At the time of this writing, however, laboratory-based attended polysomnography is still considered the "gold standard" for assessment of sleep-related physiologic and pathophysiologic processes.[4] This section focuses on normal laboratory polysomnographic findings in various developmental age groups as well as examples of characteristic sleep-related pathologic polysomnographic findings in common and uncommon pediatric diseases/disorders. It is hoped these examples will be helpful to the sleep practitioner in evaluation of polysomnographic variables in infants, children, and adolescents (Figs. 51.1, 51.2, and 51.3).

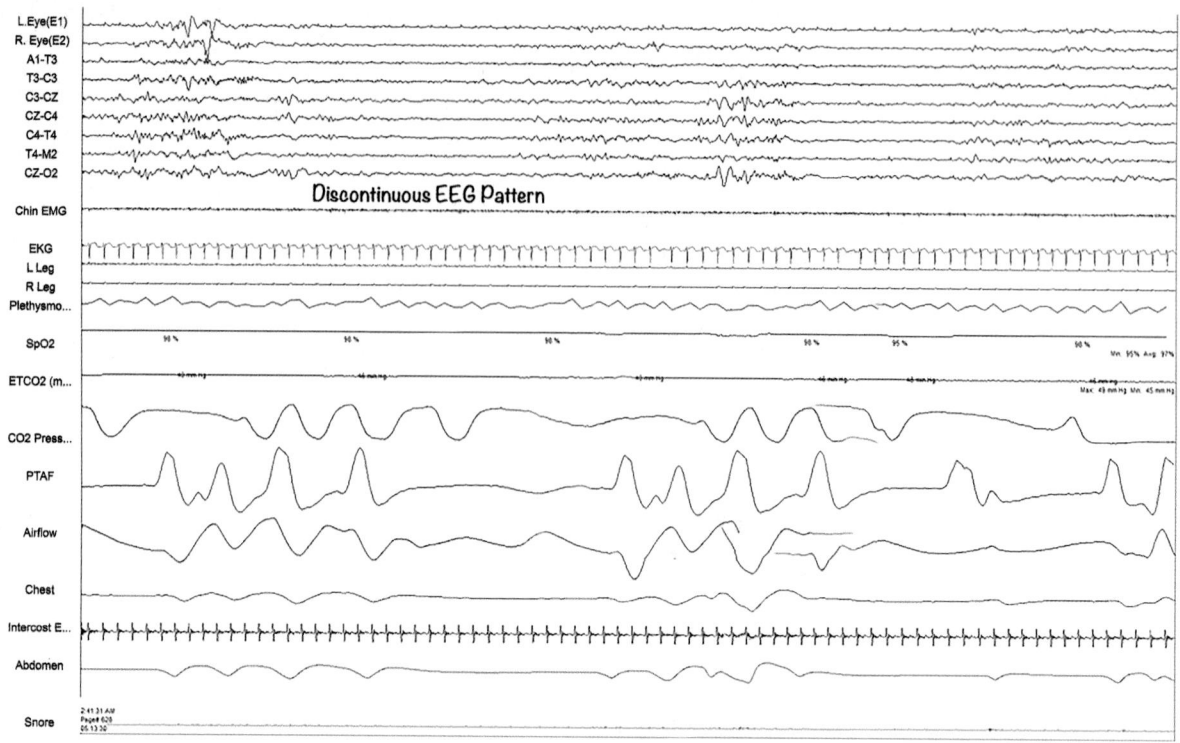

• **Fig. 51.1** Premature infant: quiet/non–rapid eye movement (NREM) sleep. This 30-second epoch was recorded from a 33-week gestation premature infant on the third day of life due to frequent oxygen desaturations and excessive periodic breathing. Prior to 28- to 32-week gestation, clearly defined sleep–wake activity cannot be electrographically identified. After this time, brain activity as monitored by electroencephalogram (EEG) consists of extended periods of relative electrical quiescence separated by bursts of bilaterally synchronous higher voltage activity at a frequency of about 4–6 Hz that may last from 1–5 seconds. This discontinuous pattern of electrical activity is termed *tracé discontinué*. Activity at a frequency of about 10–20 Hz may be superimposed on slower activity (0.5–1.0 Hz) and is termed *delta brush*. This premature pattern begins at about 28–32 weeks post-conception. This discontinuous pattern of 1–2 Hz slow wave bursts continue and is mostly concentrated over the posterior region of the head (posterior dominant rhythm). Between 32 and 36 weeks post-conception, posterior dominant rhythm with periods of relative electrical quiescence become shorter in duration and bursts of higher mixed voltage activity become longer resulting in a pattern termed *tracé alternant*. Both *tracé discontinué* and *tracé alternant* patterns are characteristic of quiet sleep, which occupies a minority of the total 24-hour sleep time in the premature infant. Between 32 weeks post-conception and term, there is continuous maturation and modification of EEG and polysomnography (PSG) patterns.

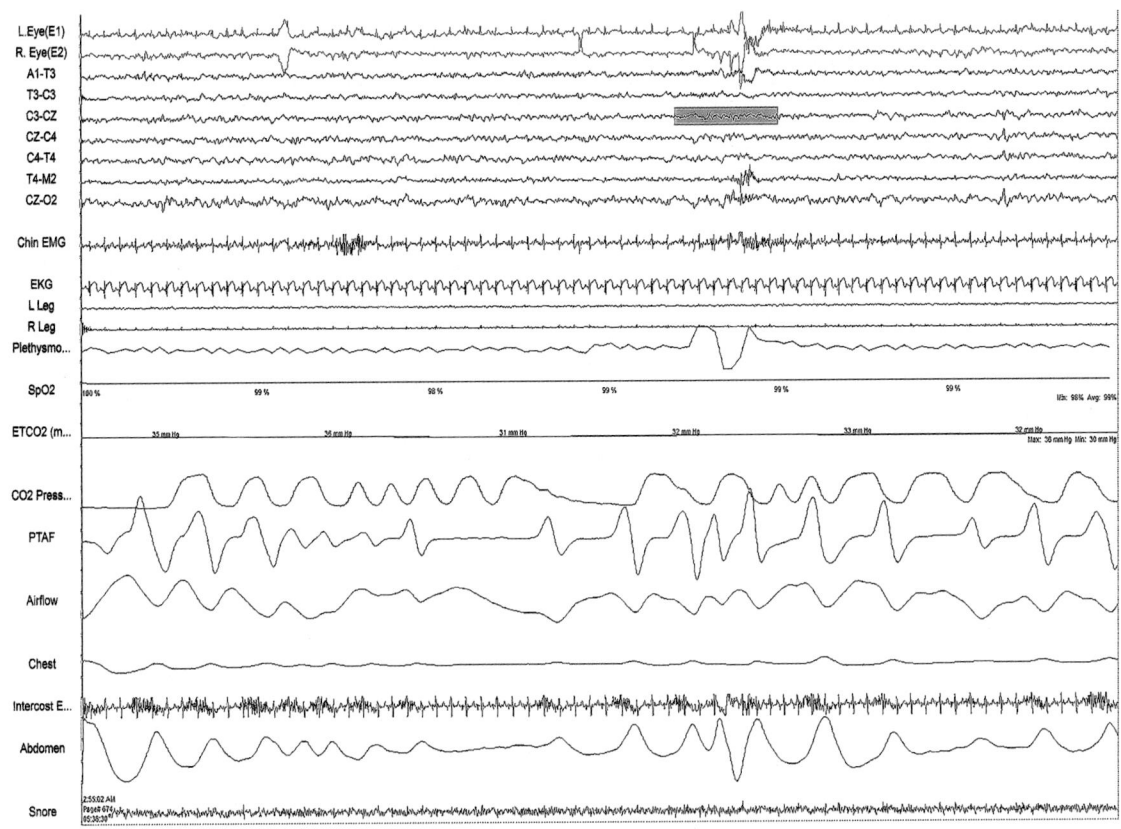

• Fig. 51.2 Premature infant: active/rapid eye movement (REM) sleep. This 30-second epoch was recorded from the previous 33-week gestation premature infant on the third day of life. It demonstrates an irregular pattern of relatively low voltage (<50 µV) mixed frequency waves in the electroencephalogram (EEG), conjugate eye movements, and chin muscle activity is generally decreased when compared with wake and quiet/NREM sleep. Phasic activity in the chin muscle electromyogram (EMG) and an irregular respiratory pattern can be noted. Brief apneas and hypopneas may be present and periodic breathing may be noted. The amount of total sleep time occupied by periodic breathing decreases as respiratory centers mature and conceptional term is reached. Gross body movements, facial and limb twitches, and vocalizations are normal during active/REM sleep. The eyes are consistently closed. This pattern is characteristic of active/REM sleep. Because EEG and motoric patterns may occur during wake and active/REM sleep, polysomnography (PSG) state determination may be difficult. Technologist notation of "eyes open" or "eyes closed" is helpful in state determination. Sustained eye closure is the most reliable determinant in assessing wake versus sleep. At about 32-weeks of gestation, active/REM sleep occupies about 90% of identifiable sleep. This gradually decreases to about 50% by conceptional term.

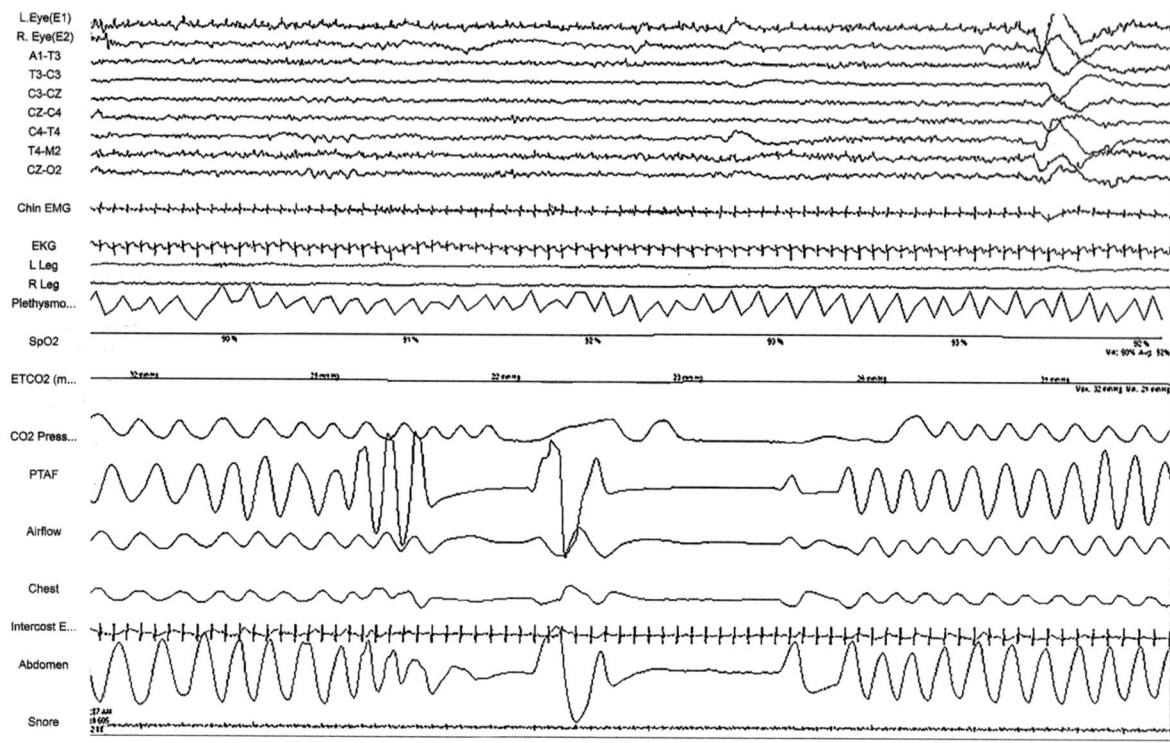

• **Fig. 51.3** Premature infant: Transitional Sleep. This 30-second epoch was recorded from the previous 33-week gestation premature infant on the third day of life. It demonstrates transitional sleep. It immediately followed a 30-second epoch of wake where eyes were open. The infant's eyes close and remained closed with the appearance of electroencephalogram (EEG) and respiratory pattern that might suggest active/rapid eye movement (REM) sleep. However, chin muscle tone remained similar to that during wakefulness, sucking movements were noted, and there are no conjugate eye movements notable in the electrooculogram (EOG).

References

1. Owens J, Kothare S, Sheldon S. PRO: "Not Just Little Adults": AASM Should Require Accreditation for Integrated Sleep medicine Programs Serving Both children (0-16 years) and Adults. *JCSM* 2012;8(5):473–476.

2. Zadra A, Stickgold R When Brains Dream: Understanding the Science and Mystery of Our Dreaming Minds. WW Norton; 2021:336.

3. Wamsley EJ, Stickgold R. Memory, Sleep, and Dreaming: Experiencing Consolidation. *Sleep Med Clin.* 2011;6(1):97–108.

4. Marcus CL, Brooks LJ, Draper KA, et al. Diagnosis and Management of Childhood Obstructive Sleep Apnea Syndrome (Clinical Practice Guideline). *Pediatrics.* 2012;130:1–9.

52
Infants 0–3 Months

Stephen H. Sheldon

Infant at Term

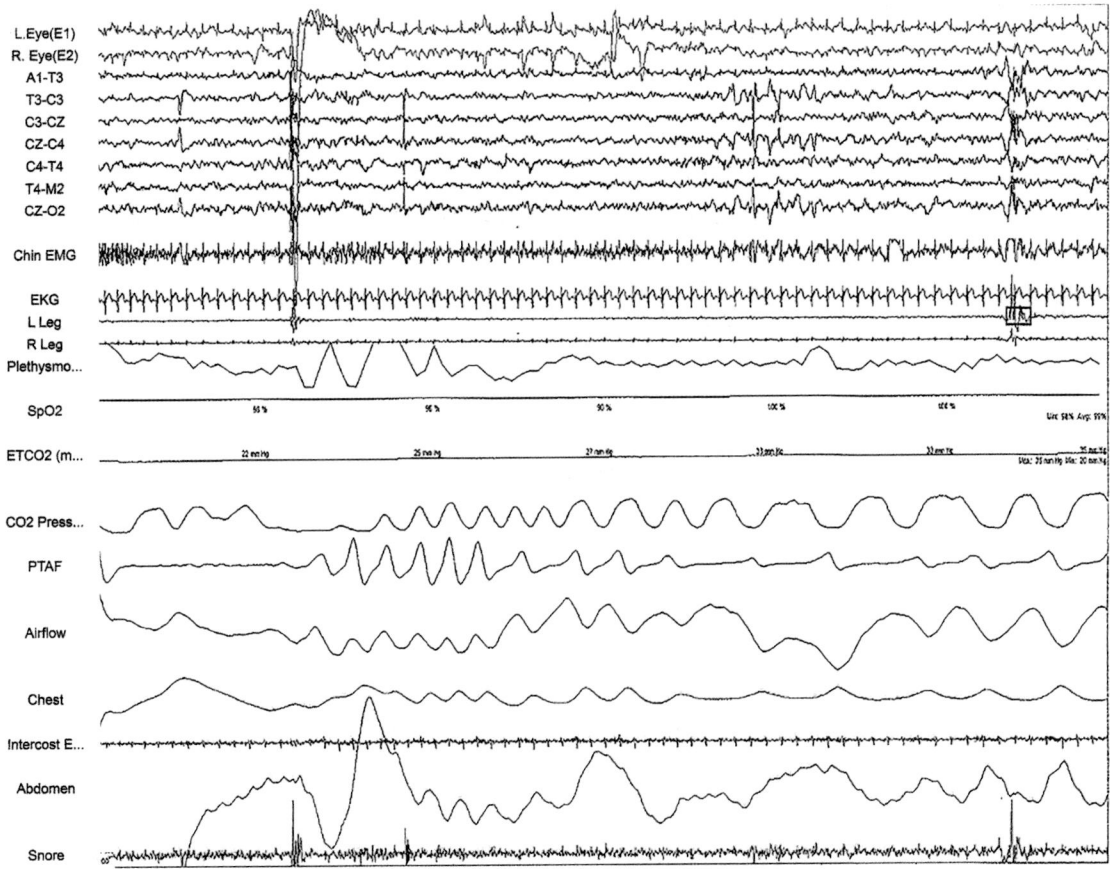

• **Fig. 52.1** Quiet/non–rapid eye movement (NREM) sleep. This 30-second epoch was recorded from a 33-week gestation premature infant on the third day of life due to frequent oxygen desaturations and excessive periodic breathing. Prior to 28- to 32-week gestation, clearly defined sleep–wake activity cannot be seen electrographically identified. After this time, brain activity as monitored by electroencephalogram (EEG) consists of extended periods of relative electrical quiescence separated by bursts of bilaterally synchronous higher voltage activity at a frequency of about 4–6 Hz that may last from 1–5 seconds. This discontinuous pattern of electrical activity is termed *tracé discontinué*. Activity at a frequency of about 10–20 Hz may be superimposed on slower activity (0.5–1.0 Hz) activity and is termed *delta brush*. This premature pattern begins at about 28–32 weeks post-conception. This discontinuous pattern of 1–2 Hz slow-wave bursts continue and is mostly concentrated over the posterior region of the head (posterior dominant rhythm). Between 32 and 36 weeks post-conception, posterior dominant rhythm with periods of relative electrical quiescence become shorter in duration and bursts of higher mixed voltage activity become longer resulting in a pattern termed *tracé alternant*. Both *tracé discontinué* and *tracé alternant* patterns are characteristic of quiet sleep, which occupies a minority of the total 24-hour sleep time in the premature infant. Between 32 weeks post-conception and term, there is continuous maturation and modification of EEG and polysomnography (PSG) patterns.

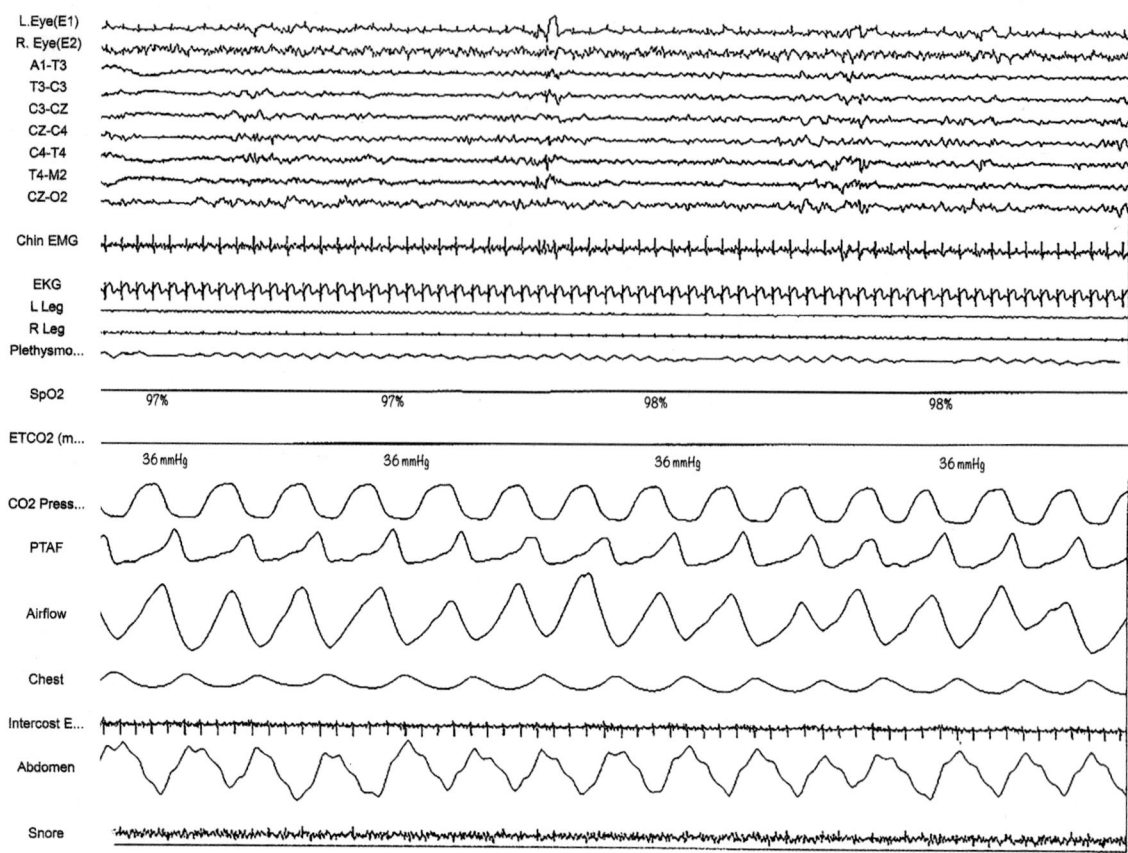

• **Fig. 52.2** Active/rapid eye movement (REM) sleep. This 30-second epoch was recorded from the previous 33-week gestation premature infant on the third day of life. It demonstrates an irregular pattern of relatively low voltage (<50 μV) mixed frequency waves in the electroencephalogram (EEG), conjugate eye movements, and chin muscle activity is generally decreased when compared with wake and quiet/non-REM sleep. Phasic activity in the chin muscle electromyogram (EMG) and an irregular respiratory pattern can be noted. Brief apneas and hypopneas may be present and periodic breathing may be noted. The amount of total sleep time occupied by periodic breathing decreases as respiratory centers mature and conceptional term is reached. Gross body movements, facial and limb twitches, and vocalizations are normal during active/REM sleep. The eyes are consistently closed. This pattern is characteristic of active/REM sleep. Because EEG and motoric patterns may occur during wake and active/REM sleep, polysomnography (PSG) state determination may be difficult. Technologist notation of "eyes open" or "eyes closed" is helpful in state determination. Sustained eye closure is the most reliable determinant in assessing wake versus sleep. At about 32-weeks of gestation, active/REM sleep occupies about 90% of identifiable sleep. This gradually decreases to about 50% by conceptional term.

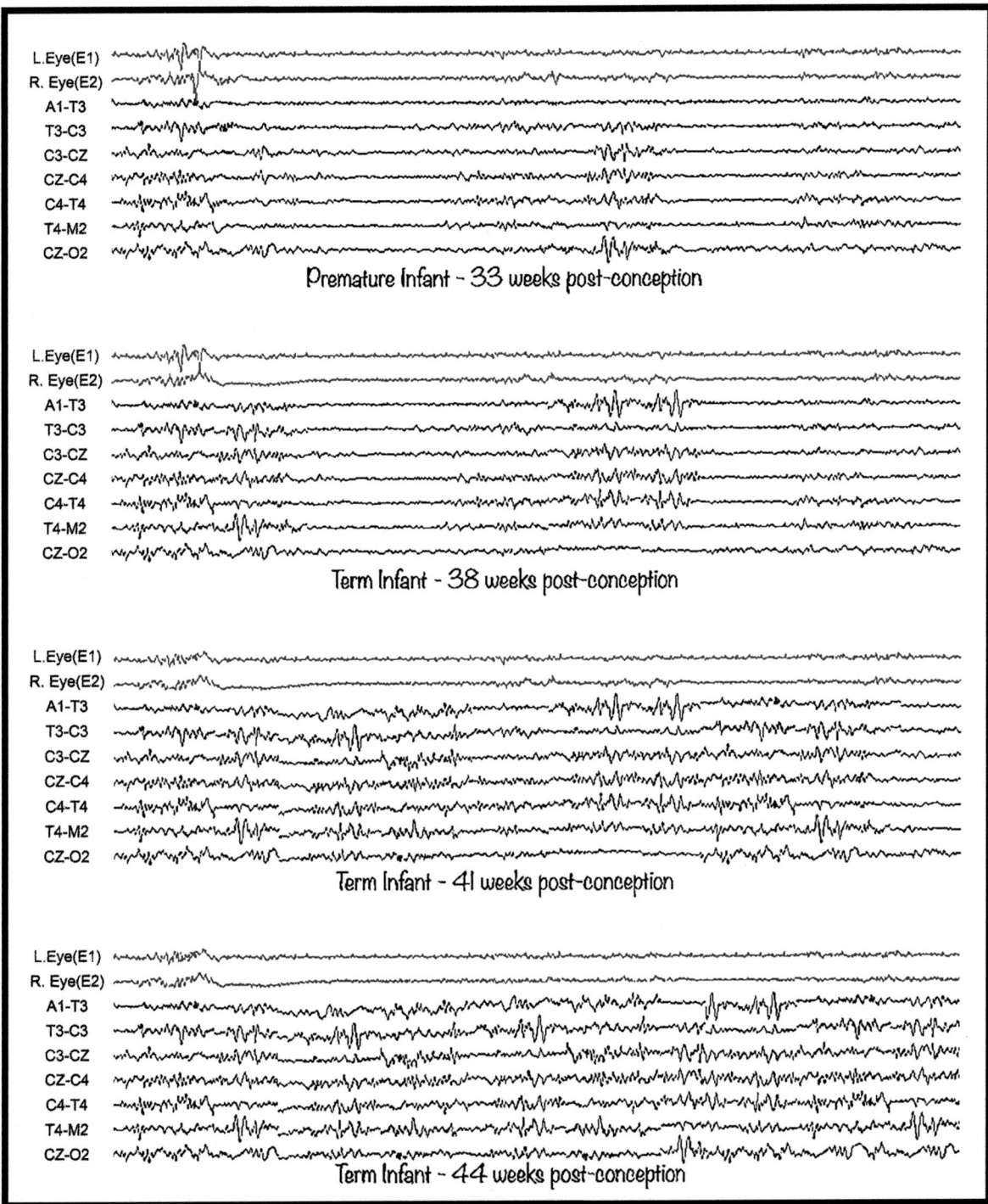

• **Fig. 52.3** Development of the electroencephalogram (EEG). These progressive figures represent development of the EEG pattern of quiet/N sleep in an infant from 33–44 weeks post-conception. Note the long periods of electrical quiescence early in development with intermittent bursts of higher voltage slow waves of mixed frequency. Periods of electrical quiescence decrease in length as the higher voltage mixed frequency activity increases until continuous synchronous activity is seen at 44 weeks post-conception.

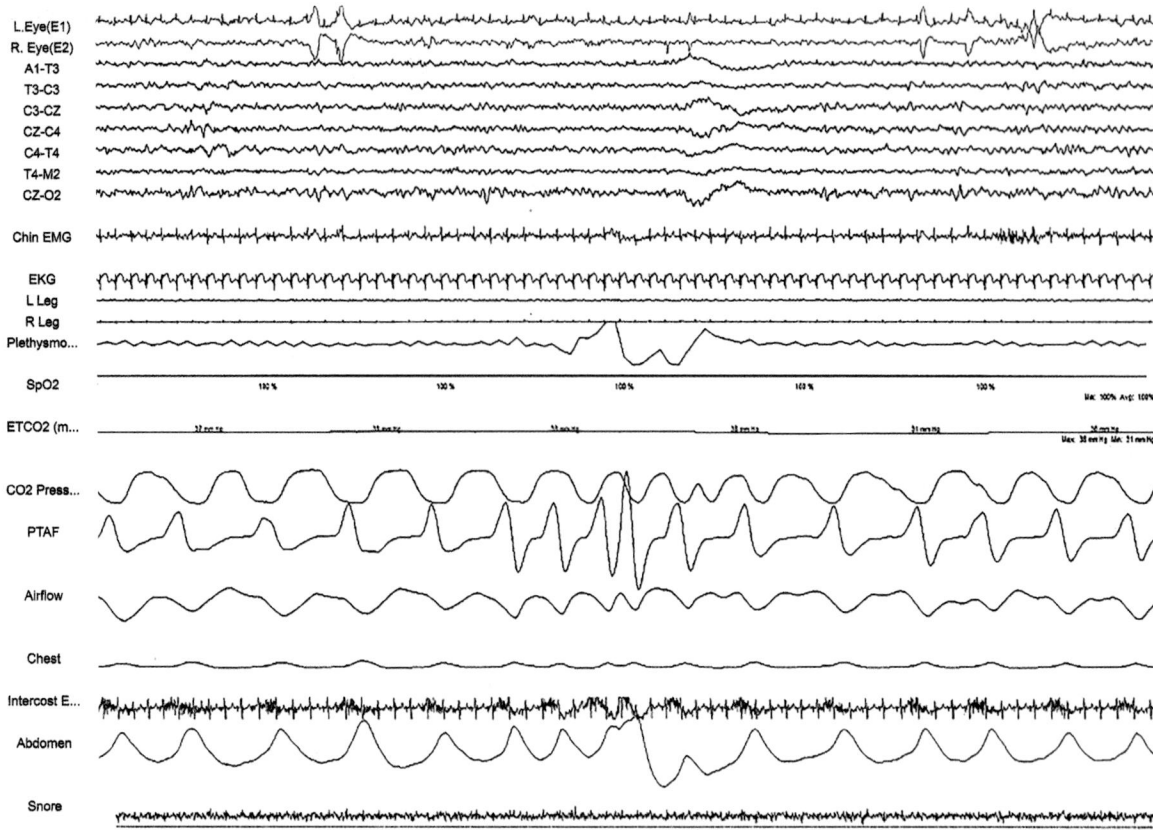

• **Fig. 52.4** Normal term infant: active/rapid eye movement (REM) (R) sleep. This 30-second polysomnographic segment was recorded from a 2-day-old infant during active (REM or R) sleep. The baby was being evaluated for unexplained periods of oxygen desaturation during sleep. Periodic breathing was noted by the nursing staff, and there were questionable perioral cyanosis during these spells. Active sleep/REM (R) sleep may appear quite similar to wakefulness polysomnographically. During wakefulness, eyes are persistently and/or intermittently open. However, during R sleep, eyes are consistently closed. There can be considerable motor activity associated with movement artifact. Behavioral vocalizations, grimaces, and twitching can be seen. In this epoch, conjugate eye movements are noted. Electroencephalogram (EEG) consists of relatively low voltage mixed frequency activity. Chin muscle tone is decreased, and phasic activity can be seen. Respiratory variability is also present.

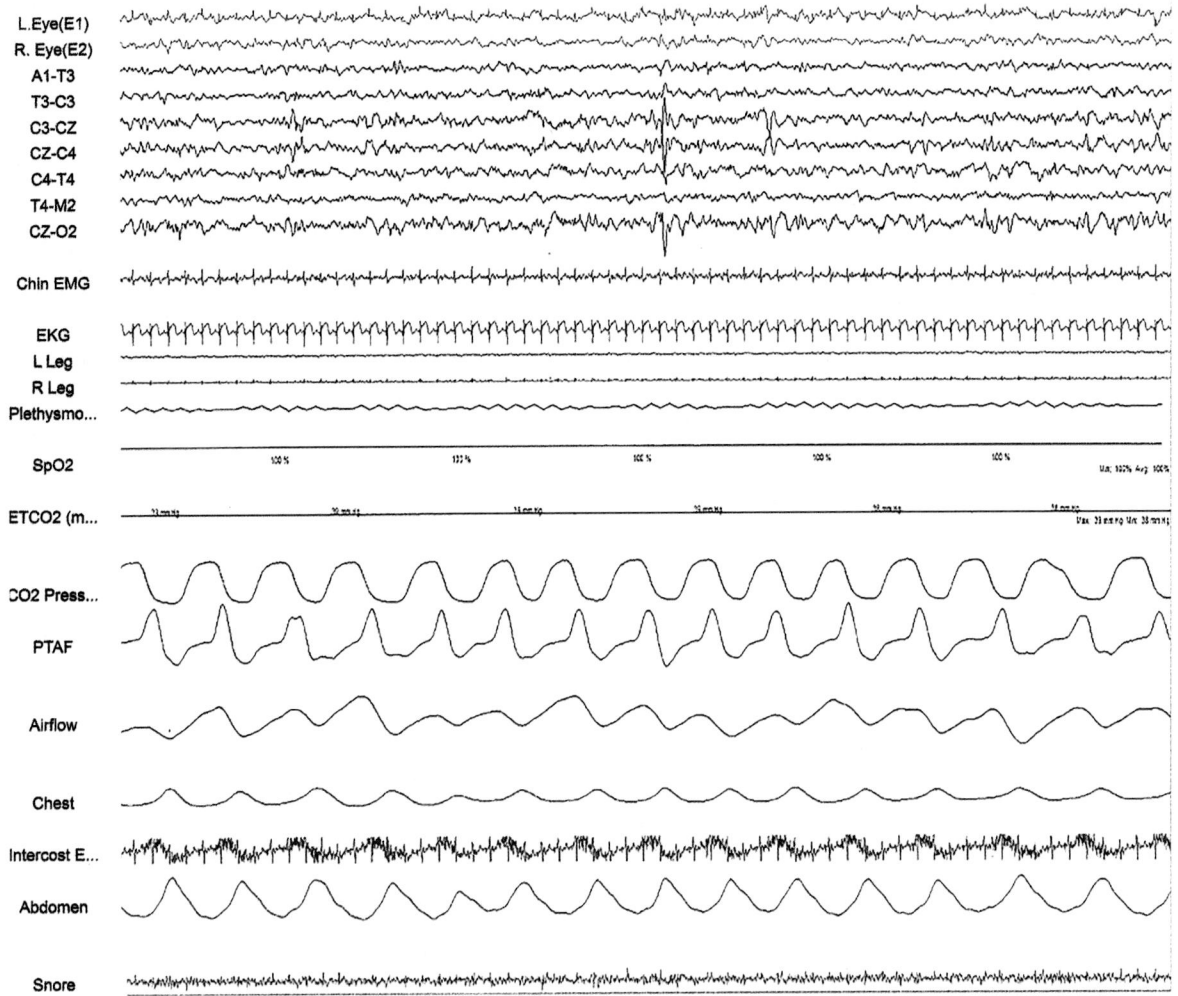

Channel labels (top to bottom): L.Eye(E1), R. Eye(E2), A1-T3, T3-C3, C3-CZ, CZ-C4, C4-T4, T4-M2, CZ-O2, Chin EMG, EKG, L Leg, R Leg, Plethysmo..., SpO2, ETCO2 (m..., CO2 Press..., PTAF, Airflow, Chest, Intercost E..., Abdomen, Snore

• **Fig. 52.5** Normal term infant: transitional sleep (indeterminate sleep). This 30-second segment was recorded from the same 2-day-old infant being evaluated for unexplained oxygen desaturations and perioral cyanosis during sleep. There seem to be characteristics of both R and N sleep. There do not appear to be characteristics of wake. According to the *American Academy of Sleep Medicine Manual for the Scoring of Sleep and Associated Events*,[ii] an epoch is considered transitional sleep (T) if it contains either three non–rapid eye movement (NREM) characteristics and two REM characteristics, or the epoch contains three REM characteristics and two NREM characteristics. In this epoch, there are questionable small eye movements noted in the electrooculogram (EOG) channels. Electroencephalogram (EEG) appears to be a mixture of low voltage mixed frequency activity and chin muscle tone is low. There is no phasic activity in the chin muscle channel noted and respiratory pattern is quite regular. According to the American Academy of Sleep Medicine (AASM) recommendations, one discordant feature noted in an epoch should not change the scoring of the preponderance of characteristics.

[ii] ASM Scoring Manual Version 2.6.

Two-Month-Old Infant

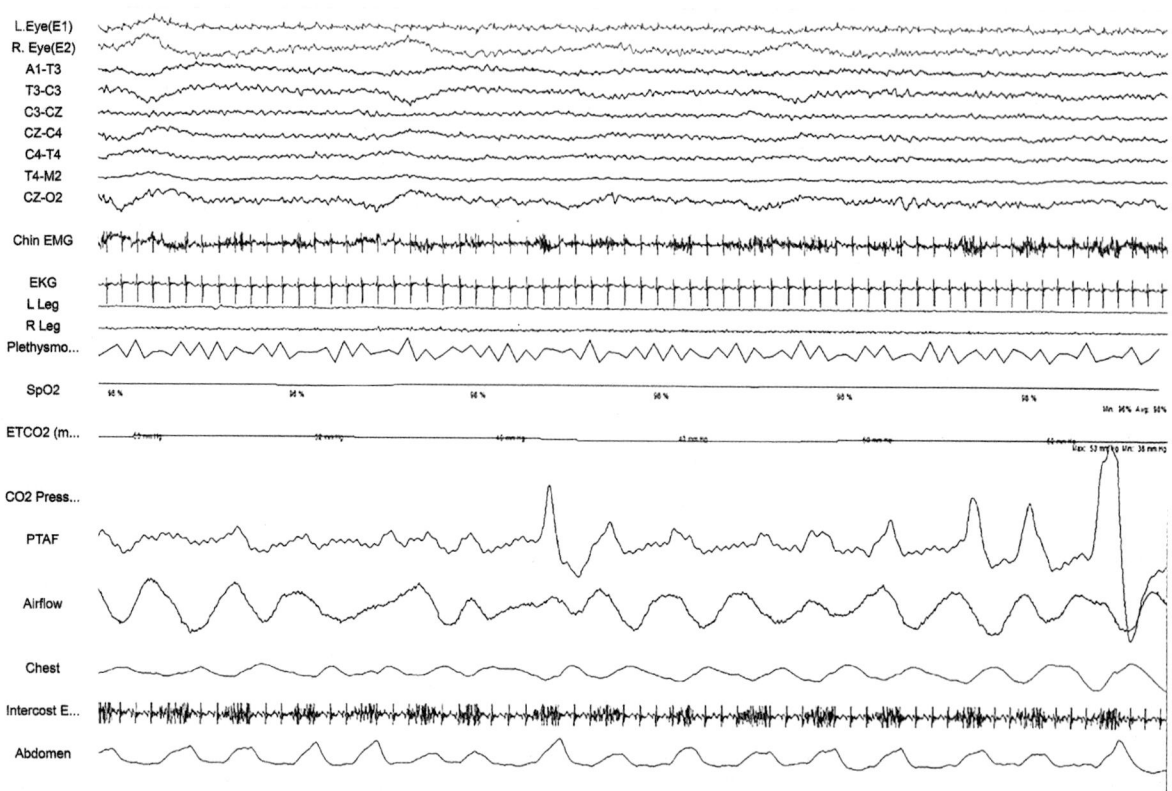

• **Fig. 52.6** Normal 2-month-old transitional sleep. This polysomnographic segment was recorded from a 2-month-old infant who was born with significant laryngomalacia and significant upper airway obstruction. The patient underwent a supraglottoplasty but symptoms of stridulous respiration, increased work of breathing, and periodic oxygen desaturations were noted. This epoch was reported to be transitional sleep. The epoch was preceded by an epoch of wake.

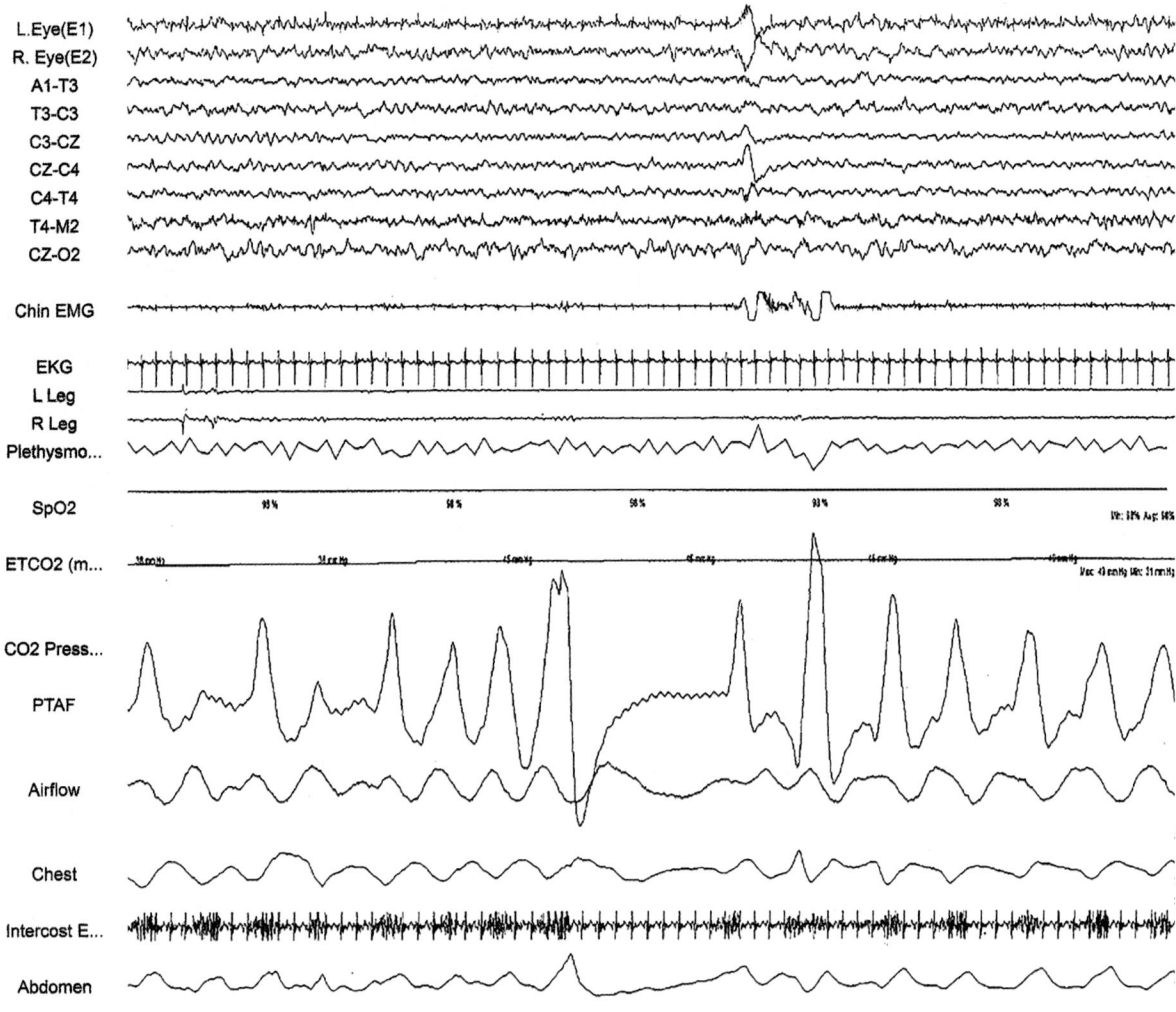

• **Fig. 52.7** Normal 2-month-old rapid eye movement (REM) (R) sleep. This is a 30-second segment from the same infant during REM/active sleep. Note that there is a slightly lower amplitude electroencephalogram (EEG) and the posterior rhythm reveals a relatively low voltage mixed frequency pattern. Heart rate is higher than during non-REM/quiet sleep and there is more heart rate variability. There is considerable irregularity and respiration noted. REM sleep respiratory instability is normal during active sleep. Gross body movements may be present. Additionally, phasic twitches, facial grimacing, arm movements, and leg movements may be seen. Sucking and vocalizations are common during REM/active sleep and infants during this developmental stage. Central respiratory pauses are also common. They are normally seen in the newborn and are typically brief in character. This epoch reveals 5-second respiratory pauses with spontaneous resolution, no oxygen desaturation, and no elevation of carbon dioxide during recovery breathing. In small infants, paradoxical breathing (180 degree phase shift between chest and abdominal efforts) is common. This is likely due to increased chest wall compliance from skeletal muscle inhibition during REM sleep.

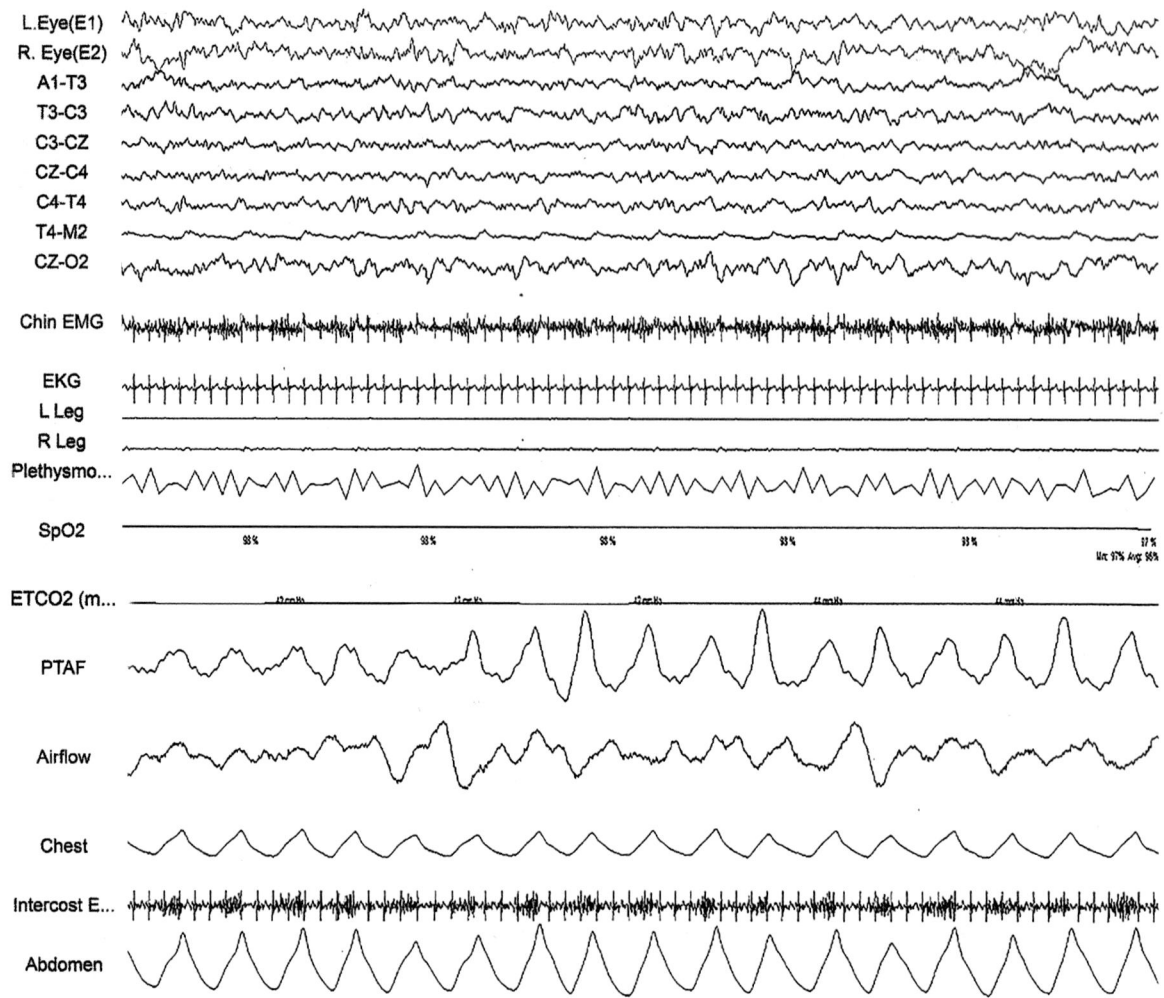

• **Fig. 52.8** Normal 2-month-old non–rapid eye movement (NREM) (N) sleep. This 30-second polysomnographic segment was recorded from the same patient during non-REM/quiet sleep. The electroencephalogram (EEG) reveals high-voltage slow-wave activity with superimposed theta frequency waves noted. The heart rate has slightly decreased from that seen during wakefulness and respiratory efforts and pattern is regular and monotonous.

53

Infants 3–6 Months

Stephen H. Sheldon

4-Month-Old Infant

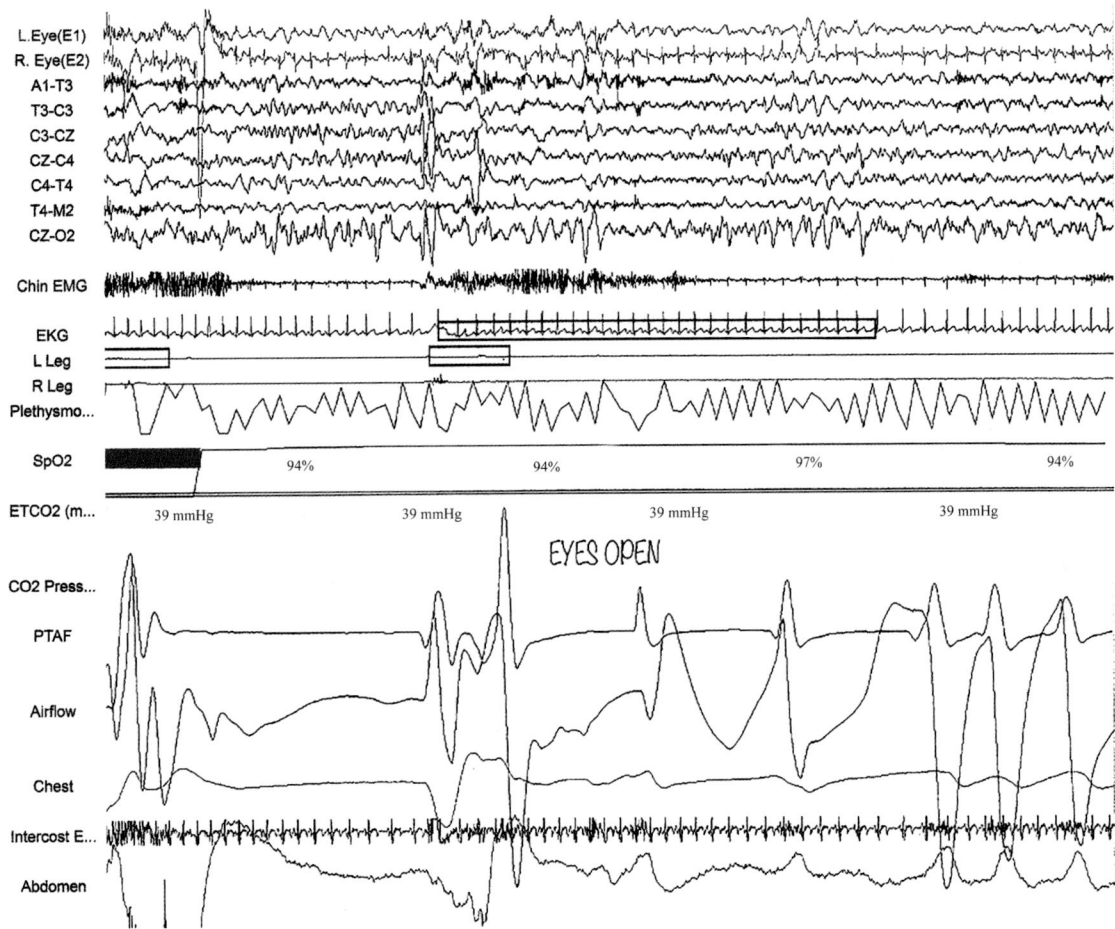

• **Fig. 53.1** Normal 4-month-old infant: wake. This 30-second polysomnographic segment was recorded from a 4-month-old infant who was studied in the laboratory due to the presence of stridulous breathing. The technical notations of eyes open signify that it is most likely wakefulness, if other characteristics of the polysomnogram are difficult to determine. There is a relatively high voltage mixed frequency posterior dominant rhythm with chin muscle activity, considerable heart rate variability, and respiratory instability. These findings are characteristic of wakefulness.

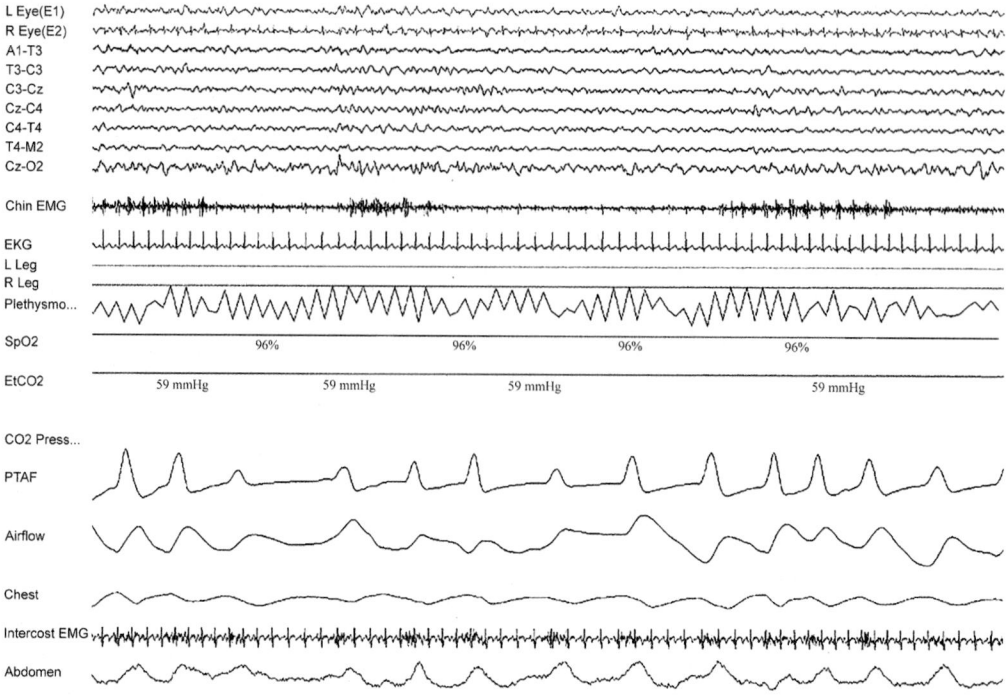

• **Fig. 53.2** Normal 4-month-old: N1. By 4 months of age, non–rapid eye movement (NREM) state differentia-tion becomes fairly clear. This polysomnographic (PSG) segment was recorded from the same infant during transitional sleep (N1). Note there is a change in electroencephalogram (EEG) pattern that reflects a relatively low voltage mixed frequency posterior dominant rhythm. Sucking artifact can be seen in the chin muscle electromyo-gram (EMG) with rhythmic movements of the genioglossus muscle. Sucking movements commonly continue from wakefulness into transitional sleep. Sucking movements may be seen in all stages of infants' sleep. In this epoch, there is noted to be some slight flow limitation in the pressure and thermal channels. However, there is no significant oxygen desaturation 3% or greater from the baseline and no hypercapnia during recovery breathing.

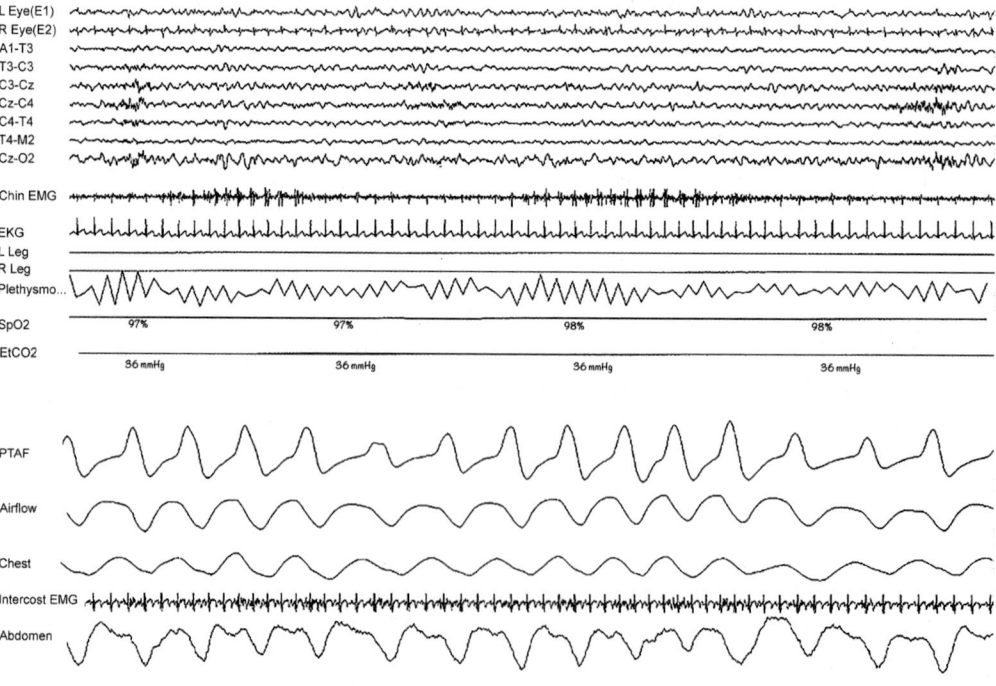

• **Fig. 53.3** Normal 4-month-old: N2. This 30-second segment was recorded from the same infant during non–rapid eye movement (NREM) sleep. Sleep spindles begin to appear between 2 and 4 months of age. Spindles may be exaggerated in length and are sometimes termed *extreme spindles*. Sleep spindles can be noted at the beginning and end of this segment. Sucking movements can still be seen in the chin muscle electromyogram (EMG). Posterior dominant background rhythm is still relatively low in voltage and mixed frequency. Mild periodic decremental airflow is present in the pressure channel. Although flow limitation lasts about two respiratory efforts, these two events do not meet criteria to be classified as hypopneas.

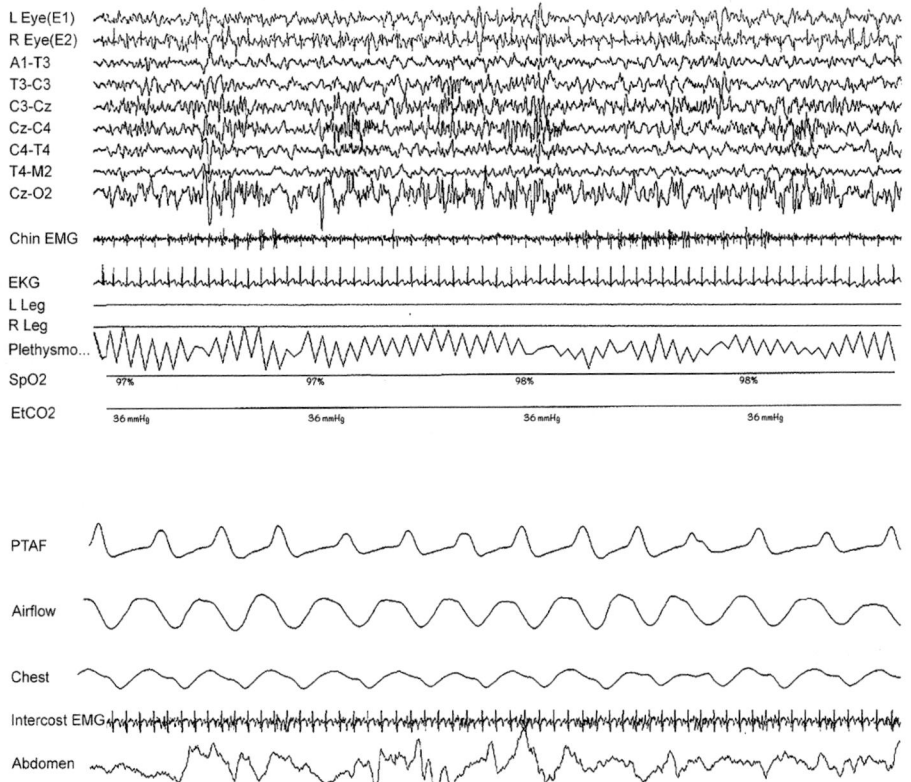

• **Fig. 53.4** Normal 4-month-old: N3. This segment was recorded from the same infant shown in Fig. 53.3 during N3 sleep. Electroencephalogram (EEG) activity in this figure reveals a slower background of greater amplitude. There continued to be noticeable spindles and there is increased EEG artifact in the electrooculogram (EOG). Heart rate is relatively steady and regular. Respiratory pattern is also regular and monotonous with normal oxygen saturation and end-tidal carbon dioxide levels. Again, sucking movements continue into N3 sleep as noted in the chin muscle electromyogram (EMG). There also continues to be some mild airflow limitation in the pressure channel during the middle portion of the epoch, but the event still does not meet criteria for classification as a hypopnea.

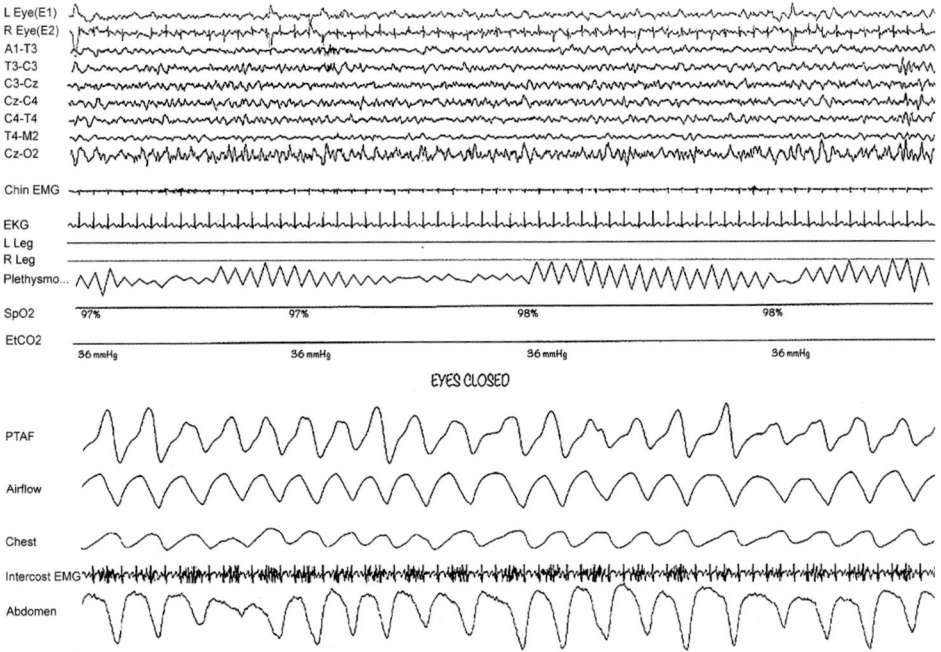

• **Fig. 53.5** Normal 4-month-old: rapid eye movement (REM). This figure shows a 30-second segment from the same patient during REM sleep. Electroencephalogram (EEG) reveals a moderate voltage with continuous activity and theta as well as delta frequency waveforms. Conjugate REMs can be seen in the electrooculogram (EOG) channels and chin tone is significantly decreased below levels seen in the previous segments. Heart rate is regular but increased variability is noted. The rate is slightly faster than noted during non-REM sleep. Respiratory pattern reveals normal REM sleep respiratory instability with irregular effort and varying airflow.

54

Infants 6–12 Months

Stephen H. Sheldon

9-Month-Old

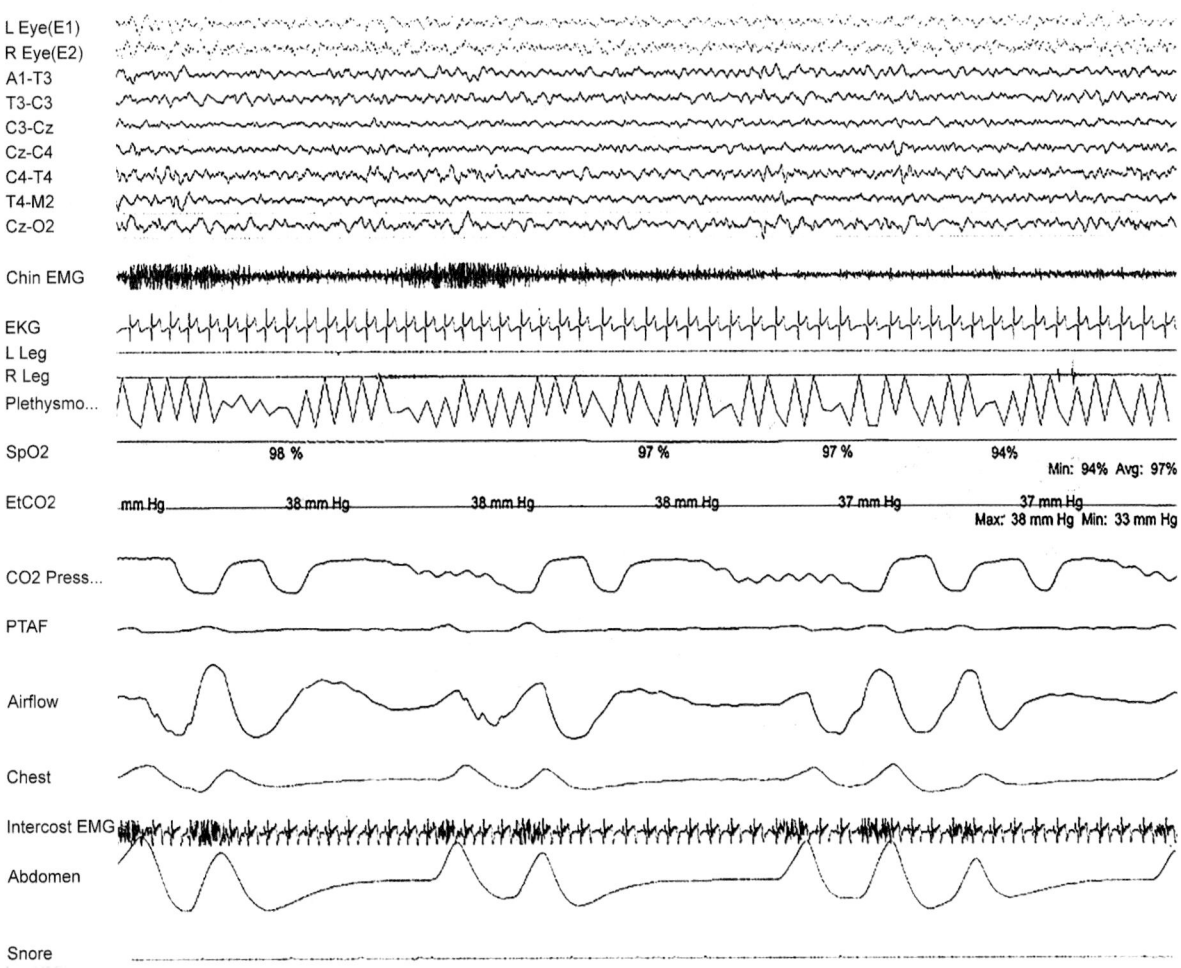

• **Fig. 54.1** Normal 9-month old infant: N1. This 30-second segment was taken from a 7-month-old with a history of reported witnessed apnea when sleeping. A polysomnogram (PSG) was conducted as part of an evaluation for a brief resolved unexplained event (BRUE). A BRUE is defined as an unexplained event in an infant <1 year of age including but not limited to witnessed apnea, change in muscle tone, experiences a color change (pallor or cyanosis), or unresponsiveness. Note the sucking artifact in the chin muscle electromyogram (EMG). There a relatively moderate voltage mixed frequency posterior dominant rhythm, and absent eye movements. Eyes are closed. Brief self-resolving central respiratory pauses can be normal during transitional sleep.

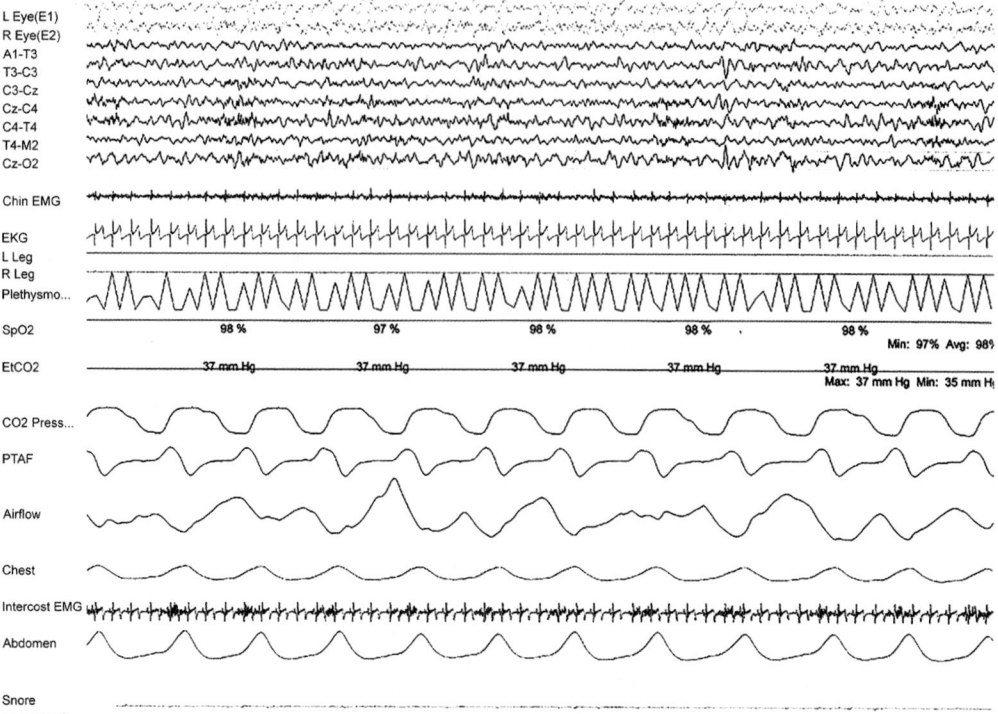

• **Fig. 54.2** Normal 9-month-old infant: N2. This 30-second segment was recorded from the same infant. Now, there is clear differentiation of N2 sleep from transitional sleep and N3 sleep. There is a relatively moderate voltage background and synchronous sleep spindles are clearly visible. Respiration is regular, carbon dioxide and oxygen saturation are normal. Electrocardiogram (ECG) reveals normal beat-to-beat variability.

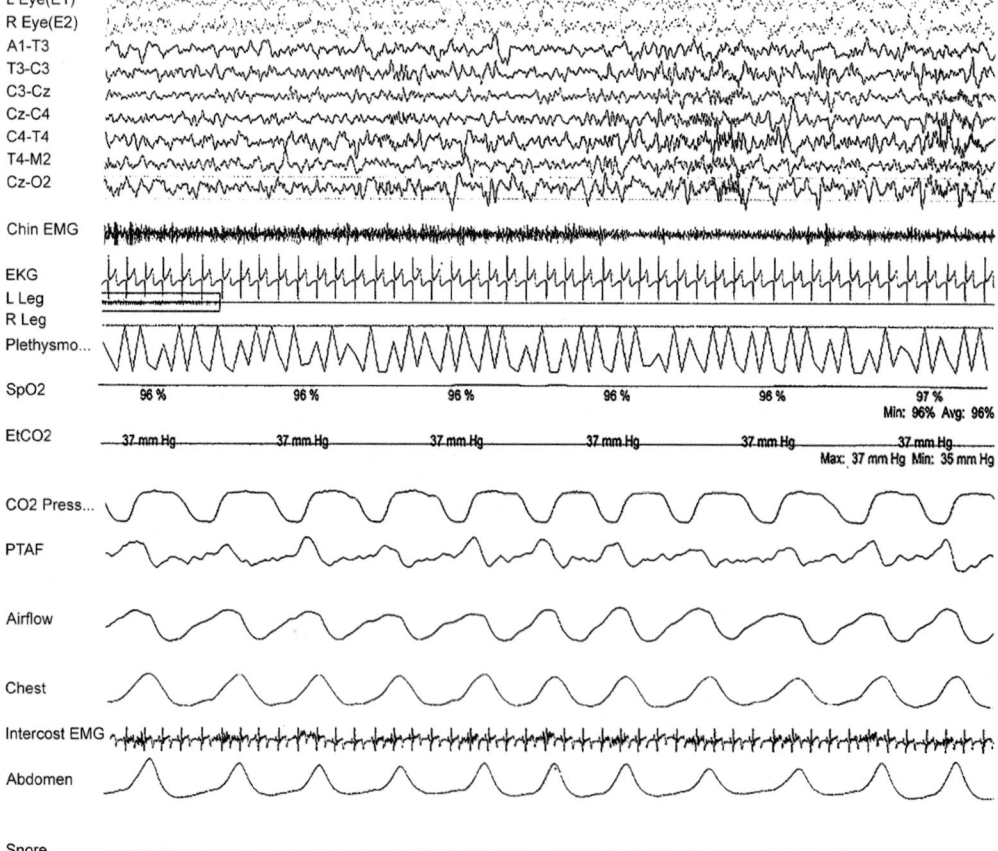

• **Fig. 54.3** Normal 9-month-old: N3. This represents a 30-second segment recorded during N3 from the same infant. High voltage slow waves predominate the epoch. Electroencephalogram (EEG) artifact is seen in the electrooculogram (EOG) channels due to high-voltage frontal activity. Heart rate is somewhat slower when compared with wake and lighter stages of sleep.

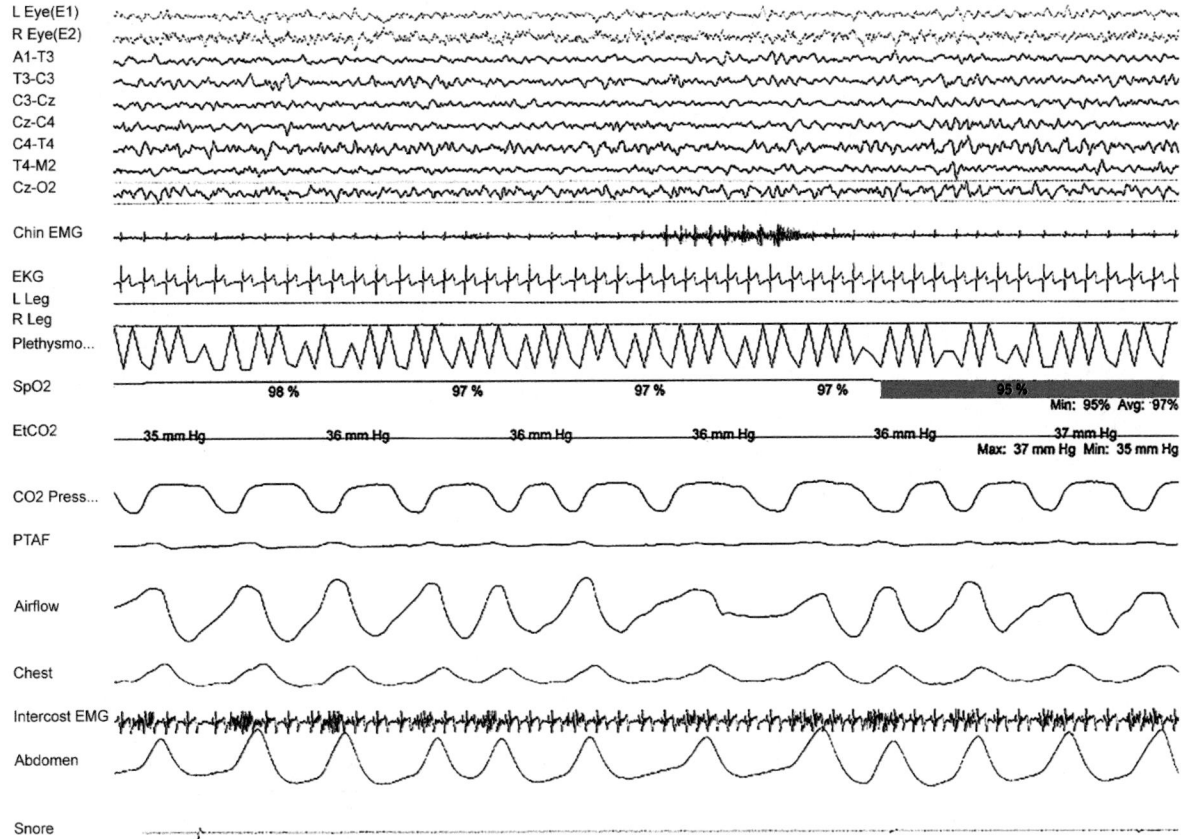

• **Fig. 54.4** Normal 9-month-old infant: rapid eye movement (REM). This 30-second segment was recorded from the same infant. Electroencephalogram (EEG) reveals high-voltage activity with frequency ranging from 0.5–3 Hz. Conjugate eye movements are noted in the electrooculogram (EOG). Respiratory pattern and heart rate variability is greater than that seen during non-REM sleep. Oxygen saturation and carbon dioxide levels continue to be normal. Red bar indicates oxygen desaturation at least 3% from baseline.

55

Toddler 12 Months to 2 Years

Stephen H. Sheldon

1-Year-Old

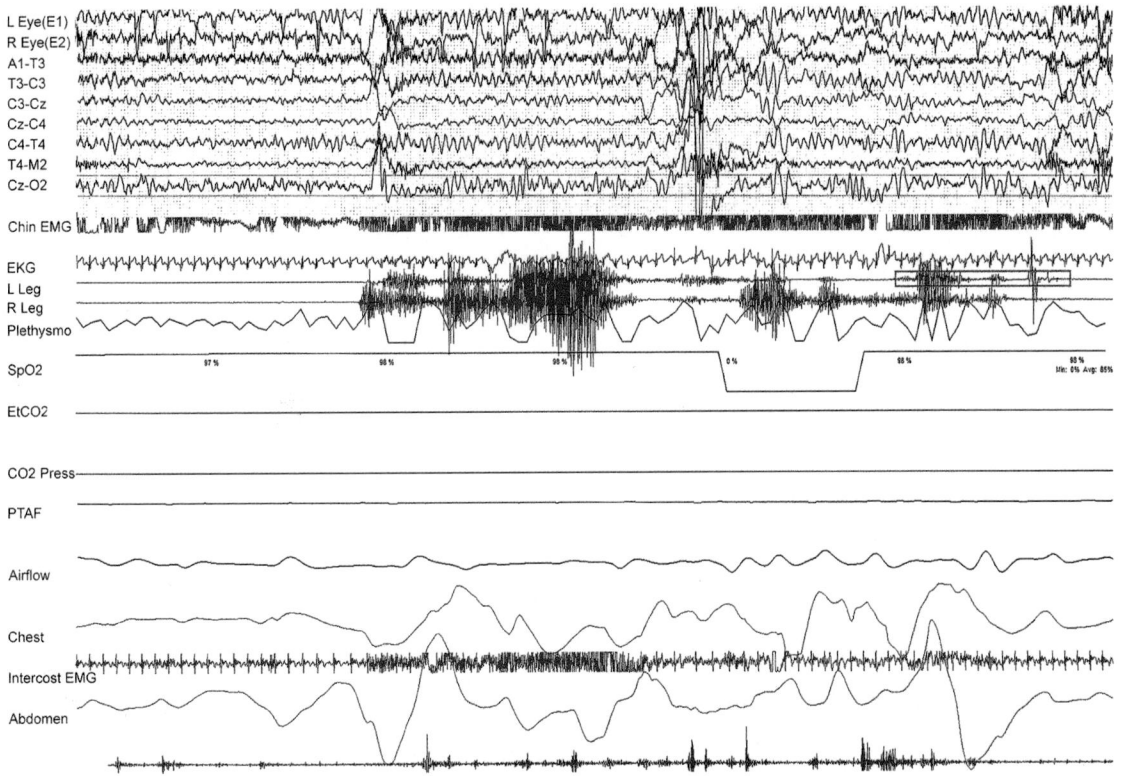

• **Fig. 55.1** Normal 1-year-old: wake. This 30-second polysomnographic (PSG) segment was recorded from a 12-month-old infant as part of a comprehensive evaluation of failure to thrive (FTT). Sleep was described as restless and there was mild intermittent snoring noted by parents. Weight was 6 kg. He woke frequently at night. In this segment, there is a moderate amplitude 5–6 Hz electroencephalogram (EEG) background rhythm. Tonic chin muscle activity is present, clear major body movements are present, limb movements are noted, and respiration is very irregular. Difficult maintaining the split-lumen nasal cannula at the beginning of the study precluded measurement of the pressure tracing and ETCO$_2$ waveform.

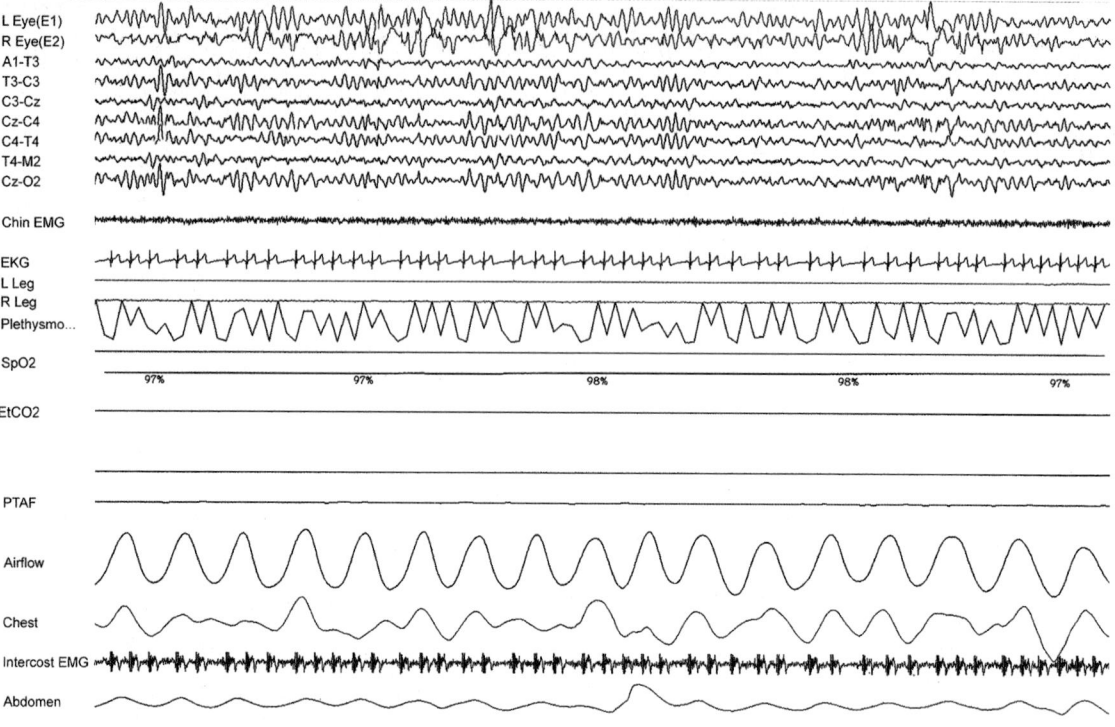

• **Fig. 55.2** Normal 1-year-old: N1. This epoch was recorded from the same infant during transition from wake to sleep. Electroencephalogram (EEG) reveals episodes of hypersynchronous 4–5 Hz moderate amplitude wave-forms. Hypersynchronous activity during transitional sleep is normal and, at times, can appear somewhat sharp in character. They are normal findings over the vertex. Electrooculogram (EOG) reveals occasional slow rolling eye movements, and somewhat higher voltage synchronous EEG artifact can be seen. Chin muscle tone is tonic. Respiratory pattern is regular. Electrocardiogram (ECG) reveals normal non–rapid eye movement (NREM) beat-to-beat variability.

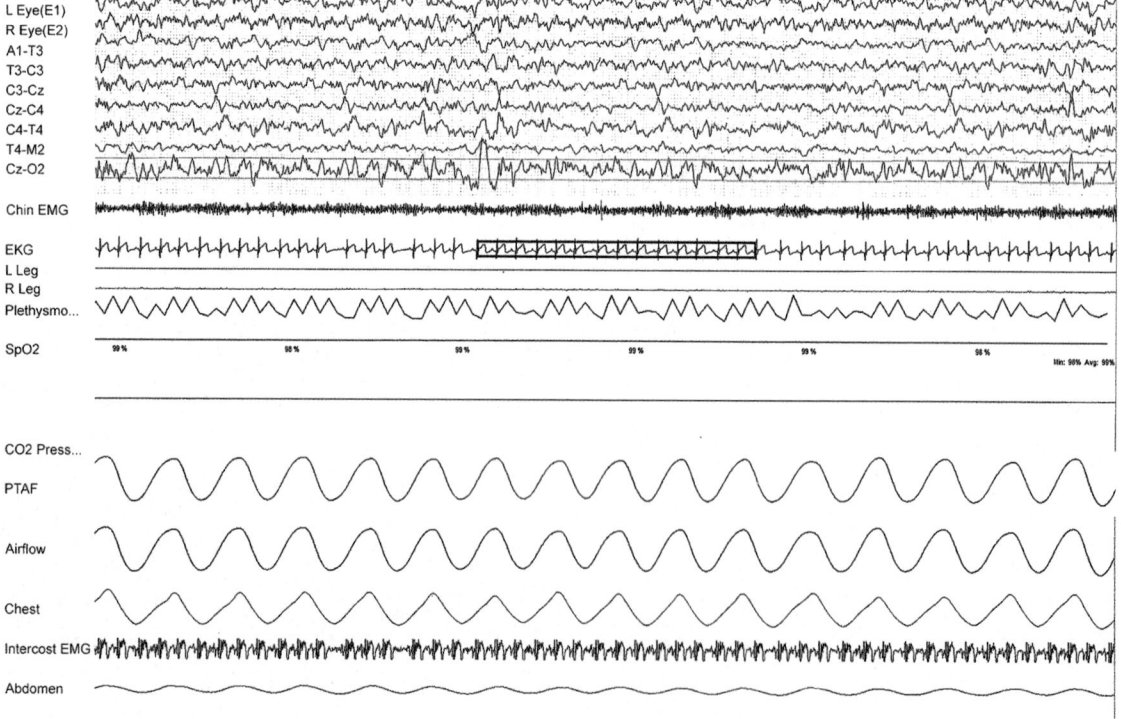

• **Fig. 55.3** Normal 1-year-old: N2. This 30-second epoch was recorded from the same patient. Relatively mixed voltage and mixed frequency pattern can be seen. Symmetrical sleep spindles are present. Chin muscle electromyogram (EMG) is tonic and heart rate has slightly slowed when compared with wake and transitional sleep. There is normal respiratory sinus variation of electrocardiogram (ECG) and respiration is stable and regular. Oxygen saturation and ETCO₂ are normal. Box indicates mild "tachydysrhythmia" (that has followed cardiac sinus deceleration).

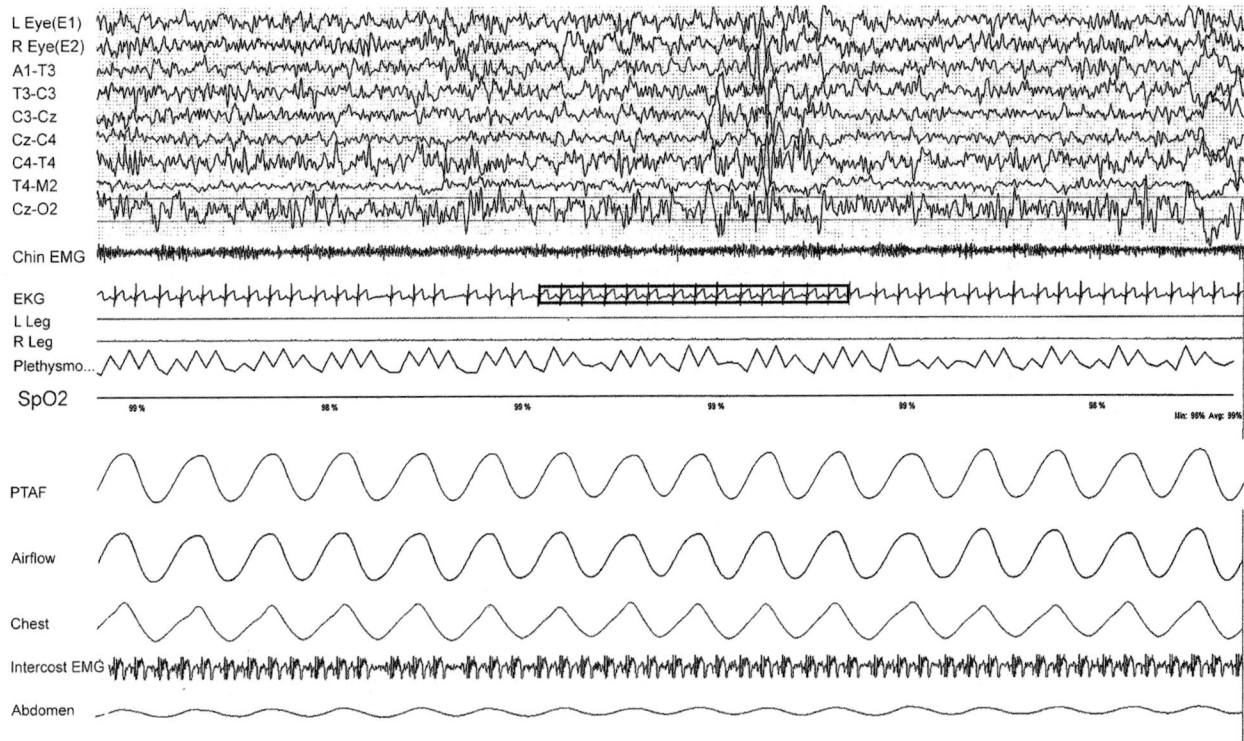

• **Fig. 55.4** Normal 1-year-old: N3. This 30-second segment was recorded from the same patient. Electroencephalogram (EEG) is dominated by high-voltage activity of about 0.5 Hz. There is also considerable superimposed activity in the theta frequency range. Sleep spindles are clear and somewhat higher voltage. Electrooculogram (EOG) reveals significant EEG artifact from high-voltage frontal activity. Heart rate shows sinus variability and respiration is extremely regular with normal gas exchange. Box indicates mild "tachydysrhythmia" (that has followed cardiac sinus deceleration).

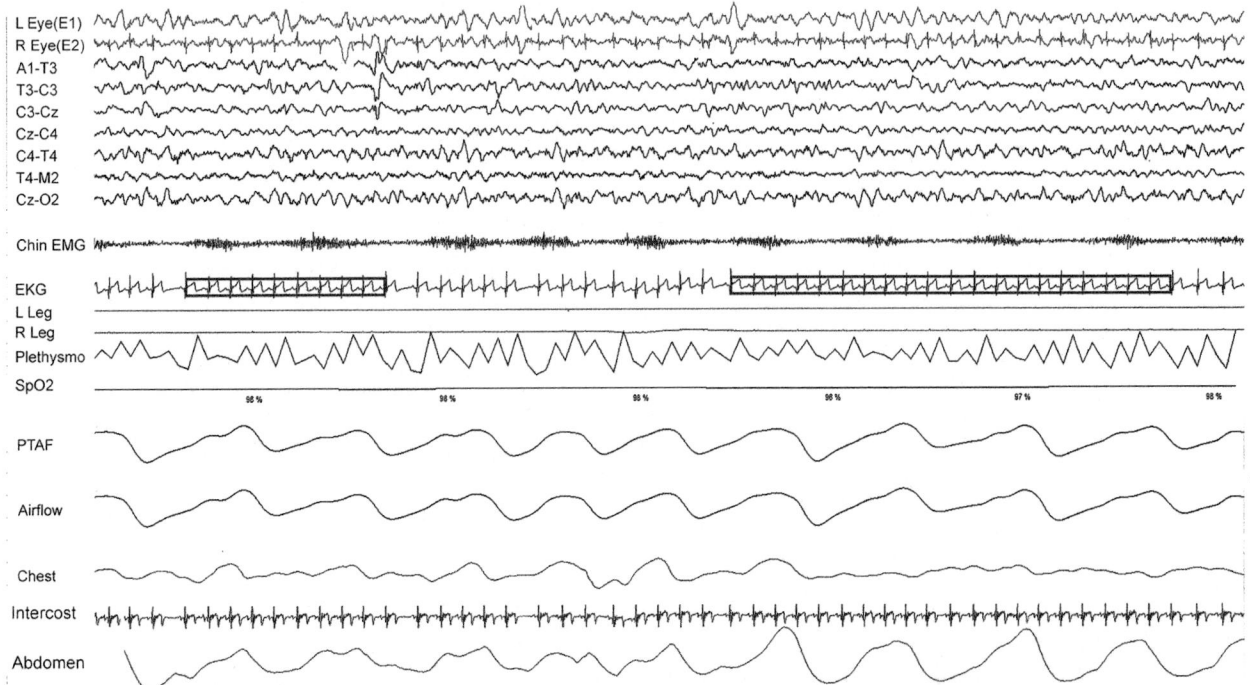

• **Fig. 55.5** Normal 1-year-old: rapid eye movement (REM). This figure demonstrates REM sleep. Electroencephalogram (EEG) consists of moderate amplitude notched theta activity, particularly over the vertex. Clearly identifiable conjugate eye movements can be seen despite the higher voltage EEG artifact noted from the frontal region. Chin muscle electromyogram (EMG) reveals decreased tone when compared with wake and non-REM (NREM) sleep. This decreased tone is interrupted by snore artifact (genioglossus muscle vibratory artifact). Heart rate and variability is similar to that of wakefulness. There is somewhat irregular respiratory pattern. Chest and abdominal movement may also appear intermittently paradoxical due to decreased skeletal muscle tone and increased chest wall compliance. Boxes indicate mild "tachydysrhythmia" (that has followed cardiac sinus deceleration).

2-Year-Old

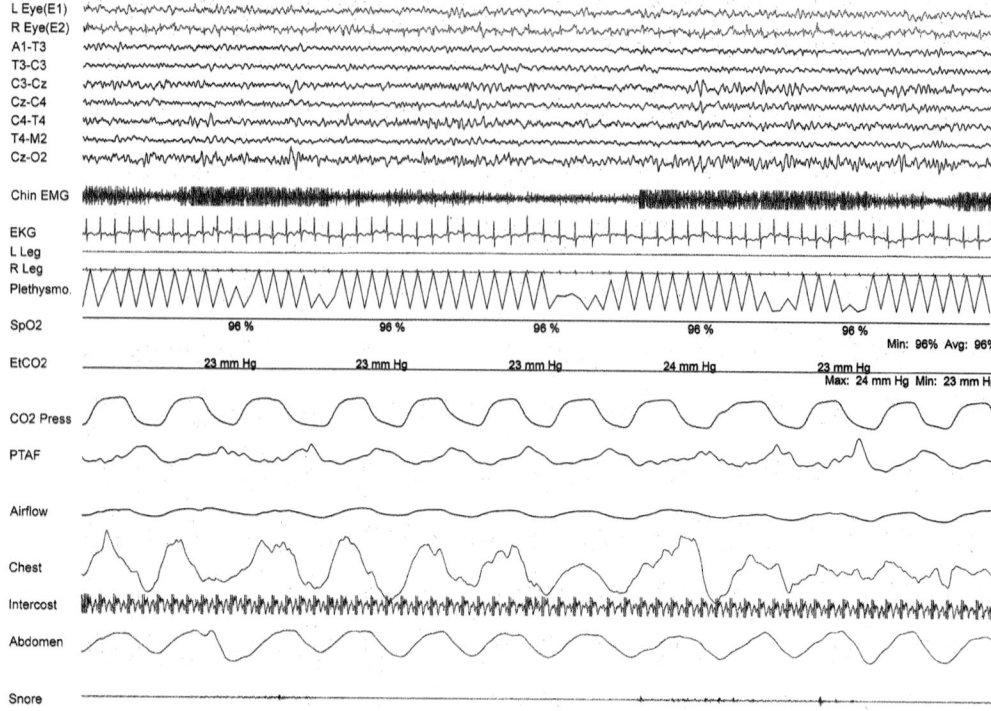

• **Fig. 55.6** Normal 2-year-old: wake-to-sleep transition. This 30-second segment was recorded during wakefulness from a 2-year-old child who had been referred for evaluation of possible sleep-disordered breathing. Waking electroencephalogram (EEG) background frequency is approximately 6–7 Hz. Some conjugate eye movements can be noted. There is slight respiratory irregularity, and chin muscle electromyogram (EMG) is quite tonic. There is some evidence near the end of this segment where eye movements become somewhat slow and rolling. EEG frequency begins to slow to approximately 4–6 Hz and amplitude increases to approximately 100 µV. Heart rate is stable, there are no limb movements, and there is some evidence of drowsiness by virtue of decremental chin muscle EMG and EEG frequency change.

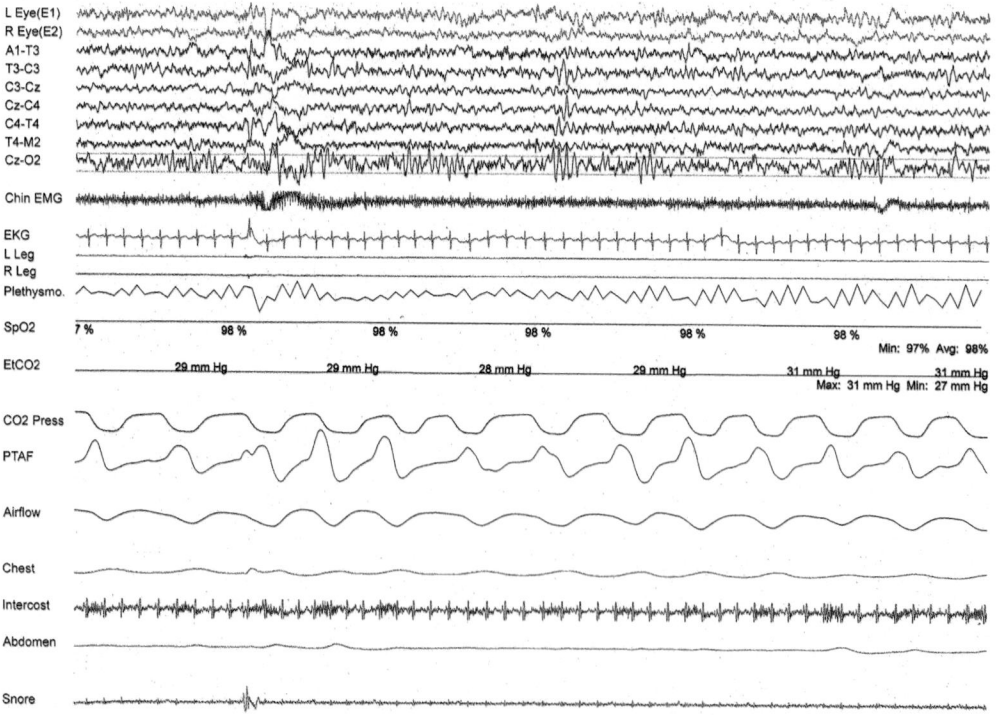

• **Fig. 55.7** Normal 2-year-old: N1 sleep. This 30-second segment was recorded from the same patient. There is clear transitional sleep noted and electroencephalogram (EEG) frequency has changed from a mixed pattern to a moderately higher voltage pattern with the majority of theta activity noted. Conjugate eye movements are absent and replaced by slow rolling movements. Electrocardiogram (ECG) is regular and respirations also remained regular when compared with wakefulness. Chin muscle tone is chronic, though somewhat decreased over the waking pattern.

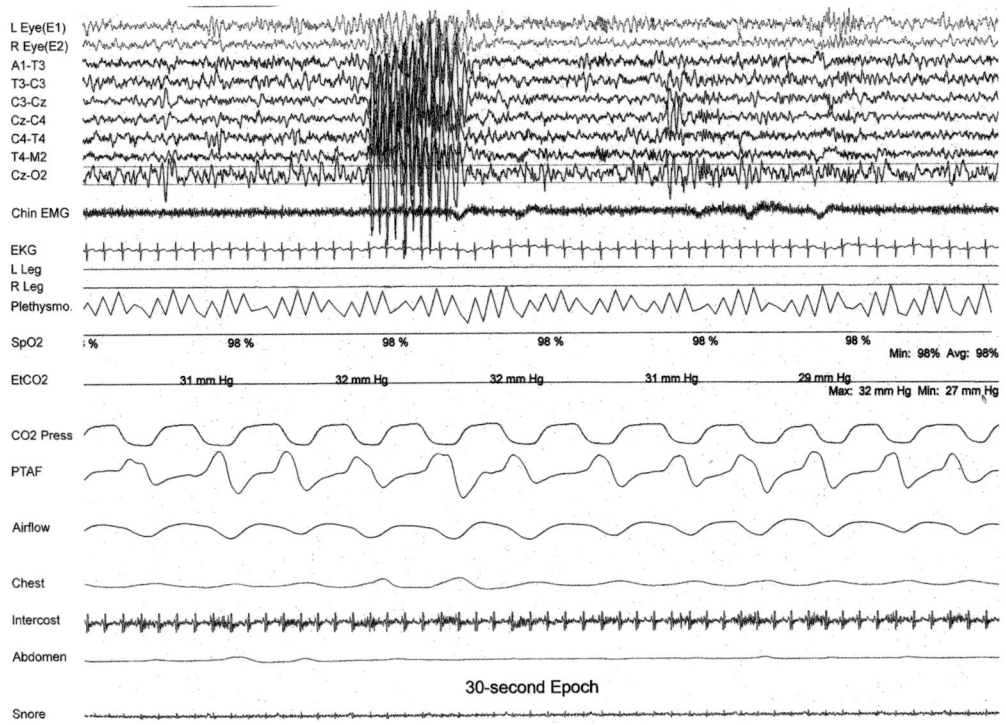

• **Fig. 55.8** Normal 2-year-old: N1-N2 with burst of hypnagogic hypersynchrony. This was recorded from the same patient and represents transition into N2 sleep. There is a mixed 2–6 Hz background electroencephalogram (EEG) activity with occasional sleep spindles noted with a frequency of approximately 14 Hz. No eye movements are noted. EEG reveals a normal sinus rhythm with a slightly slower rate than seen during wakefulness. All respiratory channels are normal and gas exchange appears to be normal. During the first half of the segment high-voltage hypersynchronous activity can be seen. This is referred to as hypnagogic hypersynchrony, which is normal during this stage of sleep and children.

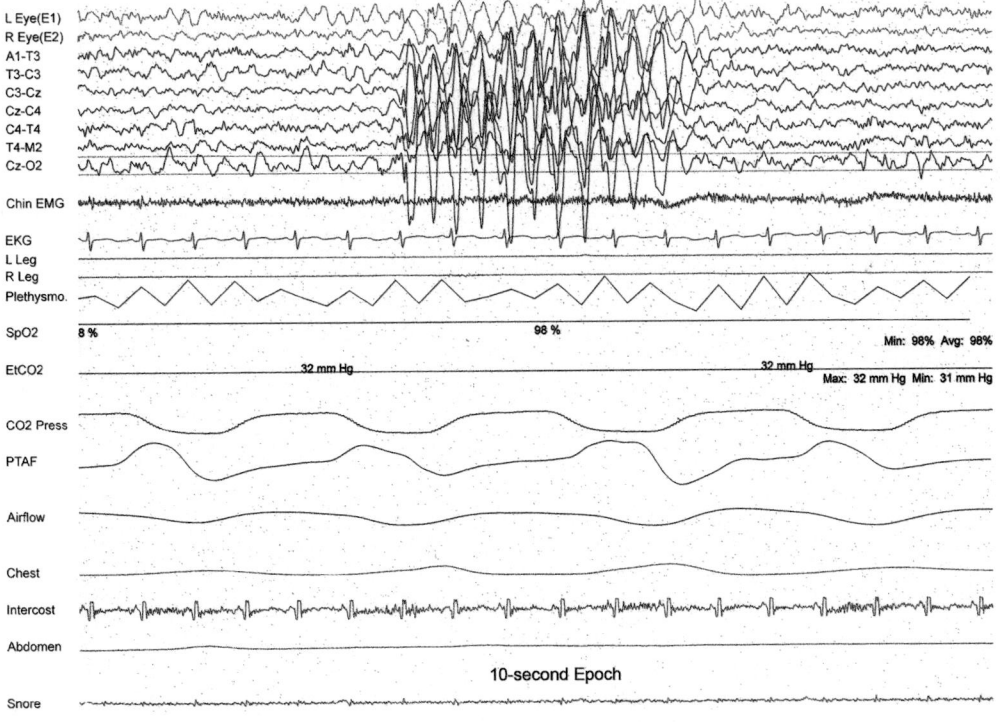

• **Fig. 55.9** Normal 2-year-old: N1-N2 with hypnagogic hypersynchrony (10-second epoch). This 10-second segment is taken from the prior 30-second episode that clearly reveals the character of hypnagogic hypersynchrony. This is not ictal activity and is normal. There is no gradual buildup to this hypersynchronous activity and there are no postictal changes noted. Hypnagogic hypersynchrony is normal during childhood and can be seen in the following epoch recorded from a 6-year-old child with a history of snoring.

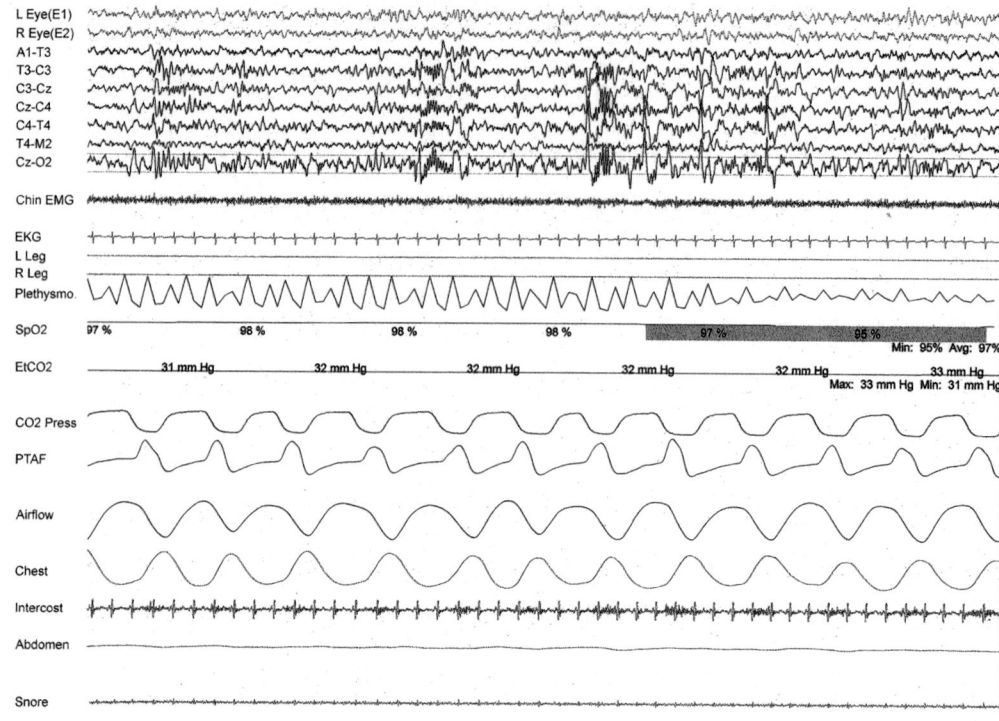

• **Fig. 55.10** Normal 2-year-old: N2. This 30-second segment demonstrates N2 sleep. It is a relatively mixed frequency background electroencephalogram (EEG) activity ranging from 2–6 Hz with notable sleep spindles that appear at a frequency of approximately 14 Hz. There are no eye movements noted on the electrooculogram (EOG). The electrocardiogram shows a normal sinus rhythm with a suggestion of a sinus arrhythmia. Heart rate is slightly slower than during wakefulness. Respiration is regular with an average rate of about 24 breaths/min. Both oxygen saturation and end-tidal carbon dioxide levels are normal. Red box indicates oxygen desaturation from baseline.

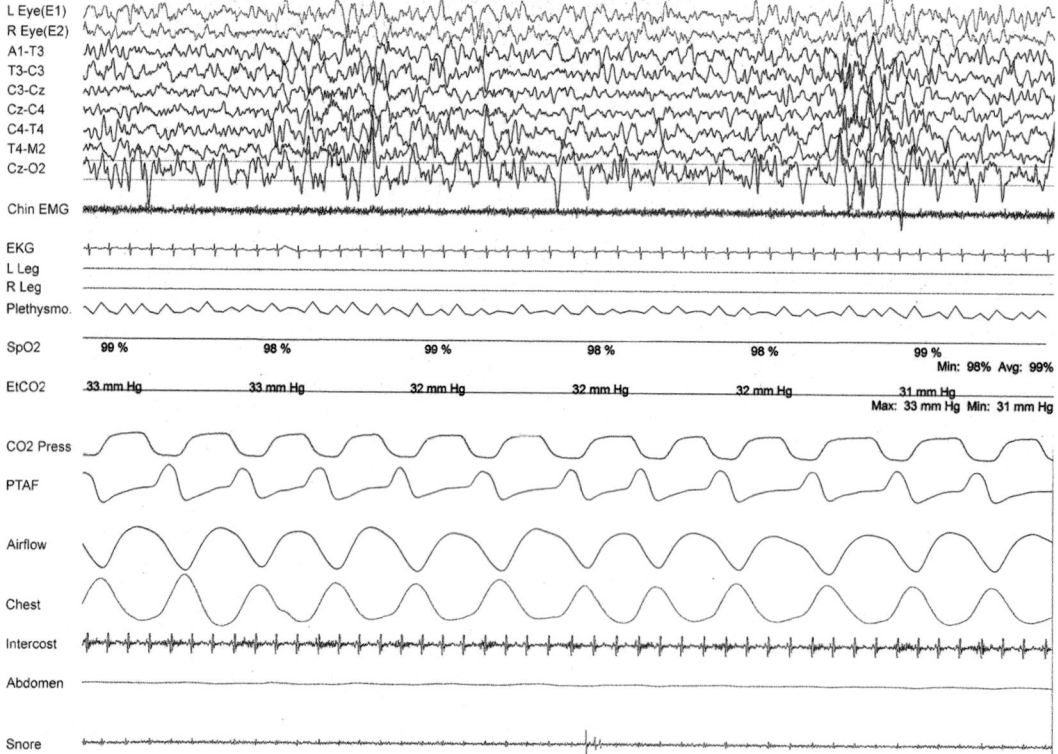

• **Fig. 55.11** Normal 2-year-old: N3. This 30-second polysomnographic segment was recorded from the same 2-year-old youngster during N3 sleep. Electroencephalogram (EEG) shows a high amplitude 0.5–2 Hz predominant background activity occupying the vast majority of this segment. There is high-voltage EEG artifact noted in the electrooculogram (EOG) leads that represents high-amplitude frontal EEG activity. Chin muscle tone is slightly lower than wakefulness. Cardiac rhythm is sinus and normal R-R interval variability is present. Respiration is regular as noted in all airflow and effort channels. Gas exchange is normal.

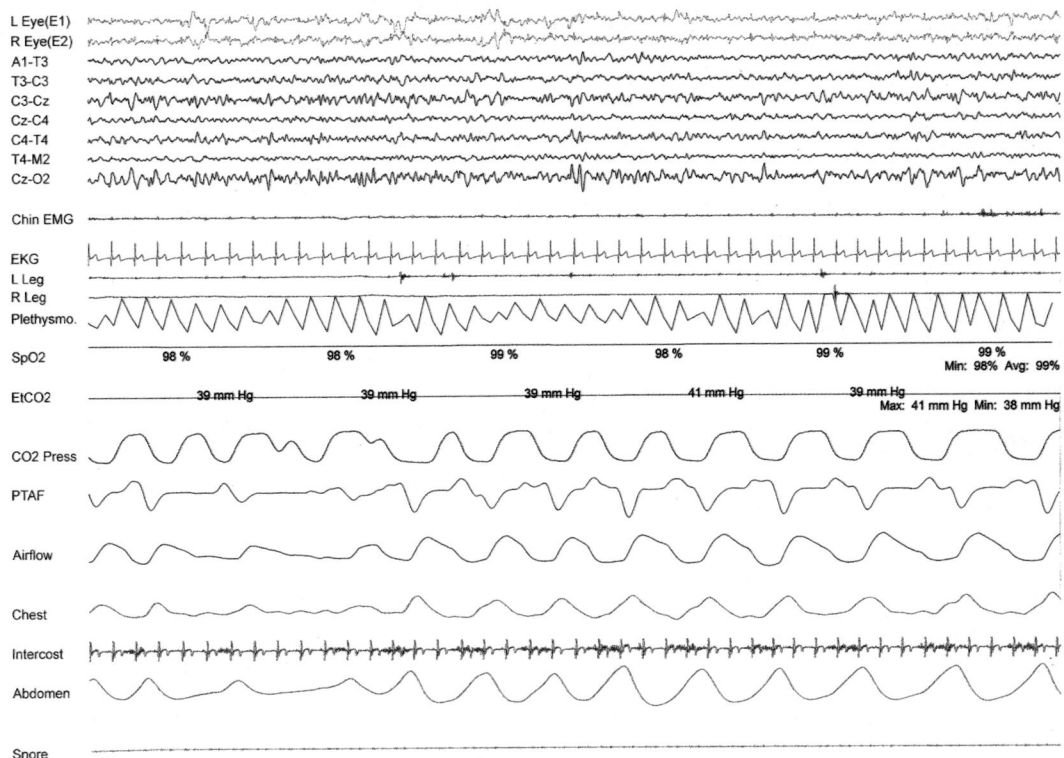

L Eye(E1)
R Eye(E2)
A1-T3
T3-C3
C3-Cz
Cz-C4
C4-T4
T4-M2
Cz-O2

Chin EMG

EKG
L Leg
R Leg
Plethysmo.

SpO2   98 %   98 %   99 %   98 %   99 %   99 %
                                              Min: 98% Avg: 99%

EtCO2   39 mm Hg   39 mm Hg   39 mm Hg   41 mm Hg   39 mm Hg
                                              Max: 41 mm Hg Min: 38 mm Hg

CO2 Press

PTAF

Airflow

Chest

Intercost

Abdomen

Snore

• **Fig. 55.12** Normal 2-year-old: rapid eye movement (REM). This figure represents REM sleep and a 2-year-old studied because of residual snoring. There is moderate amplitude theta electroencephalogram (EEG) background activity along with clearly identifiable rapid conjugate eye movements, increased heart rate, and low chin muscle tone. Phasic muscle activity can be seen in the limb leads. Respiration is somewhat irregular. Oxygen saturation remains normal and end-tidal CO_2 is also normal. Sawtooth waves can be seen particularly in the posterior $CZ-O_2$ lead.

56

Children 2–5 Years Old

Stephen H. Sheldon

4-Year-Old

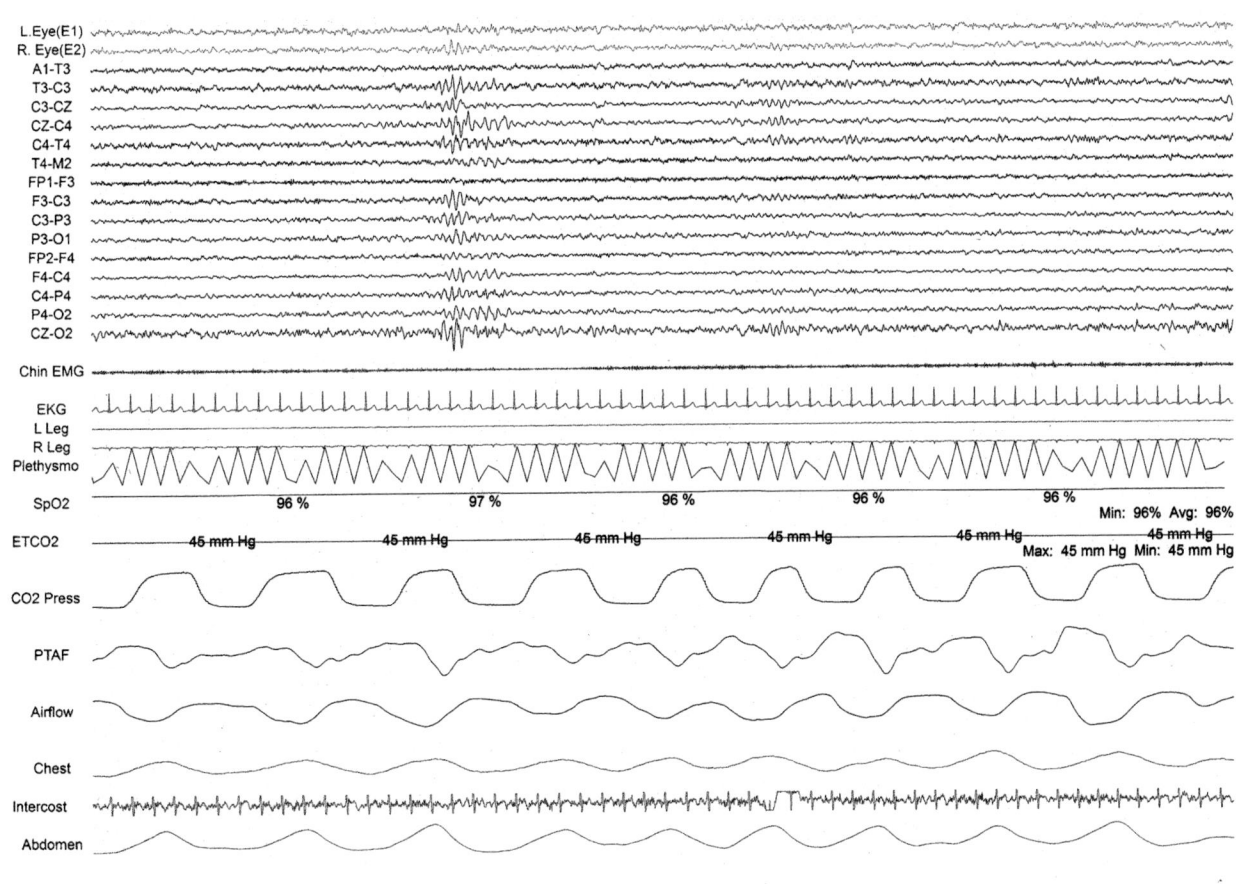

• **Fig. 56.1** Normal 4-year-old: N1. This 30-second polysomnographic segment was recorded during transitional sleep. Background electroencephalogram (EEG) rhythm has become somewhat slower and consists of mostly mixed frequency and theta activity. Alpha activity has disappeared, movements are not present, respiration has become very regular, and no conjugate eye movements can be seen. The chin muscle tone is decreased to a level lower than wakefulness but still remains tonic. At 6 years of age, a well-formed alpha rhythm at approximately 9 Hz can be demonstrated during wakefulness over the occipital region and is the posterior dominant rhythm during wakefulness. During transition this posterior dominant rhythm slows to theta frequency and ranges to approximately 5 Hz.

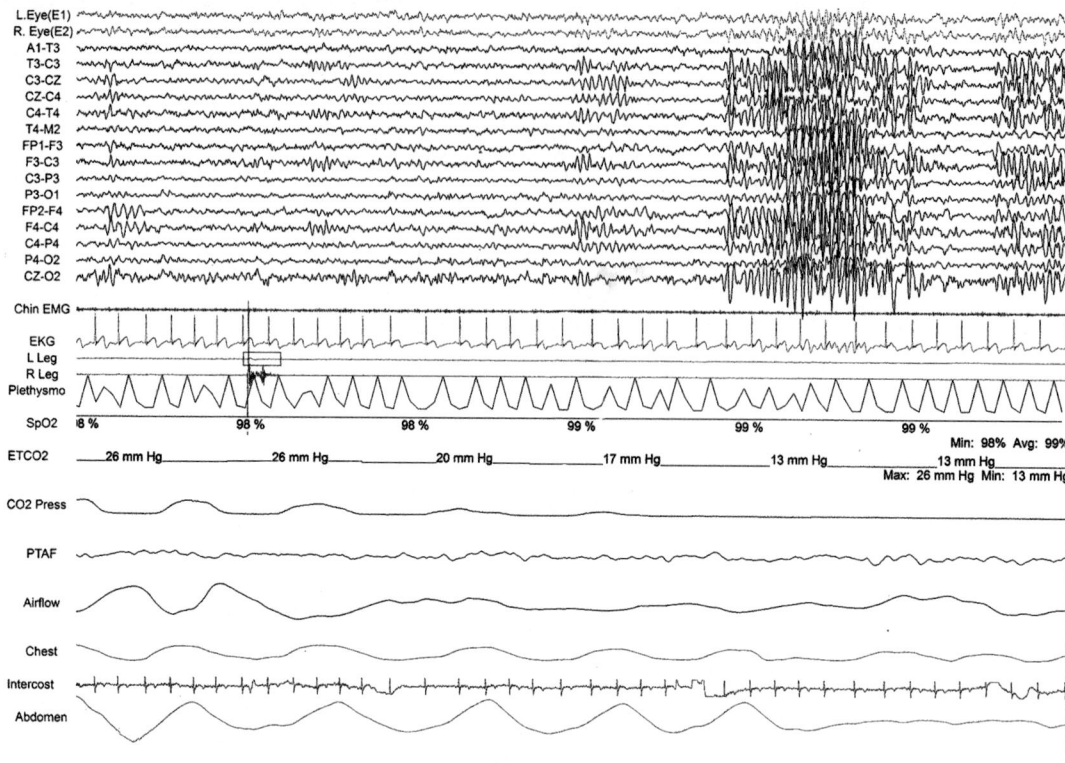

• **Fig. 56.2** Hypnagogic hypersynchrony in a 6-year-old with a history of snoring 2–3 nights per week and frequent nocturnal waking with gasps. This burst of hypersynchronous theta activity was recorded from a 6-year-old. Note the high voltage activity that is typically generalized and in the 4–6 Hz frequency range. Hypnagogic hypersynchrony is common in young children during transitional sleep as well as early non–rapid eye movement (NREM) sleep. It tends to attenuate during the second half of the recording. It sometimes can be mistaken for ictal activity. However, there is no electroencephalographic (EEG) field noted and no postictal slowing. Box identifies a limb movement in the R Leg (right anterior tibialis) channel.

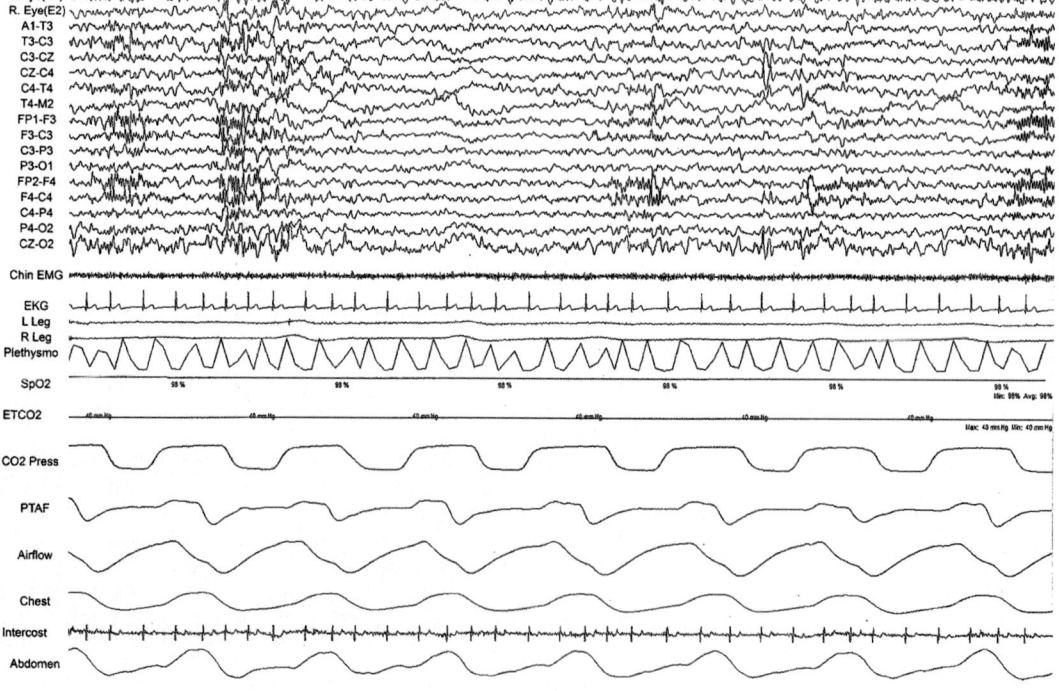

• **Fig. 56.3** Normal 4-year-old: N2. This polysomnographic segment (30 seconds) reveals clear N2 sleep in this 6-year-old. There is a relatively moderate voltage mixed frequency background with K-complexes and spindles noted. High-voltage hypersynchronous theta electroencephalographic (EEG) activity can be seen consistent with hypnagogic hypersynchrony. Respiration is regular and there is tonic chin muscle tone. No rapid eye movements can be seen in the electrooculogram (EOG).

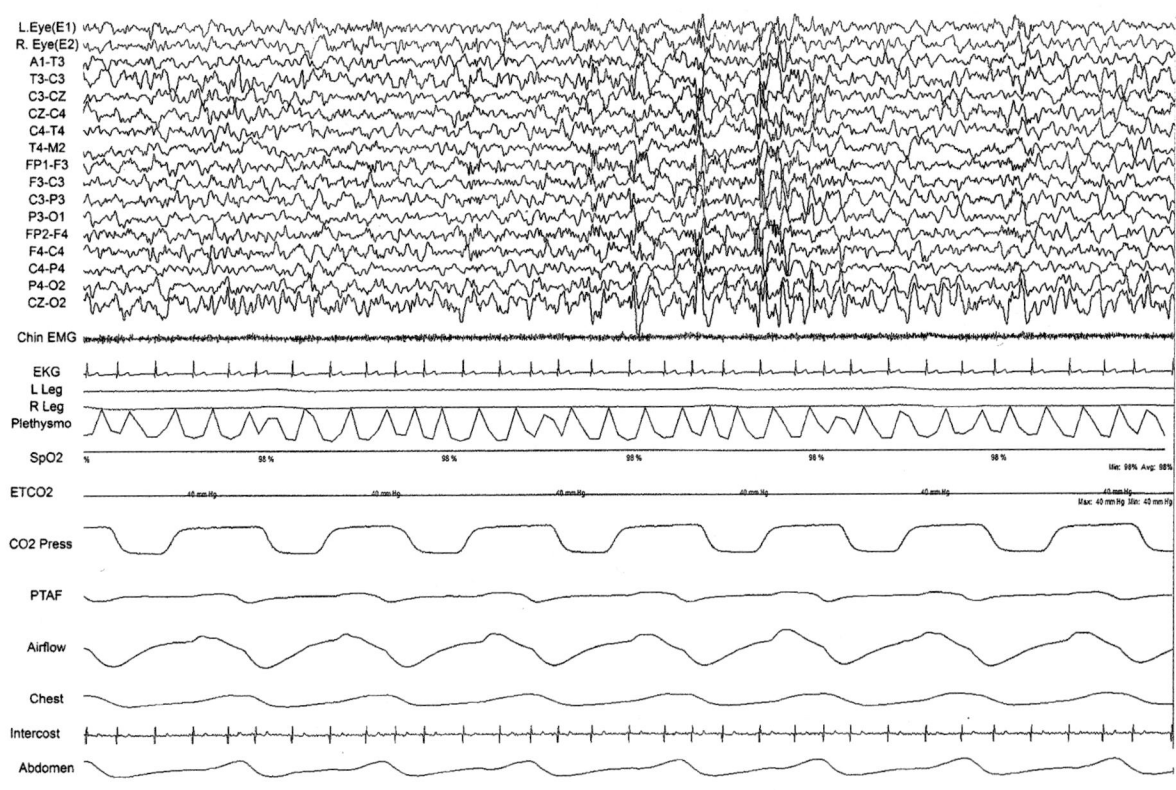

• **Fig. 56.4** Normal 4-year-old: N3. This polysomnographic segment was recorded during slow-wave sleep. The electroencephalogram (EEG) consists of very high voltage (>100 μV) activity at a frequency of about 0.5–1 Hz. In young children, moderate theta background activity superimposed on slow waves is common and normal. This theta frequency intrusion tends to resolve after 6–7 years of age. Persistence of theta intrusion (theta-delta sleep) has been noted in children with partial arousal disorders from non–rapid eye movement (NREM) sleep. Theta intrusion can make identifying N3 sleep difficult in this age group. There is normal beat-to-beat variability noted on the electrocardiogram (ECG), respiration is regular and monotonous, and no gas exchange abnormalities can be noted on this epoch.

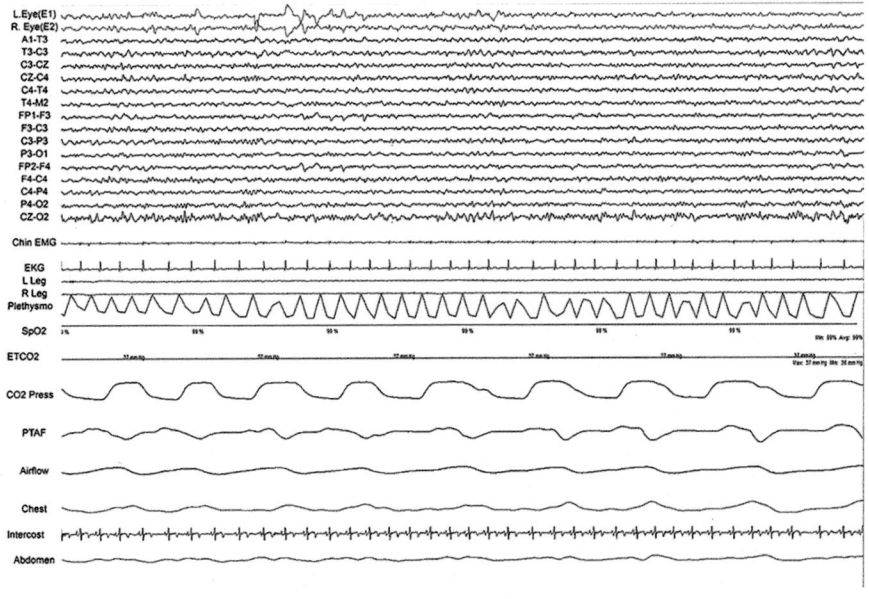

• **Fig. 56.5** Normal 4-year-old: rapid eye movement (REM). This polysomnographic segment was recorded from the same patient during REM sleep. Electroencephalogram (EEG) consists of a relatively low voltage mixed frequency background, and sawtooth waves can be seen throughout the epoch. Rapid conjugate eye movements are noted in the electrooculogram (EOG). Chin muscle tone is low and there is phasic activity noted in both the chin muscle electromyograph (EMG) and anterior tibialis EMGs. Respiration is irregular with normal oxygen saturation and normal carbon dioxide levels.

57

School-Age Children 5–10 Years Old

Stephen H. Sheldon

9-Year-Old

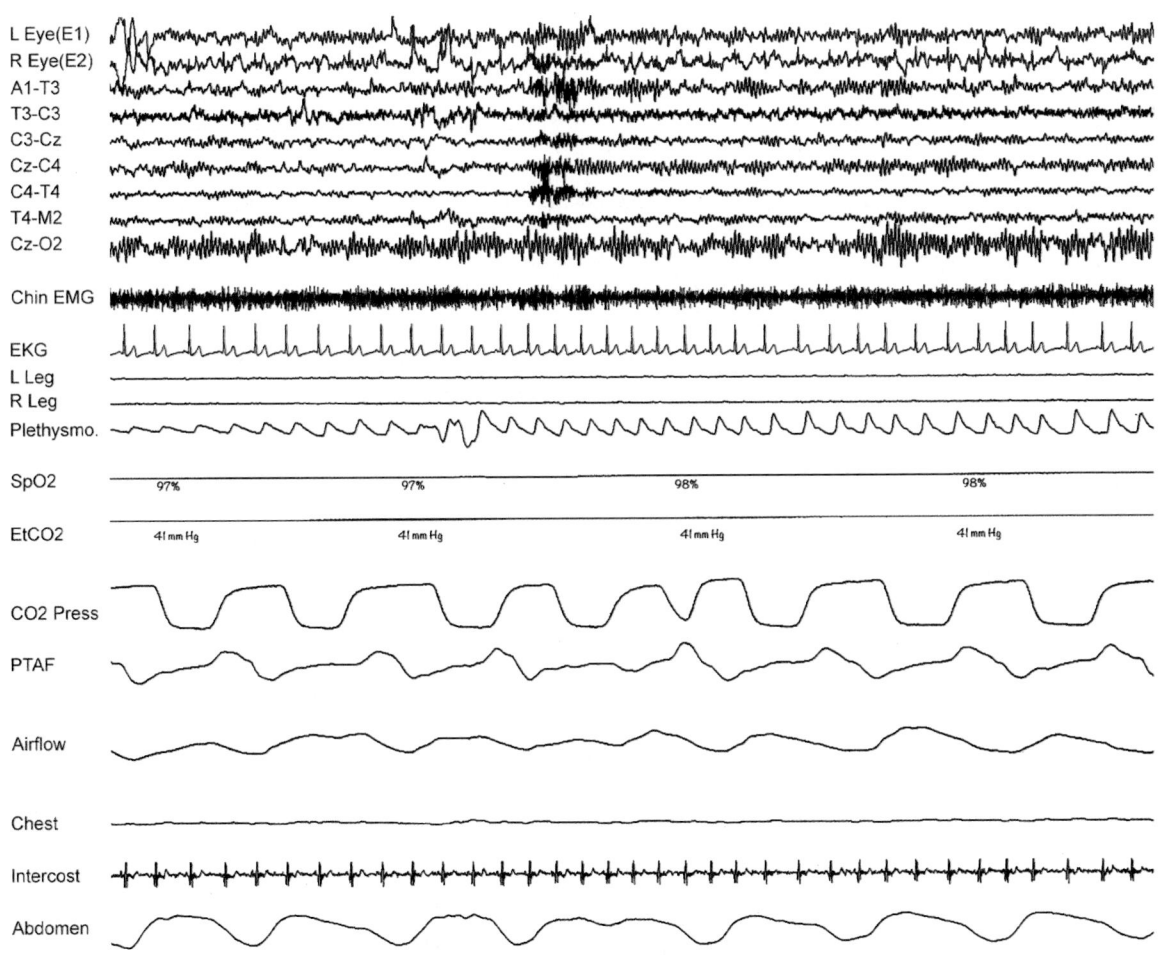

• **Fig. 57.1** 9-year-old: wake. At this age, adult polysomnographic characteristics are clearly identifiable. The American Academy of Sleep Medicine (AASM) manual of scoring sleep stages at 13 years and older may be done at the discretion of the board-certified sleep specialist. During wakefulness, eye blinks, rapid eye movements, and a posterior dominant rhythm consisting of 8–12 Hz relatively low voltage activity (alpha rhythm) is noted with the patient relaxed and eyes closed. Eye opening tends to drive the posterior dominant rhythm and low voltage and faster frequencies.

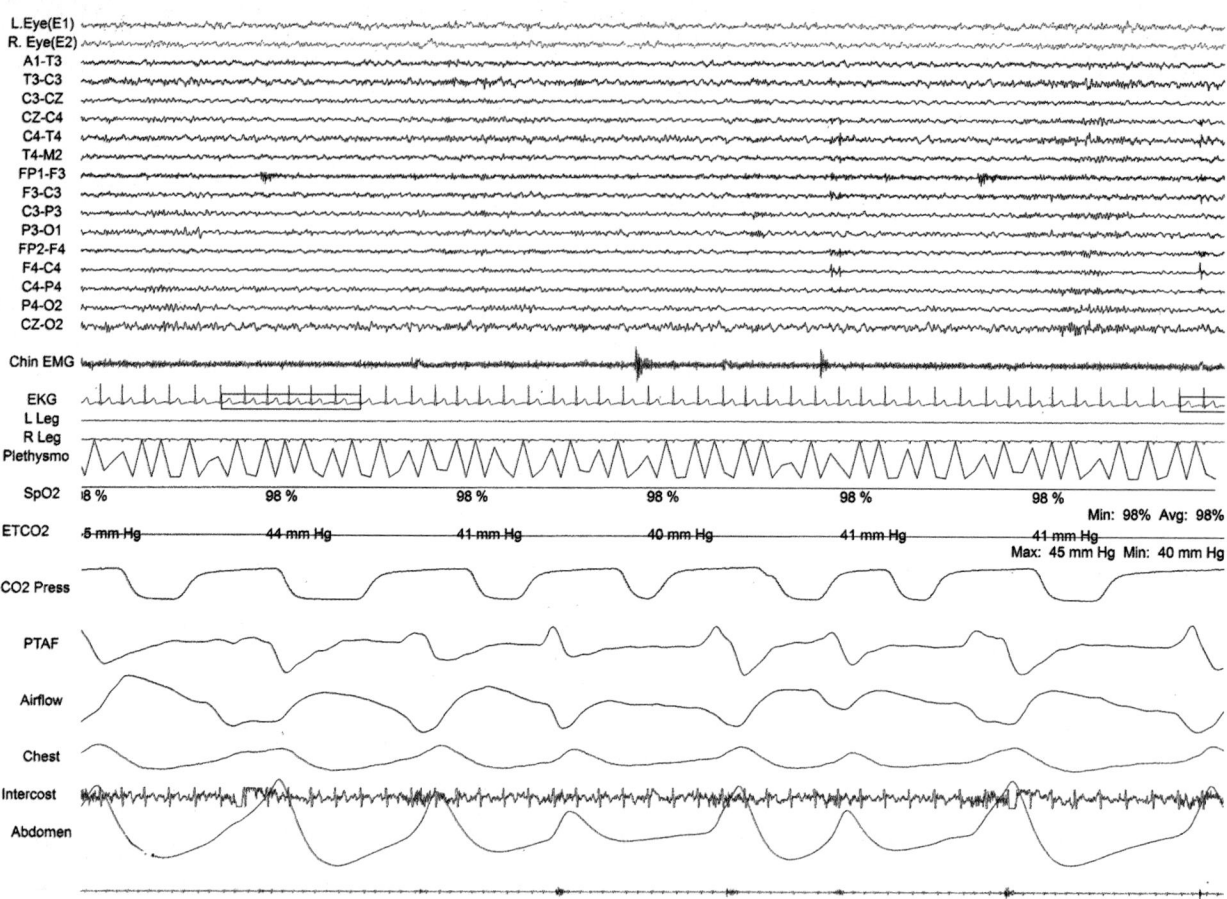

• **Fig. 57.2** Normal 9-year-old: N1. In this epoch there has been transition into N1 sleep. Eye movements have become slow and rolling, electroencephalogram (EEG) reveals a relatively low amplitude mixed frequency posterior dominant rhythm, and vertex sharp transients can be seen. Respiration is regular and monotonous, respiratory efforts become regular, and gas exchange is normal.

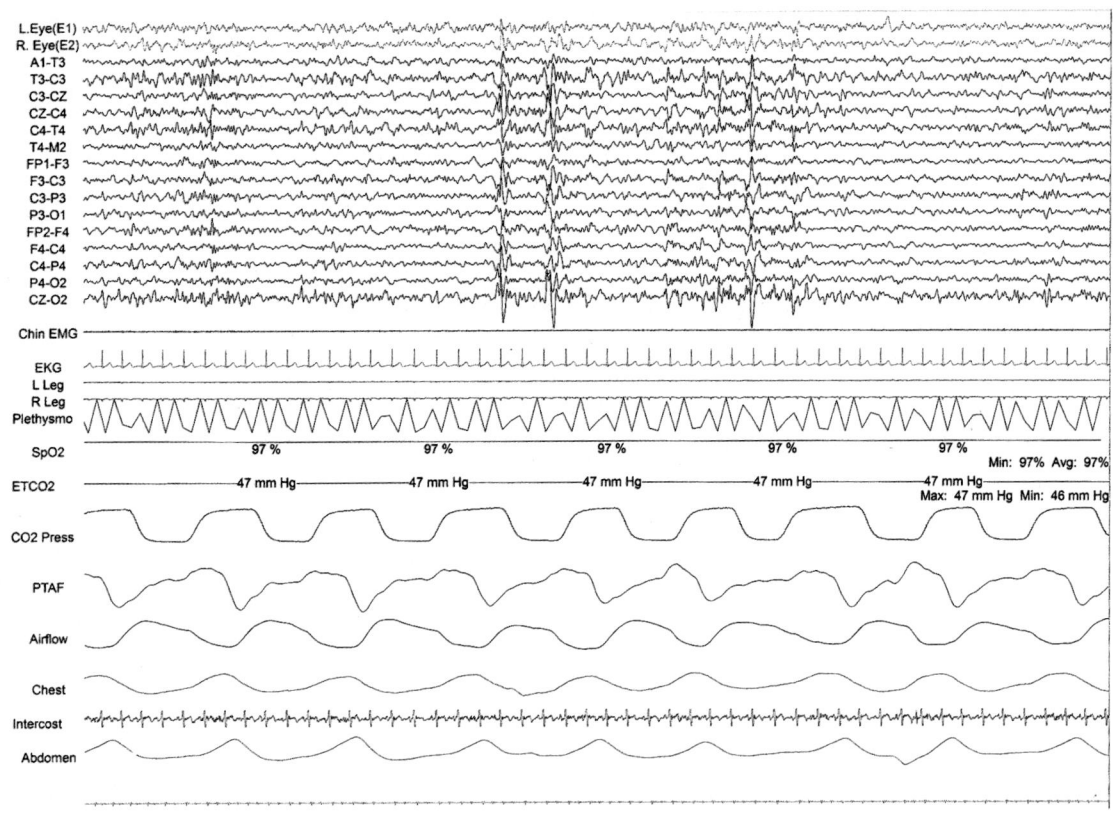

• **Fig. 57.3** Normal 9-year-old: N2. In this 30-second polysomnographic segment, the electroencephalogram (EEG) has become somewhat slower and there is a lower voltage mixed frequency background. K-complexes and sleep spindles can be seen. There is an absence of slow waves noted. Respiration is regular. Chin muscle tone is tonic, and normal respiratory sinus variation can be seen in the electrocardiogram (ECG).

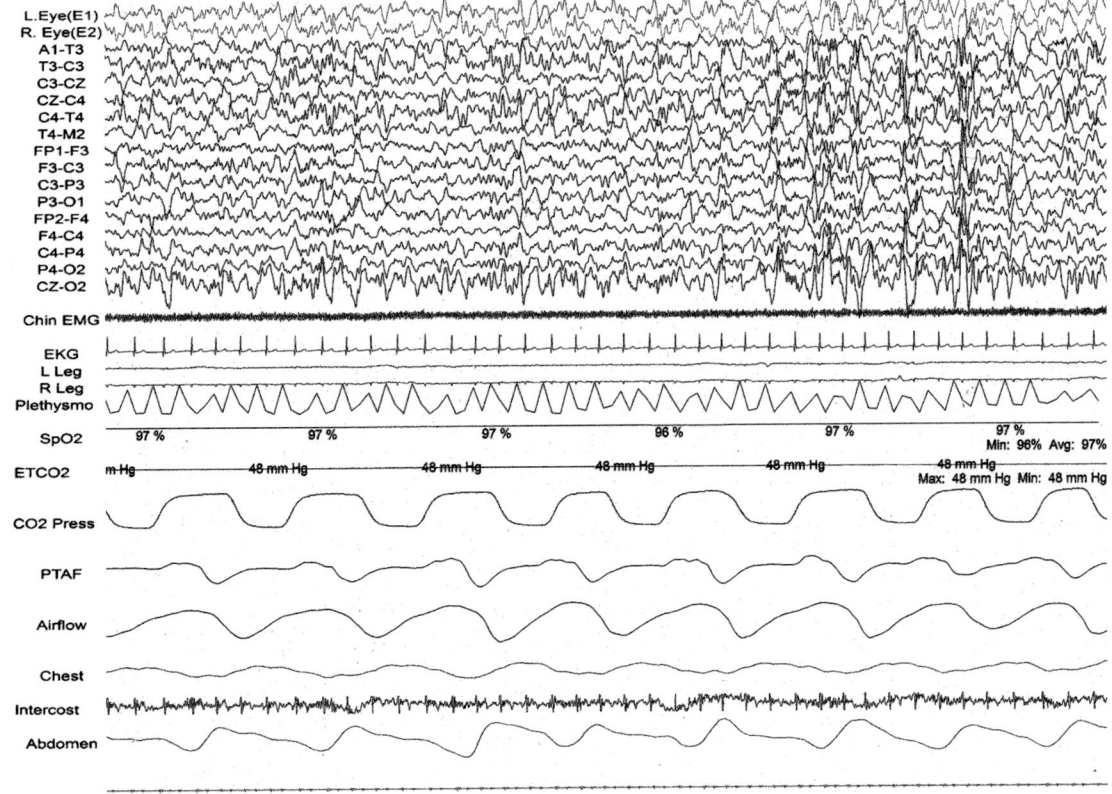

• **Fig. 57.4** Normal 9-year-old: N3. More than 50% of this polysomnographic segment is comprised of high-voltage slow waves noted with a frequency between 0.5 and 1 Hz. Spindles can still be seen; chin muscle tone remains tonic. Respirations remain regular and gas exchange is normal. There is normal respiratory sinus variation noted in the electrocardiogram (ECG).

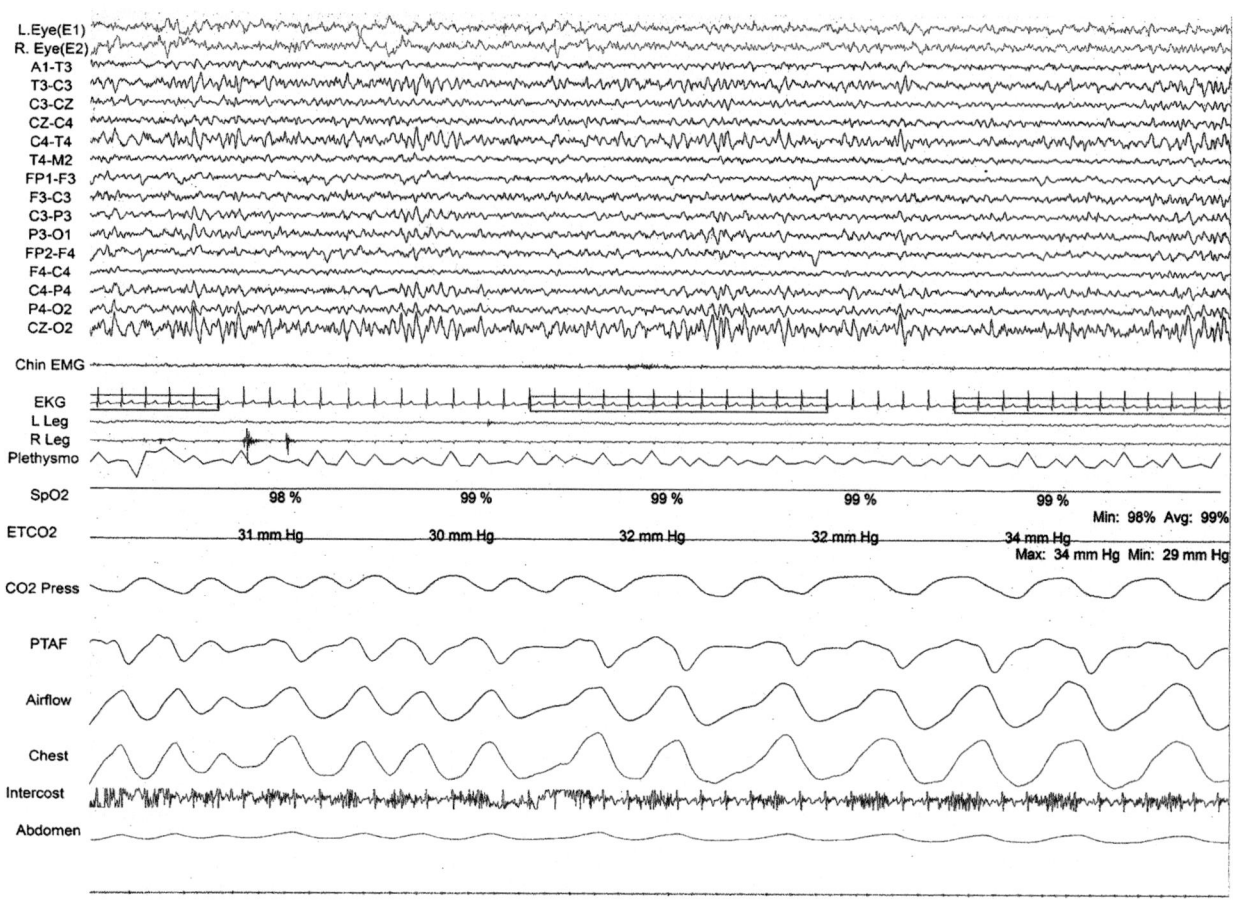

• **Fig. 57.5** Normal 9-year-old: rapid eye movement (REM). By 10 to 13 years of age, the relatively low voltage mixed frequency background is similar to adults. Chin muscle tone has decreased from levels seen in N2 and N3 sleep, phasic twitches may be noted in the chin muscle electromyogram (EMG) and limb EMGs. Notched theta activity (sawtooth waves) may be seen and respiration becomes quite irregular. This epoch is transition into REM sleep, with electroencephalogram (EEG) and EMG consistent with REM sleep, but there is still rather regular respirations. Gas exchange is normal.

Disorders

Introduction

The following polysomnographic segments are reproduced from the library of the Pediatric Sleep Medicine Center at Ann & Robert H. Lurie Children's Hospital of Chicago. Beneath each polysomnographic segment a brief history is presented. This is followed by a brief description and discussion of the recording.

Of particular note, interpretation of a pediatric polysomnogram requires comprehensive review of all epochs. Assessment of only individual epochs or pieces of segments results in an inadequate ability to confidently interpret sleep-related pathology. Presentation of complete polysomnograms is beyond the scope of this text. The interpretation is therefore based on the interpretation of the entire sleep study by the author. Complete review of the clinical history, performance of a physical examination, and comprehensive assessment of the polysomnogram, provides the best method of analysis.

To appreciate sleep-related disorders and diagnostic laboratory findings, the reader is referred to corresponding chapters in this text that provide more extensive information that will assist in evaluation and management of sleep-related disorders in infants and children.

58

Sleep-Related Breathing Disorders

STEPHEN H. SHELDON

Definitions

Obstructive Apnea

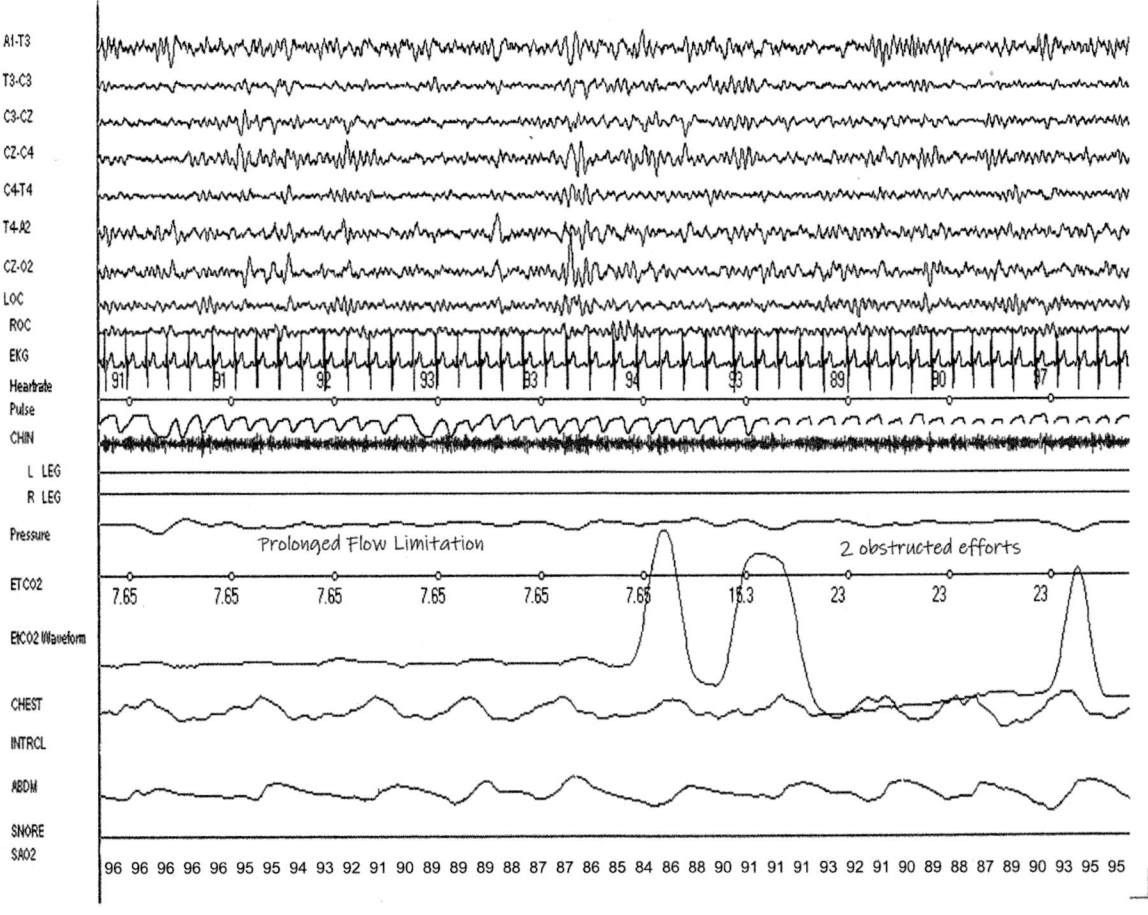

• **Fig. 58.1** This 30-second epoch was recorded from a 3-year-old in N1-N2 sleep with a history of nightly loud snoring, sleep interrupted by snorts and gasps, frequent nocturnal waking, waking feeling unrefreshed in the morning, and daytime hyperactivity alternating with fatigue and frequent napping. There was also a history of tonsillar hypertrophy (4+). Note the prolonged flow limitation during the first half of the epoch associated with paradoxical respiratory efforts and arousal. The subsequent event also meets criteria for obstructive apnea with two obstructed respiratory efforts. There was subsequent arousal and fall in oxygen saturation by >4% from the baseline. For a respiratory event to be identified as an *obstructive apnea* the following criteria must be met: 1. a drop in peak signal excursion (by 90% or greater) of the pre-event baseline using oronasal thermistor or alternative apnea thermistor, 2. duration of the (at least 90%) drop in flow signal lasts at least two breaths, 3. it is associated with a continued respiratory effort.

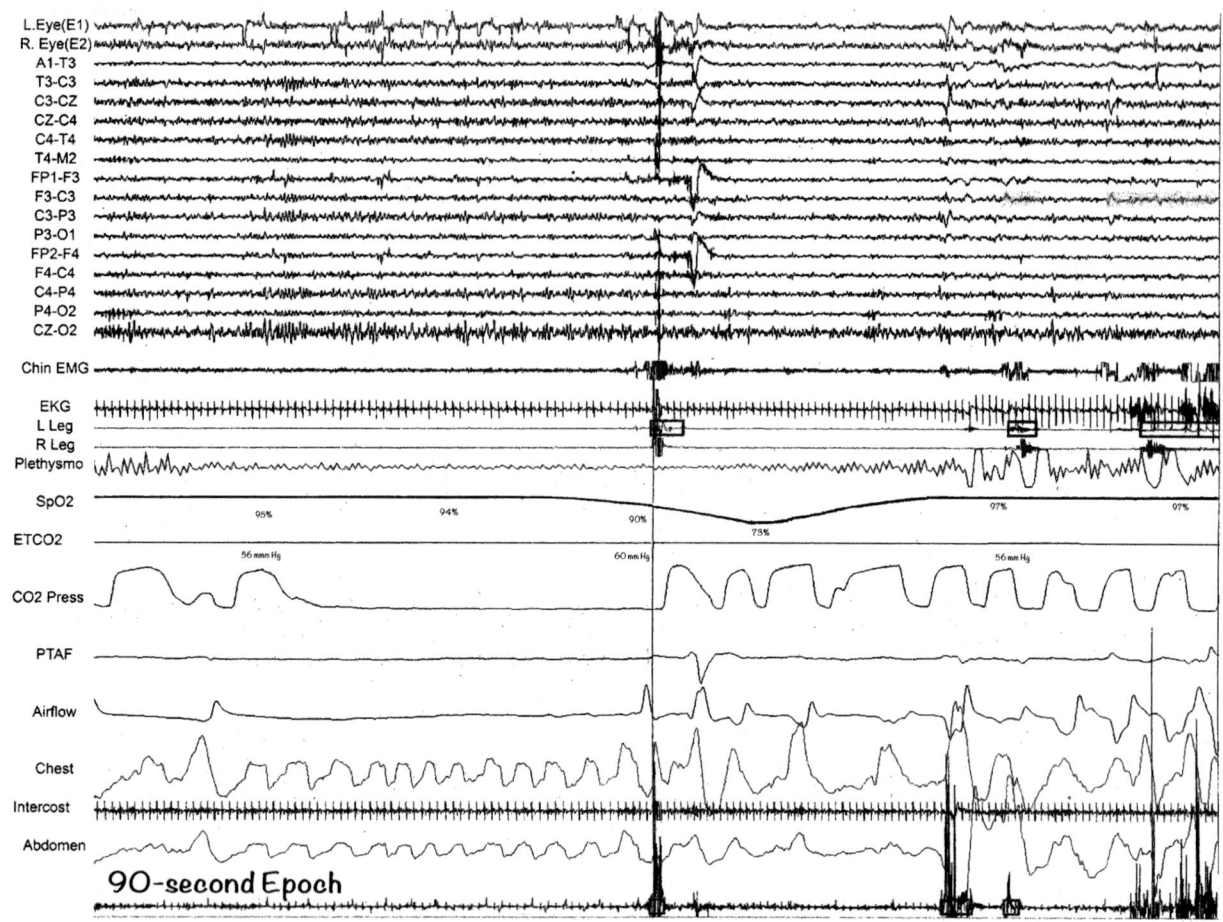

• Fig. 58.2 This is a 90-second recording of an obstructive apnea recorded during rapid eye movement (REM) sleep in a 4-year-old female with complaints of frequent nocturnal waking, daytime hyperactivity, behavior problems, and habitual snoring. Note absence of airflow in all three airflow channels (ETCO$_2$, pressure/PTAF, and thermal/airflow). Flow limitation is greater than 90% from the baseline in all three channels and there is continued respiratory effort. Oxygen saturation falls to a nadir of 73% with recovery after the arousal. Of particular note is the change in respiratory effort with increased respiratory rate and increase in effort as the obstructed event continues. These boxes represent limb movements associated with arousals.

Mixed Apnea

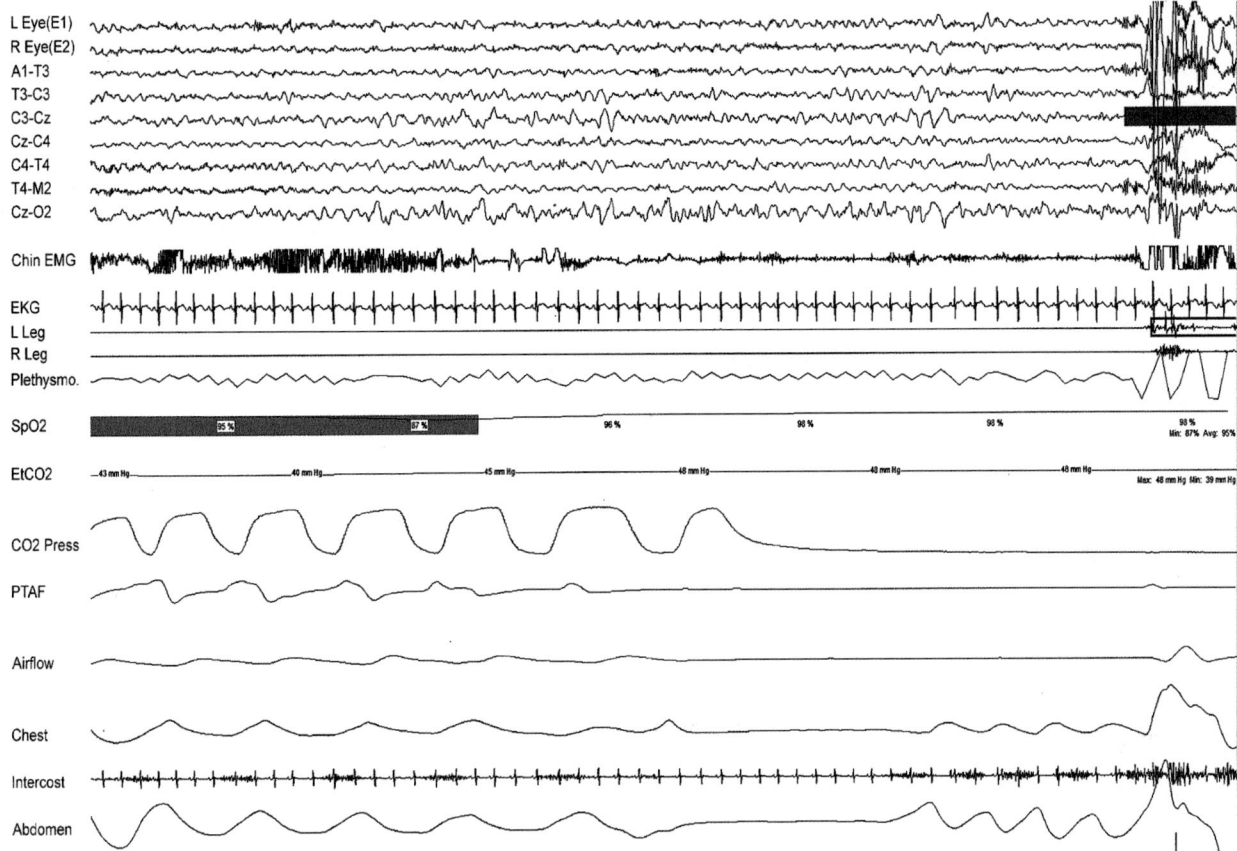

• **Fig. 58.3** This 30-second segment was recorded from a 4-year-old during rapid eye movement (REM) sleep. The parents reported a history of habitual snoring, restless sleep, and frequent nocturnal waking. It is characteristic of a mixed apnea. This event meets criteria for a pause lasting at least two baseline breaths and absence of respiratory efforts during the first half of the event, with resumption of respiratory efforts without resumption of airflow during the latter portion of the event. Interesting, the AASM scoring manual notes that mixed apneas should be scored in children (but not adults) regardless of whether the central or obstructive portion of the event comes first. Red box denotes oxygen desaturation.

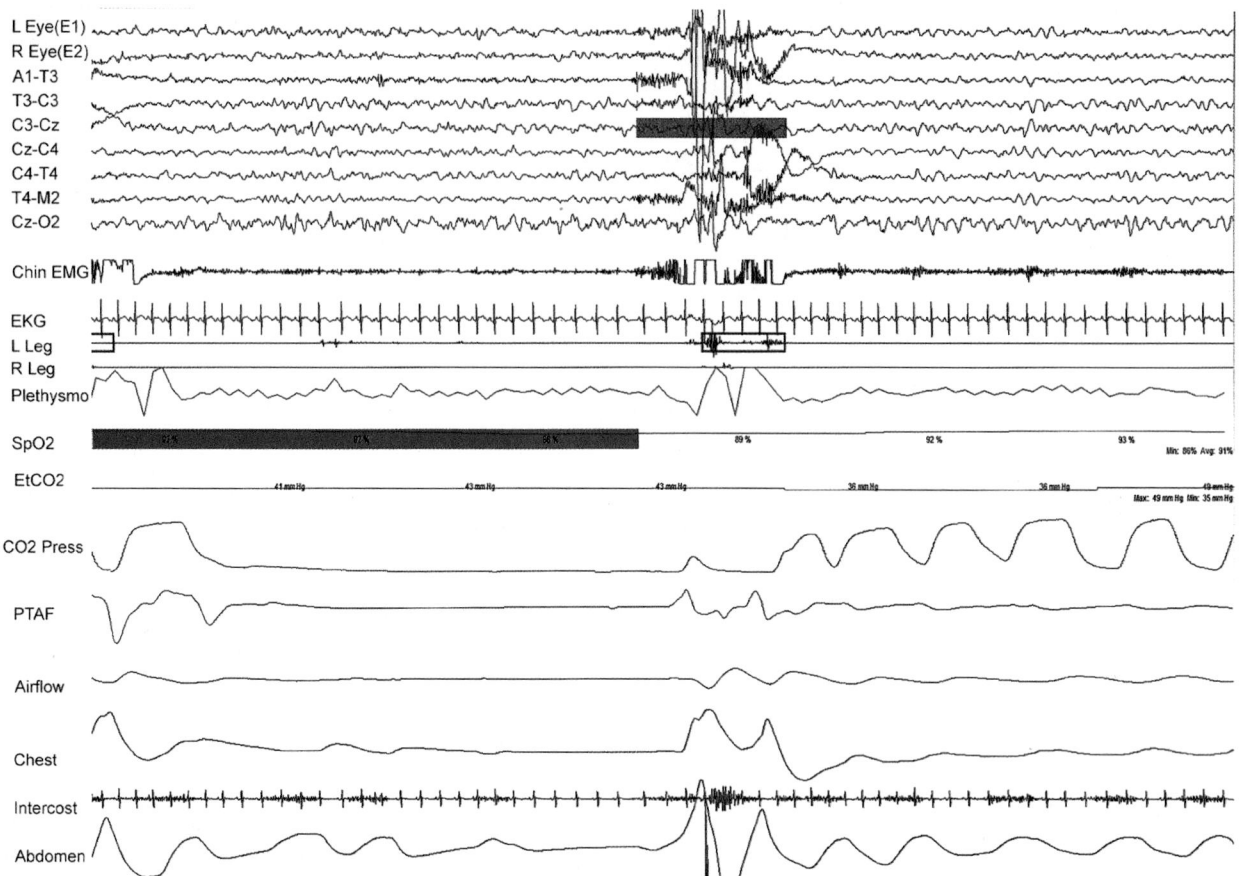

• **Fig. 58.4** This 30-second epoch was also recorded from the patient depicted in Fig. 58.3. Score an apnea as mixed if it meets apnea criteria for at least the duration of 2 breaths during baseline breathing AND is associated with absent respiratory effort during one portion of the event AND the presence of inspiratory effort in another portion, regardless of which portion comes first. As depicted in this figure, the absence of respiratory effort may occur at the end of the event as well as the beginning of the event. Blue box denotes an arousal. Red box denotes oxygen desaturation. Clear box denotes limb movement.

HYPOPNEAS

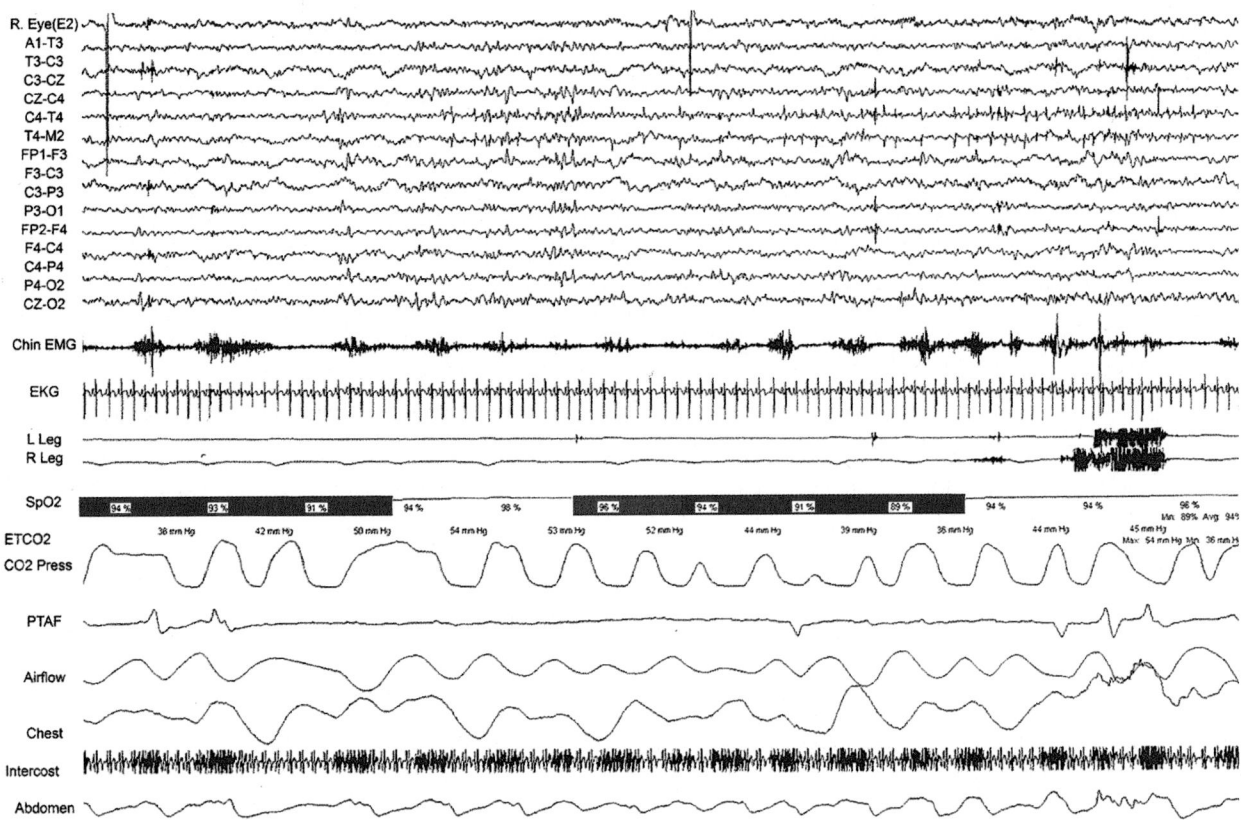

• **Fig. 58.5** This 60-second polysomnographic (PSG) segment was recorded from a 3-year-old with a history of worsening snoring following an adenoidectomy. Symptoms included nightly loud snoring, restless sleep, mouth breathing, restless sleep, screaming during sleep, and reported nightmares. There is flow limitation noted with ≥30% fall in the nasal pressure signal as well as ≥30% fall from the baseline airflow (thermal) signal with continued respiratory efforts noted in the chest and abdomen. There is also continued intercostal electromyographic (EMG) activity present. Note change in shape of the $ETCO_2$ waveform with loss of a clearly defined alveolar plateau prior to decrease in the amplitude of the waveform. Additionally, there is a fall in oxygen saturation 9% from the baseline (≥3% fall from the pre-event baseline required for hypopnea). The event is followed by an arousal. According to the American Academy of Sleep Medicine (AASM), the hypopneas should be scored if any of the following criteria are met a) snoring b) increased respiratory flattening of nasal pressure or PAP device flow signal c) there is associated thoracoabdominal paradox during the event but not prior to it. If these findings are not present, the event may be classified as obstructive hypopnea. In this segment, there is continued snoring and some change in phase angle between the chest and abdomen.

Central Apnea

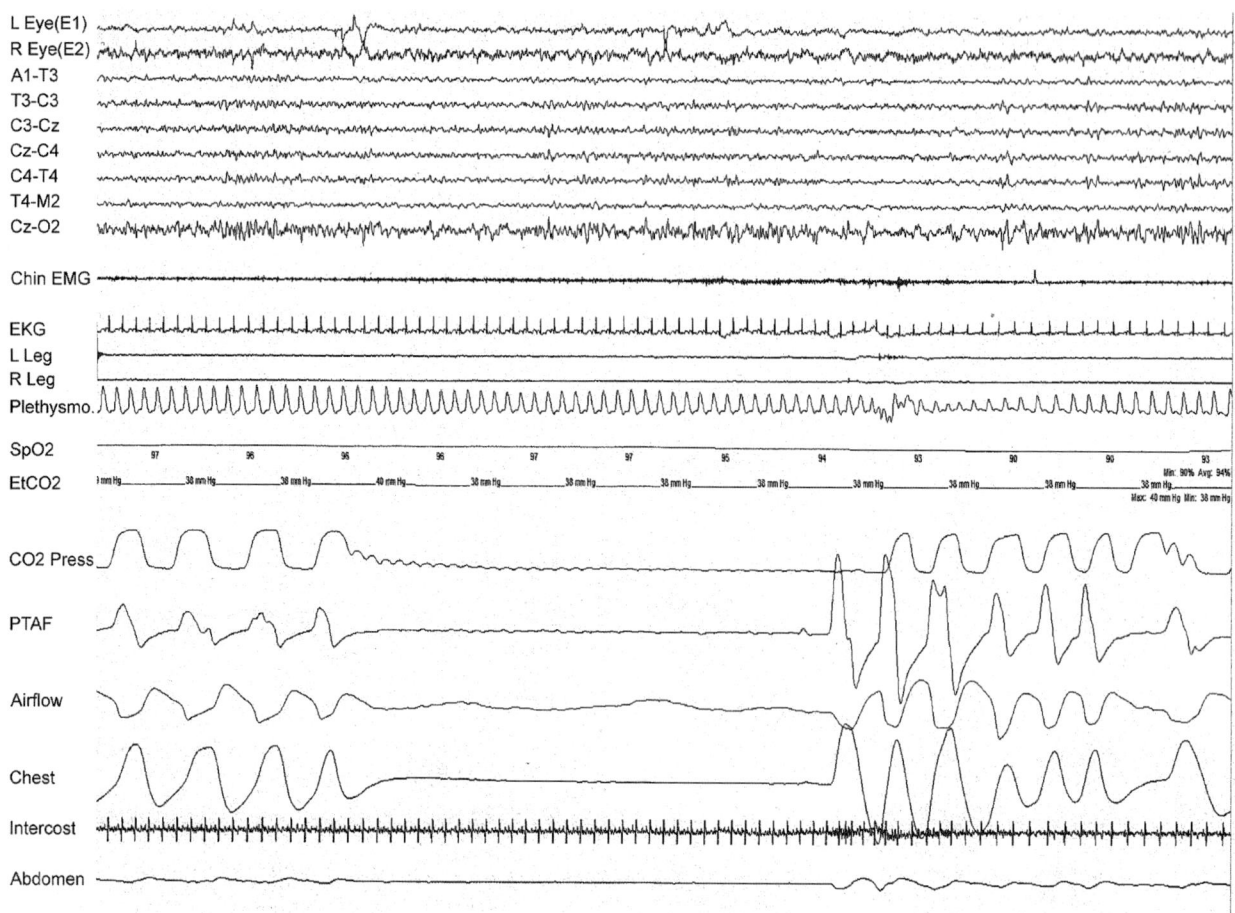

• **Fig. 58.6** This 30-second segment was recorded from a 7-year-old with a history of meningomyelocele, ventriculoperitoneal shunt, and hypotonia. There was concern of shunt malfunction and parents reported noted prolonged respiratory pauses. There was also some snoring followed by arousals noted. This respiratory event depicts a prolonged central apnea, lasting approximately 22 seconds. It is identified by the absence of both chest and abdominal respiratory effort, and absent airflow as recorded by the ETCO$_2$ waveform, airflow by thermistor, and pressure (pressure transduction). Because of the length of the event (>20 seconds), it was scored as central apnea despite no oxygen desaturation (≥3% from the pre-event baseline). Additionally, there is an associated arousal and notable cardiac deceleration during the event.

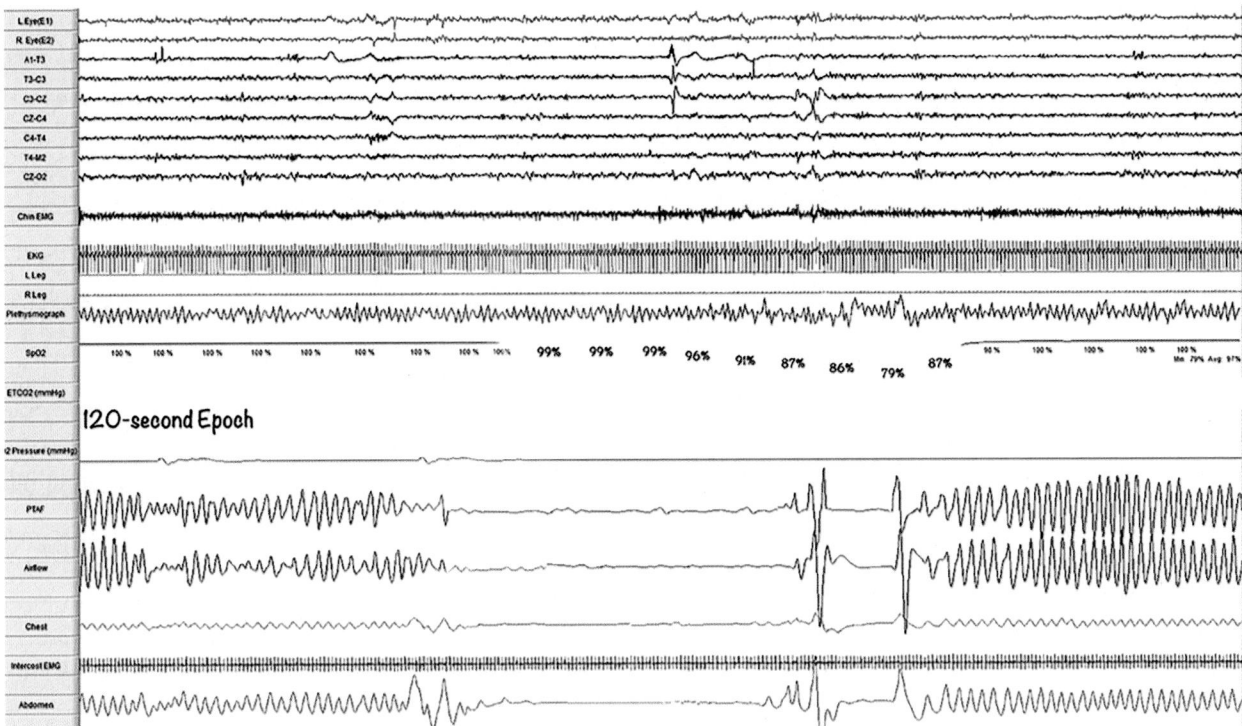

• Fig. 58.7 This 120-second polysomnographic (PSG) segment was recorded from a 6-week-old infant. It demonstrates an extended period of cessation of respiratory effort and airflow as measured by pressure transduction and thermistry. The event lasts about 33 seconds, and there are a few recovery breaths followed by a second briefer central respiratory pause. An arousal can be seen in the electroencephalogram (EEG) and chin muscle electromyogram (EMG) and oxygen desaturation into the high 70s is noted. Little to no significant cardiac deceleration was noted, even with the prolonged central apnea. A diagnosis of primary central sleep apnea of infancy was made based on the frequent presence of respiratory events such as these.

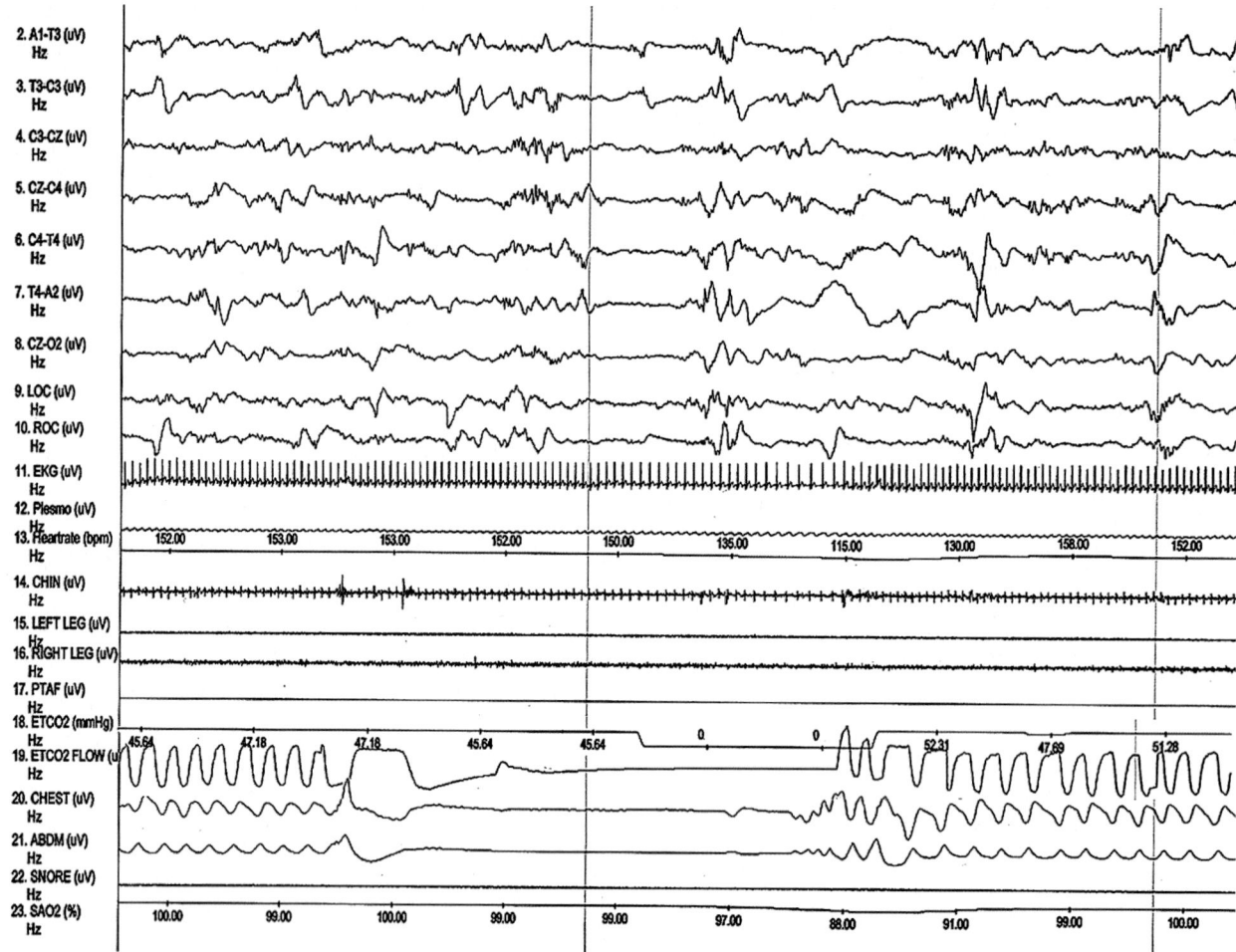

• **Fig. 58.8** This 30-second epoch was recorded from a 3-day-old infant in non–rapid eye movement (NREM) sleep who was experiencing unexplained episodes of bradycardia in the newborn nursery. Note cardiac deceleration associated with the event. The slowest heart rate (longest R-R interval) occurs during the second half to final third of the recording. Oxygen saturation falls from 100% to a nadir of 88% with rapid recovery to baseline. Also noted was an electroencephalographic (EEG) pattern of *tracé alternant* pattern characteristic of NREM sleep in a newborn infant.

Respiratory Effort–Related Arousals (RERAS)

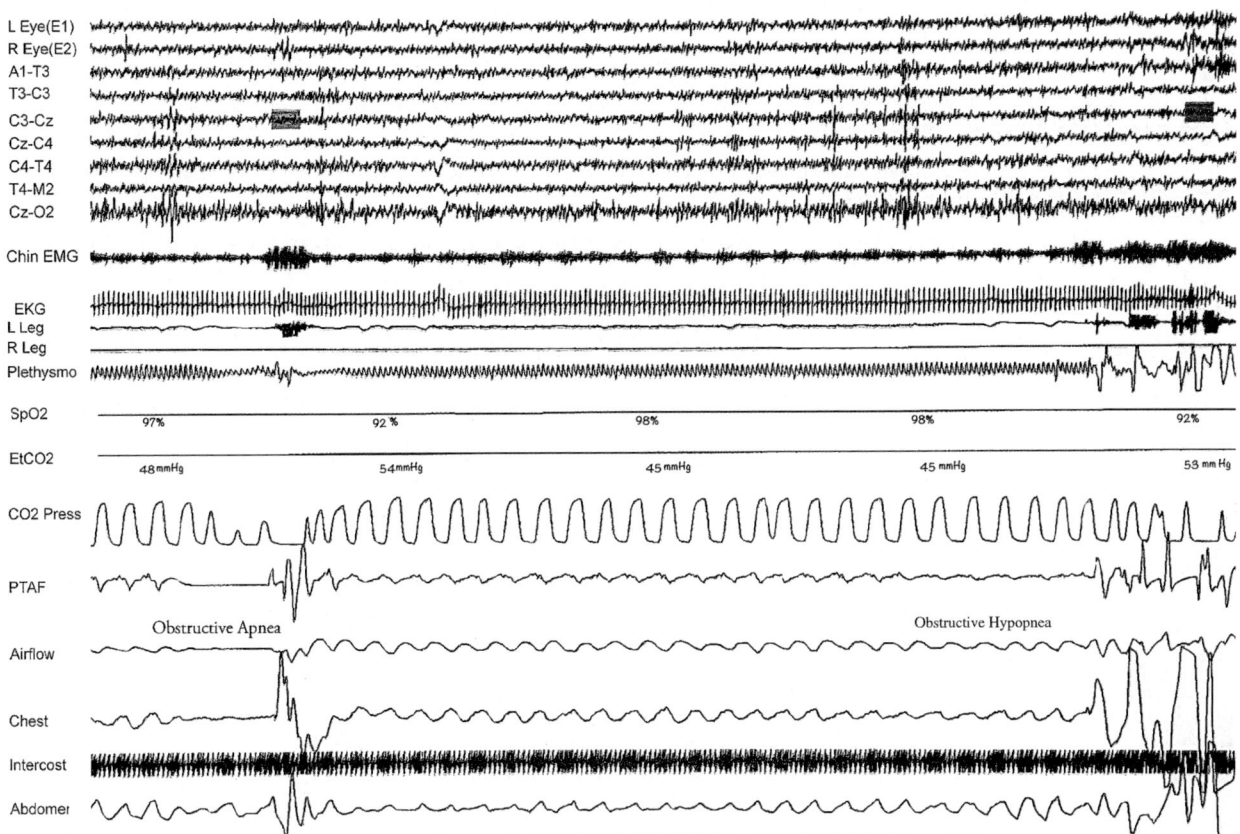

• **Fig. 58.9** This 120-second epoch was recorded from a 5-year-old with a history of habitual loud snoring, noted respiratory pauses, and increased work of breathing during sleep. A clearly defined obstructive aopnea is noted during the beginning of the epoch (marked). There is flattening of the pressure tracing (PTAF) and airflow (thermal) tracing with continued respiratory efforts throughout the event (mostly noted in the abdominal effort belt and intercostal electromyogram [EMG]). There is change in shape of the end-tidal CO_2 tracing followed by diminution of the signal, representing loss of alveolar plateau and the measurement of carbon dioxide from dead-space air. Additionally, there is oxygen desaturation at least 3% from the baseline and arousal. A hypopnea is noted at the end of the event. There is some limitation of airflow noted in the pressure channel, there is continued increasing respiratory efforts, loss of alveolar plateau on $ETCO_2$ tracing, and an arousal follows. Green box denotes arousal from respiratory event. Red box denotes movement arousal.

Obstructive Hypoventilation

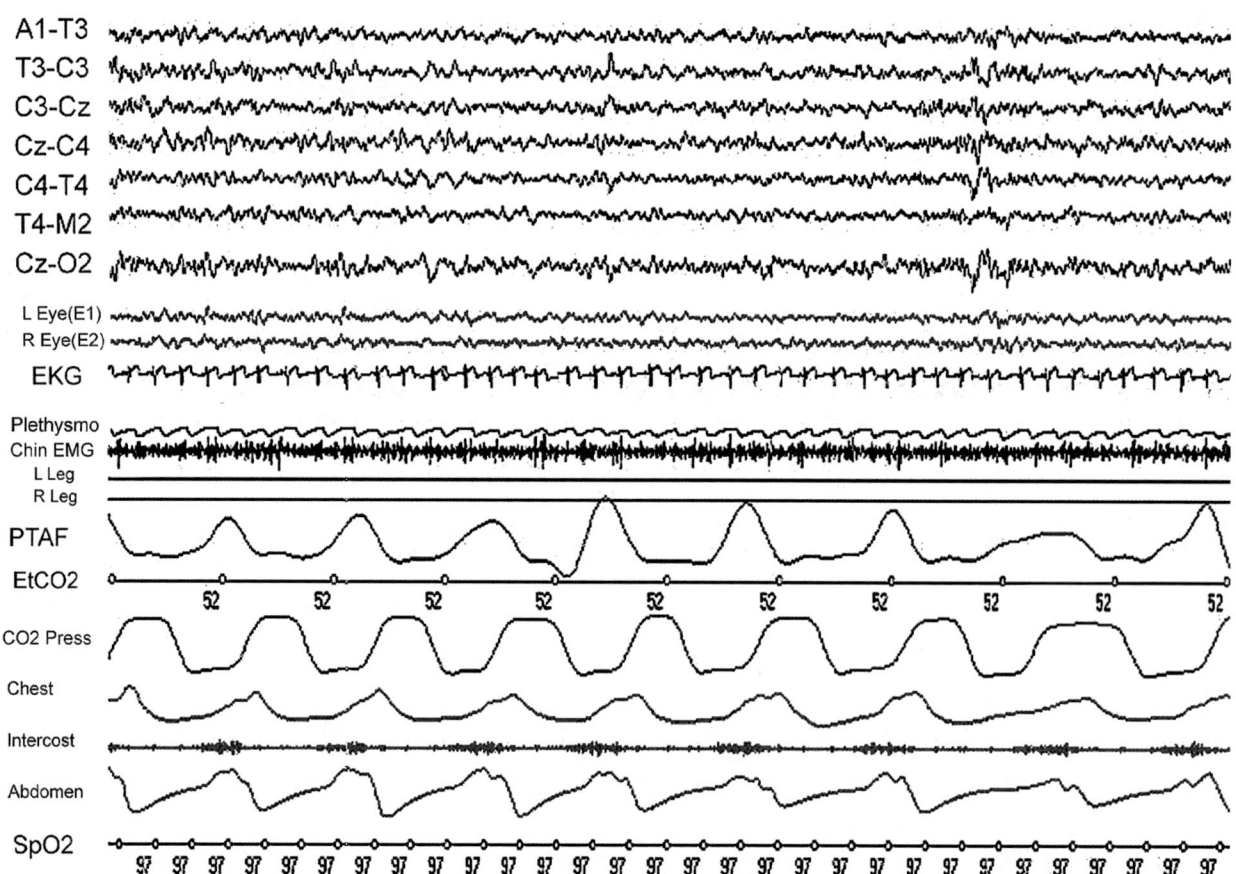

• **Fig. 58.10** This 30-second N2 segment was recorded from a 9-year-old with a history of nightly snoring, restless sleep, nightmares, sleepwalking, secondary enuresis, school learning difficulties, and excessive daytime sleepiness. He naps daily and will fall asleep in school. He has significant difficulty paying attention in school, often forgets his homework, and his grades in school have gone from As and Bs to Ds and Fs. There is no underlying pulmonary disease. In this epoch, there is no discernable evidence of airflow limitation, apneas, or hypopneas. Respiration is quite regular. Some vibratory snore artifact can be noted in the chin muscle electromyogram (EMG). Oxygen saturation baseline is 97%. Of particular note, $ETCO_2$ is >50 mm Hg for the entirety of this segment and remained >50 mm Hg for 38% of the total sleep time. This was confirmed by continuous transcutaneous monitoring of carbon dioxide. Obstructive hypoventilation is part of the continuum of pediatric obstructive sleep apnea and is present when carbon dioxide (as measured by $ETCO_2$ or $TcpCO_2$) remains >50 mm Hg for more than 25% of the total sleep time.

Periodic Breathing

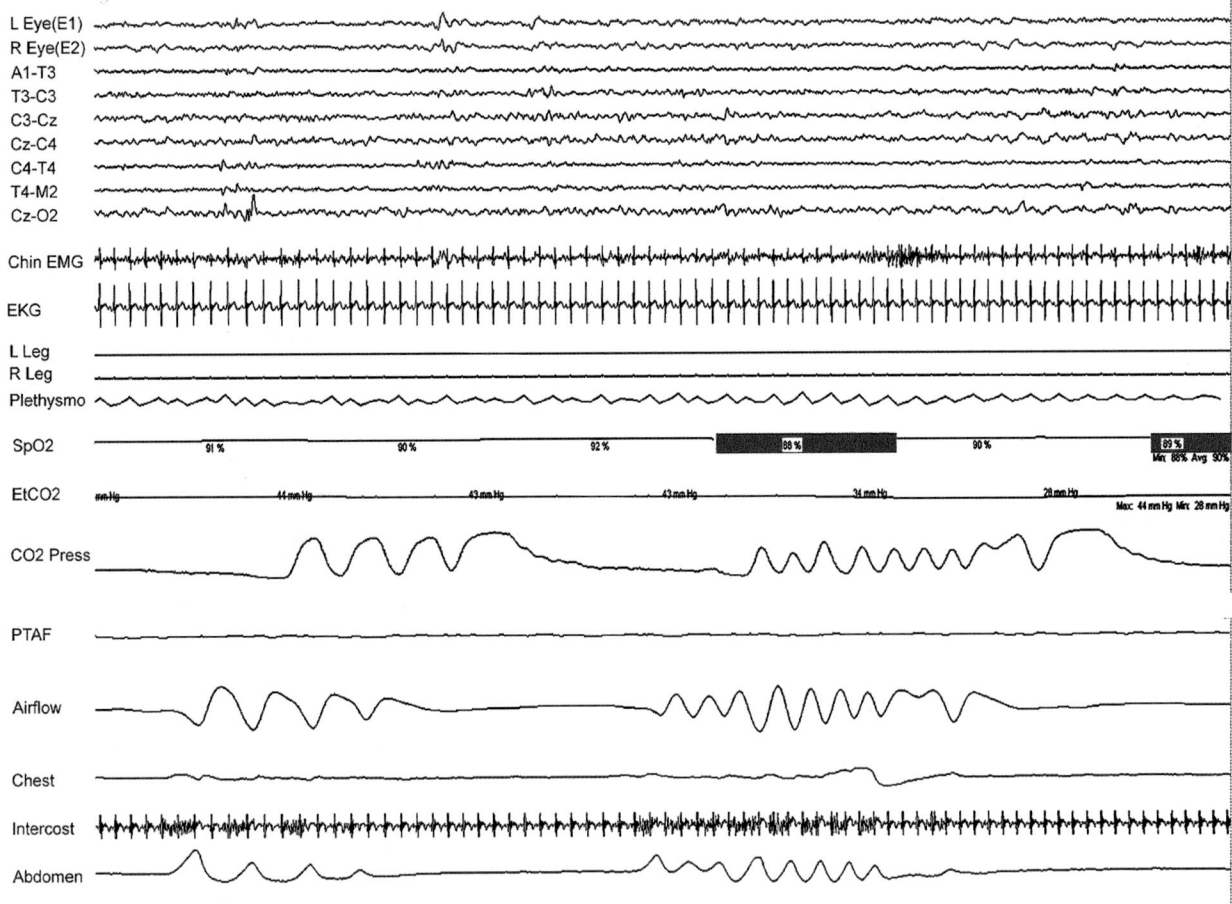

• **Fig. 58.11** This 30-second N2 epoch was recorded from a 10-year-old with a history of spina bifida, hydrocephalus, ventriculoperitoneal shunt, and Chiari II malformation. There had been episodes of nausea and sleeplessness associated with increasing daytime fatigue. Note central respiratory pauses that last approximately 10–12 seconds and about 7–10 seconds of normal breathing between pauses. There is also associated periodic oxygen desaturation >3% from the baseline with recovery when breathing resumes. These findings are likely consistent with periodic breathing. Yellow boxes denote oxygen desaturation.

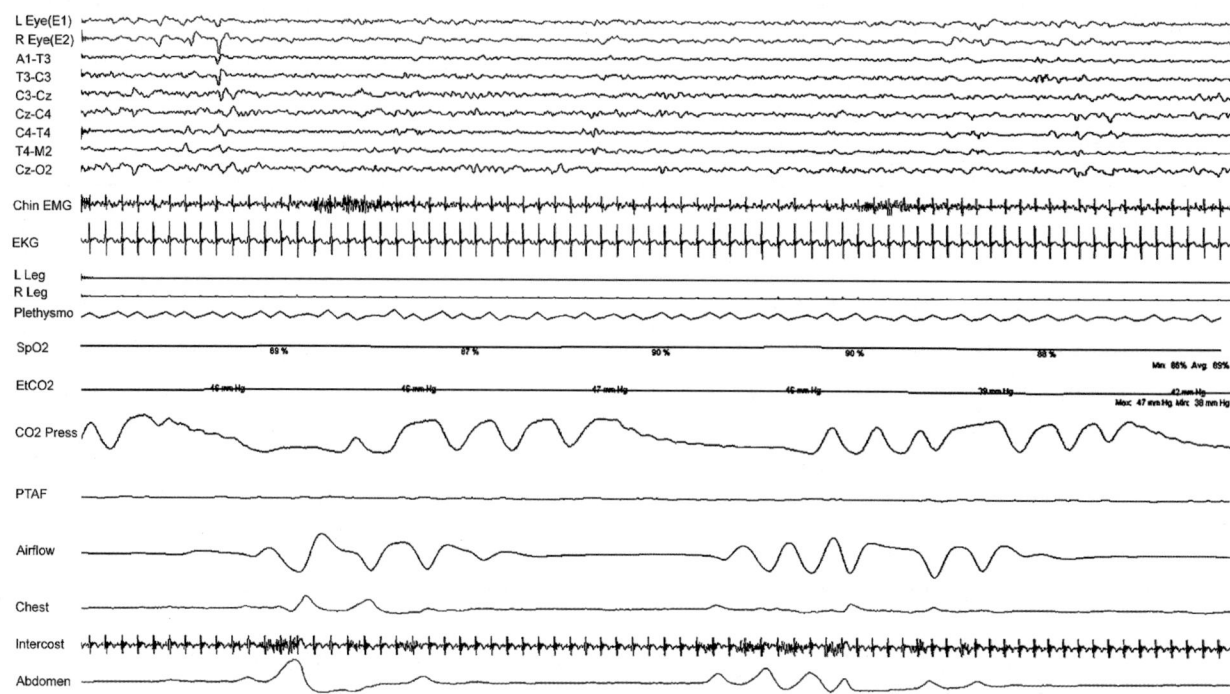

• **Fig. 58.12** This 30-second segment was recorded from the previous patient, and periodic respiratory pauses separated by normal breathing were also noted in N2 sleep.

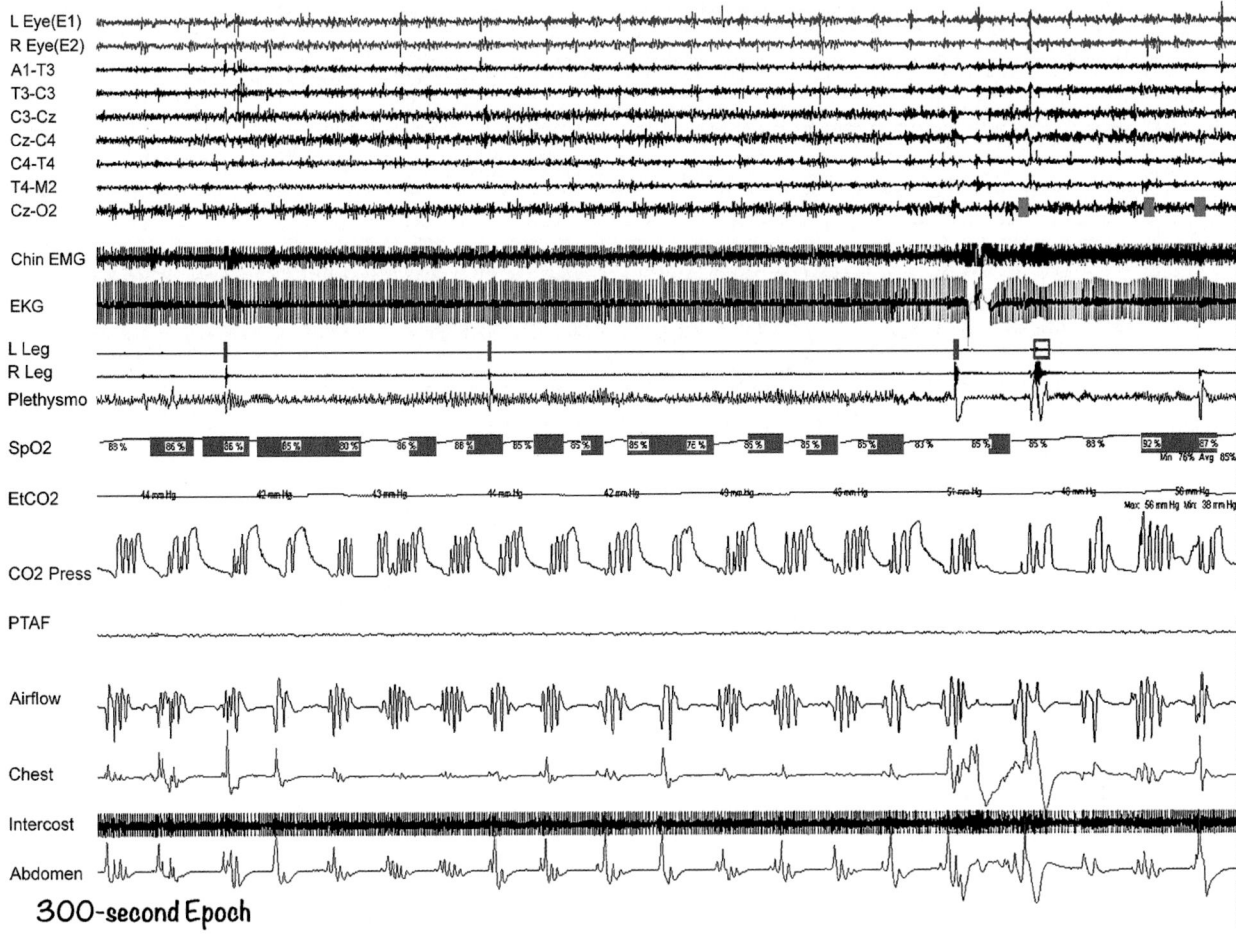

300-second Epoch

• **Fig. 58.13** This 300-second segment comes from the same patient as that in Figs. 58.11 and 58.12. It demonstrates periodic respiratory pauses that are >3 seconds in length separated by ≤20 seconds of normal breathing. This pattern of respiration is consistent with periodic breathing. Periodic breathing may be normal in premature and term infants, but typically occupies less than 5% of the total sleep time. It is an abnormal finding in older children that requires further significant diagnostic considerations. In this patient, malfunction of the ventriculoperitoneal shunt was identified. The shunt was replaced and follow-up polysomnography revealed resolution of the periodic breathing. Yellow boxes denote oxygen desaturations.

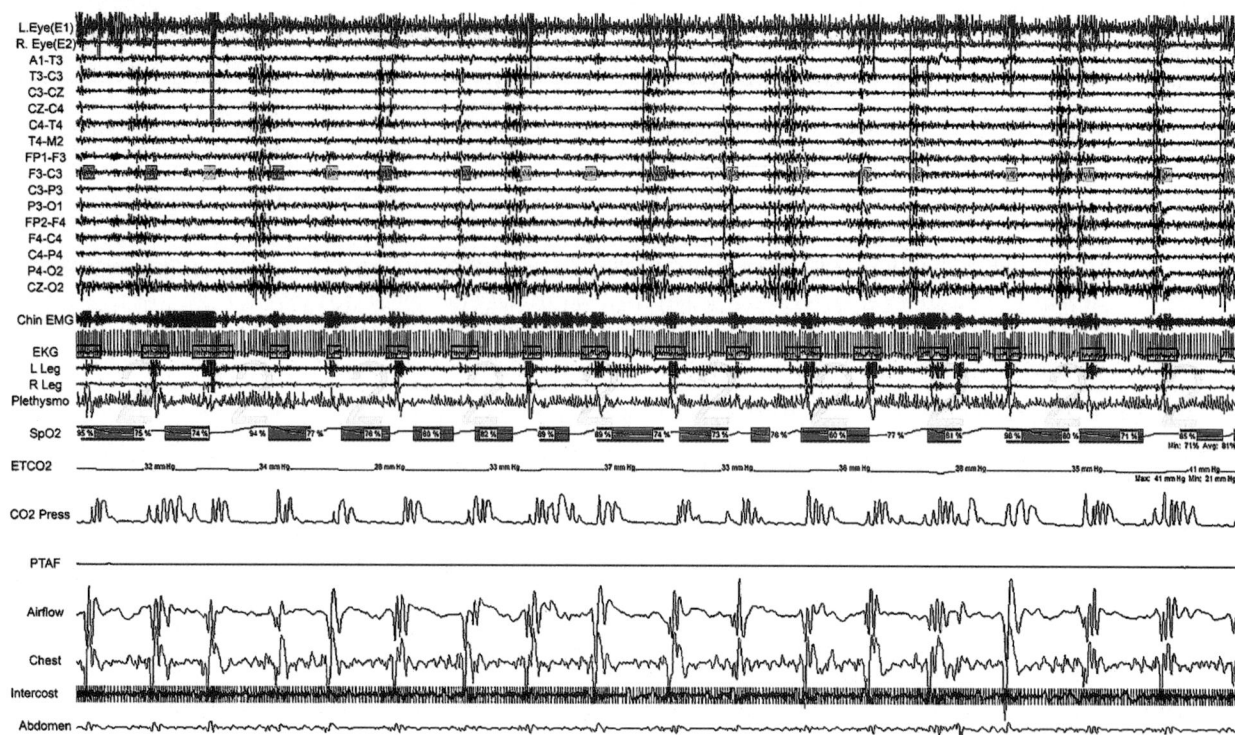

• **Fig. 58.14** This is a 300-second polysomnographic segment from an 11-year-old with a history of habitual loud snoring, restless, sleep, worsening attention problems, and increasing daytime sleepiness. Physical examination was significant for 3+ tonsillar hypertrophy, arched and elongated palate, and nasal speech, suggesting adenoidal hypertrophy. There are very frequent to almost continuous obstructive apneas with absent airflow demonstrated in the $ETCO_2$ channel and thermal channel with continued respiratory effort in chest, abdominal, and intercostal channels. There are arousals, sleep fragmentation, and significant periodic oxygen desaturation to a nadir of 71% with rapid and spontaneous return to baseline during recovery breaths. An adenotonsillectomy was performed. Red boxes denote oxygen desaturation.

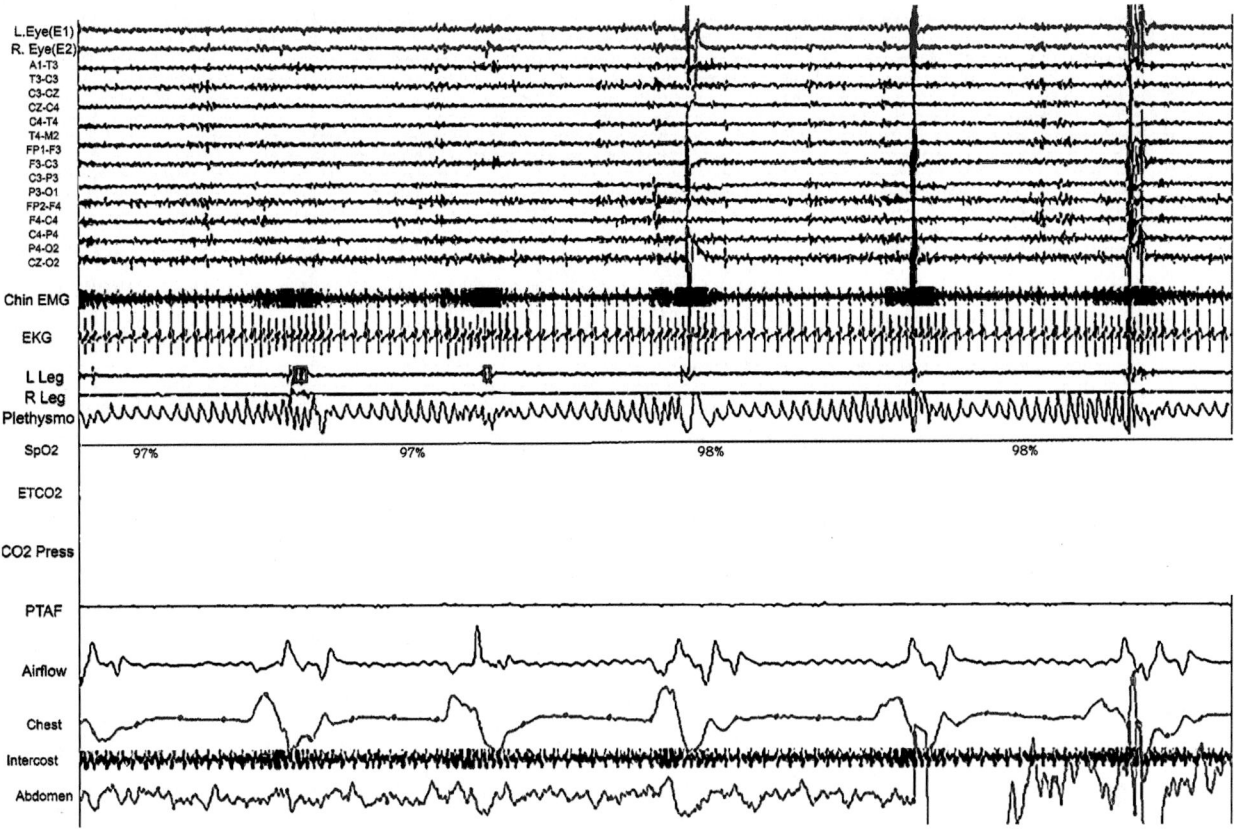

• **Fig. 58.15** Following recovery from surgery, persistent restless sleep, respiratory pauses, and continued daytime sleepiness were noted in the patient from Fig. 58.14. A sleep study was obtained three months later. This is a 120-second segment recorded from N2 sleep in the same patient 3 months following adenotonsillectomy for severe obstructive sleep apnea (OSA). Now, apparent central respiratory pauses were noted associated with cardiac decelerations, arousals, continued periodic oxygen desaturation, and sleep fragmentation. The central apnea index was 113 events per hour of sleep and a diagnosis of central sleep apnea was made. Although the neurologic examination was normal and symmetrical, this patient was then referred to a neurologist for further evaluation.

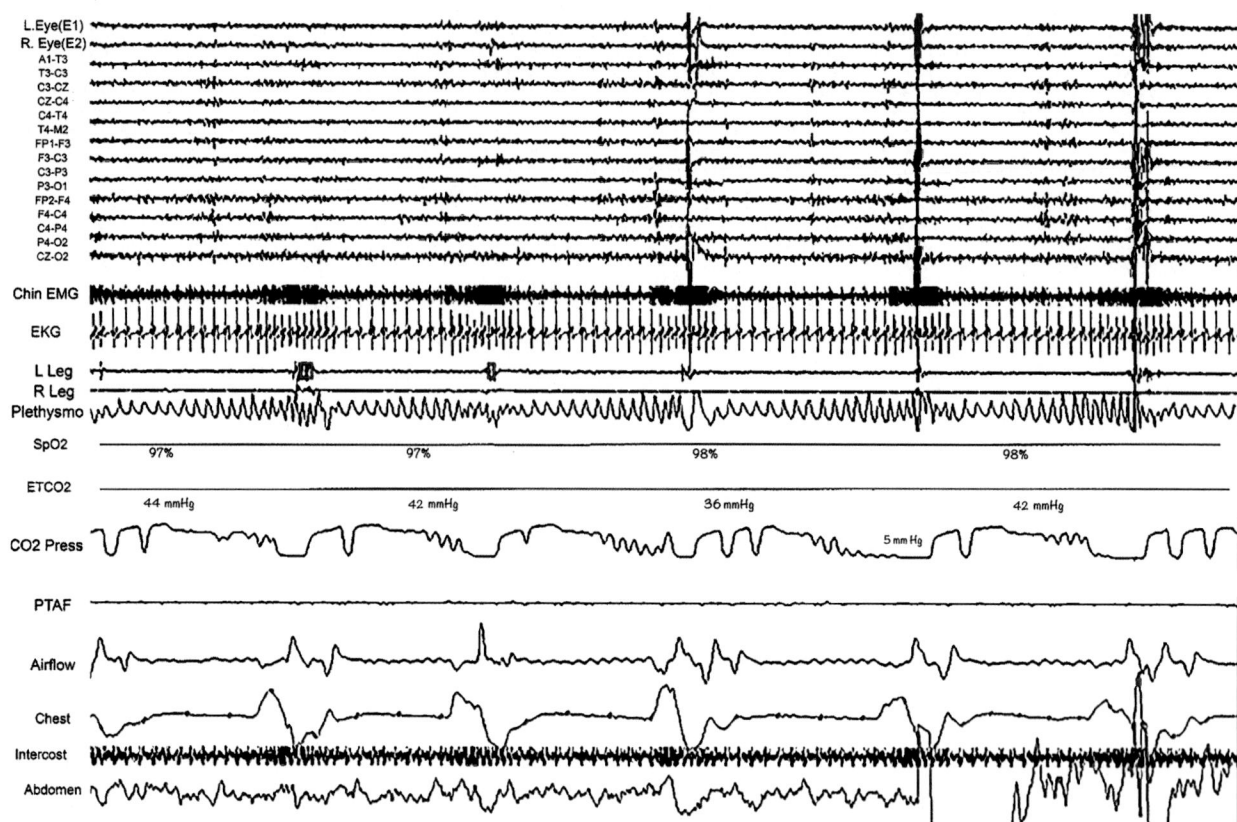

• **Fig. 58.16** This is the same 120-second epoch as depicted in Fig. 58.15. However, there has been the addition of an $ETCO_2$ waveform. This is quite illustrative of a respiratory pattern with somewhat prolonged inhalation and prolonged exhalation termed apneustic breathing. It is an abnormal breathing pattern characterized by regular deep inspirations with a pause at the end of inspiration and inadequate and prolonged exhalation. The prolonged alveolar plateau is quite notable. A magnetic resonance imaging (MRI) with particular emphasis on the posterior fossa was obtained and a Chiari I malformation was identified. The patient underwent a posterior fossa decompression and 3 months following the neurosurgical procedure respiration was normal with no significant obstructive or central apneas, hypopneas, periods of oxygen desaturation, hypercapnia, or electrocardiogram (ECG) changes noted. Daytime sleepiness resolved and there were no longer sleep-related complaints.

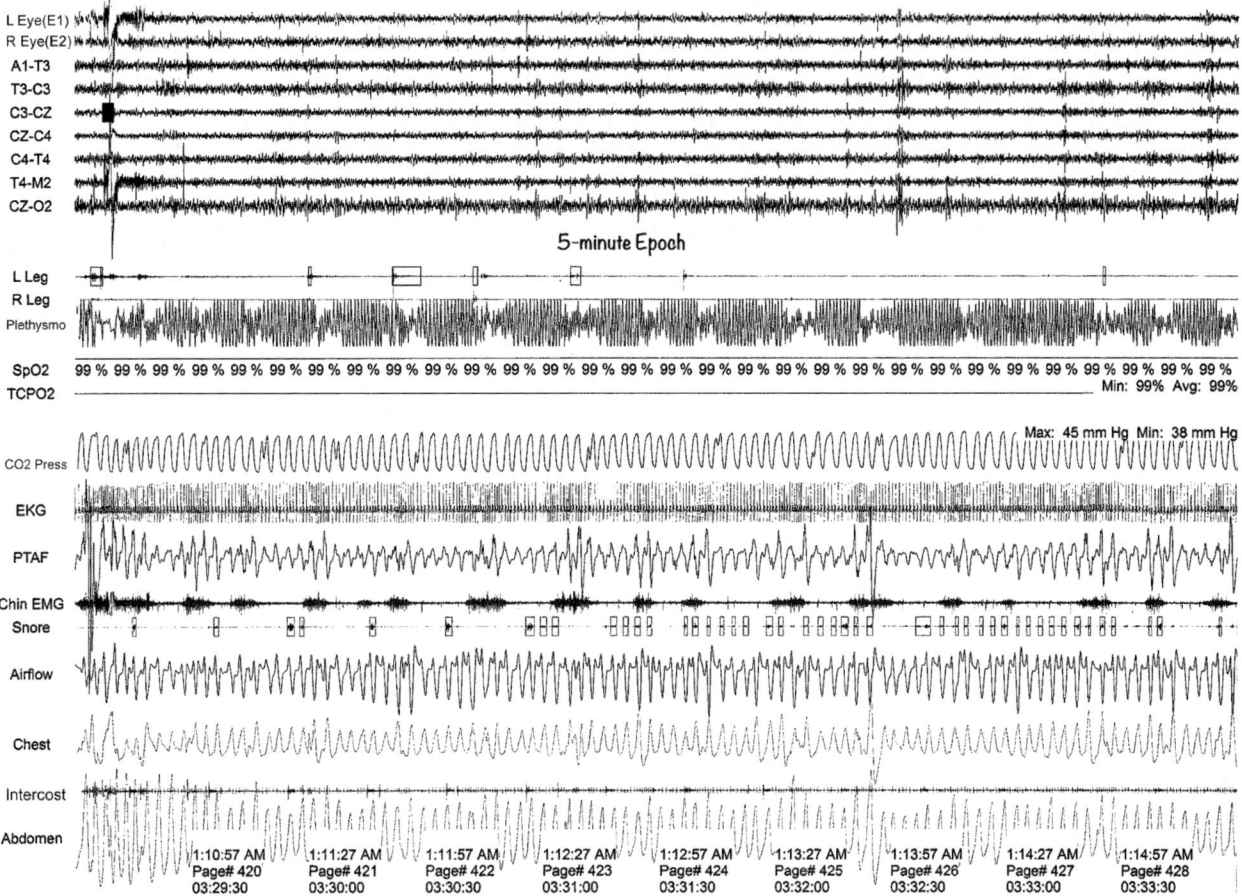

L Eye(E1)
R Eye(E2)
A1-T3
T3-C3
C3-CZ
CZ-C4
C4-T4
T4-M2
CZ-O2

5-minute Epoch

L Leg
R Leg
Plethysmo

SpO2   99 % 99 % 99 % 99 % 99 % 99 % 99 % 99 % 99 % 99 % 99 % 99 % 99 % 99 % 99 % 99 % 99 % 99 % 99 % 99 % 99 % 99 % 99 % 99 % 99 % 99 % 99 % 99 % 99 % 99 %
TCPO2   Min: 99% Avg: 99%

Max: 45 mm Hg   Min: 38 mm Hg
CO2 Press

EKG

PTAF

Chin EMG
Snore

Airflow

Chest

Intercost

Abdomen

1:10:57 AM	1:11:27 AM	1:11:57 AM	1:12:27 AM	1:12:57 AM	1:13:27 AM	1:13:57 AM	1:14:27 AM	1:14:57 AM
Page# 420	Page# 421	Page# 422	Page# 423	Page# 424	Page# 425	Page# 426	Page# 427	Page# 428
03:29:30	03:30:00	03:30:30	03:31:00	03:31:30	03:32:00	03:32:30	03:33:00	03:33:30

• **Fig. 58.17** This 5-minute polysomnographic segment was recorded from a 5-year-old female with a history of snoring four nights per week that could be heard in another room of the home. Sleep was described as restless and associated with frequent arousals and awakenings with rapid and spontaneous return to sleep. Note in the pressure transduction channel that there is periodic flow limitation. Chin muscle electromyography (EMG) revealed arousals, as did brief periods of tachycardia noted in the electrocardiogram (ECG). Although there was no change in oxygen saturation or in end-tidal CO_2, there was continued respiratory effort and periodicity of these events associated with limb movement arousals. These findings suggest the presence of increased upper airway resistance. Although these events did not meet criteria for inclusion in the apnea-hypopnea index (AHI) or respiratory disturbance index (RDI), they were associated with nocturnal and diurnal symptoms and should be reported as findings that might suggest the presence of increased upper airway resistance, even in the absence of significant pediatric obstructive sleep apnea (OSA). Typically, AHI of <1 event per hour of sleep is considered normal in children <13 years of age. An AHI between 1 and 5 events per hour suggests mild pediatric OSA, 5–10 events per hour suggests moderate pediatric OSA, and >10 events per hour suggests severe pediatric OSA. Nevertheless, the calculated frequency of respiratory events might not indicate true severity because an AHI of 3 events per hour of sleep might be associated with hypopneas (flow limitation) lasting 20 seconds, significant periodic oxygen desaturations, and/or persistent elevation of carbon dioxide during the recording. Clinically, classifying severity of obstructive sleep-disordered breathing must encompass more than simply the AHI when determining the clinical implications of sleep-disordered breathing in children.

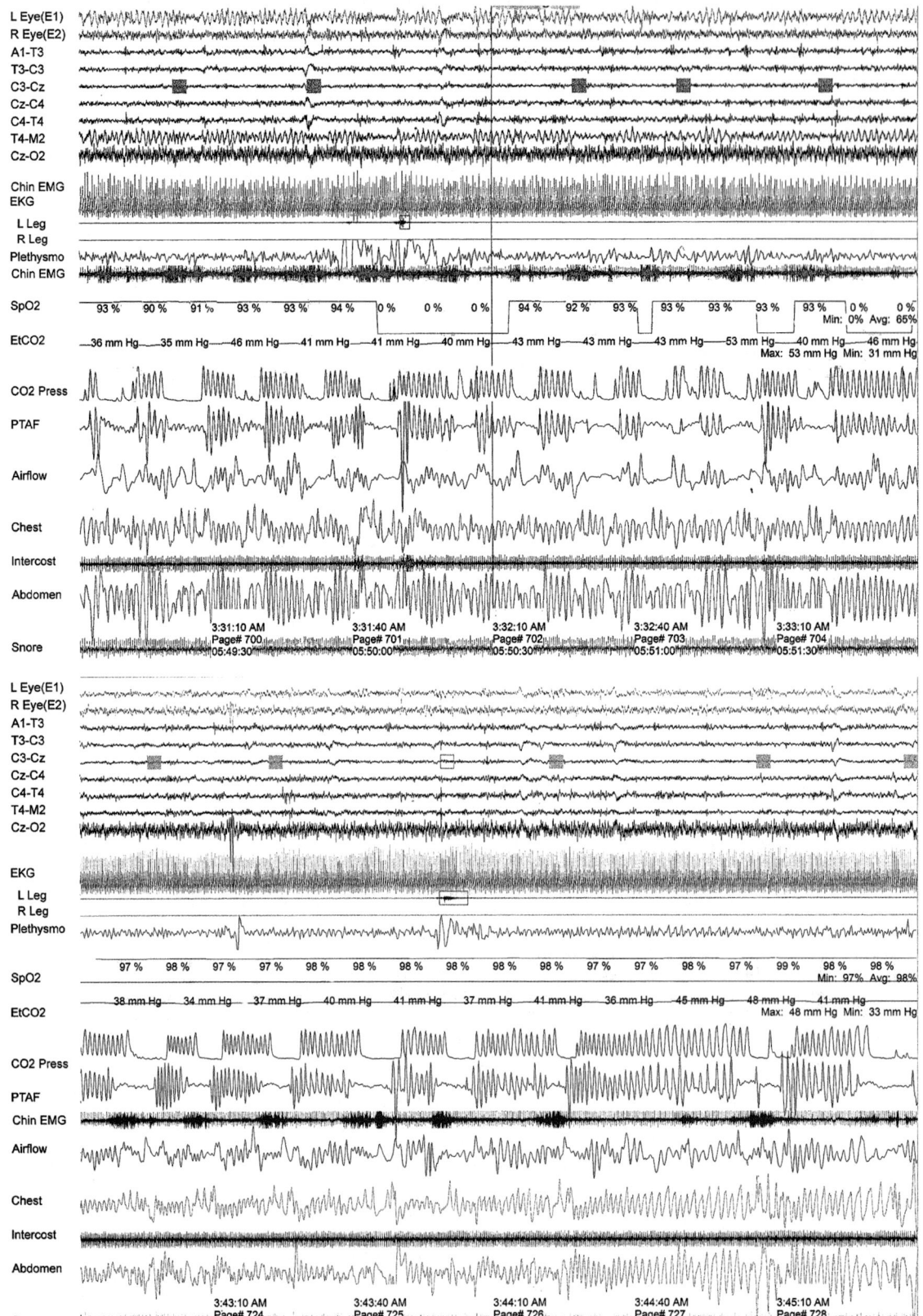

• **Fig. 58.18** (A and B) These 120-second segments were recorded from an 18-month-old with a history of restless sleep, frequent nocturnal waking, intermittent snoring (approximately 2–3 days per week), early morning waking without return to consolidated sleep, and screaming during sleep. The child required a pacifier to fall to sleep and did sleep with a pacifier. Because of the periodic decrease in airflow from the pressure tracing and what appeared to be arousals in the chin muscle electromyogram (EMG), the events were initially scored as hypopneas. This was based on the flow limitation followed by arousal, and periodicity. It was noted on video recording that the child was sleeping and sucking on a pacifier during the study. Prolonged chin muscle activation was coincident with the toddler sucking on the pacifier and swallowing. Sucking occurred during non–rapid eye movement (NREM) and REM sleep. There was movement of the nasal cannula measuring ETCO$_2$ and pressure into and out of the nasal airstream from pressure on the cannula by the pacifier. Although these events seemed to be associated with cardiac decelerations, this finding was likely due to breath holding during swallowing and a vagal response (leading to the cardiac deceleration) while sucking on the pacifier. Pacifier artifact is a unique finding in the pediatric sleep polysomnogram that may often be mistaken for hypopnea. They differ from the chin muscle findings in Fig. 58.17 by virtue of the fact that the EMG augmentation in Fig. 58.17 occurs during an arousal. Augmentation of chin muscle activity in these two epochs occurs during the apparent respiratory pause. This patient's obstructive apnea-hypopnea index (AHI) was 0.4 events per hour of sleep and the nadir oxygen saturation was 96% from a baseline of 98%. No hypercapnia was noted on the study.

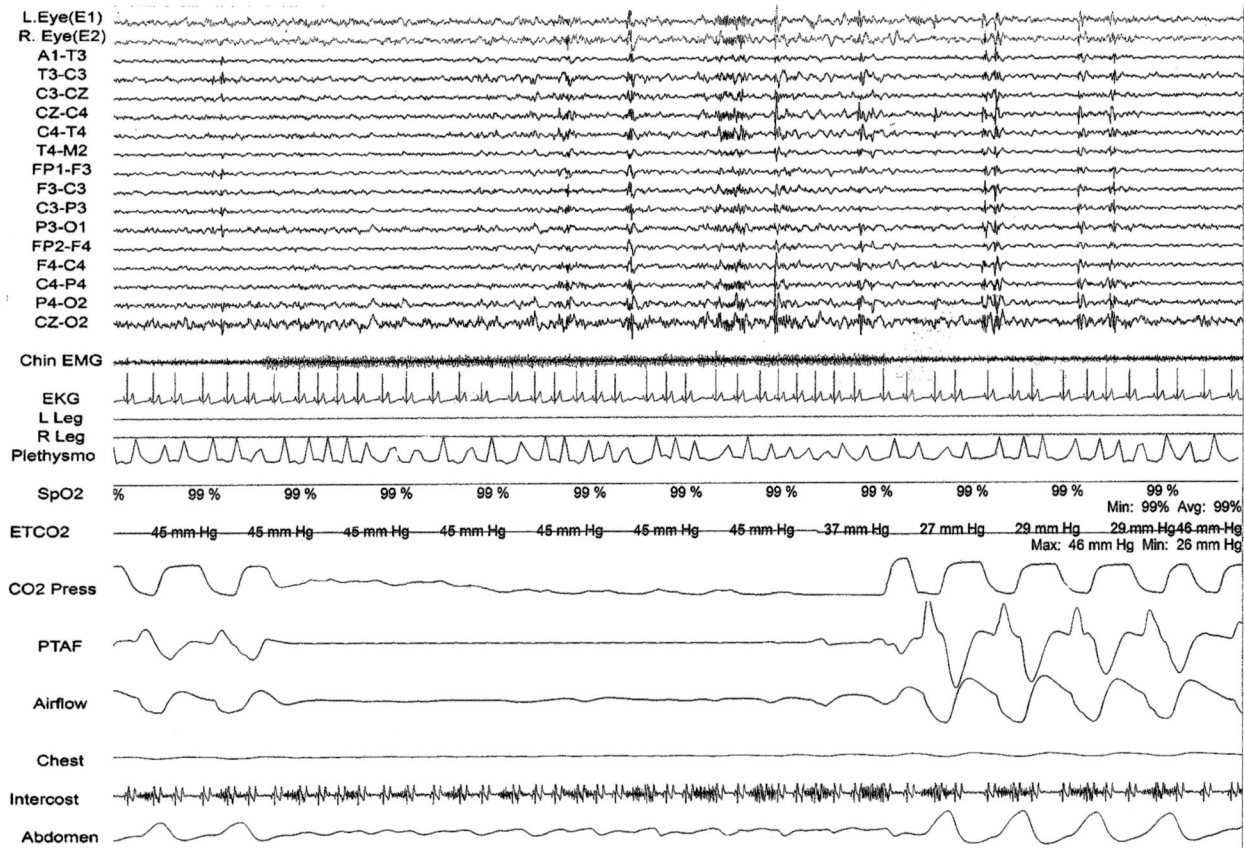

• **Fig. 58.19** Vagal nerve stimulator: 30-second segment. This 30-second epoch was recorded from a 7-year-old male with intractable epilepsy who presented with symptoms of snoring, reported witnessed apneas, restless sleep, and daytime fatigue. The patient was closely followed by an epileptologist and a vagal nerve stimulator was inserted, with good results in controlling the patient's seizures. There appears to be a scored obstructive apnea. Airflow appears absent in all three flow tracings (CO_2 waveform, pressure/PTAF, and thermal/airflow channels) and apparent continued effort in the abdominal channel and intercostal electromyogram (EMG). Note the increase in chin muscle tone during the event.

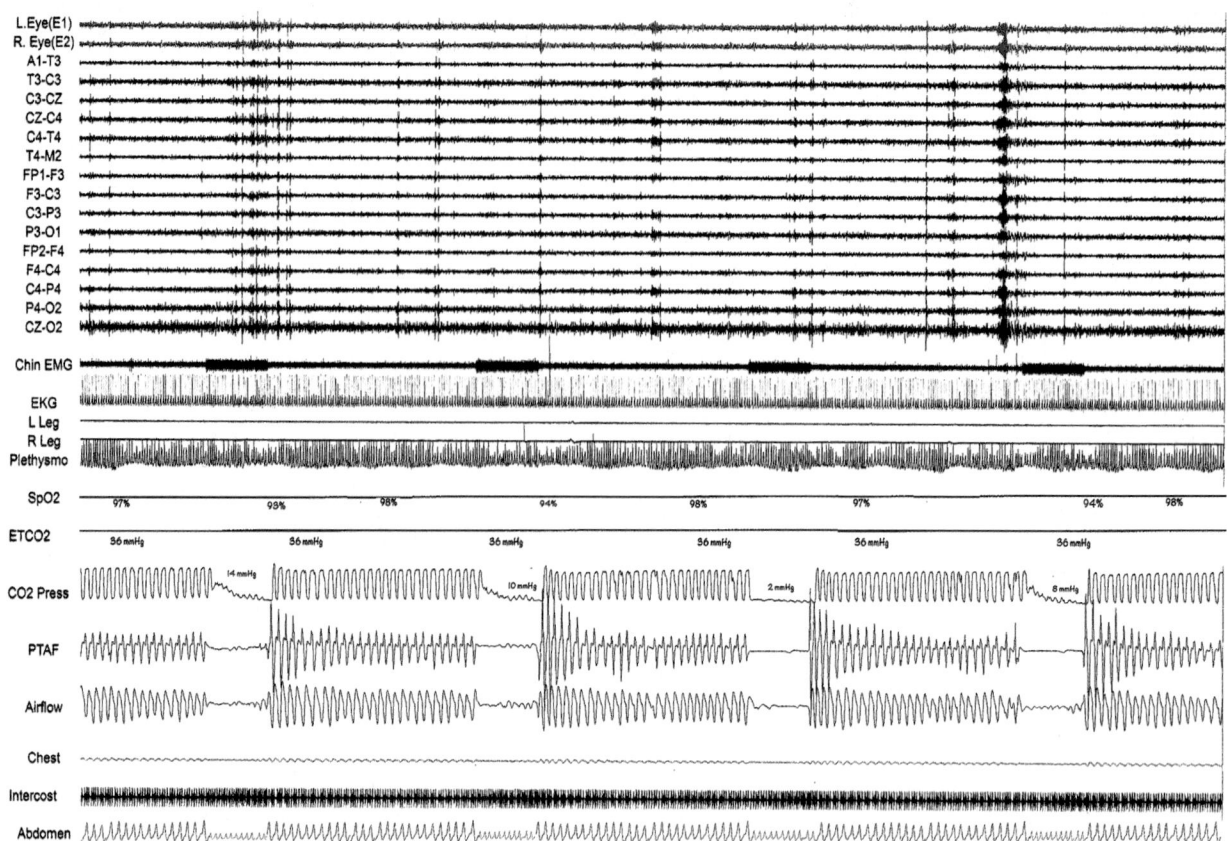

• **Fig. 58.20** Vagal nerve stimulator (VNS): 300-second segment. This is a 5-minute segment recorded from the same patient (Fig. 58.19). Four obstructive-appearing apneas are noted. These events continued throughout the recording. They were occasionally associated with oxygen desaturation. The timing of the events and the associated augmentation of chin muscle electromyogram (EMG) is mostly likely due to vagal nerve stimulation. This patient's sleep-disordered breathing was effectively managed by adjustment in the output of the VNS without resultant increased seizure activity.

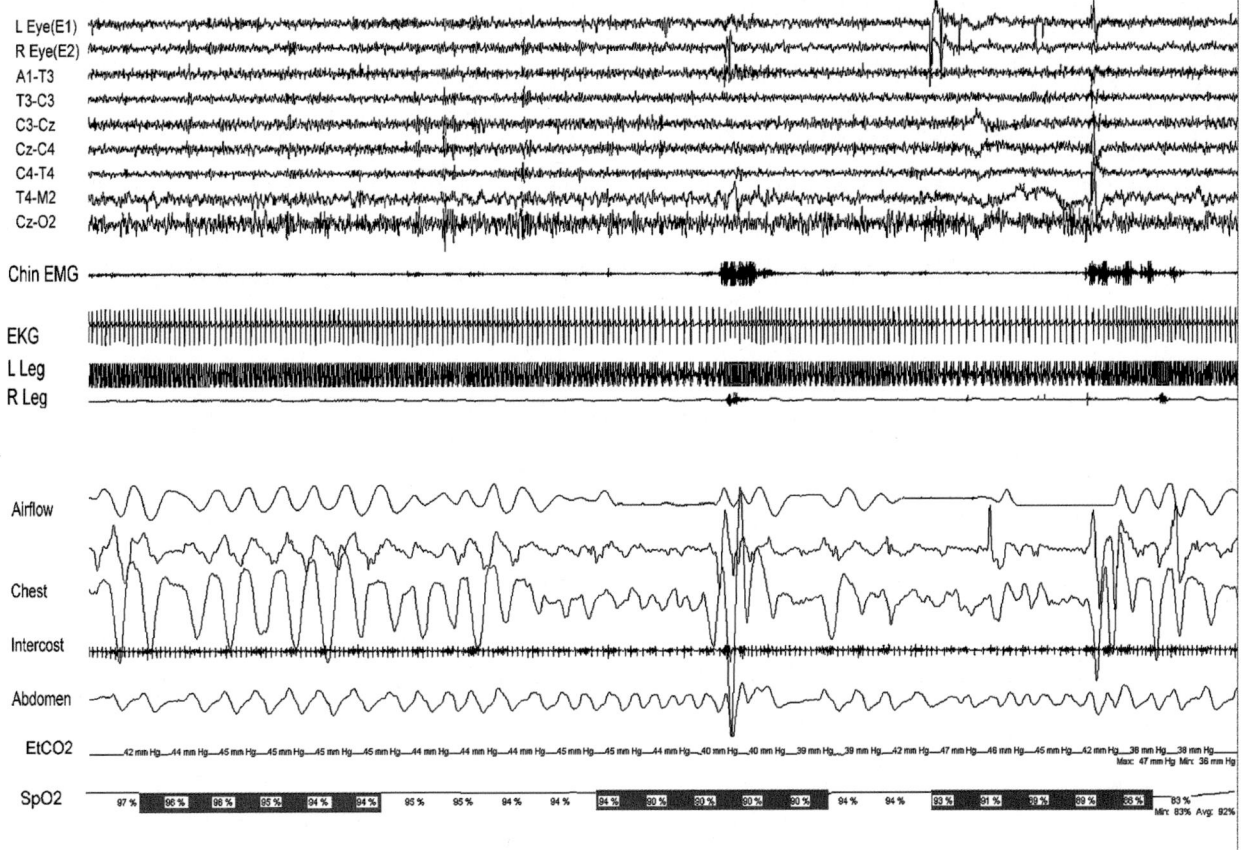

• **Fig. 58.21** Obstructive sleep apnea (OSA) with electrocardiogram (ECG) decelerations. This 120-second polysomnographic segment was recorded during rapid eye movement (REM) sleep from a 3-year-old with a history of habitual loud snoring, reported witnessed apneas, increased work of breathing, restless sleep, and sleep-related diaphoresis. There are three obstructive and partially obstructive respiratory events noted on this epoch. Of note, prior to the arousal noted in the electroencephalography (EEG) and chin muscle electromyography (EMG) cardiac decelerations are noted. With significant upper airway obstruction, cardiac decelerations during these respiratory events are common, but are not required for identification of obstructive or partially obstructive respiratory events.

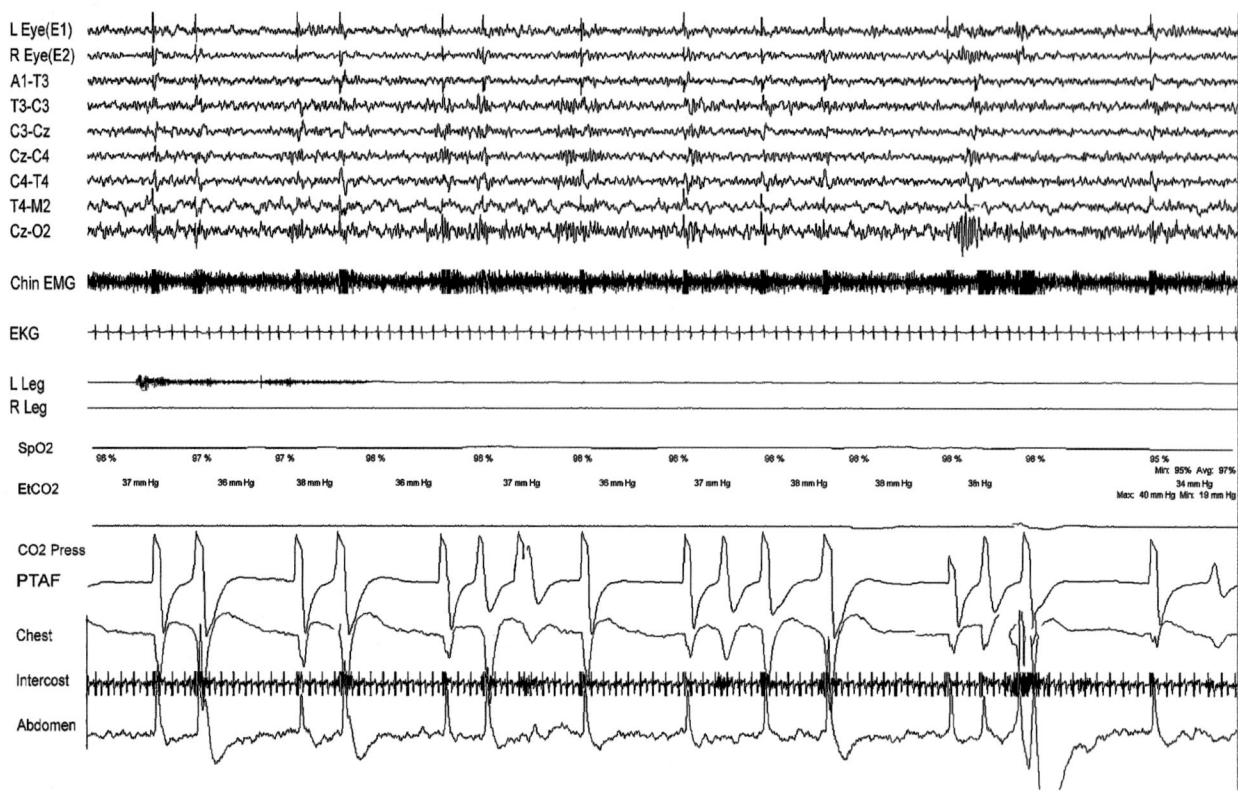

• **Fig. 58.22** Hiccups. Occasionally other respiratory phenomenon can occur during sleep that may appear as either obstructive or partially obstructive events, or they may be identified as central respiratory events. This epoch was recorded from a 2.5-year-old with a history of frequent nocturnal wakings and reported stridulous respirations during sleep. It appears during these 59 seconds of sleep that there are frequent central respiratory pauses. The respiratory pauses are followed by a chin muscle electromyography (EMG) augmentation. Vocalizations may be noted in the snore channel. It was noted by the technologist and confirmed on video recording that these episodes were associated with hiccups occurring during sleep. They were not associated with oxygen desaturation or elevation of end-tidal CO_2 or transcutaneous carbon dioxide levels. There is no change in electrocardiogram (ECG), and respiration was otherwise regular during the remainder of the recording.

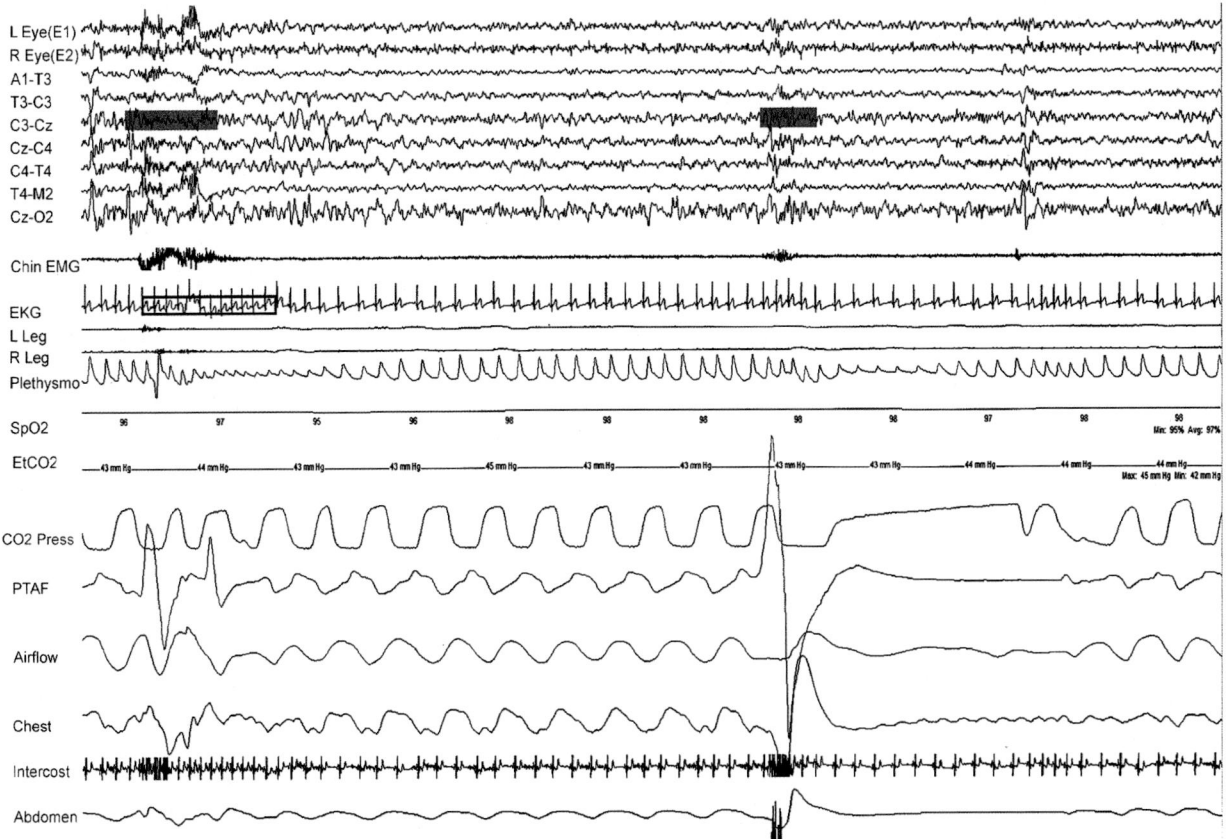

• **Fig. 58.23** Expiratory hypopnea. As previously demonstrated, a mixed apnea consists of a component that appears to be central in character followed by at least two obstructive or partially obstructed respiratory efforts. The "central" component may occur either at the beginning, middle, or end of this event. This 59-second segment was recorded from a 5-year-old with a history of significant partially obstructive sleep-disordered breathing (pediatric obstructive sleep apnea [OSA]). There appears to be no effort in the chest and abdominal channels as well as the intercostal electromyogram (EMG). Additionally, there does not appear to be airflow on the pressure channel (PTAF) or in the thermal channel. However, close assessment of the end-tidal CO_2 channel reveals a prolonged alveolar plateau with rising carbondioxide levels along with cardiac decelerations that occur at the beginning of the event rather than at the end of the event. This represents a partial expiratory obstruction with continued exhalatory airflow (not absent airflow). Often when mixed events are associated with obstructive apneas and hypopneas treatment of the obstructive sleep-disordered breathing resolves the mixed events and they are not converted to central events. Expiratory hypopneas most often follow augmented breaths (sighs). Another characteristic that differentiates these apparent physiologic events is cardiac deceleration during the first half to first third of the event with gradual return of the instantaneous heart rate to baseline. These events often are associated with arousal at the beginning of the event. Sometimes they may be quite prolonged, and the respiratory pause may last 30 seconds or more. They are not typically included in calculation of the obstructive apnea-hypopnea index (AHI) or respiratory disturbance index (RDI). Red boxes represent electrocortical arousals.

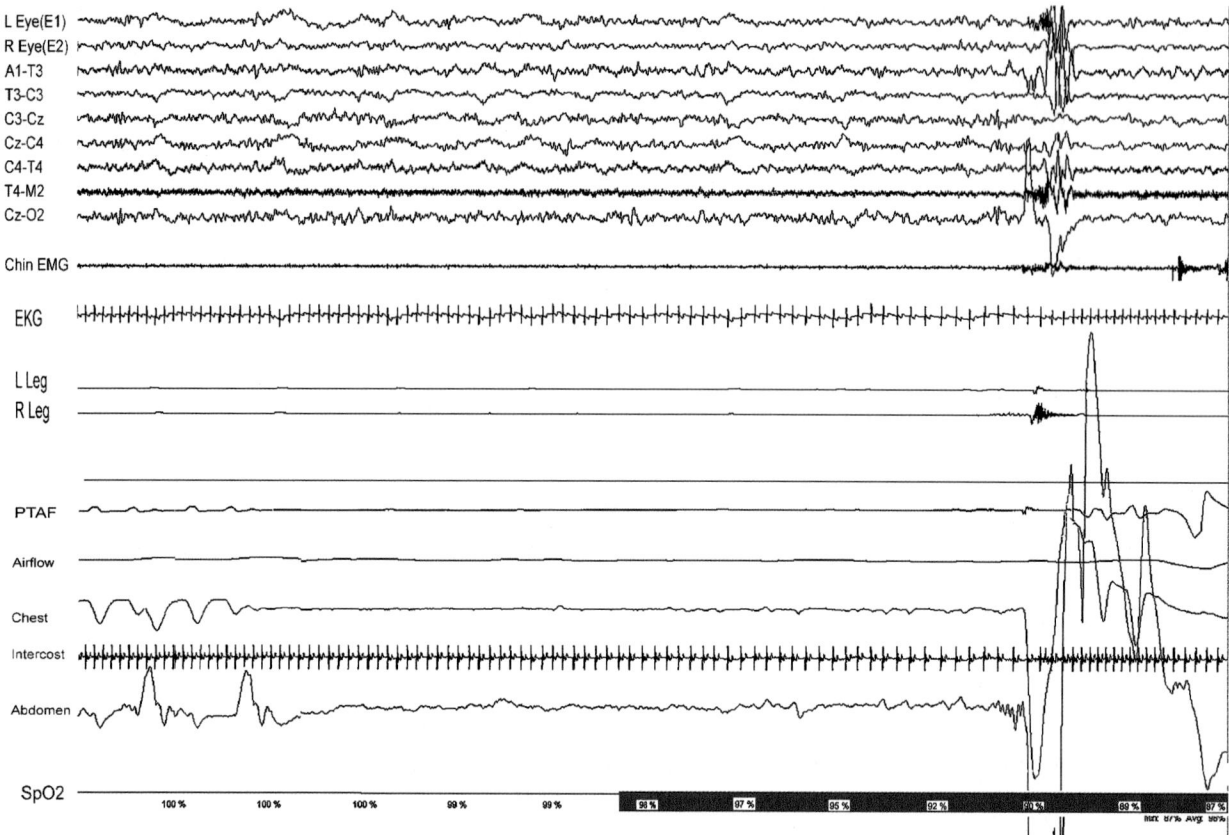

• **Fig. 58.24** Central apnea in congenital hypoventilation syndrome (CCHS). This 59-second polysomnographic segment was recorded from a 1-month-old during quiet sleep with a history of hypoxemia and hypercapnia noted during sleep. Respiratory efforts, although present, were shallow, and respiration was punctuated by somewhat prolonged central respiratory pauses. The patient had been intubated and ventilated following delivery due to cyanosis and feeble respiratory efforts. Because the patient seemed to be doing quite well on the ventilator, ventilatory support was weaned and subsequently discontinued at 1 week of age. A prolonged central apnea can be seen during the first half of the recording. Additionally, oxygen saturation fell to a nadir of 67% and there was continued rise in the end-tidal carbon dioxide level. This central apnea lasted 26 seconds with a 33% fall in the oxygen saturation. The patient was subsequently reintubated and there was difficulty removing the patient from the ventilator, with several failed attempts at extubation. Physical findings included constipation with a concern for Hirschsprung's disease, and there was noted decreased heart rate variability and decreased pupillary response to light. A *PHOX2B* analysis was sent and the results were positive. These findings are consistent with CCHS, which is typically diagnosed in the neonatal period; however, it may be diagnosed later in life. There is no available cure for CCHS, and most patients require supportive care throughout their lifespan. Treatment is focused on maintaining ventilation. Tracheostomy is usually required in infancy and older childhood, although selected older children and adults may be managed noninvasively. Mechanical ventilation is sometimes needed 24 hours a day, especially where there are more *PHOX2B* gene repeats present. Diaphragmatic pacing by a phrenic nerve stimulator is now occasionally used in some ambulatory children who require continuous ventilatory support.

59

Partial Arousal Disorders: Parasomnias

Stephen H. Sheldon

NREM PARASOMNIAS

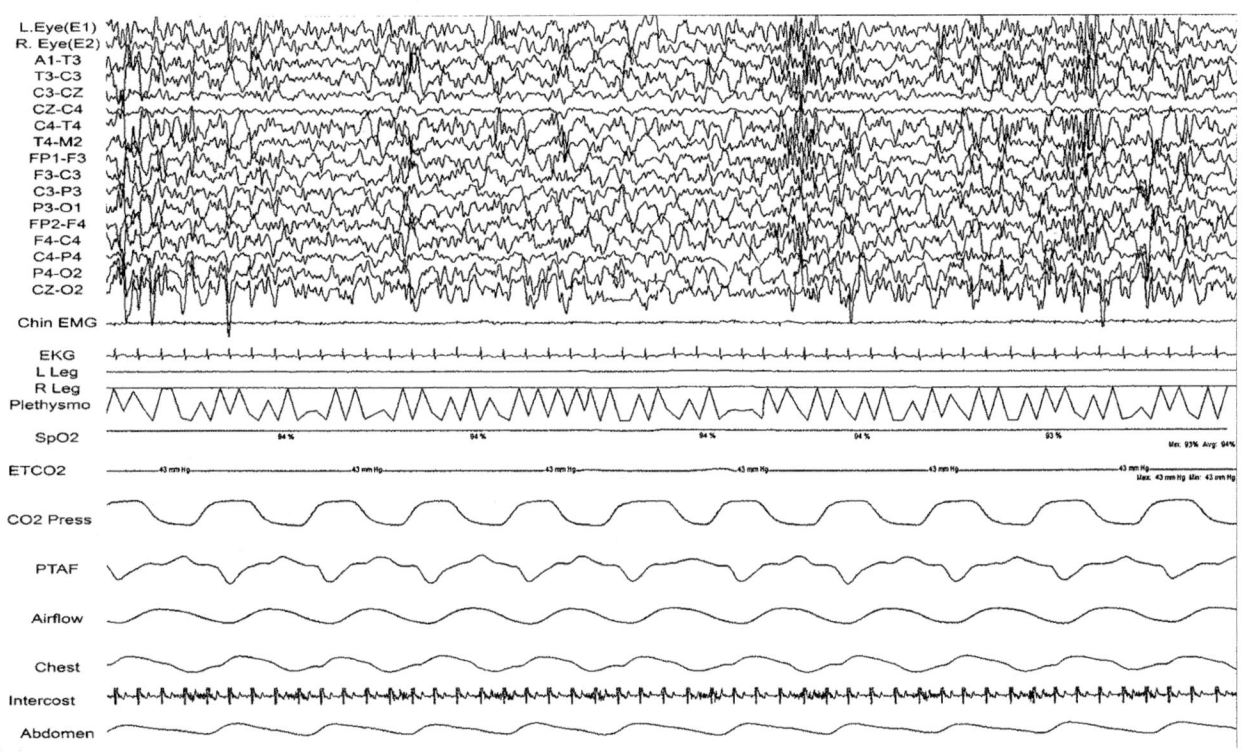

• **Fig. 59.1** Partial arousal from non–rapid eye movement (NREM) sleep, theta-delta sleep pattern. This 30-second polysomnographic segment was recorded from a 10-year-old with a history of frequent sleepwalking. Episodes occurred during the first third to first half of the sleep period, were characterized by quiet nocturnal wanderings, and there was amnesia for the events. Events occurred nightly. The patient was brought to the pediatric sleep disorders center because on several occasions he attempted to leave the home, once walking out the front door and entering a neighbor's living room. In this epoch respiration is regular and monogamous. It is recorded from N3 sleep. The predominant background rhythm is 0.5–1.0 Hz. However, it is notable for theta activity superimposed upon the background delta rhythm. This theta-delta sleep pattern is a nonspecific normal finding sometimes reported in children with partial arousal disorders from NREM sleep.

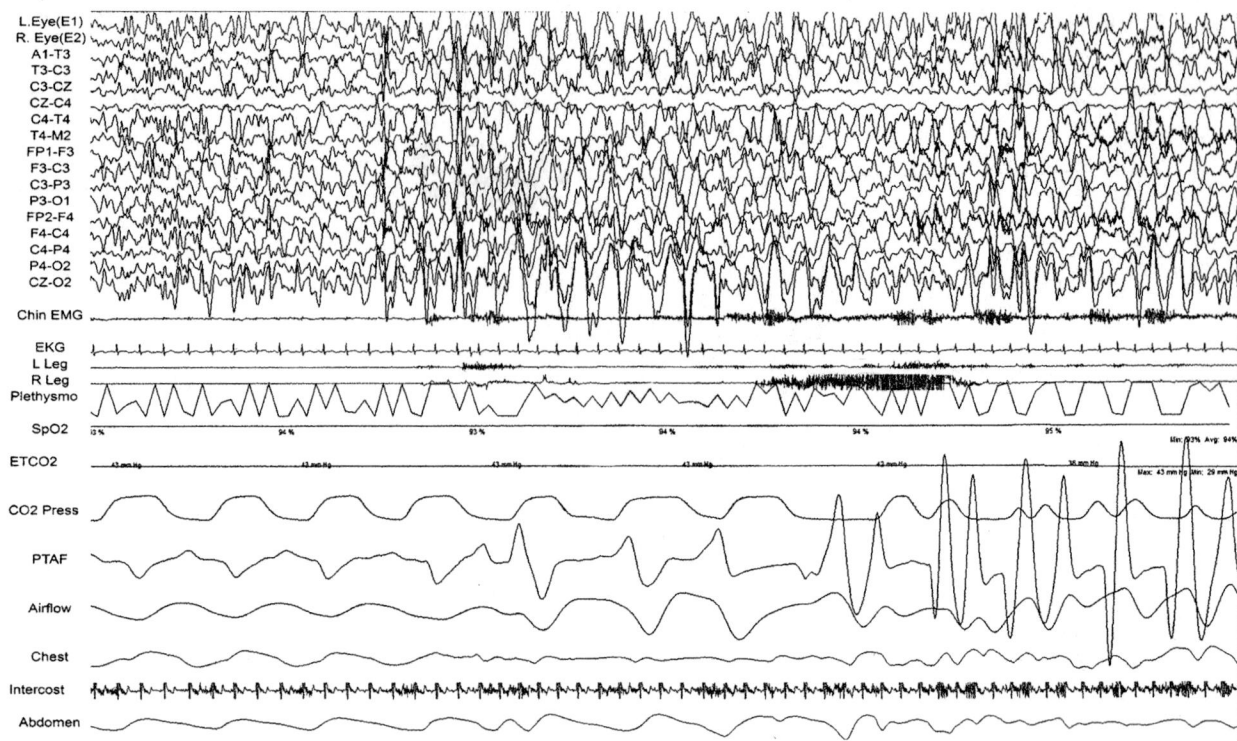

• **Fig. 59.2** Hypersynchronous delta activity and arousal rhythm in N3 sleep. Because of the movements and video revealing eye opening, the scoring technologist labeled this 30-second epoch as Wake. However, the electroencephalogram (EEG) background is clearly about 0.5 Hz.

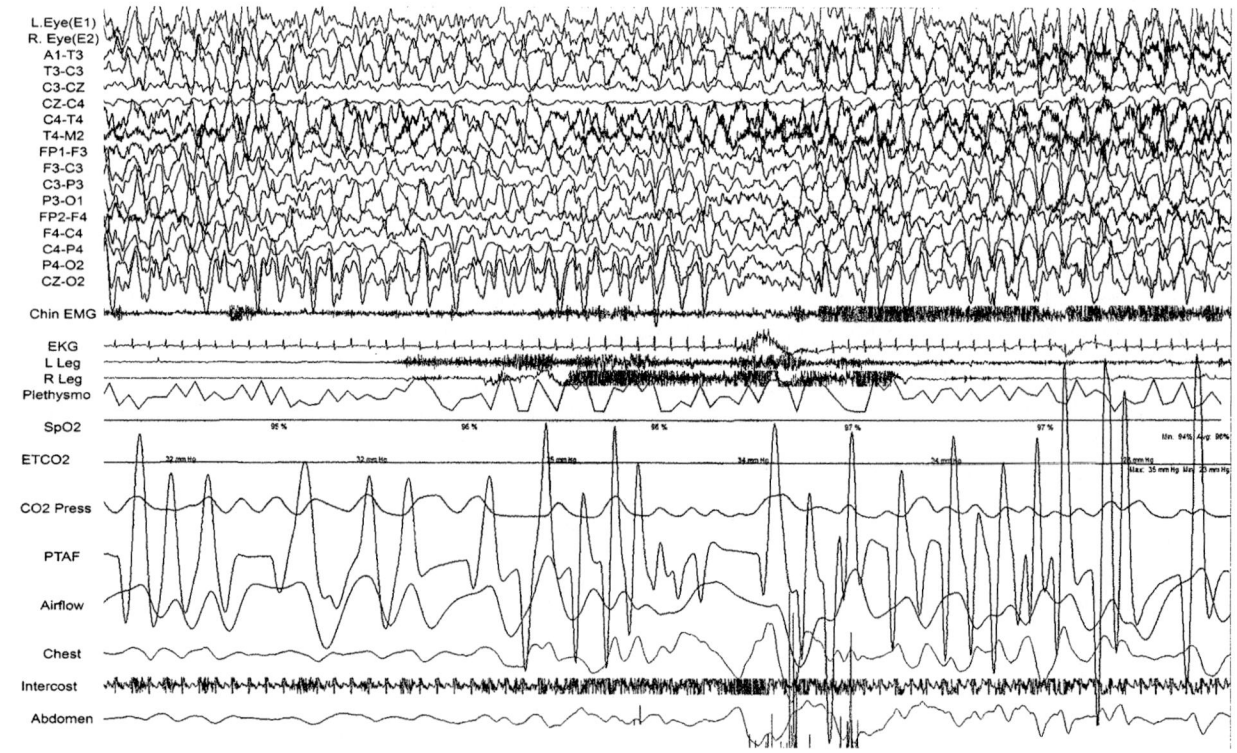

• **Fig. 59.3** Partial arousal and hypersynchronous delta activity in N3 sleep. This partial arousal in an attempt to leave the bed was noted by the technical staff. The background rhythm continues to be approximately 0.5 Hz. There is an irregular respiratory pattern, eyes open, and considerable limb movements. Augmentation of chin muscle tone can also be seen.

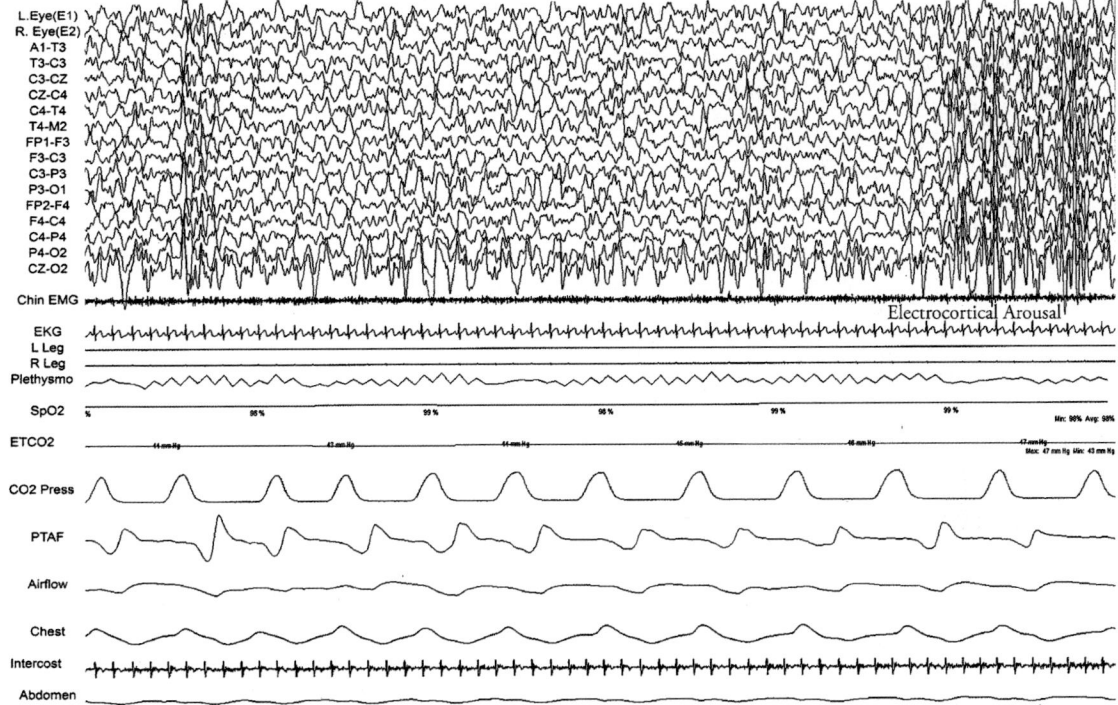

• **Fig. 59.4** Arousal rhythm in N3 sleep. In children who have partial arousal disorders, other nonspecific findings can be seen even in the absence of motor activity. There may be frequent theta arousal rhythms noted during N3 sleep as typified on this 30-second polysomnographic segment.

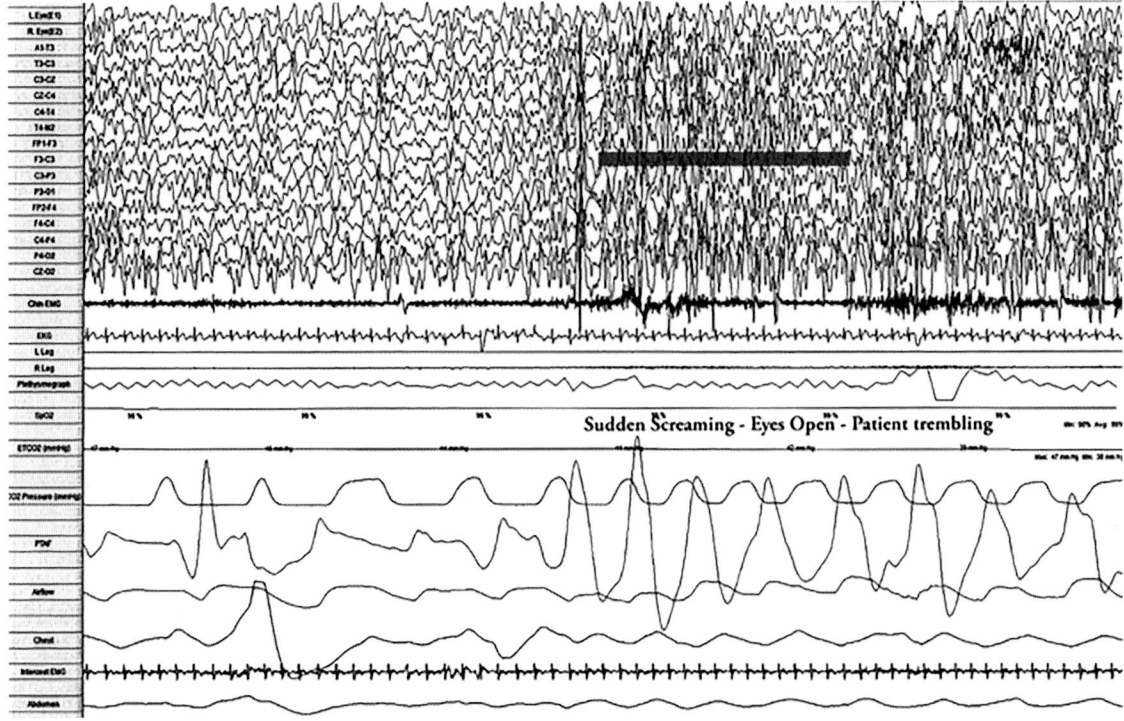

• **Fig. 59.5** Sleep terror. This 30-second polysomnographic segment was recorded from a 4-year-old child who was reported to be suffering from nightmares. Spells occurred every night during the first third of the sleep period. They were associated with abrupt onset of intense screaming, shaking, diaphoresis, pupillary dilatation, and tachycardia. Parents noted trembling during the spells. The child health care practitioner was concerned that the shaking resembled seizure activity and referred the child to a neurologist. Routine electroencephalogram (EEG) was normal and no treatment was recommended. Spells continued nightly, became more intense, and a referral to a sleep center was then made. This segment depicts the abrupt arousal and activity from N3 sleep. Of particular importance is the video recording as well as the polysomnographic technologist notations that the child abruptly sat up screaming with eyes open and trembling. A diagnosis of sleep terrors was made.

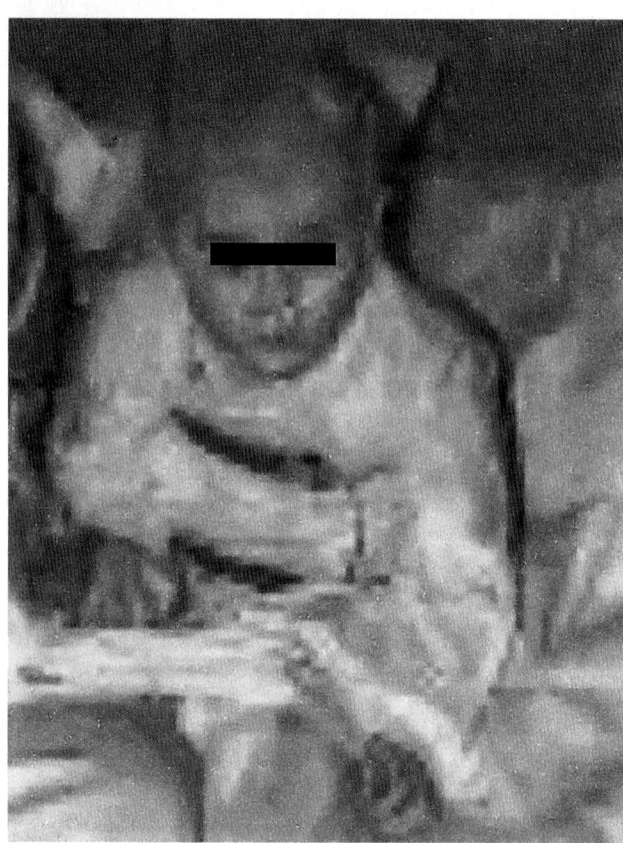

• **Fig. 59.6** Confusional arousal. This is a 3-year-old child who had been having intermittent episodes of nocturnal awakenings. Parents reported that the child would walk around the house babbling incoherently. The patient would speak in full sentences, but often these sentences did not make sense. Although the child could not remember these spells occurring, parents continued to ask if he was having nightmares and he reported that he was. He could not clearly describe a dream during the spell. His parents also asked him if he was seeing monsters, and he reported that he was. He could not describe the monsters. Starting with Fig. 59.7, this patient was recorded during nocturnal polysomnography.

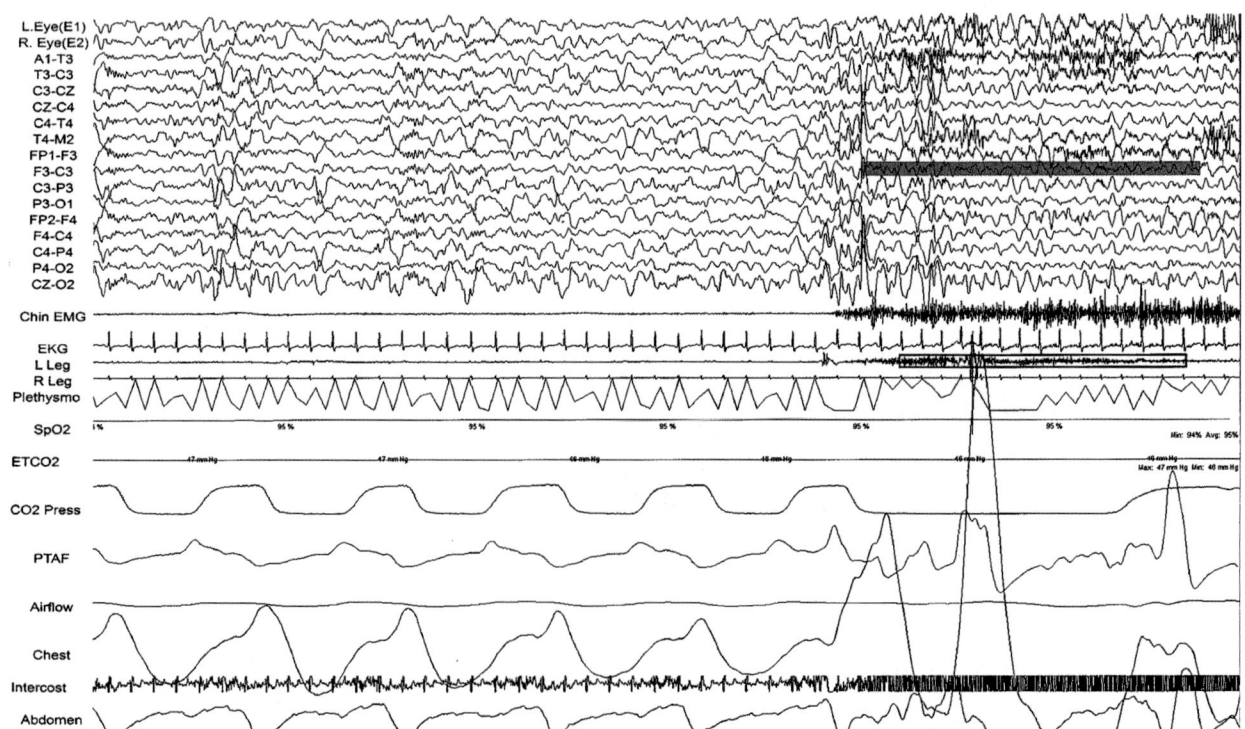

• **Fig. 59.7** Confusional arousal. This is a 30-second epoch recorded from the child described in Fig. 59.6. There is an abrupt arousal from N3 sleep with augmented chin muscle tone, respiratory variability, and increase in heart rate, but continued slow-wave background rhythm at approximately 0.5 Hz. The following 30-second segment reveals a change in the electroencephalogram (EEG) background frequency. Red highlight indicates the arousal with a delta background rhythm noted.

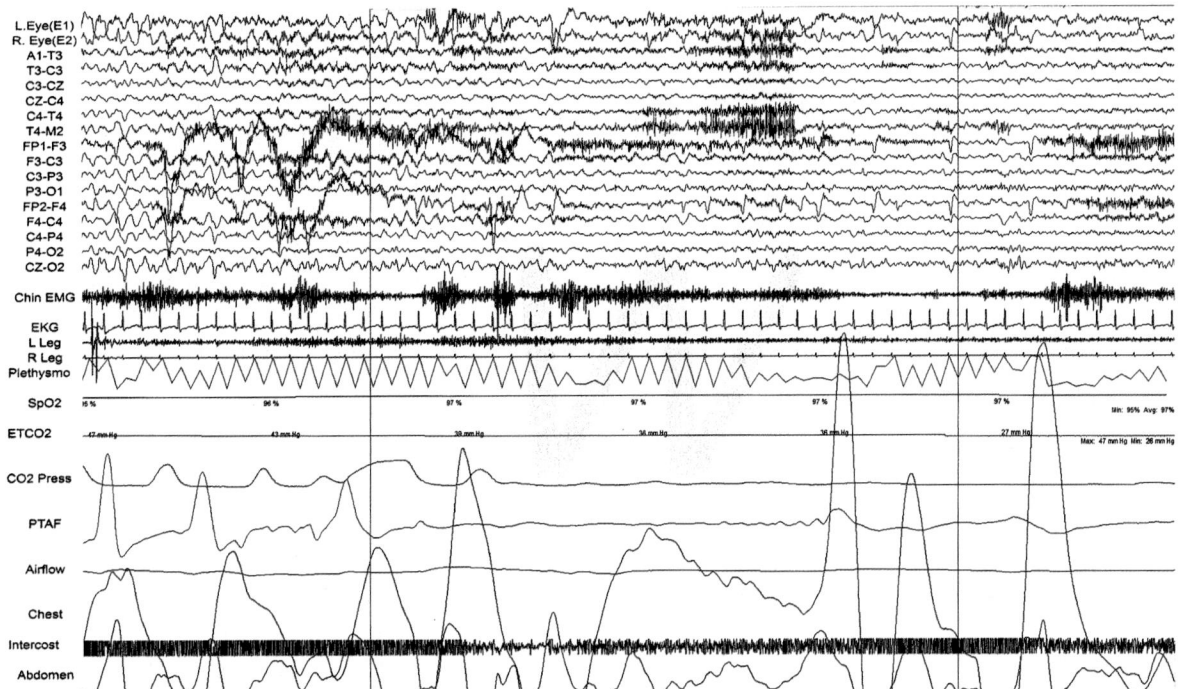

• **Fig. 59.8** Confusional arousal. The behaviors continue as in the segment from Fig. 59.7. There is continued motor activity with confusion and disorientation and a notable change in the electroencephalogram (EEG) background rhythm. No longer is delta frequency predominant, but there is a relatively low voltage mixed frequency background noted. Indeed, the EEG posterior dominant rhythm may change to a clear waking rhythm during confusional arousals.

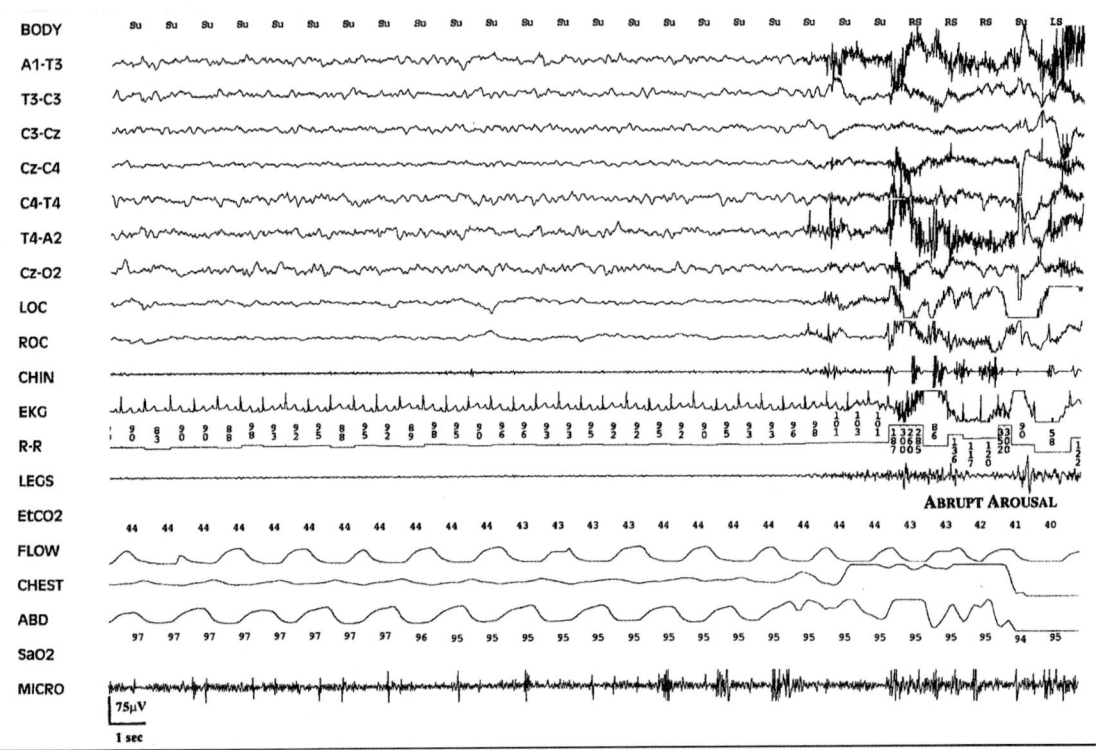

• **Fig. 59.9** Nightmare. This 30-second polysomnographic segment was recorded from a 7-year-old patient who was seen by her primary care practitioner due to frequent nightmares. She was initially referred to a psychologist because she would awaken in the early morning hours and enter her parents' bedroom crying. She would report a clearly vivid dream stating that she was being chased by children in her classroom. She had difficulty returning to sleep unless climbing into bed with her parents. Spells were becoming more frequent and there is a history of snoring. The psychologist referred the child to the sleep center for evaluation. In this segment the child is clearly in rapid eye movement (REM) sleep and there is an abrupt awakening with crying. The child did report a vivid dream and had difficulty falling back to sleep. This differed from a sleep terror by occurring during the final third of the sleep time, lack of intense autonomic discharges, and difficulty returning to sleep. Additionally, it is differentiated from sleep terror based on the vivid dream report.

REM SLEEP PARASOMNIAS

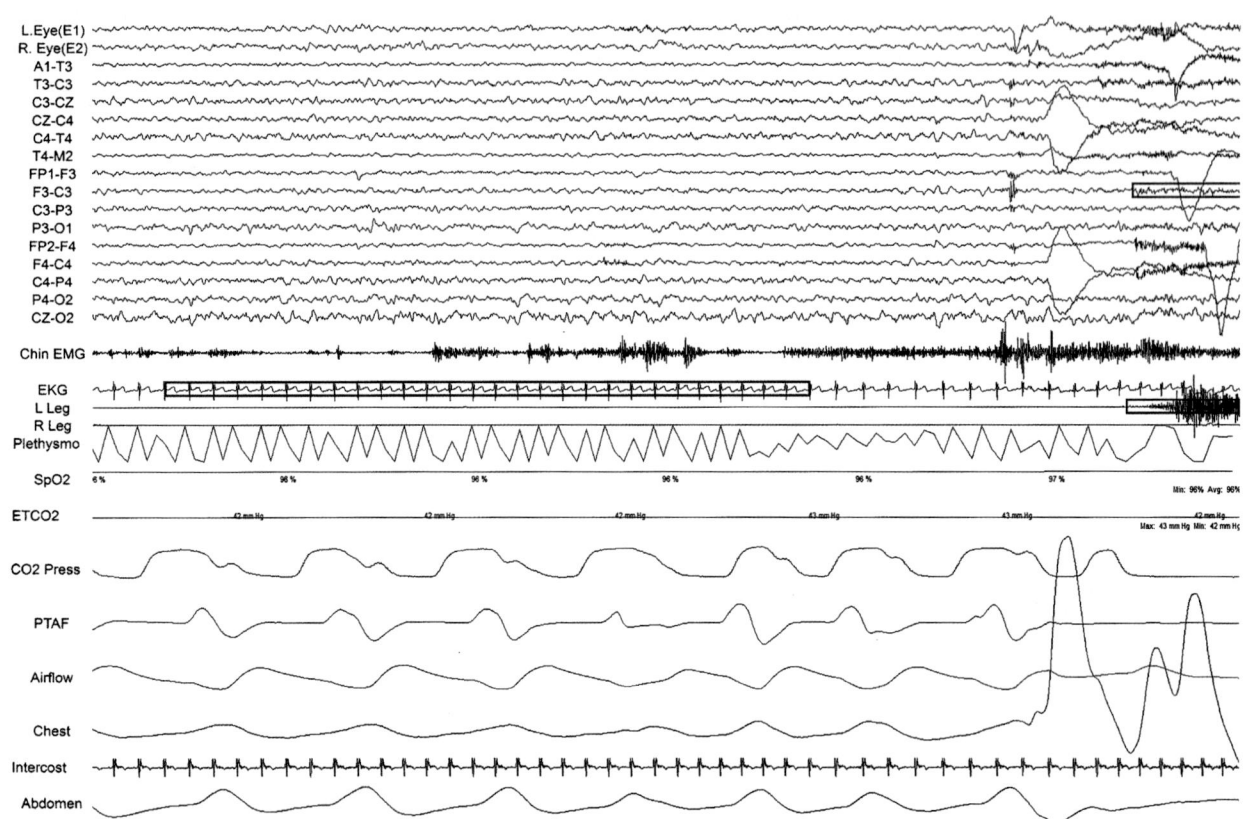

• **Fig. 59.10** Rapid eye movement (REM) sleep without atonia. This is a 30-second segment recorded from a 6-year-old who reportedly was having problems with nightmares and acting out his dreams. Parents were referred to the sleep center because during one of these dream enactments the patient kicked a wall with his feet, damaging the wall and bruising his toes. In the segment there is some respiratory instability noted, eye movements can be seen in the electrooculogram, and there is increased muscle tone in the chin and limb movements noted that are not associated with arousals due to respiratory events.

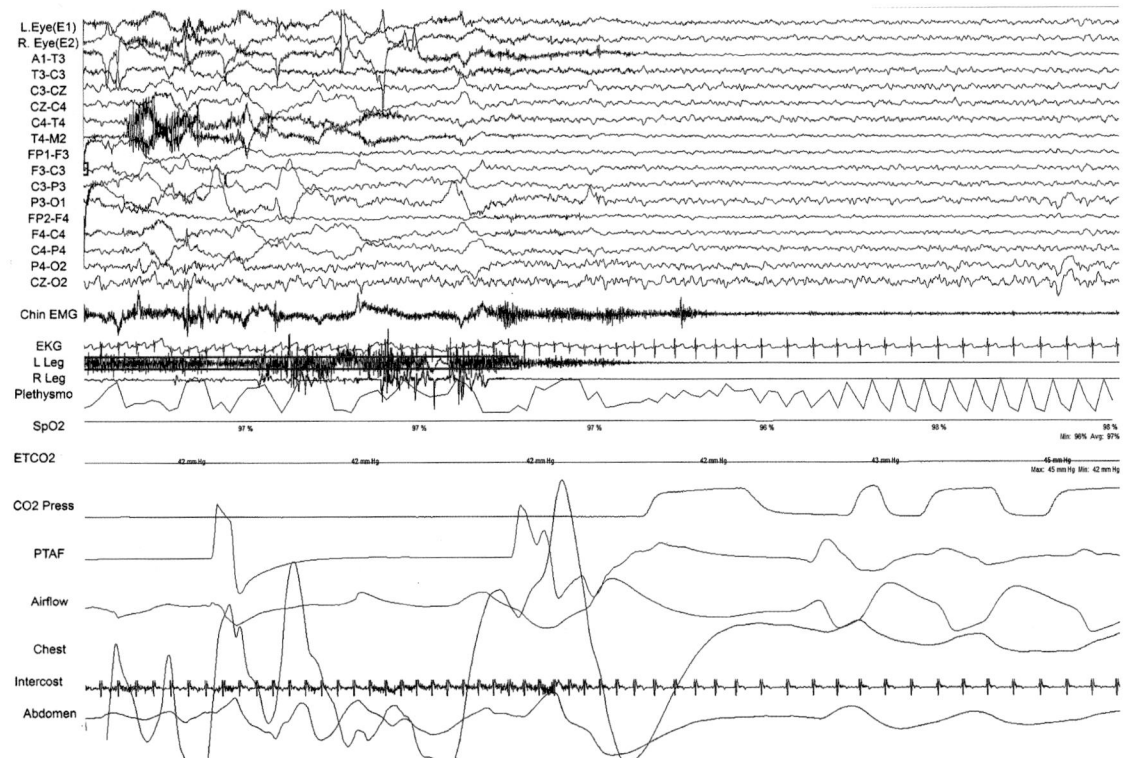

• **Fig. 59.11** Rapid eye movement (REM) sleep without atonia. This is a 30-second segment was recorded from the same patient in Fig. 59.10. Again, respiratory variability can be seen during REM sleep and there is considerable muscle activity and leg movements occurring that are episodic in character. REM sleep without atonia (RBM-sleep behavior disorder [RBD] in adults) may be seen in children with narcolepsy and has been noted in children suffering from posttraumatic stress disorder. The clinical and polysomnographic diagnosis of REM sleep without atonia in children appears to carry a different clinical significance then it does in adults with similar sleep-related phenomena. In children, progression to other sleep-related movement disorders is, at the present time, unknown but does appear to be quite unlikely.

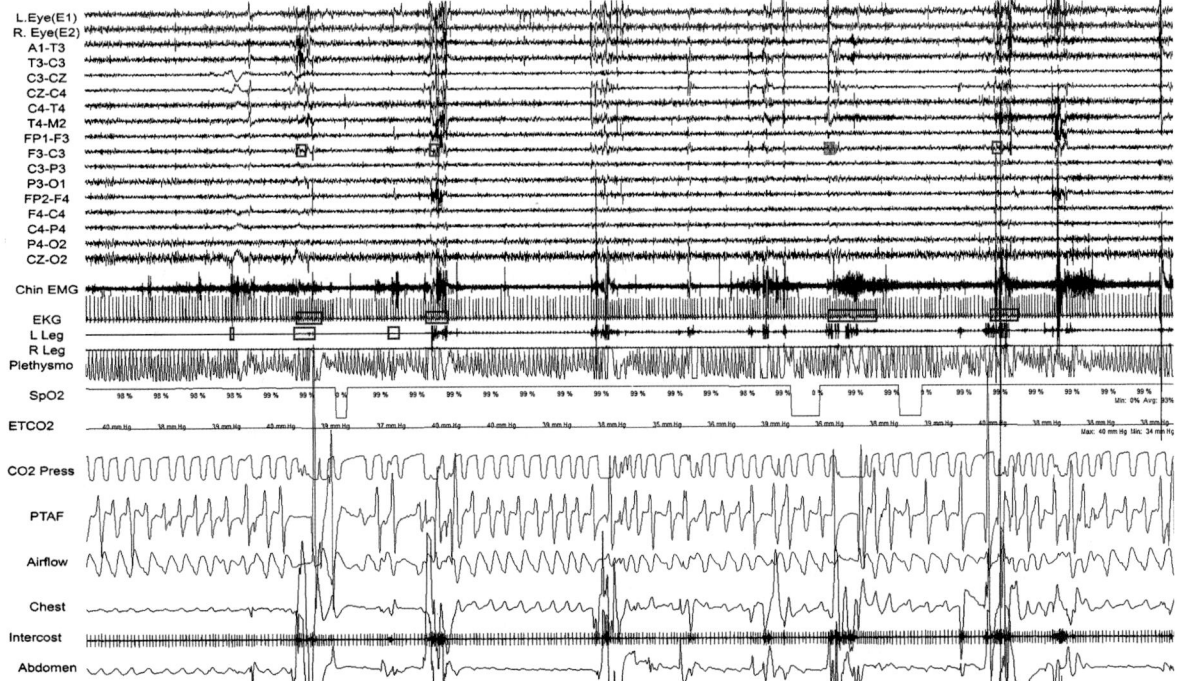

• **Fig. 59.12** Rapid eye movement (REM) sleep without atonia. This 5-minute polysomnographic segment was recorded from the same patient as in Figs. 59.10 and 59.11. The patient was yelling, "Get away! Get away!" There was also screaming and swinging arms and legs apparently attempting to "fight away" what was frightening to the patient in the dream. The patient subsequently woke, was quite frightened, and reported that he was being chased by dogs that were trying to bite him. There was no history suggestive of narcolepsy and no history of dog bites in the past. He was treated with lorazepam and the spells immediately resolved.

60
Central Hypersomnias

Stephen H. Sheldon

Central Hypersomnias

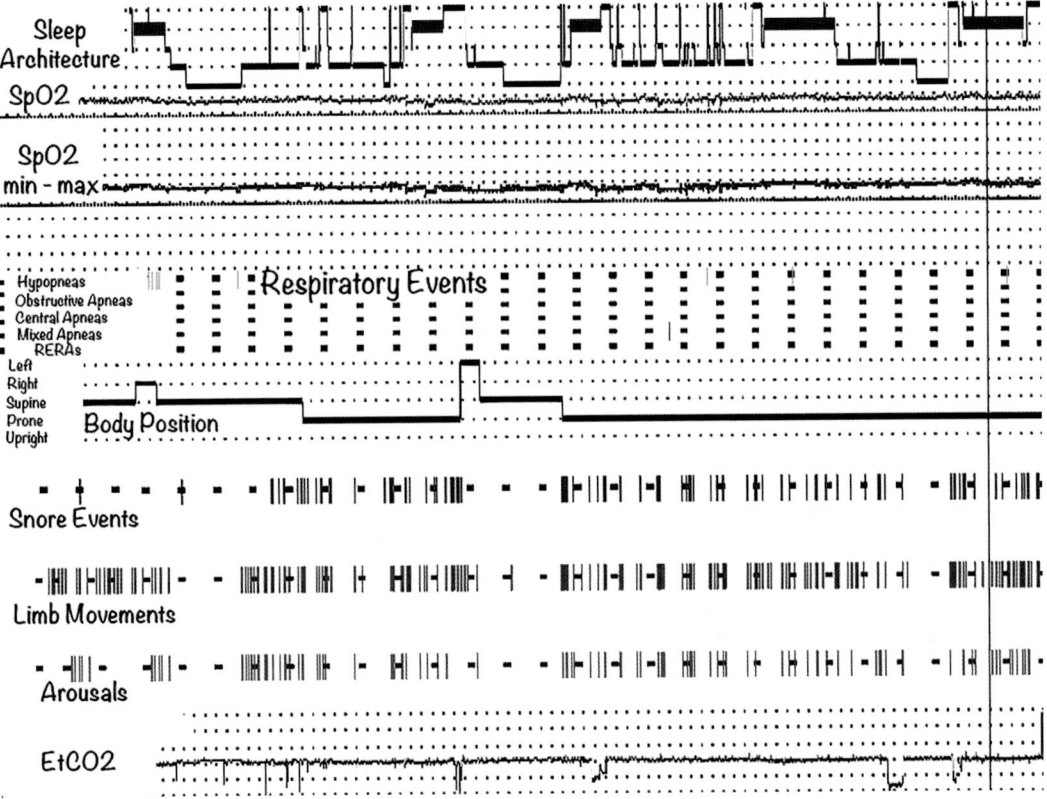

- **Fig. 60.1** Narcolepsy with sleep-onset rapid eye movement (REM) period. This patient was 8 years old when they presented with a history of attention/concentration problems, learning difficulties, motor restlessness, learning difficulties in school, forgetfulness, difficulty paying attention to assignments, and clumsiness on the playground. His parents reported that his hyperactivity alternates with sleepiness and symptoms have been getting worse over the past year. He had been an outstanding student and now he is failing most of his classes. His pediatrician stated that he had attention-deficit/hyperactivity disorder (ADHD) and believed the sleepiness was due to depression. His parents did state that his mood seemed to be quite flat all the time and he disliked playing games or watching cartoons with his friends. He has fallen asleep during meals and has fallen asleep at his birthday party. He was seen by a child psychologist for evaluation. The child psychologist noted that he was having bad dreams when he got into bed and closed his eyes resulting in fear of going to sleep. He was difficult to awaken in the morning, and when he did arouse from his not total sleep time, he was frightened and cried rather than resisting parents attempts to awaken him. The psychologist referred him to the sleep disorder center for further evaluation. He underwent a comprehensive nocturnal polysomnogram, the hypnogram of which is depicted in this figure. Please note the short sleep latency as well as the sleep-onset REM period. Sleep is quite fragmented with brief awakenings and arousals. Nevertheless, progression of sleep states seems relatively normal across the night. No sleep-disordered breathing or gas exchange abnormalities were noted on the study, although there was some considerable snoring. RERA, respiratory effort–related arousal.

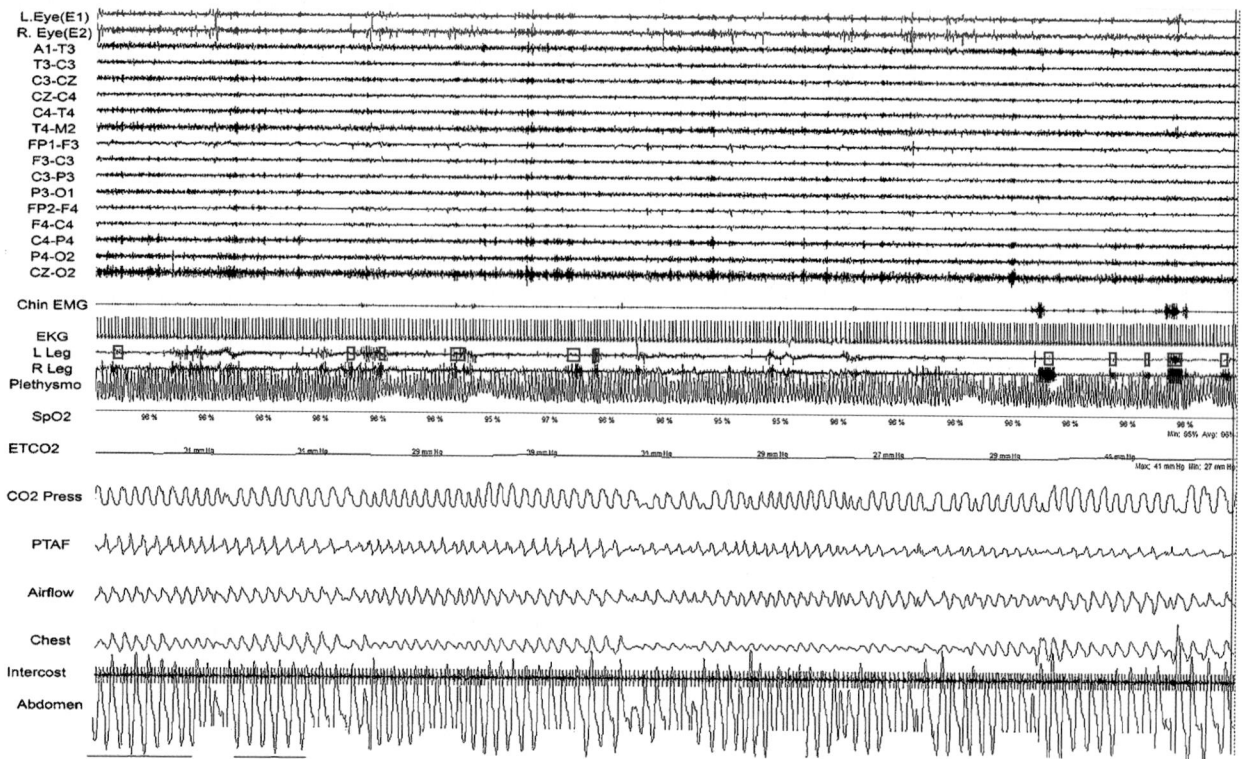

• **Fig. 60.2** Narcolepsy: rapid eye movement (REM) sleep without atonia in narcolepsy. During the nocturnal polysomnogram, REM sleep was quite active and there were many limb movements associated with augmented muscle tone of the chin noted. This 5-minute polysomnogram segment demonstrates the limb movements that were frequent during REM sleep and REM sleep respiratory instability. REM sleep without atonia is quite common in children with narcolepsy.

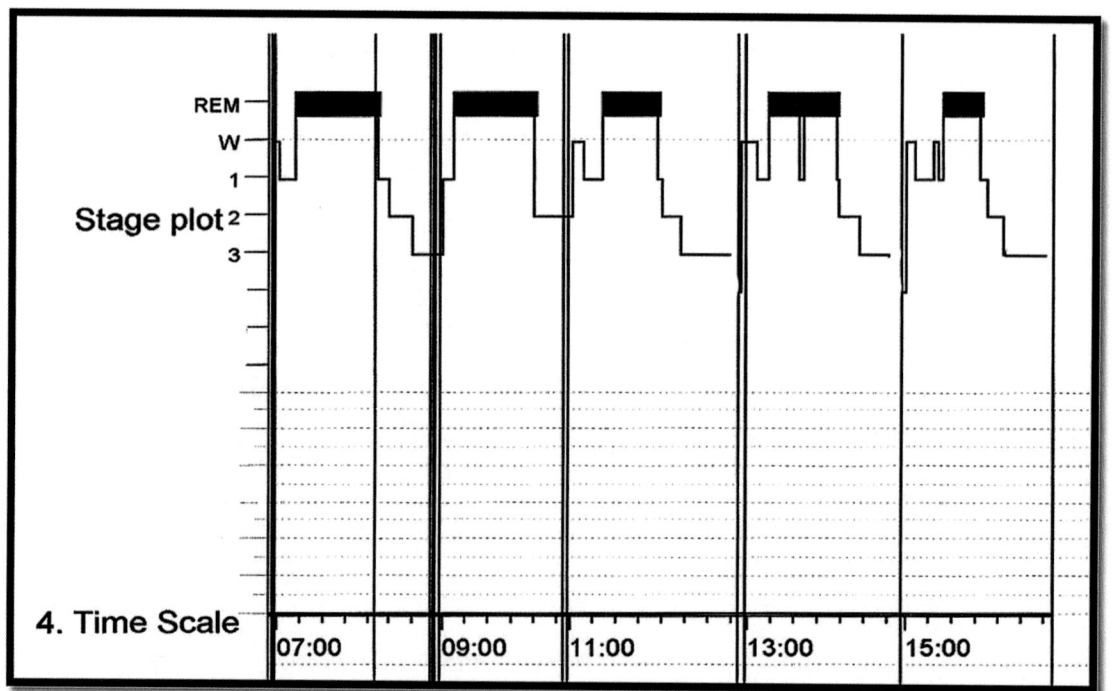

• **Fig. 60.3** Narcolepsy: multiple sleep latency test (MSLT). The patient underwent a five-nap MSLT. The mean sleep-onset latency was 3.5 minutes. Consolidated sleep was noted on 5/5 nap attempts. Rapid eye movement (REM) sleep was noted on all five naps attempts. These findings were consistent with the diagnosis of narcolepsy. The presence of cataplexy was suggested by the child being clumsy on the playground and falling when laughing, Narcolepsy (type I) was diagnosed. He was started on a regimen of methylphenidate that was titrated to an appropriate dose. Symptoms resolved, his mood improved, his schoolwork was back to baseline, and symptoms that were suggestive of attention-deficit/hyperactivity disorder (ADHD) completely resolved.

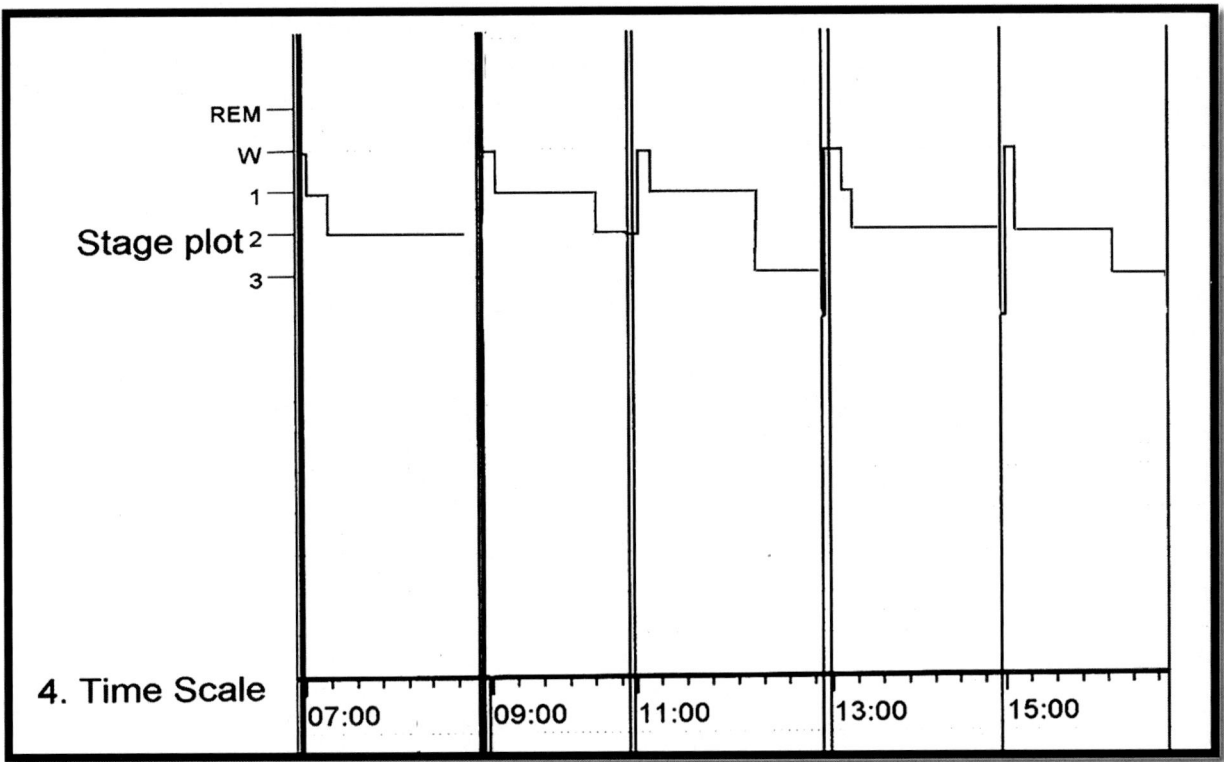

• **Fig. 60.4** Idiopathic hypersomnia. This figure represents a five-nap multiple sleep latency test (MSLT) from an 11-year-old with a history of excessive daytime sleepiness, sleep attacks, and unintentional sleep episodes. There is no history of cataplexy, hypnagogic hallucinations, or sleep paralysis. There is no family history of excessive daytime sleepiness. Symptoms have been present for 3 or more years and have been getting worse. Modified Epworth Sleepiness Scale for children was 14. The mean sleep-onset latency on this five-nap MSLT was approximately 5 minutes. Consolidated sleep was seen on 5/5 nap attempts, and no sleep-onset rapid eye movement (REM) periods were noted. The patient was notably confused and disoriented after being awakened from naps 3 and 5. This MSLT is consistent with idiopathic hypersomnia. In idiopathic hypersomnia, naps or unintentional sleep episodes may be considerably longer. The patient's naps are particularly unrefreshing. Cataplexy, hypnagogic hallucinations, and sleep paralysis are usually absent. Confusion and disorientation, which might be considered sleep drunkenness, can occur upon awakening from nocturnal sleep or from naps particularly if N3 sleep is reached.

61

Sleep-Related Movement Disorders

STEPHEN H. SHELDON

Periodic Limb Movement Disorder

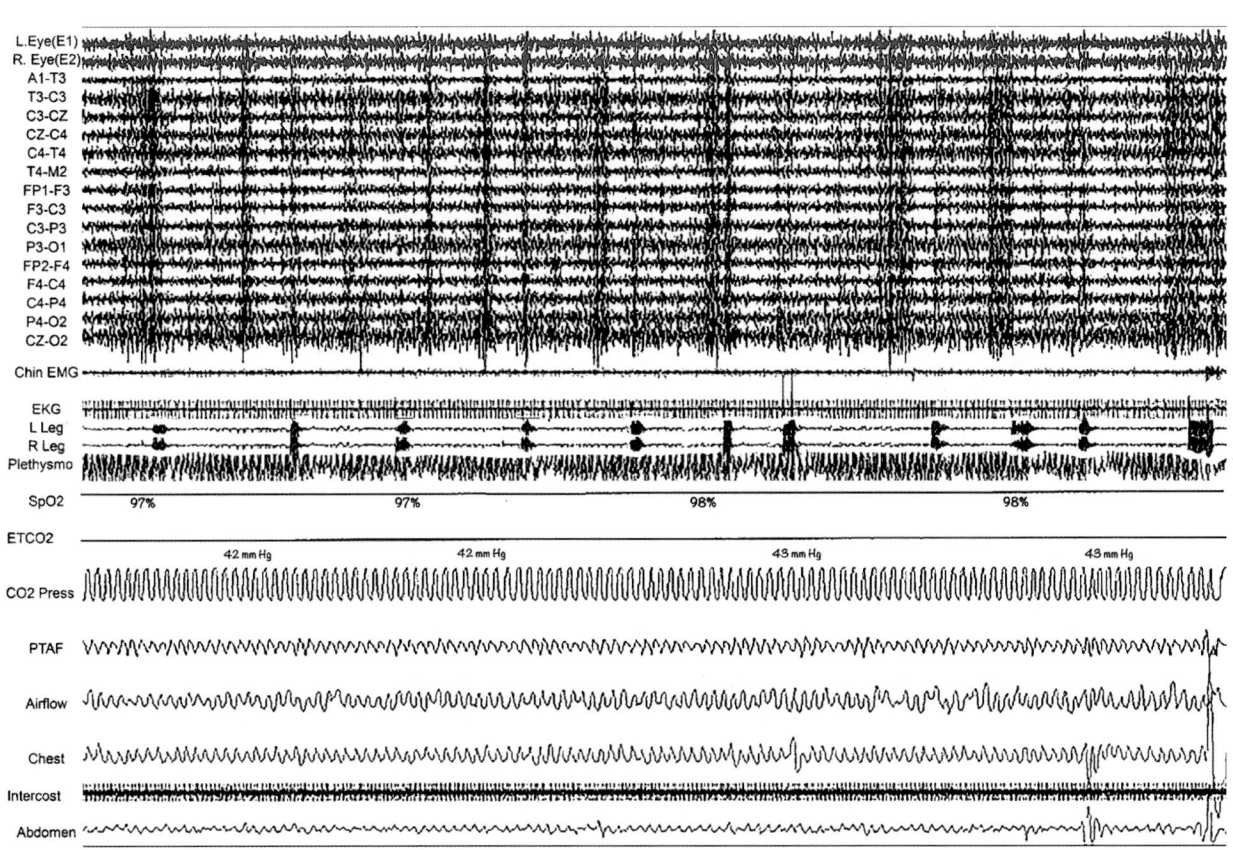

• **Fig. 61.1** Periodic limb movement disorder. This 5-minute polysomnographic epoch was recorded during N3 sleep. It is notable for a regular and monotonous respiratory pattern. No respiratory events can be seen. Note the regular and periodic limb movements associated with arousals, particularly in the right anterior tibialis electromyogram (EMG). A common presenting complaint is excessive daytime sleepiness and associated symptoms are often present. Patients may also complain of "growing pains." Sleep is often described as unrefreshing. Symptoms of leg (or arm) jerks and movements may be seen by parents and movements are repetitive and stereotypic in one or both legs. Arms may also be involved. Significant disruption of sleep architecture and continuity can occur although patients are typically unaware of these movements and partial arousals.

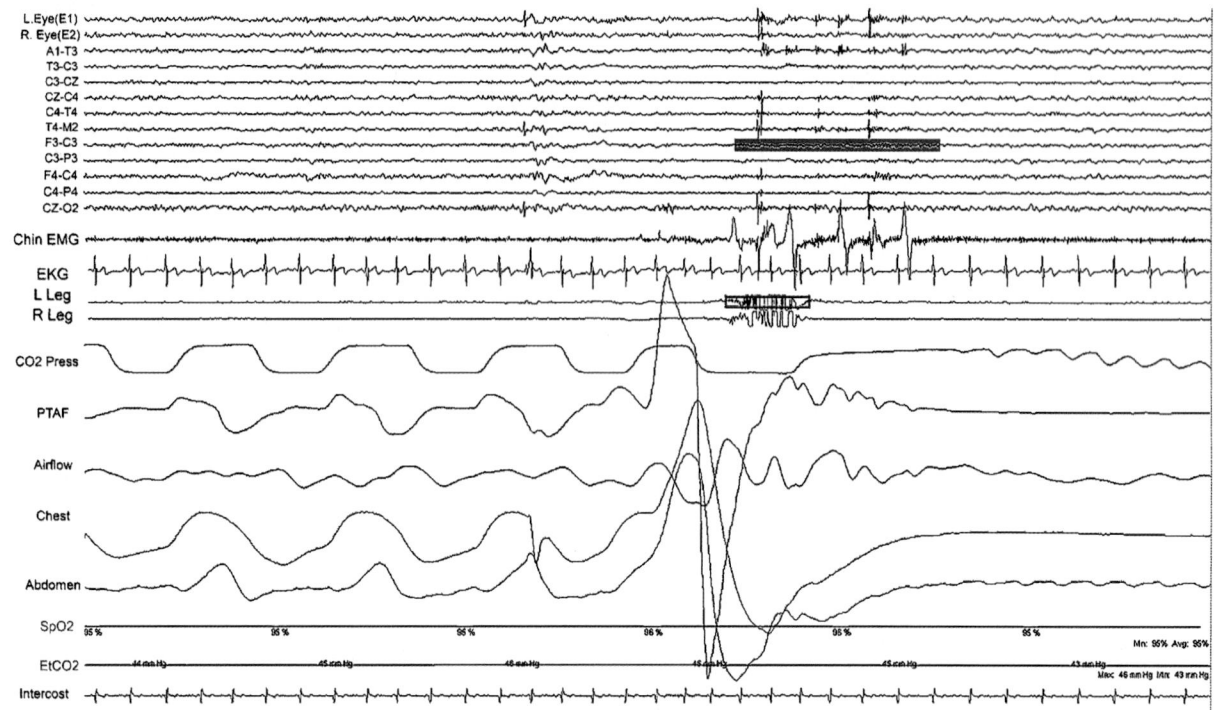

• **Fig. 61.2** Sleep-related bruxism. This 30-second polysomnographic epoch was recorded from a 9-year-old female with a history of migraine cephalgia. There were frequent morning headaches. She frequently complains of bitemporal pain that was worse in the morning and would often awaken her from sleep. The epoch demonstrates an arousal associated with an expiratory hypopnea characterized by an augmented breath (sigh) and limb movement followed by rhythmic temporalis muscle activity seen on the transcoronal electroencephalography (EEG). There is rhythmic muscle artifact noted at a frequency of approximately 1 Hz and chin muscle electromyography (EMG) reveals similar rhythmic activity. Sleep-related bruxism can occur in isolation and may result in chronic complaints of headaches. Purple box is an electrocortical arousal.

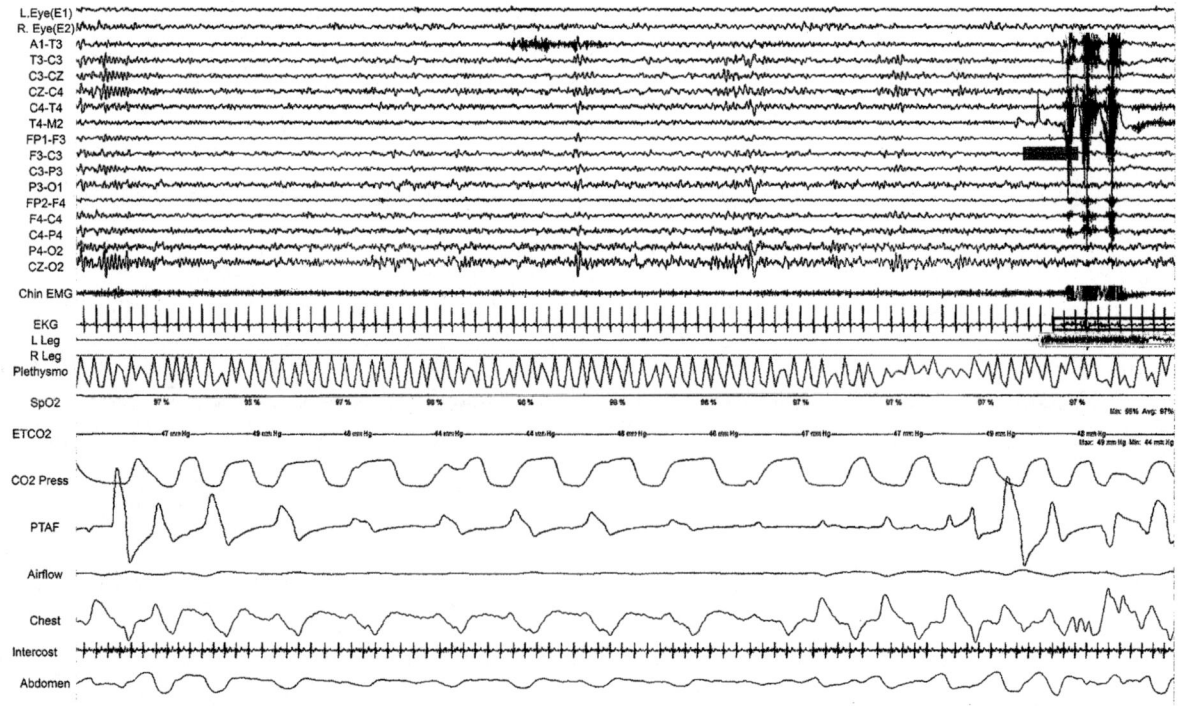

• **Fig. 61.3** Bruxism after hypopnea. This 120-second polysomnographic segment was recorded from a 4-year-old with a history of snoring, frequent nocturnal awakenings, restless sleep, and sleep-related diaphoresis. During this epoch of rapid eye movement (REM) sleep, note the flow limitation indicated in the pressure transducer airflow (PTAF), airflow, and end-tidal CO_2 waveform channels. This flow limitation is followed by an arousal and rhythmic temporalis muscle activity seen by muscle artifact obscuring the electroencephalogram (EEG) at approximately a 1-Hz frequency. Sleep-related bruxism can be independent or may be noted following occlusive or partially occlusive respiratory events.

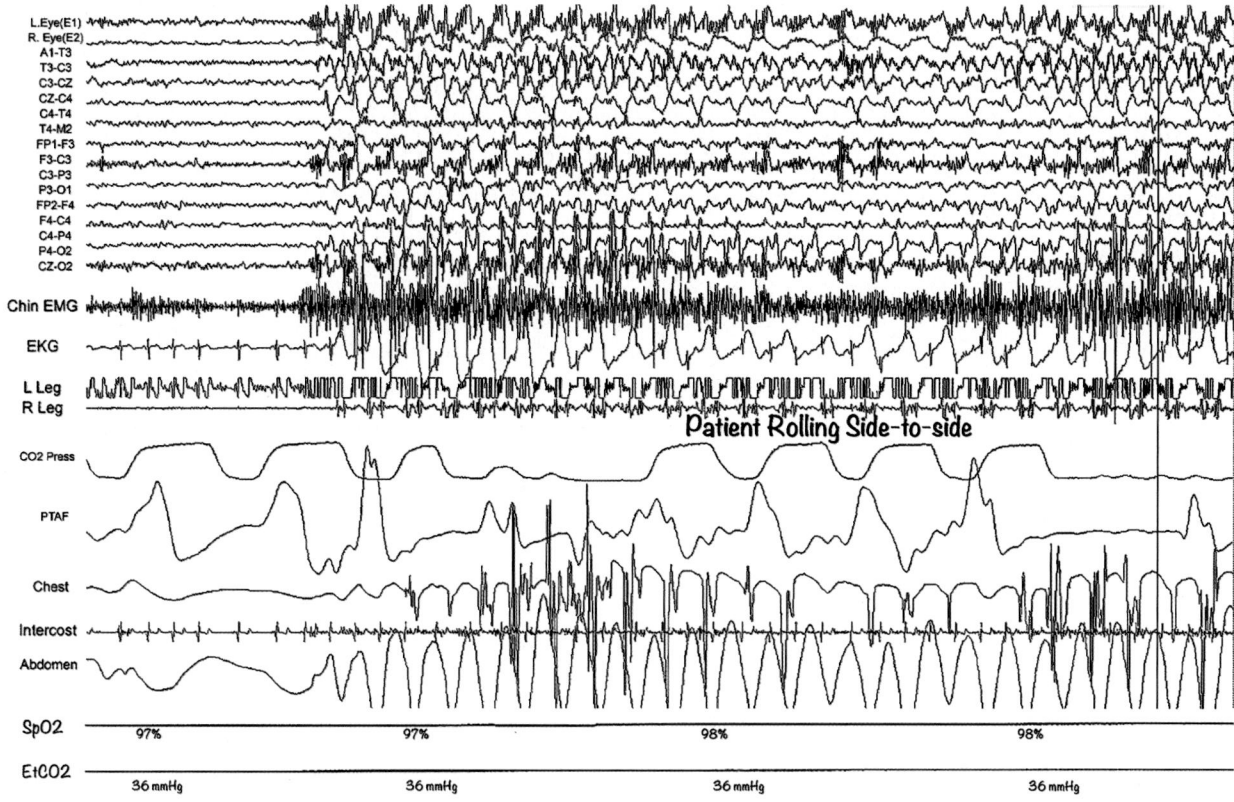

• **Fig. 61.4** Rhythmic movement disorder: head banging and body rolling. This 30-second polysomnographic segment was recorded from a 6-year-old male with a history of unusual movements during sleep. Parents reported that as an infant the patient had rhythmic head banging and now when asleep would roll back and forth from side to side. Pediatrician reported that these symptoms were "normal" and would go away as the child aged. The parents were concerned that the child may be having a seizure, because the patient's cousin suffered from a general tonic-clonic seizure disorder. Because of enlarged tonsils and habitual snoring, a sleep study was obtained. During non–rapid eye movement (NREM) sleep, episodes of rhythmic body rolling were identified and can be seen in the segment with an abrupt arousal from NREM sleep and rhythmic side-to-side movements that can be identified by movement artifact in most polysomnographic (PSG) channels.

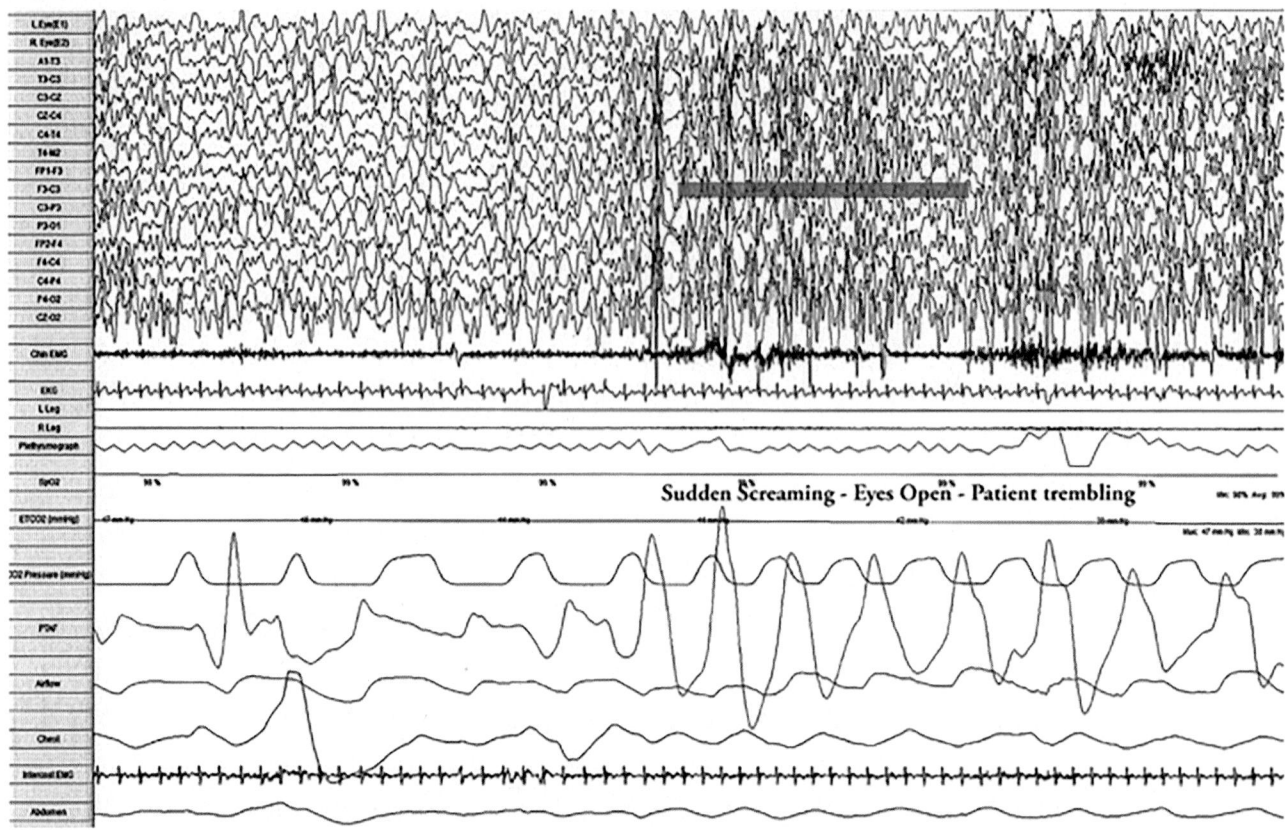

Sudden Screaming - Eyes Open - Patient trembling

• **Fig. 61.5** Rhythmic movement disorder: body rolling. This is a 30-second epoch of the same patient from Fig. 61.4 . Rhythmic body rolling can be seen after the initial arousal in four separate paroxysms. All episodes of rhythmic body rolling were stereotypic; however, they were not associated with ictal and/or postictal activity. Rhythmic head banging, body rocking, head rolling, and/or body rolling, can occur both during wake-to-sleep transition, arousals from sleep, or during sleep. The underlying etiology is unclear. Episodes may be quite violent with resultant bruising if the head banging is excessive.

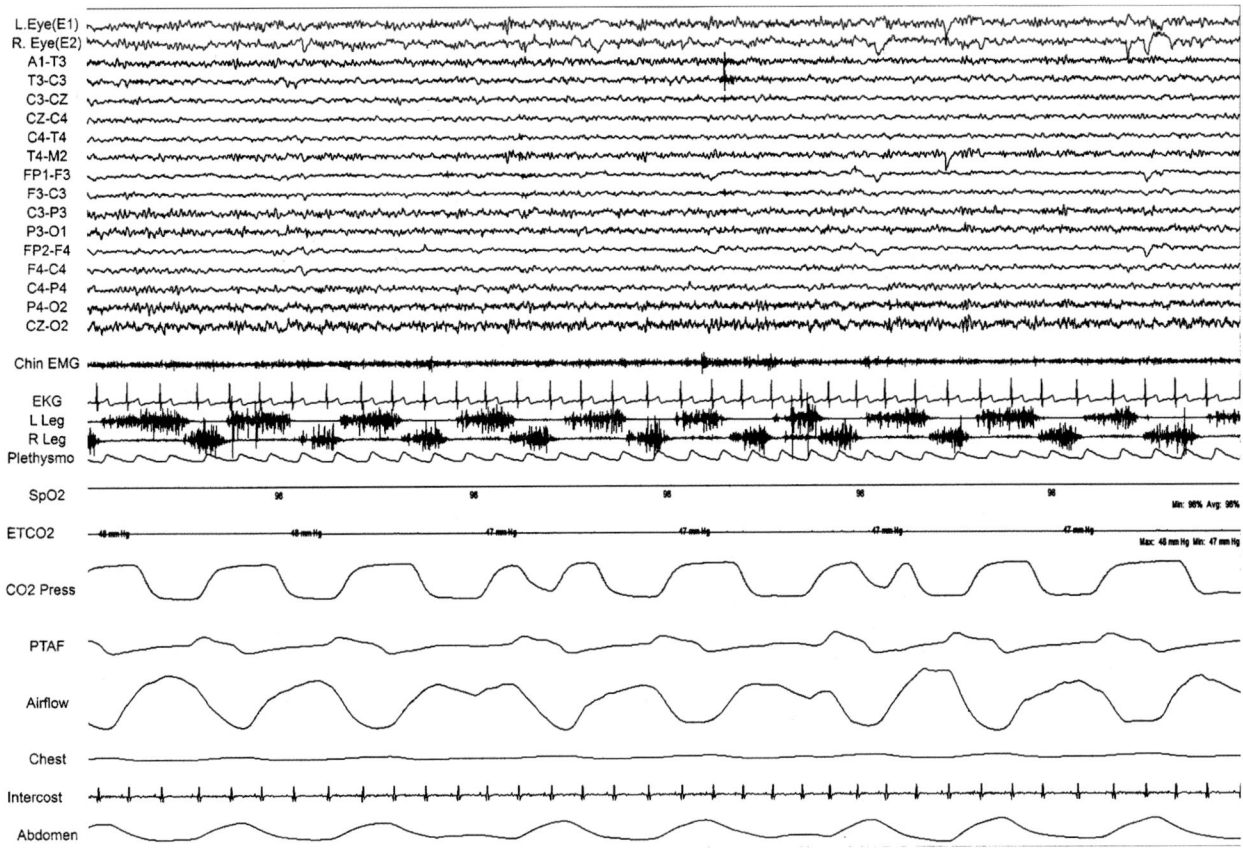

• **Fig. 61.6** Alternating limb movement activation of sleep (ALMAS). This 30-second polysomnographic segment was recorded from a 5-year-old male who was being studied in the laboratory for possible obstructive sleep-disordered breathing. There was a pattern of occasional hypopneas (apnea-hypopnea index [AHI] 5.3 events per hour) associated with arousals. During arousals, limb muscle electromyography (EMG) revealed brief activations of the anterior tibialis muscles that occasionally alternated with similar activations of the opposite leg. Anterior tibialis EMG augmentation appeared at a frequency of approximately 1 Hz and lasted between 0.1 and 0.5 seconds. In this segment the limb movement activation occurred during transitional sleep (N1). These findings of alternating leg muscle activations during sleep and arousals (ALMAS) might represent transient facilitation of a spinal central pattern generator for locomotion.

62

Sleep-Related Seizures and Epilepsy

Stephen H. Sheldon

Spike and Wave Activity

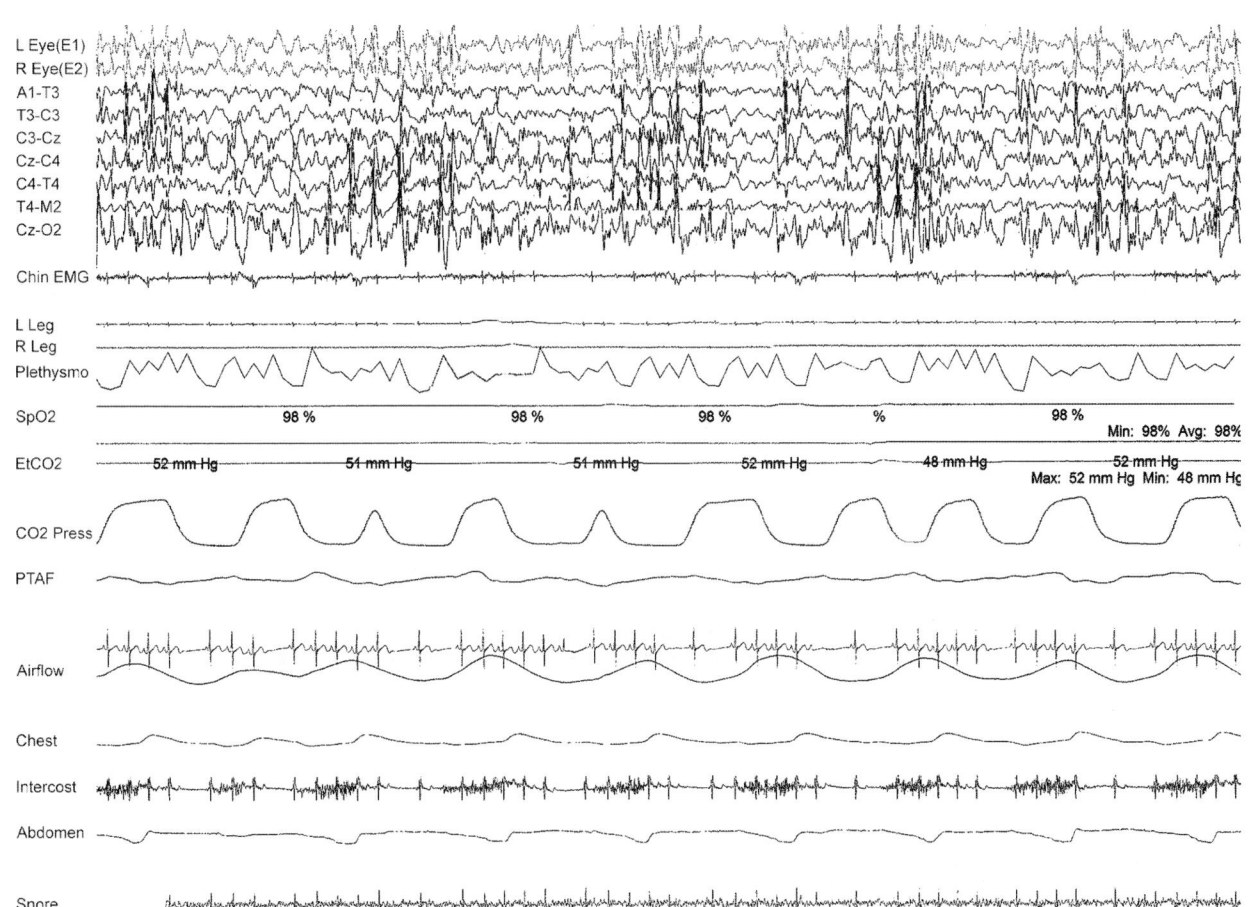

• **Fig. 62.1** Spike/wave activity. This 30-second polysomnographic segment was recorded from non–rapid eye movement (NREM) sleep in a child with a history of intermittent seizure disorder that appeared to be fairly well controlled on anticonvulsant therapy. Symptoms were daytime sleepiness and snoring. In this epoch, multifocal bilaterally independent spike and wave activity can be seen, but without clinical correlates. Respiration is regular; however, there is a somewhat significant exaggeration of respiratory sinus variation. With the single-lead electrocardiogram (ECG) juxtaposed with airflow, one can see the respiratory sinus variation clearly in this patient, although having a generalized seizure disorder had increased upper airway resistance and mild partially obstructive sleep-disordered breathing.

Generalized Tonic/Clonic Seizure

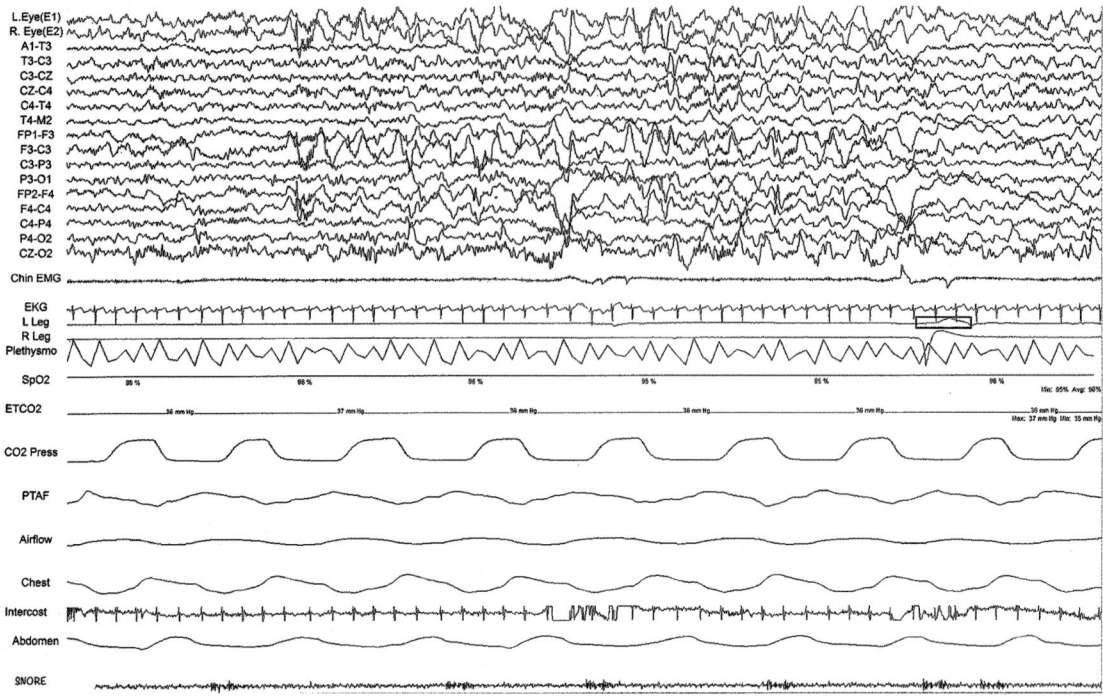

• **Fig. 62.2** Non–rapid eye movement (NREM) sleep preceding a generalized tonic-clonic seizure. This 30-second polysomnographic segment was recorded during N3 sleep from a 10-year-old male with a history of habitual loud snoring and unusual movements during sleep. Respirations are regular. There is some snoring noted in the snore channel, and there appears to be some frontal slowing as well as questionable spike activity in the frontal regions. Note the high-voltage synchronous slowing in the right and left frontal leads. This activity can also be seen in both eye channels.

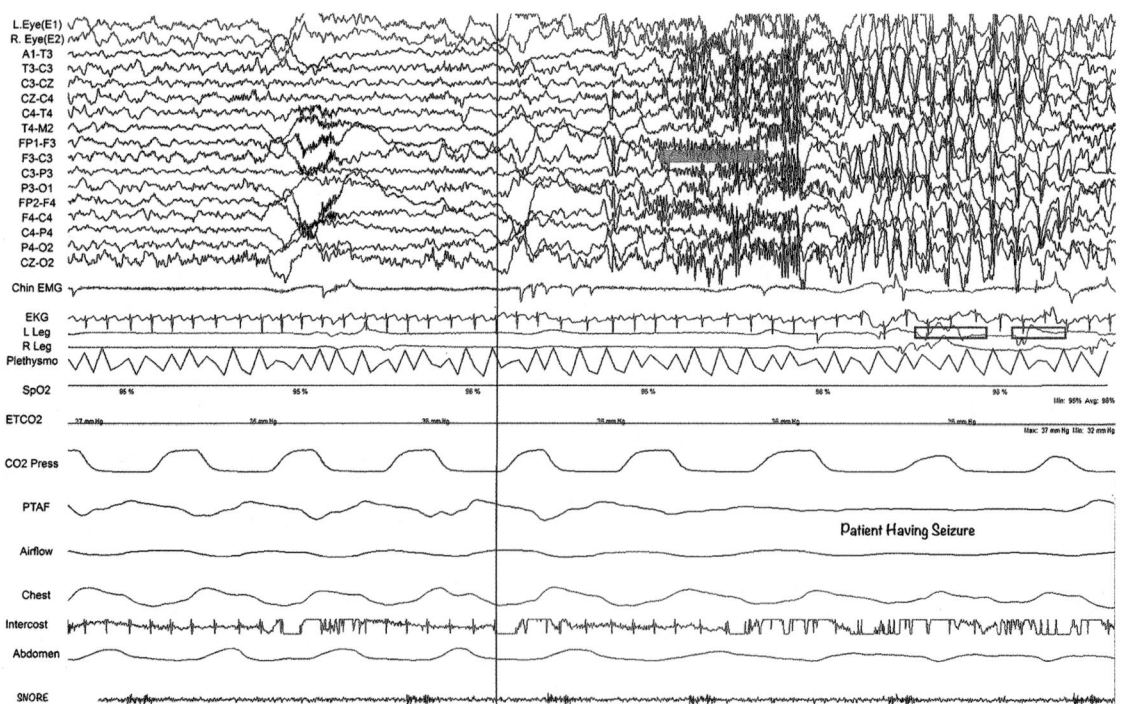

• **Fig. 62.3** Onset of generalized tonic-clonic seizure from N3 sleep. This is a subsequent 30-second epoch that shows gradual buildup of epileptiform activity that is generalized, increased motor activity as demonstrated by muscle artifact in all electroencephalographic (EEG) leads, and subsequent rhythmic spike and wave activity. Also note increased heart rate. Additionally, the technologist reported that the patient had a "seizure."

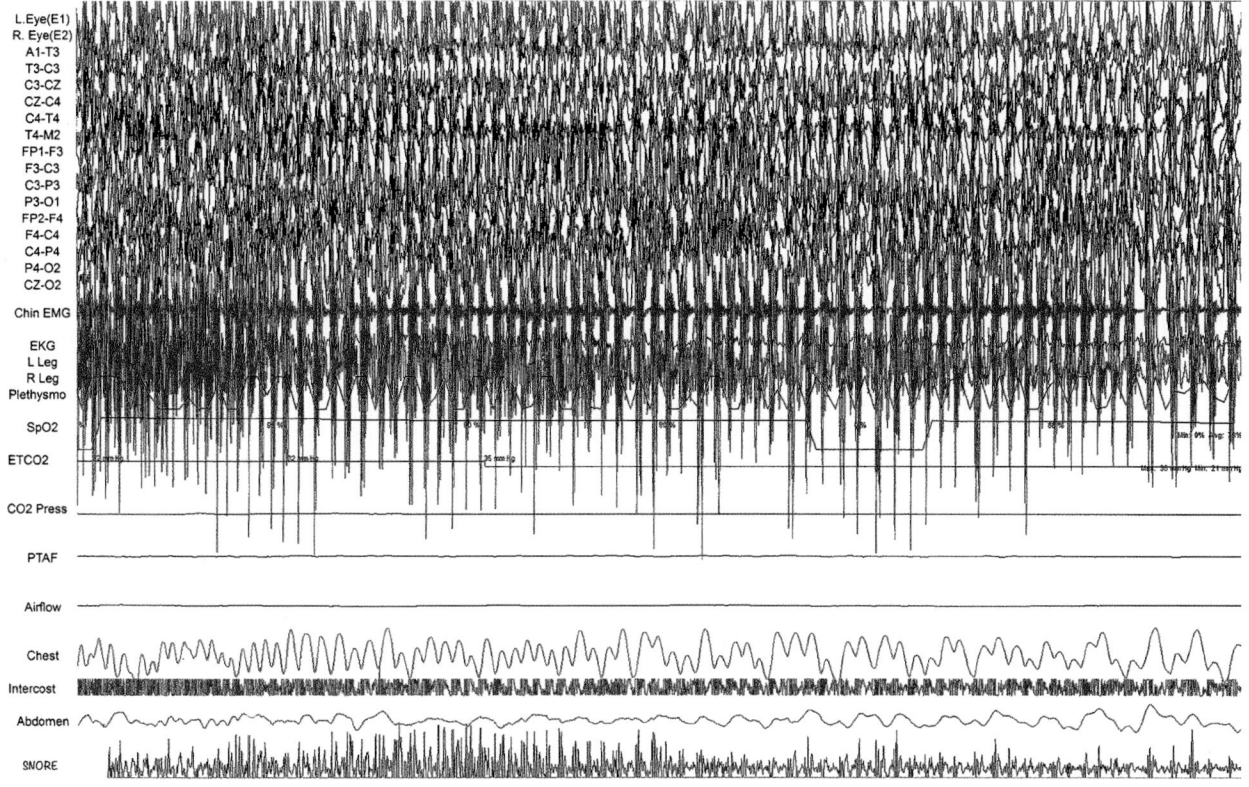

• **Fig. 62.4** Generalized tonic-clonic seizure from N3 sleep. This figure represents the following 30-second segment during a period of tonic-clonic seizure activity. Clinical tonic/clonic activity was seen on video and noted by the technologist. The technologist responded and entered the patient's room. Technologist noted the brief seizure activity that ceased upon approaching the bed (see Fig. 62.5).

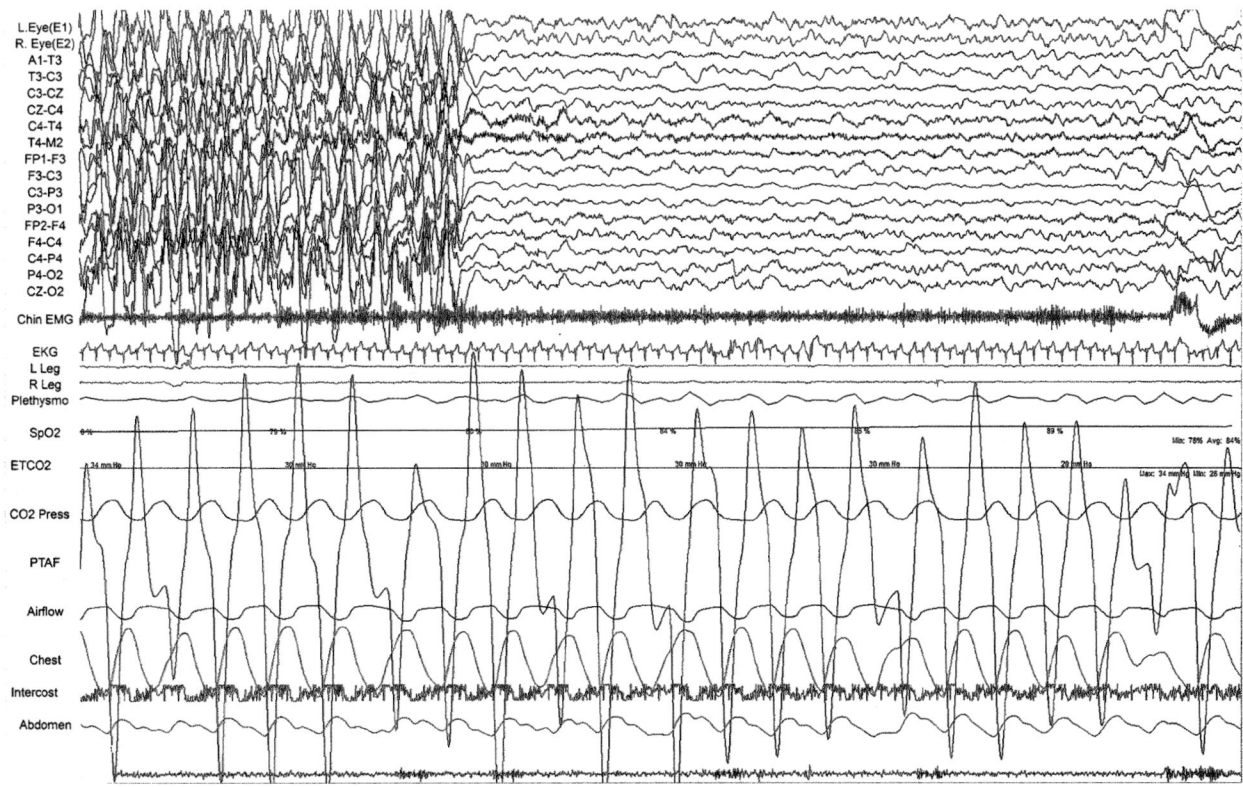

• **Fig. 62.5** Generalized tonic-clonic seizure from N3 sleep. In this segment the generalized tonic-clonic activity has subsided and there is some postictal slowing noted. Respirations and heart rate returned to baseline and snoring artifact can be seen in the chin muscle electromyogram (EMG).

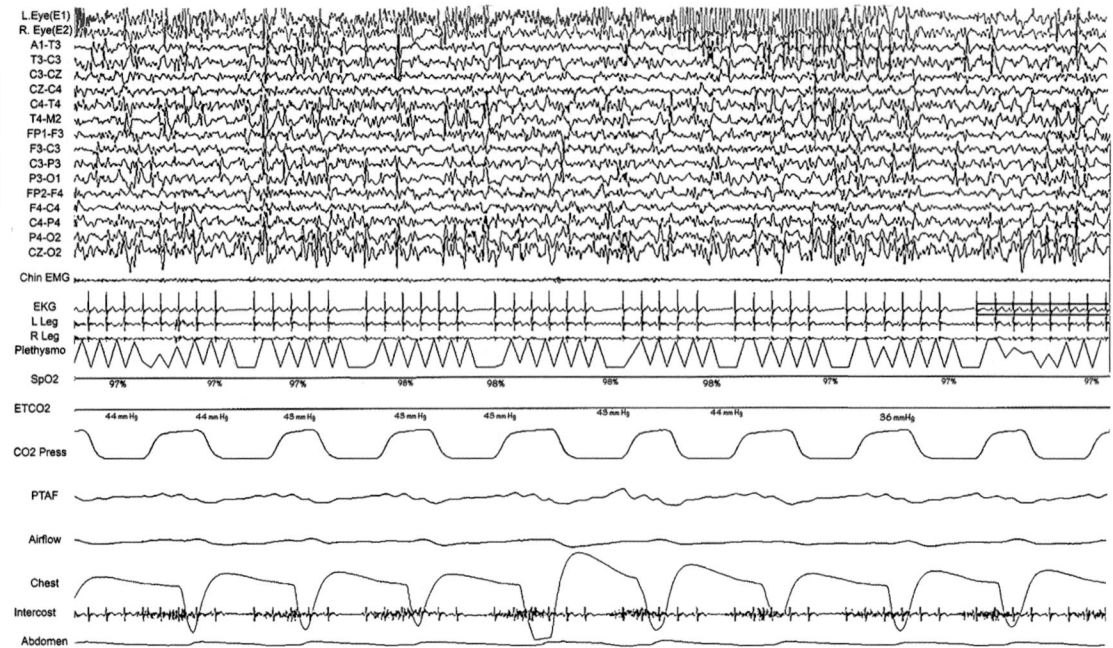

• **Fig. 62.6** Continuous epileptiform activity of sleep. This 30-second polysomnographic segment was recorded from a 4-year-old with a history of hypoxic-ischemic encephalopathy. Parents had reported the child snoring, snorting, and gasping during sleep. There had been episodes where the patient had been noted to be cyanotic, apparently stopped breathing, and aroused with a gasp. State determination is difficult due to the presence of continuous epileptiform activity as well as significant theta intrusion. During this epoch, there is significant respiratory sinus variation noted in the electrocardiogram (ECG). This, along with snoring and sleep fragmentation, might suggest the presence of increased upper airway resistance. In patients with continuous epileptiform activity, non–rapid eye movement (NREM) sleep states can be difficult to identify and are often scored as a single NREM sleep state. REM sleep tends to attenuate epileptiform activity. Therefore, in many cases REM sleep may be clearly identifiable in patients with this sleep-related electroencephalographic (EEG) abnormality. Continuous spike waves during sleep is a condition in which sequential bilaterally synchronous spike discharges present in NREM sleep.

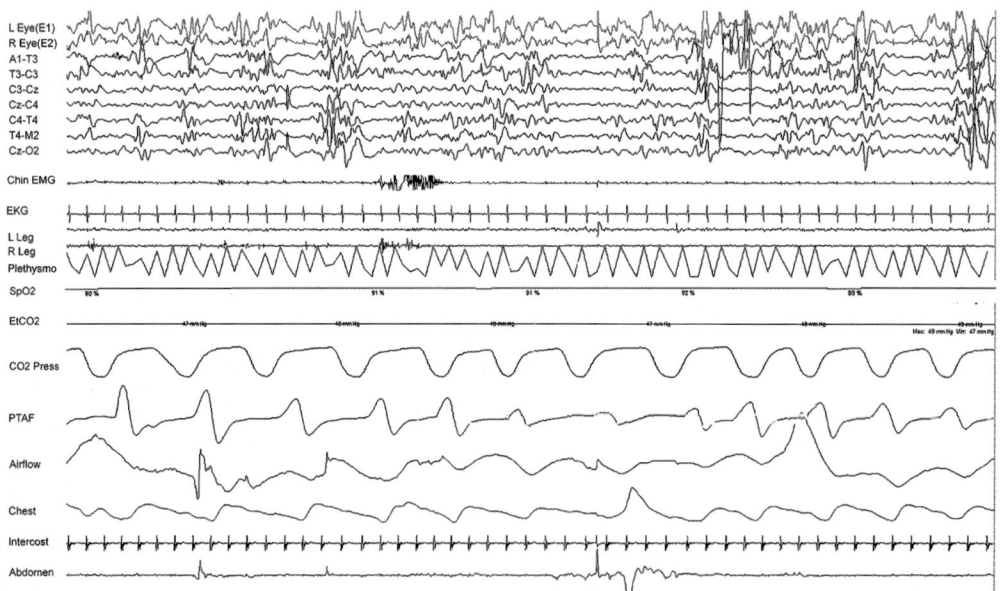

• **Fig. 62.7** Hypsarrhythmia. This 30-second segment was recorded from a 6-month-old with a complex history including infantile spasms. A pattern known as hypsarrhythmia can be noted in this bipolar transcoronal electroencephalographic (EEG) electrode array. Infantile spasms are characterized by sudden brief tonic muscular contractions that result in either flexion or extension of both the extremities and trunk. Interictal EEG reveals a chaotic mixture of high-voltage slow-wave activity including multifocal spikes and spikes/wave discharges. The pattern may be discontinuous in non–rapid eye movement (NREM) sleep. Epochs of attenuation may interrupt the hypsarrhythmic EEG tracing and asynchronous high-voltage slowing of activity can be noted. The duration of alert pro-decremental activity can last from 1 second to more than 1 minute.

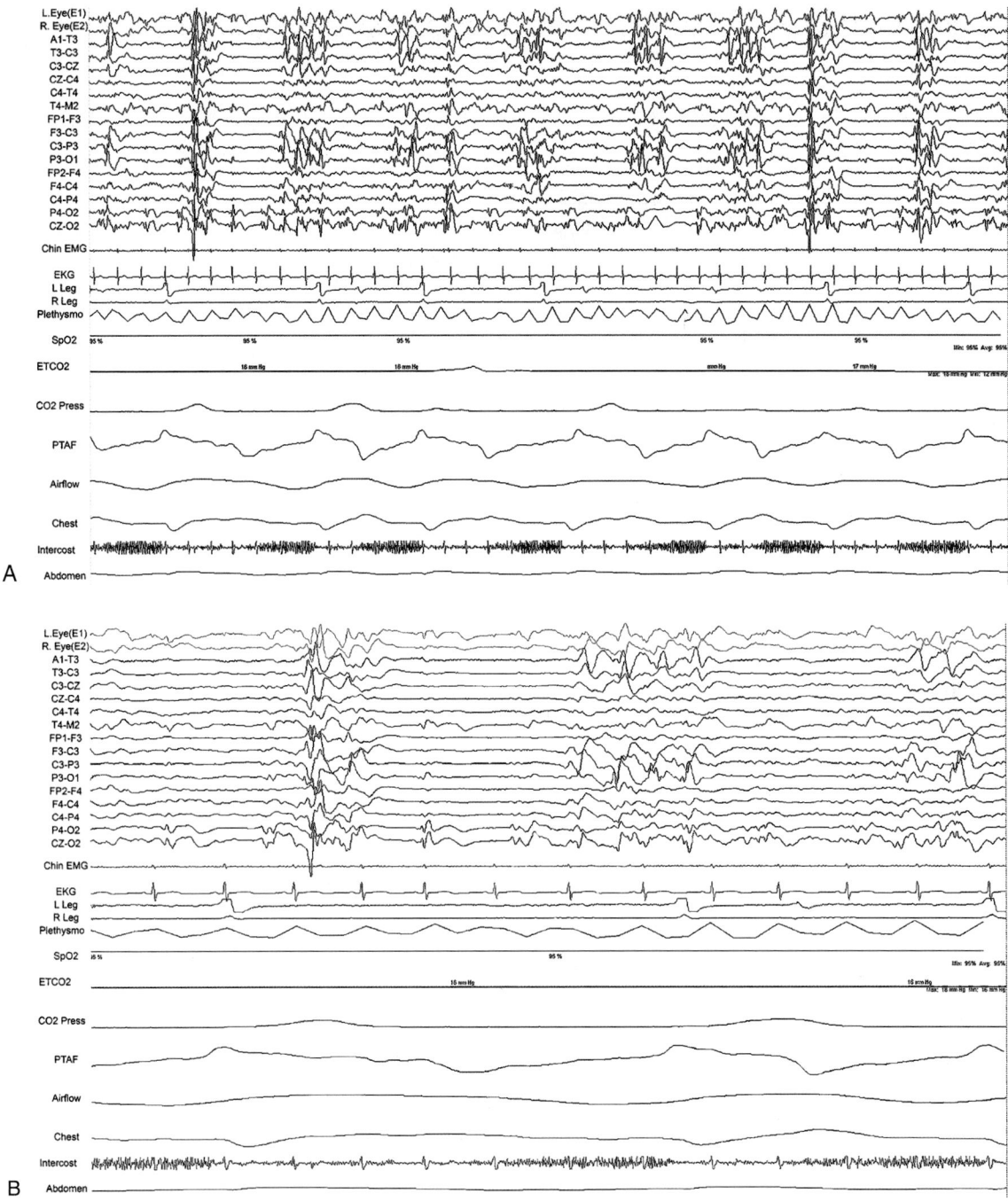

• **Fig. 62.8** Burst suppression. This 30-second polysomnographic segment was recorded from a 9-year-old who had suffered a penetrating head injury following an automobile accident. The patient was generally nonresponsive. Because of the presence of intermittent oxygen desaturations, a polysomnogram was ordered. This electroencephalographic (EEG) pattern represents bursts of brief intermittent slow waves, spikes, and theta activity separated by equal or longer periods of relative or complete electrical quiescence. This may occur either generally or may be regional in character. This pattern of burst suppression carries a very guarded prognosis and can depend on the duration of activity and the decremental changes that might occur and the EEG pattern. If any normal activity is seen, the prognosis is favorable. Most patients whose EEGs reveal a burst suppression pattern have a poor prognosis.

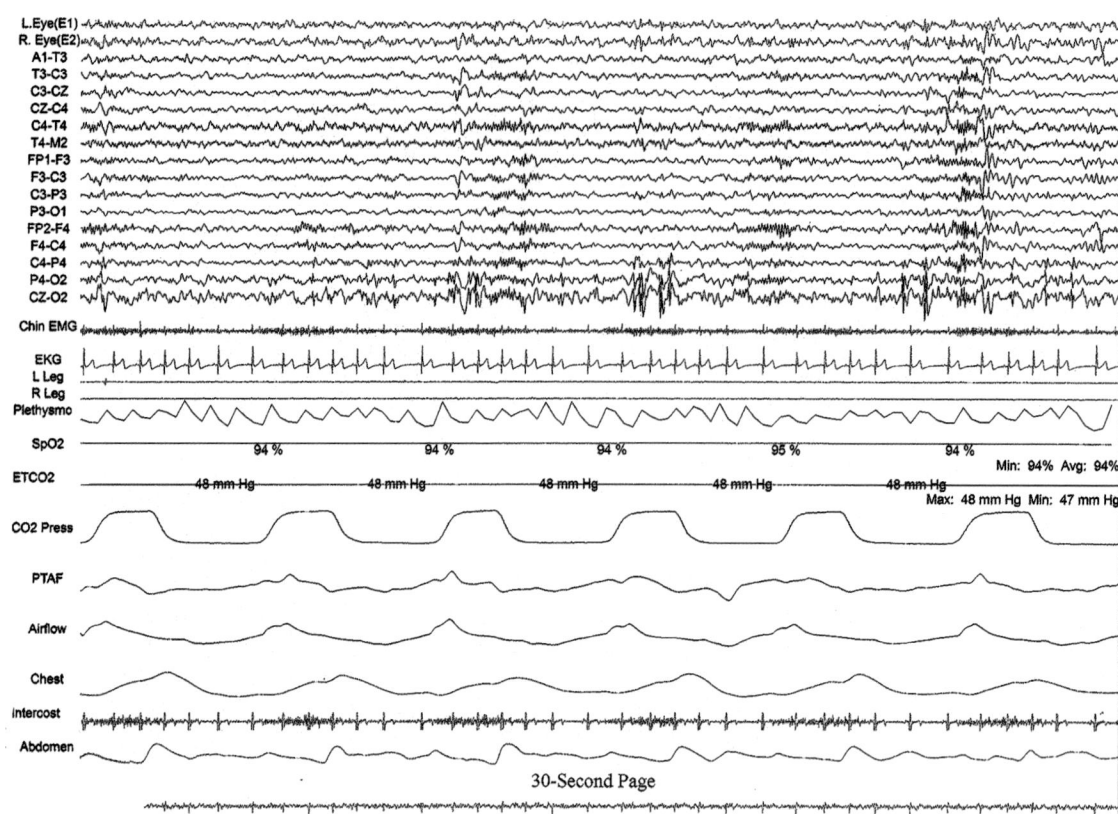

• **Fig. 62.9** Posterior occipital sharp transients of sleep (POSTS). This 30-second polysomnographic segment was recorded from a 7-year-old male. Occasionally, sharp transients are seen in posterior occipital leads. These POSTS appear during transitional sleep and N2 sleep during childhood. They may also begin during adolescence. This activity is most likely a normal phenomenon.

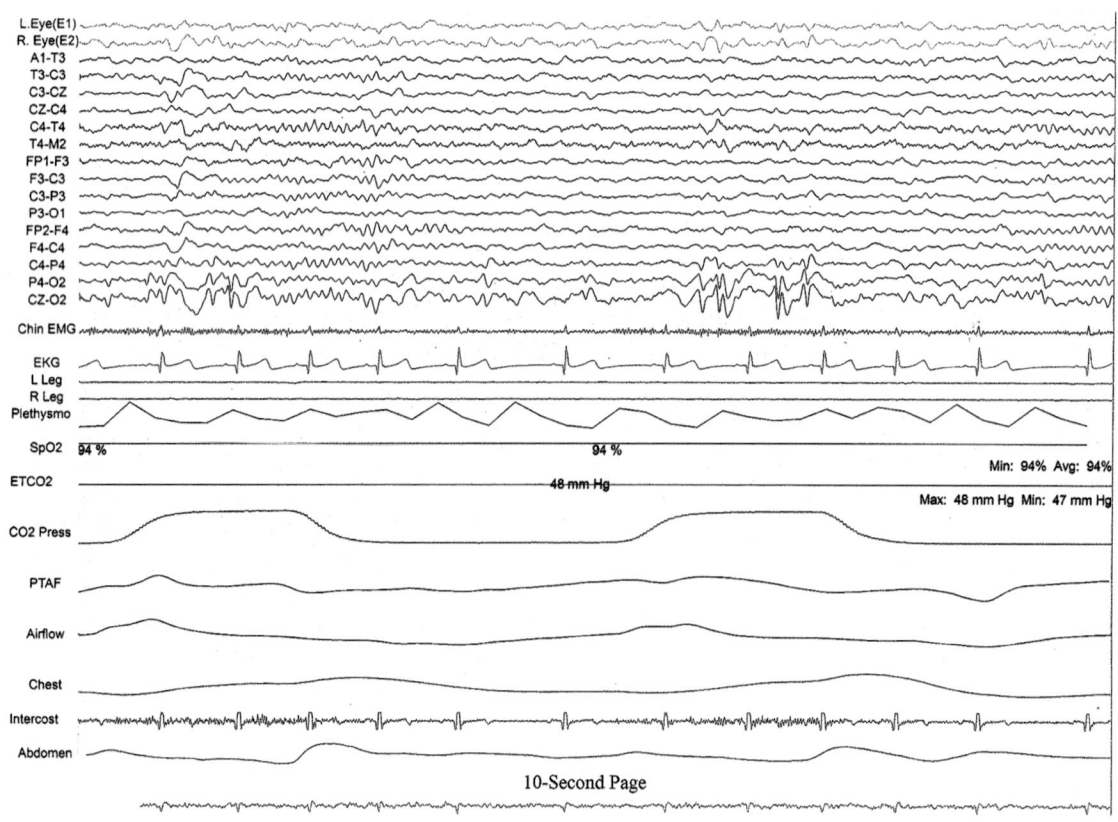

• **Fig. 62.10** Posterior occipital sharp transients of sleep (POSTS). This polysomnographic segment was recorded from the patient at 10 seconds and again demonstrates the POSTS.

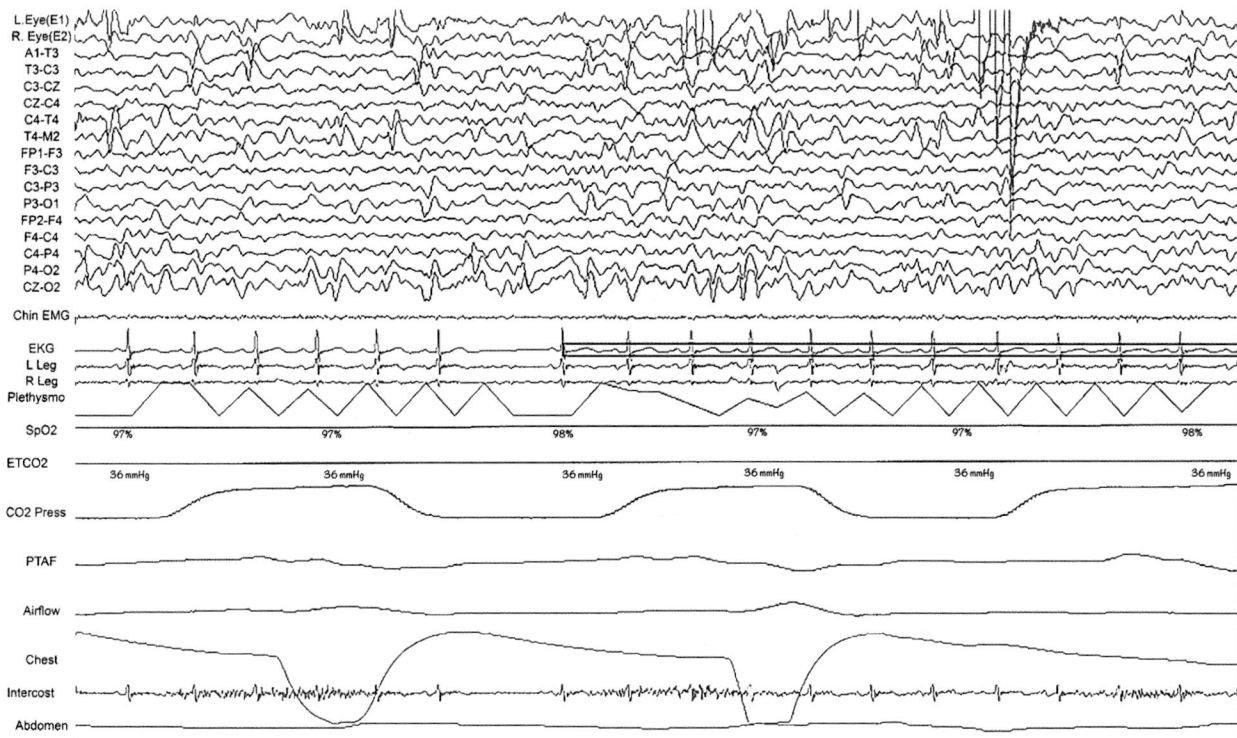

• **Fig. 62.11** Continuous epileptiform activity of sleep with electrocardiogram (ECG) sinus pauses. This 10-second polysomnographic segment was recorded from a 4-year-old with cerebral palsy. Continuous epileptiform activity of sleep was noted in non–rapid eye movement (NREM) sleep states and could not be accurately identified using standard polysomnographic (PSG) and/or electroencephalographic (EEG) criteria. There was a history of loud habitual snoring, gasping, and choking during sleep. There were 15 hypopneas per hour of sleep with questionable independent sinus pauses between breaths noted on the ECG.

Index

Page numbers followed by 'f' indicate figures, 't' indicate tables, and 'b' indicate boxes.